contexo | media

ICD-9-CM

Volumes 1 & 2, Expert for Physicians

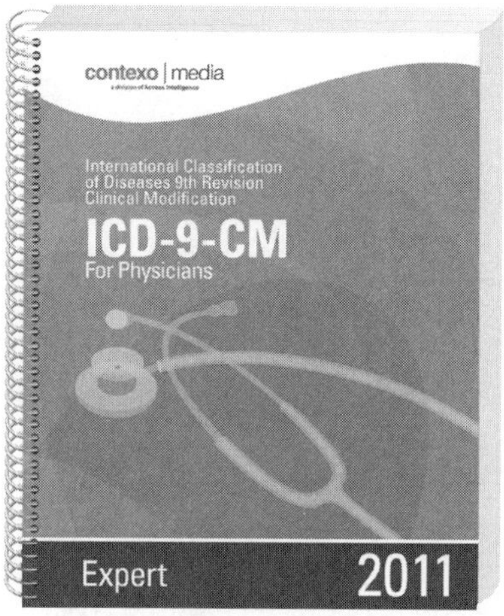

$99.95

Item ID: MICD9-11
ISBN: 978-1-58383-712-2
Spiralbound
Available September 2010

Promo Code: FOBA11

This incredibly useful resource includes coding tips, illustrations, color-coding and intuitive icons to help you find the right diagnosis code quickly, helping you code more accurately and efficiently. Decrease denials with all the helpful features included:

- NEW! ICD-10-CM documentation requirements — understand the documentation guidelines required to code for the new diagnostic coding system
- NEW! ICD-10-CM coding tips at the code level — start now to learn about the coding differences between ICD-9-CM and ICD-10-CM
- ICD-9-CM Official Coding Guidelines integrated into tabular listing with the affected code(s) — one-stop code and guideline look-up
- All 2011 new and revised codes with a summary of code changes plus official ICD-9-CM Appendixes — using updated and official information is essential to complying with HIPAA and getting paid
- Detailed, full-page anatomy illustrations plus over 500 code-specific illustrations that have been integrated into the book — allows better interpretation of clinical notes to code with more specificity
- Over 3,000 definitions of complex codes — takes the guesswork out of choosing the right code
- Intuitive icons for age and sex edits, new or revised text, 4th and 5th digit requirements — helps ensure specificity and validity
- "Unspecified" and "Other Specified" code icons — alerts you when there is insufficient information, or no specific code that fits medical record documentation
- Valid three-digit list to identify a condition or disease when an additional digit is not available — helps you speed-up coding
- V Code designation icons — recognize when V codes can be used only as primary or additional diagnoses
- AHA Coding Clinic© for ICD-9-CM references noted with applicable codes know right where to look for more guidance
- Spiralbound with color tabs for quick look-ups — find the right code quickly

Ready to order?
Call today—our friendly representatives are waiting to assist you.
800.334.5724

Contexo Media
P.O. Box 25128
SLC, UT 84125-0128

FAX
801.365.0710

PHONE
800.334.5724

ONLINE
www.codingbooks.com

contexo | media

Plain English Descriptions for ICD-9-CM and ICD-10-CM

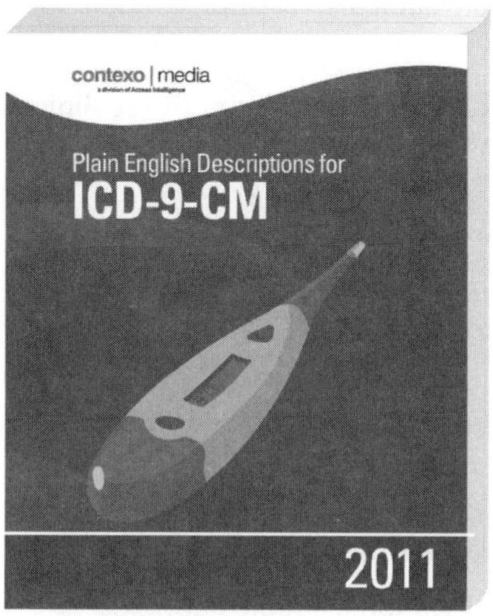

$99.95

Item ID: CDAICD-11
ISBN: 978-1-58383-691-0
Perfectbound
Available September 2010

Promo Code: FOBA11

When coders, medical staff, payers and health care professionals need more detailed information than the ICD-9-CM book provides, they turn to this comprehensive clinical, coding and documentation guide for over 11,000 ICD-9-CM codes and categories.

- NEW! Below the ICD-9-CM codes, a crosswalk to new ICD-10-CM codes is provided—enables efficient transition to the new coding system
- NEW! Plain English Descriptions for new ICD-9-CM codes—understand new codes with ease
- Detailed, full-page anatomy illustrations—helps you interpret clinical notes to code with more specificity
- Plain English Descriptions of terminology found in the medical record to provide detailed clinical explanations of the ICD-9-CM diagnosis codes—helps you assign the most appropriate code
- Plain English Descriptions for syndromes linking definitions to the applicable ICD-9-CM codes—understand what symptoms and/or diseases are included in a syndrome
- Numerically arranged just like your ICD-9-CM—easy identification and look-up
- *AHA Coding Clinic®* for ICD-9-CM references—helps you validate code choices

ICD-9-CM ASCII File

- Two sets of descriptions: short (35 characters), and full (unabbreviated)
- Fourth- or fifth-digit status field
- Keep computer systems current and up-to-date
- Import into your database or software program
- Saves time and increases accuracy
- Fixed-width and tab-delimited file formats available

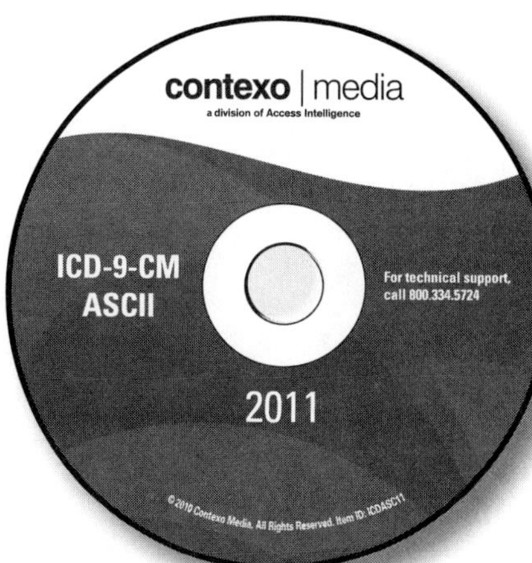

$199.95

Single User
Item ID: ICDASC-11
Available September 2010

$249.95

2-10 Users (Call for 11+ User Pricing)

Item ID: ICDASCM-11

Contexo Media
P.O. Box 25128
SLC, UT 84125-0128

FAX
801.365.0710

PHONE
800.334.5724

ONLINE
www.codingbooks.com

contexo | media

Plain English Descriptions for Procedures

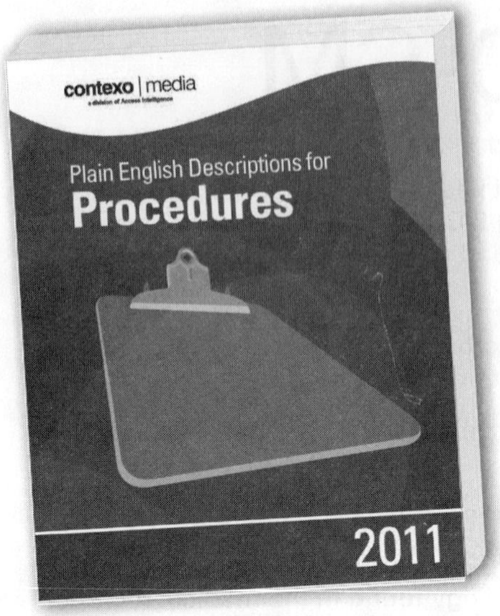

$99.95

Item ID: CDA-11
ISBN: 978-1-58383-689-7
Perfectbound
Available December 2010

Promo Code: FOBA11

This valuable resource reduces errors in code selection with plain English descriptions that help bridge the gap between practitioner notes and the language of CPT®. Master the components and details behind CPT codes, reduce the number of errors in code selection, improve understanding of the clinical meanings behind codes and check billing and coding information for Medicare for appropriate code selection.

- Detailed, full-page anatomy illustrations—helps you interpret clinical notes better to code with more specificity
- Plain English Descriptions for over 8,000 CPT codes—get the clarification you need to choose the right code
- Plain English Descriptions of CPT modifiers—ensure proper understanding and use of these important coding conventions
- E/M codes and coding guidelines—understand proper documentation and assignment of evaluation and management codes
- Easy look-up of medical prefixes/suffixes—helps you understand unfamiliar terms used in the medical record
- Eponyms, acronyms, common abbreviations, suffixes/prefixes—plain English descriptions to these critical elements help you decipher clinical notes and improve your coding knowledge

Plain English Descriptions for Coding Terms

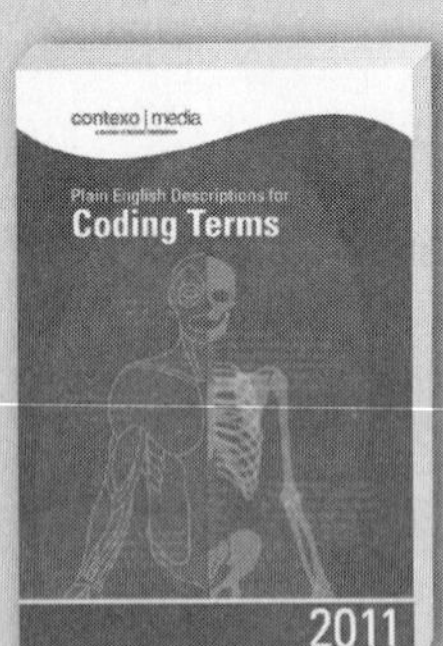

$99.95

Item ID: CDAT-11
ISBN: 978-1-58383-692-7
Compact 6 x 9
Available December 2010

Promo Code: FOBA11

More than 7,000 Plain English Descriptions for key terms including medical nomenclature, medical technology, billing and reimbursement — essential information for every coder!

- A-Z format — makes finding information easy and quick
- Anatomical illustrations — helps to crosswalk the illustrations to the plain English description for anatomy
- Coding term crosswalk — many terms are cross-referenced to the applicable CPT® and ICD-9-CM codes
- Includes drug definitions with HCPCS Level II Codes—a short cut to understanding complex drug code assignment
- Clarification of medical documentation for acronyms, eponyms, common abbreviations and suffixes/prefixes — decipher clinical notes and improve your coding knowledge

Contexo Media
P.O. Box 25128
SLC, UT 84125-0128

FAX
801.365.0710

PHONE
800.334.5724

ONLINE
www.codingbooks.com

contexo | media

Medicare Coverage Sourcebook

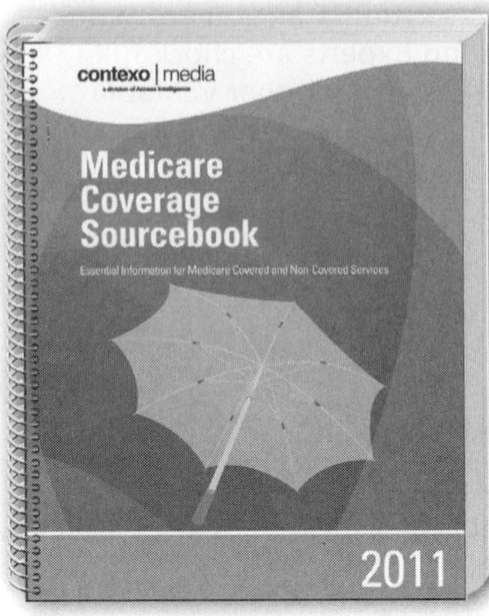

$149.95

Item ID: COVER-11
ISBN: 978-1-58383-693-4
Spiralbound
Available December 2010

Promo Code: FOBA11

We've organized Medicare's five Internet Only Manuals (IOMs) into a quick access guide to eligibility, benefit, coverage, claims processing and Medicare as secondary payer (MSP) information. Plus, we'll keep you abreast of the latest coverage policies with quarterly email alerts.

- Extensive alphabetical index — helps you locate the exact policy you need quickly
- New policy icons implemented within the past year — quickly locate this year's policies that could impact you financially
- Preventive service coverage — for all types of screenings covered by Medicare
- DME, prosthetic and orthotic guidelines — find out how and where to bill for these services, along with reimbursement data for specific items
- Billing information for nonphysician practitioners and payment methodologies — helps you bill appropriately
- Specialty-specific guidelines and regulations for Medicare coverage — identify rules targeted at your specialty
- Explanations of how and why Local Coverage Decisions (LCDs) are created and determined — helps you educate physicians and other staff
- Alert icons — easily identify services that fall under medical review policies or fraud alerts

Medicare RBRVS Sourcebook

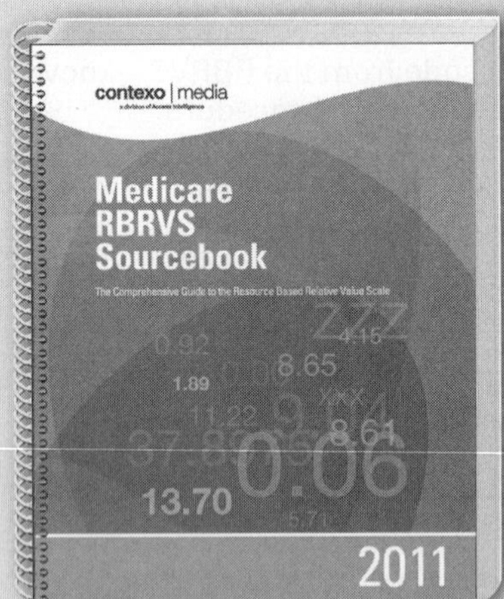

$149.95

Item ID: RBRVS-11
ISBN: 978-1-58383-716-0
Spiralbound
Available December 2010

Promo Code: FOBA11

Setting fees is not an art but a science. The way to succeed is to build a systematic approach to fee-setting with the Resource Based Relative Value Scale (RBRVS) data in the 2011 Medicare RBRVS Sourcebook. The straight-forward instructions, examples and formulas in this well-organized resource will help clarify the fee-setting process.

- NEW! Online access — e-Links to GPCI Index and other valuable tools — help determine your reimbursement
- 2011 CPT® and HCPCS Level II code changes — using updated information is key to getting the reimbursement you deserve
- Gap fill code data (RVUs not provided by Medicare) are included — helps you complete the reimbursement picture
- Instructions on conducting cost analysis and comparing fees by payer — know the reimbursement mix for your practice
- Charts detailing reimbursement of surgical package modifiers — make it easy to figure out when to use modifiers
- Modifier information integrated throughout — see at-a-glance which modifiers can or can not be used with each CPT code
- Professional component and/or technical component guidance — identifies which service or procedures have only one or both

Contexo Media
P.O. Box 25128
SLC, UT 84125-0128

FAX
801.365.0710

PHONE
800.334.5724

ONLINE
www.codingbooks.com

contexo | media

Call Today! 800.334.5724 or visit www.codingbooks.com

ITEM #	PRODUCT	PRICE	QTY	TOTAL

Thank you for your order.

Subtotal	
Sales Tax (Sales tax applies to CA, CO, MD, NJ, NY PA, TX, UT, & VA)	
Shipping	
GRAND TOTAL	

Shipping Chart

Qty	1	2-4	5-7	8-10	11+
Price	$12.95	$17.95	$22.95	$27.95	$27.95 + $5.00 each book over 10

Customer/Payment Information

Source Code: FOBA11

4 Easy Ways to Order

Contexo Media
P.O. Box 25128
SLC, UT 84125-0128

FAX
801.365.0710

PHONE
800.334.5724

ONLINE
www.codingbooks.com

Company Name: ____________________

*E-mail: ____________________
Required for confirmations

Ordered By: ____________________

❑ Check #________ Amount Enclosed $ ________

Ship to Attn: ____________________

❑ CC Card # ________________ Exp. ____ /____

Address: ____________________
(No PO boxes)

City: ____________ State: _____ ZIP: _______

Authorization: ____________________

Phone: (____) _____ - ________ *Fax: (____) _____ - ________

❑ Invoice Me PO# ____________________

Health Care Setting:

❑ Physician Office/Clinic ________# of Coders

❑ Hospital/Medical Center ________# of Beds

Specialty ____________________

❑ Payer

❑ Business/Government

❑ ASC/Lab/Home Health/SNF/Hospice

❑ Student

* "I understand that by providing a fax number or email above, I am giving Contexo Media express permission to notify me of upcoming programs and/or useful products via facsimile or email."

contexo | media
a division of Access Intelligence

Healthcare Common
Procedure Coding System

HCPCS

National Level II Codes

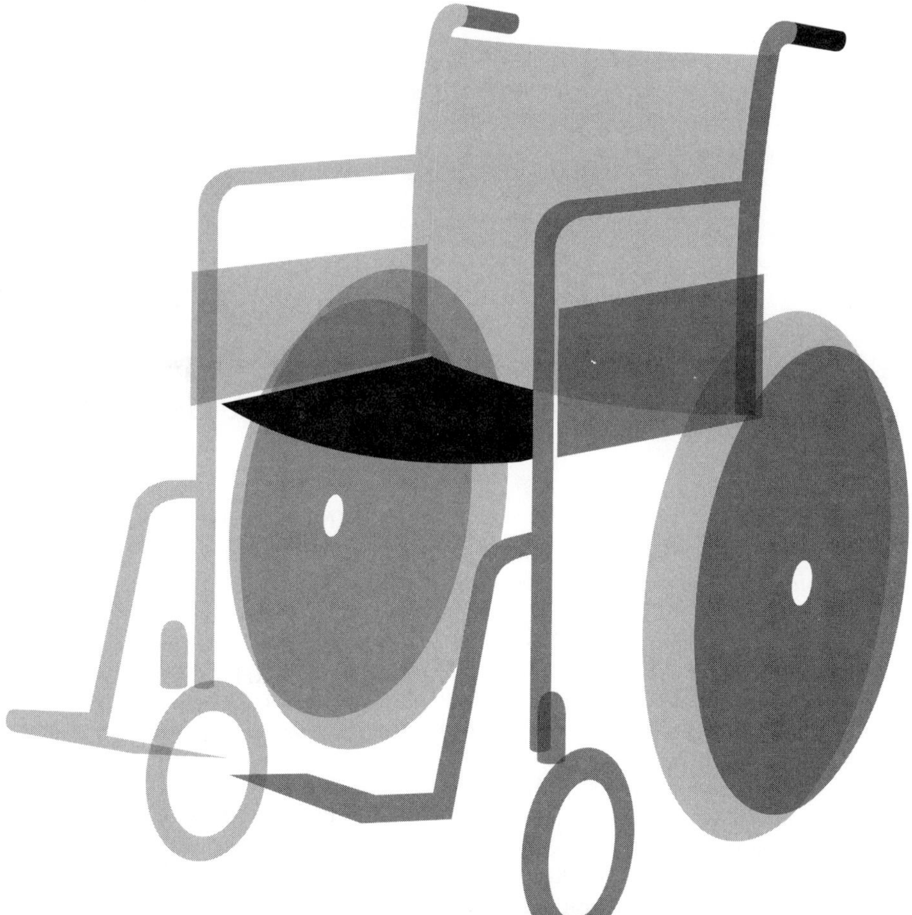

2011

Expert

2011 HCPCS Level II

Contexo Media, a division of Access Intelligence
P.O. Box 25128
Salt Lake City, UT 84125-0128
800.334.5724

ISBN: 978-1-58383-698-9
Item ID: HCPCS11

DISCLAIMER

ACKNOWLEDGEMENTS

Jerry M. Okabe, *General Manager*
Bonnie G. Schreck, CCS, CPC, CPC-H, CCS-P, COBGC, *Director, Clinical Content*
Lori Becks, RHIA, *Clinical Technical Editor*
Lauri Gray, RHIT, CPC, *Clinical Technical Editor*
Gregory A. Kemp, MA, *Desktop Publishing & Editorial Manager*
Jonas A. Croft, *Illustrator*

SUPPORT AND SOURCES

For answers to questions regarding the information contained within the pages of this manual, please call 800-334-5724, option 1. Orders for additional copies, discounted bulk pricing, and other customer service issues also can be addressed at this number. This manual contains HCPCS Level II codes effective for January 1, 2011 through December 31, 2011, as compiled and released by the Department of Health and Human Services (HHS). Many of the symbols, guidelines, and conventions used throughout are derived from the official government release of this information.

Contents

Introduction

The information provided is an abridged version of the procedures the Centers for Medicare and Medicaid Services (CMS) follows in making coding decisions for the Healthcare Common Procedure Coding System (HCPCS) Level II. To view the full text of the document, visit the CMS website at http://www.cms.hhs.gov/MedHCPCSGenInfo/02_HCPCSCODINGPROCESS.asp#TopOfPage.

A. HCPCS Background Information

Each year, in the United States, health care insurers process over 5 billion claims for payment. For Medicare and other health insurance programs to ensure that these claims are processed in an orderly and consistent manner, standardized coding systems are essential. The HCPCS Level II Code Set is one of the standard code sets used for this purpose. The HCPCS is divided into two principal subsystems, referred to as level I and level II of the HCPCS. Level I of the HCPCS is comprised of CPT (Current Procedural Terminology), a numeric coding system maintained by the American Medical Association (AMA). The CPT is a uniform coding system consisting of descriptive terms and identifying codes that are used primarily to identify medical services and procedures furnished by physicians and other health care professionals. These health care professionals use the CPT to identify services and procedures for which they bill public or private health insurance programs. Decisions regarding the addition, deletion, or revision of CPT codes are made by the AMA. The CPT codes are republished and updated annually by the AMA. Level I of the HCPCS, the CPT codes, does not include codes needed to separately report medical items or services that are regularly billed by suppliers other than physicians.

Level II of the HCPCS is a standardized coding system that is used primarily to identify products, supplies, and services not included in the CPT codes, such as ambulance services and durable medical equipment, prosthetics, orthotics, and supplies (DMEPOS) when used outside a physician's office. Because Medicare and other insurers cover a variety of services, supplies, and equipment that are not identified by CPT codes, the level II HCPCS codes were established for submitting claims for these items. The development and use of level II of the HCPCS began in the 1980's. Level II codes are also referred to as alpha-numeric codes because they consist of a single alphabetical letter followed by 4 numeric digits, while CPT codes are identified using 5 numeric digits.

In October of 2003, the Secretary of HHS delegated authority under the HIPAA legislation to CMS to maintain and distribute HCPCS Level II Codes. As stated in 42 CFR Sec. 414.40 (a) CMS establishes uniform national definitions of services, codes to represent services, and payment modifiers to the codes. Within CMS there is a CMS HCPCS Workgroup which is an internal workgroup comprised of representatives of the major components of CMS, as well as other consultants from pertinent Federal agencies. Prior to December 31, 2003, Level III HCPCS were developed and used by Medicaid State agencies, Medicare contractors, and private insurers in their specific programs or local areas of jurisdiction. For purposes of Medicare, level III codes were also referred to as local codes. Local codes were established when an insurer preferred that suppliers use a local code to identify a service, for which there is no level I or level II code, rather than use a "miscellaneous or not otherwise classified code." The Health Insurance Portability and Accountability Act of 1996 (HIPAA) required CMS to adopt standards for coding systems that are used for reporting health care transactions. We published, in the Federal Register on August 17, 2000 (65 FR 50312), regulations to implement this part of the HIPAA legislation. These regulations provided for the elimination of level III local codes by October 2002, at which time, the level I and level II code sets could be used. The elimination of local codes was postponed, as a result of section 532(a) of BIPA, which continued the use of local codes through December 31, 2003.

B. HCPCS Level II Codes

The regulation that CMS published on August 17, 2000 (45 CFR 162.10002) to implement the HIPAA requirement for standardized coding systems established the HCPCS level II codes as the standardized coding system for describing and identifying health care equipment and supplies in health care transactions that are not identified by the HCPCS level I, CPT codes. The HCPCS level II coding system was selected as the standardized coding system because of its wide acceptance among both public and private insurers. Public and private insurers were required to be in compliance with the August 2000 regulation by October 1, 2002. The purpose of this section is to provide a general description of the current HCPCS level II coding system.

The HCPCS level II coding system is a comprehensive and standardized system that classifies similar products that are medical in nature into categories for the purpose of efficient claims processing. For each alphanumeric HCPCS code, there is descriptive terminology that identifies a category of like items. These codes are used primarily for billing purposes. For example, suppliers use HCPCS level II codes to identify items on claim forms that are being billed to a private or public health insurer.

HCPCS is a system for identifying items and services. It is not a methodology or system for making coverage or payment determinations, and the existence of a code does not, of itself, determine coverage or non-coverage for an item or service. While these codes are used for billing purposes, decisions regarding the addition, deletion, or revision of HCPCS codes are made independent of the process for making determinations regarding coverage and payment.

Currently, there are national HCPCS codes representing over 4,000 separate categories of like items or services that encompass millions of products from different manufacturers. When submitting claims, suppliers are required to use one of these codes to identify the items they are billing. The descriptor that is assigned to a code represents the definition of the items and services that can be billed using that code.

In summary, the HCPCS level II coding system has the following characteristics:

- This system ensures uniform reporting on claims forms of items or services that are medical in nature. Such a standardized coding system is needed by public and private insurance programs to ensure the uniform reporting of services on claims forms by suppliers and for meaningful data collection.
- The descriptors of the codes identify a category of like items or services and typically do not identify specific products or brand/trade names.

- The coding system is not a methodology for making coverage or payment determinations. Each payer makes determinations on coverage and payment outside this coding process.

C. Types of HCPCS Level II Codes

There are several types of HCPCS level II codes depending on the purpose for the codes and who is responsible for establishing and maintaining them.

Permanent National Codes

National permanent HCPCS level II codes are maintained by the CMS HCPCS Workgroup. The Workgroup is responsible for making decisions about additions, revisions, and deletions to the permanent national alpha-numeric codes. These codes are for the use of all private and public health insurers. Since HCPCS is a national coding system all payers will be represented in the Workgroup including representatives from private insurance agencies, the Pricing, Data Analysis, and Coding (PDAC), and Medicaid will participate in the workgroup meetings and provide input as to what is necessary to meet each party's program operating needs.

The permanent national codes serve the important function of providing a standardized coding system that is managed jointly by private and public insurers. This standardized approach to developing a set of uniform codes provides a stable environment for claims submission and processing.

Dental Codes

The dental codes are a separate category of national codes. The Current Dental Terminology (CDT) is a publication copyrighted by the American Dental Association (ADA) that lists codes for billing for dental procedures and supplies. The CDT is included in HCPCS level II. Decisions regarding the revision, deletion, or addition of CDT codes are made by the ADA and not the CMS HCPCS Workgroup.

As the Department of Health and Human Services has an agreement with the AMA pertaining to the use of the Current Procedural Terminology (CPT) codes for physician services, the ADA requested that the D codes not be included in the HCPCS code set for 2011; therefore, these codes are not included in the ***2011 HCPCS Level II*** code book.

Miscellaneous Codes

National codes also include "miscellaneous/not otherwise classified" codes. These codes are used when a supplier is submitting a bill for an item or service and there is no existing national code that adequately describes the item or service being billed. The importance of miscellaneous codes is that they allow suppliers to begin billing immediately for a service or item as soon as it is allowed to be marketed by the Food and Drug Administration (FDA) even though there is no distinct code that describes the service or item. A miscellaneous code can be used during the period of time a request for a new code is being considered under the HCPCS review process. The use of miscellaneous codes also helps us to avoid the inefficiency and administrative burden of assigning distinct codes for items or services that are rarely furnished or for which we expect to receive few claims.

Because of miscellaneous codes, the absence of a specific code for a distinct category of products does not affect a supplier's ability to submit claims to private or public insurers and does not affect patient access to products. Claims with miscellaneous codes are manually reviewed, the item or service being billed must be clearly described, and pricing information must be provided along with documentation to explain why the item or service is needed by the beneficiary.

Ordinarily, before using a miscellaneous code on a claim form, a supplier should check with the entity that will receive the payment claim to determine whether there is a specific code that should be used rather than a miscellaneous code. In the case of claims that are to be submitted to one of the four Durable Medical Equipment Medicare Administrative Contractors (DME MACs), suppliers that have coding questions should check with the pricing, data analysis, and coding (PDAC), contractor to CMS. The PDAC is responsible for providing suppliers and manufacturers with assistance in determining which HCPCS code should be used to describe DMEPOS items for the purpose of billing Medicare. The PDAC has a toll free helpline for this purpose, (877) 735-1326. In addition, the PDAC publishes a product classification list on its website that lists individual items to code categories. More information about the PDAC and the PDAC's product classification list can be found at http://www.dmepdac.com.

If no code exists that describes the product category to which the item belongs, and if the item fits a Medicare Benefit Category, the PDAC may instruct the supplier to submit claims using a "miscellaneous/ not otherwise classified" code. If an item does not fit a Medicare Benefit Category, the PDAC might assign a code that indicates that the product is not covered by Medicare for example, code A9270, NON-COVERED ITEM OR SERVICE. If an item is included or bundled into another code and not separately reimbursed by Medicare, the PDAC may assign the code that includes the item or a code that indicates that the item is included as a component of another code. In those cases in which a supplier or manufacturer has been advised to use a miscellaneous code because there is no existing code that describes a given product, and the supplier or manufacturer believes that the code is needed, it should submit a request to modify the HCPCS in accordance with the established process. The process for requesting a revision to the HCPCS level II codes is explained below.

Temporary National Codes

Temporary codes are for the purpose of meeting, within a short time frame, the national program operational needs of a particular insurer that are not addressed by an already existing national code. The CMS HCPCS Workgroup has set aside certain sections of the HCPCS code set to allow the Workgroup to develop temporary codes. Decisions regarding the number and type of temporary codes and how they are used are also made by the CMS HCPCS Workgroup. These codes are used at the discretion of CMS. This means that if, before the next scheduled annual update for permanent codes, the CMS HCPCS Workgroup needs a code in order to meet specific operating needs that pertain to its particular programs, it may establish a national temporary code. In the case of Medicare, decisions regarding temporary codes are made by the CMS HCPCS workgroup. For example, Medicare may need additional codes before the next scheduled annual HCPCS update to implement newly issued coverage policies or legislative requirements. Although we establish temporary codes to meet our specific operational needs, the temporary codes we establish can be used by other insurers. Temporary codes allow insurers the flexibility to establish codes that are needed before the next January 1 annual update for permanent national codes or until consensus can be achieved on a permanent national code. Permanent national codes are only updated once a year on January 1.

The CMS HCPCS Workgroup may decide to replace temporary codes with permanent codes. However, temporary codes do not have established expiration dates. Whenever a permanent code is established by the CMS HCPCS Workgroup to replace a temporary code, the temporary code is deleted and cross-referenced to the new permanent code.

Types of temporary HCPCS codes:

The C codes were established to permit implementation of section 201 of the Balanced Budget Refinement Act of 1999. HCPCS C codes are utilized to report drugs, biologicals, magnetic resonance angiography (MRA), and devices that must be used by OPPS hospitals. HCPCS C codes are reported for device categories, new technology procedures, and drugs, biologicals and radiopharmaceuticals that do not have other HCPCS code assignments. Non-OPPS hospitals, Critical Access Hospitals (CAHs), Indian Health Service Hospitals (IHS), hospitals located in American Samoa, Guam, Saipan, or the Virgin Islands, and Maryland waiver hospitals may report these codes at their discretion. More information regarding HOPPS can be found at http://www.cms.hhs.gov/providers/hopps/.

The G codes are used to identify professional health care procedures and services that would otherwise be coded in CPT-4 but for which there are no CPT-4 codes.

The Q codes are used to identify services that would not be given a CPT-4 code, such as drugs, biologicals, and other types of medical equipment or services, and which are not identified by national level II codes but for which codes are needed for claims processing purposes.

The K codes were established for use by the DME MACs when the currently existing permanent national codes do not include the codes needed to implement a DME MAC medical review policy. For example, codes other than the permanent national codes may be needed by the DME MACs to identify certain product categories and supplies necessary for establishing appropriate regional medical review coverage policies.

The S codes are used by private insurers to report drugs, services, and supplies for which there are no national codes but for which codes are needed by the private sector to implement policies, programs, or claims processing. They are for the purpose of meeting the particular needs of the private sector. These codes are also used by the Medicaid program, but they are not payable by Medicare.

Certain H codes are used by those State Medicaid agencies that are mandated by State law to establish separate codes for identifying mental health services such as alcohol and drug treatment services.

The T codes are designated for use by Medicaid State agencies to establish codes for items for which there are no permanent national codes and for which codes are necessary to meet a national Medicaid program operating need. T codes are not used by Medicare but can be used by private insurers.

Code Modifiers

In some instances, insurers instruct suppliers that a HCPCS code must be accompanied by code modifier to provide additional information regarding the service or item identified by the HCPCS code. Modifiers are used when the information provided by a HCPCS code descriptor needs to be supplemented to identify specific circumstances that may apply to an item or service. For example, a UE modifier is used when the item identified by a HCPCS code is "used equipment," a NU modifier is used for "new equipment." The level II HCPCS modifiers are either alpha-numeric or two letters.

D. Requesting a Revision to the HCPCS Level II Codes

Anyone can submit a request for modifying the HCPCS level II national code set. A document explaining the HCPCS revision process, as well as a detailed format for submitting a request, is available on the HCPCS website at http://www.cms.hhs.gov/medicare/hcpcs. Besides the information requested in this format, a requestor should also submit any additional descriptive material, including the manufacturer's product literature and information, that it thinks would be helpful in furthering our understanding of the medical features of the item for which a coding revision is being recommended. The HCPCS coding review process is an ongoing continuous process. Requests may be submitted at any time throughout the year. Requests that are received and complete by January 4 of the current year will be considered for inclusion in the next annual update (January 1st of the following year). Requests received on or after January 5, and requests received earlier that require additional evaluation, will be included in a later HCPCS update. There are three types of coding revisions to the HCPCS that can be requested:

1. That a permanent code be added

   When there is not a distinct code that describes a product, a code may be requested (1) if the FDA allows the product to be marketed in the United States and (2) if the product is not a drug, the product has been on the market for at least 3 months; if the product is a drug, there is no requirement to submit marketing data; and (3) the product represents 3 percent or more of the outpatient use for that type of product in the national market. If a request for a new code is approved, the addition of a new HCPCS codes does not mean that the item is necessarily covered by any insurer. Whether an item identified by a new code is covered is determined by the Medicare law, regulations, and medical review policies and not by the assignment of a code.

2. That the language used to describe an existing code be changed

   When there is an existing code, a recommendation to modify the code can be made when an interested party believes that the descriptor for the code needs to be modified to provide a better description of the category of products represented by the code.

3. That an existing code be deleted

   When an existing code becomes obsolete or is duplicative of another code, a request can be made to delete the code.

When there is no currently existing code to describe a product, a miscellaneous code/not otherwise classified code may be appropriate. The use of a miscellaneous code permits a claims history to be established for an item that can be used to support the need for a national permanent code.

Requests for coding revisions should be sent to the following:

Alpha-Numeric HCPCS Coordinator
Center for Medicare Management
Centers for Medicare and Medicaid Services
C5-08-27, 7500 Security Boulevard
Baltimore, MD 21244-1850

CMS HCPCS Workgroup

The CMS HCPCS Workgroup is an internal workgroup comprised of representatives of the major components of CMS, the Medicaid State agencies, and the PDAC. The PDAC represents Medicare program operating needs with input from the four DME MACs which have responsibility for processing Durable Medical Equipment, Prosthetics, Orthotics and Supplies (DMEPOS) claims for the Medicare program. Coding decisions are coordinated with both public and private insurers. The CMS HCPCS workgroup considers each coding request, and beginning with the 2006 cycle, will determine whether HCPCS coding requests warrant a change to the national permanent codes. Prior to the 2006 cycle, the National Panel was responsible for final decisions.

When a recommendation for a revision to the HCPCS is received, it is reviewed at a regularly scheduled meeting of the CMS HCPCS Workgroup. Ordinarily, the CMS HCPCS Workgroup meets monthly to discuss whether coding requests warrant a change to the national permanent codes.

Evaluating HCPCS Coding Requests

The CMS HCPCS workgroup applies the following criteria to determine whether there is a demonstrated need for a new or modified code or the need to remove a code:

1. When an existing code adequately describes the item in a coding request, then no new or modified code is established. An existing code adequately describes an item in a coding request when the existing code describes products with the following:
   - Functions similar to the item in the coding request.
   - No significant therapeutic distinctions from the item in the coding request.
2. When an existing code describes products that are almost the same in function with only minor distinctions from the item in the coding request, the item in the coding request may be grouped with that code and the code descriptor modified to reflect the distinctions.
3. A code is not established for an item that is used only in the inpatient setting or for an item that is not diagnostic or therapeutic in nature.
4. A new or modified code is not established for an item unless the FDA allows the item to be marketed. FDA approval documentation is required to be submitted with the coding request application for all non-drug items. For drugs, FDA approval documentation will be accepted up to March 31 following the application deadline as long as the application is otherwise complete and submitted by the deadline.
5. There must be sufficient claims activity or volume, as evidenced by 3 months of marketing activity for non-drug products, so that the adding of a new or modified code enhances the efficiency of the system and justifies the administrative burden of adding or modifying a code.
6. The determination to remove a code is based on the consideration of whether a code is obsolete (for example, products no longer are used, other more specific codes have been added) or duplicative and no longer useful (for example, new codes are established that better describe items identified by existing codes). In developing its decisions, the HCPCS Workgroup uses the criteria mentioned above. In deciding upon a recommendation, the workgroup does not include cost as a factor.

Opportunity for Public Input/Public Meeting Process for HCPCS

On December 21, 2000, the Congress passed the Medicare, Medicaid, and SCHIP Benefits Improvement and Protection Act of 2000 (BIPA), Pub. L. 106-554. Section 531(b) of BIPA mandated that we establish procedures that permit public consultation for coding and payment determinations for new DME under Medicare Part B of title XVIII of the Social Security Act (the Act). As part of HCPCS reform, CMS expanded the public meeting forum to include all public requests as of the 2005-2006 coding cycle. Accordingly, CMS hosts annual public meetings that provide a forum for interested parties to make oral presentations and/or to submit written comments in response to preliminary coding and pricing recommendations for new durable medical equipment that have been submitted using the Healthcare Common Procedure Coding System coding revision process. Agenda items for the meetings will be published in advance of the public meeting on the HCPCS website at http://www.cms.hhs.gov/medicare/hcpcs. The agenda will include descriptions of the coding requests, the requestor, and the name of the product or service. This change will provide more opportunities for the public to become aware of coding changes under consideration, as well as opportunities for public input into decision-making.

The HCPCS coordinator schedules meetings with interested parties, at their request, as time permits, to discuss their recommendations regarding possible changes to the HCPCS level II codes. These meetings are held at the Central Office of CMS. In addition to representatives from the CMS HCPCS Workgroup, staff from Medicaid and Medicare coverage, payment and operations are invited to attend these meetings. These meetings are not related to the meetings mandated by section 531(b) of BIPA, they are also not decision making meetings or CMS HCPCS Workgroup meetings.

Final Decisions

The CMS HCPCS Workgroup is responsible for making the final decisions pertaining to additions, deletions, and revisions to the HCPCS codes. The CMS HCPCS Workgroup reviews all requests for coding changes and makes final decisions regarding the annual update to the national codes. The Workgroup sends letters to those who requested coding revisions to inform them of the Workgroup's decision regarding their coding requests. The decision letters include, but may not be limited to, the following types of responses:

1. A change to the national codes has been approved that reflects, completely or in part, your coding request.
2. Your request for a coding revision to this year's update has not been approved because the scope of your request necessitates that additional consideration be given to your request before the CMS HCPCS Workgroup reaches a final decision.
3. Your reported sales volume was insufficient to support your request for a revision to the national codes. To determine whether there is sufficient sales volume to warrant a permanent code, we ask requestors to submit 3 months of the most recent sales volume for non-drug items. There is not a requirement to submit marketing data for drugs.
4. Your request for a new national code has not been approved because there already is an existing permanent or temporary code that describes your product.
5. Your request for a code has not been approved because your product is not used by health care providers for diagnostic or therapeutic purposes.
6. Your request for a code has not been approved because the code you requested is for capital equipment.
7. Your request for a code has not been approved because your product is an integral part of another service and payment for that service includes payment for your product; therefore, your product may not be billed separately to Medicare.
8. Your request for a revision to the language that describes the current code has not been approved because it does not improve the code descriptor.
9. Your request for a new code has not been approved because your product is not primarily medical in nature (for example, generally not useful in the absence of an illness or injury).
10. Your request for a code has not been approved because your product is used exclusively in the inpatient hospital setting.
11. Your request for a code has not been approved because it is inappropriate for inclusion in the HCPCS Level II code set and request should be submitted independently to another coding authority (e.g. AMA for CPT coding, ADA for CDT coding, etc.)

Decision letters also inform the requestors that they may contact the entity in whose jurisdiction a claim is filed for assistance in answering any coding questions. For Medicare, contact the PDAC. Contractor to CMS, the PDAC is responsible for providing suppliers and manufacturers with assistance in determining which HCPCS code should be used to describe DMEPOS items for the purpose of billing Medicare. The PDAC has a toll free helpline for this purpose,

(877) 735-1326, which is operational during the hours of 9 AM to 4 PM (EST). For Medicaid, contact the state Medicaid agency. For private insurance, contact the individual insurer. A requestor who is dissatisfied with the final decision may submit a new request asking the CMS HCPCS Workgroup to reconsider and re-evaluate the code request. At that time, the requestor should include new information or additional explanations to support the request.

Reconsideration Process

CMS management is considering pilot-testing, a process by which denied applicants would be allowed an opportunity to have their application reconsidered during the same coding cycle. The basis for denial will be clearly delineated in a notice to the applicant and provided in a timely fashion.

E. HCPCS Updates

Permanent National Codes

The national codes are updated annually, according to the following schedule:

1. Coding requests have to be received by January 3 of the current year to be considered for the next January 1 update of the subsequent year. This means that completed requests must be received by no later than January 3 of the current year to be considered for inclusion in the January update of the following year unless January 3 falls on a weekend; then the due date is extended to the following Monday.
2. Computer tapes and instructions, that include an updated list of codes and identify which codes have been changed or deleted, are updated and sent to our contractors and Medicaid State agencies at least 60 days in advance of the January 1 implementation date for the annual update. In addition, the CMS HCPCS Workgroup's final decisions on all public requests for changes to the HCPCS coding system will be published on the official HCPCS web site at http://www.cms.hhs.gov/medicare/hcpcs in November of each year.

Temporary Codes

Temporary codes can be added, changed, or deleted on a quarterly basis. Once established, temporary codes are usually implemented within 90 days, the time needed to prepare and issue implementation instructions and to enter the new code into CMS's and the contractors' computer systems and initiate user education. This time is needed to allow for instructions such as bulletins and newsletters to be sent out to suppliers to provide them with information and assistance regarding the implementation of temporary CMS codes.

HCPCS/Medicare Website

Our website, http://www.cms.hhs.gov/medicare/hcpcs lists all of the current HCPCS codes, an alphabetical index of HCPCS codes by type of service or product, and an alphabetical table of drugs for which there are level II codes. The HCPCS Public Meeting Agendas (separated by product category) published on this website list applications submitted in the current coding cycle. Interested parties can submit comments regarding the agenda items to the CMS HCPCS Workgroup by sending an e-mail to CMS through this website. These comments are included as part of the Workgroup's review as it considers the coding requests.

The newly established temporary codes and effective dates for their use are also posted on the HCPCS website at http://www.cms.hhs.gov/medicare/hcpcs. This website enables us to quickly disseminate information on coding requests and decisions.

Code Assignment Following Medicare National Coverage Determination

Pursuant to Sec. 1862 (l) (3) (C) (iv) of the Social Security Act (added by Section 731 (a) of the Medicare Modernization Act), the Centers for Medicare and Medicaid Services (CMS), has developed a process by which the CMS HCPCS Workgroup will identify an appropriate existing code category and/or establish a new code category to describe the item that is the subject of a National Coverage Determination (NCD). If the item is considered Durable Medical Equipment, Prosthetic, Orthotic or Supply (DMEPOS), the CMS will defer to the Pricing, Data Analysis and Coding (PDAC) to determine the appropriate code category. Contractor to the CMS, the (PDAC) assigns individual DMEPOS products to HCPCS code categories for the purpose of billing Medicare.

As a matter of meeting on-going Medicare program operating needs, processes have existed for some time by which items and services that are newly covered by Medicare are assigned to a new or existing code category. Effective July 1, 2004, the process outlined below has been used by CMS to comply with the requirements of Sec. 1862 (l).

1. **Assignment of an Existing "Temporary" or "Permanent" Code:** When the CMS determines that an item is already identified by an existing "temporary" or "permanent" (as described in A and B above) HCPCS code category, but was previously not covered, the CMS will assign the item to the existing code category, and ensure that the coverage indicator assigned to the code category accurately reflects Medicare policy regarding payment for the item. Sec. 731 of the MMA does not require that a new code category or a product specific code be created for an item simply because a new coverage determination was made, without regard to codes available in the existing code set.
2. **Assignment of a new Temporary or Permanent code:** When the CMS determines that a new code category is appropriate, CMS will make every effort to establish, publish, and implement the new code at the time the final coverage determination is made.
3. **Assignment of an unclassified code:** Under certain circumstances, the assignment of an item to an unclassified code may be necessary. A number of unclassified codes already exist under various headings throughout the HCPCS Level II code set. When an item is newly covered, but usage is narrow and the item would be billed infrequently, it may be more of an administrative burden to revise the code set than to use an unclassified code along with other, existing processing methods. When a new "temporary" or "permanent" code is appropriate, but the change cannot be implemented and incorporated into billing and claims processing systems at the time the final NCD decision memorandum is released, an unclassified code may be assigned in the interim, until a new code can be implemented, in order to ensure that claims can be processed for the item. The timing of implementation of new "temporary" or "permanent" codes relative to the date of the coverage determination depends on a variety of factors, some of which are not within the direct control of the code set maintainers, for example:
   - Coding alternatives may require extensive research
   - The timing of the coverage determination may be such that the publication deadline for the next Quarterly Update is missed
   - There is insufficient time between NCD and Quarterly Update to incorporate new codes into new policy and accompanying billing instructions, and into claims processing systems along with any edits needed to operationalize the new code.

Rev. June 15, 2010

HCPCS Level II Use and Conventions

To code accurately, it is necessary to have a working knowledge of medical terminology and to understand the characteristics, terminology, and conventions of HCPCS Level II codes. Transforming verbal descriptions of diseases, injuries, conditions, and procedures into numerical designations (coding) is a complex activity. Medical codes are utilized to facilitate payment of health services, to evaluate utilization patterns, and to study the appropriateness of healthcare costs. Coding provides the basis for epidemiological studies and research into the quality of healthcare. Coding must be performed correctly and consistently to produce meaningful statistics that aid in planning for the health needs of the nation.

Basic Steps in HCPCS Level II Coding:

1. **Consult the Alphabetic Index.**
   Locate the main entry term. The Alphabetic Index is arranged by procedure, supply, drug, or service. These items and services are generally expressed as nouns. Some items and services have multiple entries under their synonyms and/or drug brand names. Select an appropriate code. If an appropriate code cannot be located, refer to the Table of Contents to locate the chapter in the Tabular List. Peruse the chapter in search of the most appropriate code.
2. **Refer to the Tabular List to locate the most appropriate code after selecting from the Alphabetical Index.**
   Be guided by any cross reference notes or other instructions that would direct the use of a different code from that selected out of the Alphabetic Index for a particular item or service.
3. **Refer to the conventions used in the Tabular List for more information.**
   Coverage and pricing information is identified with symbols in the Tabular List (see the section below titled Tabular List Conventions for more information about symbols used in this manual).
4. **Append any appropriate CPT or HCPCS Level II modifiers.**
   Certain circumstances dictate the use of a modifier to provide more complete information regarding the items or services provided. Appendix A contains a full listing of all HCPCS Level II modifiers and descriptions.

Tabular List Conventions

The HCPCS Tabular List utilizes conventions that are useful for efficient and effective coding.

Special Characters

New and Revised Text Characters

● A bullet denotes a new code (or, in a few cases, a once deleted HCPCS code that has been reinstated).

▲ The triangle denotes a revised code description.

✖ ~~word~~ A code description with a strikethrough highlights a code that has been deleted from the HCPCS Level II code set. Because the HCPCS Level II code set is updated more than once per year, the Tabular List contains all codes deleted for 2011, with a note referencing the appropriate active code.

Color-Coded Symbols

The following symbols denote Medicare coverage and payment jurisdiction for each particular item or service.

⃠ (red) **Not Covered by Medicare** – These items or services not covered by Medicare under any circumstances.

ⓘ (green) **Special Coverage Instructions Apply** – The references to the *National Coverage Determinations Manual*, additional Medicare Pub 100 manuals (***Medicare Benefit Policy Manual**, **Medicare Claims Processing Manual**, **Medicare Program Integrity Manual***), Medicare Statutes, and the Code of Federal Regulations (found in Appendix C) will give insight into the nature of the special coverage instructions.

🏛 (blue) **Coverage Carrier Determined** – There is no standard national coverage of items or services preceded by this symbol. Contact the appropriate Medicare carrier or DME MAC for more information regarding the coverage and payment for these items and services.

♀ (red) **Female** – Code is applicable for females.

♂ (red) **Male** – Code is applicable for males.

(crutch) (red) **DMEPOS** – Medicare allows billing for certain durable medical equipment, prosthetics, orthotics, and supplies (DMEPOS). Codes valid for reimbursement are noted with crutches.

PQR (green) **Physician Quality Reporting System** – Established to provide a financial incentive for those providers willing to participate in a voluntary quality reporting program. If quality measures are reported satisfactorily, providers can receive an incentive for covered Medicare physician fee schedule services, which is subject to a pre-determined cap. Applicable quality measures codes are noted in green with the letters PQR.

A2 - Z3 (blue) **ASC Indicator** – Certain HCPCS Level II codes are reimbursable when provided in an Ambulatory Surgical Center (ASC) under the Outpatient Prospective Payment System (OPPS). Under the ASC reimbursement system, a payment indicator is assigned to each HCPCS code. The payment indicator directs how payment is made or not made under OPPS for each individual code submitted.

Indicator	Payment Indicator Definition
A2	Surgical procedure on ASC list in CY 2007; payment based on OPPS relative payment weight.
D5	Deleted/discontinued code; no payment made.
F4	Corneal tissue acquisition, hepatitis B vaccine; paid at reasonable cost..
G2	Non office-based surgical procedure added in CY 2008 or later; payment based on OPPS relative payment weight.
H7	Brachytherapy source paid separately when provided integral to a surgical procedure on ASC list; payment contractor-priced.
H8	Device-intensive procedure on ASC list in CY 2007; paid at adjusted rate.

Indicator	Payment Indicator Definition
J7	OPPS pass-through device paid separately when provided integral to a surgical procedure on ASC list; payment contractor-priced.
J8	Device-intensive procedure added to ASC list in CY 2008 or later; paid at adjusted rate.
K2	Drugs and biologicals paid separately when provided integral to a surgical procedure on ASC list; payment based on OPPS rate.
K7	Unclassified drugs and biologicals; payment contractor-priced.
L1	Influenza vaccine; pneumococcal vaccine. Packaged item/service; no separate payment made.
L6	New Technology Intraocular Lens (NTIOL); special payment.
N1	Packaged service/item; no separate payment made.
P2	Office-based surgical procedure added to ASC list in CY 2008 or later with MPFS nonfacility PE RVUs; payment based on OPPS relative payment weight.
P3	Office-based surgical procedure added to ASC list in CY 2008 or later with MPFS nonfacility PE RVUs; payment based on MPFS nonfacility PE RVUs.
R2	Office-based surgical procedure added to ASC list in CY 2008 or later without MPFS nonfacility PE RVUs; payment based on OPPS relative payment weight.
Z2	Radiology service paid separately when provided integral to a surgical procedure on ASC list; payment based on OPPS relative payment weight.
Z3	Radiology service paid separately when provided integral to a surgical procedure on ASC list; payment based on MPFS nonfacility PE RVUs.

A - Y (red) **APC Indicator** – The Ambulatory Payment Classification (APC) system is a Medicare-based fee schedule for outpatient hospital reimbursement under the Outpatient Prospective Payment System (OPPS). Procedures and services are grouped, or assigned to APC codes for fee calculation. Under the APC system, a status indicator is assigned to each line item. The status indicator directs how payment is made or not made under OPPS for each individual code submitted and describes the type of service, procedure, device, or supply being reported. The same indicator applies to all codes within an APC.

Indicator	Item/Code/Service	OPPS Payment Status
A	Services furnished to a hospital outpatient that are paid under a fee schedule or payment system other than OPPS, for example: • Ambulance services • Clinical Diagnostic Laboratory Services (Not subject to deductible or coinsurance) • Non-implantble prosthetic and orthotic devices • IPO for ESRD patients • Physical, occupational, and speech therapy • Routine dialysis services for ESRD patients provided in a certified dialysis unit of a hospital • Diagnostic mammography (Not subject to deductible or coinsurance) • Screening mammography	Not paid under OPPS. Paid by fiscal intermediaries/MACs under a fee schedule or payment system other than OPPS.
B	Codes that are not recognized by OPPS when submitted on an outpatient hospital Part B bill type (12x and13x)	Not paid under OPPS. • May be paid by fiscal intermediaries/MACs when submitted on a different bill type, for example, 75x (CORF), but not paid under OPPS. • An alternate code that is recognized by OPPS when submitted on an outpatient hospital Part B bill type (12x and 13x) may be available.
C	Inpatient Procedures	Not paid under OPPS. Admit patient. Bill as inpatient.
D	Discontinued Codes	Not paid under OPPS. or any other Medicare payment system.
E	Items, Codes, and Services: • That are not covered by any Medicare outpatient benefit based on statutory exclusion. • That are not covered by any Medicare outpatient benefit for reasons other than statutory exclusion. • That are not recognized by Medicare for outpatient claims but for which an alternate code for the same item or service may be available. • For which separate payment is not provided on outpatient claims.	Not paid by Medicare when submitted on outpatient claims (any outpatient bill type).
F	Corneal Tissue Acquisition; Certain CRNA Services and Hepatitis B Vaccines	Not paid under OPPS. Paid at reasonable cost.
G	Pass-Through Drugs and Biologicals	Paid under OPPS; separate APC payment.
H	(1) Pass-Through Device Categories	Separate cost-based pass-through payment; Not subject to copayment.
K	Non-Pass-Through Drugs and Non-implantable Biologicals, including therapeutic radiopharmaceuticals.	Paid under OPPS; Separate APC payment.
L	Influenza Vaccine; Pneumococcal Pneumonia Vaccine	Not paid under OPPS. Paid at reasonable cost; not subject to deductible or coinsurance.
M	Items and Services Not Billable to the Fiscal Intermediary/MAC	Not paid under OPPS.
N	Items and Services Packaged into APC Rates	Paid under OPPS; payment is packaged into payment for other services. Therefore, there is no separate APC payment.
P	Partial Hospitalization	Paid under OPPS; per diem APC payment.
Q1	STVX-Packaged Codes	Paid under OPPS; Addendum B displays APC assignments when services are separately payable. (1) Packaged APC payment if billed on the same date of service as a HCPCS code assigned status indicator "S," "T," "V," or "X." (2) In all other circumstances, payment is made through a separate APC payment.

Indicator	Item/Code/Service	OPPS Payment Status
Q2	T-Packaged Codes	Paid under OPPS; Addendum B displays APC assignments when services are separately payable. (1) Packaged APC payment if billed on the same date of service as a HCPCS code assigned status indicator "T." (2) In all other circumstances, payment is made through a separate APC payment.
Q3	Codes that may be paid through a composite APC	Paid under OPPS; Addendum B displays APC assignments when services are separately payable.. Addendum M displays composite APC assignments when codes are paid through a composite APC. (1) Composite APC payment based on OPPS composite-specific payment criteria. Payment is packaged into a signle payment for specific combinations of service. (2) In all other circumstances, payment is made through a separate APC payment or packaged into payment of other services.
R	Blood and Blood Products	Paid under OPPS; Separate APC payment.
S	Significant Procedure, Not Discounted when Multiple	Paid under OPPS; Separate APC payment.
T	Significant Procedure, Multiple Reduction Applies	Paid under OPPS; Separate APC payment.
U	Brachytherapy Sources	Paid under OPPS; Separate APC payment.
V	Clinic or Emergency Department Visit	Paid under OPPS; Separate APC payment.
X	Ancillary Services	Paid under OPPS; Separate APC payment.
Y	Non-Implantable Durable Medical Equipment	Not paid under OPPS. All institutional providers other than home health agencies bill to DMERC.

Code Cross-References

These notes reference other HCPCS Level II codes, CPT codes, or the CPT book in general that should be reviewed before selecting that code to report a particular item or service. A cross-reference note should always be reviewed before selecting a final HCPCS Level II code to be billed.

References

Notes appearing in green under the code highlight references in the Medicare manuals that explain coverage and reimbursement guidelines about a particular item or service. A Medicare manual note references a specific section of the Medicare ***National Coverage Determinations*** (NCD) Manual, additional Medicare Pub 100 manuals, the Social Security Act (Medicare Statute), and the Code of Federal Regulations (CFR). All sections of each of these publications referenced throughout the Tabular List are reprinted in Appendix C. Italicized notes appearing in blue under the code reference the brand name of a drug or medication. References to the *AHA Coding Clinic® for HCPCS* are preceded by AHA.

HCPCS Level II Code Changes

Tabular List

The new, updated, and deleted HCPCS Level II codes for 2011 have been released. The codes and descriptors have been approved and will be available for use for dates of service on or after January 1, 2011.

New Codes

A4566 Shoulder sling or vest design, abduction restrainer, with or without swathe control, prefabricated, includes fitting and adjustment

A7020 Interface for cough stimulating device, includes all components, replacement

A9273 Hot water bottle, ice cap or collar, heat and/or cold wrap, any type

C1749 Endoscope, retrograde imaging/illumination colonoscope device (implantable)

C8931 Magnetic resonance angiography without contrast followed by contrast, spinal canal and contents

C8932 Magnetic resonance angiography without contrast, spinal canal and contents

C8933 Magnetic resonance angiography without contrast followed by with contrast, spinal canal and contents

C8934 Magnetic resonance angiography with contrast, upper extremity

C8935 Magnetic resonance angiography without contrast, upper extremity

C8936 Magnetic resonance angiography without contrast followed by with contrast, upper extremity

C9270 Injection, immune globulin (Gammaplex), intravenous, non-lyophilized (e.g. liquid), 500 mg

C9272 Injection, denosumab, 1 mg

C9273 Sipuleucel-t, minimum of 50 million autologous CD54+ cells activated with PAP-GM-CSF, including leukapheresis and all other preparatory procedures, per infusion

C9274 Crotalidae polyvalent immune fab (Ovine), 1 vial

C9275 Injection, hexaminolevulinate hydrochloride, 100 mg, per study dose

C9276 Injection, cabazitaxel, 1 mg

C9277 Injection, alglucosidase alfa (Lumizyme), 1 mg

C9278 Injection, incobotulinumtoxin a, 1 unit

C9279 Injection, ibuprofen, 100 mg

C9367 Skin substitute, endoform dermal template, per square centimeter

C9800 Dermal injection procedure(s) for facial lipodystrophy syndrome (LDS) and provision of radiesse or sculptra dermal filler, including all items and supplies

E0446 Topical oxygen delivery system, not otherwise specified, includes all supplies and accessories

E1831 Static progressive stretch toe device, extension and/or flexion, with or without range of motion adjustment, includes all components and accessories

E2622 Skin protection wheelchair seat cushion, adjustable, width less than 22 inches, any depth

E2623 Skin protection wheelchair seat cushion, adjustable, width 22 inches or greater, any depth

E2624 Skin protection and positioning wheelchair seat cushion, adjustable, width less than 22 inches, any depth

E2625 Skin protection and positioning wheelchair seat cushion, adjustable, width 22 inches or greater, any depth

G0157 Services performed by a qualified physical therapist assistant in the home health or hospice setting, each 15 minutes

G0158 Services performed by a qualified occupational therapist assistant in the home health or hospice setting, each 15 minutes

G0159 Services performed by a qualified physical therapist, in the home health setting, in the establishment or delivery of a safe and effective therapy maintenance program, each 15 minutes

G0160 Services performed by a qualified occupational therapist, in the home health setting, in the establishment or delivery of a safe and effective therapy maintenance program, each 15 minutes

G0161 Services performed by a qualified speech-language pathologist, in the home health setting, in the establishment or delivery of a safe and effective therapy maintenance program, each 15 minutes

G0162 Skilled services by a registered nurse (RN) in the delivery of management & evaluation of the plan of care; each 15 minutes (the patient's underlying condition or complication requires an rn to ensure that essential non-skilled care achieve its purpose in the home health or hospice setting)

G0163 Skilled services of a licensed nurse (LPN or RN) in the delivery of observation & assessment of the patient's condition, each 15 minutes (when the likelihood of change in the patient's condition requires skilled nursing personnel to identify and evaluate the patient's need for possible modification of treatment in the home health or hospice setting)

G0164 Skilled services of a licensed nurse, in the training and/or education of a patient or family member, in the home health or hospice setting, each 15 minutes

G0428 Collagen meniscus implant procedure for filling meniscal defects (e.g., CMI, collagen scaffold, menaflex)

G0429 Dermal filler injection(s) for the treatment of facial lipodystrophy syndrome (LDS) (e.g., as a result of highly active antiretroviral therapy)

G0432 Infectious agent antibody detection by enzyme immunoassay (EIA) technique, HIV-1 and/or HIV-2, screening

G0433 Infectious agent antibody detection by enzyme-linked immunosorbent assay (ELISA) technique, HIV-1 and/or HIV-2, screening

G0434 Drug screen, other than chromatographic; any number of drug classes, by CLIA waived test or moderate complexity test, per patient encounter

G0435 Infectious agent antibody detection by rapid antibody test, HIV-1 and/or HIV-2, screening

G0436 Smoking and tobacco cessation counseling visit for the asymptomatic patient; intermediate, greater than 3 minutes, up to 10 minutes

G0437 Smoking and tobacco cessation counseling visit for the asymptomatic patient; intensive, greater than 10 minutes

G0438 Annual wellness visit; includes a personalized prevention plan of service (PPS), initial visit

G0439 Annual wellness visit, includes a personalized prevention plan of service (PPS), subsequent visit

G0440 Application of tissue cultured allogeneic skin substitute or dermal substitute; for use on lower limb, includes the site preparation and debridement if performed; first 25 sq cm or less

G0441 Application of tissue cultured allogeneic skin substitute or dermal substitute; for use on lower limb, includes the site preparation and debridement if performed; each additional 25 sq cm

G8629 Documentation of order for prophylactic parenteral antibiotic to be given within one hour (if fluoroquinolone or vancomycin, two hours) prior to surgical incision (or start of procedure when no incision is required)

G8630 Documentation that administration of prophylactic parenteral antibiotics was initiated within one hour (if fluoroquinolone or vancomycin, two hours) prior to surgical incision (or start of procedure when no incision is required), as ordered

G8631 Clinician documented that patient was not an eligible candidate for ordering prophylactic parenteral antibiotics to be given within one hour (if fluoroquinolone or vancomycin, two hours) prior to surgical incision (or start of procedure when no incision is required)

G8632 Prophylactic parenteral antibiotics were not ordered to be given or given within one hour (if fluoroquinolone or vancomycin, two hours) prior to the surgical incision (or start of procedure when no incision is required), reason not otherwise specified)

G8633 Pharmacologic therapy (other than minierals/vitamins) for osteoporosis prescribed

G8634 Clinician documented patient not an eligible candidate to receive pharmacologic therapy for osteoporosis

G8635 Pharmacologic therapy for osteoporosis was not prescribed, reason not otherwise specified

G8636 Influenza immunization administered or previously received

G8637 Clinician documented that patient is not eligible to receive the influenza immunization

G8638 Influenza immunization not administered or previously received, reason not otherwise specified

G8639 Influenza immunization was administered or previously received

G8640 Clinician has documented that patient is not eligible to receive the influenza immunization

G8641 Influenza immunization was not administered or previously received, reason not otherwise specified

G8642 The eligible professional practices in a rural area without sufficient high speed internet access and requests a hardship exemption from the application of the payment adjustment under section 1848(a)(5)(a) of the social security act

G8643 The eligible professional practices in an area without sufficient available pharmacies for electronic prescribing and requests a hardship exemption for the application of the payment adjustment under section 1848(a)(5)(a) of the social security act

G8644 Eligible professional does not have prescribing privileges

G8645 I intend to report the asthma measures group

G8646 All quality actions for the applicable measures in the asthma measures group have been performed for this patient

G8647 Risk-adjusted functional status change residual score for the knee successfully calculated and the score was equal to zero (0) or greater than zero (>0)

G8648 Risk-adjusted functional status change residual score for the knee successfully calculated and the score was less than zero (<0)

G8649 Risk-adjusted functional status change residual scores for the knee not measured because the patient did not complete foto's functional intake on admission and/or follow up status survey near discharge, patient not eligible/not appropriate

G8650 Risk-adjusted functional status change residual scores for the knee not measured because the patient did not complete foto's functional intake on admission and/or follow up status survey near discharge, reason not specified

G8651 Risk-adjusted functional status change residual score for the hip successfully calculated and the score was equal to zero (0) or greater than zero (>0)

G8652 Risk-adjusted functional status change residual score for the hip successfully calculated and the score was less than zero (<0)

G8653 Risk-adjusted functional status change residual scores for the hip not measured because the patient did not complete foto's functional intake on admission and/or follow up status survey near discharge, patient not eligible/not appropriate

G8654 Risk-adjusted functional status change residual scores for the hip not measured because the patient did not complete foto's functional intake on admission and/or follow up status survey near discharge, reason not specified

G8655 Risk-adjusted functional status change residual score for the lower leg, foot or ankle successfully calculated and the score was equal to zero (0) or greater than zero(>0)

G8656 Risk-adjusted functional status change residual score for the lower leg, foot or ankle successfully calculated and the score was less than zero (<0)

G8657 Risk-adjusted functional status change residual scores for the lower leg, foot or ankle not measured because the patient did not complete foto's functional intake on admission and/or follow up status survey near discharge, patient not eligible/not appropriate

G8658 Risk-adjusted functional status change residual scores for the lower leg, foot or ankle not measured because the patient did not complete foto's functional intake on admission and/or follow up status survey near discharge, reason not specified

G8659 Risk-adjusted functional status change residual score for the lumbar spine successfully calculated and the score was equal to zero (0) or greater than zero (>0)

G8660 Risk-adjusted functional status change residual score for the lumbar spine successfully calculated and the score was less than zero (<0)

G8661 Risk-adjusted functional status change residual scores for the lumbar spine not measured because the patient did not complete foto's functional intake on admission and/or follow up status survey near discharge, patient not eligible/not appropriate

G8662 Risk-adjusted functional status change residual scores for the lumbar spine not measured because the patient did not complete Foto's functional intake on admission and/or follow up status survey near discharge, reason not specified

G8663 Risk-adjusted functional status change residual score for the shoulder successfully calculated and the score was equal to zero (0) or greater than zero (>0)

G8664 Risk-adjusted functional status change residual score for the shoulder successfully calculated and the score was less than zero (<0)

G8665 Risk-adjusted functional status change residual scores for the shoulder not measured because the patient did not complete foto's functional intake on admission and/or follow up status survey near discharge, patient not eligible/not appropriate

G8666 Risk-adjusted functional status change residual scores for the shoulder not measured because the patient did not complete foto's functional intake on admission and/or follow up status survey near discharge, reason not specified

G8667 Risk-adjusted functional status change residual score for the elbow, wrist or hand successfully calculated and the score was equal to zero (0) or greater than zero (>0)

G8668 Risk-adjusted functional status change residual score for the elbow, wrist or hand successfully calculated and the score was less than zero (<0)

G8669 Risk-adjusted functional status change residual scores for the elbow, wrist or hand not measured because the patient did not complete foto's functional intake on admission and/or follow up status survey near discharge, patient not eligible/not appropriate

G8670 Risk-adjusted functional status change residual scores for the elbow, wrist or hand not measured because the patient did not complete foto's functional intake on admission and/or follow up status survey near discharge, reason not specified

G8671 Risk-adjusted functional status change residual score for the neck, cranium, mandible, thoracic spine, ribs, or other general orthopedic impairment successfully calculated and the score was equal to zero (0) or greater than zero (>0)

G8672 Risk-adjusted functional status change residual score for the neck, cranium, mandible, thoracic spine, ribs, or other general orthopedic impairment successfully calculated and the score was less than zero (<0)

G8673 Risk-adjusted functional status change residual scores for the neck, cranium, mandible, thoracic spine, ribs, or other general orthopedic impairment not measured because the patient did not complete foto's functional intake on admission and/or follow up status survey near discharge, patient not eligible/not appropriate

G8674 Risk-adjusted functional status change residual scores for the neck, cranium, mandible, thoracic spine, ribs, or other general orthopedic impairment not measured because the patient did not complete foto's functional intake on admission and/or follow up status survey near discharge, reason not specified

G8675 Most recent systolic blood pressure >= 140 mm hg

G8676 Most recent diastolic blood pressure >= 90 mm hg

G8677 Most recent systolic blood pressure < 130 mm hg

G8678 Most recent systolic blood pressure 130 to 139 mm hg

G8679 Most recent diastolic blood pressure < 80 mm hg

G8680 Most recent diastolic blood pressure 80 – 89 mm hg

G8681 Patient hospitalized with principal diagnosis of heart failure during the measurement period

G8682 Left ventricular function testing performed during the measurement period

G8683 Clinician documented that patient is not an eligible candidate for left ventricular function testing during the measurement period

G8684 Patient not hospitalized with principal diagnosis of heart failure during the measurement period

G8685 Left ventricular function testing not performed during the measurement period, reason not specified

G8686 Currently a tobacco smoker or current exposure to secondhand smoke

G8687 Currently a tobacco non-user and no exposure to secondhand smoke

G8688 Currently a smokeless tobacco user (eg, chew, snuff) and no exposure to secondhand smoke

G8689 Tobacco use not assessed, reason not otherwise specified

G8690 Current tobacco smoker or current exposure to secondhand smoke

G8691 Current tobacco non-user and no exposure to secondhand smoke

G8692 Current smokeless tobacco user (eg, chew, snuff) and no exposure to secondhand smoke

G8693 Tobacco use not assessed, reason not specified

G9147 Outpatient intravenous insulin treatment (Oivit) either pulsatile or continuous, by any means, guided by the results of measurements for: respiratory quotient; and/or, urine urea nitrogen (UUN); and/or, arterial, venous or capillary glucose; and/or potassium concentration

J0171 Injection, adrenalin, epinephrine, 0.1 mg

J0558 Injection, penicillin G benzathine and penicillin G procaine, 100,000 units

J0561 Injection, penicillin G benzathine, 100,000 units

J0597 Injection, C-1 esterase inhibitor (human), Berinert, 10 units

J0638 Injection, Canakinumab, 1 mg

J0775 Injection, Collagenase, clostridium histolyticum, 0.01 mg

J1290 Injection, Ecallantide, 1 mg

J1559 Injection, immune globulin (hizentra), 100 mg

J1599 Injection, immune globulin, intravenous, non-lyophilized (e.g. liquid), not otherwise specified, 500 mg

J1786 Injection, Imiglucerase, 10 units

J1826 Injection, Interferon beta-1A, 30 mcg

J2358 Injection, Olanzapine, long-acting, 1 mg

J2426 Injection, Paliperidone palmitate extended release, 1 mg

J3095 Injection, Televancin, 10 mg

J3262 Injection, Tocilizumab, 1 mg

J3357 Injection, Ustekinumab, 1 mg

J3385 Injection, Velaglucerase alfa, 100 units

J7184 Injection, von Willebrand factor complex (human), Wilate, per 100 IU VWF:RCO

J7196 Injection, antithrombin recombinant, 50 i.u.

J7309 Methyl aminolevulinate (MAL) for topical administration, 16.8%, 1 gram

J7312 Injection, Dexamethasone, intravitreal implant, 0.1 mg

J7335 Capsaicin 8% patch, per 10 square centimeters

J7686 Treprostinil, inhalation solution, FDA-approved final product, non-compounded, administered through DME, unit dose form, 1.74 mg

J8562 Fludarabine phosphate, oral, 10 mg

J9302 Injection, Oatumumab, 10 mg

J9307 Injection, Pralatrexate, 1 mg

J9315 Injection, Romidepsin, 1 mg

J9351 Injection, Topotecan, 0.1 mg

L3674 Shoulder orthosis, abduction positioning (airplane design), thoracic component and support bar, with or without nontorsion joint/turnbuckle, may include soft interface, straps, custom fabricated, includes fitting and adjustment

L4631 Ankle foot orthosis, walking boot type, varus/valgus correction, rocker bottom, anterior tibial shell, soft interface, custom arch support, plastic or other material, includes straps and closures, custom fabricated

L5961 Addition, endoskeletal system, polycentric hip joint, pneumatic or hydraulic control, rotation control, with or without flexion and/or extension control

L8693 Auditory osseointegrated device abutment, any length, replacement only

Q0478 Power adapter for use with electric or electric/ pneumatic ventricular assist device, vehicle type

Q0479 Power module for use with electric or electric/ pneumatic ventricular assist device, replacement only

Q2026 Injection, Radiesse, 0.1 ml

Q2027 Injection, Sculptra, 0.1 ml

Q2035 Influenza virus vaccine, split virus, when administered to individuals 3 years of age and older, for intramuscular use (Afluria)

Q2036 Influenza virus vaccine, split virus, when administered to individuals 3 years of age and older, for intramuscular use (Fulaval)

Q2037 Influenza virus vaccine, split virus, when administered to individuals 3 years of age and older, for intramuscular use (Fluvirin)

Q2038 Influenza virus vaccine, split virus, when administered to individuals 3 years of age and older, for intramuscular use (Fluzone)

Q2039 Influenza virus vaccine, split virus, when administered to individuals 3 years of age and older, for intramuscular use (not otherwise specified)

Q4117 Hyalomatrix, per square centimeter

Q4118 Matristem micromatrix, 1 mg

Q4119 Matristem wound matrix, per square centimeter

Q4120 Matristem burn matrix, per square centimeter

Q4121 Theraskin, per square centimeter

Q5010 Hospice home care provided in a hospice facility

S0148 Injection, Pegylated interferon Alfa-2B, 10 mcg

S0169 Calcitrol, 0.25 microgram

T1505 Electronic medication compliance management device, includes all components and accessories, not otherwise classified

New Modifiers

AY Item or service furnished to an esrd patient that is not for the treatment of ESRD

AZ Physician providing a service in a dental health professional shortage area for the purpose of an electronic health record incentive payment

CS Item or service related, in whole or in part, to an illness, injury, or condition that was caused by or exacerbated by the effects, direct or indirect, of the 2010 oil spill in the gulf of mexico, including but not limited to subsequent clean-up activities

DA Oral health assessment by a licensed health professional other than a dentist

GU Waiver of liability statement issued as required by payer policy, routine notice

GX Notice of liability issued, voluntary under payer policy

NB Nebulizer system, any type, FDA-cleared for use with specific drug

PT Colorectal cancer screening test; converted to diagnostic test or other procedure

Revised Codes

A4399 Ostomy irrigation supply; cone/catheter, with or without brush

A5112 Urinary drainage bag, leg or abdomen, latex, with or without tube, with straps, each

A6011 Collagen based wound filler, gel/paste, per gram of collagen

A6248 Hydrogel dressing, wound filler, gel, per fluid ounce

A6260 Wound cleansers, any type, any size

A6261 Wound filler, gel/paste, per fluid ounce, not otherwise specified

A6262 Wound filler, dry form, per gram, not otherwise specified

A7013 Filter, disposable, used with aerosol compressor or ultrasonic generator

B4034 Enteral feeding supply kit; syringe fed, per day, includes but not limited to feeding/flushing syringe, administration set tubing, dressings, tape

B4035 Enteral feeding supply kit; pump fed, per day, includes but not limited to feeding/flushing syringe, administration set tubing, dressings, tape

B4036 Enteral feeding supply kit; gravity fed, per day, includes but not limited to feeding/flushing syringe, administration set tubing, dressings, tape

C8923 Transthoracic echocardiography with contrast, or without contrast followed by contrast, real-time, with image documentation (2D), includes M-mode recording, when performed, complete, without spectral or color doppler echocardiography

C8924 Transthoracic echocardiography with contrast, or without contrast, followed by with contrast, real-time with image documentation (2D), includes M-mode recording, when performed, follow-up or limited study

C8928 Transthoracic echocardiography with contrast, or without contrast followed by with contrast, real-time with image documentation (2D), includes M-mode recording, when performed, during rest and cardiovascular stress test using treadmill, bicycle exercise and/or pharmacologically induced stress, with interpretation and report

G0151 Services performed by a qualified physical therapist in the home health or hospice setting, each 15 minutes

G0152 Services performed by a qualified occupational therapist in the home health or hospice setting, each 15 minutes

G0153 Services performed by a qualified speech-language pathologist in the home health or hospice setting, each 15 minutes

G0154 Direct skilled nursing services of a licensed nurse (lpn or rn) in the home health or hospice setting, each 15 minutes

G0431 Drug screen, qualitative; multiple drug classes by high complexity test method (e.g., immunoassay, enzyme assay), per patient encounter

G8427 List of current medications (includes prescription, over-the-counter, herbals, vitamin/mineral/dietary [nutritional] supplements) documented by the provider, including drug name, dosage, frequency and route

G8428 Current medications (includes prescription, over-the-counter, herbals, vitamin/mineral/dietary [nutritional] supplements) with drug name, dosage, frequency and route not documented by the provider, reason not specified

G8440 Documentation of pain assessment (including location, intensity and description) prior to initiation of therapy or documentation of the absence of pain as a result of assessment through discussion with the patient including the use of a standardized tool and a follow-up plan is documented

G8441 No documentation of pain assessment (including location, intensity and description) prior to initiation of therapy

G8447 Patient encounter was documented using an ehr system that has been certified by an authorized testing and certification body (ATCB)

G8448 Patient encounter was documented using a PQRI qualified ehr or other acceptable systems

G8508 Documentation of pain assessment (including location, intensity and description) prior to initiation of therapy or documentation of the absence of pain as a result of assessment through discussion with the patient including the use of a standardized tool; no documentation of a follow-up plan, patient not eligible

G8509 Documentation of pain assessment (including location, intensity and description) prior to initiation of therapy or documentation of the absence of pain as a result of assessment through discussion with the patient including the use of a standardized tool; no documentation of a follow-up plan, reason not specified

J0598 Injection, C-1 Esterase inhibitor (human), Cinryze, 10 units

J9060 Injection, cisplatin, powder or sOlution, 10 mg

L3671 Shoulder orthosis, shoulder joint design, without joints, may include soft interface, straps, custom fabricated, includes fitting and adjustment

L3677 Shoulder orthosis, shoulder joint design, without joints, may include soft interface, straps, prefabricated, includes fitting and adjustment

Q0499 Belt/vest/bag for use to carry external peripheral components of any type ventricular assist device, replacement only

Q4101 Apligraf, per square centimeter

Q4102 Oasis wound matrix, per square centimeter

Q4103 Oasis burn matrix, per square centimeter

Q4104 Integra bilayer matrix wound dressing (BMWD), per square centimeter

Q4105 Integra dermal regeneration template (DRT), per square centimeter

Q4106 Dermagraft, per square centimeter

Q4107 Graftjacket, per square centimeter

Q4108 Integra matrix, per square centimeter

Q4110 Primatrix, per square centimeter

Q4111 Gammagraft, per square centimeter

Q4112 Cymetra, injectable, 1cc

Q4113 Graftjacket Xpress, injectable, 1cc

Q4115 Alloskin, per square centimeter

Q4116 Alloderm, per square centimeter

Revised Modifiers

GA Waiver of liability statement issued as required by payer policy, individual case

RA Replacement of a DME, orthotic or prosthetic item

RB Replacement of a part of a DME, orthotic or prosthetic item furnished as part of a repair

V5 Vascular catheter (alone or with any other vascular access)

V6 Arteriovenous graft (or other vascular access not including a vascular catheter)

V7 Arteriovenous fistula only (in use with two needles)

Deleted Code(s) List

C9255 Injection, Paliperidone palmitate, 1 mg

C9256 Injection, Dexamethasone intravitreal implant, 0.1 mg

C9258 Injection, Telavancin, 10 mg

C9259 Injection, Pralatrexate, 1 mg

C9260 Injection, Ofatumumab, 10 mg

C9261 Injection, Ustekinumab, 1 mg

C9262 Fludarabine phosphate, oral, 1 mg

C9263 Injection, Ecallantide, 1 mg

C9264 Injection, Tocilizumab, 1 mg

C9265 Injection, Romidepsin, 1 mg

C9266 Injection, Collagenase clostridium histolyticum, 0.1 mg

C9267 Injection, von Willebrand factor complex (human), Wilate, per 100 IU VWF: RCO

C9268 Capsaicin, patch, 10cm2

C9269 Injection, C-1 Esterase inhibitor (human), Berinert, 10 units

C9271 Injection, Velaglucerase Alfa, 100 units

G0430 Drug screen, qualitative; multiple drug classes other than chromatographic method, each procedure

G8006 Acute myocardial infarction: patient documented to have received aspirin at arrival

G8007 Acute myocardial infarction: patient not documented to have received aspirin at arrival

G8008 Clinician documented that acute myocardial infarction patient was not an eligible candidate to receive aspirin at arrival measure

G8009 Acute myocardial infarction: patient documented to have received beta-blocker arrival

G8010 Acute myocardial infarction: patient not documented to have received beta-blocker at arrival

G8011 Clinician documented that acute myocardial infarction patient was not an eligible candidate for beta-blocker at arrival measure

G8012 Pneumonia: patient documented to have received antibiotic within 4 hours of presentation

G8013 Pneumonia: patient not documented to have received antibiotic within 4 hours of presentation

G8014 Clinician documented that pneumonia patient was not an eligible candidate for antibiotic within 4 hours of presentation measure

G8015 Diabetic patient with most recent hemoglobin A1c level (within the last 6 months) documented as greater than 9%

G8016 Diabetic patient with most recent hemoglobin A1c level (within the last 6 months) documented as less than or equal to 9%

G8017 Clinician documented that diabetic patient was not eligible candidate for hemoglobin a1c measure

G8018 Clinician has not provided care for the diabetic patient for the required time for hemoglobin a1c measure (6 months)

G8019 Diabetic patient with most recent low-density lipoprotein (within the last 12 months) documented as greater than or equal to 100 mg/dl

G8020 Diabetic patient with most recent low-density lipoprotein (within the last 12 months) documented as less than 100 mg/dl

G8021 Clinician documented that diabetic patient was not eligible candidate for

G8022 Clinician has not provided care for the diabetic patient for the required time for low-density lipoprotein measure (12 months)

G8023 Diabetic patient with most recent blood pressure (within the last 6 months) documented as equal to or greater than 140 systolic or equal to or greater than 80 mmhg diastolic

G8024 Diabetic patient with most recent blood pressure (within the last 6 months) documented as less than 140 systolic and less than 80 diastolic

G8025 Clinician documented that the diabetic patient was not eligible candidate for blood pressure measure

G8026 Clinician has not provided care for the diabetic patient for the required time for blood pressure measure (within the last 6 months)

G8027 Heart failure patient with left ventricular systolic dysfunction (LVSD) documented to be on either angiotensin-converting enzyme inhibitor or angiotensin-receptor blocker (ACE-I or ARB) therapy

G8028 Heart failure patient with left ventricular systolic dysfunction (LVSD) not documented to be on either angiotensin-converting enzyme inhibitor or angiotensin-receptor blocker (ACE-I or ARB) therapy

G8029 Clinician documented that heart failure patient was not an eligible candidate for either angiotensin-converting enzyme inhibitor or angiotensin-receptor blocker (ACE-I or ARB) therapy measure

G8030 Heart failure patient with left ventricular systolic dysfunction (LVSD) documented to be on beta-blocker therapy

G8031 Heart failure patient with left ventricular systolic dysfunction (LVSD) not documented to be on beta-blocker therapy

G8032 Clinician documented that heart failure patient was not eligible candidate for beta-blocker therapy measure

G8033 Prior myocardial infarction – coronary artery disease patient documented to be on beta-blocker therapy

G8034 Prior myocardial infarction – coronary artery disease patient not documented to be on beta-blocker therapy

G8035 Clinician documented that prior myocardial infarction – coronary artery disease patient was not eligible candidate for beta-blocker therapy measure

G8036 Coronary artery disease patient documented to be on antiplatelet therapy

G8037 Coronary artery disease patient not documented to be on antiplatelet therapy

G8038 Clinician documented that coronary artery disease patient was not eligible candidate for antiplatelet therapy measure

G8039 Coronary artery disease – patient with low-density lipoprotein documented to be greater than 100mg/dl

G8040 Coronary artery disease – patient with low-density lipoprotein documented to be less than or equal to 100mg/dl

G8041 Clinician documented that coronary artery disease patient was not eligible candidate for low-density lipoprotein measure

G8051 Patient (female) documented to have been assessed for osteoporosis

G8052 Patient (female) not documented to have been assessed for osteoporosis

G8053 Clinician documented that (female) patient was not an eligible candidate for osteoporosis assessment measure

G8054 Patient not documented for the assessment for falls within last 12 months

G8055 Patient documented for the assessment for falls within last 12 months

G8056 Clinician documented that patient was not an eligible candidate for the falls assessment measure within the last 12 months

G8057 Patient documented to have received hearing assessment

G8058 Patient not documented to have received hearing assessment

G8059 Clinician documented that patient was not an eligible candidate for hearing assessment measure

G8060 Patient documented for the assessment of urinary incontinence

G8061 Patient not documented for the assessment of urinary incontinence

G8062 Clinician documented that patient was not an eligible candidate for urinary incontinence assessment measure

G8075 End stage renal disease patient with documented dialysis dose of URR greater than or equal to 65% (or kt/v greater than or equal to 1.2)

G8076 End stage renal disease patient with documented dialysis dose of URR less than 65% (or kt/v less than 1.2)

G8077 Clinician documented that end stage renal disease patient was not an eligible candidate for URR or kt/v measure

G8078 End stage renal disease patient with documented hematocrit greater than or equal to 33 (or hemoglobin greater than or equal to 11)

G8079 End stage renal disease patient with documented hematocrit less than 33 (or hemoglobin less than 11)

G8080 Clinician documented that end stage renal disease patient was not an eligible candidate for hematocrit (hemoglobin) measure

G8081 End stage renal disease patient requiring hemodialysis vascular access documented to have received autogenous av fistula

G8082 End stage renal disease patient requiring hemodialysis documented to have received vascular access other than autogenous av fistula

G8085 End-stage renal disease patient requiring hemodialysis vascular access was not an eligible candidate for autogenous av fistula

G8093 Newly diagnosed chronic obstructive pulmonary disease (COPD) patient documented to have received smoking cessation intervention, within 3 months of diagnosis

G8094 Newly diagnosed chronic obstructive pulmonary disease (COPD) patient not documented to have received smoking cessation intervention, within 3 months of diagnosis

G8099 Osteoporosis patient documented to have been prescribed calcium and vitamin D supplements

G8100 Clinician documented that osteoporosis patient was not an eligible candidate for calcium and vitamin D supplement measure

G8103 Newly diagnosed osteoporosis patients documented to have been treated with antiresorptive therapy and/or pth within 3 months of diagnosis

G8104 Clinician documented that newly diagnosed osteoporosis patient was not an eligible candidate for within 3 months of diagnosis antiresorptive therapy and/or PTH treatment measure

G8106 Within 6 months of suffering a nontraumatic fracture, female patient 65 years of age or older documented have been prescribed a drug to treat or prevent osteoporosis to have undergone bone mineral density testing or to

G8107 Clinician documented that female patient 65 years of age or older who suffered a nontraumatic fracture for measure to test bone mineral density or drug to treat or prevent within the last 6 months was not an eligible candidate osteoporosis

G8108 Patient documented to have received influenza vaccination during influenza season

G8109 Patient not documented to have received influenza vaccination during influenza season

G8110 Clinician documented that patient was not an eligible candidate for influenza vaccination measure

G8111 Patient (female) documented to have received a mammogram during the measurement year or prior year to the measurement year

G8112 Patient (female) not documented to have received a mammogram during the measurement year or prior year to the measurement year

G8113 Clinician documented that female patient was not an eligible candidate for mammography measure

G8114 Clinician did not provide care to patient for the required time of mammography measure (i.e., measurement year or prior year)

G8115 Patient documented to have received pneumococcal vaccination

G8116 Patient not documented to have received pneumococcal vaccination

G8117 Clinician documented that patient was not an eligible candidate for pneumococcal vaccination measure

G8129 Patient documented as being treated with antidepressant medication for at least

G8130 Patient not documented as being treated with antidepressant medication for at least 6 months continuous treatment phase

G8131 Clinician documented that patient was not an eligible candidate for antidepressant medication for continuous treatment phase

G8152 Patient documented to have received antibiotic prophylaxis one hour prior to incision time (two hours for vancomycin)

G8153 Patient not documented to have received antibiotic prophylaxis one hour prior to incision time (two hours for vancomycin)

G8154 Clinician documented that patient was not an eligible candidate for antibiotic prophylaxis one hour prior to incision time (two hours for vancomycin) measure

G8155 Patient with documented receipt of thromboembolism prophylaxis

G8156 Patient without documented receipt of thromboembolism prophylaxis

G8157 Clinician documented that patient was not an eligible candidate for

G8159 Patient documented to have received coronary artery bypass graft without use of internal mammary artery

G8162 Patient with isolated coronary artery bypass graft not documented to have received pre-operative beta-blockade

G8164 Patient with isolated coronary artery bypass graft documented to have prolonged intubation

G8165 Patient with isolated coronary artery bypass graft not documented to have prolonged intubation

G8166 Patient with isolated coronary artery bypass graft documented to have required surgical re-exploration

G8167 Patient with isolated coronary artery bypass graft did not require surgical re-exploration

G8170 Patient with isolated coronary artery bypass graft documented to have been discharged on aspirin or clopidogrel

G8171 Patient with isolated coronary artery bypass graft not documented to have been discharged on aspirin or clopidogrel

G8172 Clinician documented that patient with isolated coronary artery bypass graft was not an eligible candidate for antiplatelet therapy at discharge measure

G8182 Clinician has not provided care for the cardiac patient for the required time for low-density lipoprotein measure (6 months)

G8183 Patient with heart failure and atrial fibrillation documented to be on warfarin therapy

G8184 Clinician documented that patient with heart failure and atrial fibrillation was not an eligible candidate for warfarin therapy measure

G8185 Patients diagnosed with symptomatic osteoarthritis with documented annual assessment of function and pain

G8186 Clinician documented that symptomatic osteoarthritis patient was not an eligible candidate for annual assessment of function and pain measure

G8193 Clinician did not document that an order for prophylactic antibiotic to be given within one hour (if vancomycin, two hours) prior to surgical incision (or start of procedure when no incision is required) was given

G8196 Clinician did not document a prophylactic antibiotic was administered within one hour (if Vancomycin, two hours) prior to surgical incision (or start of procedure when no incision is required)

G8200 Order for Cefazolin or Cefuroxime for antimicrobial prophylaxis not documented

G8204 Clinician did not document an order was given to discontinue prophylactic antibiotics within 24 hours of surgical end time

G8209 Clinician did not document an order was given to discontinue prophylactic antibiotics within 48 hours of surgical end time

G8214 Clinician did not document an order was given for appropriate venous thromboembolism (VTE) prophylaxis to be given within 24 hrs prior to incision time or 24 hours after surgery end time

G8217 Patient not documented to have received DVT prophylaxis by end of hospital day 2

G8219 Patient documented to have received DVT prophylaxis by end of hospital day 2

G8220 Patient not documented to have received DVT prophylaxis by end of hospital day 2

G8221 Clinician documented that patient was not an eligible candidate for DVT prophylaxis by the end of hospital day 2, including physician documentation that patient is ambulatory

G8223 Patient not documented to have received prescription for antiplatelet therapy at discharge

G8226 Patient not documented to have received prescription for anticoagulant therapy at discharge

G8231 Patient not documented to have received t-PA or not documented to have been considered a candidate for t-PA administration

G8234 Patient not documented to have received dysphagia screening

G8238 Patient not documented to have received order for or consideration for rehabilitation services

G8240 Internal carotid stenosis patient in the 30-99% range, and no documentation of reference to measurements of distal internal carotid diameter as the denominator for stenosis measurement

G8243 Patient not documented to have received CT or MRI and the presence or absence of hemorrhage, mass lesion and acute infarction not documented in the final report

G8246 Patient was not an eligible candidate for medical history review with assessment of new or changing moles

G8248 Patient with at least one alarm symptom not documented to have had upper endoscopy or referral for upper endoscopy

G8251 Patient not documented to have received an esophageal biopsy when suspicion of Barrett's esophagus is indicated in the endoscopy report

G8254 Patient with no documentation order for barium swallow test

G8257 Clinician has not documented reconciliation of discharge medications with current medication list in medical record

G8260 Patient not documented to have surrogate decision maker or advance care plan in

G8263 Patient not documented to have been assessed for presence or absence of urinary incontinence

G8266 Patient not documented to have received characterization of urinary incontinence

G8268 Patient not documented to have received plan of care for urinary incontinence

G8271 Patient with no documentation of screening for fall risks (2 or more falls in the past year or any fall with injury in the past year)

G8274 Clinician has not documented presence or absence of alarm symptoms

G8276 Patient not documented to have received medical history with assessment of new or changing moles

G8279 Patient not documented to have received a complete physical skin exam

G8282 Patient not documented to have received counseling to perform a self-examination

G8285 Patient not documented to have received pharmacologic therapy

G8289 Patient with no documentation of calcium and vitamin D use or counseling regarding both calcium and vitamin D use, or exercise

G8293 COPD patient without spirometry results documented

G8296 COPD patient not documented to have inhaled bronchodilator therapy prescribed

G8298 Patient documented to have received optic nerve head evaluation

G8299 Patient not documented to have received optic nerve head evaluation

G8302 Patient documented to have a specific target intraocular pressure range goal

G8303 Patient not documented to have a specific target intraocular pressure range goal

G8304 Clinician documented that patient was not an eligible candidate for a specific target intraocular pressure range goal

G8305 Clinician has not provided care for the primary open-angle glaucoma patient for the required time for treatment range goal documentation measurement

G8306 Primary open-angle glaucoma patient with intraocular pressure above the target range goal documented to have received plan of care

G8307 Primary open-angle glaucoma patient with intraocular pressure at or below goal, no plan of care necessary

G8308 Primary open-angle glaucoma patient with intraocular pressure above the target range goal, and not documented to have received plan of care during the reporting year

G8310 Patient not documented to have been prescribed/ recommended at least one antioxidant vitamin or mineral supplement during the reporting year

G8314 Patient not documented to have received macular exam with documentation of presence or absence of macular thickening or hemorrhage and no documentation of level of macular degeneration severity

G8318 Patient documented not to have visual functional status assessed

G8322 Patient not documented to have had pre-surgical axial length, corneal power measurement and method of intraocular lens power calculation

G8326 Patient not documented to have received fundus evaluation within six months prior to cataract surgery

G8330 Patient not documented to have received dilated macular or fundus exam with level of severity of retinopathy and the presence or absence of macular edema not documented

G8334 Documentation of findings of macular or fundus exam not communicated to the physician managing the patient's ongoing diabetes care

G8338 Clinician has not documented that communication was sent to the physician managing ongoing care of patient that a fracture occurred and that the patient was or should be tested or treated for osteoporosis

G8341 Patient not documented to have had central dexa measurement or pharmacologic therapy

G8345 Patient not documented to have had central dexa measurement ordered or performed or pharmacologic therapy

G8351 Patient not documented to have had ecg

G8354 Patient not documented to have received or taken aspirin 24 hours before emergency department arrival or during emergency department stay

G8357 Patient not documented to have had ecg

G8360 Patient not documented to have vital signs recorded and reviewed

G8362 Patient not documented to have oxygen saturation assessed

G8365 Patient not documented to have mental status assessed

G8367 Patient not documented to have appropriate empiric antibiotic prescribed

G8370 Asthma patients with numeric frequency of symptoms or patient completion of an asthma assessment tool/ survey/questionnaire not documented

G8371 Chemotherapy documented as not received or prescribed for stage iii colon cancer patients

G8372 Chemotherapy documented as received or prescribed for stage iii colon cancer patients

G8373 Chemotherapy plan documented prior to chemotherapy administration

G8374 Chemotherapy plan not documented prior to chemotherapy administration

G8375 Chronic lymphocytic leukemia (CLL) patient with no documentation of baseline flow cytometry performed

G8376 Clinician documentation that breast cancer patient was not eligible for tamoxifen or aromatase inhibitor therapy measure

G8377 Clinician documentation that colon cancer patient is not eligible for chemotherapy measure

G8378 Clinician documentation that patient was not an eligible candidate for radiation therapy measure

G8379 Documentation of radiation therapy recommended within 12 months of first office visit

G8380 For patients with ER or PR positive, stage IC-iii breast cancer, clinician did not document that the patient received or was prescribed tamoxifen or aromatase inhibitor

G8381 For patients with ER or PR positive, stage IC-iii breast cancer, clinician documented or prescribed that the patient is receiving tamoxifen or aromatase inhibitor

G8382 Multiple myeloma patients with no documentation of prescribed or received intravenous bisphosphonate therapy

G8383 No documentation of radiation therapy recommended within 12 months of first office visit

G8384 Baseline cytogenetic testing not performed in patients with myelodysplastic syndrome (MDS) or acute leukemias

G8385 Diabetic patients with no documentation of hemoglobin A1c level (within the last 12 months)

G8386 Diabetic patients with no documentation of low-density lipoprotein (within the last 12 months)

G8387 End-stage renal disease patient with a hematocrit or hemoglobin not documented

G8388 End-stage renal disease patient with URR or kt/v value not documented, but otherwise eligible for measure

G8389 Myelodysplastic syndrome (MDS) patients with no documentation of iron stores prior to receiving erythropoietin therapy

G8390 Diabetic patients with no documentation of blood pressure measurement (within the last 12 months)

G8391 Patients with persistent asthma, no documentation of preferred long term control medication or acceptable alternative treatment prescribed

G8402 Tobacco (smoke) use cessation intervention, counseling

G8403 Tobacco (smoke) use cessation intervention not counseled

G8407 Abi measured and documented

G8408 Abi measurement was not obtained

G8409 Clinician documented that patient was not an eligible candidate for abi measurement measure

G8423 Documented that patient was screened and either influenza vaccination status is current or patient was counseled

G8424 Influenza vaccine status was not screened

G8425 Influenza vaccine status screened, patient not current and counseling was not provided

G8426 Documented that patient was not appropriate for screening and/or counseling about the influenza vaccine (e.g., allergy to eggs)

G8429 Incomplete or no provider documentation that patient's current medications with dosages (includes prescription, over-the-counter, herbals, vitamin/mineral/dietary [nutritional] supplements) were assessed

G8434 Documentation of cognitive impairment screening using a standardized tool

G8435 No documentation of cognitive impairment screening using a standardized tool

G8436 Patient not eligible/not appropriate for cognitive impairment screening

G8437 Documentation of clinician and patient involvement with the development of a plan of care including signature by the practitioner/therapist and either a co-signature by the patient or documented verbal agreement obtained from the patient or, when necessary, an authorized representative

G8438 No documentation of clinician and patient involvement with the development of a plan of care including signature by the practitioner/therapist and either a co-signature by the patient or documented verbal agreement obtained from the patient or, when necessary, an authorized representative

G8439 Documentation that patient is not eligible for co-developing a plan of care including signature by the practitioner/therapist and either a co-signature by the patient or documented verbal agreement obtained from the patient or, when necessary, an authorized representative

G8443 All prescriptions created during the encounter were generated using a qualified e-prescribing system

G8445 No prescriptions were generated during the encounter, provider does have access to a qualified e-prescribing system

G8446 Provider does have access to a qualified e-prescribing system and some or all of the prescriptions generated during the encounter were printed or phoned in as required by state or federal law or regulations, patient request or pharmacy system being unable to receive electronic transmission; or because they were for narcotics or other controlled substances

G8449 Patient encounter was not documented using an emr due to system reasons such as, the system being inoperable at the time of the visit; use of this code implies that an emr is in place and generally available

G8453 Tobacco use cessation intervention, counseling

G8454 Tobacco use cessation intervention not counseled, reason not specified

G8455 Current tobacco smoker

G8456 Current smokeless tobacco user

G8457 Current tobacco non-user

G8466 Clinician documented that patient is not an eligible candidate for suicide risk assessment; major depressive disorder, in remission

G8467 Documentation of new diagnosis of initial or recurrent episode of major depressive disorder

G8479 Clinician prescribed angiotensin converting enzyme (ACE) inhibitor or angiotensin receptor blocker (ARB) therapy

G8480 Clinician documented that patient was not an eligible candidate for angiotensin converting enzyme (ACE) inhibitor or angiotensin receptor blocker (ARB) therapy

G8481 Clinician did not prescribe angiotensin converting enzyme (ACE) inhibitor or angiotensin receptor blocker (ARB) therapy, reason not specified

G8488 Clinician intends to report the end stage renal disease (ESRD) measure group

G8507 Provider documentation that patient is not eligible for patient verification of current medications

G8518 Clinical stage prior to surgery for lung cancer and esophageal cancer resection was recorded

G8519 Clinician documented that patient was not eligible for clinical stage prior to surgery for lung cancer and esophageal cancer resection measure

G8520 Clinician stage prior to surgery for lung cancer and esophageal cancer resection was not recorded, reason not specified
J0128 Injection, Abarelix, 10 mg
J0170 Injection, adrenalin, epinephrine, up to 1 ml ampule
J0559 Injection, penicillin F benzathine and penicillin G procaine, 2500 units
J0560 Injection, penicillin G benzathine, up to 600,000 units
J0570 Injection, penicillin G benzathine, up to 1,200,000 units
J0580 Injection, penicillin G benzathine, up to 2,400,000 units
J0704 Injection, betamethasone sodium phosphate, per 4 mg
J0970 Injection, Estradiol valerate, up to 40 mg
J1390 Injection, Estradiol valerate, up to 20 mg
J1470 Injection, gamma globulin, intramuscular, 2 cc
J1480 Injection, gamma globulin, intramuscular, 3 cc
J1490 Injection, gamma globulin, intramuscular, 4 cc
J1500 Injection, gamma globulin, intramuscular, 5 cc
J1510 Injection, gamma globulin, intramuscular, 6 cc
J1520 Injection, gamma globulin, intramuscular, 7 cc
J1530 Injection, gamma globulin, intramuscular, 8 cc
J1540 Injection, gamma globulin, intramuscular, 9 cc
J1550 Injection, gamma globulin, intramuscular, 10 cc
J1785 Injection, Imiglucerase, per unit
J1825 Injection, Interferon beta-1A, 33 mcg
J2321 Injection, Nandrolone decanoate, up to 100 mg
J2322 Injection, Nandrolone decanoate, up to 200 mg
J9062 Cisplatin, 50 mg
J9080 Cyclophosphamide, 200 mg
J9090 Cyclophosphamide, 500 mg
J9091 Cyclophosphamide, 1.0 gram
J9092 Cyclophosphamide, 2.0 gram
J9093 Cyclophosphamide, lyophilized, 100 mg
J9094 Cyclophosphamide, lyophilized, 200 mg
J9095 Cyclophosphamide, lyophilized, 500 mg
J9096 Cyclophosphamide, lyophilized, 1.0 gram
J9097 Cyclophosphamide, lyophilized, 2.0 gram
J9110 Injection, Cytarabine, 500 mg
J9140 Dacarbazine, 200 mg
J9290 Mitomycin, 20 mg
J9291 Mitomycin, 40 mg
J9350 Injection, Topotecan, 4 mg
J9375 Vincristine sulfate, 2 mg
J9380 Vincristine sulfate, 5 mg
K0734 Skin protection wheelchair seat cushion, adjustable, width less than 22 inches, any depth
K0735 Skin protection wheelchair seat cushion, adjustable, width 22 inches or greater, any depth
K0736 Skin protection and positioning wheelchair seat cushion, adjustable, width less than 22 inches, any depth
K0737 Skin protection and positioning wheelchair seat cushion, adjustable, width 22 inches or greater, any depth
L3660 Shoulder orthosis, figure of eight design abduction restrainer, canvas and webbing, prefabricated, includes fitting and adjustment
L3670 Shoulder orthosis, acromio/clavicular (canvas and webbing type), prefabricated, includes fitting and adjustment
L3672 Shoulder orthosis, abduction positioning (airplane design), thoracic component and support bar, without joints, may inlcude soft interface, straps, custom fabricated, includes fitting and adjustment
L3673 Shoulder orthosis, abduction positioning (airplane design), thoracic component and support bar, includes nontorsion joint/turnbuckle, may include soft interface, straps, custom fabricated, includes fitting and adjustment
L3675 Shoulder orthosis, vest type abduction restrainer, canvas webbing type or equal, prefabricated, includes fitting and adjustment
Q2025 Fludarabine phosphate, oral, 1 mg
Q4109 Skin substitute, tissuemend, per square centimeter
S0146 Injection, Pegylated interferon alfa-2B, 10 mcg per 0.5 ml
S0161 Calcitrol, 0.25 mg
S0196 Injectable Poly-L-Lactic acid, restorative implant, 1 ml, face (deep dermis, subcutaneous layers)

HCPCS Level II Deleted Codes Crosswalk

The codes below have been deleted for 2011. Replacement codes have been noted, where applicable.

Deleted Code	Replacement Code(s)
C9255	J2426
C9256	J7312
C9258	J3095
C9259	J9307
C9260	J9302
C9261	J3357
C9262	J8562
C9263	J1290
C9264	J3262
C9265	J9315
C9266	J0775
C9267	J7184
C9268	J7335
C9269	J0597
C9271	J3385
G0430	80104
J0128	N/A
J0170	J0171
J0559	J0558
J0560	J0561
J0570	J0561
J0580	J1561
J0704	J0702

Deleted Code	Replacement Code(s)
J0970	J1380
J1390	J1380
J1470	J1560
J1480	J1560
J1490	J1560
J1500	J1560
J1510	J1560
J1520	J1560
J1530	J1560
J1540	J1560
J1550	J1560
J1785	J1786
J1825	J1825, Q3025, Q3026
J2321	J2320
J2322	J2320
J9062	J9060
J9080	J9070
J9090	J9070
J9091	J9070
J9092	J9070
J9093	J9070
J9094	J9070
J9095	J9070
J9096	J9070
J9097	J9070
J9110	J9100

Deleted Code	Replacement Code(s)
J9140	J9130
J9290	J9280
J9291	J9280
J9350	J9351
J9375	J9370
J9380	J9370
K0734	E2603
K0735	E2604
K0736	E2607
K0737	E2608
L3660	L3650
L3670	L3671, L3677
L3672	L3674
L3673	L3674
L3675	N/A
Q2025	J8562
Q4109	N/A
S0146	S0148
S0161	A0169
S0196	C9800, Q2027
E0220	A9273
E0230	A9273
E0238	A9273
C9801	G0436, G0437
C9802	G0436, G0437
C9271	J3385

A

B

C

Blood – Cast

E

F

G

H

I

J

K

L

M

N

Monitor – Northwestern Suspension, socket prosthesis

O

P

Q

R

S

- **Shoes** — *continued*
  - orthopedic footwear, L3201-L3265
  - positioning device, L3140-L3170
  - transfer, L3600-L3649
  - wedge, L3340-L3485
- **Shoulder**
  - arthroscopy, S2300
  - cast supplies, Q4003-Q4004
  - disarticulation, prosthetic, L6300-L6320, L6550
  - harness, L5699
  - orthosis (SO), L3650-L3677
  - sling, A4566
  - spinal, cervical, L0112-L0200
- **Shoulder abduction kit**, L3674
- **Shoulder-elbow-wrist-hand orthosis**, L3960-L3971, L3973, L3975-L3978
- **Shunt**
  - accessory for dialysis, A4740
  - aqueous, L8612
- **Sigmoidoscopy, cancer screening**, G0104, G0106
- **Sildenafil citrate**, S0090
- **Simulect**, J0480
- **Sincalide injection**, J2805
- **Sinusol-B**, J0945
- **Sipuleucel-T**, C9273
- **Sirolimus**, J7520
- **Sitz bath**, E0160-E0161
  - chair, E0162
- **Skin**
  - anchoring device, urinary catheter, A4333
  - barrier, ostomy, A4362, A4369-A4373, A4385, A4405-A4411, A5120-A5122
  - bond or cement, ostomy, A4364
  - sealant, protectant, moisturizer, A6250
  - substitute, C9363, C9367, G0440-G0441, Q4100-Q4116
  - support, breast prosthesis, A4280
  - test, collagen, Q3031
  - tissue (human), Q4100-Q4111
  - wipes, A5120
- **Sleeve, elastic/stretchable material,** A4466
- **Sling**, A4565
  - axilla, L1010
  - Legg-Perthes, A4565
  - lumbar, L1090
  - patient lift, E0621, E0630, E0635
  - pelvic, L2580
  - Sam Brown, A4565
  - trapezius, L1070
- **Slow Fe**, A4565
- **Smith & Nephew®**
  - dressings
    - AlgiSite® M Alginate Dressing
      - wound cover, A6196-A6198
      - wound filler, A6199
    - ALGOSTERIL® Alginate Dressing
      - wound cover, A6196-A6198
      - wound filler, A6199
    - Allevyn®
      - adhesive dressings, A6212-A6214
      - adhesive sacrum, A6213
      - cavity, A6215
      - heel, A6210
      - hydrocellular foam dressings, A6209-A6211
      - island dressings, A6212
      - sacrum, A6213
      - wound cover, A6209-A6214
      - wound filler, A6215
    - Conformant® 2 Wound Veil, A6206-A6208
    - CovRSite®
      - dressing, A6219
      - plus composite dressing, A6203
- **Smith & Nephew®** — *continued*
  - dressings — *continued*
    - CUTINOVA®
      - hydro hydrocolloid dressing, A6234-A6239
      - thin, A6209-A6211
    - EXU-DRY®
      - incision dressings, A6252
      - infant boot/foot dressing, A6253
      - large burn jacket, vest, A6253
      - pad, non-permeable, A6253
      - slit tube dressings, A6251-A6252
      - wound dressings, A6251-A6253
    - FlexiGel®
      - hydrogel sheet dressing, A6242-A6243
      - island dressing, A6245
    - Hypafix® dressing retention sheets, A4452
    - IntraSite® gel, A6248
    - OpSite®, A6257-A6259
      - Flexifix, A6257-A6259
      - Post-Op, A6203-A6205
    - Primapore®, A6251-A6256
    - SoloSite® wound gel, A6248
    - TransiGel® conformable gel dressing, A6231
    - UniFlex®, A6257-A6258
    - Uni-Solve®
      - adhesive remover, A4455
        - wipes, A4456
    - Viscopaste® PB7 zinc paste bandage, A6456
- **Smoking cessation**
  - classes, S9453
  - gum, S4995
  - treatment, S9075
- **SMZ-TMP**, S0039
- **Social worker**
  - CORF-qualified, G0409
  - home health setting, G0155
  - hospice referral visit, S0255
  - nonemergency transport, A0160
- **Sock**
  - body, L0984
  - prosthetic, L8420-L8435, L8470-L8485
  - stump, L8470-L8485
- **Sodium**
  - chromate Cr-51, A9553
  - ferric gluconate complex in sucrose, J2916
  - fluoride F-18, A9580
  - hyaluronate
    - Euflexxa, J7324
    - Hyalgan, J7321
    - Orthovisc, J7323
    - Supartz, J7321
    - Synvisc, J7325
  - iodide I-123, A9516
  - iodide I-131, A9517, A9528-A9531
  - iothalamate I-125, A9554
  - phosphate P-32, A9563
  - succinate, J1720
- **Solgaal**, J2910
- **SoloSite® Wound Gel**, A6248
- **Solu-Cortef**, J1720
- **Solu-Medrol**, J2920, J2930
- **Solurex**, J1100
  - LA, J1094
- **Solution**
  - calibrator, A4256
  - dialysate, A4760
  - Elliott's B, J9175
  - enteral formulae, B4149-B4162
  - irrigation, A4217
  - parenteral nutrition, B4164-B5200
  - saline, J7030, J7040, J7050, J7130
- **Somatrem**, J2940
- **Somatropin**, J2941
- **Somatuline Depot**, J1930
- **SOMI brace**, L0190
- **Sominex**, J1200, Q0163
- **Sorbent cartridge**, **ESRD**, E1636
- **Sparine**, J2950
- **Spasmoject**, J0500
- **Specialist™ J-Splint™ Plaster Roll Immobilizer**, A4580
- **Specialist™ Plaster Bandages**, A4580
- **Specialties™ C/Up Splint W/Stay**, L3908
- **Specialty absorptive dressing**, A6251-A6256
- **Spectinomycin HCl**, J3320
- **Speech and language pathologist, home health setting**, G0153, G0161
- **Speech assessment**, V5362-V5364
- **Speech generating device**
  - accessory, E2512, E2599
  - digitized, E2500-E2506
  - software, E2511
  - synthesized, E2508, E2510
- **Speech therapy**, S9128
  - home health, G0161
  - re-evaluation, S9152
- **Sperm procurement and cryopreservation**, S4026, S4030-S4031
  - donor service, S4025
- **Spinal orthosis**
  - anterior-posterior, L0450-L0490, L0632
  - anterior-posterior-lateral-rotary, L0450-L0490
  - cervical, L0112-L0200
  - cervical-thoracic-lumbar-sacral orthosis (CTLSO), L0700, L0710, L1000
  - halo, L0810-L0830
    - addition, L0859
  - lumbar flexion, L0635-L0636
  - lumbar-sacral (LSO), L0628-L0640
  - Milwaukee, L1000
  - multiple post collar, L0180-L0200
  - sacroiliac, L0621-L0624
  - scoliosis, L1000-L1499
- **Spirometer**
  - electronic, E0487
  - non-electronic, A9284
- **Splint**, A4570, L3100, L4350-L4380
  - ankle, L4396-L4398
  - arm
    - long, Q4017-Q4020
    - short, Q4021-Q4024
  - Dennis-Browne, L3640
  - digit, prefabricated, S8450
  - dynamic, E1800, E1805, E1810, E1815, E1825, E1830, E1840
  - elbow, S8452
  - finger, Q4049
  - footdrop, L4398
  - Hallus-Valgus night dynamic, L3100
  - knee, L4380
  - leg
    - full, pneumatic, L4370
    - long, Q4041-Q4044
    - short, Q4045-Q4048
  - supplies, Q4051
  - wrist, S8451
- **Spoke protectors**, K0065
- **Spoken language comprehension measure score**
  - higher at discharge than atadmission, G8603
  - not higher at discharge than at admission, G8604
  - not scored, either at admission or discharge, G8605

Shoes – Spoken language comprehension measure score

T

U

V

Y

Z

Transportation Services Including Ambulance A0021–A0999

Modifiers to Identify Ambulance Place of Origin and Destination

Modifiers to identify ambulance place of origin and destination for use in items 12 and 13 of CMS form 1491. These are one-digit codes to be used in combination. The first place alpha code = origin; the second place alpha code = destination.

D Diagnostic or therapeutic site other than "P" or "H" when these are used as origin codes

E Residential, domiciliary, custodial facility (other than an 1819 facility)

G Hospital based dialysis facility (hospital or hospital related)

H Hospital

I Site of transfer (e.g., airport or helicopter pad) between modes of ambulance transport

J Non-hospital based dialysis facility

N Skilled nursing facility (SNF) (1819 facility)

P Physician's office (includes HMO non-hospital facility, clinic, etc.)

R Residence

S Scene of accident or acute event

X (Destination code only) intermediate stop at physician's office enroute to the hospital (includes HMO non-hospital facility, clinic, etc.)

Transportation Services Including Ambulance

⊘ A0021 Ambulance service, outside state per mile, transport (Medicaid only) E

⊘ A0080 Non-emergency transportation, per mile – vehicle provided by volunteer (individual or organization), with no vested interest E

⊘ A0090 Non-emergency transportation, per mile – vehicle provided by individual (family member, self, neighbor) with vested interest E

⊘ A0100 Non-emergency transportation; taxi

⊘ A0110 Non-emergency transportation and bus, intra or inter state carrier E

⊘ A0120 Non-emergency transportation: mini-bus, mountain area transports, or other transportation systems E

⊘ A0130 Non-emergency transportation: wheelchair van E

⊘ A0140 Non-emergency transportation and air travel (private or commercial) intra or inter state E

⊘ A0160 Non-emergency transportation: per mile – case worker or social worker E

⊘ A0170 Transportation; ancillary: parking fees, tolls, other E

⊘ A0180 Non-emergency transportation: ancillary; lodging recipient E

⊘ A0190 Non-emergency transportation: ancillary: meals recipient E

⊘ A0200 Non-emergency transportation: ancillary: lodging escort E

⊘ A0210 Non-emergency transportation: ancillary: meals escort E

⊘ A0225 Ambulance service, neonatal transport, base rate, emergency transport, one way E

⊘ A0380 BLS mileage (per mile) E
Cross reference A0425

A0382 BLS routine disposable supplies A

A0384 BLS specialized service disposable supplies; defibrillation (used by ALS ambulances and BLS ambulances in jurisdictions where defibrillation is permitted in BLS ambulances) A

⊘ A0390 ALS mileage (per mile) E
Cross reference A0425

A0392 ALS specialized service disposable supplies; defibrillation (to be used only in jurisdictions where defibrillation cannot be performed in BLS ambulances) A

A0394 ALS specialized service disposable supplies; IV drug therapy A

A0396 ALS specialized service disposable supplies; esophageal intubation A

A0398 ALS routine disposable supplies A

A0420 Ambulance waiting time (ALS or BLS), one half (1/2) hour increments A

A0422 Ambulance (ALS or BLS) oxygen and oxygen supplies, life sustaining situation A

A0424 Extra ambulance attendant, ground (ALS or BLS) or air (fixed or rotary winged); (requires medical review) A

A0425 Ground mileage, per statute mile A

A0426 Ambulance service, advanced life support, non-emergency transport, level 1 (ALS 1) A

A0427 Ambulance service, advanced life support, emergency transport, level 1 (ALS 1-emergency) A

A0428 Ambulance service, basic life support, non-emergency transport (BLS) A

A0429 Ambulance service, basic life support, emergency transport (BLS-emergency) A

A0430 Ambulance service, conventional air services, transport, one way (fixed wing) A

A0431 Ambulance service, conventional air services, transport, one way (rotary wing) A

A0432 Paramedic intercept (PI), rural area, transport furnished by a volunteer ambulance company which is prohibited by state law from billing third party payers A

A0433 Advanced life support, level 2 (ALS 2) A

A0434 Specialty care transport (SCT) A

A0435 Fixed wing air mileage, per statute mile A

A0436 Rotary wing air mileage, per statute mile A

⊘ A0888 Non-covered ambulance mileage, per mile (e.g., for miles traveled beyond closest appropriate facility) E
Pub 100-02, 10, 20

⊘ A0998 Ambulance response and treatment, no transport E

ⓘ A0999 Unlisted ambulance service A
Pub 100-02, 10, 10.1-10.1.5; 100-2, 10, 20

Medical and Surgical Supplies A4206–A8004

Note: These procedure codes should be used in lieu of CPT® code 99070.

- A4206 Syringe with needle, sterile 1 cc or less, each E
- A4207 Syringe with needle, sterile 2 cc, each E
- A4208 Syringe with needle, sterile 3 cc, each E
- A4209 Syringe with needle, sterile 5 cc or greater, each E
- A4210 Needle-free injection device, each E
  NCD 280.1
- A4211 Supplies for self-administered injections E
  Pub 100-02, 15, 50; 100-4, 17, 10
- A4212 Non-coring needle or stylet with or without catheter B
- A4213 Syringe, sterile, 20 cc or greater, each E

Syringe

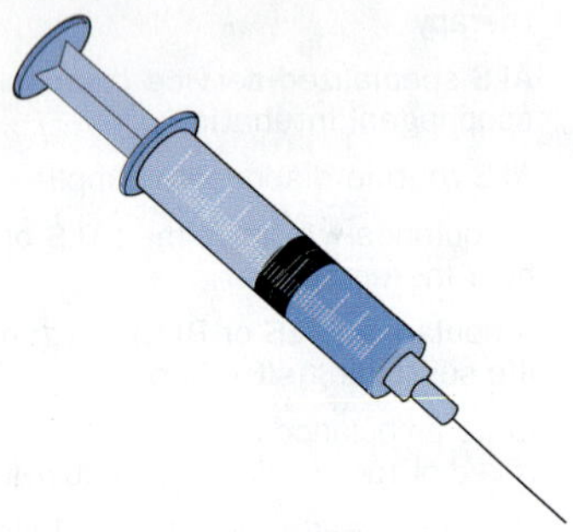

- A4215 Needle, sterile, any size, each E
- A4216 Sterile water, saline and/or dextrose, diluent/flush, 10 ml A
  Pub 100-02, 15, 50; 100-4, 17, 10
- A4217 Sterile water/saline, 500 ml A
  Pub 100-02, 15, 50; 100-4, 17, 10
- A4218 Sterile saline or water, metered dose dispenser, 10 ml N NI
  Pub 100-02, 15, 50; 100-4, 17, 10
- A4220 Refill kit for implantable infusion pump N NI
  NCD 40.2
- A4221 Supplies for maintenance of drug infusion catheter, per week (list drug separately) Y
- A4222 Infusion supplies for external drug infusion pump, per cassette or bag (list drugs separately) Y
- A4223 Infusion supplies not used with external infusion pump, per cassette or bag (list drugs separately) E
- A4230 Infusion set for external insulin pump, non-needle cannula type Y
  NCD 40.2
- A4231 Infusion set for external insulin pump, needle type Y
  NCD 40.2
- A4232 Syringe with needle for external insulin pump, sterile, 3 cc E
  NCD 40.2
- A4233 Replacement battery, alkaline (other than J cell), for use with medically necessary home blood glucose monitor owned by patient, each Y
- A4234 Replacement battery, alkaline, J cell, for use with medically necessary home blood glucose monitor owned by patient, each Y
- A4235 Replacement battery, lithium, for use with medically necessary home blood glucose monitor owned by patient, each Y
- A4236 Replacement battery, silver oxide, for use with medically necessary home blood glucose monitor owned by patient, each Y
- A4244 Alcohol or peroxide, per pint E
- A4245 Alcohol wipes, per box E
- A4246 Betadine or pHisoHex solution, per pint E
- A4247 Betadine or iodine swabs/wipes, per box E
- A4248 Chlorhexidine containing antiseptic, 1 ml N NI
- A4250 Urine test or reagent strips or tablets (100 tablets or strips) E
  Pub 100-02, 15, 110; 100-4, 20-10
- A4252 Blood ketone test or reagent strip, each E
  Medicare statute 1861(n)

Blood ketone/reagent test strip

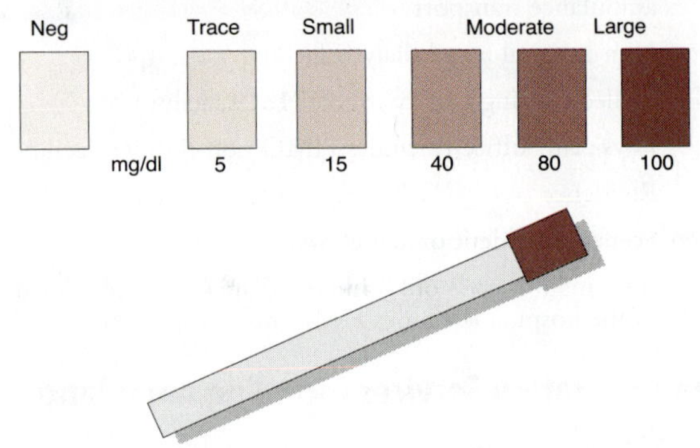

- A4253 Blood glucose test or reagent strips for home blood glucose monitor, per 50 strips Y
  NCD 40.2

Blood glucose/reagent test strip

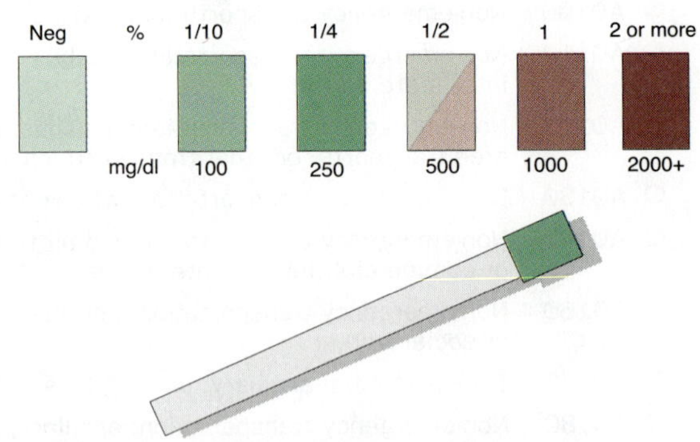

- A4255 Platforms for home blood glucose monitor, 50 per box Y
  NCD 40.2
- A4256 Normal, low and high calibrator solution/chips Y
  NCD 40.2
- A4257 Replacement lens shield cartridge for use with laser skin piercing device, each Y
- A4258 Spring-powered device for lancet, each Y
  NCD 40.2

ⓘ A4259 Lancets, per box of 100 Y
NCD 40.2

⊘ A4261 Cervical cap for contraceptive use ♀ E
Medicare Statute 1862(a)(1)

ⓘ A4262 Temporary, absorbable lacrimal duct implant, each N NI

ⓘ A4263 Permanent, long-term, non-dissolvable lacrimal duct implant, each N NI
Pub 100-04, 12, 20.4.4

⊘ A4264 Permanent implantable contraceptive intratubal occlusion device(s) and delivery system ♀ E

ⓘ A4265 Paraffin, per pound Y
NCD 280.1

⊘ A4266 Diaphragm for contraceptive use ♀ E

⊘ A4267 Contraceptive supply, condom, male, each ♂ E

⊘ A4268 Contraceptive supply, condom, female, each ♀ E

⊘ A4269 Contraceptive supply, spermicide (e.g., foam, gel), each ♀ E

A4270 Disposable endoscope sheath, each N NI

A4280 Adhesive skin support attachment for use with external breast prosthesis, each A

A4281 Tubing for breast pump, replacement ♀ E

A4282 Adapter for breast pump, replacement ♀ E

A4283 Cap for breast pump bottle, replacement ♀ E

A4284 Breast shield and splash protector for use with breast pump, replacement ♀ E

A4285 Polycarbonate bottle for use with breast pump, replacement ♀ E

A4286 Locking ring for breast pump, replacement ♀ E

A4290 Sacral nerve stimulation test lead, each B
Pub 100-04, 32, 40-40.5

Vascular Catheters

ⓘ A4300 Implantable access catheter, (e.g., venous, arterial, epidural subarachnoid, or peritoneal, etc.) external access N NI
Pub 100-02, 15, 120; 100-04, 12, 20.4.4

Implantable access catheter

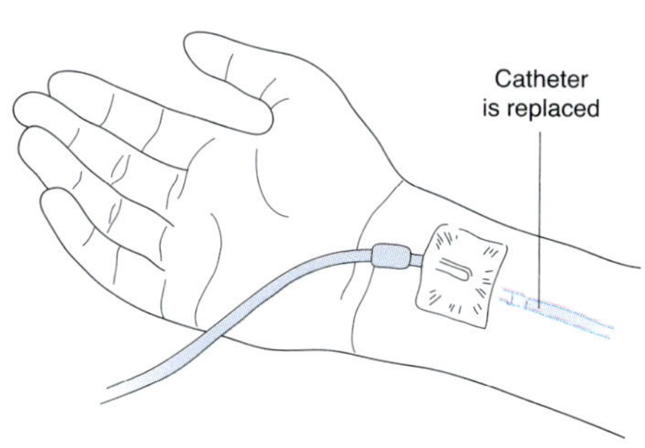

A4301 Implantable access total catheter, port/reservoir (e.g., venous, arterial, epidural, subarachnoid, peritoneal, etc.) N NI

A4305 Disposable drug delivery system, flow rate of 50 ml or greater per hour N NI

A4306 Disposable drug delivery system, flow rate of less than 50 ml per hour N NI

Incontinence Appliances and Care Supplies

ⓘ A4310 Insertion tray without drainage bag and without catheter (accessories only) A
Pub 100-02, 15, 120

ⓘ A4311 Insertion tray without drainage bag with indwelling catheter, Foley type, two-way latex with coating (Teflon, silicone, silicone elastomer or hydrophilic, etc.) A
Pub 100-02, 15, 120

ⓘ A4312 Insertion tray without drainage bag with indwelling catheter, Foley type, two-way, all silicone A
Pub 100-02, 15, 120

ⓘ A4313 Insertion tray without drainage bag with indwelling catheter, Foley type, three-way, for continuous irrigation A
Pub 100-02, 15, 120

ⓘ A4314 Insertion tray with drainage bag with indwelling catheter, Foley type, two-way latex with coating (Teflon, silicone, silicone elastomer or hydrophilic, etc.) A
Pub 100-02, 15, 120

ⓘ A4315 Insertion tray with drainage bag with indwelling catheter, Foley type, two-way, all silicone A
Pub 100-02, 15, 120

ⓘ A4316 Insertion tray with drainage bag with indwelling catheter, Foley type, three-way, for continuous irrigation A
Pub 100-02, 15, 120

Urinary Catheters

ⓘ A4320 Irrigation tray with bulb or piston syringe, any purpose A
Pub 100-02, 15, 120

ⓘ A4321 Therapeutic agent for urinary catheter irrigation A
Pub 100-02, 15, 120

ⓘ A4322 Irrigation syringe, bulb or piston, each A
Pub 100-02, 15, 120

ⓘ A4326 Male external catheter with integral collection chamber, any type, each ♂ A
Pub 100-02, 15, 120

ⓘ A4327 Female external urinary collection device; metal cup, each ♀ A
Pub 100-02, 15, 120

ⓘ A4328 Female external urinary collection device; pouch, each ♀ A
Pub 100-02, 15, 120

ⓘ A4330 Perianal fecal collection pouch with adhesive, each A
Pub 100-02, 15, 120

ⓘ A4331 Extension drainage tubing, any type, any length, with connector/adaptor, for use with urinary leg bag or urostomy pouch, each A
Pub 100-02, 15, 120

ⓘ A4332 Lubricant, individual sterile packet, each A
Pub 100-02, 15, 120

ⓘ A4333 Urinary catheter anchoring device, adhesive skin attachment, each A
Pub 100-02, 15, 120

ⓘ A4334 Urinary catheter anchoring device, leg strap, each A
Pub 100-02, 15, 120

ⓘ A4335 Incontinence supply; miscellaneous A
Pub 100-02, 15, 120

ⓘ A4336 Incontinence supply, urethral insert, any type, each

ⓘ A4338 Indwelling catheter; Foley type, two-way latex with coating (Teflon, silicone, silicone elastomer, or hydrophilic, etc.), each
Pub 100-02, 15, 120

ⓘ A4340 Indwelling catheter; specialty type, eg; coude, mushroom, wing, etc.), each
Pub 100-02, 15, 120

ⓘ A4344 Indwelling catheter, Foley type, two-way, all silicone, each
Pub 100-02, 15, 120

ⓘ A4346 Indwelling catheter; Foley type, three way for continuous irrigation, each
Pub 100-02, 15, 120

ⓘ A4349 Male external catheter, with or without adhesive, disposable, each ♂
Pub 100-02, 15, 120

ⓘ A4351 Intermittent urinary catheter; straight tip, with or without coating (Teflon, silicone, silicone elastomer, or hydrophilic, etc.), each
Pub 100-02, 15, 120

ⓘ A4352 Intermittent urinary catheter; coude (curved) tip, with or without coating (Teflon, silicone, silicone elastomeric, or hydrophilic, etc.), each
Pub 100-02, 15, 120

ⓘ A4353 Intermittent urinary catheter, with insertion supplies
Pub 100-02, 15, 120

ⓘ A4354 Insertion tray with drainage bag but without catheter
Pub 100-02, 15, 120

ⓘ A4355 Irrigation tubing set for continuous bladder irrigation through a three-way indwelling Foley catheter, each
Pub 100-02, 15, 120

External Urinary Supplies

ⓘ A4356 External urethral clamp or compression device (not to be used for catheter clamp), each
Pub 100-02, 15, 120

ⓘ A4357 Bedside drainage bag, day or night, with or without anti-reflux device, with or without tube, each
Pub 100-02, 15, 120

Drainage bag

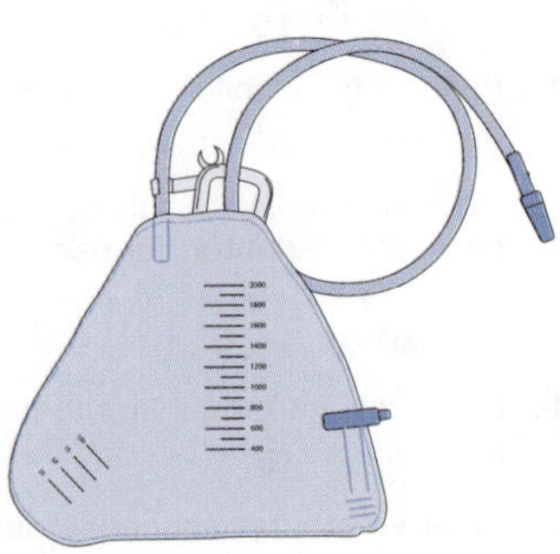

ⓘ A4358 Urinary drainage bag, leg or abdomen, vinyl, with or without tube, with straps, each
Pub 100-02, 15, 120

ⓘ A4360 Disposable external urethral clamp or compression device, with pad and/or pouch, each

Ostomy Supplies

ⓘ A4361 Ostomy faceplate, each
Pub 100-02, 15, 120

ⓘ A4362 Skin barrier; solid, 4 x 4 or equivalent; each
Pub 100-02, 15, 120

ⓘ A4363 Ostomy clamp, any type, replacement only, each
Pub 100-02, 15, 50; 100-4, 17, 10

ⓘ A4364 Adhesive, liquid or equal, any type, per oz
Pub 100-02, 15, 120

A4366 Ostomy vent, any type, each

ⓘ A4367 Ostomy belt, each
Pub 100-02, 15, 120

A4368 Ostomy filter, any type, each

ⓘ A4369 Ostomy skin barrier, liquid (spray, brush, etc), per oz
Pub 100-02, 15, 120

ⓘ A4371 Ostomy skin barrier, powder, per oz
Pub 100-02, 15, 120

ⓘ A4372 Ostomy skin barrier, solid 4x4 or equivalent, standard wear, with built-in convexity, each
Pub 100-02, 15, 120

ⓘ A4373 Ostomy skin barrier, with flange (solid, flexible or accordian), with built-in convexity, any size, each
Pub 100-02, 15, 120

ⓘ A4375 Ostomy pouch, drainable, with faceplate attached, plastic, each
Pub 100-02, 15, 120

ⓘ A4376 Ostomy pouch, drainable, with faceplate attached, rubber, each
Pub 100-02, 15, 120

ⓘ A4377 Ostomy pouch, drainable, for use on faceplate, plastic, each
Pub 100-02, 15, 120

ⓘ A4378 Ostomy pouch, drainable, for use on faceplate, rubber, each
Pub 100-02, 15, 120

ⓘ A4379 Ostomy pouch, urinary, with faceplate attached, plastic, each
Pub 100-02, 15, 120

ⓘ A4380 Ostomy pouch, urinary, with faceplate attached, rubber, each
Pub 100-02, 15, 120

ⓘ A4381 Ostomy pouch, urinary, for use on faceplate, plastic, each
Pub 100-02, 15, 120

ⓘ A4382 Ostomy pouch, urinary, for use on faceplate, heavy plastic, each
Pub 100-02, 15, 120

ⓘ A4383 Ostomy pouch, urinary, for use on faceplate, rubber, each
Pub 100-02, 15, 120

ⓘ A4384 Ostomy faceplate equivalent, silicone ring, each
Pub 100-02, 15, 120

ⓘ A4385 Ostomy skin barrier, solid 4x4 or equivalent, extended wear, without built-in convexity, each
Pub 100-02, 15, 120

Ⓘ A4387 Ostomy pouch, closed, with barrier attached, with built-in convexity (1 piece), each DMEPOS A
Pub 100-02, 15, 120

Ⓘ A4388 Ostomy pouch, drainable, with extended wear barrier attached, (1 piece), each DMEPOS A
Pub 100-02, 15, 120

Ⓘ A4389 Ostomy pouch, drainable, with barrier attached, with built-in convexity (1 piece), each DMEPOS A
Pub 100-02, 15, 120

Ⓘ A4390 Ostomy pouch, drainable, with extended wear barrier attached, with built-in convexity (1 piece), each DMEPOS A
Pub 100-02, 15, 120

Ⓘ A4391 Ostomy pouch, urinary, with extended wear barrier attached (1 piece), each DMEPOS A
Pub 100-02, 15, 120

Ⓘ A4392 Ostomy pouch, urinary, with standard wear barrier attached, with built-in convexity (1 piece), each DMEPOS A
Pub 100-02, 15, 120

Ⓘ A4393 Ostomy pouch, urinary, with extended wear barrier attached, with built-in convexity (1 piece), each DMEPOS A
Pub 100-02, 15, 120

Ⓘ A4394 Ostomy deodorant, with or without lubricant, for use in ostomy pouch, per fluid ounce DMEPOS A
Pub 100-02, 15, 120

Ⓘ A4395 Ostomy deodorant for use in ostomy pouch, solid, per tablet DMEPOS A
Pub 100-02, 15, 120

Ⓘ A4396 Ostomy belt with peristomal hernia support DMEPOS A
Pub 100-02, 15, 120

Ⓘ A4397 Irrigation supply; sleeve, each DMEPOS A
Pub 100-02, 15, 120

Ⓘ A4398 Ostomy irrigation supply; bag, each DMEPOS A
Pub 100-02, 15, 120

▲ Ⓘ A4399 Ostomy irrigation supply; cone/catheter, with or without brush DMEPOS A
Pub 100-02, 15, 120

Ⓘ A4400 Ostomy irrigation set DMEPOS A
Pub 100-02, 15, 120

Ⓘ A4402 Lubricant, per ounce DMEPOS A
Pub 100-02, 15, 120

Ⓘ A4404 Ostomy ring, each DMEPOS A
Pub 100-02, 15, 120

Ⓘ A4405 Ostomy skin barrier, non-pectin based, paste, per ounce DMEPOS A
Pub 100-02, 15, 120

Ⓘ A4406 Ostomy skin barrier, pectin-based, paste, per ounce DMEPOS A
Pub 100-02, 15, 120

Ⓘ A4407 Ostomy skin barrier, with flange (solid, flexible, or accordion), extended wear, with built-in convexity, 4 x 4 inches or smaller, each DMEPOS A
Pub 100-02, 15, 120

Ⓘ A4408 Ostomy skin barrier, with flange (solid, flexible or accordion), extended wear, with built-in convexity, larger than 4 x 4 inches, each DMEPOS A
Pub 100-02, 15, 120

Ⓘ A4409 Ostomy skin barrier, with flange (solid, flexible or accordion), extended wear, without built-in convexity, 4 x 4 inches or smaller, each DMEPOS A
Pub 100-02, 15, 120

Ⓘ A4410 Ostomy skin barrier, with flange (solid, flexible or accordion), extended wear, without built-in convexity, larger than 4 x 4 inches, each DMEPOS A
Pub 100-02, 15, 120

Ⓘ A4411 Ostomy skin barrier, solid 4x4 or equivalent, extended wear, with built-in convexity, each DMEPOS A
Pub 100-02, 15, 120

Ⓘ A4412 Ostomy pouch, drainable, high output, for use on a barrier with flange (2 piece system), without filter, each DMEPOS A
Pub 100-02, 15, 120

Ⓘ A4413 Ostomy pouch, drainable, high output, for use on a barrier with flange (2 piece system), with filter, each DMEPOS A
Pub 100-02, 15, 120

Ⓘ A4414 Ostomy skin barrier, with flange (solid, flexible or accordion), without built-in convexity, 4 x 4 inches or smaller, each DMEPOS A
Pub 100-02, 15, 120

Ⓘ A4415 Ostomy skin barrier, with flange (solid, flexible or accordion), without built-in convexity, larger than 4x4 inches, each DMEPOS A
Pub 100-02, 15, 120

Coverage Carrier Determined A4416 Ostomy pouch, closed, with barrier attached, with filter (1 piece), each DMEPOS A

Coverage Carrier Determined A4417 Ostomy pouch, closed, with barrier attached, with built-in convexity, with filter (1 piece), each DMEPOS A

Coverage Carrier Determined A4418 Ostomy pouch, closed; without barrier attached, with filter (1 piece), each DMEPOS A

Coverage Carrier Determined A4419 Ostomy pouch, closed; for use on barrier with non-locking flange, with filter (2 piece), each DMEPOS A

Coverage Carrier Determined A4420 Ostomy pouch, closed; for use on barrier with locking flange (2 piece), each DMEPOS A

⃠ A4421 Ostomy supply; miscellaneous E
Pub 100-02, 15, 120

Ⓘ A4422 Ostomy absorbent material (sheet/pad/crystal packet)
for use in ostomy pouch to thicken liquid stomal output, each DMEPOS A
Pub 100-02, 15, 120

Coverage Carrier Determined A4423 Ostomy pouch, closed; for use on barrier with locking flange, with filter (2 piece), each DMEPOS A

Coverage Carrier Determined A4424 Ostomy pouch, drainable, with barrier attached, with filter (1 piece), each DMEPOS A

Coverage Carrier Determined A4425 Ostomy pouch, drainable; for use on barrier with non-locking flange, with filter (2 piece system), each DMEPOS A

Coverage Carrier Determined A4426 Ostomy pouch, drainable; for use on barrier with locking flange (2 piece system), each DMEPOS A

Coverage Carrier Determined A4427 Ostomy pouch, drainable; for use on barrier with locking flange, with filter (2 piece system), each DMEPOS A

Coverage Carrier Determined A4428 Ostomy pouch, urinary, with extended wear barrier attached, with faucet-type tap with valve (1 piece), each DMEPOS A

Coverage Carrier Determined A4429 Ostomy pouch, urinary, with barrier attached, with built-in convexity, with faucet-type tap with valve (1 piece), each DMEPOS A

Coverage Carrier Determined A4430 Ostomy pouch, urinary, with extended wear barrier attached, with built-in convexity, with faucet-type tap with valve (1 piece), each DMEPOS A

Coverage Carrier Determined A4431 Ostomy pouch, urinary; with barrier attached, with faucet-type tap with valve (1 piece), each DMEPOS A

Coverage Carrier Determined A4432 Ostomy pouch, urinary; for use on barrier with non-locking flange, with faucet-type tap with valve (2 piece), each DMEPOS A

A4433 Ostomy pouch, urinary; for use on barrier with locking flange (2 piece), each A

A4434 Ostomy pouch, urinary; for use on barrier with locking flange, with faucet-type tap with valve (2 piece), each A

Additional Miscellaneous Supplies

A4450 Tape, non-waterproof, per 18 square inches A
Pub 100-02, 15, 120

A4452 Tape, waterproof, per 18 square inches A
Pub 100-02, 15, 120

A4455 Adhesive remover or solvent (for tape, cement or other adhesive), per ounce A
Pub 100-02, 15, 120

A4456 Adhesive remover, wipes, any type, each A

A4458 Enema bag with tubing, reusable E

A4461 Surgical dressing holder, non-reusable, each A

A4463 Surgical dressing holder, reusable, each A

A4465 Non-elastic binder for extremity A

A4466 Garment, belt, sleeve or other covering, elastic or similar stretchable material, any type, each E

A4470 Gravlee jet washer A
NCD 230.5; Pub 100-02, 16, 90

A4480 Vabra aspirator A
NCD 230.6; Pub 100-02, 16, 90

A4481 Tracheostoma filter, any type, any size, each A
Pub 100-02, 15, 120

A4483 Moisture exchanger, disposable, for use with invasive mechanical ventilation A
Pub 100-02, 15, 120

A4490 Surgical stockings above knee length, each E
NCD 280.1; Pub 100-02, 15, 100; 100-2, 15, 110; 100-4, 20-10

A4495 Surgical stockings thigh length, each E
NCD 280.1; Pub 100-02, 15, 100; 100-2, 15, 110; 100-4, 20-10

A4500 Surgical stockings below knee length, each E
NCD 280.1; Pub 100-02, 15, 100; 100-2, 15, 110; 100-4, 20-10

A4510 Surgical stockings full length, each E
NCD 280.1; Pub 100-02, 15, 100; 100-2, 15, 110; 100-4, 20-10

A4520 Incontinence garment, any type, (e.g. brief, diaper), each E
NCD 280.1

A4550 Surgical trays B
Pub 100-04, 12, 20.4.4

A4554 Disposable underpads, all sizes E
NCD 280.1

A4556 Electrodes, (e.g., apnea monitor), per pair Y

A4557 Lead wires, (e.g., apnea monitor), per pair Y

A4558 Conductive gel or paste, for use with electrical device (e.g., TENS, NMES), per oz Y

A4559 Coupling gel or paste, for use with ultrasound device, per oz Y

A4561 Pessary, rubber, any type ♀ N

A4562 Pessary, non rubber, any type ♀ N

A4565 Slings A

Arm sling

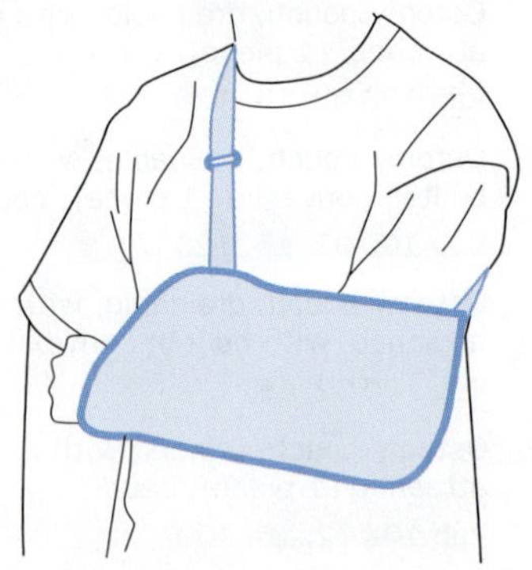

● A4566 Shoulder sling or vest design, abduction restrainer, with or without swathe control, prefabricated, includes fitting and adjustment E
This code is effective January 1, 2011

A4570 Splint E
Pub 100-02, 15, 100

A4575 Topical hyperbaric oxygen chamber, disposable E
NCD 20.29

A4580 Cast supplies (e.g. plaster) E
Pub 100-02, 15, 100

A4590 Special casting material (e.g. fiberglass) E
Pub 100-02, 15, 100

A4595 Electrical stimulator supplies, 2 lead, per month (e.g. TENS, NMES) Y
NCD 160.13

A4600 Sleeve for intermittent limb compression device, replacement only, each Y

A4601 Lithium ion battery for non-prosthetic use, replacement Y

A4604 Tubing with integrated heating element for use with positive airway pressure device Y

A4605 Tracheal suction catheter, closed system, each Y

A4606 Oxygen probe for use with oximeter device, replacement A

A4608 Transtracheal oxygen catheter, each Y

Supplies for Oxygen and Related Respiratory Equipment

A4611 Battery, heavy duty; replacement for patient-owned ventilator Y

A4612 Battery cables; replacement for patient-owned ventilator Y

A4613 Battery charger; replacement for patient-owned ventilator Y

A4614 Peak expiratory flow rate meter, hand held N

A4615 Cannula, nasal Y
NCD 240.2; Pub 100-04, 20, 100.2

A4616 Tubing (oxygen), per foot Y
NCD 240.2; Pub 100-04, 20, 100.2

A4617 Mouthpiece Y
NCD 240.2; Pub 100-04, 20, 100.2

A4618 Breathing circuits Y
NCD 240.2; Pub 100-04, 20, 100.2

A4619 Face tent
NCD 240.2; Pub 100-04, 20, 100.2

A4620 Variable concentration mask
NCD 240.2; Pub 100-04, 20, 100.2

A4623 Tracheostomy, inner cannula
NCD 20.9; Pub 100-02, 15, 120

A4624 Tracheal suction catheter, any type other than closed system, each

A4625 Tracheostomy care kit for new tracheostomy
Pub 100-02, 15, 120

A4626 Tracheostomy cleaning brush, each
Pub 100-02, 15, 120

A4627 Spacer, bag or reservoir, with or without mask, for use with metered dose inhaler
Pub 100-02, 15, 110; 100-4, 20-10

A4628 Oropharyngeal suction catheter, each

A4629 Tracheostomy care kit for established tracheostomy
Pub 100-02, 15, 120

Supplies for Other Durable Medical Equipment

A4630 Replacement batteries, medically necessary, transcutaneous electrical stimulator, owned by patient
NCD 160.7

A4633 Replacement bulb/lamp for ultraviolet light therapy system, each

A4634 Replacement bulb for therapeutic light box, tabletop model

A4635 Underarm pad, crutch, replacement, each
NCD 280.1

A4636 Replacement, handgrip, cane, crutch, or walker, each
NCD 280.1

A4637 Replacement, tip, cane, crutch, walker, each
NCD 280.1

A4638 Replacement battery for patient-owned ear pulse generator, each

Ear pulse generator

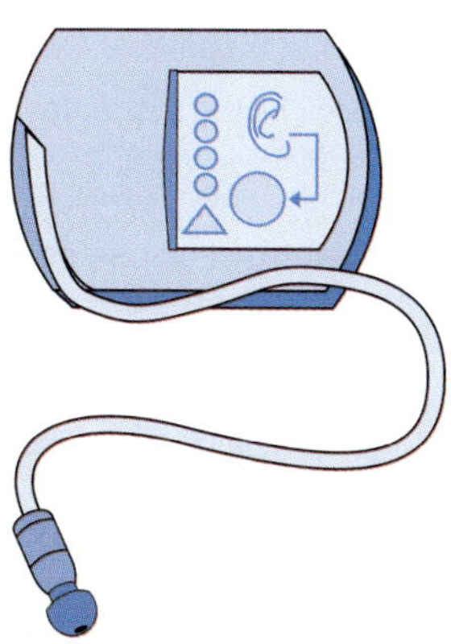

A4639 Replacement pad for infrared heating pad system, each

A4640 Replacement pad for use with medically necessary alternating pressure pad owned by patient
NCD 280.1; Pub 100-8, 5, 5.3

Supplies for Radiological Procedures

A4641 Radiopharmaceutical, diagnostic, not otherwise classified
Pub 100-04, 13, 60.3.2; 100-4, 12, 20.4.4

A4642 Indium In-111 satumomab pendetide, diagnostic, per study dose, up to 6 millicuries
Pub 100-04, 12, 20.4.4

A4648 Tissue marker, implantable, any type, each

A4649 Surgical supply; miscellaneous

A4650 Implantable radiation dosimeter, each

Supplies for ESRD

Note: For DME items for ESRD, see procedure codes E1500-E1699.

A4651 Calibrated microcapillary tube, each
Pub 100-04, 8, 60.1; 100-4, 8, 80; 100-4, 8, 90; 100-4, 8, 90.3.2; 100-4, 8, 130

A4652 Microcapillary tube sealant
Pub 100-04, 8, 60.1; 100-4, 8, 80; 100-4, 8, 90; 100-4, 8, 90.3.2; 100-4, 8, 130

A4653 Peritoneal dialysis catheter anchoring device, belt, each

A4657 Syringe, with or without needle, each
Pub 100-04, 8, 60.1; 100-4, 8, 80; 100-4, 8, 90; 100-4, 8, 90.3.2; 100-4, 8, 130

A4660 Sphygmomanometer/blood pressure apparatus with cuff and stethoscope
Pub 100-04, 8, 60.1; 100-4, 8, 80; 100-4, 8, 90; 100-4, 8, 90.3.2; 100-4, 8, 130

A4663 Blood pressure cuff only
Pub 100-04, 8, 60.1; 100-4, 8, 80; 100-4, 8, 90; 100-4, 8, 90.3.2; 100-4, 8, 130

A4670 Automatic blood pressure monitor
NCD 20.19; Pub 100-04, 8, 60.1; 100-4, 8, 80; 100-4, 8, 90; 100-4, 8, 90.3.2; 100-4, 8, 130

A4671 Disposable cycler set used with cycler dialysis machine, each
Pub 100-04, 8, 60.1; 100-4, 8, 80; 100-4, 8, 90; 100-4, 8, 90.3.2; 100-4, 8, 130

A4672 Drainage extension line, sterile, for dialysis, each
Pub 100-04, 8, 60.1; 100-4, 8, 80; 100-4, 8, 90; 100-4, 8, 90.3.2; 100-4, 8, 130

A4673 Extension line with easy lock connectors, used with dialysis
Pub 100-04, 8, 60.1; 100-4, 8, 80; 100-4, 8, 90; 100-4, 8, 90.3.2; 100-4, 8, 130

A4674 Chemicals/antiseptics solution used to clean/sterilize dialysis equipment, per 8 oz
Pub 100-04, 8, 60.1; 100-4, 8, 80; 100-4, 8, 90; 100-4, 8, 90.3.2; 100-4, 8, 130

A4680 Activated carbon filter for hemodialysis, each
NCD 230.7; Pub 100-04, 8, 60.1; 100-4, 8, 80; 100-4, 8, 90; 100-4, 8, 90.3.2; 100-4, 8, 130

A4690 Dialyzer (artificial kidneys), all types, all sizes, for hemodialysis, each
Pub 100-04, 8, 60.1; 100-4, 8, 80; 100-4, 8, 90; 100-4, 8, 90.3.2; 100-4, 8, 130

A4706 Bicarbonate concentrate, solution, for hemodialysis, per gallon
Pub 100-04, 8, 60.1; 100-4, 8, 80; 100-4, 8, 90; 100-4, 8, 90.3.2; 100-4, 8, 130

ⓘ **A4707** Bicarbonate concentrate, powder, for hemodialysis, per packet N
Pub 100-04, 8, 60.1; 100-4, 8, 80; 100-4, 8, 90; 100-4, 8, 90.3.2; 100-4, 8, 130

ⓘ **A4708** Acetate concentrate solution, for hemodialysis, per gallon N
Pub 100-04, 8, 60.1; 100-4, 8, 80; 100-4, 8, 90; 100-4, 8, 90.3.2; 100-4, 8, 130

ⓘ **A4709** Acid concentrate, solution, for hemodialysis, per gallon N
Pub 100-04, 8, 60.1; 100-4, 8, 80; 100-4, 8, 90; 100-4, 8, 90.3.2; 100-4, 8, 130

ⓘ **A4714** Treated water (deionized, distilled, or reverse osmosis) for peritoneal dialysis, per gallon N
NCD 230.7; Pub 100-04, 8, 60.1; 100-4, 8, 80; 100-4, 8, 90; 100-4, 8, 90.3.2; 100-4, 8, 130

ⓘ **A4719** Y-set tubing for peritoneal dialysis N
Pub 100-04, 8, 60.1; 100-4, 8, 80; 100-4, 8, 90; 100-4, 8, 90.3.2; 100-4, 8, 130

Y-set tubing

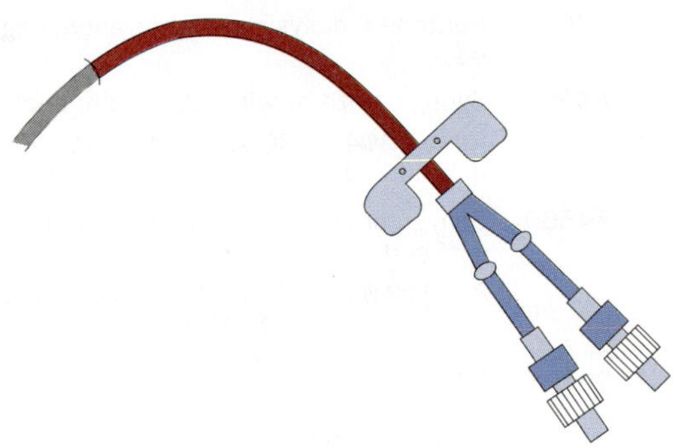

ⓘ **A4720** Dialysate solution, any concentration of dextrose, fluid volume greater than 249 cc, but less than or equal to 999 cc, for peritoneal dialysis N
Pub 100-04, 8, 60.1; 100-4, 8, 80; 100-4, 8, 90; 100-4, 8, 90.3.2; 100-4, 8, 130

ⓘ **A4721** Dialysate solution, any concentration of dextrose, fluid volume greater than 999 cc, but less than or equal to 1999 cc, for peritoneal dialysis N
Pub 100-04, 8, 60.1; 100-4, 8, 80; 100-4, 8, 90; 100-4, 8, 90.3.2; 100-4, 8, 130

ⓘ **A4722** Dialysate solution, any concentration of dextrose, fluid volume greater than 1999 cc, but less than or equal to 2999 cc, for peritoneal dialysis N
Pub 100-04, 8, 60.1; 100-4, 8, 80; 100-4, 8, 90; 100-4, 8, 90.3.2; 100-4, 8, 130

ⓘ **A4723** Dialysate solution, any concentration of dextrose, fluid volume greater than 2999 cc, but less than or equal to 3999 cc, for peritoneal dialysis N
Pub 100-04, 8, 60.1; 100-4, 8, 80; 100-4, 8, 90; 100-4, 8, 90.3.2; 100-4, 8, 130

ⓘ **A4724** Dialysate solution, any concentration of dextrose, fluid volume greater than 3999 cc, but less than or equal to 4999 cc, for peritoneal dialysis N
Pub 100-04, 8, 60.1; 100-4, 8, 80; 100-4, 8, 90; 100-4, 8, 90.3.2; 100-4, 8, 130

ⓘ **A4725** Dialysate solution, any concentration of dextrose, fluid volume greater than 4999 cc, but less than or equal to 5999 cc, for peritoneal dialysis N
Pub 100-04, 8, 60.1; 100-4, 8, 80; 100-4, 8, 90; 100-4, 8, 90.3.2; 100-4, 8, 130

ⓘ **A4726** Dialysate solution, any concentration of dextrose, fluid volume greater than 5999 cc, for peritoneal dialysis N
Pub 100-04, 8, 60.1; 100-4, 8, 80; 100-4, 8, 90; 100-4, 8, 90.3.2; 100-4, 8, 130

A4728 Dialysate solution, non-dextrose containing, 500 ml B

ⓘ **A4730** Fistula cannulation set for hemodialysis, each N
Pub 100-04, 8, 60.1; 100-4, 8, 80; 100-4, 8, 90; 100-4, 8, 90.3.2; 100-4, 8, 130

ⓘ **A4736** Topical anesthetic, for dialysis, per gram N
Pub 100-04, 8, 60.1; 100-4, 8, 80; 100-4, 8, 90; 100-4, 8, 90.3.2; 100-4, 8, 130

ⓘ **A4737** Injectable anesthetic, for dialysis, per 10 ml N
Pub 100-04, 8, 60.1; 100-4, 8, 80; 100-4, 8, 90; 100-4, 8, 90.3.2; 100-4, 8, 130

ⓘ **A4740** Shunt accessory, for hemodialysis, any type, each N
Pub 100-04, 8, 60.1; 100-4, 8, 80; 100-4, 8, 90; 100-4, 8, 90.3.2; 100-4, 8, 130

ⓘ **A4750** Blood tubing, arterial or venous, for hemodialysis, each N
Pub 100-04, 8, 60.1; 100-4, 8, 80; 100-4, 8, 90; 100-4, 8, 90.3.2; 100-4, 8, 130

ⓘ **A4755** Blood tubing, arterial and venous combined, for hemodialysis, each N
Pub 100-04, 8, 60.1; 100-4, 8, 80; 100-4, 8, 90; 100-4, 8, 90.3.2; 100-4, 8, 130

ⓘ **A4760** Dialysate solution test kit, for peritoneal dialysis, any type, each N
Pub 100-04, 8, 60.1; 100-4, 8, 80; 100-4, 8, 90; 100-4, 8, 90.3.2; 100-4, 8, 130

ⓘ **A4765** Dialysate concentrate, powder, additive for peritoneal dialysis, per packet N
Pub 100-04, 8, 60.1; 100-4, 8, 80; 100-4, 8, 90; 100-4, 8, 90.3.2; 100-4, 8, 130

ⓘ **A4766** Dialysate concentrate, solution, additive for peritoneal dialysis, per 10 ml N
Pub 100-04, 8, 60.1; 100-4, 8, 80; 100-4, 8, 90; 100-4, 8, 90.3.2; 100-4, 8, 130

ⓘ **A4770** Blood collection tube, vacuum, for dialysis, per 50 N
Pub 100-04, 8, 60.1; 100-4, 8, 80; 100-4, 8, 90; 100-4, 8, 90.3.2; 100-4, 8, 130

ⓘ **A4771** Serum clotting time tube, for dialysis, per 50 N
Pub 100-04, 8, 60.1; 100-4, 8, 80; 100-4, 8, 90; 100-4, 8, 90.3.2; 100-4, 8, 130

ⓘ **A4772** Blood glucose test strips, for dialysis, per 50 N
Pub 100-04, 8, 60.1; 100-4, 8, 80; 100-4, 8, 90; 100-4, 8, 90.3.2; 100-4, 8, 130

ⓘ **A4773** Occult blood test strips, for dialysis, per 50 N
Pub 100-04, 8, 60.1; 100-4, 8, 80; 100-4, 8, 90; 100-4, 8, 90.3.2; 100-4, 8, 130

ⓘ **A4774** Ammonia test strips, for dialysis, per 50 N
Pub 100-04, 8, 60.1; 100-4, 8, 80; 100-4, 8, 90; 100-4, 8, 90.3.2; 100-4, 8, 130

ⓘ **A4802** Protamine sulfate, for hemodialysis, per 50 mg N
Pub 100-04, 8, 60.1; 100-4, 8, 80; 100-4, 8, 90; 100-4, 8, 90.3.2; 100-4, 8, 130

ⓘ **A4860** Disposable catheter tips for peritoneal dialysis, per 10 N
Pub 100-04, 8, 60.1; 100-4, 8, 80; 100-4, 8, 90; 100-4, 8, 90.3.2; 100-4, 8, 130

A4870 Plumbing and/or electrical work for home hemodialysis equipment N
Pub 100-04, 8, 60.1; 100-4, 8, 80; 100-4, 8, 90; 100-4, 8, 90.3.2; 100-4, 8, 130

A4890 Contracts, repair and maintenance, for hemodialysis equipment N
Pub 100-02, 15, 110.2

A4911 Drain bag/bottle, for dialysis, each N

A4913 Miscellaneous dialysis supplies, not otherwise specified N

A4918 Venous pressure clamp, for hemodialysis, each N

A4927 Gloves, non-sterile, per 100 N

A4928 Surgical mask, per 20 N

A4929 Tourniquet for dialysis, each N

A4930 Gloves, sterile, per pair N

A4931 Oral thermometer, reusable, any type, each N

A4932 Rectal thermometer, reusable, any type, each E

Additional Ostomy Supplies

A5051 Ostomy pouch, closed; with barrier attached (1 piece), each A
Pub 100-02, 15, 120

A5052 Ostomy pouch, closed; without barrier attached (1 piece), each A
Pub 100-02, 15, 120

A5053 Ostomy pouch, closed; for use on faceplate, each A
Pub 100-02, 15, 120

A5054 Ostomy pouch, closed; for use on barrier with flange (2 piece), each A
Pub 100-02, 15, 120

A5055 Stoma cap A
Pub 100-02, 15, 120

A5061 Ostomy pouch, drainable; with barrier attached (1 piece), each A

A5062 Ostomy pouch, drainable; without barrier attached (1 piece), each A
Pub 100-02, 15, 120

A5063 Ostomy pouch, drainable; for use on barrier with flange (2 piece system), each A
Pub 100-02, 15, 120

A5071 Ostomy pouch, urinary; with barrier attached (1 piece), each A
Pub 100-02, 15, 120

A5072 Ostomy pouch, urinary; without barrier attached (1 piece), each A
Pub 100-02, 15, 120

A5073 Ostomy pouch, urinary; for use on barrier with flange (2 piece), each A
Pub 100-02, 15, 120

A5081 Continent device; plug for continent stoma A
Pub 100-02, 15, 120

A5082 Continent device; catheter for continent stoma A
Pub 100-02, 15, 120

A5083 Continent device, stoma absorptive cover for continent stoma A

A5093 Ostomy accessory; convex insert A
Pub 100-02, 15, 120

Additional Incontinence Appliances/Supplies

A5102 Bedside drainage bottle with or without tubing, rigid or expandable, each A
Pub 100-02, 15, 120

A5105 Urinary suspensory with leg bag, with or without tube, each A
Pub 100-02, 15, 120

▲ A5112 Urinary drainage bag, leg or abdomen, latex, with or without tube, with straps, each A
Pub 100-02, 15, 120

A5113 Leg strap; latex, replacement only, per set A
Pub 100-02, 15, 120

A5114 Leg strap; foam or fabric, replacement only, per set A
Pub 100-02, 15, 120

Supplies for Either Incontinence or Ostomy Appliances

A5120 Skin barrier, wipes or swabs, each A
Pub 100-02, 15, 120

A5121 Skin barrier; solid, 6 x 6 or equivalent, each A
Pub 100-02, 15, 120

A5122 Skin barrier; solid, 8 x 8 or equivalent, each A
Pub 100-02, 15, 120

A5126 Adhesive or non-adhesive; disk or foam pad A
Pub 100-02, 15, 120

A5131 Appliance cleaner, incontinence and ostomy appliances, per 16 oz A
Pub 100-02, 15, 120

A5200 Percutaneous catheter/tube anchoring device, adhesive skin attachment A
Pub 100-02, 15, 120

Diabetic Shoes, Fitting, and Modifications

A5500 For diabetics only, fitting (including follow-up), custom preparation and supply of off-the-shelf depth-inlay shoe manufactured to accommodate multi-density insert(s), per shoe Y
Pub 100-02, 15, 140

A5501 For diabetics only, fitting (including follow-up), custom preparation and supply of shoe molded from cast(s) of patient's foot (custom-molded shoe), per shoe Y
Pub 100-02, 15, 140

A5503 For diabetics only, modification (including fitting) of off-the-shelf depth-inlay shoe or custom-molded shoe with roller or rigid rocker bottom, per shoe Y
Pub 100-02, 15, 140

A5504 For diabetics only, modification (including fitting) of off-the-shelf depth-inlay shoe or custom-molded shoe with wedge(s), per shoe Y
Pub 100-02, 15, 140

A5505 For diabetics only, modification (including fitting) of off-the-shelf depth-inlay shoe or custom-molded shoe with metatarsal bar, per shoe Y
Pub 100-02, 15, 140

A5506 For diabetics only, modification (including fitting) of off-the-shelf depth-inlay shoe or custom-molded shoe with off-set heel(s), per shoe Y
Pub 100-02, 15, 140

A5507 For diabetics only, not otherwise specified modification (including fitting) of off-the-shelf depth-inlay shoe or custom-molded shoe, per shoe
Pub 100-02, 15, 140

A5508 For diabetics only, deluxe feature of off-the-shelf depth-inlay shoe or custom-molded shoe, per shoe
Pub 100-02, 15, 140

A5510 For diabetics only, direct formed, compression-molded to patient's foot without external heat source, multiple-density insert(s) prefabricated, per shoe
Pub 100-02, 15, 140

A5512 For diabetics only, multiple density insert, direct formed, molded to foot after external heat source of 230 degrees Fahrenheit or higher, total contact with patient's foot, including arch, base layer minimum of 1/4 inch material of shore a 35 durometer or 3/16 inch material of shore a 40 durometer (or higher), prefabricated, each

A5513 For diabetics only, multiple density insert, custom-molded from model of patient's foot, total contact with patient's foot, including arch, base layer minimum of 3/16 inch material of shore a 35 durometer (or higher), includes arch filler and other shaping material, custom fabricated, each

Dressings, Wound Care, and Burn Supplies

A6000 Non-contact wound warming wound cover for use with the non-contact wound warming device and warming card
Pub 100-02, 16, 20

A6010 Collagen based wound filler, dry form, sterile, per gram of collagen
Pub 100-02, 15, 100

▲ A6011 Collagen based wound filler, gel/paste, per gram of collagen
Pub 100-02, 15, 100

A6021 Collagen dressing, sterile, pad size 16 sq. in. or less, each
Pub 100-02, 15, 100

A6022 Collagen dressing, sterile, pad size more than 16 sq. in. but less than or equal to 48 sq. in., each
Pub 100-02, 15, 100

A6023 Collagen dressing, sterile, pad size more than 48 sq. in., each
Pub 100-02, 15, 100

A6024 Collagen dressing wound filler, sterile, per 6 inches
Pub 100-02, 15, 100

A6025 Gel sheet for dermal or epidermal application, (e.g., silicone, hydrogel, other), each

A6154 Wound pouch, each
Pub 100-02, 15, 100

A6196 Alginate or other fiber gelling dressing, wound cover, sterile, pad size 16 sq. in. or less, each dressing
Pub 100-02, 15, 100

A6197 Alginate or other fiber gelling dressing, wound cover, sterile, pad size more than 16 sq. in. but less than or equal to 48 sq. in., each dressing
Pub 100-02, 15, 100

A6198 Alginate or other fiber gelling dressing, wound cover, sterile, pad size more than 48 sq. in., each dressing
Pub 100-02, 15, 100

A6199 Alginate or other fiber gelling dressing, wound filler, sterile, per 6 inches
Pub 100-02, 15, 100

A6203 Composite dressing, sterile, pad size 16 sq. in. or less, with any size adhesive border, each dressing
Pub 100-02, 15, 100

A6204 Composite dressing, sterile, pad size more than 16 sq. in. but less than or equal to 48 sq. in., with any size adhesive border, each dressing
Pub 100-02, 15, 100

A6205 Composite dressing, sterile, pad size more than 48 sq. in., with any size adhesive border, each dressing
Pub 100-02, 15, 100

A6206 Contact layer, sterile, 16 sq. in. or less, each dressing
Pub 100-02, 15, 100

A6207 Contact layer, sterile, more than 16 sq. in. but less than or equal to 48 sq. in., each dressing
Pub 100-02, 15, 100

A6208 Contact layer, sterile, more than 48 sq. in., each dressing
Pub 100-02, 15, 100

A6209 Foam dressing, wound cover, sterile, pad size 16 sq. in. or less, without adhesive border, each dressing
Pub 100-02, 15, 100

A6210 Foam dressing, wound cover, sterile, pad size more than 16 sq. in. but less than or equal to 48 sq. in., without adhesive border, each dressing
Pub 100-02, 15, 100

A6211 Foam dressing, wound cover, sterile, pad size more than 48 sq. in., without adhesive border, each dressing
Pub 100-02, 15, 100

A6212 Foam dressing, wound cover, sterile, pad size 16 sq. in. or less, with any size adhesive border, each dressing
Pub 100-02, 15, 100

A6213 Foam dressing, wound cover, sterile, pad size more than 16 sq. in. but less than or equal to 48 sq. in., with any size adhesive border, each dressing
Pub 100-02, 15, 100

A6214 Foam dressing, wound cover, sterile, pad size more than 48 sq. in., with any size adhesive border, each dressing
Pub 100-02, 15, 100

A6215 Foam dressing, wound filler, sterile, per gram
Pub 100-02, 15, 100

A6216 Gauze, non-impregnated, non-sterile, pad size 16 sq. in. or less, without adhesive border, each dressing
Pub 100-02, 15, 100

A6217 Gauze, non-impregnated, non-sterile, pad size more than 16 sq. in. but less than or equal to 48 sq. In., without adhesive border, each dressing
Pub 100-02, 15, 100

A6218 Gauze, non-impregnated, non-sterile, pad size more than 48 sq. in., without adhesive border, each dressing
Pub 100-02, 15, 100

A6219 Gauze, non-impregnated, sterile, pad size 16 sq. in. or less, with any size adhesive border, each dressing
Pub 100-02, 15, 100

A6220 Gauze, non-impregnated, sterile, pad size more than 16 sq. in. but less than or equal to 48 sq. in., with any size adhesive border, each dressing
Pub 100-02, 15, 100

Ⓘ A6221 Gauze, non-impregnated, sterile, pad size more than 48 sq. in., with any size adhesive border, each dressing A
Pub 100-02, 15, 100

Ⓘ A6222 Gauze, impregnated with other than water, normal saline, or hydrogel, sterile, pad size 16 sq. in. or less, without adhesive border, each dressing A
Pub 100-02, 15, 100

Ⓘ A6223 Gauze, impregnated with other than water, normal saline, or hydrogel, sterile, pad size more than 16 sq. in., but less than or equal to 48 sq. in., without adhesive border, each dressing A
Pub 100-02, 15, 100

Ⓘ A6224 Gauze, impregnated with other than water, normal saline, or hydrogel, sterile, pad size more than 48 sq. in., without adhesive border, each dressing A
Pub 100-02, 15, 100

Ⓘ A6228 Gauze, impregnated, water or normal saline, sterile, pad size 16 sq. in. or less, without adhesive border, each dressing A
Pub 100-02, 15, 100

Ⓘ A6229 Gauze, impregnated, water or normal saline, sterile, pad size more than 16 sq. in. but less than or equal to 48 sq. in., without adhesive border, each dressing A
Pub 100-02, 15, 100

Ⓘ A6230 Gauze, impregnated, water or normal saline, sterile, pad size more than 48 sq. in., without adhesive border, each dressing A
Pub 100-02, 15, 100

Ⓘ A6231 Gauze, impregnated, hydrogel, for direct wound contact, sterile, pad size 16 sq. in. or less, each dressing A
Pub 100-02, 15, 100

Ⓘ A6232 Gauze, impregnated, hydrogel, for direct wound contact, sterile, pad size greater than 16 sq. in., but less than or equal to 48 sq. in., each dressing A
Pub 100-02, 15, 100

Ⓘ A6233 Gauze, impregnated, hydrogel, for direct wound contact, sterile, pad size more than 48 sq. in., each dressing A
Pub 100-02, 15, 100

Ⓘ A6234 Hydrocolloid dressing, wound cover, sterile, pad size 16 sq. in. or less, without adhesive border, each dressing A
Pub 100-02, 15, 100

Ⓘ A6235 Hydrocolloid dressing, wound cover, sterile, pad size more than 16 sq. in. but less than or equal to 48 sq. in., without adhesive border, each dressing A
Pub 100-02, 15, 100

Ⓘ A6236 Hydrocolloid dressing, wound cover, sterile, pad size more than 48 sq. in., without adhesive border, each dressing A
Pub 100-02, 15, 100

Ⓘ A6237 Hydrocolloid dressing, wound cover, sterile, pad size 16 sq. in. or less, with any size adhesive border, each dressing A
Pub 100-02, 15, 100

Ⓘ A6238 Hydrocolloid dressing, wound cover, sterile, pad size more than 16 sq. in. but less than or equal to 48 sq. in., with any size adhesive border, each dressing A
Pub 100-02, 15, 100

Ⓘ A6239 Hydrocolloid dressing, wound cover, sterile, pad size more than 48 sq. in., with any size adhesive border, each dressing A
Pub 100-02, 15, 100

Ⓘ A6240 Hydrocolloid dressing, wound filler, paste, sterile, per ounce A
Pub 100-02, 15, 100

Ⓘ A6241 Hydrocolloid dressing, wound filler, dry form, sterile, per gram A
Pub 100-02, 15, 100

Ⓘ A6242 Hydrogel dressing, wound cover, sterile, pad size 16 sq. in. or less, without adhesive border, each dressing A
Pub 100-02, 15, 100

Ⓘ A6243 Hydrogel dressing, wound cover, sterile, pad size more than 16 sq. in. but less than or equal to 48 sq. in., without adhesive border, each dressing A
Pub 100-02, 15, 100

Ⓘ A6244 Hydrogel dressing, wound cover, sterile, pad size more than 48 sq. in., without adhesive border, each dressing A
Pub 100-02, 15, 100

Ⓘ A6245 Hydrogel dressing, wound cover, sterile, pad size 16 sq. in. or less, with any size adhesive border, each dressing A
Pub 100-02, 15, 100

Ⓘ A6246 Hydrogel dressing, wound cover, sterile, pad size more than 16 sq. in. but less than or equal to 48 sq. in., with any size adhesive border, each dressing A
Pub 100-02, 15, 100

Ⓘ A6247 Hydrogel dressing, wound cover, sterile, pad size more than 48 sq. in., with any size adhesive border, each dressing A
Pub 100-02, 15, 100

▲ Ⓘ A6248 Hydrogel dressing, wound filler, gel, per fluid ounce A
Pub 100-02, 15, 100

Ⓘ A6250 Skin sealants, protectants, moisturizers, ointments, any type, any size A
Pub 100-02, 15, 100

Ⓘ A6251 Specialty absorptive dressing, wound cover, sterile, pad size 16 sq. in. or less, without adhesive border, each dressing A
Pub 100-02, 15, 100

Ⓘ A6252 Specialty absorptive dressing, wound cover, sterile, pad size more than 16 sq. in. but less than or equal to 48 sq. in., without adhesive border, each dressing A
Pub 100-02, 15, 100

Ⓘ A6253 Specialty absorptive dressing, wound cover, sterile, pad size more than 48 sq. in., without adhesive border, each dressing A
Pub 100-02, 15, 100

Ⓘ A6254 Specialty absorptive dressing, wound cover, sterile, pad size 16 sq. in. or less, with any size adhesive border, each dressing A
Pub 100-02, 15, 100

Ⓘ A6255 Specialty absorptive dressing, wound cover, sterile, pad size more than 16 sq. in. but less than or equal to 48 sq. in., with any size adhesive border, each dressing A
Pub 100-02, 15, 100

Ⓘ A6256 Specialty absorptive dressing, wound cover, sterile, pad size more than 48 sq. in., with any size adhesive border, each dressing A
Pub 100-02, 15, 100

Ⓘ A6257 Transparent film, sterile, 16 sq. in. or less, each dressing A
Pub 100-02, 15, 100

ⓘ A6258 Transparent film, sterile, more than 16 sq. in. but less than or equal to 48 sq. in., each dressing A
Pub 100-02, 15, 100

ⓘ A6259 Transparent film, sterile, more than 48 sq. in., each dressing A
Pub 100-02, 15, 100

▲ ⓘ A6260 Wound cleansers, any type, any size A
Pub 100-02, 15, 100

▲ ⓘ A6261 Wound filler, gel/paste, per fluid ounce, not otherwise specified A
Pub 100-02, 15, 100

▲ ⓘ A6262 Wound filler, dry form, per gram, not otherwise specified A
Pub 100-02, 15, 100

ⓘ A6266 Gauze, impregnated, other than water, normal saline, or zinc paste, sterile, any width, per linear yard A
Pub 100-02, 15, 100

ⓘ A6402 Gauze, non-impregnated, sterile, pad size 16 sq. in. or less, without adhesive border, each dressing A
Pub 100-02, 15, 100

ⓘ A6403 Gauze, non-impregnated, sterile, pad size more than 16 sq. in. but less than or equal to 48 sq. in., without adhesive border, each dressing A
Pub 100-02, 15, 100

ⓘ A6404 Gauze, non-impregnated, sterile, pad size more than 48 sq. in., without adhesive border, each dressing A
Pub 100-02, 15, 100

A6407 Packing strips, non-impregnated, sterile, up to 2 inches in width, per linear yard A

ⓘ A6410 Eye pad, sterile, each A
Pub 100-02, 15, 100

ⓘ A6411 Eye pad, non-sterile, each A
Pub 100-02, 15, 100

A6412 Eye patch, occlusive, each E

⊘ A6413 Adhesive bandage, first-aid type, any size, each E
Medicare statute 1861(s)(5)

A6441 Padding bandage, non-elastic, non-woven/non-knitted, width greater than or equal to three inches and less than five inches, per yard A

A6442 Conforming bandage, non-elastic, knitted/woven, non-sterile, width less than three inches, per yard A

A6443 Conforming bandage, non-elastic, knitted/woven, non-sterile, width greater than or equal to three inches and less than five inches, per yard A

A6444 Conforming bandage, non-elastic, knitted/woven, non-sterile, width greater than or equal to 5 inches, per yard A

A6445 Conforming bandage, non-elastic, knitted/woven, sterile, width less than three inches, per yard A

A6446 Conforming bandage, non-elastic, knitted/woven, sterile, width greater than or equal to three inches and less than five inches, per yard A

A6447 Conforming bandage, non-elastic, knitted/woven, sterile, width greater than or equal to five inches, per yard A

A6448 Light compression bandage, elastic, knitted/woven, width less than three inches, per yard A

A6449 Light compression bandage, elastic, knitted/woven, width greater than or equal to three inches and less than five inches, per yard A

A6450 Light compression bandage, elastic, knitted/woven, width greater than or equal to five inches, per yard A

A6451 Moderate compression bandage, elastic, knitted/woven, load resistance of 1.25 to 1.34 foot pounds at 50% maximum stretch, width greater than or equal to three inches and less than five inches, per yard A

A6452 High compression bandage, elastic, knitted/woven, load resistance greater than or equal to 1.35 foot pounds at 50% maximum stretch, width greater than or equal to three inches and less than five inches, per yard A

A6453 Self-adherent bandage, elastic, non-knitted/non-woven, width less than three inches, per yard A

A6454 Self-adherent bandage, elastic, non-knitted/non-woven, width greater than or equal to three inches and less than five inches, per yard A

A6455 Self-adherent bandage, elastic, non-knitted/non-woven, width greater than or equal to five inches, per yard A

A6456 Zinc paste impregnated bandage, non-elastic, knitted/woven, width greater than or equal to three inches and less than five inches, per yard A

A6457 Tubular dressing with or without elastic, any width, per linear yard A

ⓘ A6501 Compression burn garment, bodysuit (head to foot), custom fabricated A
Pub 100-02, 15, 100

ⓘ A6502 Compression burn garment, chin strap, custom fabricated A
Pub 100-02, 15, 100

ⓘ A6503 Compression burn garment, facial hood, custom fabricated A
Pub 100-02, 15, 100

ⓘ A6504 Compression burn garment, glove to wrist, custom fabricated A
Pub 100-02, 15, 100

ⓘ A6505 Compression burn garment, glove to elbow, custom fabricated A
Pub 100-02, 15, 100

ⓘ A6506 Compression burn garment, glove to axilla, custom fabricated A
Pub 100-02, 15, 100

ⓘ A6507 Compression burn garment, foot to knee length, custom fabricated A
Pub 100-02, 15, 100

ⓘ A6508 Compression burn garment, foot to thigh length, custom fabricated A
Pub 100-02, 15, 100

ⓘ A6509 Compression burn garment, upper trunk to waist including arm openings (vest), custom fabricated A
Pub 100-02, 15, 100

ⓘ A6510 Compression burn garment, trunk, including arms down to leg openings (leotard), custom fabricated A
Pub 100-02, 15, 100

ⓘ A6511 Compression burn garment, lower trunk including leg openings (panty), custom fabricated A
Pub 100-02, 15, 100

ⓘ A6512 Compression burn garment, not otherwise classified A
Pub 100-02, 15, 100

A6513 Compression burn mask, face and/or neck, plastic or equal, custom fabricated B

⊘ A6530 Gradient compression stocking, below knee, 18-30 mmHg, each E
NCD 280.1

	Code	Description	Indicator
ⓘ	A6531	Gradient compression stocking, below knee, 30-40 mmHg, each Pub 100-02, 15, 100	A
ⓘ	A6532	Gradient compression stocking, below knee, 40-50 mmHg, each Pub 100-02, 15, 100	A
⊘	A6533	Gradient compression stocking, thigh length, 18-30 mmHg, each NCD 280.1; Pub 100-02, 15, 130	E
⊘	A6534	Gradient compression stocking, thigh length, 30-40 mmHg, each NCD 280.1; Pub 100-02, 15, 130	E
⊘	A6535	Gradient compression stocking, thigh length, 40-50 mmHg, each NCD 280.1; Pub 100-02, 15, 130	E
⊘	A6536	Gradient compression stocking, full length/chap style, 18-30 mmHg, each NCD 280.1; Pub 100-02, 15, 130	E
⊘	A6537	Gradient compression stocking, full length/chap style, 30-40 mmHg, each NCD 280.1; Pub 100-02, 15, 130	E
⊘	A6538	Gradient compression stocking, full length/chap style, 40-50 mmHg, each NCD 280.1; Pub 100-02, 15, 130	E
⊘	A6539	Gradient compression stocking, waist length, 18-30 mmHg, each NCD 280.1; Pub 100-02, 15, 130	E
⊘	A6540	Gradient compression stocking, waist length, 30-40 mmHg, each NCD 280.1; Pub 100-02, 15, 130	E
⊘	A6541	Gradient compression stocking, waist length, 40-50 mmHg, each NCD 280.1; Pub 100-02, 15, 130	E
⊘	A6544	Gradient compression stocking, garter belt NCD 280.1; Pub 100-02, 15, 130	E
ⓘ	A6545	Gradient compression wrap, non-elastic, below knee, 30-50 mm hg, each	A
⊘	A6549	Gradient compression stocking/sleeve, not otherwise specified NCD 280.1; Pub 100-02, 15, 130	E
	A6550	Wound care set, for negative pressure wound therapy electrical pump, includes all supplies and accessories	Y

Respiratory Supplies

	Code	Description	Indicator
	A7000	Canister, disposable, used with suction pump, each	Y
	A7001	Canister, non-disposable, used with suction pump, each	Y
	A7002	Tubing, used with suction pump, each	Y
	A7003	Administration set, with small volume nonfiltered pneumatic nebulizer, disposable	Y
	A7004	Small volume nonfiltered pneumatic nebulizer, disposable	Y
	A7005	Administration set, with small volume nonfiltered pneumatic nebulizer, non-disposable	Y
	A7006	Administration set, with small volume filtered pneumatic nebulizer	Y
	A7007	Large volume nebulizer, disposable, unfilled, used with aerosol compressor	Y
	A7008	Large volume nebulizer, disposable, prefilled, used with aerosol compressor	Y
	A7009	Reservoir bottle, non-disposable, used with large volume ultrasonic nebulizer	Y
	A7010	Corrugated tubing, disposable, used with large volume nebulizer, 100 feet	Y
	A7011	Corrugated tubing, non-disposable, used with large volume nebulizer, 10 feet	Y
	A7012	Water collection device, used with large volume nebulizer	Y
▲	A7013	Filter, disposable, used with aerosol compressor or ultrasonic generator	Y
	A7014	Filter, non-disposable, used with aerosol compressor or ultrasonic generator	Y
	A7015	Aerosol mask, used with DME nebulizer	Y

Aerosol mask

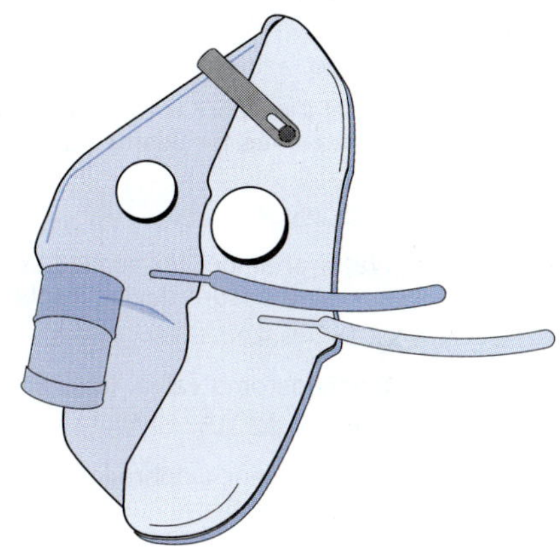

	Code	Description	Indicator
	A7016	Dome and mouthpiece, used with small volume ultrasonic nebulizer	Y
ⓘ	A7017	Nebulizer, durable, glass or autoclavable plastic, bottle type, not used with oxygen NCD 280.1	Y
	A7018	Water, distilled, used with large volume nebulizer, 1000 ml	Y
●	A7020	Interface for cough stimulating device, includes all components, replacement **This code is effective January 1, 2011**	Y
	A7025	High frequency chest wall oscillation system vest, replacement for use with patient owned equipment, each	Y
	A7026	High frequency chest wall oscillation system hose, replacement for use with patient owned equipment, each	Y
	A7027	Combination oral/nasal mask, used with continuous positive airway pressure device, each	Y
	A7028	Oral cushion for combination oral/nasal mask, replacement only, each	Y
	A7029	Nasal pillows for combination oral/nasal mask, replacement only, pair	Y
	A7030	Full face mask used with positive airway pressure device, each	Y
	A7031	Face mask interface, replacement for full face mask, each	Y
	A7032	Cushion for use on nasal mask interface, replacement only, each	Y
	A7033	Pillow for use on nasal cannula type interface, replacement only, pair	Y

A7034 Nasal interface (mask or cannula type) used with positive airway pressure device, with or without head strap Y

A7035 Headgear used with positive airway pressure device Y

A7036 Chinstrap used with positive airway pressure device Y

A7037 Tubing used with positive airway pressure device Y

A7038 Filter, disposable, used with positive airway pressure device Y

A7039 Filter, non disposable, used with positive airway pressure device Y

A7040 One way chest drain valve A

A7041 Water seal drainage container and tubing for use with implanted chest tube A

A7042 Implanted pleural catheter, each N

A7043 Vacuum drainage bottle and tubing for use with implanted catheter A

A7044 Oral interface used with positive airway pressure device, each Y

A7045 Exhalation port with or without swivel used with accessories for positive airway devices, replacement only Y
NCD 240.4

A7046 Water chamber for humidifier, used with positive airway pressure device, replacement, each Y
NCD 240.4

A7501 Tracheostoma valve, including diaphragm, each A
Pub 100-02, 15, 120

A7502 Replacement diaphragm/faceplate for tracheostoma valve, each A
Pub 100-02, 15, 120

A7503 Filter holder or filter cap, reusable, for use in a tracheostoma heat and moisture exchange system, each A
Pub 100-02, 15, 120

A7504 Filter for use in a tracheostoma heat and moisture exchange system, each A
Pub 100-02, 15, 120

A7505 Housing, reusable without adhesive, for use in a heat and moisture exchange system and/or with a tracheostoma valve, each A
Pub 100-02, 15, 120

A7506 Adhesive disc for use in a heat and moisture exchange system and/or with tracheostoma valve, any type each A
Pub 100-02, 15, 120

A7507 Filter holder and integrated filter without adhesive, for use in a tracheostoma heat and moisture exchange system, each A
Pub 100-02, 15, 120

A7508 Housing and integrated adhesive, for use in a tracheostoma heat and moisture exchange system and/or with a tracheostoma valve, each A
Pub 100-02, 15, 120

A7509 Filter holder and integrated filter housing, and adhesive, for use as a tracheostoma heat and moisture exchange system, each A
Pub 100-02, 15, 120

A7520 Tracheostomy/laryngectomy tube, non-cuffed, polyvinylchloride (PVC), silicone or equal, each A

A7521 Tracheostomy/laryngectomy tube, cuffed, polyvinylchloride (PVC), silicone or equal, each A

A7522 Tracheostomy/laryngectomy tube, stainless steel or equal (sterilizable and reusable), each A

A7523 Tracheostomy shower protector, each A

Tracheostomy shower protector

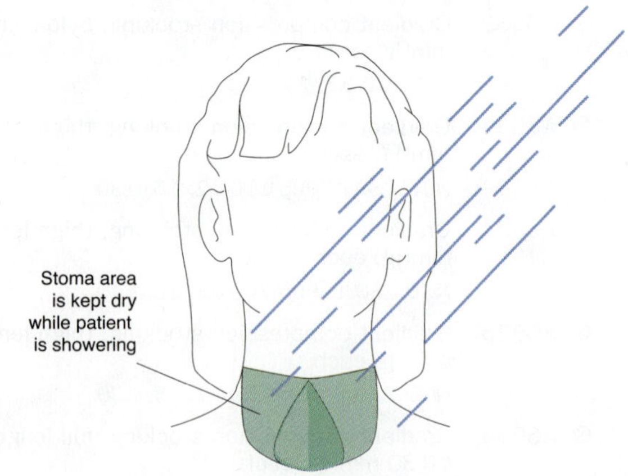

A7524 Tracheostoma stent/stud/button, each A

A7525 Tracheostomy mask, each A

A7526 Tracheostomy tube collar/holder, each A

A7527 Tracheostomy/laryngectomy tube plug/stop, each A

A8000 Helmet, protective, soft, prefabricated, includes all components and accessories Y

A8001 Helmet, protective, hard, prefabricated, includes all components and accessories Y

A8002 Helmet, protective, soft, custom fabricated, includes all components and accessories Y

A8003 Helmet, protective, hard, custom fabricated, includes all components and accessories Y

A8004 Soft interface for helmet, replacement only Y

Administrative, Miscellaneous, and Investigational A9150–A9999

A9150 Non-prescription drugs B
Pub 100-02, 15, 50

A9152 Single vitamin/mineral/trace element, oral, per dose, not otherwise specified E

A9153 Multiple vitamins, with or without minerals and trace elements, oral, per dose, not otherwise specified E

A9155 Artificial saliva, 30 ml B

A9180 Pediculosis (lice infestation) treatment, topical, for administration by patient/caretaker E

A9270 Non-covered item or service E
Pub 100-02, 16, 20

● A9273 Hot water bottle, ice cap or collar, heat and/or cold wrap, any type E
This code is effective January 1, 2011

A9274 External ambulatory insulin delivery system, disposable, each, includes all supplies and accessories E

A9275 Home glucose disposable monitor, includes test strips E

A9276 Sensor; invasive (e.g. subcutaneous), disposable, for use with interstitial continuous glucose monitoring system, one unit = 1 day supply E
Medicare statute 1861(n)

A9277 Transmitter; external, for use with interstitial continuous glucose monitoring system E
Medicare statute 1861(n)

⊘ A9278 Receiver (monitor); external, for use with interstitial continuous glucose monitoring system E
Medicare statute 1861(n)

⊘ A9279 Monitoring feature/device, stand-alone or integrated, any type, includes all accessories, components and electronics, not otherwise classified E

⊘ A9280 Alert or alarm device, not otherwise classified E
Medicare Statute 1861

⊘ A9281 Reaching/grabbing device, any type, any length, each E
Medicare Statute 1862

Reaching/grabbing device

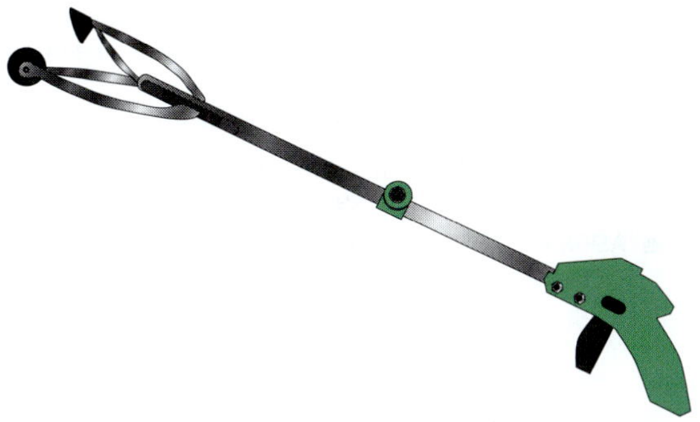

⊘ A9282 Wig, any type, each E
Medicare Statute 1861

⊘ A9283 Foot pressure off loading/supportive device, any type, each E
Medicare statute 1862a(i)13

Ⓘ A9284 Spirometer, non-electronic, includes all accessories N

⊘ A9300 Exercise equipment E
NCD 280.1; Pub 100-02, 15, 110.1; 100-4, 20, 10.1-10.1.4.2

A9500 Technetium TC-99m sestamibi, diagnostic, per study dose N
Cardiolite
AHA: 2Q 2006, 5

A9501 Technetium Tc-99m teboroxime, diagnostic, per study dose N
AHA: 1Q 2008, 6

A9502 Technetium Tc-99m tetrofosmin, diagnostic, per study dose N
AHA: 2Q 2006, 5

A9503 Technetium Tc-99m medronate, diagnostic, per study dose, up to 30 millicuries N
CIS-MDP

A9504 Technetium Tc-99m apcitide, diagnostic, per study dose, up to 20 millicuries N

A9505 Thallium Tl-201 thallous chloride, diagnostic, per millicurie N

A9507 Indium In-111 capromab pendetide, diagnostic, per study dose, up to 10 millicuries N
Prosta-Scint

A9508 Iodine I-131 iobenguane sulfate, diagnostic, per 0.5 millicurie N

A9509 Iodine I-123 sodium iodide, diagnostic, per millicurie N
AHA: 1Q 2008, 6

A9510 Technetium Tc-99m disofenin, diagnostic, per study dose, up to 15 millicuries N

A9512 Technetium Tc-99m pertechnetate, diagnostic, per millicurie N

A9516 Iodine I-123 sodium iodide, diagnostic, per 100 microcuries, up to 999 microcuries N

A9517 Iodine I-131 sodium iodide capsule(s), therapeutic, per millicurie N
AHA: 3Q 2008, 6

A9521 Technetium Tc-99m exametazime, diagnostic, per study dose, up to 25 millicuries N
Ceretec

A9524 Iodine I-131 iodinated serum albumin, diagnostic, per 5 microcuries N

A9526 Nitrogen N-13 ammonia, diagnostic, per study dose, up to 40 millicuries N
Pub 100-04, 13, 60.3.2; 100-4, 13, 60.11

A9527 Iodine I-125, sodium iodide solution, therapeutic, per millicurie U H2

A9528 Iodine I-131 sodium iodide capsule(s), diagnostic, per millicurie N

A9529 Iodine I-131 sodium iodide solution, diagnostic, per millicurie N

A9530 Iodine I-131 sodium iodide solution, therapeutic, per millicurie H

A9531 Iodine I-131 sodium iodide, diagnostic, per microcurie (up to 100 microcuries) N

A9532 Iodine I-125 serum albumin, diagnostic, per 5 microcuries N

A9536 Technetium Tc-99m depreotide, diagnostic, per study dose, up to 35 millicuries H

A9537 Technetium Tc-99m mebrofenin, diagnostic, per study dose, up to 15 millicuries N
Choletec

A9538 Technetium Tc-99m pyrophosphate, diagnostic, per study dose, up to 25 millicuries N
TechneScan PYP

A9539 Technetium Tc-99m pentetate, diagnostic, per study dose, up to 25 millicuries H
AN-DTPA

A9540 Technetium Tc-99m macroaggregated albumin, diagnostic, per study dose, up to 10 millicuries N

A9541 Technetium Tc-99m sulfur colloid, diagnostic, per study dose, up to 20 millicuries N

A9542 Indium In-111 ibritumomab tiuxetan, diagnostic, per study dose, up to 5 millicuries N
In-111 Zevalin

A9543 Yttrium Y-90 ibritumomab tiuxetan, therapeutic, per treatment dose, up to 40 millicuries H
Y-90 Zevalin

A9544 Iodine I-131 tositumomab, diagnostic, per study dose N

A9545 Iodine I-131 tositumomab, therapeutic, per treatment dose H
Bexxar

A9546 Cobalt Co-57/58, cyanocobalamin, diagnostic, per study dose, up to 1 microcurie N

A9547 Indium In-111 oxyquinoline, diagnostic, per 0.5 millicuries N

A9548 Indium In-111 pentetate, diagnostic, per 0.5 millicuries N
Indium DTPA

A9550 Technetium Tc-99m sodium gluceptate, diagnostic, per study dose, up to 25 millicuries N

A9551 Technetium Tc-99m succimer, diagnostic, per study dose, up to 10 millicuries N

A9552 Fluorodeoxyglucose F-18 FDG, diagnostic, per study dose, up to 45 millicuries N
Pub 100-04, 13, 60.3.2
AHA: 3Q 2008, 7

A9553 Chromium Cr-51 sodium chromate, diagnostic, per study dose, up to 250 microcurie N
Chromitope

A9554 Iodine I-125 sodium iothalamate, diagnostic, per study dose, up to 10 microcurie N
Glofil-125

A9555 Rubidium Rb-82, diagnostic, per study dose, up to 60 millicuries N
Cardiogen-82
Pub 100-04, 13, 60.3.2; 100-4, 13, 60.4

A9556 Gallium Ga-67 citrate, diagnostic, per millicuries N

A9557 Technetium Tc-99m bicisate, diagnostic, per study dose, up to 25 millicuries N

A9558 Xenon Xe-133 gas, diagnostic, per 10 millicuries N

A9559 Cobalt Co-57 cyanocobalamin, oral, diagnostic, per study dose, up to 1 microcurie N
Rubratope-57

A9560 Technetium Tc-99m labeled red blood cells, diagnostic, per study dose, up to 30 millicuries N
AHA: 3Q 2008, 7

A9561 Technetium Tc-99m oxidronate, diagnostic, per study dose, up to 30 millicuries N

A9562 Technetium Tc-99m mertiatide, diagnostic, per study dose, up to 15 millicuries N
TechneScan MAG3

A9563 Sodium phosphate P-32, therapeutic, per millicuries

A9564 Chromic phosphate P-32 suspension, therapeutic, per millicuries H
Phosphocol P 32

A9566 Technetium Tc-99m fanolesomab, diagnostic, per study dose, up to 25 millicuries H
NeutroSpec

A9567 Technetium Tc-99m pentetate, diagnostic, aerosol, per study dose, up to 75 millicuries N

A9568 Technetium TC-99m arcitumomab, diagnostic, per study dose, up to 45 millicuries N

A9569 Technetium Tc-99m exametazime labeled autologous white blood cells, diagnostic, per study dose N
AHA: 1Q 2008, 6

A9570 Indium In-111 labeled autologous white blood cells, diagnostic, per study dose N
AHA: 1Q 2008, 6

A9571 Indium In-111 labeled autologous platelets, diagnostic, per study dose N
AHA: 1Q 2008, 6

A9572 Indium In-111 pentetreotide, diagnostic, per study dose, up to 6 millicuries N
OctreoScan
AHA: 1Q 2008, 6

A9576 Injection, gadoteridol, (ProHance multipack), per ml N N1
AHA: 1Q 2008, 6

A9577 Injection, gadobenate dimeglumine (MultiHance), per ml N N1
AHA: 1Q 2008, 6

A9578 Injection, gadobenate dimeglumine (MultiHance multipack), per ml N N1
AHA: 1Q 2008, 6

A9579 Injection, gadolinium-based magnetic resonance contrast agent, not otherwise specified (NOS), per ml N N1
AHA: 1Q 2008, 6

A9580 Sodium fluoride F-18, diagnostic, per study dose, up to 30 millicuries N N1

A9581 Injection, gadoxetate disodium, 1 ml G K2
Eovist

A9582 Iodine I-123 iobenguane, diagnostic, per study dose, up to 15 millicuries G K2
AdreView

A9583 Injection, gadofosveset trisodium, 1 ml G K2
Vasovist

A9600 Strontium Sr-89 chloride, therapeutic, per millicurie H
Metastron

A9604 Samarium Sm-153 lexidronam, therapeutic, per treatment dose, up to 150 millicuries K
Quadramet

ⓘ A9698 Non-radioactive contrast imaging material, not otherwise classified, per study N N1
Pub 100-04, 13, 20; 100-4, 13, 90

A9699 Radiopharmaceutical, therapeutic, not otherwise classified N

ⓘ A9700 Supply of injectable contrast material for use in echocardiography, per study B
Pub 100-04, 12, 30.4

A9900 Miscellaneous DME supply, accessory, and/or service component of another HCPCS code Y

A9901 DME delivery, set up, and/or dispensing service component of another HCPCS code A

A9999 Miscellaneous DME supply or accessory, not otherwise specified Y

Enteral and Parenteral Therapy B4034–B9999

Enteral Formulae Supplies

▲ ⓘ B4034 Enteral feeding supply kit; syringe fed, per day, includes but not limited to feeding/flushing syringe, administration set tubing, dressings, tape Y
NCD 180.2; Pub 100-02, 15, 120; 100-4, 20; 100.2.2.3; 100-8, 5, 5.3

▲ ⓘ B4035 Enteral feeding supply kit; pump fed, per day, includes but not limited to feeding/flushing syringe, administration set tubing, dressings, tape Y
NCD 180.2; Pub 100-02, 15, 120; 100-4, 20; 100.2.2.3; 100-8, 5, 5.3

▲ ⓘ B4036 Enteral feeding supply kit; gravity fed, per day, includes but not limited to feeding/flushing syringe, administration set tubing, dressings, tape Y
NCD 180.2; Pub 100-02, 15, 120; 100-4, 20; 100.2.2.3; 100-8, 5, 5.3

ⓘ B4081 Nasogastric tubing with stylet Y
NCD 180.2; Pub 100-02, 15, 120; 100-4, 20; 100.2.2.3; 100-8, 5, 5.3

Naso/oro gastric tube

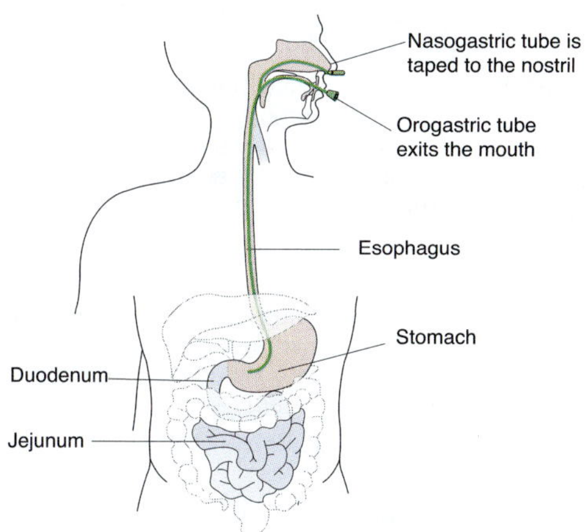

ⓘ B4082 Nasogastric tubing without stylet Y
NCD 180.2; Pub 100-02, 15, 120; 100-4, 20; 100.2.2.3; 100-8, 5, 5.3

ⓘ B4083 Stomach tube – Levine type Y
NCD 180.2; Pub 100-02, 15, 120; 100-4, 20; 100.2.2.3; 100-8, 5, 5.3

B4087 Gastrostomy/jejunostomy tube, standard, any material, any type, each A

Gastrostomy

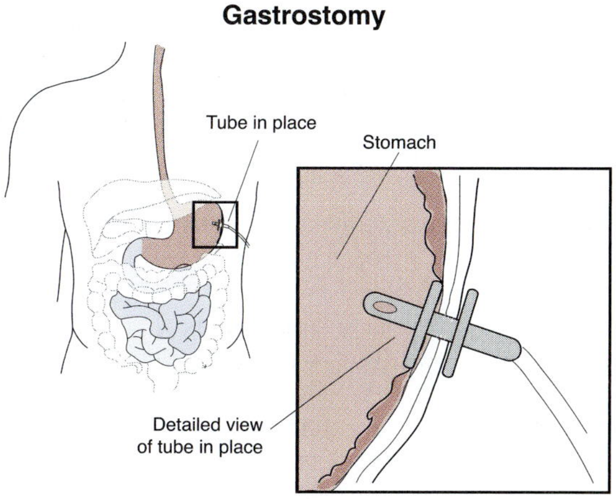

B4088 Gastrostomy/jejunostomy tube, low-profile, any material, any type, each A

⊘ B4100 Food thickener, administered orally, per ounce E
NCD 180.1

ⓘ B4102 Enteral formula, for adults, used to replace fluids and electrolytes (e.g. clear liquids), 500 ml = 1 unit Y
NCD 180.2

ⓘ B4103 Enteral formula, for pediatrics, used to replace fluids and electrolytes (e.g. clear liquids), 500 ml = 1 unit Y
NCD 180.2

ⓘ B4104 Additive for enteral formula (e.g. fiber) E
NCD 180.2

ⓘ B4149 Enteral formula, manufactured blenderized natural foods with intact nutrients, includes proteins, fats, carbohydrates, vitamins and minerals, may include fiber, administered through an enteral feeding tube, 100 calories = 1 unit Y
NCD 180.2; Pub 100-02, 15, 120; 100-4, 20; 100.2.2.3; 100-8, 5, 5.3

ⓘ B4150 Enteral formula, nutritionally complete with intact nutrients, includes proteins, fats, carbohydrates, vitamins and minerals, may include fiber, administered through an enteral feeding tube, 100 calories = 1 unit Y
NCD 180.2; Pub 100-02, 15, 120; 100-4, 20; 100.2.2.3; 100-8, 5, 5.3

ⓘ B4152 Enteral formula, nutritionally complete, calorically dense (equal to or greater than 1.5 kcal/ml) with intact nutrients, includes proteins, fats, carbohydrates, vitamins and minerals, may include fiber, administered through an enteral feeding tube, 100 calories = 1 unit Y
NCD 180.2; Pub 100-02, 15, 120; 100-4, 20; 100.2.2.3; 100-8, 5, 5.3

ⓘ B4153 Enteral formula, nutritionally complete, hydrolyzed proteins (amino acids and peptide chain), includes fats, carbohydrates, vitamins and minerals, may include fiber, administered through an enteral feeding tube, 100 calories = 1 unit Y
NCD 180.2; Pub 100-02, 15, 120; 100-4, 20; 100.2.2.3; 100-8, 5, 5.3

ⓘ B4154 Enteral formula, nutritionally complete, for special metabolic needs, excludes inherited disease of metabolism, includes altered composition of proteins, fats, carbohydrates, vitamins and/or minerals, may include fiber, administered through an enteral feeding tube, 100 calories = 1 unit Y
NCD 180.2; Pub 100-02, 15, 120; 100-4, 20; 100.2.2.3; 100-8, 5, 5.3

ⓘ B4155 Enteral formula, nutritionally incomplete/modular nutrients, includes specific nutrients, carbohydrates (e.g., glucose polymers), proteins/amino acids (e.g., glutamine, arginine), fat (e.g., medium chain triglycerides) or combination, administered through an enteral feeding tube, 100 calories = 1 unit Y
NCD 180.2; Pub 100-02, 15, 120; 100-4, 20; 100.2.2.3; 100-8, 5, 5.3

ⓘ B4157 Enteral formula, nutritionally complete, for special metabolic needs for inherited disease of metabolism, includes proteins, fats, carbohydrates, vitamins and minerals, may include fiber, administered through an enteral feeding tube, 100 calories = 1 unit Y
NCD 180.2

ⓘ B4158 Enteral formula, for pediatrics, nutritionally complete with intact nutrients, includes proteins, fats, carbohydrates, vitamins and minerals, may include fiber and/or iron, administered through an enteral feeding tube, 100 calories = 1 unit Y
NCD 180.2

B4034 – B4158

Ⓘ B4159 Enteral formula, for pediatrics, nutritionally complete soy based with intact nutrients, includes proteins, fats, carbohydrates, vitamins and minerals, may include fiber and/or iron, administered through an enteral feeding tube, 100 calories = 1 unit Y

NCD 180.2

Ⓘ B4160 Enteral formula, for pediatrics, nutritionally complete calorically dense (equal to or greater than 0.7 kcal/ml) with intact nutrients, includes proteins, fats, carbohydrates, vitamins and minerals, may include fiber, administered through an enteral feeding tube, 100 calories = 1 unit Y

NCD 180.2

Ⓘ B4161 Enteral formula, for pediatrics, hydrolyzed/amino acids and peptide chain proteins, includes fats, carbohydrates, vitamins and minerals, may include fiber, administered through an enteral feeding tube, 100 calories = 1 unit Y

NCD 180.2

Ⓘ B4162 Enteral formula, for pediatrics, special metabolic needs for inherited disease of metabolism, includes proteins, fats, carbohydrates, vitamins and minerals, may include fiber, administered through an enteral feeding tube, 100 calories = 1 unit Y

NCD 180.2

Parenteral Nutrition Solutions and Supplies

Ⓘ B4164 Parenteral nutrition solution; carbohydrates (dextrose), 50% or less (500 ml = 1 unit) – home mix Y

NCD 180.2; Pub 100-02, 15, 120; 100-4, 20; 100.2.2.3; 100-8, 5, 5.3

Ⓘ B4168 Parenteral nutrition solution; amino acid, 3.5%, (500 ml = 1 unit) – home mix Y

NCD 180.2; Pub 100-02, 15, 120; 100-4, 20; 100.2.2.3; 100-8, 5, 5.3

Ⓘ B4172 Parenteral nutrition solution; amino acid, 5.5% through 7%, (500 ml = 1 unit) – home mix Y

NCD 180.2; Pub 100-02, 15, 120; 100-4, 20; 100.2.2.3; 100-8, 5, 5.3

Ⓘ B4176 Parenteral nutrition solution; amino acid, 7% through 8.5%, (500 ml = 1 unit) – home mix Y

NCD 180.2; Pub 100-02, 15, 120; 100-4, 20; 100.2.2.3; 100-8, 5, 5.3

Ⓘ B4178 Parenteral nutrition solution; amino acid, greater than 8.5% (500 ml = 1 unit) – home mix Y

NCD 180.2; Pub 100-02, 15, 120; 100-4, 20; 100.2.2.3; 100-8, 5, 5.3

Ⓘ B4180 Parenteral nutrition solution; carbohydrates (dextrose), greater than 50% (500 ml=1 unit) – home mix Y

NCD 180.2; Pub 100-02, 15, 120; 100-4, 20; 100.2.2.3; 100-8, 5, 5.3

Ⓘ B4185 Parenteral nutrition solution, per 10 grams lipids B

Ⓘ B4189 Parenteral nutrition solution; compounded amino acid and carbohydrates with electrolytes, trace elements, and vitamins, including preparation, any strength, 10 to 51 grams of protein – premix Y

NCD 180.2; Pub 100-02, 15, 120; 100-4, 20; 100.2.2.3; 100-8, 5, 5.3

Ⓘ B4193 Parenteral nutrition solution; compounded amino acid and carbohydrates with electrolytes, trace elements, and vitamins, including preparation, any strength, 52 to 73 grams of protein – premix Y

NCD 180.2; Pub 100-02, 15, 120; 100-4, 20; 100.2.2.3; 100-8, 5, 5.3

Ⓘ B4197 Parenteral nutrition solution; compounded amino acid and carbohydrates with electrolytes, trace elements and vitamins, including preparation, any strength, 74 to 100 grams of protein – premix Y

NCD 180.2; Pub 100-02, 15, 120; 100-4, 20; 100.2.2.3; 100-8, 5, 5.3

Ⓘ B4199 Parenteral nutrition solution; compounded amino acid and carbohydrates with electrolytes, trace elements and vitamins, including preparation, any strength, over 100 grams of protein – premix Y

NCD 180.2; Pub 100-02, 15, 120; 100-4, 20; 100.2.2.3; 100-8, 5, 5.3

Ⓘ B4216 Parenteral nutrition; additives (vitamins, trace elements, heparin, electrolytes) home mix per day Y

NCD 180.2; Pub 100-02, 15, 120; 100-4, 20; 100.2.2.3; 100-8, 5, 5.3

Ⓘ B4220 Parenteral nutrition supply kit; premix, per day Y

NCD 180.2; Pub 100-02, 15, 120; 100-4, 20; 100.2.2.3; 100-8, 5, 5.3

Ⓘ B4222 Parenteral nutrition supply kit; home mix, per day Y

NCD 180.2; Pub 100-02, 15, 120; 100-4, 20; 100.2.2.3; 100-8, 5, 5.3

Ⓘ B4224 Parenteral nutrition administration kit, per day Y

NCD 180.2; Pub 100-02, 15, 120; 100-4, 20; 100.2.2.3; 100-8, 5, 5.3

Ⓘ B5000 Parenteral nutrition solution: compounded amino acid and carbohydrates with electrolytes, trace elements, and vitamins, including preparation, any strength, renal – amirosyn RF, nephramine, renamine – premix Y

NCD 180.2; Pub 100-02, 15, 120; 100-4, 20; 100.2.2.3; 100-8, 5, 5.3

Ⓘ B5100 Parenteral nutrition solution: compounded amino acid and carbohydrates with electrolytes, trace elements, and vitamins, including preparation, any strength, hepatic – freamine HBC, hepatamine – premix Y

NCD 180.2; Pub 100-02, 15, 120; 100-4, 20; 100.2.2.3; 100-8, 5, 5.3

Ⓘ B5200 Parenteral nutrition solution: compounded amino acid and carbohydrates with electrolytes, trace elements, and vitamins, including preparation, any strength, stress – branch chain amino acids – premix Y

NCD 180.2; Pub 100-02, 15, 120; 100-4, 20; 100.2.2.3; 100-8, 5, 5.3

Enteral and Parenteral Pumps

Ⓘ B9000 Enteral nutrition infusion pump – without alarm Y

NCD 180.2; Pub 100-02, 15, 120; 100-4, 20; 100.2.2.3; 100-8, 5, 5.3

Ⓘ B9002 Enteral nutrition infusion pump – with alarm Y

NCD 180.2; Pub 100-02, 15, 120; 100-4, 20; 100.2.2.3; 100-8, 5, 5.3

Ⓘ B9004 Parenteral nutrition infusion pump, portable Y

NCD 180.2; Pub 100-02, 15, 120; 100-4, 20; 100.2.2.3; 100-8, 5, 5.3

Ⓘ B9006 Parenteral nutrition infusion pump, stationary Y

NCD 180.2; Pub 100-02, 15, 120; 100-4, 20; 100.2.2.3; 100-8, 5, 5.3

Ⓘ B9998 NOC for enteral supplies Y

NCD 180.2; Pub 100-02, 15, 120; 100-4, 20; 100.2.2.3; 100-8, 5, 5.3

Ⓘ B9999 NOC for parenteral supplies Y

NCD 180.2; Pub 100-02, 15, 120; 100-4, 20; 100.2.2.3; 100-8, 5, 5.3

Pass-Through Items C1300–C9728

Note: These codes should only be used by hospital outpatient departments under the prospective payment system.

ⓘ C1300 Hyperbaric oxygen under pressure, full body chamber, per 30 minute interval S
Medicare Statute 1833(t)
AHA: 1Q 2005, 6
Pub 100-04, 32, 30.1

ⓘ C1713 Anchor/screw for opposing bone-to-bone or soft tissue-to-bone (implantable) N N1
Medicare Statute 1833(t)

ⓘ C1714 Catheter, transluminal atherectomy, directional N N1
Medicare Statute 1833(t)

ⓘ C1715 Brachytherapy needle N N1
Medicare Statute 1833(t)

ⓘ C1716 Brachytherapy source, non-stranded, gold 198, per source U H2
Medicare Statute 1833(t)

ⓘ C1717 Brachytherapy source, non-stranded, high dose rate iridium-192, per source U H2

ⓘ C1719 Brachytherapy source, non-stranded, non-high dose rate iridium-192, per source U H2
Medicare Statute 1833(t)

ⓘ C1721 Cardioverter-defibrillator, dual chamber (implantable) N N1
Medicare Statute 1833(t)

ⓘ C1722 Cardioverter-defibrillator, single chamber (implantable) N N1
Medicare Statute 1833(t)
AHA: 2Q 2006, 9

ⓘ C1724 Catheter, transluminal atherectomy, rotational N N1
Medicare Statute 1833(t)

ⓘ C1725 Catheter, transluminal angioplasty, non-laser (may include guidance, infusion/perfusion capability) N N1
Medicare Statute 1833(t)

ⓘ C1726 Catheter, balloon dilatation, non-vascular N N1
Medicare Statute 1833(t)

ⓘ C1727 Catheter, balloon tissue dissector, non-vascular (insertable) N N1
Medicare Statute 1833(t)

ⓘ C1728 Catheter, brachytherapy seed administration N N1
Medicare Statute 1833(t)

ⓘ C1729 Catheter, drainage N N1
Medicare Statute 1833(t)

ⓘ C1730 Catheter, electrophysiology, diagnostic, other than 3D mapping (19 or fewer electrodes) N N1
Medicare Statute 1833(t)

ⓘ C1731 Catheter, electrophysiology, diagnostic, other than 3D mapping (20 or more electrodes) N N1
Medicare Statute 1833(t)

ⓘ C1732 Catheter, electrophysiology, diagnostic/ ablation, 3D or vector mapping N N1
Medicare Statute 1833(t)

ⓘ C1733 Catheter, electrophysiology, diagnostic/ ablation, other than 3D or vector mapping, other than cool-tip N N1
Medicare Statute 1833(t)

● ⓘ C1749 Endoscope, retrograde imaging/illumination colonoscope device (implantable) N N1
This code was effective October 1, 2010

ⓘ C1750 Catheter, hemodialysis/peritoneal, long-term N N1
Medicare Statute 1833(t)

ⓘ C1751 Catheter, infusion, inserted peripherally, centrally or midline (other than hemodialysis) N N1
Medicare Statute 1833(t)

ⓘ C1752 Catheter, hemodialysis/peritoneal, short-term N N1
Medicare Statute 1833(t)

ⓘ C1753 Catheter, intravascular ultrasound N N1
Medicare Statute 1833(t)

ⓘ C1754 Catheter, intradiscal N N1
Medicare Statute 1833(t)

ⓘ C1755 Catheter, intraspinal N N1
Medicare Statute 1833(t)

ⓘ C1756 Catheter, pacing, transesophageal N N1
Medicare Statute 1833(t)

ⓘ C1757 Catheter, thrombectomy/embolectomy N N1
Medicare Statute 1833(t)

ⓘ C1758 Catheter, ureteral N N1
Medicare Statute 1833(t)

ⓘ C1759 Catheter, intracardiac echocardiography N N1
Medicare Statute 1833(t)

ⓘ C1760 Closure device, vascular (implantable/ insertable) N N1
Medicare Statute 1833(t)

ⓘ C1762 Connective tissue, human (includes fascia lata) N N1
Medicare Statute 1833(t)

ⓘ C1763 Connective tissue, non-human (includes synthetic) N N1
Medicare Statute 1833(t)

ⓘ C1764 Event recorder, cardiac (implantable) N N1
Medicare Statute 1833(t)

ⓘ C1765 Adhesion barrier N N1
Medicare Statute 1833(t)

ⓘ C1766 Introducer/sheath, guiding, intracardiac electrophysiological, steerable, other than peel-away N N1
Medicare Statute 1833(t)

ⓘ C1767 Generator, neurostimulator (implantable), non-rechargeable N N1
Medicare Statute 1833(t)
AHA: 1Q 2007, 8
Pub 100-04, 32, 40-40.5

ⓘ C1768 Graft, vascular N N1
Medicare Statute 1833(t)

ⓘ C1769 Guide wire N N1
Medicare Statute 1833(t)
AHA: 2Q 2007, 7

ⓘ C1770 Imaging coil, magnetic resonance (insertable) N N1
Medicare Statute 1833(t)

ⓘ C1771 Repair device, urinary, incontinence, with sling graft N N1
Medicare Statute 1833(t)
AHA: 2Q 2008, 9

ⓘ C1772 Infusion pump, programmable (implantable) N N1
Medicare Statute 1833(t)

C1300 – C1772

Ⓘ C1773 Retrieval device, insertable (used to retrieve fractured medical devices) N NI
Medicare Statute 1833(t)

Ⓘ C1776 Joint device (implantable) N NI
Medicare Statute 1833(t)

Ⓘ C1777 Lead, cardioverter-defibrillator, endocardial single coil (implantable) N NI
Medicare Statute 1833(t)
AHA: 2Q 2006, 9

Ⓘ C1778 Lead, neurostimulator (implantable) N NI
Medicare Statute 1833(t)
AHA: 1Q 2007, 8
Pub 100-04, 32, 40-40.5

Ⓘ C1779 Lead, pacemaker, transvenous VDD single pass N NI
Medicare Statute 1833(t)

Ⓘ C1780 Lens, intraocular (new technology) N NI
Medicare Statute 1833(t)

Ⓘ C1781 Mesh (implantable) N NI
Medicare Statute 1833(t)

Ⓘ C1782 Morcellator N NI
Medicare Statute 1833(t)

Ⓘ C1783 Ocular implant, aqueous drainage assist device N NI
Medicare Statute 1833(t)

Ⓘ C1784 Ocular device, intraoperative, detached retina N NI
Medicare Statute 1833(t)

Ⓘ C1785 Pacemaker, dual chamber, rate-responsive (implantable) N NI
Medicare Statute 1833(t)

Ⓘ C1786 Pacemaker, single chamber, rate-responsive (implantable) N NI
Medicare Statute 1833(t)

Pacemaker Implantation

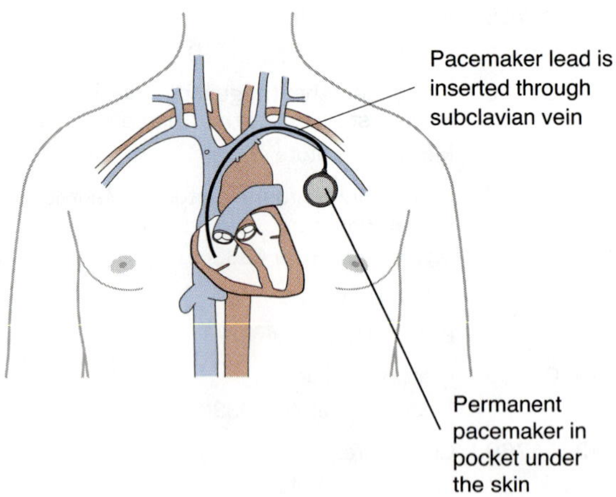

Ⓘ C1787 Patient programmer, neurostimulator N NI
Medicare Statute 1833(t)

Ⓘ C1788 Port, indwelling (implantable) N NI
Medicare Statute 1833(t)

Ⓘ C1789 Prosthesis, breast (implantable) N NI
Medicare Statute 1833(t)

Breast prosthesis (implantable)

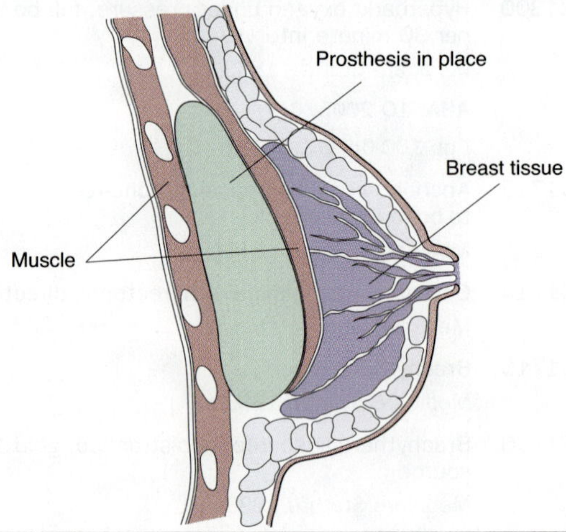

Ⓘ C1813 Prosthesis, penile, inflatable ♂ N NI
Medicare Statute 1833(t)

Ⓘ C1814 Retinal tamponade device, silicone oil N NI
Medicare Statute 1833(t)
AHA: 2Q 2006, 9

Ⓘ C1815 Prosthesis, urinary sphincter (implantable) N NI
Medicare Statute 1833(t)

Ⓘ C1816 Receiver and/or transmitter, neurostimulator (implantable) N NI
Medicare Statute 1833(t)

Ⓘ C1817 Septal defect implant system, intracardiac N NI
Medicare Statute 1833(t)

Ⓘ C1818 Integrated keratoprosthesis N NI
Medicare Statute 1833(t)

Ⓘ C1819 Surgical tissue localization and excision device (implantable) N NI
Medicare Statute 1833(t)

Ⓘ C1820 Generator, neurostimulator (implantable), with rechargeable battery and charging system N NI
Medicare Statute 1833(t)

Ⓘ C1821 Interspinous process distraction device (implantable) N J7
Medicare Statute 1833(t)

Ⓘ C1874 Stent, coated/covered, with delivery system N NI
Medicare Statute 1833(t)
AHA: 3Q 2002, 9

Ⓘ C1875 Stent, coated/covered, without delivery system N NI
Medicare Statute 1833(t)
AHA: 3Q 2002, 9

Ⓘ C1876 Stent, non-coated/non-covered, with delivery system N NI
Medicare Statute 1833(t)
AHA: 3Q 2002, 9

Ⓘ C1877 Stent, non-coated/non-covered, without delivery system N NI
Medicare Statute 1833(t)
AHA: 3Q 2002, 9

Ⓘ C1878 Material for vocal cord medialization, synthetic (implantable) N N1
Medicare Statute 1833(t)

Ⓘ C1880 Vena cava filter N N1
Medicare Statute 1833(t)

Ⓘ C1881 Dialysis access system (implantable) N N1
Medicare Statute 1833(t)

Ⓘ C1882 Cardioverter-defibrillator, other than single or dual chamber (implantable) N N1
Medicare Statute 1833(t)
AHA: 3Q 2002, 9

Ⓘ C1883 Adaptor/extension, pacing lead or neurostimulator lead (implantable) N N1
Medicare Statute 1833(t)
AHA: 1Q 2007, 8
Pub 100-04, 32, 40-40.5

Ⓘ C1884 Embolization protective system N N1
Medicare Statute 1833(t)

Ⓘ C1885 Catheter, transluminal angioplasty, laser N N1
Medicare Statute 1833(t)

Ⓘ C1887 Catheter, guiding (may include infusion/perfusion capability) N N1
Medicare Statute 1833(t)

Ⓘ C1888 Catheter, ablation, non-cardiac, endovascular (implantable) N N1
Medicare Statute 1833(t)

Ⓘ C1891 Infusion pump, non-programmable, permanent (implantable) N N1
Medicare Statute 1833(t)

Ⓘ C1892 Introducer/sheath, guiding, intracardiac electrophysiological, fixed-curve, peel-away N N1
Medicare Statute 1833(t)

Ⓘ C1893 Introducer/sheath, guiding, intracardiac electrophysiological, fixed-curve, other than peel-away N N1
Medicare Statute 1833(t)

Ⓘ C1894 Introducer/sheath, other than guiding, other than intracardiac electrophysiological, non-laser N N1
Medicare Statute 1833(t)

Ⓘ C1895 Lead, cardioverter-defibrillator, endocardial dual coil (implantable) N N1
Medicare Statute 1833(t)
AHA: 2Q 2006, 9

Ⓘ C1896 Lead, cardioverter-defibrillator, other than endocardial single or dual coil (implantable) N N1
Medicare Statute 1833(t)
AHA: 2Q 2006, 9

Ⓘ C1897 Lead, neurostimulator test kit (implantable) N N1
Medicare Statute 1833(t)
AHA: 1Q 2007, 8
Pub 100-04, 32, 40-40.5

Ⓘ C1898 Lead, pacemaker, other than transvenous VDD single pass N N1
Medicare Statute 1833(t)
AHA: 3Q 2002, 8

Ⓘ C1899 Lead, pacemaker/cardioverter-defibrillator combination (implantable) N N1
Medicare Statute 1833(t)

Ⓘ C1900 Lead, left ventricular coronary venous system N N1
Medicare Statute 1833(t)

Ⓘ C2614 Probe, percutaneous lumbar discectomy N N1
Medicare Statute 1833(t)

Percutaneous lumbar discectomy probe

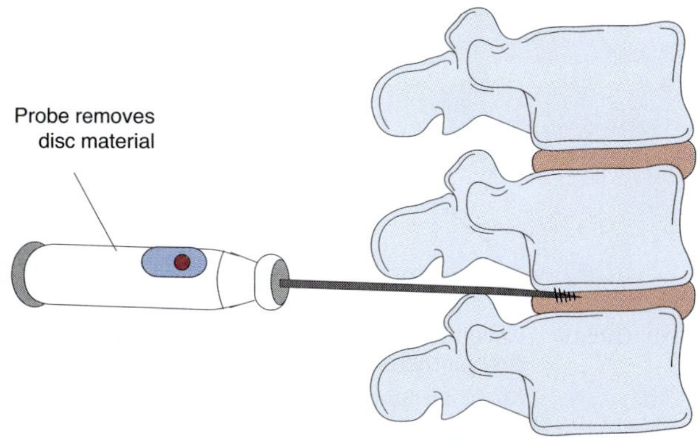

Ⓘ C2615 Sealant, pulmonary, liquid N N1
Medicare Statute 1833(t)

Ⓘ C2616 Brachytherapy source, non-stranded, yttrium-90, per source U H2
Medicare Statute 1833(t)

Ⓘ C2617 Stent, non-coronary, temporary, without delivery system N N1
Medicare Statute 1833(t)

Transcatheter placement of an intravascular stent

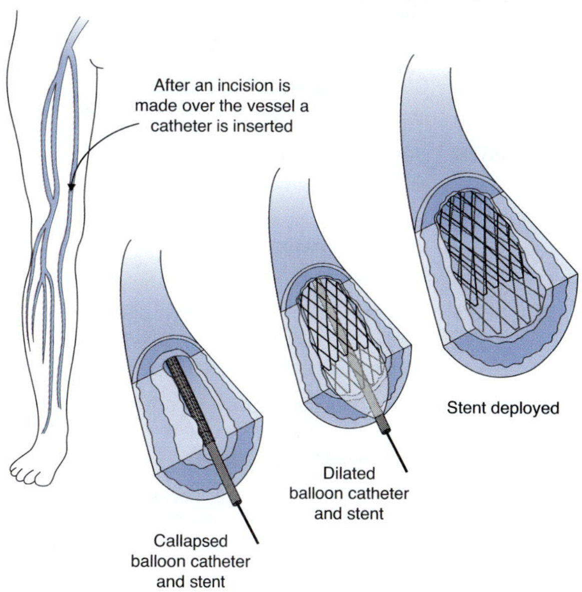

C1878 – C2617

ⓘ C2618 Probe, cryoablation N N1
Medicare Statute 1833(t)

Cryoablation probe

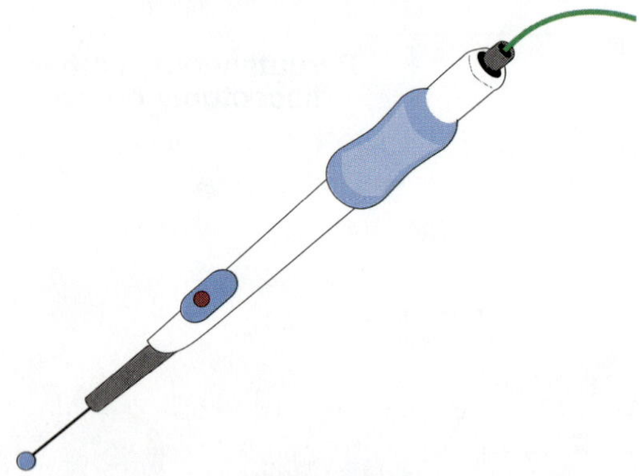

ⓘ C2619 Pacemaker, dual chamber, non rate-responsive (implantable) N N1
Medicare Statute 1833(t)

ⓘ C2620 Pacemaker, single chamber, non rate-responsive (implantable) N N1
Medicare Statute 1833(t)

ⓘ C2621 Pacemaker, other than single or dual chamber (implantable) N N1
Medicare Statute 1833(t)
AHA: 3Q 2002, 8

ⓘ C2622 Prosthesis, penile, non-inflatable ♂ N N1
Medicare Statute 1833(t)

ⓘ C2625 Stent, non-coronary, temporary, with delivery system N N1
Medicare Statute 1833(t)

ⓘ C2626 Infusion pump, non-programmable, temporary (implantable) N N1
Medicare Statute 1833(t)

ⓘ C2627 Catheter, suprapubic/cystoscopic N N1
Medicare Statute 1833(t)

ⓘ C2628 Catheter, occlusion N N1
Medicare Statute 1833(t)

ⓘ C2629 Introducer/sheath, other than guiding, intracardiac electrophysiological, laser N N1
Medicare Statute 1833(t)

ⓘ C2630 Catheter, electrophysiology, diagnostic/ ablation, other than 3D or vector mapping, cool-tip N N1
Medicare Statute 1833(t)

ⓘ C2631 Repair device, urinary, incontinence, without sling graft N N1
Medicare Statute 1833(t)

ⓘ C2634 Brachytherapy source, non-stranded, high activity, iodine-125, greater than 1.01 mCi (NIST), per source U H2
Medicare Statute 1833(t)

ⓘ C2635 Brachytherapy source, non-stranded, high activity, paladium-103, greater than 2.2 mCi (NIST), per source U H2
Medicare Statute 1833(t)

ⓘ C2636 Brachytherapy linear source, non-stranded, paladium-103, per 1 mm U H2
Medicare Statute 1833(t)

ⓘ C2637 Brachytherapy source, non-stranded, ytterbium-169, per source B
Medicare Statute 1833(t)

ⓘ C2638 Brachytherapy source, stranded, iodine-125, per source U H2
Medicare statute 1833(t)(2)

ⓘ C2639 Brachytherapy source, non-stranded, iodine-125, per source U H2
Medicare statute 1833(t)(2)

ⓘ C2640 Brachytherapy source, stranded, palladium-103, per source U H2
Medicare statute 1833(t)(2)

ⓘ C2641 Brachytherapy source, non-stranded, palladium-103, per source U H2
Medicare statute 1833(t)(2)

ⓘ C2642 Brachytherapy source, stranded, cesium-131, per source U H2
Medicare statute 1833(t)(2)

ⓘ C2643 Brachytherapy source, non-stranded, cesium-131, per source U H2
Medicare statute 1833(t)(2)

ⓘ C2698 Brachytherapy source, stranded, not otherwise specified, per source U H2
Medicare statute 1833(t)(2)

ⓘ C2699 Brachytherapy source, non-stranded, not otherwise specified, per source U H2
Medicare statute 1833(t)(2)

ⓘ C8900 Magnetic resonance angiography with contrast, abdomen Q3 Z2
Pub 100-03, 1, 220.2
Medicare Statute 1833(t)(2)

ⓘ C8901 Magnetic resonance angiography without contrast, abdomen Q3 Z2
Pub 100-03, 1, 220.2
Medicare Statute 1833(t)(2)

ⓘ C8902 Magnetic resonance angiography without contrast followed by with contrast, abdomen Q3 Z2
Pub 100-03, 1, 220.2
Medicare Statute 1833(t)(2)

ⓘ C8903 Magnetic resonance imaging with contrast, breast; unilateral Q3 Z2
Pub 100-03, 1, 220.2
Medicare Statute 1833(t)(2)

ⓘ C8904 Magnetic resonance imaging without contrast, breast; unilateral Q3 Z2
Pub 100-03, 1, 220.2
Medicare Statute 1833(t)(2)

ⓘ C8905 Magnetic resonance imaging without contrast followed by with contrast, breast; unilateral Q3 Z2
Pub 100-03, 1, 220.2
Medicare Statute 1833(t)(2)

ⓘ C8906 Magnetic resonance imaging with contrast, breast; bilateral Q3 Z2
Pub 100-03, 1, 220.2
Medicare Statute 1833(t)(2)

ⓘ C8907 Magnetic resonance imaging without contrast, breast; bilateral Q3 Z2
Pub 100-03, 1, 220.2
Medicare Statute 1833(t)(2)

Ⓣ C8908 Magnetic resonance imaging without contrast followed by with contrast, breast; bilateral Q3 Z2
Pub 100-03, 1, 220.2
Medicare Statute 1833(t)(2)

Ⓣ C8909 Magnetic resonance angiography with contrast, chest (excluding myocardium) Q3 Z2
Pub 100-03, 1, 220.2
Medicare Statute 1833(t)(2)

Ⓣ C8910 Magnetic resonance angiography without contrast, chest (excluding myocardium) Q3 Z2
Pub 100-03, 1, 220.2
Medicare Statute 1833(t)(2)

Ⓣ C8911 Magnetic resonance angiography without contrast followed by with contrast, chest (excluding myocardium) Q3 Z2
Pub 100-03, 1, 220.2
Medicare Statute 1833(t)(2)

Ⓣ C8912 Magnetic resonance angiography with contrast, lower extremity Q3 Z2
Pub 100-03, 1, 220.2
Medicare Statute 1833(t)(2)

Ⓣ C8913 Magnetic resonance angiography without contrast, lower extremity Q3 Z2
Pub 100-03, 1, 220.2
Medicare Statute 1833(t)(2)

Ⓣ C8914 Magnetic resonance angiography without contrast followed by with contrast, lower extremity Q3 Z2
Pub 100-03, 1, 220.2
Medicare Statute 1833(t)(2)

Ⓣ C8918 Magnetic resonance angiography with contrast, pelvis Q3 Z2
Pub 100-03, 1, 220.2
Medicare Statute 1833(t)(2)

Ⓣ C8919 Magnetic resonance angiography without contrast, pelvis Q3 Z2
Pub 100-03, 1, 220.2
Medicare Statute 1833(t)(2)

Ⓣ C8920 Magnetic resonance angiography without contrast followed by with contrast, pelvis Q3 Z2
Pub 100-03, 1, 220.2
Medicare Statute 1833(t)(2)

Ⓣ C8921 Transthoracic echocardiography with contrast, or without contrast followed by with contrast, for congenital cardiac anomalies; complete S
Medicare statute 1833(t)(2)
AHA: 2Q 2008, 9

Ⓣ C8922 Transthoracic echocardiography with contrast, or without contrast followed by with contrast, for congenital cardiac anomalies; follow-up or limited study S
Medicare statute 1833(t)(2)
AHA: 2Q 2008, 9

▲ Ⓣ C8923 Transthoracic echocardiography with contrast, or without contrast followed by contrast, real-time, with image documentation (2D), includes M-mode recording, when performed, complete, without spectral or color doppler echocardiography S
Medicare statute 1833(t)(2)
AHA: 2Q 2008, 9

▲ Ⓣ C8924 Transthoracic echocardiography with contrast, or without contrast, followed by with contrast, real-time with image documentation (2D), includes M-mode recording, when performed, follow-up or limited study S
Medicare statute 1833(t)(2)
AHA: 2Q 2008, 9

Ⓣ C8925 Transesophageal echocardiography (TEE) with contrast, or without contrast followed by with contrast, real time with image documentation (2D) (with or without M-mode recording); including probe placement, image acquisition, interpretation and report S
Medicare statute 1833(t)(2)
AHA: 2Q 2008, 9

Ⓣ C8926 Transesophageal echocardiography (TEE) with contrast, or without contrast followed by with contrast, for congenital cardiac anomalies; including probe placement, image acquisition, interpretation and report S
Medicare statute 1833(t)(2)
AHA: 2Q 2008, 9

Ⓣ C8927 Transesophageal echocardiography (TEE) with contrast, or without contrast followed by with contrast, for monitoring purposes, including probe placement, real time 2-dimensional image acquisition and interpretation leading to ongoing (continuous) assessment of (dynamically changing) cardiac pumping function and to therapeutic measures on an immediate time basis S
Medicare statute 1833(t)(2)
AHA: 2Q 2008, 9

▲ Ⓣ C8928 Transthoracic echocardiography with contrast, or without contrast followed by with contrast, real-time with image documentation (2d), includes M-mode recording, when performed, during rest and cardiovascular stress test using treadmill, bicycle exercise and/or pharmacologically induced stress, with interpretation and report S
Medicare statute 1833(t)(2)
AHA: 2Q 2008, 9

Ⓣ C8929 Transthoracic echocardiography with contrast, or without contrast followed by with contrast, real-time with image documentation (2D), includes M-mode recording, when performed, complete, with spectral doppler echocardiography, and with color flow doppler echocardiography S

Ⓣ C8930 Transthoracic echocardiography, with contrast, or without contrast followed by with contrast, real-time with image documentation (2D), includes M-mode recording, when performed, during rest and cardiovascular stress test using treadmill, bicycle exercise and/or pharmacologically induced stress, with interpretation and report; including performance of continuous electrocardiographic monitoring, with physician supervision S

● Ⓣ C8931 Magnetic resonance angiography without contrast followed by contrast, spinal canal and contents S
This code was effective October 1, 2010
Pub 100-03, 1, 220.2

● Ⓣ C8932 Magnetic resonance angiography without contrast, spinal canal and contents S
This code was effective October 1, 2010
Pub 100-03, 1, 220.2

● Ⓣ C8933 Magnetic resonance angiography without contrast followed by with contrast, spinal canal and contents S
This code was effective October 1, 2010
Pub 100-03, 1, 220.2

C8908 – C8933

● Ⓘ C8934 Magnetic resonance angiography with contrast, upper extremity S
This code was effective October 1, 2010
Pub 100-03, 1, 220.2

● Ⓘ C8935 Magnetic resonance angiography without contrast, upper extremity S
This code was effective October 1, 2010
Pub 100-03, 1, 220.2

● Ⓘ C8936 Magnetic resonance angiography without contrast followed by with contrast, upper extremity S
This code was effective October 1, 2010
Pub 100-03, 1, 220.2

C8957 Intravenous infusion for therapy/diagnosis; initiation of prolonged infusion (more than 8 hours), requiring use of portable or implantable pump S

Ⓘ C9113 Injection, pantoprazole sodium, per vial N N1
Medicare Statute 1833(t)
Protonix

Ⓘ C9121 Injection, argatroban, per 5 mg K K2
Medicare Statute 1833(t)

Ⓘ C9248 Injection, clevidipine butyrate, 1 mg G K2
Cleviprex

Ⓘ C9250 Human plasma fibrin sealant, vapor-heated, solvent-detergent (ARTISS), 2ml

Ⓘ C9254 Injection, lacosamide, 1 mg K K2
Vimpat

✖ ~~C9255 Injection, paliperidone palmitate, 1 mg~~
This code is deleted as of December 31, 2010
See code(s) J2426

✖ ~~C9256 Injection, dexamethasone intravitreal implant, 0.1 mg~~
This code is deleted as of December 31, 2010
See code(s) J7312

Ⓘ C9257 Injection, bevacizumab, 0.25 mg K K2
Avastin

✖ ~~C9258 Injection, telavancin, 10 mg~~
This code was new and effective April 1, 2010
This code is deleted as of December 31, 2010
See code(s) J3095

✖ ~~C9259 Injection, pralatrexate, 1 mg~~
This code was new and effective April 1, 2010
This code is deleted as of December 31, 2010
See code(s) J9307

✖ ~~C9260 Injection, ofatumumab, 10 mg~~
This code was new and effective April 1, 2010
This code is deleted as of December 31, 2010
See code(s) J9302

✖ ~~C9261 Injection, ustekinumab, 1 mg~~
This code was new and effective April 1, 2010
This code is deleted as of December 31, 2010
See code(s) J3357

✖ ~~C9262 Fludarabine phosphate, oral, 1 mg~~
This code was new and effective April 1, 2010
This code was deleted July 1, 2010
See code(s) J8562

✖ ~~C9263 Injection, ecallantide, 1 mg~~
This code was new and effective April 1, 2010
This code is deleted as of December 31, 2010
See code(s) J1290

✖ ~~C9264 Injection, tocilizumab, 1 mg~~
This code was new and effective July 1, 2010
This code is deleted as of December 31, 2010
See code(s) J3262

✖ ~~C9265 Injection, romidepsin, 1 mg~~
This code was new and effective July 1, 2010
This code is deleted as of December 31, 2010
See code(s) J9315

✖ ~~C9266 Injection, collagenase clostridium histolyticum, 0.1 mg~~
This code was new and effective July 1, 2010
This code is deleted as of December 31, 2010
See code(s) J0775

✖ ~~C9267 Injection, von Willebrand factor complex (human), Wilate, per 100 IU VWF: RCO~~
This code was new and effective July 1, 2010
This code is deleted as of December 31, 2010
See code(s) J7184

✖ ~~C9268 Capsaicin, patch, 10cm2~~
This code was new and effective July 1, 2010
This code is deleted as of December 31, 2010
See code(s) J3335

✖ ~~C9269 Injection, C-1 esterase inhibitor (human), Berinert, 10 units~~
This code was new and effective October 1, 2010
This code is deleted as of December 31, 2010
See code(s) J0597

● Ⓘ C9270 Injection, immune globulin (gammaplex), intravenous, non-lyophilized (e.g. liquid), 500 mg
Gammaplex
This code was new and effective October 1, 2010

✖ ~~C9271 Injection, velaglucerase alfa, 100 units~~
This code was new and effective October 1, 2010
This code is deleted as of December 31, 2010
See code(s) J3385

● Ⓘ C9272 Injection, denosumab, 1 mg
Prolia
This code was new and effective October 1, 2010

● Ⓘ C9273 Sipuleucel-t, minimum of 50 million autologous CD54+ cells activated with PAP-GM-CSF, including leukapheresis and all other preparatory procedures, per infusion
This code was new and effective October 1, 2010

● Ⓘ C9274 Crotalidae polyvalent immune fab (Ovine), 1 vial
This code is effective January 1, 2011

● Ⓘ C9275 Injection, hexaminolevulinate hydrochloride, 100 mg, per study dose
Cysview
This code is effective January 1, 2011

● Ⓘ C9276 Injection, cabazitaxel, 1 mg
Jevtana
This code is effective January 1, 2011

● Ⓘ C9277 Injection, alglucosidase alfa (Lumizyme), 1 mg
This code is effective January 1, 2011

● Ⓘ C9278 Injection, incobotulinumtoxin A, 1 unit
Xeomin
This code is effective January 1, 2011

● Ⓘ C9279 Injection, ibuprofen, 100 mg
NeoProfen, Caldolor
This code is effective January 1, 2011

Ⓘ C9352 Microporous collagen implantable tube (NeuraGen nerve guide), per centimeter length N K2
Medicare statute 1833(t)
AHA: 1Q 2008, 6

Ⓘ C9353 Microporous collagen implantable slit tube (NeuraWrap nerve protector), per centimeter length N K2
Medicare statute 1833(t)
AHA: 1Q 2008, 6

C9354 Acellular pericardial tissue matrix of nonhuman origin (Veritas), per square centimeter G
AHA: 1Q 2008, 6

C9355 Collagen nerve cuff (NeuroMatrix), per 0.5 centimeter length G
AHA: 1Q 2008, 6

Ⓘ C9356 Tendon, porous matrix of cross-linked collagen and glycosaminoglycan matrix (TenoGlide Tendon Protector Sheet), per square centimeter G
AHA: 3Q 2008, 6

C9358 Dermal substitute, native, non-denatured collagen, fetal bovine origin (Surgimend Collagen Matrix), per 0.5 square centimeters G K2

AHA: 1Q 2008, 6

C9359 Porous purified collagen matrix bone void filler (Integra Mozaik Osteoconductive Scaffold Putty, Integra Os Osteoconductive Scaffold Putty), per 0.5 cc G N1

C9360 Dermal substitute, native, non-denatured collagen, neonatal bovine origin (Surgimend Collagen Matrix), per 0.5 square centimeters G K2

C9361 Collagen matrix nerve wrap (Neuromend Collagen Nerve Wrap), per 0.5 centimeter length G K2

C9362 Porous purified collagen matrix bone void filler (Integra Mozaik Osteoconductive Scaffold Strip), per 0.5 cc G K2

C9363 Skin substitute, Integra Meshed Bilayer Wound Matrix, per square centimeter G K2

C9364 Porcine implant, permacol, per square centimeter G K2

● C9367 Skin substitute, endoform dermal template, per square centimeter K2

This code was new and effective July 1, 2010

C9399 Unclassified drugs or biologicals A K7

Medicare Statute 1833(t)

C9716 Creations of thermal anal lesions by radiofrequency energy T G2

Medicare Statute 1833(t)

C9724 Endoscopic full-thickness plication in the gastric cardia using endoscopic plication system (EPS); includes endoscopy T G2

Medicare Statute 1833(t)

C9725 Placement of endorectal intracavitary applicator for high intensity brachytherapy T G2

Medicare Statute 1833(t)

C9726 Placement and removal (if performed) of applicator into breast for radiation therapy T G2

Medicare Statute 1833(t)

C9727 Insertion of implants into the soft palate; minimum of three implants T G2

Medicare Statute 1833(t)

C9728 Placement of interstitial device(s) for radiation therapy/surgery guidance (eg, fiducial markers, dosimeter), for other than the following sites (any approach): abdomen, pelvis, prostate, retroperitoneum, thorax, single or multiple X R2

Medicare statute 1833(t)

● C9800 Dermal injection procedure(s) for facial lipodystrophy syndrome (lds) and provision of Radiesse or Sculptra dermal filler, including all items and supplies R2

This code was effective July 1, 2010

× ~~C9801 Smoking and tobacco cessation counseling visit for the asymptomatic patient; intermediate, greater than 3 minutes, up to 10 minutes~~

This code was effective August 25, 2010

This code is deleted as of December 31, 2010

See code(s) G0436

× ~~C9802 Smoking and tobacco cessation counseling visit for the asymptomatic patient; intensive, greater than 10 minutes~~

This code was effective August 25, 2010

This code is deleted as of December 31, 2010

See code(s) G0437

C9898 Radiolabeled product provided during a hospital inpatient stay N

C9899 Implanted prosthetic device, payable only for inpatients who do not have inpatient coverage A

Durable Medical Equipment E0100–E8002

Ambulation Devices

Canes

E0100 Cane, includes canes of all materials, adjustable or fixed, with tip Y

NCD 280.2, 280.1; Pub 100-02, 15, 110.1; 100-4, 20, 10.1-10.1.4.2

E0105 Cane, quad or three-prong, includes canes of all materials, adjustable or fixed, with tips Y

NCD 280.3, 280.1; Pub 100-02, 15, 110.1; 100-4, 20, 10.1-10.1.4.2

Crutches

E0110 Crutches, forearm, includes crutches of various materials, adjustable or fixed, pair, complete with tips and handgrips Y

NCD 280.1; Pub 100-02, 15, 110.1; 100-4, 20, 10.1-10.1.4.2

E0111 Crutch forearm, includes crutches of various materials, adjustable or fixed, each, with tip and handgrips Y

NCD 280.1; Pub 100-02, 15, 110.1; 100-4, 20, 10.1-10.1.4.2

Crutch, forearm

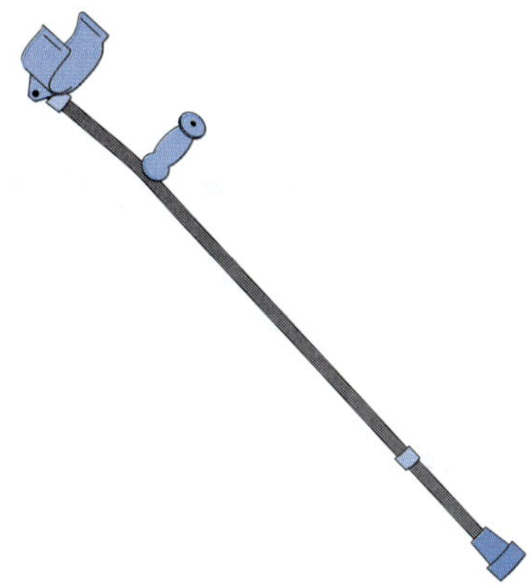

E0112 Crutches underarm, wood, adjustable or fixed, pair, with pads, tips and handgrips Y

NCD 280.1; Pub 100-02, 15, 110.1; 100-4, 20, 10.1-10.1.4.2

E0113 Crutch underarm, wood, adjustable or fixed, each, with pad, tip and handgrip Y

NCD 280.1; Pub 100-02, 15, 110.1; 100-4, 20, 10.1-10.1.4.2

E0114 Crutches underarm, other than wood, adjustable or fixed, pair, with pads, tips and handgrips Y

NCD 280.1; Pub 100-02, 15, 110.1; 100-4, 20, 10.1-10.1.4.2

E0116 Crutch, underarm, other than wood, adjustable or fixed, with pad, tip, handgrip, with or without shock absorber, each Y

NCD 280.1; Pub 100-02, 15, 110.1; 100-4, 20, 10.1-10.1.4.2

E0117 Crutch, underarm, articulating, spring assisted, each Y

Pub 100-02, 15, 110.1; 100-4, 20, 10.1-10.1.4.2

E0118 Crutch substitute, lower leg platform, with or without wheels, each E

Walkers

E0130 Walker, rigid (pickup), adjustable or fixed height
NCD 280.1; Pub 100-02, 15, 110.1; 100-4, 20, 10.1-10.1.4.2

E0135 Walker, folding (pickup), adjustable or fixed height
NCD 280.1; Pub 100-02, 15, 110.1; 100-4, 20, 10.1-10.1.4.2

E0140 Walker, with trunk support, adjustable or fixed height, any type
NCD 280.1; Pub 100-02, 15, 110.1; 100-4, 20, 10.1-10.1.4.2

E0141 Walker, rigid, wheeled, adjustable or fixed height
NCD 280.1; Pub 100-02, 15, 110.1; 100-4, 20, 10.1-10.1.4.2

E0143 Walker, folding, wheeled, adjustable or fixed height
NCD 280.1; Pub 100-02, 15, 110.1; 100-4, 20, 10.1-10.1.4.2

E0144 Walker, enclosed, four sided framed, rigid or folding, wheeled with posterior seat
NCD 280.1; Pub 100-02, 15, 110.1; 100-4, 20, 10.1-10.1.4.2

E0147 Walker, heavy duty, multiple braking system, variable wheel resistance
NCD 280.3; Pub 100-02, 15, 110.1; 100-4, 20, 10.1-10.1.4.2

E0148 Walker, heavy duty, without wheels, rigid or folding, any type, each

E0149 Walker, heavy duty, wheeled, rigid or folding, any type

Walker; rolled with seat

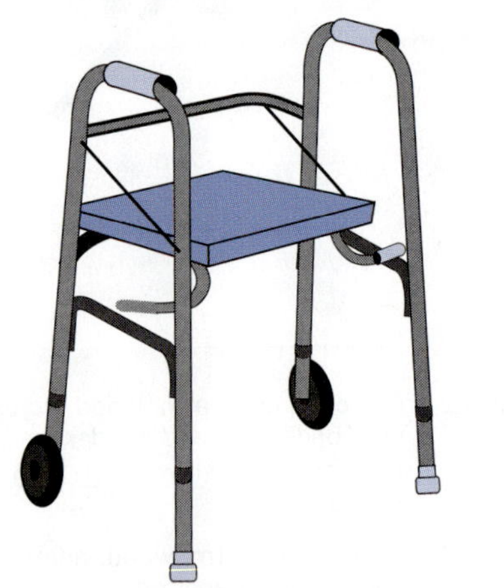

Accessories for Ambulation Devices

E0153 Platform attachment, forearm crutch, each

E0154 Platform attachment, walker, each

E0155 Wheel attachment, rigid pick-up walker, per pair

Attachments

E0156 Seat attachment, walker

E0157 Crutch attachment, walker, each

E0158 Leg extensions for walker, per set of four (4)

E0159 Brake attachment for wheeled walker, replacement, each

Commodes

E0160 Sitz type bath or equipment, portable, used with or without commode
NCD 280.1

E0161 Sitz type bath or equipment, portable, used with or without commode, with faucet attachment(s)
NCD 280.1

E0162 Sitz bath chair
NCD 280.1

E0163 Commode chair, mobile or stationary, with fixed arms
NCD 280.1; Pub 100-02, 15, 110.1; 100-4, 20, 10.1-10.1.4.2

E0165 Commode chair, mobile or stationary, with detachable arms
NCD 280.1; Pub 100-02, 15, 110.1; 100-4, 20, 10.1-10.1.4.2

E0167 Pail or pan for use with commode chair, replacement only
NCD 280.1

E0168 Commode chair, extra wide and/or heavy duty, stationary or mobile, with or without arms, any type, each

E0170 Commode chair with integrated seat lift mechanism, electric, any type

E0171 Commode chair with integrated seat lift mechanism, non-electric, any type

E0172 Seat lift mechanism placed over or on top of toilet, any type   E
Medicare Statute 1861

E0175 Foot rest, for use with commode chair, each

Decubitis Care Equipment

E0181 Powered pressure reducing mattress overlay/pad, alternating, with pump, includes heavy duty
NCD 280.1; Pub 100-8, 5, 5.3

E0182 Pump for alternating pressure pad, for replacement only
NCD 280.1; Pub 100-8, 5, 5.3

E0184 Dry pressure mattress
NCD 280.1; Pub 100-8, 5, 5.3

E0185 Gel or gel-like pressure pad for mattress, standard mattress length and width
NCD 280.1; Pub 100-8, 5, 5.3

E0186 Air pressure mattress
NCD 280.1

E0187 Water pressure mattress
NCD 280.1

E0188 Synthetic sheepskin pad
NCD 280.1; Pub 100-8, 5, 5.3

E0189 Lambswool sheepskin pad, any size
NCD 280.1; Pub 100-8, 5, 5.3

E0190 Positioning cushion/pillow/wedge, any shape or size, includes all components and accessories   E
Pub 100-02, 15, 110.1; 100-4, 20, 10.1-10.1.4.2

E0191 Heel or elbow protector, each

E0193 Powered air flotation bed (low air loss therapy)

E0194 Air fluidized bed
Cross-reference Q0049
NCD 280.8

ⓘ **E0196** Gel pressure mattress Y
NCD 280.1

ⓘ **E0197** Air pressure pad for mattress, standard mattress length and width Y
NCD 280.1

ⓘ **E0198** Water pressure pad for mattress, standard mattress length and width Y
NCD 280.1

ⓘ **E0199** Dry pressure pad for mattress, standard mattress length and width Y
NCD 280.1

Heat/Cold Application

ⓘ **E0200** Heat lamp, without stand (table model), includes bulb, or infrared element Y
NCD 280.1; Pub 100-02, 15, 110.1; 100-4, 20, 10.1-10.1.4.2

E0202 Phototherapy (bilirubin) light with photometer Y

⊘ **E0203** Therapeutic lightbox, minimum 10,000 lux, table top model A
NCD 180.1

ⓘ **E0205** Heat lamp, with stand, includes bulb, or infrared element Y
NCD 280.1; Pub 100-02, 15, 110.1; 100-4, 20, 10.1-10.1.4.2

ⓘ **E0210** Electric heat pad, standard Y
NCD 280.1

ⓘ **E0215** Electric heat pad, moist Y
NCD 280.1

ⓘ **E0217** Water circulating heat pad with pump Y
NCD 280.1

ⓘ **E0218** Water circulating cold pad with pump Y
NCD 280.1

✖ ~~E0220 Hot water bottle~~
This code is deleted as of December 31, 2010
See code(s) A9273

E0221 Infrared heating pad system E
NCD 270.2

ⓘ **E0225** Hydrocollator unit, includes pads Y
NCD 280.1; Pub 100-02, 15, 230

✖ ~~E0230 Ice cap or collar~~
This code is deleted as of December 31, 2010
See code(s) A9273

⊘ **E0231** Non-contact wound warming device (temperature control unit, AC adapter and power cord) for use with warming card and wound cover E
Pub 100-02, 16, 20

⊘ **E0232** Warming card for use with the non-contact wound warming device and non-contact wound warming wound cover E
Pub 100-02, 16, 20

ⓘ **E0235** Paraffin bath unit, portable (see medical supply code A4265 for paraffin) Y
NCD 280.1; Pub 100-02, 15, 230

ⓘ **E0236** Pump for water circulating pad Y
NCD 280.1

✖ ~~E0238 Non-electric heat pad, moist~~
This code is deleted as of December 31, 2010
See code(s) A9273

ⓘ **E0239** Hydrocollator unit, portable Y
NCD 280.1; Pub 100-02, 15, 230

Bath and Toilet Aids

⊘ **E0240** Bath/shower chair, with or without wheels, any size E
NCD 280.1

Bathtub transfer chair

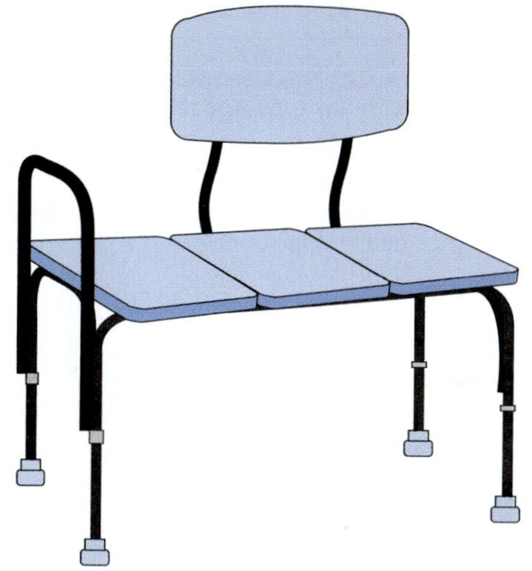

⊘ **E0241** Bath tub wall rail, each E
NCD 280.1; Pub 100-02, 15, 110.1; 100-4, 20, 10.1-10.1.4.2

⊘ **E0242** Bath tub rail, floor base E
NCD 280.1; Pub 100-02, 15, 110.1; 100-4, 20, 10.1-10.1.4.2

⊘ **E0243** Toilet rail, each E
NCD 280.1; Pub 100-02, 15, 110.1; 100-4, 20, 10.1-10.1.4.2

⊘ **E0244** Raised toilet seat E
NCD 280.1

⊘ **E0245** Tub stool or bench E
NCD 280.1

E0246 Transfer tub rail attachment E

ⓘ **E0247** Transfer bench for tub or toilet with or without commode opening E
NCD 280.1

ⓘ **E0248** Transfer bench, heavy duty, for tub or toilet with or without commode opening E
NCD 280.1

ⓘ **E0249** Pad for water circulating heat unit, for replacement only Y
NCD 280.1

ⓘ **E0250** Hospital bed, fixed height, with any type side rails, with mattress E
NCD 280.7; Pub 100-02, 15, 110.1; 100-4, 20, 10.1-10.1.4.2

ⓘ **E0251** Hospital bed, fixed height, with any type side rails, without mattress E
NCD 280.7; Pub 100-02, 15, 110.1; 100-4, 20, 10.1-10.1.4.2

ⓘ **E0255** Hospital bed, variable height, hi-lo, with any type side rails, with mattress E
NCD 280.7; Pub 100-02, 15, 110.1; 100-4, 20, 10.1-10.1.4.2

ⓘ E0256 Hospital bed, variable height, hi-lo, with any type side rails, without mattress E
NCD 280.7; Pub 100-02, 15, 110.1; 100-4, 20, 10.1-10.1.4.2

ⓘ E0260 Hospital bed, semi-electric (head and foot adjustment), with any type side rails, with mattress E
NCD 280.7; Pub 100-02, 15, 110.1; 100-4, 20, 10.1-10.1.4.2

ⓘ E0261 Hospital bed, semi-electric (head and foot adjustment), with any type side rails, without mattress E
NCD 280.7; Pub 100-02, 15, 110.1; 100-4, 20, 10.1-10.1.4.2

ⓘ E0265 Hospital bed, total electric (head, foot and height adjustments), with any type side rails, with mattress E
NCD 280.7; Pub 100-02, 15, 110.1; 100-4, 20, 10.1-10.1.4.2

ⓘ E0266 Hospital bed, total electric (head, foot and height adjustments), with any type side rails, without mattress E
NCD 280.7; Pub 100-02, 15, 110.1; 100-4, 20, 10.1-10.1.4.2

⊘ E0270 Hospital bed, institutional type includes: oscillating, circulating and stryker frame, with mattress E
NCD 280.1

ⓘ E0271 Mattress, innerspring E
NCD 280.7, NCD 280.1

ⓘ E0272 Mattress, foam rubber E
NCD 280.7, NCD 280.1

⊘ E0273 Bed board E
NCD 280.1

⊘ E0274 Over-bed table E
NCD 280.1

ⓘ E0275 Bed pan, standard, metal or plastic Y
NCD 280.1

ⓘ E0276 Bed pan, fracture, metal or plastic Y
NCD 280.1

ⓘ E0277 Powered pressure-reducing air mattress Y
NCD 280.1

E0280 Bed cradle, any type Y

ⓘ E0290 Hospital bed, fixed height, without side rails, with mattress E
NCD 280.7; Pub 100-02, 15, 110.1; 100-4, 20, 10.1-10.1.4.2

ⓘ E0291 Hospital bed, fixed height, without side rails, without mattress Y
NCD 280.7; Pub 100-02, 15, 110.1; 100-4, 20, 10.1-10.1.4.2

ⓘ E0292 Hospital bed, variable height, hi-lo, without side rails, with mattress E
NCD 280.7; Pub 100-02, 15, 110.1; 100-4, 20, 10.1-10.1.4.2

ⓘ E0293 Hospital bed, variable height, hi-lo, without side rails, without mattress Y
NCD 280.7; Pub 100-02, 15, 110.1; 100-4, 20, 10.1-10.1.4.2

ⓘ E0294 Hospital bed, semi-electric (head and foot adjustment), without side rails, with mattress E
NCD 280.7; Pub 100-02, 15, 110.1; 100-4, 20, 10.1-10.1.4.2

ⓘ E0295 Hospital bed, semi-electric (head and foot adjustment), without side rails, without mattress Y
NCD 280.7; Pub 100-02, 15, 110.1; 100-4, 20, 10.1-10.1.4.2

ⓘ E0296 Hospital bed, total electric (head, foot and height adjustments). Without side rails, with mattress E
NCD 280.7; Pub 100-02, 15, 110.1; 100-4, 20, 10.1-10.1.4.2

ⓘ E0297 Hospital bed, total electric (head, foot and height adjustments), without side rails, without mattress Y
NCD 280.7; Pub 100-02, 15, 110.1; 100-4, 20, 10.1-10.1.4.2

E0300 Pediatric crib, hospital grade, fully enclosed Y

ⓘ E0301 Hospital bed, heavy duty, extra wide, with weight capacity greater than 350 pounds, but less than or equal to 600 pounds, with any type side rails, without mattress Y
NCD 280.7

ⓘ E0302 Hospital bed, extra heavy duty, extra wide, with weight capacity greater than 600 pounds, with any type side rails, without mattress Y
NCD 280.7

ⓘ E0303 Hospital bed, heavy duty, extra wide, with weight capacity greater than 350 pounds, but less than or equal to 600 pounds, with any type side rails, with mattress E
NCD 280.7

ⓘ E0304 Hospital bed, extra heavy duty, extra wide, with weight capacity greater than 600 pounds, with any type side rails, with mattress E
NCD 280.7

Hospital Bed Accessories

ⓘ E0305 Bedside rails, half-length D
NCD 280.7

ⓘ E0310 Bedside rails, full-length D
NCD 280.7

⊘ E0315 Bed accessory: board, table, or support device, any type E
NCD 280.1

E0316 Safety enclosure frame/canopy for use with hospital bed, any type Y

ⓘ E0325 Urinal; male, jug-type, any material ♂ Y
NCD 280.1

ⓘ E0326 Urinal; female, jug-type, any material ♀ Y
NCD 280.1

E0328 Hospital bed, pediatric, manual, 360 degree side enclosures, top of headboard, footboard and side rails up to 24 inches above the spring, includes mattress Y

E0329 Hospital bed, pediatric, electric or semi-electric, 360 degree side enclosures, top of headboard, footboard and side rails up to 24 inches above the spring, includes mattress Y

E0350 Control unit for electronic bowel irrigation/ evacuation system E

E0352 Disposable pack (water reservoir bag, speculum, valving mechanism and collection bag/box) for use with the electronic bowel irrigation/evacuation system E

E0370 Air pressure elevator for heel E

E0371 Nonpowered advanced pressure reducing overlay for mattress, standard mattress length and width Y

E0372 Powered air overlay for mattress, standard mattress length and width Y

E0373 Nonpowered advanced pressure reducing mattress Y

Oxygen and Related Respiratory Equipment

E0424 Stationary compressed gaseous oxygen system, rental; includes container, contents, regulator, flowmeter, humidifier, nebulizer, cannula or mask, and tubing Y
NCD 240.2; Pub 100-8, 5, 5.3

E0425 Stationary compressed gas system, purchase; includes regulator, flowmeter, humidifier, nebulizer, cannula or mask, and tubing E
NCD 240.2; Pub 100-8, 5, 5.3

E0430 Portable gaseous oxygen system, purchase; includes regulator, flowmeter, humidifier, cannula or mask, and tubing E
NCD 240.2; Pub 100-8, 5, 5.3

E0431 Portable gaseous oxygen system, rental; includes portable container, regulator, flowmeter, humidifier, cannula or mask, and tubing Y
NCD 240.2; Pub 100-8, 5, 5.3

E0433 Portable liquid oxygen system, rental; home liquefier used to fill portable liquid oxygen containers, includes portable containers, regulator, flowmeter, humidifier, cannula or mask and tubing, with or without supply reservoir and contents gauge Y

E0434 Portable liquid oxygen system, rental; includes portable container, supply reservoir, humidifier, flowmeter, refill adaptor, contents gauge, cannula or mask, and tubing Y
NCD 240.2; Pub 100-8, 5, 5.3

E0435 Portable liquid oxygen system, purchase; includes portable container, supply reservoir, flowmeter, humidifier, contents gauge, cannula or mask, tubing and refill adaptor E
NCD 240.2; Pub 100-8, 5, 5.3

E0439 Stationary liquid oxygen system, rental; includes container, contents, regulator, flowmeter, humidifier, nebulizer, cannula or mask, & tubing Y
NCD 240.2; Pub 100-8, 5, 5.3

E0440 Stationary liquid oxygen system, purchase; includes use of reservoir, contents indicator, regulator, flowmeter, humidifier, nebulizer, cannula or mask, and tubing E
NCD 240.2; Pub 100-8, 5, 5.3

E0441 Stationary oxygen contents, gaseous, 1 month's supply = 1 unit Y
NCD 240.2; Pub 100-8, 5, 5.3

E0442 Stationary oxygen contents, liquid, 1 month's supply = 1 unit Y
NCD 240.2; Pub 100-8, 5, 5.3

E0443 Portable oxygen contents, gaseous, 1 month's supply = 1 unit Y
NCD 240.2; Pub 100-8, 5, 5.3

E0444 Portable oxygen contents, liquid, 1 month's supply = 1 unit Y
NCD 240.2; Pub 100-8, 5, 5.3

E0445 Oximeter device for measuring blood oxygen levels non-invasively A

● E0446 Topical oxygen delivery system, not otherwise specified, includes all supplies and accessories Y
This code is effective January 1, 2011

E0450 Volume control ventilator, without pressure support mode, may include pressure control mode, used with invasive interface (e.g., tracheostomy tube) Y
NCD 280.1

E0455 Oxygen tent, excluding croup or pediatric tents Y
NCD 240.2; Pub 100-8, 5, 5.3

E0457 Chest shell (cuirass) Y

E0459 Chest wrap Y

E0460 Negative pressure ventilator; portable or stationary Y
NCD 280.1

E0461 Volume control ventilator, without pressure support mode, may include pressure control mode, used with non-invasive interface (e.g., mask) Y
NCD 280.1

E0462 Rocking bed, with or without side rails Y

E0463 Pressure support ventilator with volume control mode, may include pressure control mode, used with invasive interface (e.g. tracheostomy tube) Y

E0464 Pressure support ventilator with volume control mode, may include pressure control mode, used with non-invasive interface (e.g. mask) Y

E0470 Respiratory assist device, bi-level pressure capability, without backup rate feature, used with noninvasive interface, e.g., nasal or facial mask (intermittent assist device with continuous positive airway pressure device) Y
NCD 280.1

E0471 Respiratory assist device, bi-level pressure capability, with back-up rate feature, used with noninvasive interface, e.g., nasal or facial mask (intermittent assist device with continuous positive airway pressure device) Y
NCD 280.1

E0472 Respiratory assist device, bi-level pressure capability, with backup rate feature, used with invasive interface, e.g., tracheostomy tube (intermittent assist device with continuous positive airway pressure device) Y
NCD 280.1

E0480 Percussor, electric or pneumatic, home model Y
NCD 280.1

E0481 Intrapulmonary percussive ventilation system and related accessories E
NCD 240.5

E0482 Cough stimulating device, alternating positive and negative airway pressure Y

E0483 High frequency chest wall oscillation air-pulse generator system, (includes hoses and vest), each Y

High frequency chest wall air-pulse generator system

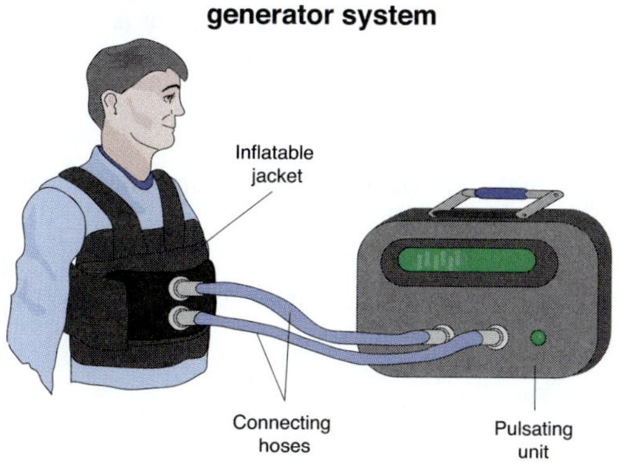

E0484 Oscillatory positive expiratory pressure device, non-electric, any type, each Y

E0485 Oral device/appliance used to reduce upper airway collapsibility, adjustable or non-adjustable, prefabricated, includes fitting and adjustment Y

E0486 Oral device/appliance used to reduce upper airway collapsibility, adjustable or non-adjustable, custom fabricated, includes fitting and adjustment Y

E0487 Spirometer, electronic, includes all accessories N

IPPB Machines

E0500 IPPB machine, all types, with built-in nebulization; manual or automatic valves; internal or external power source Y
NCD 280.1

Humidifiers/Compressors/Nebulizers for Use With Oxygen IPPB Equipment

E0550 Humidifier, durable for extensive supplemental humidification during IPPB treatments or oxygen delivery Y
NCD 280.1

E0555 Humidifier, durable, glass or autoclavable plastic bottle type, for use with regulator or flowmeter Y
NCD 280.1; Pub 100-8, 5, 5.3

E0560 Humidifier, durable for supplemental humidification during IPPB treatment or oxygen delivery Y
NCD 280.1

E0561 Humidifier, non-heated, used with positive airway pressure device Y

E0562 Humidifier, heated, used with positive airway pressure device Y

E0565 Compressor, air power source for equipment which is not self- contained or cylinder driven Y

E0570 Nebulizer, with compressor Y
NCD 280.1; Pub 100-8, 5, 5.3

E0571 Aerosol compressor, battery powered, for use with small volume nebulizer Y
NCD 280.1

E0572 Aerosol compressor, adjustable pressure, light duty for intermittent use Y

E0574 Ultrasonic/electronic aerosol generator with small volume nebulizer Y

E0575 Nebulizer, ultrasonic, large volume Y
NCD 280.1

E0580 Nebulizer, durable, glass or autoclavable plastic, bottle type, for use with regulator or flowmeter Y
NCD 280.1; Pub 100-8, 5, 5.3

E0585 Nebulizer, with compressor and heater Y
NCD 280.1; Pub 100-8, 5, 5.3

Suction Pump/Room Vaporizers

E0600 Respiratory suction pump, home model, portable or stationary, electric Y
NCD 280.1

E0601 Continuous airway pressure (CPAP) device Y
NCD 240.4

E0602 Breast pump, manual, any type ♀ Y

Breast pump; manual

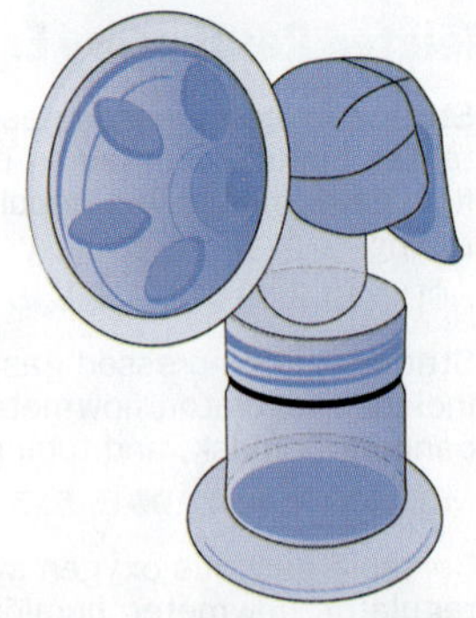

E0603 Breast pump, electric (AC and/or DC), any type ♀ A

E0604 Breast pump, hospital grade, electric (AC and/or DC), any type ♀ A

E0605 Vaporizer, room type Y
NCD 280.1

E0606 Postural drainage board Y
NCD 280.1

Monitoring Equipment

E0607 Home blood glucose monitor Y
NCD 40.2

Blood glucose meter

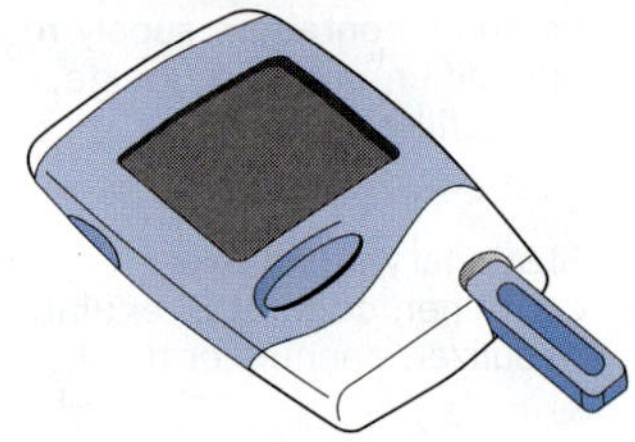

Pacemaker Monitor

E0610 Pacemaker monitor, self-contained, (checks battery depletion, includes audible and visible check systems) Y
NCD 20.8.1.2, 20.8.1

E0615 Pacemaker monitor, self contained, checks battery depletion and other pacemaker components, includes digital/visible check systems Y
NCD 20.8.1.2, 20.8.1

E0616 Implantable cardiac event recorder with memory, activator and programmer N N1

E0617 External defibrillator with integrated electrocardiogram analysis Y

E0618 Apnea monitor, without recording feature A

E0619 Apnea monitor, with recording feature A

E0620 Skin piercing device for collection of capillary blood, laser, each Y

Medicare Non-Coverage | Special Coverage Instructions | Coverage Carrier Determined | A – Y APC Status Indicators | ● New Code | ▲ Revised Code | ✖ Deleted Code
AHA *AHA Coding Clinic for HCPCS* | A2 – Z3 ASC Payment Indicators | DMEPOS | ♂ Male | ♀ Female | PQR PQRI

E0484 – E0620

Patient Lifts

- ⓘ E0621 Sling or seat, patient lift, canvas or nylon DMEPOS Y
  NCD 280.1
- ⊘ E0625 Patient lift, bathroom or toilet, not otherwise classified E
  NCD 280.1
- ⓘ E0627 Seat lift mechanism incorporated into a combination lift-chair mechanism DMEPOS Y
  NCD 280.4; Pub 100-04, 20, 100; 100-4, 20, 130.2-130.5; 100-8, 5, 5.3
- ⓘ E0628 Separate seat lift mechanism for use with patient owned furniture-electric DMEPOS Y
  NCD 280.4; Pub 100-04, 20, 100; 100-4, 20, 130.2-130.5; 100-8, 5, 5.3
- ⓘ E0629 Separate seat lift mechanism for use with patient owned furniture-non-electric DMEPOS Y
  Pub 100-04, 20, 100; 100-4, 20, 130.2-130.5; 100-8, 5, 5.3
- ⓘ E0630 Patient lift, hydraulic or mechanical, includes any seat, sling, strap(s) or pad(s) DMEPOS Y
  NCD 280.1
- ⓘ E0635 Patient lift, electric with seat or sling DMEPOS Y
  NCD 280.1
- Coverage Carrier Determined E0636 Multipositional patient support system, with integrated lift, patient accessible controls DMEPOS Y
- ⓘ E0637 Combination sit to stand system, any size including pediatric, with seatlift feature, with or without wheels E
  NCD 280.1
- ⊘ E0638 Standing frame system, one position (e.g. upright, supine or prone stander), any size including pediatric, with or without wheels E
  NCD 280.1
- ⊘ E0639 Patient lift, moveable from room to room with disassembly and reassembly, includes all components/accessories E
- ⊘ E0640 Patient lift, fixed system, includes all components/accessories E
- ⊘ E0641 Standing frame system, multi-position (e.g. three-way stander), any size including pediatric, with or without wheels E
  NCD 280.1
- ⊘ E0642 Standing frame system, mobile (dynamic stander), any size including pediatric E
  NCD 280.1

Pneumatic Compressor and Appliances

- ⓘ E0650 Pneumatic compressor, non-segmental home model DMEPOS Y
  NCD 280.6; Pub 100-8, 5, 5.3
- ⓘ E0651 Pneumatic compressor, segmental home model without calibrated gradient pressure DMEPOS Y
  NCD 280.6; Pub 100-8, 5, 5.3
- ⓘ E0652 Pneumatic compressor, segmental home model with calibrated gradient pressure DMEPOS Y
  NCD 280.6; Pub 100-8, 5, 5.3
- ⓘ E0655 Non-segmental pneumatic appliance for use with pneumatic compressor, half arm DMEPOS Y
  NCD 280.6; Pub 100-8, 5, 5.3
- ⓘ E0656 Segmental pneumatic appliance for use with pneumatic compressor, trunk DMEPOS Y
- ⓘ E0657 Segmental pneumatic appliance for use with pneumatic compressor, chest DMEPOS Y
- ⓘ E0660 Non-segmental pneumatic appliance for use with pneumatic compressor, full leg DMEPOS Y
  NCD 280.6; Pub 100-8, 5, 5.3
- ⓘ E0665 Non-segmental pneumatic appliance for use with pneumatic compressor, full arm DMEPOS Y
  NCD 280.6; Pub 100-8, 5, 5.3
- ⓘ E0666 Non-segmental pneumatic appliance for use with pneumatic compressor, half leg DMEPOS Y
  NCD 280.6; Pub 100-8, 5, 5.3
- ⓘ E0667 Segmental pneumatic appliance for use with pneumatic compressor, full leg DMEPOS Y
  NCD 280.6; Pub 100-8, 5, 5.3
- ⓘ E0668 Segmental pneumatic appliance for use with pneumatic compressor, full arm DMEPOS Y
  NCD 280.6; Pub 100-8, 5, 5.3
- ⓘ E0669 Segmental pneumatic appliance for use with pneumatic compressor, half leg DMEPOS Y
  NCD 280.6; Pub 100-8, 5, 5.3
- ⓘ E0671 Segmental gradient pressure pneumatic appliance, full leg DMEPOS Y
  NCD 280.6; Pub 100-8, 5, 5.3
- ⓘ E0672 Segmental gradient pressure pneumatic appliance, full arm DMEPOS Y
  NCD 280.6; Pub 100-8, 5, 5.3
- ⓘ E0673 Segmental gradient pressure pneumatic appliance, half leg DMEPOS Y
  NCD 280.6; Pub 100-8, 5, 5.3
- Coverage Carrier Determined E0675 Pneumatic compression device, high pressure, rapid inflation/deflation cycle, for arterial insufficiency (unilateral or bilateral system) DMEPOS Y
  Pub 100-8, 5, 5.3
- Coverage Carrier Determined E0676 Intermittent limb compression device (includes all accessories), not otherwise specified Y

Ultraviolet Cabinet

- Coverage Carrier Determined E0691 Ultraviolet light therapy system panel, includes bulbs/lamps, timer and eye protection; treatment area 2 square feet or less DMEPOS Y
- Coverage Carrier Determined E0692 Ultraviolet light therapy system panel, includes bulbs/lamps, timer and eye protection, 4 foot panel DMEPOS Y
- Coverage Carrier Determined E0693 Ultraviolet light therapy system panel, includes bulbs/lamps, timer and eye protection, 6 foot panel DMEPOS Y
- Coverage Carrier Determined E0694 Ultraviolet multidirectional light therapy system in 6 foot cabinet, includes bulbs/lamps, timer and eye protection DMEPOS Y

Safety Equipment

- Coverage Carrier Determined E0700 Safety equipment, device or accessory, any type E
- ⓘ E0705 Transfer device, any type, each B

Restraints

- Coverage Carrier Determined E0710 Restraints, any type (body, chest, wrist or ankle) E

Transcutaneous and/or Neuromuscular Electrical Nerve Stimulators – TENS

ⓘ **E0720** Transcutaneous electrical nerve stimulation (TENS) device, two lead, localized stimulation Y
NCD 160.2, 160.3; Pub 100-8, 5, 5.3

Transcutaneous neurostimulator

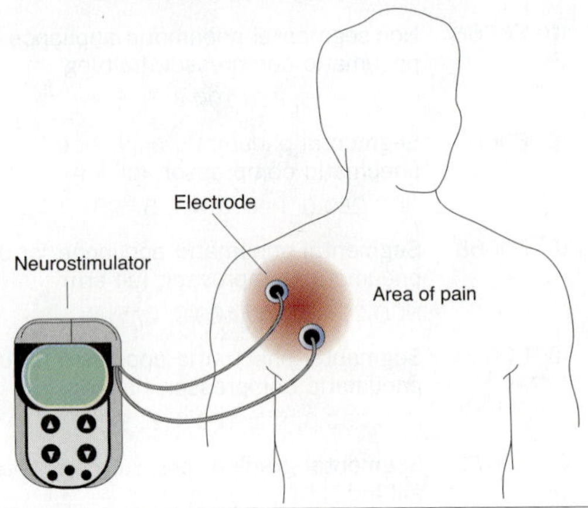

ⓘ **E0730** Transcutaneous electrical nerve stimulation (TENS) device, four or more leads, for multiple nerve stimulation Y
NCD 160.2, 160.3; Pub 100-8, 5, 5.3

ⓘ **E0731** Form-fitting conductive garment for delivery of TENS or NMES (with conductive fibers separated from the patient's skin by layers of fabric) Y
NCD 160.13

ⓘ **E0740** Incontinence treatment system, pelvic floor stimulator, monitor, sensor and/or trainer Y
NCD 230.8

E0744 Neuromuscular stimulator for scoliosis Y

ⓘ **E0745** Neuromuscular stimulator, electronic shock unit Y
NCD 160.12

ⓘ **E0746** Electromyography (EMG), biofeedback device A
NCD 30.1.1

ⓘ **E0747** Osteogenesis stimulator, electrical, non-invasive, other than spinal applications Y
NCD 150.2; Pub 100-8, 5, 5.3

ⓘ **E0748** Osteogenesis stimulator, electrical, non-invasive, spinal applications Y
NCD 150.2; Pub 100-8, 5, 5.3

ⓘ **E0749** Osteogenesis stimulator, electrical, surgically implanted N N1
NCD 150.2; Pub 100-8, 5, 5.3

E0755 Electronic salivary reflex stimulator (intra-oral/non-invasive) E

E0760 Ostogenesis stimulator, low intensity ultrasound, non-invasive Y
NCD 150.2; Pub 100-04, 32, 110-110.5

ⓘ **E0761** Non-thermal pulsed high frequency radiowaves, high peak power electromagnetic energy treatment device E
NCD 270.1

E0762 Transcutaneous electrical joint stimulation device system, includes all accessories B

ⓘ **E0764** Functional neuromuscular stimulation, transcutaneous stimulation of sequential muscle groups of ambulation with computer control, used for walking by spinal cord injured, entire system, after completion of training program Y
NCD 160.12

E0765 FDA-approved nerve stimulator, with replaceable batteries, for treatment of nausea and vomiting Y

ⓘ **E0769** Electrical stimulation or electromagnetic wound treatment device, not otherwise classified B
NCD 160.13

ⓘ **E0770** Functional electrical stimulator, transcutaneous stimulation of nerve and/or muscle groups, any type, complete system, not otherwise specified Y

Infusion Pump Equipment and Accessories

E0776 IV pole Y

E0779 Ambulatory infusion pump, mechanical, reusable, for infusion 8 hours or greater

E0780 Ambulatory infusion pump, mechanical, reusable, for infusion less than 8 hours Y

ⓘ **E0781** Ambulatory infusion pump, single or multiple channels, electric or battery operated, with administrative equipment, worn by patient Y
NCD 40.2

ⓘ **E0782** Infusion pump, implantable, non-programmable (includes all components, e.g., pump, catheter, connectors, etc.) N N1
NCD 40.2

ⓘ **E0783** Infusion pump system, implantable, programmable (includes all components, e.g., pump, catheter, connectors, etc.) N N1
NCD 40.2

ⓘ **E0784** External ambulatory infusion pump, insulin Y
NCD 40.2; Pub 100-8, 5, 5.3

ⓘ **E0785** Implantable intraspinal (epidural/intrathecal) catheter used with implantable infusion pump, replacement N N1
NCD 40.2

ⓘ **E0786** Implantable programmable infusion pump, replacement (excludes implantable intraspinal catheter) N N1
NCD 40.2

ⓘ **E0791** Parenteral infusion pump, stationary, single or multi-channel Y
NCD 180.2; Pub 100-02, 15, 120; 100-4, 20; 100.2.2.3; 100-8, 5, 5.3

ⓘ **E0830** Ambulatory traction device, all types, each N
NCD 280.1

Traction-Equipment

ⓘ **E0840** Traction frame, attached to headboard, cervical traction Y
NCD 280.1

E0849 Traction equipment, cervical, free-standing stand/frame, pneumatic, applying traction force to other than mandible Y

ⓘ **E0850** Traction stand, free standing, cervical traction Y
NCD 280.1

E0855 Cervical traction equipment not requiring additional stand or frame Y

E0856 Cervical traction device, cervical collar with inflatable air bladder Y

- E0860 Traction equipment, overdoor, cervical Y
  NCD 280.1
- E0870 Traction frame, attached to footboard, extremity traction, (e.g. Buck's) Y
  NCD 280.1
- E0880 Traction stand, free standing, extremity traction, (e.g., Buck's) Y
  NCD 280.1
- E0890 Traction frame, attached to footboard, pelvic traction Y
  NCD 280.1
- E0900 Traction stand, free standing, pelvic traction, (e.g., Buck's) Y
  NCD 280.1

Trapeze Equipment, Fracture Frame and Other Orthopedic Devices

- E0910 Trapeze bars, a/k/a patient helper, attached to bed, with grab bar Y
  NCD 280.1
- E0911 Trapeze bar, heavy duty, for patient weight capacity greater than 250 pounds, attached to bed, with grab bar Y
  NCD 280.1
- E0912 Trapeze bar, heavy duty, for patient weight capacity greater than 250 pounds, free standing, complete with grab bar Y
  NCD 280.1
- E0920 Fracture frame, attached to bed, includes weights Y
  NCD 280.1
- E0930 Fracture frame, free standing, includes weights Y
  NCD 280.1
- E0935 Continuous passive motion exercise device for use on knee only Y
  NCD 280.1
- E0936 Continuous passive motion exercise device for use other than knee E
- E0940 Trapeze bar, free standing, complete with grab bar Y
  NCD 280.1
- E0941 Gravity assisted traction device, any type Y
  NCD 280.1
- E0942 Cervical head harness/halter Y
- E0944 Pelvic belt/harness/boot Y
- E0945 Extremity belt/harness Y
- E0946 Fracture, frame, dual with cross bars, attached to bed, (e.g. Balken, 4 poster) Y
  NCD 280.1
- E0947 Fracture frame, attachments for complex pelvic traction Y
  NCD 280.1
- E0948 Fracture frame, attachments for complex cervical traction Y
  NCD 280.1

Wheelchair Accessories

- E0950 Wheelchair accessory, tray, each A
  NCD 280.1
- E0951 Heel loop/holder, any type, with or without ankle strap, each A
- E0952 Toe loop/holder, any type, each A
  NCD 280.1
- E0955 Wheelchair accessory, headrest, cushioned, any type, including fixed mounting hardware, each Y
- E0956 Wheelchair accessory, lateral trunk or hip support, any type, including fixed mounting hardware, each Y
- E0957 Wheelchair accessory, medial thigh support, any type, including fixed mounting hardware, each Y
- E0958 Manual wheelchair accessory, one-arm drive attachment, each A
  NCD 280.1
- E0959 Manual wheelchair accessory, adapter for amputee, each B
  NCD 280.1
- E0960 Wheelchair accessory, shoulder harness/straps or chest strap, including any type mounting hardware Y
- E0961 Manual wheelchair accessory, wheel lock brake extension (handle), each B
  NCD 280.1
- E0966 Manual wheelchair accessory, headrest extension, each B
  NCD 280.1
- E0967 Manual wheelchair accessory, hand rim with projections, any type, each Y
  NCD 280.1
- E0968 Commode seat, wheelchair Y
  NCD 280.1
- E0969 Narrowing device, wheelchair Y
  NCD 280.1
- E0970 No.2 footplates, except for elevating leg rest B
  Cross-reference K0037, K0042
  NCD 280.1
- E0971 Manual wheelchair accessory, anti-tipping device, each B
  Cross-reference K0021
  NCD 280.1
- E0973 Wheelchair accessory, adjustable height, detachable armrest, complete assembly, each B
  NCD 280.1
- E0974 Manual wheelchair accessory, anti-rollback device, each B
  Cross-reference K0080
- E0978 Wheelchair accessory, positioning belt/safety belt/pelvic strap, each B
- E0980 Safety vest, wheelchair Y
- E0981 Wheelchair accessory, seat upholstery, replacement only, each Y
- E0982 Wheelchair accessory, back upholstery, replacement only, each Y
- E0983 Manual wheelchair accessory, power add-on to convert manual wheelchair to motorized wheelchair, joystick control Y
- E0984 Manual wheelchair accessory, power add-on to convert manual wheelchair to motorized wheelchair, tiller control Y
- E0985 Wheelchair accessory, seat lift mechanism Y
- E0986 Manual wheelchair accessory, push activated power assist, each Y

E0990 Wheelchair accessory, elevating leg rest, complete assembly, each B
Cross-reference K0048
NCD 280.1

E0992 Manual wheelchair accessory, solid seat insert B

E0994 Arm rest, each Y
NCD 280.1

E0995 Wheelchair accessory, calf rest/pad, each B
NCD 280.1

E1002 Wheelchair accessory, power seating system, tilt only Y

E1003 Wheelchair accessory, power seating system, recline only, without shear reduction Y

E1004 Wheelchair accessory, power seating system, recline only, with mechanical shear reduction Y

E1005 Wheelchair accessory, power seating system, recline only, with power shear reduction Y

E1006 Wheelchair accessory, power seating system, combination tilt and recline, without shear reduction Y

E1007 Wheelchair accessory, power seating system, combination tilt and recline, with mechanical shear reduction Y

E1008 Wheelchair accessory, power seating system, combination tilt and recline, with power shear reduction Y

E1009 Wheelchair accessory, addition to power seating system, mechanically linked leg elevation system, including pushrod and leg rest, each Y

E1010 Wheelchair accessory, addition to power seating system, power leg elevation system, including leg rest, pair Y

E1011 Modification to pediatric size wheelchair, width adjustment package (not to be dispensed with initial chair) Y
NCD 280.1

E1014 Reclining back, addition to pediatric size wheelchair Y
NCD 280.1

E1015 Shock absorber for manual wheelchair, each Y
NCD 280.1

E1016 Shock absorber for power wheelchair, each Y
NCD 280.1

E1017 Heavy duty shock absorber for heavy duty or extra heavy duty manual wheelchair, each Y
NCD 280.1

E1018 Heavy duty shock absorber for heavy duty or extra heavy duty power wheelchair, each Y
NCD 280.1

E1020 Residual limb support system for wheelchair Y
NCD 280.3

E1028 Wheelchair accessory, manual swingaway, retractable or removable mounting hardware for joystick, other control interface or positioning accessory Y

E1029 Wheelchair accessory, ventilator tray, fixed Y

E1030 Wheelchair accessory, ventilator tray, gimbaled Y

Rollabout Chair

E1031 Rollabout chair, any and all types with casters 5" or greater Y
NCD 280.1

E1035 Multi-positional patient transfer system, with integrated seat, operated by care giver, patient weight capacity up to and including 300 lbs Y
Pub 100-02, 15, 110; 100-4, 20-10

E1036 Multi-positional patient transfer system, extra-wide, with integrated seat, operated by caregiver, patient weight capacity greater than 300 lbs Y

E1037 Transport chair, pediatric size Y
NCD 280.1

E1038 Transport chair, adult size, patient weight capacity up to and including 300 pounds Y
NCD 280.1

E1039 Transport chair, adult size, heavy duty, patient weight capacity greater than 300 pounds Y

Wheelchair – Fully-Reclining

E1050 Fully-reclining wheelchair, fixed full-length arms, swing away, detachable, elevating leg rests A
NCD 280.1

E1060 Fully-reclining wheelchair, detachable arms, desk or full length, swing away detachable elevating legrests A
NCD 280.1

E1070 Fully-reclining wheelchair, detachable arms (desk or full-length) swing-away, detachable footrest A
NCD 280.1

E1083 Hemi-wheelchair, fixed full-length arms, swing-away, detachable, elevating leg rest A
NCD 280.1

E1084 Hemi-wheelchair, detachable arms desk or full-length arms, swing-away, detachable, elevating leg rests A
NCD 280.1

E1085 Hemi-wheelchair, fixed full length arms, swing-away, detachable footrests A
Cross-reference K0002
NCD 280.1

E1086 Hemi-wheelchair detachable arms, desk or full-length, swing-away, detachable footrests A
Cross-reference K0002
NCD 280.1

E1087 High-strength lightweight wheelchair, fixed full-length arms, swing-away, detachable elevating leg rests A
NCD 280.1

E1088 High-strength lightweight wheelchair, detachable arms desk or full-length, swing-away, detachable, elevating leg rests A
NCD 280.1

E1089 High-strength lightweight wheelchair, fixed-length arms, swing-away detachable footrest A
Cross-reference K0004
NCD 280.1

E1090 High-strength lightweight wheelchair, detachable arms, desk or full-length, swing-away, detachable footrests A
Cross-reference K0004
NCD 280.1

E1092 Wide, heavy-duty wheelchair, detachable arms (desk or full-length), swing-away, detachable, elevating leg rests A
NCD 280.1

E1093 Wide, heavy-duty wheelchair, detachable arms desk or full-length arms, swing-away, detachable footrests A
NCD 280.1

Wheelchair – Semi-Reclining

E1100 Semi-reclining wheelchair; fixed full-length arms, swing-away, detachable, elevating leg rests
NCD 280.1

E1110 Semi-reclining wheelchair; detachable arms (desk or full- length), elevating leg rest
NCD 280.1

Wheelchair – Standard

E1130 Standard wheelchair; fixed full-length arms, fixed or swing-away, detachable footrests
Cross-reference K0001
NCD 280.1

E1140 Wheelchair; detachable arms, desk or full-length, swing-away, detachable footrests
Cross-reference K0001
NCD 280.1

E1150 Wheelchair; detachable arms, desk or full-length, swing-away, detachable, elevating legrests
NCD 280.1

E1160 Wheelchair, fixed full-length arms, swing-away, detachable, elevating legrests
NCD 280.1

E1161 Manual adult size wheelchair, includes tilt in space

Wheelchair – Amputee

E1170 Amputee wheelchair; fixed full-length arms, swing-away, detachable, elevating legrests
NCD 280.1

E1171 Amputee wheelchair; fixed full-length arms, without footrests or legrests
NCD 280.1

E1172 Amputee wheelchair; detachable arms (desk or full-length) without footrests or legrests
NCD 280.1

E1180 Amputee wheelchair, detachable arms (desk or full-length) swing-away, detachable footrests
NCD 280.1

E1190 Amputee wheelchair; detachable arms (desk or full-length) swing-away, detachable, elevating legrests
NCD 280.1

E1195 Heavy duty wheelchair; fixed full-length arms, swing-away, detachable, elevating legrests
NCD 280.1

E1200 Amputee wheelchair, fixed full-length arms, swing-away, detachable footrests
NCD 280.1

Wheelchair – Special Size

E1220 Wheelchair; specially sized or constructed, (indicate brand name, model number, if any, and justification)
NCD 280.3

E1221 Wheelchair with fixed arm, footrests
NCD 280.3

E1222 Wheelchair with fixed arm, elevating legrests
NCD 280.3

E1223 Wheelchair with detachable arms, footrests
NCD 280.3

E1224 Wheelchair with detachable arms, elevating legrests
NCD 280.3

E1225 Wheelchair accessory, manual semi-reclining back, (recline greater than 15 degrees, but less than 80 degrees), each
NCD 280.3

E1226 Wheelchair accessory, manual fully-reclining back, (recline greater than 80 degrees), each
NCD 280.3

E1227 Special height arms for wheelchair
NCD 280.3

E1228 Special back height for wheelchair
NCD 280.3

E1229 Wheelchair, pediatric size, not otherwise specified

E1230 Power operated vehicle (three or four wheel nonhighway), specify brand name and model number
NCD 280.9; Pub 100-8, 5, 5.3

E1231 Wheelchair, pediatric size, tilt-in-space, rigid, adjustable, with seating system
NCD 280.1

E1232 Wheelchair, pediatric size, tilt-in-space, folding, adjustable, with seating system
NCD 280.1

E1233 Wheelchair, pediatric size, tilt-in-space, rigid, adjustable, without seating system
NCD 280.1

E1234 Wheelchair, pediatric size, tilt-in-space, folding, adjustable, without seating system
NCD 280.1

E1235 Wheelchair, pediatric size, rigid, adjustable, with seating system
NCD 280.1

E1236 Wheelchair, pediatric size, folding, adjustable, with seating system
NCD 280.1

E1237 Wheelchair, pediatric size, rigid, adjustable, without seating system
NCD 280.1

E1238 Wheelchair, pediatric size, folding, adjustable, without seating system
NCD 280.1

E1239 Power wheelchair, pediatric size, not otherwise specified

Wheelchair – Lightweight

E1240 Lightweight wheelchair; detachable arms, (desk or full-length) swing away, detachable, elevating legrest
NCD 280.1

E1250 Lightweight wheelchair; fixed full-length arms, swing-away, detachable footrest
Cross-reference K0003
NCD 280.1

E1260 Lightweight wheelchair, detachable arms (desk or full length) swing-away, detachable footrest
Cross-reference K0003
NCD 280.1

E1270 Lightweight wheelchair, fixed full length arms, swing-away, detachable, elevating legrests
NCD 280.1

Wheelchair – Heavy Duty

ⓘ E1280 Heavy duty wheelchair, detachable arms (desk or full length) elevating legrest A
NCD 280.1

⊘ E1285 Heavy duty wheelchair, fixed full length arms, swing-away, detachable footrest A
Cross-reference K0006
NCD 280.1

⊘ E1290 Heavy duty wheelchair, detachable arms (desk or full length) swing-away, detachable footrest A
Cross-reference K0006
NCD 280.1

ⓘ E1295 Heavy duty wheelchair, fixed-full-length arms, elevating legrest A
NCD 280.1

ⓘ E1296 Special wheelchair seat height from floor Y
NCD 280.3

ⓘ E1297 Special wheelchair seat depth, by upholstery Y
NCD 280.3

ⓘ E1298 Special wheelchair seat depth and/or width, by construction Y
NCD 280.3

Whirlpool-Equipment

⊘ E1300 Whirlpool, portable (overtub type) E
NCD 280.1

ⓘ E1310 Whirlpool, non-portable (built-in type) Y
NCD 280.1

Additional Oxygen Related Equipment

ⓘ E1353 Regulator Y
NCD 240.2; Pub 100-8, 5, 5.3

E1354 Oxygen accessory, wheeled cart for portable cylinder or portable concentrator, any type, replacement only, each Y

ⓘ E1355 Stand/rack Y
NCD 240.2

E1356 Oxygen accessory, battery pack/cartridge for portable concentrator, any type, replacement only, each Y

E1357 Oxygen accessory, battery charger for portable concentrator, any type, replacement only, each Y

⊘ E1358 Oxygen accessory, DC power adapter for portable concentrator, any type, replacement only, each Y

ⓘ E1372 Immersion external heater for nebulizer Y
NCD 240.2

ⓘ E1390 Oxygen concentrator, single delivery port, capable of delivering 85 percent or greater oxygen concentration at the prescribed flow rate Y
NCD 240.2

ⓘ E1391 Oxygen concentrator, dual delivery port, capable of delivering 85 percent or greater oxygen concentration at the prescribed flow rate, each Y
NCD 240.2

ⓘ E1392 Portable oxygen concentrator, rental Y
NCD 240.2

E1399 Durable medical equipment, miscellaneous Y

ⓘ E1405 Oxygen and water vapor enriching system with heated delivery Y
NCD 240.2, Pub 100-8, 5, 5.3

ⓘ E1406 Oxygen and water vapor enriching system without heated delivery Y
NCD 240.2, Pub 100-8, 5, 5.3

Artificial Kidney Machines and Accessories

Note: For supplies for ESRD see codes A4651 – A4999

ⓘ E1500 Centrifuge, for dialysis A

ⓘ E1510 Kidney, dialysate delivery syst. Kidney machine, pump recirculating, air removal syst, flowrate meter, power off, heater and temperature control with alarm, I.V. poles, pressure gauge, concentrate container A

ⓘ E1520 Heparin infusion pump for hemodialysis A

ⓘ E1530 Air bubble detector for hemodialysis, each, replacement A

ⓘ E1540 Pressure alarm for hemodialysis, each, replacement A

ⓘ E1550 Bath conductivity meter for hemodialysis, each A

ⓘ E1560 Blood leak detector for hemodialysis, each, replacement A

ⓘ E1570 Adjustable chair, for ESRD patients A

ⓘ E1575 Transducer protectors/fluid barriers, for hemodialysis, any size, per 10 A

ⓘ E1580 Unipuncture control system for hemodialysis A

ⓘ E1590 Hemodialysis machine A

ⓘ E1592 Automatic intermittent peritioneal dialysis system A

ⓘ E1594 Cycler dialysis machine for peritoneal dialysis A

ⓘ E1600 Delivery and/or installation charges for hemodialysis equipment A

ⓘ E1610 Reverse osmosis water purification system, for hemodialysis A
NCD 230.7

ⓘ E1615 Deionizer water purification system, for hemodialysis A
NCD 230.7

ⓘ E1620 Blood pump for hemodialysis, replacement A

ⓘ E1625 Water softening system, for hemodialysis A
NCD 230.7

E1630 Reciprocating peritoneal dialysis system A

ⓘ E1632 Wearable artificial kidney, each A

ⓘ E1634 Peritoneal dialysis clamps, each B
Pub 100-04, 8, 60.1; 100-4, 8, 80; 100-4, 8, 90; 100-4, 8, 90.3.2; 100-4, 8, 130

ⓘ E1635 Compact (portable) travel hemodialyzer system A

ⓘ E1636 Sorbent cartridges, for hemodialysis, per 10 A

ⓘ E1637 Hemostats, each A

ⓘ E1639 Scale, each A

ⓘ E1699 Dialysis equipment, not otherwise specified A

Jaw Motion Rehabilitation System and Accessories

E1700 Jaw motion rehabilitation system Y

E1701 Replacement cushions for jaw motion rehabilitation system, pkg. of 6 Y

E1702 Replacement measuring scales for jaw motion rehabilitation system, pkg. of 200 Y

Other Orthopedic Devices

E1800 Dynamic adjustable elbow extension/flexion device, includes soft interface material Y

E1801 Static progressive stretch elbow device, extension and/or flexion, with or without range of motion adjustment, includes all components and accessories Y

E1802 Dynamic adjustable forearm pronation/supination device, includes soft interface material Y

E1805 Dynamic adjustable wrist extension/flexion device, includes soft interface material Y

E1806 Static progressive stretch wrist device, flexion and/or extension, with or without range of motion adjustment, includes all components and accessories Y

E1810 Dynamic adjustable knee extension/flexion device, includes soft interface material Y

E1811 Static progressive stretch knee device, extension and/or flexion, with or without range of motion adjustment, includes all components and accessories Y

E1812 Dynamic knee, extension/flexion device with active resistance control Y

E1815 Dynamic adjustable ankle extension/flexion device, includes soft interface material Y

E1816 Static progressive stretch ankle device, flexion and/or extension, with or without range of motion adjustment, includes all components and accessories Y

E1818 Static progressive stretch forearm pronation/supination device, with or without range of motion adjustment, includes all components and accessories Y

E1820 Replacement soft interface material, dynamic adjustable extension/flexion device Y

E1821 Replacement soft interface material/cuffs for bi-directional static progressive stretch device Y

E1825 Dynamic adjustable finger extension/flexion device, includes soft interface material Y

E1830 Dynamic adjustable toe extension/flexion device, includes soft interface material Y

● E1831 Static progressive stretch toe device, extension and/or flexion, with or without range of motion adjustment, includes all components and accessories Y
This code is effective January 1, 2011

E1840 Dynamic adjustable shoulder flexion/abduction/rotation device, includes soft interface material Y

E1841 Static progressive stretch shoulder device, with or without range of motion adjustment, includes all components and accessories Y

E1902 Communication board, non-electronic augmentative or alternative communication device Y

Gastric Suction Pumps

E2000 Gastric suction pump, home model, portable or stationary, electric Y

Blood Glucose Monitors

ⓘ E2100 Blood glucose monitor with integrated voice synthesizer Y
NCD 40.2

ⓘ E2101 Blood glucose monitor with integrated lancing/blood sample Y
NCD 40.2

Pulse Generator Systems

E2120 Pulse generator system for tympanic treatment of inner ear endolymphatic fluid Y

Manual Wheelchair Accessory

E2201 Manual wheelchair accessory, nonstandard seat frame, width greater than or equal to 20 inches and less than 24 inches Y

E2202 Manual wheelchair accessory, nonstandard seat frame width, 24-27 inches Y

E2203 Manual wheelchair accessory, nonstandard seat frame depth, 20 to less than 22 inches Y

E2204 Manual wheelchair accessory, nonstandard seat frame depth, 22 to 25 inches Y

E2205 Manual wheelchair accessory, handrim without projections (includes ergonomic or contoured), any type, replacement only, each Y

E2206 Manual wheelchair accessory, wheel lock assembly, complete, each Y

E2207 Wheelchair accessory, crutch and cane holder, each Y

E2208 Wheelchair accessory, cylinder tank carrier, each Y

E2209 Accessory, arm trough, with or without hand support, each Y

E2210 Wheelchair accessory, bearings, any type, replacement only, each Y

E2211 Manual wheelchair accessory, pneumatic propulsion tire, any size, each Y

E2212 Manual wheelchair accessory, tube for pneumatic propulsion tire, any size, each Y

E2213 Manual wheelchair accessory, insert for pneumatic propulsion tire (removable), any type, any size, each Y

E2214 Manual wheelchair accessory, pneumatic caster tire, any size, each Y

E2215 Manual wheelchair accessory, tube for pneumatic caster tire, any size, each Y

E2216 Manual wheelchair accessory, foam filled propulsion tire, any size, each Y

E2217 Manual wheelchair accessory, foam filled caster tire, any size, each Y

E2218 Manual wheelchair accessory, foam propulsion tire, any size, each Y

E2219 Manual wheelchair accessory, foam caster tire, any size, each Y

E2220 Manual wheelchair accessory, solid (rubber/plastic) propulsion tire, any size, each Y

E2221 Manual wheelchair accessory, solid (rubber/plastic) caster tire (removable), any size, each Y

E2222 Manual wheelchair accessory, solid (rubber/plastic) caster tire with integrated wheel, any size, each Y

E2224 Manual wheelchair accessory, propulsion wheel excludes tire, any size, each Y

E2225 Manual wheelchair accessory, caster wheel excludes tire, any size, replacement only, each Y

E2226 Manual wheelchair accessory, caster fork, any size, replacement only, each Y

E2227 Manual wheelchair accessory, gear reduction drive wheel, each Y

E2228 Manual wheelchair accessory, wheel braking system and lock, complete, each Y

⊘ E2230 Manual wheelchair accessory, manual standing system E

E2231 Manual wheelchair accessory, solid seat support base (replaces sling seat), includes any type mounting hardware Y

E2291 Back, planar, for pediatric size wheelchair including fixed attaching hardware Y

E2292 Seat, planar, for pediatric size wheelchair including fixed attaching hardware Y

E2293 Back, contoured, for pediatric size wheelchair including fixed attaching hardware Y

E2294 Seat, contoured, for pediatric size wheelchair including fixed attaching hardware

E2295 Manual wheelchair accessory, for pediatric size wheelchair, dynamic seating frame, allows coordinated movement of multiple positioning features

Power Wheelchair Accessory

E2300 Power wheelchair accessory, power seat elevation system

E2301 Power wheelchair accessory, power standing system

E2310 Power wheelchair accessory, electronic connection between wheelchair controller and one power seating system motor, including all related electronics, indicator feature, mechanical function selection switch, and fixed mounting hardware

E2311 Power wheelchair accessory, electronic connection between wheelchair controller and two or more power seating system motors, including all related electronics, indicator feature, mechanical function selection switch, and fixed mounting hardware

E2312 Power wheelchair accessory, hand or chin control interface, mini-proportional remote joystick, proportional, including fixed mounting hardware

E2313 Power wheelchair accessory, harness for upgrade to expandable controller, including all fasteners, connectors and mounting hardware, each

E2321 Power wheelchair accessory, hand control interface, remote joystick, nonproportional, including all related electronics, mechanical stop switch, and fixed mounting hardware

E2322 Power wheelchair accessory, hand control interface, multiple mechanical switches, nonproportional, including all related electronics, mechanical stop switch, and fixed mounting hardware

E2323 Power wheelchair accessory, specialty joystick handle for hand control interface, prefabricated

E2324 Power wheelchair accessory, chin cup for chin control interface

E2325 Power wheelchair accessory, sip and puff interface, nonproportional, including all related electronics, mechanical stop switch, and manual swingaway mounting hardware

E2326 Power wheelchair accessory, breath tube kit for sip and puff interface

E2327 Power wheelchair accessory, head control interface, mechanical, proportional, including all related electronics, mechanical direction change switch, and fixed mounting hardware

E2328 Power wheelchair accessory, head control or extremity control interface, electronic, proportional, including all related electronics and fixed mounting hardware

E2329 Power wheelchair accessory, head control interface, contact switch mechanism, nonproportional, including all related electronics, mechanical stop switch, mechanical direction change switch, head array, and fixed mounting hardware

E2330 Power wheelchair accessory, head control interface, proximity switch mechanism, nonproportional, including all related electronics, mechanical stop switch, mechanical direction change switch, head array, and fixed mounting hardware

E2331 Power wheelchair accessory, attendant control, proportional, including all related electronics and fixed mounting hardware

E2340 Power wheelchair accessory, nonstandard seat frame width, 20-23 inches

E2341 Power wheelchair accessory, nonstandard seat frame width, 24-27 inches

E2342 Power wheelchair accessory, nonstandard seat frame depth, 20 or 21 inches

E2343 Power wheelchair accessory, nonstandard seat frame depth, 22-25 inches

E2351 Power wheelchair accessory, electronic interface to operate speech generating device using power wheelchair control interface

E2360 Power wheelchair accessory, 22NF non-sealed lead acid battery, each

E2361 Power wheelchair accessory, 22NF sealed lead acid battery, each, (e.g. Gel Cell, Absorbed Glassmat)

E2362 Power wheelchair accessory, group 24 non-sealed lead acid battery, each

E2363 Power wheelchair accessory, group 24 sealed lead acid battery, each (e.g. Gel Cell, Absorbed Glassmat)

E2364 Power wheelchair accessory, U-1 non-sealed lead acid battery, each

E2365 Power wheelchair accessory, U-1 sealed lead acid battery, each (e.g. Gel Cell, Absorbed Glassmat)

E2366 Power wheelchair accessory, battery charger, single mode, for use with only one battery type, sealed or non-sealed, each

E2367 Power wheelchair accessory, battery charger, dual mode, for use with either battery type, sealed or non-sealed, each

E2368 Power wheelchair component, motor, replacement only

E2369 Power wheelchair component, gear box, replacement only

E2370 Power wheelchair component, motor and gear box combination, replacement only

E2371 Power wheelchair accessory, group 27 sealed lead acid battery, (e.g. Gel Cell, Absorbed Glassmat), each

E2372 Power wheelchair accessory, group 27 non-sealed lead acid battery, each

E2373 Power wheelchair accessory, hand or chin control interface, compact remote joystick, proportional, including fixed mounting hardware

E2374 Power wheelchair accessory, hand or chin control interface, standard remote joystick (not including controller), proportional, including all related electronics and fixed mounting hardware, replacement only

E2375 Power wheelchair accessory, non-expandable controller, including all related electronics and mounting hardware, replacement only

E2376 Power wheelchair accessory, expandable controller, including all related electronics and mounting hardware, replacement only

E2377 Power wheelchair accessory, expandable controller, including all related electronics and mounting hardware, upgrade provided at initial issue

E2381 Power wheelchair accessory, pneumatic drive wheel tire, any size, replacement only, each

E2382 Power wheelchair accessory, tube for pneumatic drive wheel tire, any size, replacement only, each

E2383 Power wheelchair accessory, insert for pneumatic drive wheel tire (removable), any type, any size, replacement only, each

E2384 Power wheelchair accessory, pneumatic caster tire, any size, replacement only, each

Ⓘ E2385 Power wheelchair accessory, tube for pneumatic caster tire, any size, replacement only, each

Ⓘ E2386 Power wheelchair accessory, foam filled drive wheel tire, any size, replacement only, each

Ⓘ E2387 Power wheelchair accessory, foam filled caster tire, any size, replacement only, each

Ⓘ E2388 Power wheelchair accessory, foam drive wheel tire, any size, replacement only, each

Ⓘ E2389 Power wheelchair accessory, foam caster tire, any size, replacement only, each

Ⓘ E2390 Power wheelchair accessory, solid (rubber/plastic) drive wheel tire, any size, replacement only, each

Ⓘ E2391 Power wheelchair accessory, solid (rubber/plastic) caster tire (removable), any size, replacement only, each

Ⓘ E2392 Power wheelchair accessory, solid (rubber/plastic) caster tire with integrated wheel, any size, replacement only, each

Ⓘ E2394 Power wheelchair accessory, drive wheel excludes tire, any size, replacement only, each

Ⓘ E2395 Power wheelchair accessory, caster wheel excludes tire, any size, replacement only, each

Ⓘ E2396 Power wheelchair accessory, caster fork, any size, replacement only, each

E2397 Power wheelchair accessory, lithium-based battery, each

Negative Pressure Electrical Pump

E2402 Negative pressure wound therapy electrical pump, stationary or portable

Speech Generating Equipment

Ⓘ E2500 Speech generating device, digitized speech, using pre-recorded messages, less than or equal to 8 minutes recording time

NCD 50.1

Ⓘ E2502 Speech generating device, digitized speech, using pre-recorded messages, greater than 8 minutes but less than or equal to 20 minutes recording time

NCD 50.1

Ⓘ E2504 Speech generating device, digitized speech, using pre-recorded messages, greater than 20 minutes but less than or equal to 40 minutes recording time

NCD 50.1

Ⓘ E2506 Speech generating device, digitized speech, using pre-recorded messages, greater than 40 minutes recording time

NCD 50.1

Ⓘ E2508 Speech generating device, synthesized speech, requiring message formulation by spelling and access by physical contact with the device

NCD 50.1

Ⓘ E2510 Speech generating device, synthesized speech, permitting multiple methods of message formulation and multiple methods of device access

NCD 50.1

Ⓘ E2511 Speech generating software program, for personal computer or personal digital assistant

NCD 50.1

Ⓘ E2512 Accessory for speech generating device, mounting system

NCD 50.1

Ⓘ E2599 Accessory for speech generating device, not otherwise classified

NCD 50.1

Additional Wheelchair Accessory

E2601 General use wheelchair seat cushion, width less than 22 inches, any depth

E2602 General use wheelchair seat cushion, width 22 inches or greater, any depth

E2603 Skin protection wheelchair seat cushion, width less than 22 inches, any depth

E2604 Skin protection wheelchair seat cushion, width 22 inches or greater, any depth

E2605 Positioning wheelchair seat cushion, width less than 22 inches, any depth

E2606 Positioning wheelchair seat cushion, width 22 inches or greater, any depth

E2607 Skin protection and positioning wheelchair seat cushion, width less than 22 inches, any depth

E2608 Skin protection and positioning wheelchair seat cushion, width 22 inches or greater, any depth

E2609 Custom fabricated wheelchair seat cushion, any size

E2610 Wheelchair seat cushion, powered

E2611 General use wheelchair back cushion, width less than 22 inches, any height, including any type mounting hardware

E2612 General use wheelchair back cushion, width 22 inches or greater, any height, including any type mounting hardware

E2613 Positioning wheelchair back cushion, posterior, width less than 22 inches, any height, including any type mounting hardware

E2614 Positioning wheelchair back cushion, posterior, width 22 inches or greater, any height, including any type mounting hardware

E2615 Positioning wheelchair back cushion, posterior-lateral, width less than 22 inches, any height, including any type mounting hardware

E2616 Positioning wheelchair back cushion, posterior-lateral, width 22 inches or greater, any height, including any type mounting hardware

E2617 Custom fabricated wheelchair back cushion, any size, including any type mounting hardware

E2619 Replacement cover for wheelchair seat cushion or back cushion, each

E2620 Positioning wheelchair back cushion, planar back with lateral supports, width less than 22 inches, any height, including any type mounting hardware

E2621 Positioning wheelchair back cushion, planar back with lateral supports, width 22 inches or greater, any height, including any type mounting hardware

● E2622 Skin protection wheelchair seat cushion, adjustable, width less than 22 inches, any depth

This code is effective January 1, 2011

● E2623 Skin protection wheelchair seat cushion, adjustable, width 22 inches or greater, any depth

This code is effective January 1, 2011

● E2624 Skin protection and positioning wheelchair seat cushion, adjustable, width less than 22 inches, any depth

This code is effective January 1, 2011

● E2625 Skin protection and positioning wheelchair seat cushion, adjustable, width 22 inches or greater, any depth

This code is effective January 1, 2011

Gait Trainer

⊘ E8000 Gait trainer, pediatric size, posterior support, includes all accessories and components E

⊘ E8001 Gait trainer, pediatric size, upright support, includes all accessories and components E

⊘ E8002 Gait trainer, pediatric size, anterior support, includes all accessories and components E

Procedures/Professional Services G0008–G9140

G0008 Administration of influenza virus vaccine S
Pub 100-04, 18, 10-10.5

G0009 Administration of pneumococcal vaccine S
Pub 100-04, 18, 10-10.5

G0010 Administration of hepatitis B vaccine B
Pub 100-04, 18, 10-10.5

G0027 Semen analysis; presence and/or motility of sperm excluding Huhner ♂ A
Pub 100-02 , 15, 80

ⓘ G0101 Cervical or vaginal cancer screening; pelvic and clinical breast examination ♀ V PQR
Pub 100-02 , 15, 80; Pub 100-03, 1, 210.2; Pub 100-04, 18, 40-40.8

Cervical or vaginal cancer screening

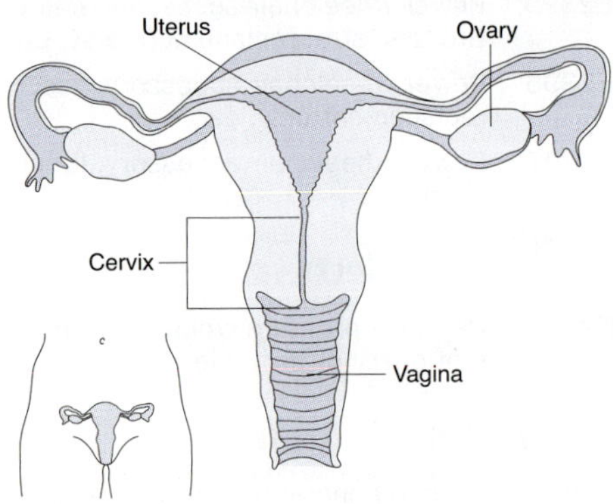

ⓘ G0102 Prostate cancer screening; digital rectal examination ♂ N
NCD 210.1; Pub 100-02, 15, 80; Pub 100-03, 1, 210.1; Pub 100-04, 18, 50-50.8

ⓘ G0103 Prostate cancer screening; prostate specific antigen test (PSA) ♂ A
NCD 210.1; Pub 100-02 , 15, 80; Pub 100-03, 1, 210.1; Pub 100-04, 18, 50-50.8

ⓘ G0104 Colorectal cancer screening; flexible sigmoidoscopy S P3
Pub 100-02, 15, 80, 280.2; Pub 100-03, 1, 210.3; Pub 100-04, 18, 60-60.8

ⓘ G0105 Colorectal cancer screening; colonoscopy on individual at high risk T A2 PQR
Pub 100-02, 15, 80, 280.2; Pub 100-03, 1, 210.3; Pub 100-04, 18, 60-60.8

ⓘ G0106 Colorectal cancer screening; alternative to G0104, screening sigmoidoscopy, barium enema S PQR
Pub 100-02, 15, 80, 280.2; Pub 100-03, 1, 210.3; Pub 100-04, 18, 60-60.8

G0108 Diabetes outpatient self-management training services, individual, per 30 minutes A PQR
Pub 100-03, 1, 210.3; Pub 100-04, 18, 120-120.2.2

G0109 Diabetes outpatient self-management training services, group session (2 or more), per 30 minutes A PQR

G0117 Glaucoma screening for high risk patients furnished by an optometrist or ophthalmologist S
AHA: 3Q 2001, 12
Pub 100-04, 18, 70-70.5

G0118 Glaucoma screening for high risk patient furnished under the direct supervision of an optometrist or ophthalmologist S
AHA: 3Q 2001, 12

G0120 Colorectal cancer screening; alternative to G0105, screening colonoscopy, barium enema S PQRI
Pub 100-02, 15, 80, 280.2; Pub 100-03, 1, 210.3; Pub 100-04, 18, 60-60.8

G0121 Colorectal cancer screening; colonoscopy on individual not meeting criteria for high risk T A2
Pub 100-02, 15, 80, 280.2; Pub 100-03, 1, 210.3; Pub 100-04, 18, 60-60.8

G0122 Colorectal cancer screening; barium enema E
Pub 100-02, 15, 80; Pub 100-04, 18, 60-60.8

G0123 Screening cytopathology, cervical or vaginal (any reporting system), collected in preservative fluid, automated thin layer preparation, screening by cytotechnologist under physician supervision ♀ A
NCD 190.2; Pub 100-02, 15, 280.4; Pub 100-03, 1, 210.2

G0124 Screening cytopathology, cervical or vaginal (any reporting system), collected in preservative fluid, automated thin layer preparation, requiring interpretation by physician ♀ B
NCD 190.2; Pub 100-02, 15, 80, 280.4; Pub 100-03, 1, 210.2; Pub 100-04, 18, 30-30.9

G0127 Trimming of dystrophic nails, any number T P3
Pub 100-02, 15, 290; 100-2, 15, 290

Trimming of dystrophic nails

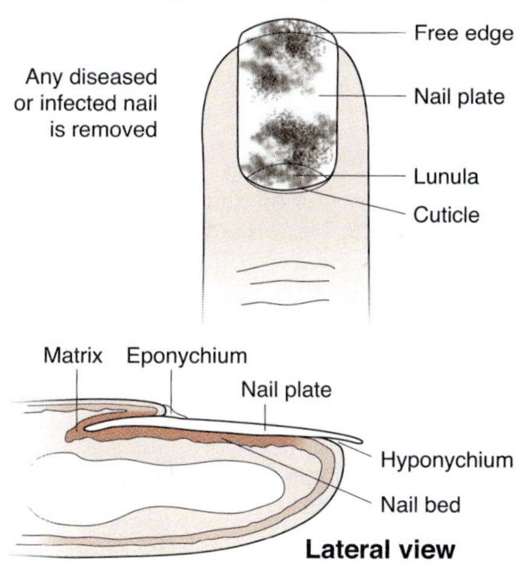

G0128 Direct (face-to-face with patient) skilled nursing services of a registered nurse provided in a comprehensive outpatient rehabilitation facility, each 10 minutes beyond the first 5 minutes B
Medicare Statute 1833(a)

G0129 Occupational therapy services requiring the skills of a qualified occupational therapist, furnished as a component of a partial hospitalization treatment program, per session (45 minutes or more) P

G0130 Single energy x-ray absorptiometry (SEXA) bone density study, one or more sites; appendicular skeleton (peripheral) (e.g., radius, wrist, heel) X Z3
NCD 150.3; Pub 100-02 , 15, 80

G0141 Screening cytopathology smears, cervical or vaginal, performed by automated system, with manual rescreening, requiring interpretation by physician ♀ B
Pub 100-02, 15, 80, 280.4; Pub 100-03, 1, 210.2; Pub 100-04, 18, 30-30.9

G0143 Screening cytopathology, cervical or vaginal (any reporting system), collected in preservative fluid, automated thin layer preparation, with manual screening and rescreening by cytotechnologist under physician supervision ♀ A
Pub 100-02, 15, 80, 280.4; Pub 100-03, 1, 210.2; Pub 100-04, 18, 30-30.9

G0144 Screening cytopathology, cervical or vaginal (any reporting system), collected in preservative fluid, automated thin layer preparation, with screening by automated system, under physician supervision ♀ A
Pub 100-02, 15, 80, 280.4; Pub 100-03, 1, 210.2; Pub 100-04, 18, 30-30.9

G0145 Screening cytopathology, cervical or vaginal (any reporting system), collected in preservative fluid, automated thin layer preparation, with screening by automated system and manual rescreening under physician supervision ♀ A
Pub 100-02, 15, 80, 280.4; Pub 100-03, 1, 210.2; Pub 100-04, 18, 30-30.9

G0147 Screening cytopathology smears, cervical or vaginal, performed by automated system under physician supervision ♀ A
Pub 100-02, 15, 80, 280.4; Pub 100-03, 1, 210.2; Pub 100-04, 18, 30-30.9

G0148 Screening cytopathology smears, cervical or vaginal, performed by automated system with manual rescreening ♀ A
Pub 100-02, 15, 80, 280.4; Pub 100-03, 1, 210.2; Pub 100-04, 18, 30-30.9

▲ G0151 Services performed by a qualified physical therapist in the home health or hospice setting, each 15 minutes B

▲ G0152 Services performed by a qualified occupational therapist in the home health or hospice setting, each 15 minutes B

▲ G0153 Services performed by a qualified speech-language pathologist in the home health or hospice setting, each 15 minutes B

▲ G0154 Direct skilled nursing services of a licensed nurse (LPN or RN) in the home health or hospice setting, each 15 minutes B

G0155 Services of clinical social worker in home health or hospice settings, each 15 minutes B

G0156 Services of home health/hospice aide in home health or hospice settings, each 15 minutes B

● G0157 Services performed by a qualified physical therapist assistant in the home health or hospice setting, each 15 minutes B
This code is effective January 1, 2011

● G0158 Services performed by a qualified occupational therapist assistant in the home health or hospice setting, each 15 minutes B
This code is effective January 1, 2011

● G0159 Services performed by a qualified physical therapist, in the home health setting, in the establishment or delivery of a safe and effective therapy maintenance program, each 15 minutes B
This code is effective January 1, 2011

● G0160 Services performed by a qualified occupational therapist, in the home health setting, in the establishment or delivery of a safe and effective therapy maintenance program, each 15 minutes B
This code is effective January 1, 2011

● G0161 Services performed by a qualified speech-language pathologist, in the home health setting, in the establishment or delivery of a safe and effective therapy maintenance program, each 15 minutes B
This code is effective January 1, 2011

● G0162 Skilled services by a registered nurse (RN) in the delivery of management & evaluation of the plan of care; each 15 minutes (the patient's underlying condition or complication requires an rn to ensure that essential non-skilled care achieve its purpose in the home health or hospice setting) B
This code is effective January 1, 2011

● G0163 Skilled services of a licensed nurse (LPN or RN) in the delivery of observation & assessment of the patient's condition, each 15 minutes (when the likelihood of change in the patient's condition requires skilled nursing personnel to identify and evaluate the patient's need for possible modification of treatment in the home health or hospice setting) B
This code is effective January 1, 2011

● G0164 Skilled services of a licensed nurse, in the training and/or education of a patient or family member, in the home health or hospice setting, each 15 minutes B
This code is effective January 1, 2011

G0166 External counterpulsation, per treatment session T
NCD 20.20; Pub 100-04, 32, 130-130.2

G0168 Wound closure utilizing tissue adhesive(s) only B
AHA: 1Q 2005, 5; 4Q 2001, 12; 3Q 2001, 13

G0173 Linear accelerator based stereotactic radiosurgery, complete course of therapy in one session S Z2

G0175 Scheduled interdisciplinary team conference (minimum of three exclusive of patient care nursing staff) with patient present V

G0176 Activity therapy, such as music, dance, art or play therapies not for recreation, related to the care and treatment of patient's disabling mental health problems, per session (45 minutes or more) P

G0177 Training and educational services related to the care and treatment of patient's disabling mental health problems per session (45 minutes or more) P

G0179 Physician re-certification for Medicare-covered home health services under a home health plan of care (patient not present), including contacts with home health agency and review of reports of patient status required by physicians to affirm the initial implementation of the plan of care that meets patient's needs, per re-certification period M

G0180 Physician certification for Medicare-covered home health services under a home health plan of care (patient not present), including contacts with home health agency and review of reports of patient status required by physicians to affirm the initial implementation of the plan of care that meets patient's needs, per certification period M

G0181 Physician supervision of a patient receiving Medicare-covered services provided by a participating home health agency (patient not present) requiring complex and multidisciplinary care modalities involving regular physician development and/or revision of care plans, review of subsequent reports of patient status, review of laboratory and other studies, communication (including telephone calls) with other health care professionals involved in the patient's care, integration of new information into the medical treatment plan and/or adjustment of medical therapy, within a calendar month, 30 minutes or more M

G0182 Physician supervision of a patient under a Medicare-approved hospice (patient not present) requiring complex and multidisciplinary care modalities involving regular physician development and/or revision of care plans, review of subsequent reports of patient status, review of laboratory and other studies, communication (including telephone calls) with other health care professionals involved in the patient's care, integration of new information into the medical treatment plan and/or adjustment of medical therapy, within a calendar month, 30 minutes or more M

G0186 Destruction of localized lesion of choroid (for example, choroidal neovascularization); photocoagulation, feeder vessel technique (one or more sessions) T R2

Destruction of locolized lesion of choroid

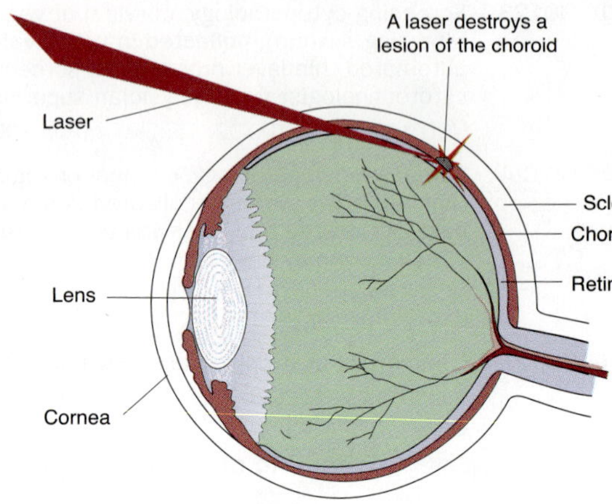

G0202 Screening mammography, producing direct digital image, bilateral, all views PQR
Pub 100-02, 15, 80; Pub 100-04, 18, 20-20.8.2

G0204 Diagnostic mammography, producing direct digital image, bilateral, all views A
NCD 220.4; Pub 100-02, 15, 80; Pub 100-04, 18, 20-20.8.2

G0206 Diagnostic mammography, producing direct digital image, unilateral, all views A
NCD 220.4; Pub 100-02, 15, 80; Pub 100-04, 18, 20-20.8.2

G0219 PET imaging whole body; melanoma for non-covered indications E
NCD 220.6; Pub 100-02, 15, 80; Pub 100-03, 1, 220.6, 220.6.17; Pub 100-04, 13, 60.3

G0235 PET imaging, any site, not otherwise specified E
NCD 220.6; Pub 100-02, 15, 80; Pub 100-04, 13, 60.3; 100-4, 13, 60.14
AHA: 1Q 2007, 6

G0237 Therapeutic procedures to increase strength or endurance of respiratory muscles, face to face, one on one, each 15 minutes (includes monitoring) S

G0238 Therapeutic procedures to improve respiratory function, other than described by G0237, one on one, face to face, per 15 minutes (includes monitoring) S

G0239 Therapeutic procedures to improve respiratory function or increase strength or endurance of respiratory muscles, two or more individuals (includes monitoring) S

G0245 Initial physician evaluation and management of a diabetic patient with diabetic sensory neuropathy resulting in a loss of protective sensation (LOPS) which must include: (1) the diagnosis of LOPS, (2) a patient history, (3) a physical examination that consists of at least the following elements: (a) visual inspection of the forefoot, hindfoot and toe web spaces, (b) evaluation of a protective sensation, (c) evaluation of foot structure and biomechanics, (d) evaluation of vascular status and skin integrity, and (e) evaluation and recommendation of footwear and (4) patient education V

NCD 70.2; Pub 100-04, 32, 80-80.8

G0246 Follow-up physician evaluation and management of a diabetic patient with diabetic sensory neuropathy resulting in a loss of protective sensation (LOPS) to include at least the following: (1) a patient history, (2) a physical examination that includes: (a) visual inspection of the forefoot, hindfoot and toe web spaces, (b) evaluation of protective sensation, (c) evaluation of foot structure and biomechanics, (d) evaluation of vascular status and skin integrity, and (e) evaluation and recommendation of footwear, and (3) patient education V

NCD 70.2; Pub 100-04, 32, 80-80.8

G0247 Routine foot care by a physician of a diabetic patient with diabetic sensory neuropathy resulting in a loss of protective sensation (LOPS) to include, the local care of superficial wounds (i.e. superficial to muscle and fascia) and at least the following if present: (1) local care of superficial wounds, (2) debridement of corns and calluses, and (3) trimming and debridement of nails T P3

NCD 70.2; Pub 100-04, 32, 80-80.8

G0248 Demonstration, prior to initial use, of home INR monitoring for patient with either mechanical heart valve(s), chronic atrial fibrillation, or venous thromboembolism who meets Medicare coverage criteria, under the direction of a physician; includes: face-to-face demonstration of use and care of the INR monitor, obtaining at least one blood sample, provision of instructions for reporting home INR test results, and documentation of patient ability to perform testing prior to its use X

NCD 210.1; Pub 100-04, 32, 60-60.8.2

G0249 Provision of test materials and equipment for home INR monitoring of patient with either mechanical heart valve(s), chronic atrial fibrillation, or venous thromboembolism who meets Medicare coverage criteria; includes provision of materials for use in the home and reporting of test results to physician; not occurring more frequently than once a week X

NCD 210.1

G0250 Physician review, interpretation, and patient management of home INR testing for a patient with either mechanical heart valve(s), chroic atrial fibrillation, or venous thromboembolism who meets Medicare coverage criteria; includes face-to-face verification by the physician at least once a year (e.g. during an evaluation and management service) that the patient uses the device in the context of the management of the anticoagulation therapy following initiation of the home INR monitoring; not occurring more frequently than once a week M

NCD 210.1

G0251 Linear accelerator based stereotactic radiosurgery, delivery including collimator changes and custom plugging, fractionated treatment, all lesions, per session, maximum five sessions per course of treatment S Z2

G0252 PET imaging, full and partial-ring PET scanners only, for initial diagnosis of breast cancer and/or surgical planning for breast cancer (e.g. initial staging of axillary lymph nodes) E

Pub 100-03, 1, 220.6, 220.6.17, 220.6.19

G0255 Current perception threshold/sensory nerve conduction test, (SNCT) per limb, any nerve E

NCD 160.23

G0257 Unscheduled or emergency dialysis treatment for an ESRD patient in a hospital outpatient department that is not certified as an ESRD facility S

AHA: 1Q 2003, 9

G0259 Injection procedure for sacroiliac joint; arthrograpy N N1 PQR

G0260 Injection procedure for sacroiliac joint; provision of anesthetic, steroid and/or other therapeutic agent, with or without arthrography T A2 PQR

G0268 Removal of impacted cerumen (one or both ears) by physician on same date of service as audiologic function testing X N1

AHA: 1Q 2003, 12

G0269 Placement of occlusive device into either a venous or arterial access site, post surgical or interventional procedure (e.g. angioseal plug, vascular plug) N N1

G0270 Medical nutrition therapy; reassessment and subsequent intervention(s) following second referral in same year for change in diagnosis, medical condition or treatment regimen (including additional hours needed for renal disease), individual, face to face with the patient, each 15 minutes A PQR

G0271 Medical nutrition therapy, reassessment and subsequent intervention(s) following second referral in same year for change in diagnosis, medical condition, or treatment regimen (including additional hours needed for renal disease), group (2 or more individuals), each 30 minutes A PQR

G0275 Renal angiography, non-selective, one or both kidneys, performed at the same time as cardiac catheterization and/or coronary angiography, includes positioning or placement of any catheter in the abdominal aorta at or near the origins (ostia) of the renal arteries, injection of dye, flush aortogram, production of permanent images, and radiologic supervision and interpretation (list separately in addition to primary procedure) N PQR

G0278 Iliac and/or femoral artery angiography, non-selective, bilateral or ipsilateral to catheter insertion, performed at the same time as cardiac catheterization and/or coronary angiography, includes positioning or placement of the catheter in the distal aorta or ipsilateral femoral or iliac artery, injection of dye, production of permanent images, and radiologic supervision and interpretation (list separately in addition to primary procedure) N PQR

G0281 Electrical stimulation, (unattended), to one or more areas, for chronic stage III and stage IV pressure ulcers, arterial ulcers, diabetic ulcers, and venous statsis ulcers not demonstrating measurable signs of healing after 30 days of conventional care, as part of a therapy plan of care A

Pub 100-04, 32, 11.1

G0282 Electrical stimulation, (unattended), to one or more areas, for wound care other than described in G0281 E

NCD 270.1

G0283 Electrical stimulation (unattended), to one or more areas for indication(s) other than wound care, as part of a therapy plan of care A

G0288 Reconstruction, computed tomographic angiography of aorta for surgical planning for vascular surgery S

G0289 Arthroscopy, knee, surgical, for removal of loose body, foreign body, debridement/shaving of articular cartilage (chrondroplasty) at the time of other surgical knee arthroscopy in a different compartment of the same knee N N1

G0290 Transcatheter placement of a drug eluting intracoronary stent(s), percutaneous, with or without other therapeutic intervention, any method; single vessel T

AHA: 1Q 2007, 7; 3Q 2003, 11

G0291 Transcatheter placement of a drug eluting intracoronary stent(s), percutaneous, with or without other therapeutic intervention, any method; each additional vessel T

AHA: 3Q 2003, 11

G0293 Noncovered surgical procedure(s) using conscious sedation, regional, general or spinal anesthesia in a Medicare qualifying clinical trial, per day X

G0294 Noncovered procedure(s) using either no anesthesia or local anesthesia only, in a Medicare qualifying clinical trial, per day X

G0295 Electromagnetic therapy, to one or more areas, for wound care other than described in G0329 or for other uses E

NCD 270.1

G0302 Pre-operative pulmonary surgery services for preparation for LVRS, complete course of services, to include a minimum of 16 days of services S

G0303 Pre-operative pulmonary surgery services for preparation for LVRS, 10 to 15 days of services S

G0304 Pre-operative pulmonary surgery services for preparation for LVRS, 1 to 9 days of services S

G0305 Post-discharge pulmonary surgery services after LVRS, minimum of 6 days of services S

G0306 Complete CBC, automated (Hgb, Hct, RBC, WBC, without platelet count) and automated WBC differential count A

G0307 Complete (CBC), automated (Hgb, Hct, RBC, WBC; without platelet count) A

G0328 Colorectal cancer screening; fecal occult blood test, immunoassay, 1-3 simultaneous A

Pub 100-02, 15, 80; Pub 100-04, 18, 60-60.8

G0329 Electromagnetic therapy, to one or more areas for chronic stage III and stage IV pressure ulcers, arterial ulcers, diabetic ulcers and venous stasis ulcers not demonstrating measurable signs of healing after 30 days of conventional care as part of a therapy plan of care A

Pub 100-04, 32, 11.2

G0333 Pharmacy dispensing fee for inhalation drug(s); initial 30-day supply as a beneficiary M

Medicare Statute 1842(o)(6)

G0337 Hospice evaluation and counseling services, pre-election B

G0339 Image-guided robotic linear-accelerator-based stereotactic radiosurgery, complete course of therapy in one session or first session of fractionated treatment S Z2

G0340 Image-guided robotic linear-accelerator-based stereotactic radiosurgery, delivery including collimator change and custom plugging, fractionated treatment, all lesions, per session, second through fifth sessions, maximum five sessions per course of treatment S Z2

G0341 Percutaneous islet cell transplant, includes portal vein catheterization and infusion C

NCD 260.3; Pub 100-04, 32, 70-70.5

G0342 Laparoscopy for islet cell transplant, includes portal vein catheterization and infusion C

NCD 260.3; Pub 100-04, 32, 70-70.5

G0343 Laparotomy for islet cell transplant, includes portal vein catheterization and infusion C

NCD 260.3; Pub 100-04, 32, 70-70.5

G0364 Bone marrow aspiration performed with bone marrow biopsy through the same incision on the same date of service X P3

Bone marrow aspiration

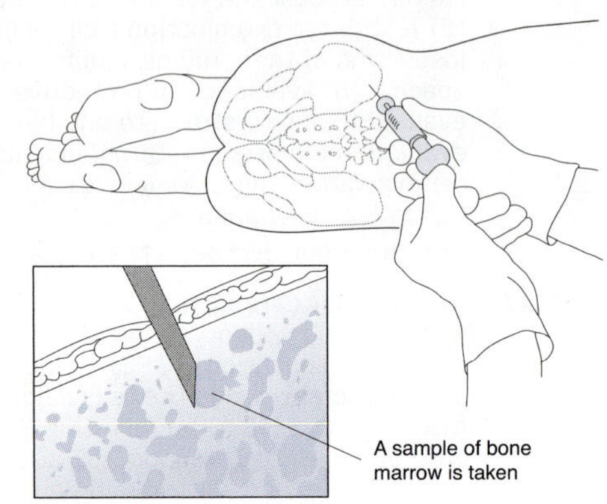

G0365 Vessel mapping of vessels for hemodialysis access (services for preoperative vessel mapping prior to creation of hemodialysis access using an autogenous hemodialysis conduit, including arterial inflow and venous outflow) S PQR

G0372 Physician service required to establish and document the need for a power mobility device M

G0378 Hospital observation service, per hour Q

AHA: 1Q 2007, 10

G0379 Direct admission of patient for hospital observation care Q

G0380 Level 1 hospital emergency department visit provided in a type B emergency department; (the ED must meet at least one of the following requirements: (1) it is licensed by the state in which it is located under applicable state law as an emergency room or emergency department; (2) it is held out to the public (by name, posted signs, advertising, or other means) as a place that provides care for emergency medical conditions on an urgent basis without requiring a previously scheduled appointment; or (3) during the calendar year immediately preceding the calendar year in which a determination under 42 CFR §489.24 is being made, based on a representative sample of patient visits that occurred during that calendar year, it provides at least one-third of all of its outpatient visits for the treatment of emergency medical conditions on an urgent basis without requiring a previously scheduled appointment) V

G0381 Level 2 hospital emergency department visit provided in a type B emergency department; (the ED must meet at least one of the following requirements: (1) it is licensed by the state in which it is located under applicable state law as an emergency room or emergency department; (2) it is held out to the public (by name, posted signs, advertising, or other means) as a place that provides care for emergency medical conditions on an urgent basis without requiring a previously scheduled appointment; or (3) during the calendar year immediately preceding the calendar year in which a determination under 42 CFR §489.24 is being made, based on a representative sample of patient visits that occurred during that calendar year, it provides at least one-third of all of its outpatient visits for the treatment of emergency medical conditions on an urgent basis without requiring a previously scheduled appointment) V

G0382 Level 3 hospital emergency department visit provided in a type B emergency department; (the ED must meet at least one of the following requirements: (1) it is licensed by the state in which it is located under applicable state law as an emergency room or emergency department; (2) it is held out to the public (by name, posted signs, advertising, or other means) as a place that provides care for emergency medical conditions on an urgent basis without requiring a previously scheduled appointment; or (3) during the calendar year immediately preceding the calendar year in which a determination under 42 CFR §489.24 is being made, based on a representative sample of patient visits that occurred during that calendar year, it provides at least one-third of all of its outpatient visits for the treatment of emergency medical conditions on an urgent basis without requiring a previously scheduled appointment) V

G0383 Level 4 hospital emergency department visit provided in a type B emergency department; (the ED must meet at least one of the following requirements: (1) it is licensed by the state in which it is located under applicable state law as an emergency room or emergency department; (2) it is held out to the public (by name, posted signs, advertising, or other means) as a place that provides care for emergency medical conditions on an urgent basis without requiring a previously scheduled appointment; or (3) during the calendar year immediately preceding the calendar year in which a determination under 42 CFR §489.24 is being made, based on a representative sample of patient visits that occurred during that calendar year, it provides at least one-third of all of its outpatient visits for the treatment of emergency medical conditions on an urgent basis without requiring a previously scheduled appointment) V

G0384 Level 5 hospital emergency department visit provided in a type B emergency department; (the ED must meet at least one of the following requirements: (1) it is licensed by the state in which it is located under applicable state law as an emergency room or emergency department; (2) it is held out to the public (by name, posted signs, advertising, or other means) as a place that provides care for emergency medical conditions on an urgent basis without requiring a previously scheduled appointment; or (3) during the calendar year immediately preceding the calendar year in which a determination under 42 CFR §489.24 is being made, based on a representative sample of patient visits that occurred during that calendar year, it provides at least one-third of all of its outpatient visits for the treatment of emergency medical conditions on an urgent basis without requiring a previously scheduled appointment) V

G0389 Ultrasound B-scan and/or real time with image documentation; for abdominal aortic aneurysm (AAA) screening S

Pub 100-02, 15, 80; Pub 100-04, 18, 110-110.3.3

G0390 Trauma response team associated with hospital critical care service S

G0396 Alcohol and/or substance (other than tobacco) abuse structured assessment (e.g., AUDIT, DAST), and brief intervention 15 to 30 minutes S

G0397 Alcohol and/or substance (other than tobacco) abuse structured assessment (e.g., AUDIT, DAST), and intervention, greater than 30 minutes S

G0398 Home sleep study test (HST) with type II portable monitor, unattended; minimum of 7 channels: EEG, EOG, EMG, ECG/heart rate, airflow, respiratory effort and oxygen saturation S

AHA:3Q 2008, 5

G0399 Home sleep test (HST) with type III portable monitor, unattended; minimum of 4 channels: 2 respiratory movement/airflow, 1 ECG/heart rate and 1 oxygen saturation S

AHA: 3Q 2008, 5

G0400 Home sleep test (HST) with type IV portable monitor, unattended; minimum of 3 channels S

AHA: 3Q 2008, 5

G0402 Initial preventive physical examination; face-to-face visit, services limited to new beneficiary during the first 12 months of Medicare enrollment V

G0403 Electrocardiogram, routine ECG with 12 leads; performed as a screening for the initial preventive physical examination with interpretation and report M

G0404 Electrocardiogram, routine ECG with 12 leads; tracing only, without interpretation and report, performed as a screening for the initial preventive physical examination S

G0405 Electrocardiogram, routine ECG with 12 leads; interpretation and report only, performed as a screening for the initial preventive physical examination B

G0406 Follow-up inpatient telehealth consultation, limited, physicians typically spend 15 minutes communicating with the patient via telehealth C

Pub 100-02, 15, 270.2; Pub 100-04, 12, 190.3.1, 190.3.3

G0407 Follow-up inpatient telehealth consultation, intermediate, physicians typically spend 25 minutes communicating with the patient via telehealth C

Pub 100-02, 15, 270.2; Pub 100-04, 12, 190.3.1, 190.3.3

G0408 Follow-up inpatient telehealth consultation, complex, physicians typically spend 35 minutes or more communicating with the patient via telehealth C

Pub 100-02, 15, 270.2; Pub 100-04, 12, 190.3.1, 190.3.3

G0409 Social work and psychological services, directly relating to and/or furthering the patient's rehabilitation goals, each 15 minutes, face-to-face; individual (services provided by a CORF-qualified social worker or psychologist in a CORF) M

G0410 Group psychotherapy other than of a multiple-family group, in a partial hospitalization setting, approximately 45 to 50 minutes P

G0411 Interactive group psychotherapy, in a partial hospitalization setting, approximately 45 to 50 minutes P

G0412 Open treatment of iliac spine(s), tuberosity avulsion, or iliac wing fracture(s), unilateral or bilateral for pelvic bone fracture patterns which do not disrupt the pelvic ring includes internal fixation, when performed C

G0413 Percutaneous skeletal fixation of posterior pelvic bone fracture and/or dislocation, for fracture patterns which disrupt the pelvic ring, unilateral or bilateral, (includes ilium, sacroiliac joint and/or sacrum) T

G0414 Open treatment of anterior pelvic bone fracture and/or dislocation for fracture patterns which disrupt the pelvic ring, unilateral or bilateral, includes internal fixation when performed (includes pubic symphysis and/or superior/inferior rami) C

G0415 Open treatment of posterior pelvic bone fracture and/or dislocation, for fracture patterns which disrupt the pelvic ring, unilateral or bilateral, includes internal fixation, when performed (includes ilium, sacroiliac joint and/or sacrum) C

G0416 Surgical pathology, gross and microscopic examination for prostate needle saturation biopsy sampling, 1-20 specimens ♂ S

G0417 Surgical pathology, gross and microscopic examination for prostate needle saturation biopsy sampling, 21-40 specimens ♂ S

G0418 Surgical pathology, gross and microscopic examination for prostate needle saturation biopsy sampling, 41-60 specimens ♂ S

G0419 Surgical pathology, gross and microscopic examination for prostate needle saturation biopsy sampling, greater than 60 specimens ♂ S

G0420 Face-to-face educational services related to the care of chronic kidney disease; individual, per session, per one hour A

G0421 Face-to-face educational services related to the care of chronic kidney disease; group, per session, per one hour A

G0422 Intensive cardiac rehabilitation; with or without continuous ECG monitoring with exercise, per session S

G0423 Intensive cardiac rehabilitation; with or without continuous ECG monitoring; without exercise, per session S

G0424 Pulmonary rehabilitation, including exercise (includes monitoring), one hour, per session, up to two sessions per day S

G0425 Initial inpatient telehealth consultation, typically 30 minutes communicating with the patient via telehealth C

Pub 100-02, 15, 270.2; Pub 100-04, 12, 190.3.1, 190.3.2

G0426 Initial inpatient telehealth consultation, typically 50 minutes communicating with the patient via telehealth C

Pub 100-02, 15, 270.2; Pub 100-04, 12, 190.3.1, 190.3.2

G0427 Initial inpatient telehealth consultation, typically 70 minutes or more communicating with the patient via telehealth C

Pub 100-02, 15, 270.2; Pub 100-04, 12, 190.3.1, 190.3.2

● ⃠ G0428 Collagen meniscus implant procedure for filling meniscal defects (e.g., CMI, collagen scaffold, menaflex) A

This code was effective May 25, 2010

● G0429 Dermal filler injection(s) for the treatment of facial lipodystrophy syndrome (LDS) (e.g., as a result of highly active antiretroviral therapy) A

This code was effective March 23, 2010

✖ ~~G0430 Drug screen, qualitative; multiple drug classes other than chromatographic method, each procedure~~

This code is deleted as of December 31, 2010

See CPT© code(s) 80104

▲ G0431 Drug screen, qualitative; multiple drug classes by high complexity test method (e.g., immunoassay, enzyme assay), per patient encounter A

● G0432 Infectious agent antibody detection by enzyme immunoassay (EIA) technique, HIV-1 and/or HIV-2, screening A

This code was effective December 8, 2010

● G0433 Infectious agent antibody detection by enzyme-linked immunosorbent assay (ELISA) technique, HIV-1 and/or HIV-2, screening A

This code was effective December 8, 2010

● G0434 Drug screen, other than chromatographic; any number of drug classes, by CLIA waived test or moderate complexity test, per patient encounter A

This code is effective January 1, 2011

● G0435 Infectious agent antibody detection by rapid antibody test, HIV-1 and/or HIV-2, screening A

This code was effective December 8, 2010

● G0436 Smoking and tobacco cessation counseling visit for the asymptomatic patient; intermediate, greater than 3 minutes, up to 10 minutes A

This code is effective January 1, 2011

● G0437 Smoking and tobacco cessation counseling visit for the asymptomatic patient; intensive, greater than 10 minutes A

This code is effective January 1, 2011

● G0438 Annual wellness visit; includes a personalized prevention plan of service (PPS), initial visit A

This code is effective January 1, 2011

● G0439 Annual wellness visit, includes a personalized prevention plan of service (PPS), subsequent visit A

This code is effective January 1, 2011

● G0440 Application of tissue cultured allogeneic skin substitute or dermal substitute; for use on lower limb, includes the site preparation and debridement if performed; first 25 sq cm or less A

This code is effective January 1, 2011

● G0441 Application of tissue cultured allogeneic skin substitute or dermal substitute; for use on lower limb, includes the site preparation and debridement if performed; each additional 25 sq cm A

This code is effective January 1, 2011

G3001 Administration and supply of tositumomab, 450 mg S

Performance Measures

✖ ~~G8006 Acute myocardial infarction: patient documented to have received aspirin at arrival~~

This code is deleted as of December 31, 2010

✖ ~~G8007 Acute myocardial infarction: patient not documented to have received aspirin at arrival~~

This code is deleted as of December 31, 2010

✖ ~~G8008 Clinician documented that acute myocardial infarction patient was not an eligible candidate to receive aspirin at arrival measure~~

This code is deleted as of December 31, 2010

✖ ~~G8009 Acute myocardial infarction: patient documented to have received beta-blocker at arrival~~

This code is deleted as of December 31, 2010

✖ ~~G8010 Acute myocardial infarction: patient not documented to have received beta-blocker at arrival~~

This code is deleted as of December 31, 2010

✖ ~~G8011 Clinician documented that acute myocardial infarction patient was not an eligible candidate for beta-blocker at arrival measure~~

This code is deleted as of December 31, 2010

✖ ~~G8012 Pneumonia: patient documented to have received antibiotic within 4 hours of presentation~~

This code is deleted as of December 31, 2010

⃠ Medicare Non-Coverage ⓘ Special Coverage Instructions Coverage Carrier Determined A – Y APC Status Indicators ● New Code ▲ Revised Code ✖ Deleted Code
AHA AHA Coding Clinic for HCPCS A2 – Z3 ASC Payment Indicators DMEPOS ♂ Male ♀ Female PQRI PQRI

✖ ~~G8013 Pneumonia: patient not documented to have received antibiotic within 4 hours of presentation~~
This code is deleted as of December 31, 2010

✖ ~~G8014 Clinician documented that pneumonia patient was not an eligible candidate for antibiotic within 4 hours of presentation measure~~
This code is deleted as of December 31, 2010

✖ ~~G8015 Diabetic patient with most recent hemoglobin A1c level (within the last 6 months) documented as greater than 9%~~
This code is deleted as of December 31, 2010

✖ ~~G8016 Diabetic patient with most recent hemoglobin A1c level (within the last 6 months) documented as less than or equal to 9%~~
This code is deleted as of December 31, 2010

✖ ~~G8017 Clinician documented that diabetic patient was not eligible candidate for hemoglobin A1c measure~~
This code is deleted as of December 31, 2010

✖ ~~G8018 Clinician has not provided care for the diabetic patient for the required time for hemoglobin A1c measure (6 months)~~
This code is deleted as of December 31, 2010

✖ ~~G8019 Diabetic patient with most recent low-density lipoprotein (within the last 12 months) documented as greater than or equal to 100 mg/dL~~
This code is deleted as of December 31, 2010

✖ ~~G8020 Diabetic patient with most recent low-density lipoprotein (within the last 12 months) documented as less than 100 mg/dL~~
This code is deleted as of December 31, 2010

✖ ~~G8021 Clinician documented that diabetic patient was not eligible candidate for low-density lipoprotein measure~~
This code is deleted as of December 31, 2010

✖ ~~G8022 Clinician has not provided care for the diabetic patient for the required time for low-density lipoprotein measure (12 months)~~
This code is deleted as of December 31, 2010

✖ ~~G8023 Diabetic patient with most recent blood pressure (within the last 6 months) documented as equal to or greater than 140 systolic or equal to or greater than 80 mmHg diastolic~~
This code is deleted as of December 31, 2010

✖ ~~G8024 Diabetic patient with most recent blood pressure (within the last 6 months) documented as less than 140 systolic and less than 80 diastolic~~
This code is deleted as of December 31, 2010

✖ ~~G8025 Clinician documented that the diabetic patient was not eligible candidate for blood pressure measure~~
This code is deleted as of December 31, 2010

✖ ~~G8026 Clinician has not provided care for the diabetic patient for the required time for blood pressure measure (within the last 6 months)~~
This code is deleted as of December 31, 2010

✖ ~~G8027 Heart failure patient with left ventricular systolic dysfunction (LVSD) documented to be on either angiotensin-converting enzyme inhibitor or angiotensin-receptor blocker (ACE-I or ARB) therapy~~
This code is deleted as of December 31, 2010

✖ ~~G8028 Heart failure patient with left ventricular systolic dysfunction (LVSD) not documented to be on either angiotensin-converting enzyme inhibitor or angiotensin-receptor blocker (ACE-I or ARB) therapy~~
This code is deleted as of December 31, 2010

✖ ~~G8029 Clinician documented that heart failure patient was not an eligible candidate for either angiotensin-converting enzyme inhibitor or angiotensin-receptor blocker (ACE-I or ARB) therapy measure~~
This code is deleted as of December 31, 2010

✖ ~~G8030 Heart failure patient with left ventricular systolic dysfunction (LVSD) documented to be on beta-blocker therapy~~
This code is deleted as of December 31, 2010

✖ ~~G8031 Heart failure patient with left ventricular systolic dysfunction (LVSD) not documented to be on beta-blocker therapy~~
This code is deleted as of December 31, 2010

✖ ~~G8032 Clinician documented that heart failure patient was not eligible candidate for beta-blocker therapy measure~~
This code is deleted as of December 31, 2010

✖ ~~G8033 Prior myocardial infarction – coronary artery disease patient documented to be on beta-blocker therapy~~
This code is deleted as of December 31, 2010

✖ ~~G8034 Prior myocardial infarction – coronary artery disease patient not documented to be on beta-blocker therapy~~
This code is deleted as of December 31, 2010

✖ ~~G8035 Clinician documented that prior myocardial infarction – coronary artery disease patient was not eligible candidate for beta-blocker therapy measure~~
This code is deleted as of December 31, 2010

✖ ~~G8036 Coronary artery disease patient documented to be on antiplatelet therapy~~
This code is deleted as of December 31, 2010

✖ ~~G8037 Coronary artery disease patient not documented to be on antiplatelet therapy~~
This code is deleted as of December 31, 2010

✖ ~~G8038 Clinician documented that coronary artery disease patient was not eligible candidate for antiplatelet therapy measure~~
This code is deleted as of December 31, 2010

✖ ~~G8039 Coronary artery disease – patient with low-density lipoprotein documented to be greater than 100mg/dL~~
This code is deleted as of December 31, 2010

✖ ~~G8040 Coronary artery disease – patient with low-density lipoprotein documented to be less than or equal to 100mg/dL~~
This code is deleted as of December 31, 2010

✖ ~~G8041 Clinician documented that coronary artery disease patient was not eligible candidate for low-density lipoprotein measure~~
This code is deleted as of December 31, 2010

✖ ~~G8051 Patient (female) documented to have been assessed for osteoporosis~~
This code is deleted as of December 31, 2010

✖ ~~G8052 Patient (female) not documented to have been assessed for osteoporosis~~
This code is deleted as of December 31, 2010

✖ ~~G8053 Clinician documented that (female) patient was not an eligible candidate for osteoporosis assessment measure~~
This code is deleted as of December 31, 2010

✖ ~~G8054 Patient not documented for the assessment for falls within last 12 months~~
This code is deleted as of December 31, 2010

✖ ~~G8055 Patient documented for the assessment for falls within last 12 months~~
This code is deleted as of December 31, 2010

✖ ~~G8056 Clinician documented that patient was not an eligible candidate for the falls assessment measure within the last 12 months~~
This code is deleted as of December 31, 2010

✖ ~~G8057 Patient documented to have received hearing assessment~~
This code is deleted as of December 31, 2010

✖ ~~G8058 Patient not documented to have received hearing assessment~~
This code is deleted as of December 31, 2010

✖ ~~G8059 Clinician documented that patient was not an eligible candidate for hearing assessment measure~~
This code is deleted as of December 31, 2010

✖ ~~G8060 Patient documented for the assessment of urinary incontinence~~
This code is deleted as of December 31, 2010

× ~~G8061 Patient not documented for the assessment of urinary incontinence~~
This code is deleted as of December 31, 2010

× ~~G8062 Clinician documented that patient was not an eligible candidate for urinary incontinence assessment measure~~
This code is deleted as of December 31, 2010

× ~~G8075 End stage renal disease patient with documented dialysis dose of URR greater than or equal to 65% (or Kt/V greater than or equal to 1.2)~~
This code is deleted as of December 31, 2010

× ~~G8076 End stage renal disease patient with documented dialysis dose of URR less than 65% (or Kt/V less than 1.2)~~
This code is deleted as of December 31, 2010

× ~~G8077 Clinician documented that end stage renal disease patient was not an eligible candidate for URR or Kt/V measure~~
This code is deleted as of December 31, 2010

× ~~G8078 End stage renal disease patient with documented hematocrit greater than or equal to 33 (or hemoglobin greater than or equal to 11)~~
This code is deleted as of December 31, 2010

× ~~G8079 End stage renal disease patient with documented hematocrit less than 33 (or hemoglobin less than 11)~~
This code is deleted as of December 31, 2010

× ~~G8080 Clinician documented that end stage renal disease patient was not an eligible candidate for hematocrit (hemoglobin) measure~~
This code is deleted as of December 31, 2010

× ~~G8081 End stage renal disease patient requiring hemodialysis vascular access documented to have received autogenous AV fistula~~
This code is deleted as of December 31, 2010

× ~~G8082 End stage renal disease patient requiring hemodialysis documented to have received vascular access other than autogenous AV fistula~~
This code is deleted as of December 31, 2010

× ~~G8085 End-stage renal disease patient requiring hemodialysis vascular access was not an eligible candidate for autogenous AV fistula~~
This code is deleted as of December 31, 2010

× ~~G8093 Newly diagnosed chronic obstructive pulmonary disease (COPD) patient documented to have received smoking cessation intervention, within 3 months of diagnosis~~
This code is deleted as of December 31, 2010

× ~~G8094 Newly diagnosed chronic obstructive pulmonary disease (COPD) patient not documented to have received smoking cessation intervention, within 3 months of diagnosis~~
This code is deleted as of December 31, 2010

× ~~G8099 Osteoporosis patient documented to have been prescribed calcium and vitamin D supplements~~
This code is deleted as of December 31, 2010

× ~~G8100 Clinician documented that osteoporosis patient was not an eligible candidate for calcium and vitamin D supplement measure~~
This code is deleted as of December 31, 2010

× ~~G8103 Newly diagnosed osteoporosis patients documented to have been treated with antiresorptive therapy and/or PTH within 3 months of diagnosis~~
This code is deleted as of December 31, 2010

× ~~G8104 Clinician documented that newly diagnosed osteoporosis patient was not an eligible candidate for antiresorptive therapy and/or PTH treatment measure within 3 months of diagnosis~~
This code is deleted as of December 31, 2010

× ~~G8106 Within 6 months of suffering a nontraumatic fracture, female patient 65 years of age or older documented to have undergone bone mineral density testing or to have been prescribed a drug to treat or prevent osteoporosis~~
This code is deleted as of December 31, 2010

× ~~G8107 Clinician documented that female patient 65 years of age or older who suffered a nontraumatic fracture within the last 6 months was not an eligible candidate for measure to test bone mineral density or drug to treat or prevent osteoporosis~~
This code is deleted as of December 31, 2010

× ~~G8108 Patient documented to have received influenza vaccination during influenza season~~
This code is deleted as of December 31, 2010

× ~~G8109 Patient not documented to have received influenza vaccination during influenza season~~
This code is deleted as of December 31, 2010

× ~~G8110 Clinician documented that patient was not an eligible candidate for influenza vaccination measure~~
This code is deleted as of December 31, 2010

× ~~G8111 Patient (female) documented to have received a mammogram during the measurement year or prior year to the measurement year~~
This code is deleted as of December 31, 2010

× ~~G8112 Patient (female) not documented to have received a mammogram during the measurement year or prior year to the measurement year~~
This code is deleted as of December 31, 2010

× ~~G8113 Clinician documented that female patient was not an eligible candidate for mammography measure~~
This code is deleted as of December 31, 2010

× ~~G8114 Clinician did not provide care to patient for the required time of mammography measure (i.e., measurement year or prior year)~~
This code is deleted as of December 31, 2010

× ~~G8115 Patient documented to have received pneumococcal vaccination~~
This code is deleted as of December 31, 2010

× ~~G8116 Patient not documented to have received pneumococcal vaccination~~
This code is deleted as of December 31, 2010

× ~~G8117 Clinician documented that patient was not an eligible candidate for pneumococcal vaccination measure~~
This code is deleted as of December 31, 2010

G8126 Patient documented as being treated with antidepressant medication during the entire 12 week acute treatment phase PQR M

G8127 Patient not documented as being treated with antidepressant medication during the entire 12 weeks acute treatment phase PQR M

G8128 Clinician documented that patient was not an eligible candidate for antidepressant medication during the entire 12 week acute treatment phase measure PQR M

× ~~G8129 Patient documented as being treated with antidepressant medication for at least 6 months continuous treatment phase~~
This code is deleted as of December 31, 2010

× ~~G8130 Patient not documented as being treated with antidepressant medication for at least 6 months continuous treatment phase~~
This code is deleted as of December 31, 2010

× ~~G8131 Clinician documented that patient was not an eligible candidate for antidepressant medication for continuous treatment phase~~
This code is deleted as of December 31, 2010

× ~~G8152 Patient documented to have received antibiotic prophylaxis one hour prior to incision time (two hours for vancomycin)~~
This code is deleted as of December 31, 2010

✖ ~~G8153 Patient not documented to have received antibiotic prophylaxis one hour prior to incision time (two hours for vancomycin)~~
This code is deleted as of December 31, 2010

✖ ~~G8154 Clinician documented that patient was not an eligible candidate for antibiotic prophylaxis one hour prior to incision time (two hours for vancomycin) measure~~
This code is deleted as of December 31, 2010

✖ ~~G8155 Patient with documented receipt of thromboembolism prophylaxis~~
This code is deleted as of December 31, 2010

✖ ~~G8156 Patient without documented receipt of thromboembolism prophylaxis~~
This code is deleted as of December 31, 2010

✖ ~~G8157 Clinician documented that patient was not an eligible candidate for thromboembolism prophylaxis measure~~
This code is deleted as of December 31, 2010

✖ ~~G8159 Patient documented to have received coronary artery bypass graft without use of internal mammary artery~~
This code is deleted as of December 31, 2010

✖ ~~G8162 Patient with isolated coronary artery bypass graft not documented to have received pre-operative beta blockade~~
This code is deleted as of December 31, 2010

✖ ~~G8164 Patient with isolated coronary artery bypass graft documented to have prolonged intubation~~
This code is deleted as of December 31, 2010

✖ ~~G8165 Patient with isolated coronary artery bypass graft not documented to have prolonged intubation~~
This code is deleted as of December 31, 2010

✖ ~~G8166 Patient with isolated coronary artery bypass graft documented to have required surgical re-exploration~~
This code is deleted as of December 31, 2010

✖ ~~G8167 Patient with isolated coronary artery bypass graft did not require surgical re-exploration~~
This code is deleted as of December 31, 2010

✖ ~~G8170 Patient with isolated coronary artery bypass graft documented to have been discharged on aspirin or clopidogrel~~
This code is deleted as of December 31, 2010

✖ ~~G8171 Patient with isolated coronary artery bypass graft not documented to have been discharged on aspirin or clopidogrel~~
This code is deleted as of December 31, 2010

✖ ~~G8172 Clinician documented that patient with isolated coronary artery bypass graft was not an eligible candidate for antiplatelet therapy at discharge measure~~
This code is deleted as of December 31, 2010

✖ ~~G8182 Clinician has not provided care for the cardiac patient for the required time for low-density lipoprotein measure (6 months)~~
This code is deleted as of December 31, 2010

✖ ~~G8183 Patient with heart failure and atrial fibrillation documented to be on warfarin therapy~~
This code is deleted as of December 31, 2010

✖ ~~G8184 Clinician documented that patient with heart failure and atrial fibrillation was not an eligible candidate for warfarin therapy measure~~
This code is deleted as of December 31, 2010

✖ ~~G8185 Patients diagnosed with symptomatic osteoarthritis with documented annual assessment of function and pain~~
This code is deleted as of December 31, 2010

✖ ~~G8186 Clinician documented that symptomatic osteoarthritis patient was not an eligible candidate for annual assessment of function and pain measure~~
This code is deleted as of December 31, 2010

✖ ~~G8193 Clinician did not document that an order for prophylactic antibiotic to be given within one hour (if vancomycin, two hours) prior to surgical incision (or start of procedure when no incision is required) was given~~
This code is deleted as of December 31, 2010

✖ ~~G8196 Clinician did not document a prophylactic antibiotic was administered within one hour (if vancomycin, two hours) prior to surgical incision (or start of procedure when no incision is required)~~
This code is deleted as of December 31, 2010

✖ ~~G8200 Order for cefazolin or cefuroxime for antimicrobial prophylaxis not documented~~
This code is deleted as of December 31, 2010

✖ ~~G8204 Clinician did not document an order was given to discontinue prophylactic antibiotics within 24 hours of surgical end time~~
This code is deleted as of December 31, 2010

✖ ~~G8209 Clinician did not document an order was given to discontinue prophylactic antibiotics within 48 hours of surgical end time~~
This code is deleted as of December 31, 2010

✖ ~~G8214 Clinician did not document an order was given for appropriate venous thromboembolism (VTE) prophylaxis to be given within 24 hrs prior to incision time or 24 hours after surgery end time~~
This code is deleted as of December 31, 2010

✖ ~~G8217 Patient not documented to have received DVT prophylaxis by end of hospital day 2~~
This code is deleted as of December 31, 2010

✖ ~~G8219 Patient documented to have received DVT prophylaxis by end of hospital day 2~~
This code is deleted as of December 31, 2010

✖ ~~G8220 Patient not documented to have received DVT prophylaxis by end of hospital day 2~~
This code is deleted as of December 31, 2010

✖ ~~G8221 Clinician documented that patient was not an eligible candidate for DVT prophylaxis by the end of hospital day 2, including physician documentation that patient is ambulatory~~
This code is deleted as of December 31, 2010

✖ ~~G8223 Patient not documented to have received prescription for antiplatelet therapy at discharge~~
This code is deleted as of December 31, 2010

✖ ~~G8226 Patient not documented to have received prescription for anticoagulant therapy at discharge~~
This code is deleted as of December 31, 2010

✖ ~~G8231 Patient not documented to have received t-PA or not documented to have been considered a candidate for t-PA administration~~
This code is deleted as of December 31, 2010

✖ ~~G8234 Patient not documented to have received dysphagia screening~~
This code is deleted as of December 31, 2010

✖ ~~G8238 Patient not documented to have received order for or consideration for rehabilitation services~~
This code is deleted as of December 31, 2010

✖ ~~G8240 Internal carotid stenosis patient in the 30-99% range, and no documentation of reference to measurements of distal internal carotid diameter as the denominator for stenosis measurement~~
This code is deleted as of December 31, 2010

✖ ~~G8243 Patient not documented to have received CT or MRI and the presence or absence of hemorrhage, mass lesion and acute infarction not documented in the final report~~
This code is deleted as of December 31, 2010

✖ ~~G8246 Patient was not an eligible candidate for medical history review with assessment of new or changing moles~~
This code is deleted as of December 31, 2010

✖ ~~G8248 Patient with at least one alarm symptom not documented to have had upper endoscopy or referral for upper endoscopy~~
This code is deleted as of December 31, 2010

✖ ~~G8251 Patient not documented to have received an esophageal biopsy when suspicion of Barrett's esophagus is indicated in the endoscopy report~~
This code is deleted as of December 31, 2010

✖ ~~G8254 Patient with no documentation order for barium swallow test~~
This code is deleted as of December 31, 2010

✖ ~~G8257 Clinician has not documented reconciliation of discharge medications with current medication list in medical record~~
This code is deleted as of December 31, 2010

✖ ~~G8260 Patient not documented to have surrogate decision maker or advance care plan in medical record~~
This code is deleted as of December 31, 2010

✖ ~~G8263 Patient not documented to have been assessed for presence or absence of urinary incontinence~~
This code is deleted as of December 31, 2010

✖ ~~G8266 Patient not documented to have received characterization of urinary incontinence~~
This code is deleted as of December 31, 2010

✖ ~~G8268 Patient not documented to have received plan of care for urinary incontinence~~
This code is deleted as of December 31, 2010

✖ ~~G8271 Patient with no documentation of screening for fall risks (2 or more falls in the past year or any fall with injury in the past year)~~
This code is deleted as of December 31, 2010

✖ ~~G8274 Clinician has not documented presence or absence of alarm symptoms~~
This code is deleted as of December 31, 2010

✖ ~~G8276 Patient not documented to have received medical history with assessment of new or changing moles~~
This code is deleted as of December 31, 2010

✖ ~~G8279 Patient not documented to have received a complete physical skin exam~~
This code is deleted as of December 31, 2010

✖ ~~G8282 Patient not documented to have received counseling to perform a self-examination~~
This code is deleted as of December 31, 2010

✖ ~~G8285 Patient not documented to have received pharmacologic therapy~~
This code is deleted as of December 31, 2010

✖ ~~G8289 Patient with no documentation of calcium and vitamin D use or counseling regarding both calcium and vitamin D use, or exercise~~
This code is deleted as of December 31, 2010

✖ ~~G8293 COPD patient without spirometry results documented~~
This code is deleted as of December 31, 2010

✖ ~~G8296 COPD patient not documented to have inhaled bronchodilator therapy prescribed~~
This code is deleted as of December 31, 2010

✖ ~~G8298 Patient documented to have received optic nerve head evaluation~~
This code is deleted as of December 31, 2010

✖ ~~G8299 Patient not documented to have received optic nerve head evaluation~~
This code is deleted as of December 31, 2010

✖ ~~G8302 Patient documented to have a specific target intraocular pressure range goal~~
This code is deleted as of December 31, 2010

✖ ~~G8303 Patient not documented to have a specific target intraocular pressure range goal~~
This code is deleted as of December 31, 2010

✖ ~~G8304 Clinician documented that patient was not an eligible candidate for a specific target intraocular pressure range goal~~
This code is deleted as of December 31, 2010

✖ ~~G8305 Clinician has not provided care for the primary open-angle glaucoma patient for the required time for treatment range goal documentation measurement~~
This code is deleted as of December 31, 2010

✖ ~~G8306 Primary open-angle glaucoma patient with intraocular pressure above the target range goal documented to have received plan of care~~
This code is deleted as of December 31, 2010

✖ ~~G8307 Primary open-angle glaucoma patient with intraocular pressure at or below goal, no plan of care necessary~~
This code is deleted as of December 31, 2010

✖ ~~G8308 Primary open-angle glaucoma patient with intraocular pressure above the target range goal, and not documented to have received plan of care during the reporting year~~
This code is deleted as of December 31, 2010

✖ ~~G8310 Patient not documented to have been prescribed/recommended at least one antioxidant vitamin or mineral supplement during the reporting year~~
This code is deleted as of December 31, 2010

✖ ~~G8314 Patient not documented to have received macular exam with documentation of presence or absence of macular thickening or hemorrhage and no documentation of level of macular degeneration severity~~
This code is deleted as of December 31, 2010

✖ ~~G8318 Patient documented not to have visual functional status assessed~~
This code is deleted as of December 31, 2010

✖ ~~G8322 Patient not documented to have had pre-surgical axial length, corneal power measurement and method of intraocular lens power calculation~~
This code is deleted as of December 31, 2010

✖ ~~G8326 Patient not documented to have received fundus evaluation within six months prior to cataract surgery~~
This code is deleted as of December 31, 2010

✖ ~~G8330 Patient not documented to have received dilated macular or fundus exam with level of severity of retinopathy and the presence or absence of macular edema not documented~~
This code is deleted as of December 31, 2010

✖ ~~G8334 Documentation of findings of macular or fundus exam not communicated to the physician managing the patient's ongoing diabetes care~~
This code is deleted as of December 31, 2010

✖ ~~G8338 Clinician has not documented that communication was sent to the physician managing ongoing care of patient that a fracture occurred and that the patient was or should be tested or treated for osteoporosis~~
This code is deleted as of December 31, 2010

✖ ~~G8341 Patient not documented to have had central DEXA measurement or pharmacologic therapy~~
This code is deleted as of December 31, 2010

✖ ~~G8345 Patient not documented to have had central DEXA measurement ordered or performed or pharmacologic therapy~~
This code is deleted as of December 31, 2010

✖ ~~G8351 Patient not documented to have had ECG~~
This code is deleted as of December 31, 2010

✖ ~~G8354 Patient not documented to have received or taken aspirin 24 hours before emergency department arrival or during emergency department stay~~
This code is deleted as of December 31, 2010

✖ ~~G8357 Patient not documented to have had ECG~~
This code is deleted as of December 31, 2010

× ~~G8360 Patient not documented to have vital signs recorded and reviewed~~
This code is deleted as of December 31, 2010

× ~~G8362 Patient not documented to have oxygen saturation assessed~~
This code is deleted as of December 31, 2010

× ~~G8365 Patient not documented to have mental status assessed~~
This code is deleted as of December 31, 2010

× ~~G8367 Patient not documented to have appropriate empiric antibiotic prescribed~~
This code is deleted as of December 31, 2010

× ~~G8370 Asthma patients with numeric frequency of symptoms or patient completion of an asthma assessment tool/survey/questionnaire not documented~~
This code is deleted as of December 31, 2010

× ~~G8371 Chemotherapy documented as not received or prescribed for stage III colon cancer patients~~
This code is deleted as of December 31, 2010

× ~~G8372 Chemotherapy documented as received or prescribed for stage III colon cancer patients~~
This code is deleted as of December 31, 2010

× ~~G8373 Chemotherapy plan documented prior to chemotherapy administration~~
This code is deleted as of December 31, 2010

× ~~G8374 Chemotherapy plan not documented prior to chemotherapy administration~~
This code is deleted as of December 31, 2010

× ~~G8375 Chronic lymphocytic leukemia (CLL) patient with no documentation of baseline flow cytometry performed~~
This code is deleted as of December 31, 2010

× ~~G8376 Clinician documentation that breast cancer patient was not eligible for tamoxifen or aromatase inhibitor therapy measure~~
This code is deleted as of December 31, 2010

× ~~G8377 Clinician documentation that colon cancer patient is not eligible for chemotherapy measure~~
This code is deleted as of December 31, 2010

× ~~G8378 Clinician documentation that patient was not an eligible candidate for radiation therapy measure~~
This code is deleted as of December 31, 2010

× ~~G8379 Documentation of radiation therapy recommended within 12 months of first office visit~~
This code is deleted as of December 31, 2010

× ~~G8380 For patients with ER or PR positive stage IC-III breast cancer, clinician did not document that the patient received or was prescribed tamoxifen or aromatase inhibitor~~
This code is deleted as of December 31, 2010

× ~~G8381 For patients with ER or PR positive stage IC-III breast cancer, clinician documented or prescribed that the patient is receiving tamoxifen or aromatase inhibitor~~
This code is deleted as of December 31, 2010

× ~~G8382 Multiple myeloma patients with no documentation of prescribed or received intravenous bisphosphonate therapy~~
This code is deleted as of December 31, 2010

× ~~G8383 No documentation of radiation therapy recommended within 12 months of first office visit~~
This code is deleted as of December 31, 2010

× ~~G8384 Baseline cytogenetic testing not performed in patients with myelodysplastic syndrome (MDS) or acute l eukemias~~
This code is deleted as of December 31, 2010

× ~~G8385 Diabetic patients with no documentation of hemoglobin A1c level (within the last 12 months)~~
This code is deleted as of December 31, 2010

× ~~G8386 Diabetic patients with no documentation of low-density lipoprotein (within the last 12 months)~~
This code is deleted as of December 31, 2010

× ~~G8387 End-stage renal disease patient with a hematocrit or hemoglobin not documented~~
This code is deleted as of December 31, 2010

× ~~G8388 End-stage renal disease patient with URR or Kt/V value not documented, but otherwise eligible for measure~~
This code is deleted as of December 31, 2010

× ~~G8389 Myelodysplastic syndrome (MDS) patients with no documentation of iron stores prior to receiving erythropoietin therapy~~
This code is deleted as of December 31, 2010

× ~~G8390 Diabetic patients with no documentation of blood pressure measurement (within the last 12 months)~~
This code is deleted as of December 31, 2010

× ~~G8391 Patients with persistent asthma, no documentation of preferred long term control medication or acceptable alternative treatment prescribed~~
This code is deleted as of December 31, 2010

G8395 Left ventricular ejection fraction (LVEF) ≥ 40% or documentation as normal or mildly depressed left ventricular systolic function PQR M

G8396 Left ventricular ejection fraction (LVEF) not performed or documented PQR M

G8397 Dilated macular or fundus exam performed, including documentation of the presence or absence of macular edema and level of severity of retinopathy PQR M

G8398 Dilated macular or fundus exam not performed PQR M

G8399 Patient with central dual-energy x-ray absorptiometry (DXA) results documented or ordered or pharmacologic therapy (other than minerals/vitamins) for osteoporosis prescribed PQR M

G8400 Patient with central dual-energy x-ray absorptiometry (DXA) results not documented or not ordered or pharmacologic therapy (other than minerals/vitamins) for osteoporosis not prescribed PQR M

G8401 Clinician documented that patient was not an eligible candidate for screening or therapy for osteoporosis for women measure PQR M

× ~~G8402 Tobacco (smoke) use cessation intervention, counseling~~
This code is deleted as of December 31, 2010

× ~~G8403 Tobacco (smoke) use cessation intervention not counseled~~
This code is deleted as of December 31, 2010

G8404 Lower extremity neurological exam performed and documented PQR M

G8405 Lower extremity neurological exam not performed PQR M

G8406 Clinician documented that patient was not an eligible candidate for lower extremity neurological exam measure PQR M

× ~~G8407 ABI measured and documented~~
This code is deleted as of December 31, 2010

× ~~G8408 ABI measurement was not obtained~~
This code is deleted as of December 31, 2010

× ~~G8409 Clinician documented that patient was not an eligible candidate for ABI measurement measure~~
This code is deleted as of December 31, 2010

G8410 Footwear evaluation performed and documented PQR M

G8415 Footwear evaluation was not performed PQR M

G8416 Clinician documented that patient was not an eligible candidate for footwear evaluation measure PQR M

G8417 Calculated BMI above the upper parameter and a follow-up plan was documented in the medical record PQR M

G8418 Calculated BMI below the lower parameter and a follow-up plan was documented in the medical record PQRI M

G8419 Calculated BMI outside normal parameters, no follow-up plan was documented in the medical record PQRI M

G8420 Calculated BMI within normal parameters and documented PQRI M

G8421 BMI not calculated PQRI M

G8422 Patient not eligible for BMI calculation PQRI M

× ~~G8423 Documented that patient was screened and either influenza vaccination status is current or patient was counseled~~
This code is deleted as of December 31, 2010

× ~~G8424 Influenza vaccine status was not screened~~
This code is deleted as of December 31, 2010

× ~~G8425 Influenza vaccine status screened, patient not current and counseling was not provided~~
This code is deleted as of December 31, 2010

× ~~G8426 Documented that patient was not appropriate for screening and/or counseling about the influenza vaccine (e.g., allergy to eggs)~~
This code is deleted as of December 31, 2010

▲ G8427 List of current medications (includes prescription, over-the-counter, herbals, vitamin/mineral/dietary [nutritional] supplements) documented by the provider, including drug name, dosage, frequency and route PQRI M

▲ G8428 Current medications (includes prescription, over-the-counter, herbals, vitamin/mineral/dietary [nutritional] supplements) with drug name, dosage, frequency and route not documented by the provider, reason not specified PQRI M

× ~~G8429 Incomplete or no provider documentation that patient's current medications with dosages (includes prescription, over-the-counter, herbals, vitamin/mineral/dietary [nutritional] supplements) were assessed~~
This code is deleted as of December 31, 2010

G8430 Provider documentation that patient is not eligible for medication assessment PQRI M

G8431 Positive screen for clinical depression using a standardized tool and a follow-up plan documented PQRI M

G8432 No documentation of clinical depression screening using a standardized tool PQRI M

G8433 Screening for clinical depression using a standardized tool not documented, patient not eligible/appropriate PQRI M

× ~~G8434 Documentation of cognitive impairment screening using a standardized tool~~
This code is deleted as of December 31, 2010

× ~~G8435 No documentation of cognitive impairment screening using a standardized tool~~
This code is deleted as of December 31, 2010

× ~~G8436 Patient not eligible/not appropriate for cognitive impairment screening~~
This code is deleted as of December 31, 2010

× ~~G8437 Documentation of clinician and patient involvement with the development of a plan of care including signature by the practitioner/therapist and either a co-signature by the patient or documented verbal agreement obtained from the patient or, when necessary, an authorized representative~~
This code is deleted as of December 31, 2010

× ~~G8438 No documentation of clinician and patient involvement with the development of a plan of care including signature by the practitioner/therapist and either a co-signature by the patient or documented verbal agreement obtained from the patient or, when necessary, an authorized representative~~
This code is deleted as of December 31, 2010

× ~~G8439 Documentation that patient is not eligible for co-developing a plan of care including signature by the practitioner/therapist and either a co-signature by the patient or documented verbal agreement obtained from the patient or, when necessary, an authorized representative~~
This code is deleted as of December 31, 2010

▲ G8440 Documentation of pain assessment (including location, intensity and description) prior to initiation of therapy or documentation of the absence of pain as a result of assessment through discussion with the patient including the use of a standardized tool and a follow-up plan is documented PQRI M

▲ G8441 No documentation of pain assessment (including location, intensity and description) prior to initiation of therapyt PQRI M

G8442 Documentation that patient is not eligible for pain assessment PQRI M

× ~~G8443 All prescriptions created during the encounter were generated using a qualified e-prescribing system~~
This code is deleted as of December 31, 2010

× ~~G8445 No prescriptions were generated during the encounter, provider does have access to a qualified e-prescribing system~~
This code is deleted as of December 31, 2010

× ~~G8446 Provider does have access to a qualified e-prescribing system and some or all of the prescriptions generated during the encounter were printed or phoned in as required by state or federal law or regulations, patient request or pharmacy system being unable to receive electronic transmission; or because they were for narcotics or other controlled substances~~
This code is deleted as of December 31, 2010

▲ G8447 Patient encounter was documented using an ehr system that has been certified by an authorized testing and certification body (ATCB) PQRI M

▲ G8448 Patient encounter was documented using a PQRI qualified ehr or other acceptable systems PQRI M

× ~~G8449 Patient encounter was not documented using an EMR due to system reasons such as, the system being inoperable at the time of the visit; use of this code implies that an EMR is in place and generally available~~
This code is deleted as of December 31, 2010

G8450 Beta-blocker therapy prescribed for patients with left ventricular ejection fraction (LVEF) <40% or documentation as moderately or severely depressed left ventricular systolic function PQRI M

G8451 Clinician documented patient with left ventricular ejection fraction (LVEF) <40% or documentation as moderately or severely depressed left ventricular systolic function was not eligible candidate for beta-blocker therapy PQRI M

G8452 Beta-blocker therapy not prescribed for patients with left ventricular ejection fraction (LVEF) <40% or documentation as moderately or severely depressed left ventricular systolic function PQRI M

× ~~G8453 Tobacco use cessation intervention, counseling~~
This code is deleted as of December 31, 2010

× ~~G8454 Tobacco use cessation intervention not counseled, reason not specified~~
This code is deleted as of December 31, 2010

× ~~G8455 Current tobacco smoker~~
This code is deleted as of December 31, 2010

× ~~G8456 Current smokeless tobacco user~~
This code is deleted as of December 31, 2010

× ~~G8457 Current tobacco non-user~~
This code is deleted as of December 31, 2010

G8458 Clinician documented that patient is not an eligible candidate for genotype testing; patient not receiving antiviral treatment for hepatitis C PQRI M

Medicare Non-Coverage | Special Coverage Instructions | Coverage Carrier Determined | A – Y APC Status Indicators | ● New Code | ▲ Revised Code | × Deleted Code
AHA AHA Coding Clinic for HCPCS | A2 – Z3 ASC Payment Indicators | DMEPOS | ♂ Male | ♀ Female | PQRI PQRI

G8459 Clinician documented that patient is receiving antiviral treatment for hepatitis C PQR M

G8460 Clinician documented that patient is not an eligible candidate for quantitative RNA testing at week 12; patient not receiving antiviral treatment for hepatitis C PQR M

G8461 Patient receiving antiviral treatment for hepatitis C PQR M

G8462 Clinician documented that patient is not an eligible candidate for counseling regarding contraception prior to antiviral treatment; patient not receiving antiviral treatment for hepatitis C PQR M

G8463 Patient receiving antiviral treatment for hepatitis C documented PQR M

G8464 Clinician documented that prostate cancer patient is not an eligible candidate for adjuvant hormonal therapy; low or intermediate risk of recurrence or risk of recurrence not determined PQR M

G8465 High risk of recurrence of prostate cancer PQR M

× ~~G8466 Clinician documented that patient is not an eligible candidate for suicide risk assessment; major depressive disorder, in remission~~

This code is deleted as of December 31, 2010

× ~~G8467 Documentation of new diagnosis of initial or recurrent episode of major depressive disorder~~

This code is deleted as of December 31, 2010

G8468 Angiotensin converting enzyme (ACE) inhibitor or angiotensin receptor blocker (ARB) therapy prescribed for patients with a left ventricular ejection fraction (LVEF) <40% or documentation of moderately or severely depressed left ventricular systolic function PQR M

G8469 Clinician documented that patient with a left ventricular ejection fraction (LVEF) <40% or documentation of moderately or severely depressed left ventricular systolic function was not an eligible candidate for angiotensin converting enzyme (ACE) inhibitor or angiotensin receptor blocker (ARB) therapy PQR M

G8470 Patient with left ventricular ejection fraction (LVEF) ≥40% or documentation as normal or mildly depressed left ventricular systolic function PQR M

G8471 Left ventricular ejection fraction (LVEF) was not performed or documented PQR M

G8472 Angiotensin converting enzyme (ACE) inhibitor or angiotensin receptor blocker (ARB) therapy not prescribed for patients with a left ventricular ejection fraction (LVEF) <40% or documentation of moderately or severely depressed left ventricular systolic function, reason not specified PQR M

G8473 Angiotensin converting enzyme (ACE) inhibitor or angiotensin receptor blocker (ARB) therapy prescribed PQR M

G8474 Angiotensin converting enzyme (ACE) inhibitor or angiotensin receptor blocker (ARB) therapy not prescribed for reasons documented by the clinician PQR M

G8475 Angiotensin converting enzyme (ACE)inhibitor or angiotensin receptor blocker (ARB) therapy not prescribed, reason not specified PQR M

G8476 Most recent blood pressure has a systolic measurement of <130 mm/Hg and a diastolic measurement of <80 mm/Hg PQR M

G8477 Most recent blood pressure has a systolic measurement of ≥130 mm/Hg and/or a diastolic measurement of ≥80 mm/Hg PQR M

G8478 Blood pressure measurement not performed or documented, reason not specified PQR M

× ~~G8479 Clinician prescribed angiotensin converting enzyme (ACE) inhibitor or angiotensin receptor blocker (ARB) therapy~~

This code is deleted as of December 31, 2010

× ~~G8480 Clinician documented that patient was not an eligible candidate for angiotensin converting enzyme (ACE) inhibitor or angiotensin receptor blocker (ARB) therapy~~

This code is deleted as of December 31, 2010

× ~~G8481 Clinician did not prescribe angiotensin converting enzyme (ACE) inhibitor or angiotensin receptor blocker (ARB) therapy, reason not specified~~

This code is deleted as of December 31, 2010

G8482 Influenza immunization was ordered or administered PQR M

G8483 Influenza immunization was not ordered or administered for reasons documented by clinician PQR M

G8484 Influenza immunization was not ordered or administered, reason not specified PQR M

G8485 I intend to report the diabetes mellitus measures group PQR M

G8486 I intend to report the preventive care measures group PQR M

G8487 I intend to report the chronic kidney disease (CKD) measures group PQR M

× G8488 ~~Clinician intends to report the end stage renal disease (ESRD) measure group~~

This code is deleted as of December 31, 2010

G8489 I intend to report the coronary artery disease (CAD) measures group PQR M

G8490 I intend to report the rheumatoid arthritis measures group PQR M

G8491 I intend to report the HIV/AIDS measures group PQR M

G8492 I intend to report the perioperative care measures group PQR M

G8493 I intend to report the back pain measures group PQR M

G8494 All quality actions for the applicable measures in the diabetes mellitus measures group have been performed for this patient PQR M

G8495 All quality actions for the applicable measures in the CKD measures group have been performed for this patient PQR M

G8496 All quality actions for the applicable measures in the preventive care measures group have been performed for this patient PQR M

G8497 All quality actions for the applicable measures in the coronary artery bypass graft (CABG) measures group have been performed for this patient PQR M

G8498 All quality actions for the applicable measures in the coronary artery disease (CAD) measures group have been performed for this patient PQR M

G8499 All quality actions for the applicable measures in the rheumatoid arthritis measures group have been performed for this patient PQR M

G8500 All quality actions for the applicable measures in the HIV/AIDS measures group have been performed for this patient PQR M

G8501 All quality actions for the applicable measures in the perioperative care measures group have been performed for this patient PQR M

G8502 All quality actions for the applicable measures in the back pain measures group have been performed for this patient PQR M

G8506 Patient receiving angiotensin converting enzyme (ACE) inhibitor or angiotensin receptor blocker (ARB) therapy PQR M

× ~~G8507 Provider documentation that patient is not eligible for patient verification of current medications~~
This code is deleted as of December 31, 2010

▲ G8508 Documentation of pain assessment (including location, intensity and description) prior to initiation of therapy or documentation of the absence of pain as a result of assessment through discussion with the patient including the use of a standardized tool; no documentation of a follow-up plan, patient not eligible PQR M

▲ G8509 Documentation of pain assessment (including location, intensity and description) prior to initiation of therapy or documentation of the absence of pain as a result of assessment through discussion with the patient including the use of a standardized tool; no documentation of a follow-up plan, reason not specified PQR M

G8510 Negative screen for clinical depression using a standardized tool, patient not eligible/appropriate for follow-up plan documented PQR M

G8511 Screen for clinical depression using a standardized tool documented, follow up plan not documented, reason not specified PQR M

× ~~G8518 Clinical stage prior to surgery for lung cancer and esophageal cancer resection was recorded~~
This code is deleted as of December 31, 2010

× ~~G8519 Clinician documented that patient was not eligible for clinical stage prior to surgery for lung cancer and esophageal cancer resection measure~~
This code is deleted as of December 31, 2010

× ~~G8520 Clinician stage prior to surgery for lung cancer and esophageal cancer resection was not recorded, reason not specified~~
This code is deleted as of December 31, 2010

G8524 Patch closure used for patient undergoing conventional CEA PQR M

G8525 Clinician documented that patient did not receive conventional CEA PQR M

G8526 Patch closure not used for patient undergoing conventional CEA, reason not specified PQR M

G8530 Autogenous AV fistula received PQR M

G8531 Clinician documented that patient was not an eligible candidate for autogenous AV fistula PQR M

G8532 Clinician documented that patient received vascular access other than autogenous AV fistula, reason not specified PQR M

G8534 Documentation of an elder maltreatment screen and follow-up plan PQR M

G8535 No documentation of an elder maltreatment screen, patient not eligible PQR M

G8536 No documentation of an elder maltreatment screen, reason not specified PQR M

G8537 Elder maltreatment screen documented, follow-up plan not documented, patient not eligible PQR M

G8538 Elder maltreatment screen documented, follow-up plan not documented, reason not specified PQR M

G8539 Documentation of a current functional outcome assessment using a standardized tool and care plan based on identified deficiencies PQR M

G8540 Documentation that the patient is not eligible for a functional outcome assessment using a standardized tool PQR M

G8541 No documentation of a current functional outcome assessment using a standardized tool, reason not specified PQR M

G8542 Documentation of a current functional outcome assessment using a standardized tool; no documentation of a care plan, patient not eligible PQR M

G8543 Documentation of a current functional outcome assessment using a standardized tool; no documentation of a care plan, reason not specified PQR M

G8544 I intend to report the coronary artery bypass graft (CABG) measures group PQR M

G8545 I intend to report the hepatitis C measures group PQR M

G8546 I intend to report the community-acquired pneumonia (CAP) measures group PQR M

G8547 I intend to report the ischemic vascular disease (IVD) measures group PQR M

G8548 I intend to report the heart failure (HF) measures group PQR M

G8549 All quality actions for the applicable measures in the hepatitis C measures group have been performed for this patient PQR M

G8550 All quality actions for the applicable measures in the community-acquired pneumonia (CAP) measures group have been performed for this patient PQR M

G8551 All quality actions for the applicable measures in the heart failure (HF) measures group have been performed for this patient PQR M

G8552 All quality actions for the applicable measures in the ischemic vascular disease (IVD) measures group have been performed for this patient PQR M

G8553 At least one prescription created during the encounter was generated and transmitted electronically using a qualified ERX system PQR M

G8556 Referred to a physician (preferably a physician with training in disorders of the ear) for an otologic evaluation PQR M

G8557 Patient is not eligible for the referral for otologic evaluation measure PQR M

G8558 Not referred to a physician (preferably a physician with training in disorders PQR M

G8559 Patient referred to a physician (preferably a physician with training in of the ear) for an otologic evaluation, reason not specified PQR M

G8560 Patient has a history of active drainage from the ear within the previous 90 days PQR M

G8561 Patient is not eligible for the referral for otologic evaluation for patients with a history of active drainage measure PQR M

G8562 Patient does not have a history of active drainage from the ear within the previous 90 days PQR M

G8563 Patient not referred to a physician (preferably a physician with training in disorders of the ear) for an otologic evaluation, reason not specified PQR M

G8564 Patient was referred to a physician (preferably a physician with training in disorders of the ear) for an otologic evaluation, reason not specified) PQR M

G8565 Verification and documentation of sudden or rapidly progressive hearing loss PQR M

G8566 Patient is not eligible for the referral for otologic evaluation for sudden or rapidly progressive hearing loss measure PQR M

G8567 Patient does not have verification and documentation of sudden or rapidly progressive hearing loss PQR M

G8568 Patient was not referred to a physician (preferably a physician with training in disorders of the ear) for an otologic evaluation, reason not specified) PQR M

G8569 Prolonged intubation (>24 hrs) required PQR M

G8570 Prolonged intubation (>24 hrs) not required PQR M

G8571 Development of deep sternal wound infection within 30 days postoperatively PQR M

G8572 No deep sternal wound infection PQR M

G8573 Stroke/CVA following isolated CABG surgery PQR M

G8574 No stroke/CVA following isolated CABG surgery PQR M

G8575 Developed postoperative renal insufficiency or required dialysis PQR M

G8576 No postoperative renal insufficiency/dialysis not required PQR M

G8577 Reoperation required due to bleeding/tamponade, graft occlusion or other cardiac reason PQR M

G8578 Reoperation not required due to bleeding/tamponade, graft occlusion or other cardiac reason PQR M

G8579 Antiplatelet medication at discharge PQR M

G8580 Antiplatelet medication contraindicated/not indicated PQR M

G8581 No antiplatelet medication at discharge PQR M

G8582 Beta-blocker at discharge PQR M

G8583 Beta-blocker contraindicated/not indicated PQR M

G8584 No beta-blocker at discharge PQR M

G8585 Anti-lipid treatment at discharge PQR M

G8586 Anti-lipid treatment contraindicated/not indicated PQR M

G8587 No anti-lipid treatment at discharge PQR M

G8588 Most recent systolic blood pressure < 140 mmHg PQR M

G8589 Most recent systolic blood pressure >= 140 mmHg PQR M

G8590 Most recent diastolic blood pressure < 90 mmHg PQR M

G8591 Most recent diastolic blood pressure >= 90 mmHg PQR M

G8592 No documentation of blood pressure measurement PQR M

G8593 Lipid profile results documented and reviewed (must include total cholesterol, HDL-C, triglycerides and calculated LDL-C) PQR M
Pub 100-03, 1, 190.23

G8594 Lipid profile not performed, reason not otherwise specified PQR M

G8595 Most recent LDL-C < 100 mg/dl PQR M
Pub 100-03, 1, 190.23

G8596 LDL-C was not performed PQR M

G8597 Most recent LDL-C >= 100 mg/dl PQR M
Pub 100-03, 1, 190.23

G8598 Aspirin or another antithrombotic therapy used PQR M

G8599 Aspirin or another antithrombotic therapy not used, reason not otherwise specified PQR M

G8600 IV t-PA initiated within three hours (<= 180 minutes) of time last known well PQR M

G8601 IV t-PA not initiated within three hours (<= 180 minutes) of time last known well for reasons documented by clinician PQR M

G8602 IV t-PA not initiated within three hours (<= 180 minutes) of time last known well, reason not specified PQR M

G8603 Score on the spoken language comprehension functional communication measure at discharge was higher than at admission PQR M

G8604 Score on the spoken language comprehension functional communication measure at discharge was not higher than at admission, reason not specified PQR M

G8605 Patient was not scored on the spoken language comprehension functional communication measure either at admission or at discharge PQR M

G8606 Score on the attention functional communication measure at discharge was higher than at admission PQR M

G8607 Score on the attention functional communication measure at discharge was not higher than at admission, reason not specified PQR M

G8608 Patient was not scored on the attention functional communication measure either at admission or at discharge PQR M

G8609 Score on the memory functional communication measure at discharge was higher than at admission PQR M

G8610 Score on the memory functional communication measure at discharge was not higher than at admission, reason not specified PQR M

G8611 Patient was not scored on the memory functional communication measure at either admission or at discharge PQR M

G8612 Score on the motor speech functional communication measure at discharge was higher than at admission PQR M

G8613 Score on the motor speech functional communication measure at discharge was not higher than at admission, reason not specified PQR M

G8614 Patient was not scored on the motor speech functional communication measure either at admission or at discharge PQR M

G8615 Score on the reading functional communication measure at discharge was higher than at admission PQR M

G8616 Score on the reading functional communication measure at discharge was not higher than at admission, reason not specified PQR M

G8617 Patient was not scored on the reading functional communication measure either at admission or at discharge PQR M

G8618 Score on the spoken language expression functional communication measure at discharge was higher than at admission PQR M

G8619 Score on the spoken language expression functional communication measure at discharge was not higher than at admission, reason not specified PQR M

G8620 Patient was not scored on the spoken language expression functional communication measure either at admission or at discharge PQR M

G8621 Score on the writing functional communication measure at discharge was higher than at admission PQR M

G8622 Score on the writing functional communication measure at discharge was not higher than at admission, reason not specified PQR M

G8623 Patient was not scored on the writing functional communication measure either at admission or at discharge PQR M

G8624 Score on the swallowing functional communication measure at discharge was higher than at admission PQR M

G8625 Score on the swallowing functional communication measure at discharge was not higher than at admission, reason not specified PQR M

G8626 Patient was not scored on the swallowing functional communication measure at admission or at discharge PQR M

G8627 Surgical procedure performed within 30 days following cataract surgery for major complications (e.g. retained nuclear fragments, endophthalmitis, dislocated or wrong power IOL, retinal detachment, or wound dehiscence) PQR M

G8628 Surgical procedure not performed within 30 days following cataract surgery for major complications (e.g. retained nuclear fragments, endophthalmitis, dislocated or wrong power IOL, retinal detachment, or wound dehiscence) PQR M

● G8629 Documentation of order for prophylactic parenteral antibiotic to be given within one hour (if fluoroquinolone or vancomycin, two hours) prior to surgical incision (or start of procedure when no incision is required) PQR M
This code is effective January 1, 2011

● G8630 Documentation that administration of prophylactic parenteral antibiotics was initiated within one hour (if fluoroquinolone or vancomycin, two hours) prior to surgical incision (or start of procedure when no incision is required), as ordered PQR M
This code is effective January 1, 2011

● G8631 Clinician documented that patient was not an eligible candidate for ordering prophylactic parenteral antibiotics to be given within one hour (if fluoroquinolone or vancomycin, two hours) prior to surgical incision (or start of procedure when no incision is required) PQR M
This code is effective January 1, 2011

● G8632 Prophylactic parenteral antibiotics were not ordered to be given or given within one hour (if fluoroquinolone or vancomycin, two hours) prior to the surgical incision (or start of procedure when no incision is required), reason not otherwise specified) PQR M
This code is effective January 1, 2011

● G8633 Pharmacologic therapy (other than minierals/vitamins) for osteoporosis prescribed PQR M
This code is effective January 1, 2011

● G8634 Clinician documented patient not an eligible candidate to receive pharmacologic therapy for osteoporosis PQR M
This code is effective January 1, 2011

● G8635 Pharmacologic therapy for osteoporosis was not prescribed, reason not otherwise specified PQR M
This code is effective January 1, 2011

● G8636 Influenza immunization administered or previously received PQR M
This code is effective January 1, 2011

● G8637 Clinician documented that patient is not eligible to receive the influenza immunization PQR M
This code is effective January 1, 2011

● G8638 Influenza immunization not administered or previously received, reason not otherwise specified PQR M
This code is effective January 1, 2011

● G8639 Influenza immunization was administered or previously received PQR M
This code is effective January 1, 2011

● G8640 Clinician has documented that patient is not eligible to receive the influenza immunization PQR M
This code is effective January 1, 2011

● G8641 Influenza immunization was not administered or previously received, reason not otherwise specified PQR M
This code is effective January 1, 2011

● G8642 The eligible professional practices in a rural area without sufficient high speed internet access and requests a hardship exemption from the application of the payment adjustment under section 1848(a)(5)(a) of the social security act PQR M
This code is effective January 1, 2011

● G8643 The eligible professional practices in an area without sufficient available pharmacies for electronic prescribing and requests a hardship exemption for the application of the payment adjustment under section 1848(a)(5)(a) of the social security act PQR M
This code is effective January 1, 2011

● G8644 Eligible professional does not have prescribing privileges PQR M
This code is effective January 1, 2011

● G8645 I intend to report the asthma measures group PQR M
This code is effective January 1, 2011

● G8646 All quality actions for the applicable measures in the asthma measures group have been performed for this patient PQR M
This code is effective January 1, 2011

● G8647 Risk-adjusted functional status change residual score for the knee successfully calculated and the score was equal to zero (0) or greater than zero (>0) PQR M
This code is effective January 1, 2011

● G8648 Risk-adjusted functional status change residual score for the knee successfully calculated and the score was less than zero (<0) PQR M
This code is effective January 1, 2011

● G8649 Risk-adjusted functional status change residual scores for the knee not measured because the patient did not complete foto's functional intake on admission and/or follow up status survey near discharge, patient not eligible/not appropriate PQR M
This code is effective January 1, 2011

● G8650 Risk-adjusted functional status change residual scores for the knee not measured because the patient did not complete foto's functional intake on admission and/or follow up status survey near discharge, reason not specified PQR M
This code is effective January 1, 2011

● G8651 Risk-adjusted functional status change residual score for the hip successfully calculated and the score was equal to zero (0) or greater than zero (>0) PQR M
This code is effective January 1, 2011

● G8652 Risk-adjusted functional status change residual score for the hip successfully calculated and the score was less than zero (<0) PQR M
This code is effective January 1, 2011

● G8653 Risk-adjusted functional status change residual scores for the hip not measured because the patient did not complete foto's functional intake on admission and/or follow up status survey near discharge, patient not eligible/not appropriate PQR M
This code is effective January 1, 2011

● G8654 Risk-adjusted functional status change residual scores for the hip not measured because the patient did not complete foto's functional intake on admission and/or follow up status survey near discharge, reason not specified PQR M
This code is effective January 1, 2011

● G8655 Risk-adjusted functional status change residual score for the lower leg, foot or ankle successfully calculated and the score was equal to zero (0) or greater than zero(>0) PQR M
This code is effective January 1, 2011

● G8656 Risk-adjusted functional status change residual score for the lower leg, foot or ankle successfully calculated and the score was less than zero (<0) PQR M
This code is effective January 1, 2011

● G8657 Risk-adjusted functional status change residual scores for the lower leg, foot or ankle not measured because the patient did not complete foto's functional intake on admission and/or follow up status survey near discharge, patient not eligible/not appropriate PQR M
This code is effective January 1, 2011

● G8658 Risk-adjusted functional status change residual scores for the lower leg, foot or ankle not measured because the patient did not complete foto's functional intake on admission and/or follow up status survey near discharge, reason not specified PQR M
This code is effective January 1, 2011

● G8659 Risk-adjusted functional status change residual score for the lumbar spine successfully calculated and the score was equal to zero (0) or greater than zero (>0) PQR M
This code is effective January 1, 2011

● G8660 Risk-adjusted functional status change residual score for the lumbar spine successfully calculated and the score was less than zero (<0) PQR M
This code is effective January 1, 2011

● G8661 Risk-adjusted functional status change residual scores for the lumbar spine not measured because the patient did not complete foto's functional intake on admission and/or follow up status survey near discharge, patient not eligible/not appropriate PQR M
This code is effective January 1, 2011

● G8662 Risk-adjusted functional status change residual scores for the lumbar spine not measured because the patient did not complete foto's functional intake on admission and/or follow up status survey near discharge, reason not specified PQR M
This code is effective January 1, 2011

● G8663 Risk-adjusted functional status change residual score for the shoulder successfully calculated and the score was equal to zero (0) or greater than zero (>0) PQR M
This code is effective January 1, 2011

● G8664 Risk-adjusted functional status change residual score for the shoulder successfully calculated and the score was less than zero (<0) PQR M
This code is effective January 1, 2011

● G8665 Risk-adjusted functional status change residual scores for the shoulder not measured because the patient did not complete foto's functional intake on admission and/or follow up status survey near discharge, patient not eligible/not appropriate PQR M
This code is effective January 1, 2011

● G8666 Risk-adjusted functional status change residual scores for the shoulder not measured because the patient did not complete foto's functional intake on admission and/or follow up status survey near discharge, reason not specified PQR M
This code is effective January 1, 2011

● G8667 Risk-adjusted functional status change residual score for the elbow, wrist or hand successfully calculated and the score was equal to zero (0) or greater than zero (>0) PQR M
This code is effective January 1, 2011

● G8668 Risk-adjusted functional status change residual score for the elbow, wrist or hand successfully calculated and the score was less than zero (<0) PQR M
This code is effective January 1, 2011

● G8669 Risk-adjusted functional status change residual scores for the elbow, wrist or hand not measured because the patient did not complete foto's functional intake on admission and/or follow up status survey near discharge, patient not eligible/not appropriate PQR M
This code is effective January 1, 2011

● G8670 Risk-adjusted functional status change residual scores for the elbow, wrist or hand not measured because the patient did not complete foto's functional intake on admission and/or follow up status survey near discharge, reason not specified PQR M
This code is effective January 1, 2011

● G8671 Risk-adjusted functional status change residual score for the neck, cranium, mandible, thoracic spine, ribs, or other general orthopedic impairment successfully calculated and the score was equal to zero (0) or greater than zero (>0) PQR M
This code is effective January 1, 2011

● G8672 Risk-adjusted functional status change residual score for the neck, cranium, mandible, thoracic spine, ribs, or other general orthopedic impairment successfully calculated and the score was less than zero (<0) PQR M
This code is effective January 1, 2011

● G8673 Risk-adjusted functional status change residual scores for the neck, cranium, mandible, thoracic spine, ribs, or other general orthopedic impairment not measured because the patient did not complete foto's functional intake on admission and/or follow up status survey near discharge, patient not eligible/not appropriate PQR M
This code is effective January 1, 2011

● G8674 Risk-adjusted functional status change residual scores for the neck, cranium, mandible, thoracic spine, ribs, or other general orthopedic impairment not measured because the patient did not complete foto's functional intake on admission and/or follow up status survey near discharge, reason not specified PQR M
This code is effective January 1, 2011

● G8675 Most recent systolic blood pressure >= 140 mm hg PQR M
This code is effective January 1, 2011

● G8676 Most recent diastolic blood pressure >= 90 mm hg PQR M
This code is effective January 1, 2011

● G8677 Most recent systolic blood pressure < 130 mm hg PQR M
This code is effective January 1, 2011

● G8678 Most recent systolic blood pressure 130 to 139 mm hg PQR M
This code is effective January 1, 2011

● G8679 Most recent diastolic blood pressure < 80 mm hg PQR M
This code is effective January 1, 2011

● G8680 Most recent diastolic blood pressure 80 - 89 mm hg PQR M
This code is effective January 1, 2011

● G8681 Patient hospitalized with principal diagnosis of heart failure during the measurement period PQR M
This code is effective January 1, 2011

● G8682 Left ventricular function testing performed during the measurement period PQR M
This code is effective January 1, 2011

● G8683 Clinician documented that patient is not an eligible candidate for left ventricular function testing during the measurement period PQR M
This code is effective January 1, 2011

● G8684 Patient not hospitalized with principal diagnosis of heart failure during the measurement period PQR M
This code is effective January 1, 2011

● G8685 Left ventricular function testing not performed during the measurement period, reason not specified PQR M
This code is effective January 1, 2011

● G8686 Currently a tobacco smoker or current exposure to secondhand smoke PQR M
This code is effective January 1, 2011

● G8687 Currently a tobacco non-user and no exposure to secondhand smoke PQR M
This code is effective January 1, 2011

● G8688 Currently a smokeless tobacco user (eg, chew, snuff) and no exposure to secondhand smoke PQR M
This code is effective January 1, 2011

● G8689 Tobacco use not assessed, reason not otherwise specified PQR M
This code is effective January 1, 2011

● G8690 Current tobacco smoker or current exposure to secondhand smoke PQR M
This code is effective January 1, 2011

G8659 – G8690

- G8691 Current tobacco non-user and no exposure to secondhand smoke PQR M
  This code is effective January 1, 2011
- G8692 Current smokeless tobacco user (eg, chew, snuff) and no exposure to secondhand smoke PQR M
  This code is effective January 1, 2011
- G8693 Tobacco use not assessed, reason not specified PQR M
  This code is effective January 1, 2011

Coordination of Care/Demonstration Project Items and Services

G9001 Coordinated care fee, initial rate B

G9002 Coordinated care fee, maintenance rate B

G9003 Coordinated care fee, risk adjusted high, initial B

G9004 Coordinated care fee, risk adjusted low, initial B

G9005 Coordinated care fee, risk adjusted maintenance B

G9006 Coordinated care fee, home monitoring B

G9007 Coordinated care fee, scheduled team conference B

G9008 Coordinated care fee, physician coordinated care oversight services B

G9009 Coordinated care fee, risk adjusted maintenance, level 3 B

G9010 Coordinated care fee, risk adjusted maintenance, level 4 B

G9011 Coordinated care fee, risk adjusted maintenance, level 5 B

G9012 Other specified case management service not elsewhere classified B

G9013 ESRD demo basic bundle level I E

G9014 ESRD demo expanded bundle including venous access and related services E

G9016 Smoking cessation counseling, individual, in the absence of or in addition to any other evaluation and management service, per session (6-10 minutes) [demo project code only] E

G9017 Amantadine hydrochloride, oral, per 100 mg (for use in a Medicare-approved demonstration project) A

G9018 Zanamivir, inhalation powder, administered through inhaler, per 10 mg (for use in a Medicare-approved demonstration project) A

G9019 Oseltamivir phosphate, oral, per 75 mg (for use in a Medicare-approved demonstration project) A

G9020 Rimantadine hydrochloride, oral, per 100 mg (for use in a Medicare-approved demonstration project) A

G9033 Amantadine hydrochloride, oral brand, per 100 mg (for use in a Medicare-approved demonstration project) A

G9034 Zanamivir, inhalation powder, administered through inhaler, brand, per 10 mg (for use in a Medicare-approved demonstration project) A

G9035 Oseltamivir phosphate, oral, brand, per 75 mg (for use in a Medicare-approved demonstration project) A

G9036 Rimantadine hydrochloride, oral, brand, per 100 mg (for use in a Medicare-approved demonstration project) A

G9041 Rehabilitation services for low vision by qualified occupational therapist, direct one-on-one contact, each 15 minutes A

G9042 Rehabilitation services for low vision by certified orientation and mobility specialists, direct one-on-one contact, each 15 minutes A

G9043 Rehabilitation services for low vision by certified low vision rehabilitation therapist, direct one-on-one contact, each 15 minutes A

G9044 Rehabilitation services for low vision by certified low vision rehabilitation teacher, direct one-on-one contact, each 15 minutes A

G9050 Oncology; primary focus of visit; work-up, evaluation, or staging at the time of cancer diagnosis or recurrence (for use in a Medicare-approved demonstration project) E

G9051 Oncology; primary focus of visit; treatment decision-making after disease is staged or restaged, discussion of treatment options, supervising/coordinating active cancer directed therapy or managing consequences of cancer directed therapy (for use in a Medicare-approved demonstration project) E

G9052 Oncology; primary focus of visit; surveillance for disease recurrence for patient who has completed definitive cancer-directed therapy and currently lacks evidence of recurrent disease; cancer directed therapy might be considered in the future (for use in a Medicare-approved demonstration project) E

G9053 Oncology; primary focus of visit; expectant management of patient with evidence of cancer for whom no cancer directed therapy is being administered or arranged at present; cancer directed therapy might be considered in the future (for use in a Medicare-approved demonstration project) E

G9054 Oncology; primary focus of visit; supervising, coordinating or managing care of patient with terminal cancer or for whom other medical illness prevents further cancer treatment; includes symptom management, end-of-life care planning, management of palliative therapies (for use in a Medicare-approved demonstration project) E

G9055 Oncology; primary focus of visit; other, unspecified service not otherwise listed (for use in a Medicare-approved demonstration project) E

G9056 Oncology; practice guidelines; management adheres to guidelines (for use in a Medicare-approved demonstration project) E

G9057 Oncology; practice guidelines; management differs from guidelines as a result of patient enrollment in an institutional review board approved clinical trial (for use in a Medicare-approved demonstration project) E

G9058 Oncology; practice guidelines; management differs from guidelines because the treating physician disagrees with guideline recommendations (for use in a Medicare-approved demonstration project) E

G9059 Oncology; practice guidelines; management differs from guidelines because the patient, after being offered treatment consistent with guidelines, has opted for alternative treatment or management, including no treatment (for use in a Medicare-approved demonstration project) E

G9060 Oncology; practice guidelines; management differs from guidelines for reason(s) associated with patient comorbid illness or performance status not factored into guidelines (for use in a Medicare-approved demonstration project) E

G9061 Oncology; practice guidelines; patient's condition not addressed by available guidelines (for use in a Medicare-approved demonstration project) M

G9062 Oncology; practice guidelines; management differs from guidelines for other reason(s) not listed (for use in a Medicare-approved demonstration project) E

G9063 Oncology; disease status; limited to non-small cell lung cancer; extent of disease initially established as stage I (prior to neo-adjuvant therapy, if any) with no evidence of disease progression, recurrence, or metastases (for use in a Medicare-approved demonstration project) E

G9064 Oncology; disease status; limited to non-small cell lung cancer; extent of disease initially established as stage II (prior to neo-adjuvant therapy, if any) with no evidence of disease progression, recurrence, or metastases (for use in a Medicare-approved demonstration project) M

G9065 Oncology; disease status; limited to non-small cell lung cancer; extent of disease initially established as stage IIIA (prior to neo-adjuvant therapy, if any) with no evidence of disease progression, recurrence, or metastases (for use in a Medicare-approved demonstration project) M

G9066 Oncology; disease status; limited to non-small cell lung cancer; stage IIIB-IV at diagnosis, metastatic, locally recurrent, or progressive (for use in a Medicare-approved demonstration project) M

G9067 Oncology; disease status; limited to non-small cell lung cancer; extent of disease unknown, staging in progress, or not listed (for use in a Medicare-approved demonstration project) M

G9068 Oncology; disease status; limited to small cell and combined small cell/non-small cell; extent of disease initially established as limited with no evidence of disease progression, recurrence, or metastases (for use in a Medicare-approved demonstration project) M

G9069 Oncology; disease status; small cell lung cancer, limited to small cell and combined small cell/non-small cell; extensive stage at diagnosis, metastatic, locally recurrent, or progressive (for use in a Medicare-approved demonstration project) M

G9070 Oncology; disease status; small cell lung cancer, limited to small cell and combined small cell/non-small; extent of disease unknown, staging in progress, or not listed (for use in a Medicare-approved demonstration project) M

G9071 Oncology; disease status; invasive female breast cancer (does not include ductal carcinoma in situ); adenocarcinoma as predominant cell type; stage I or stage IIA-IIB; or T3, N1, M0; and ER and/or PR positive; with no evidence of disease progression, recurrence, or metastases (for use in a Medicare-approved demonstration project) ♀ M

G9072 Oncology; disease status; invasive female breast cancer (does not include ductal carcinoma in situ); adenocarcinoma as predominant cell type; stage I, or stage IIA-IIB; or T3, N1, M0; and ER and PR negative; with no evidence of disease progression, recurrence, or metastases (for use in a Medicare-approved demonstration project) ♀ M

G9073 Oncology; disease status; invasive female breast cancer (does not include ductal carcinoma in situ); adenocarcinoma as predominant cell type; stage IIIA-IIIB; and not T3, N1, M0; and ER and/or PR positive; with no evidence of disease progression, recurrence, or metastases (for use in a Medicare-approved demonstration project) ♀ M

G9074 Oncology; disease status; invasive female breast cancer (does not include ductal carcinoma in situ); adenocarcinoma as predominant cell type; stage IIIA-IIIB; and not T3, N1, M0; and ER and PR negative; with no evidence of disease progression, recurrence, or metastases (for use in a Medicare-approved demonstration project) ♀ M

G9075 Oncology; disease status; invasive female breast cancer (does not include ductal carcinoma in situ); adenocarcinoma as predominant cell type; M1 at diagnosis, metastatic, locally recurrent, or progressive (for use in a Medicare-approved demonstration project) ♀ M

G9077 Oncology; disease status; prostate cancer, limited to adenocarcinoma as predominant cell type; T1-T2C and Gleason 2-7 and PSA < or equal to 20 at diagnosis with no evidence of disease progression, recurrence, or metastases (for use in a Medicare-approved demonstration project) ♂ M

G9078 Oncology; disease status; prostate cancer, limited to adenocarcinoma as predominant cell type; T2 or T3 Gleason 8-10 or PSA > 20 at diagnosis with no evidence of disease progression, recurrence, or metastases (for use in a Medicare-approved demonstration project) ♂ M

G9079 Oncology; disease status; prostate cancer, limited to adenocarcinoma as predominant cell type; T3B-T4, any N; any T, N1 at diagnosis with no evidence of disease progression, recurrence, or metastases (for use in a Medicare-approved demonstration project) ♂ M

G9080 Oncology; disease status; prostate cancer, limited to adenocarcinoma; after initial treatment with rising PSA or failure of PSA decline (for use in a Medicare-approved demonstration project) ♂ M

G9081 Oncology; disease status; prostate cancer, limited to adenocarcinoma; non-castrate, incompletely castrate; clinical metastases or M1 at diagnosis (for use in a Medicare-approved demonstration project) ♂ M

G9082 Oncology; disease status; prostate cancer, limited to adenocarcinoma; castrate; clinical metastases or M1 at diagnosis (for use in a Medicare-approved demonstration project) ♂ M

G9083 Oncology; disease status; prostate cancer, limited to adenocarcinoma; extent of disease unknown, staging in progress, or not listed (for use in a Medicare-approved demonstration project) ♂ M

G9084 Oncology; disease status; colon cancer, limited to invasive cancer, adenocarcinoma as predominant cell type; extent of disease initially established as T1-3, N0, M0 with no evidence of disease progression, recurrence, or metastases (for use in a Medicare-approved demonstration project) M

G9085 Oncology; disease status; colon cancer, limited to invasive cancer, adenocarcinoma as predominant cell type; extent of disease initially established as T4, N0, M0 with no evidence of disease progression, recurrence, or metastases (for use in a Medicare-approved demonstration project) M

G9086 Oncology; disease status; colon cancer, limited to invasive cancer, adenocarcinoma as predominant cell type; extent of disease initially established as T1-4, N1-2, M0 with no evidence of disease progression, recurrence, or metastases (for use in a Medicare-approved demonstration project) M

G9087 Oncology; disease status; colon cancer, limited to invasive cancer, adenocarcinoma as predominant cell type; M1 at diagnosis, metastatic, locally recurrent, or progressive with current clinical, radiologic, or biochemical evidence of disease (for use in a Medicare-approved demonstration project) M

G9088 Oncology; disease status; colon cancer, limited to invasive cancer, adenocarcinoma as predominant cell type; M1 at diagnosis, metastatic, locally recurrent, or progressive without current clinical, radiologic, or biochemical evidence of disease (for use in a Medicare-approved demonstration project) M

G9089 Oncology; disease status; colon cancer, limited to invasive cancer; adenocarcinoma as predominant cell type; extent of disease unknown, staging in progress, or not listed (for use in a Medicare-approved demonstration project) M

G9090 Oncology; disease status; rectal cancer, limited to invasive cancer, adenocarcinoma as predominant cell type; extent of disease initially established as T1-2, N0, M0 (prior to neo-adjuvant therapy, if any) with no evidence of disease progression, recurrence, or metastases (for use in a Medicare-approved demonstration project) M

G9091 Oncology; disease status; rectal cancer, limited to invasive cancer, adenocarcinoma as predominant cell type; extent of disease initially established as T3, N0, M0 (prior to neo-adjuvant therapy, if any) with no evidence of disease progression, recurrence, or metastases (for use in a Medicare-approved demonstration project) M

G9092 Oncology; disease status; rectal cancer, limited to invasive cancer, adenocarcinoma as predominant cell type; extent of disease initially established as T1-3, N1-2, M0 (prior to neo-adjuvant therapy, if any) with no evidence of disease progression, recurrence or metastases (for use in a Medicare-approved demonstration project) M

G9093 Oncology; disease status; rectal cancer, limited to invasive cancer, adenocarcinoma as predominant cell type; extent of disease initially established as T4, any N, M0 (prior to neo-adjuvant therapy, if any) with no evidence of disease progression, recurrence, or metastases (for use in a Medicare-approved demonstration project) M

G9094 Oncology; disease status; rectal cancer, limited to invasive cancer, adenocarcinoma as predominant cell type; M1 at diagnosis, metastatic, locally recurrent, or progressive (for use in a Medicare-approved demonstration project) M

G9095 Oncology; disease status; rectal cancer, limited to invasive cancer; adenocarcinoma as predominant cell type; extent of disease unknown, staging in progress, or not listed (for use in a Medicare-approved demonstration project) M

G9096 Oncology; disease status; esophageal cancer, limited to adenocarcinoma or squamous cell carcinoma as predominant cell type; extent of disease initially established as T1-T3, N0-N1 or NX (prior to neo-adjuvant therapy, if any) with no evidence of disease progression, recurrence, or metastases (for use in a Medicare-approved demonstration project) M

G9097 Oncology; disease status; esophageal cancer, limited to adenocarcinoma or squamous cell carcinoma as predominant cell type; extent of disease initially established as T4, any N, M0 (prior to neo-adjuvant therapy, if any) with no evidence of disease progression, recurrence, or metastases (for use in a Medicare-approved demonstration project) M

G9098 Oncology; disease status; esophageal cancer, limited to adenocarcinoma or squamous cell carcinoma as predominant cell type; M1 at diagnosis, metastatic, locally recurrent, or progressive (for use in a Medicare-approved demonstration project) M

G9099 Oncology; disease status; esophageal cancer, limited to adenocarcinoma or squamous cell carcinoma as predominant cell type; extent of disease unknown, staging in progress, or not listed (for use in a Medicare-approved demonstration project) M

G9100 Oncology; disease status; gastric cancer, limited to adenocarcinoma as predominant cell type; post R0 resection (with or without neoadjuvant therapy) with no evidence of disease recurrence, progression, or metastases (for use in a Medicare-approved demonstration project) M

G9101 Oncology; disease status; gastric cancer, limited to adenocarcinoma as predominant cell type; post R1 or R2 resection (with or without neoadjuvant therapy) with no evidence of disease progression, or metastases (for use in a Medicare-approved demonstration project) M

G9102 Oncology; disease status; gastric cancer, limited to adenocarcinoma as predominant cell type; clinical or pathologic M0, unresectable with no evidence of disease progression, or metastases (for use in a Medicare-approved demonstration project) M

G9103 Oncology; disease status; gastric cancer, limited to adenocarcinoma as predominant cell type; clinical or pathologic M1 at diagnosis, metastatic, locally recurrent, or progressive (for use in a Medicare-approved demonstration project) M

G9104 Oncology; disease status; gastric cancer, limited to adenocarcinoma as predominant cell type; extent of disease unknown, staging in progress, or not listed (for use in a Medicare-approved demonstration project) M

G9105 Oncology; disease status; pancreatic cancer, limited to adenocarcinoma as predominant cell type; post R0 resection without evidence of disease progression, recurrence, or metastases (for use in a Medicare-approved demonstration project) M

G9106 Oncology; disease status; pancreatic cancer, limited to adenocarcinoma; post R1 or R2 resection with no evidence of disease progression, or metastases (for use in a Medicare-approved demonstration project) M

G9107 Oncology; disease status; pancreatic cancer, limited to adenocarcinoma; unresectable at diagnosis, M1 at diagnosis, metastatic, locally recurrent, or progressive (for use in a Medicare-approved demonstration project) M

G9108 Oncology; disease status; pancreatic cancer, limited to adenocarcinoma; extent of disease unknown, staging in progress, or not listed (for use in a Medicare-approved demonstration project) M

G9109 Oncology; disease status; head and neck cancer, limited to cancers of oral cavity, pharynx and larynx with squamous cell as predominant cell type; extent of disease initially established as T1-T2 and N0, M0 (prior to neo-adjuvant therapy, if any) with no evidence of disease progression, recurrence, or metastases (for use in a Medicare-approved demonstration project) M

G9110 Oncology; disease status; head and neck cancer, limited to cancers of oral cavity, pharynx and larynx with squamous cell as predominant cell type; extent of disease initially established as T3-4 and/or N1-3, M0 (prior to neo-adjuvant therapy, if any) with no evidence of disease progression, recurrence, or metastases (for use in a Medicare-approved demonstration project) M

G9111 Oncology; disease status; head and neck cancer, limited to cancers of oral cavity, pharynx and larynx with squamous cell as predominant cell type; M1 at diagnosis, metastatic, locally recurrent, or progressive (for use in a Medicare-approved demonstration project) M

G9112 Oncology; disease status; head and neck cancer, limited to cancers of oral cavity, pharynx and larynx with squamous cell as predominant cell type; extent of disease unknown, staging in progress, or not listed (for use in a Medicare-approved demonstration project) M

G9113 Oncology; disease status; ovarian cancer, limited to epithelial cancer; pathologic stage IA-B (grade 1) without evidence of disease progression, recurrence, or metastases (for use in a Medicare-approved demonstration project) ♀ M

G9114 Oncology; disease status; ovarian cancer, limited to epithelial cancer; pathologic stage IA-B (grade 2-3); or stage IC (all grades); or stage II; without evidence of disease progression, recurrence, or metastases (for use in a Medicare-approved demonstration project) ♀ M

G9115 Oncology; disease status; ovarian cancer, limited to epithelial cancer; pathologic stage III-IV; without evidence of progression, recurrence, or metastases (for use in a Medicare-approved demonstration project) ♀ M

G9116 Oncology; disease status; ovarian cancer, limited to epithelial cancer; evidence of disease progression, or recurrence, and/or platinum resistance (for use in a Medicare-approved demonstration project) ♀ M

G9117 Oncology; disease status; ovarian cancer, limited to epithelial cancer; extent of disease unknown, staging in progress, or not listed (for use in a Medicare-approved demonstration project) ♀ M

G9123 Oncology; disease status; chronic myelogenous leukemia, limited to philadelphia chromosome positive and/or BCR-ABL positive; chronic phase not in hematologic, cytogenetic, or molecular remission (for use in a medicare-approved demonstration project) M

G9124 Oncology; disease status; chronic myelogenous leukemia, limited to philadelphia chromosome positive and/or BCR-ABL positive; accelerated phase not in hematologic cytogenetic, or molecular remission (for use in a medicare-approved demonstration project M

G9125 Oncology; disease status; chronic myelogenous leukemia, limited to philadelphia chromosome positive and/or BCR-ABL positive; blast phase not in hematologic, cytogenetic, or molecular remission (for use in a medicare-approved demonstration project) M

G9126 Oncology; disease status; chronic myelogenous leukemia, limited to Philadelphia chromosome positive and/or BCR-ABL positive; in hematologic, cytogenetic, or molecular remission (for use in a Medicare-approved demonstration project) M

G9128 Oncology; disease status; limited to multiple myeloma, systemic disease; smoldering, stage I (for use in a medicare-approved demonstration project) M

G9129 Oncology; disease status; limited to multiple myeloma, systemic disease; stage II or higher (for use in a Medicare-approved demonstration project) M

G9130 Oncology; disease status; limited to multiple myeloma, systemic disease; extent of disease unknown, staging in progress, or not listed (for use in a Medicare-approved demonstration project) M

G9131 Oncology; disease status; invasive female breast cancer (does not include ductal carcinoma in situ); adenocarcinoma as predominant cell type; extent of disease unknown, staging in progress, or not listed (for use in a Medicare-approved demonstration project) ♀ M

G9132 Oncology; disease status; prostate cancer, limited to adenocarcinoma; hormone-refractory/androgen-independent (e.g., rising PSA on anti-androgen therapy or post-orchiectomy); clinical metastases (for use in a Medicare-approved demonstration project) ♂ M

G9133 Oncology; disease status; prostate cancer, limited to adenocarcinoma; hormone-responsive; clinical metastases or M1 at diagnosis (for use in a Medicare-approved demonstration project) ♂ M

G9134 Oncology; disease status; non-Hodgkin's lymphoma, any cellular classification; stage I, II at diagnosis, not relapsed, not refractory (for use in a Medicare-approved demonstration project) M

G9135 Oncology; disease status; non-Hodgkin's lymphoma, any cellular classification; stage III, IV, not relapsed, not refractory (for use in a Medicare-approved demonstration project) M

G9136 Oncology; disease status; non-Hodgkin's lymphoma, transformed from original cellular diagnosis to a second cellular classification (for use in a Medicare-approved demonstration project) M

G9137 Oncology; disease status; non-Hodgkin's lymphoma, any cellular classification; relapsed/refractory (for use in a Medicare-approved demonstration project) M

G9138 Oncology; disease status; non-Hodgkin's lymphoma, any cellular classification; diagnostic evaluation, stage not determined, evaluation of possible relapse or non-response to therapy, or not listed (for use in a Medicare-approved demonstration project) M

G9139 Oncology; disease status; chronic myelogenous leukemia, limited to Philadelphia chromosome positive and/or BCR-ABL positive; extent of disease unknown, staging in progress, not listed (for use in a Medicare-approved demonstration project) M

G9140 Frontier extended stay clinic demonstration; for a patient stay in a clinic approved for the CMS demonstration project; the following measures should be present: the stay must be equal to or greater than 4 hours; weather or other conditions must prevent transfer or the case falls into a category of monitoring and observation cases that are permitted by the rules of the demonstration; there is a maximum frontier extended stay clinic (FESC) visit of 48 hours, except in the case when weather or other conditions prevent transfer; payment is made on each period up to 4 hours, after the first 4 hours A

G9141 Influenza a (H1N1) immunization administration (includes the physician counseling the patient/family) S

G9142 Influenza a (H1N1) vaccine, any route of administration E

G9143 Warfarin responsiveness testing by genetic technique using any method, any number of specimen(s) A

● ⊘ G9147 Outpatient intravenous insulin treatment (oivit) either pulsatile or continuous, by any means, guided by the results of measurements for: respiratory quotient; and/or, urine urea nitrogen (uun); and/or, arterial, venous or capillary glucose; and/or potassium concentration A

This code was effective April 1, 2010

Alcohol and Drug Abuse Treatment Services H0001–H2037

- ⊘ H0001 Alcohol and/or drug assessment
- ⊘ H0002 Behavioral health screening to determine eligibility for admission to treatment program
- ⊘ H0003 Alcohol and/or drug screening; laboratory analysis of specimens for presence of alcohol and/or drugs
- ⊘ H0004 Behavioral health counseling and therapy, per 15 minutes
- ⊘ H0005 Alcohol and/or drug services; group counseling by a clinician
- ⊘ H0006 Alcohol and/or drug services; case management
- ⊘ H0007 Alcohol and/or drug services; crisis intervention (outpatient)
- ⊘ H0008 Alcohol and/or drug services; sub-acute detoxification (hospital inpatient)
- ⊘ H0009 Alcohol and/or drug services; acute detoxification (hospital inpatient)
- ⊘ H0010 Alcohol and/or drug services; sub-acute detoxification (residential addiction program inpatient)
- ⊘ H0011 Alcohol and/or drug services; acute detoxification (residential addiction program inpatient)
- ⊘ H0012 Alcohol and/or drug services; sub-acute detoxification (residential addiction program outpatient)
- ⊘ H0013 Alcohol and/or drug services; acute detoxification (residential addiction program outpatient)
- ⊘ H0014 Alcohol and/or drug services; ambulatory detoxification
- ⊘ H0015 Alcohol and/or drug services; intensive outpatient (treatment program that operates at least 3 hours/day and at least 3 days/week and is based on an individualized treatment plan), including assessment, counseling; crisis intervention, and activity therapies or education
- ⊘ H0016 Alcohol and/or drug services; medical/somatic (medical intervention in ambulatory setting)
- ⊘ H0017 Behavioral health; residential (hospital residential treatment program), without room and board, per diem
- ⊘ H0018 Behavioral health; short-term residential (non-hospital residential treatment program), without room and board, per diem
- ⊘ H0019 Behavioral health; long-term residential (non-medical, non-acute care in a residential treatment program where stay is typically longer than 30 days), without room and board, per diem
- ⊘ H0020 Alcohol and/or drug services; methadone administration and/or service (provision of the drug by a licensed program)
- ⊘ H0021 Alcohol and/or drug training service (for staff and personnel not employed by providers)
- ⊘ H0022 Alcohol and/or drug intervention service (planned facilitation)
- ⊘ H0023 Behavioral health outreach service (planned approach to reach a targeted population)
- ⊘ H0024 Behavioral health prevention information dissemination service (one-way direct or non-direct contact with service audiences to affect knowledge and attitude)
- ⊘ H0025 Behavioral health prevention education service (delivery of services with target population to affect knowledge, attitude and/or behavior)
- ⊘ H0026 Alcohol and/or drug prevention process service, community-based (delivery of services to develop skills of impactors)
- ⊘ H0027 Alcohol and/or drug prevention environmental service (broad range of external activities geared toward modifying systems in order to mainstream prevention through policy and law)
- ⊘ H0028 Alcohol and/or drug prevention problem identification and referral service (e.g. student assistance and employee assistance programs), does not include assessment
- ⊘ H0029 Alcohol and/or drug prevention alternatives service (services for populations that exclude alcohol and other drug use e.g. alcohol free social events)
- ⊘ H0030 Behavioral health hotline service
- ⊘ H0031 Mental health assessment, by non-physician
- ⊘ H0032 Mental health service plan development by non-physician
- ⊘ H0033 Oral medication administration, direct observation
- ⊘ H0034 Medication training and support, per 15 minutes
- ⊘ H0035 Mental health partial hospitalization, treatment, less than 24 hours
- ⊘ H0036 Community psychiatric supportive treatment, face-to-face, per 15 minutes
- ⊘ H0037 Community psychiatric supportive treatment program, per diem
- ⊘ H0038 Self-help/peer services, per 15 minutes
- ⊘ H0039 Assertive community treatment, face-to-face, per 15 minutes
- ⊘ H0040 Assertive community treatment program, per diem
- ⊘ H0041 Foster care, child, non-therapeutic, per diem
- ⊘ H0042 Foster care, child, non-therapeutic, per month
- ⊘ H0043 Supported housing, per diem
- ⊘ H0044 Supported housing, per month
- ⊘ H0045 Respite care services, not in the home, per diem
- ⊘ H0046 Mental health services, not otherwise specified
- ⊘ H0047 Alcohol and/or other drug abuse services, not otherwise specified
- ⊘ H0048 Alcohol and/or other drug testing: collection and handling only, specimens other than blood
- ⊘ H0049 Alcohol and/or drug screening
- ⊘ H0050 Alcohol and/or drug services, brief intervention, per 15 minutes
- ⊘ H1000 Prenatal care, at-risk assessment ♀
- ⊘ H1001 Prenatal care, at-risk enhanced service; antepartum management ♀
- ⊘ H1002 Prenatal care, at risk enhanced service; care coordination ♀
- ⊘ H1003 Prenatal care, at-risk enhanced service; education ♀
- ⊘ H1004 Prenatal care, at-risk enhanced service; follow-up home visit ♀
- ⊘ H1005 Prenatal care, at-risk enhanced service package (includes H1001-H1004) ♀
- ⊘ H1010 Non-medical family planning education, per session
- ⊘ H1011 Family assessment by licensed behavioral health professional for state defined purposes
- ⊘ H2000 Comprehensive multidisciplinary evaluation
- ⊘ H2001 Rehabilitation program, per 1/2 day
- ⊘ H2010 Comprehensive medication services, per 15 minutes
- ⊘ H2011 Crisis intervention service, per 15 minutes
- ⊘ H2012 Behavioral health day treatment, per hour
- ⊘ H2013 Psychiatric health facility service, per diem
- ⊘ H2014 Skills training and development, per 15 minutes

H2015 Comprehensive community support services, per 15 minutes

H2016 Comprehensive community support services, per diem

H2017 Psychosocial rehabilitation services, per 15 minutes

H2018 Psychosocial rehabilitation services, per diem

H2019 Therapeutic behavioral services, per 15 minutes

H2020 Therapeutic behavioral services, per diem

H2021 Community-based wrap-around services, per 15 minutes

H2022 Community-based wrap-around services, per diem

H2023 Supported employment, per 15 minutes

H2024 Supported employment, per diem

H2025 Ongoing support to maintain employment, per 15 minutes

H2026 Ongoing support to maintain employment, per diem

H2027 Psychoeducational service, per 15 minutes

H2028 Sexual offender treatment service, per 15 minutes

H2029 Sexual offender treatment service, per diem

H2030 Mental health clubhouse services, per 15 minutes

H2031 Mental health clubhouse services, per diem

H2032 Activity therapy, per 15 minutes

H2033 Multisystemic therapy for juveniles, per 15 minutes

H2034 Alcohol and/or drug abuse halfway house services, per diem

H2035 Alcohol and/or other drug treatment program, per hour

H2036 Alcohol and/or other drug treatment program, per diem

H2037 Developmental delay prevention activities, dependent child of client, per 15 minutes

Drugs Administered Other Than Oral Method J0120–J8999

(Exception: Oral Immunosuppressive Drugs)

Injections

The following list of drugs can be administered subcutaneously, intramuscularly, or intravenously.

J0120 Injection, tetracycline, up to 250 mg N N1
Ala-Tet, Brodspec, Emtet-500, Panmycin, Robitet 500, Sumycin, Tetracap, Tetracon
Pub 100-02, 15, 50; 100-4, 17, 10

✖ ~~J0128 Injection, abarelix, 10 mg~~
This code is deleted as of December 31, 2010

J0129 Injection, abatacept, 10 mg K K2
Orencia

J0130 Injection abciximab, 10 mg K K2
ReoPro
Pub 100-02, 15, 50; 100-4, 17, 10

J0132 Injection, acetylcysteine, 100 mg K N1

J0133 Injection, acyclovir, 5 mg N N1
Zovirax

J0135 Injection, adalimumab, 20 mg K K2
Humira

J0150 Injection, adenosine for therapeutic use, 6 mg (not to be used to report any adenosine phosphate compounds, instead use A9270) K K2
Adenocard, Adenoscan
Pub 100-02, 15, 50; 100-4, 17, 10
AHA: 2Q 2002, 10

J0152 Injection, adenosine for diagnostic use, 30 mg (not to be used to report any adenosine phosphate compounds; instead use A9270) K K2
Adenocard, Adenoscan

~~J0170 Injection, adrenalin, epinephrine, up to 1 ml ampule~~
This code is deleted as of December 31, 2010
See code(s) J0171

● J0171 Injection, adrenalin, epinephrine, 0.1 mg K N1
This code is effective January 1, 2011

J0180 Injection, agalsidase beta, 1 mg K K2
Fabrazyme

J0190 Injection, biperiden lactate, per 5 mg N K2
Akineton
Pub 100-02, 15, 50; 100-4, 17, 10

J0200 Injection, alatrofloxacin mesylate, 100 mg N N1
Pub 100-02, 15, 50.5; 100-2, 15, 50.5.2.1; 100-4, 17, 80.3-80.3.2
Trovan IV

J0205 Injection, alglucerase, per 10 units K K2
Pub 100-02, 15, 50; 100-4, 17, 10
Ceredase

J0207 Injection, amifostine, 500 mg K K2
Ethyol, Ethiofos, Gammaphos, WR-2721
Pub 100-02, 15, 50; 100-4, 17, 10

J0210 Injection, methyldopate HCl, up to 250 mg K K2
Aldomet
Pub 100-02, 15, 50; 100-4, 17, 10

J0215 Injection, alefacept, 0.5 mg K K2
Amevive

J0220 Injection, alglucosidase alfa, 10 mg K K2
Myozyme
AHA: 1Q 2008, 7

H2015 – J0220

Ⓘ J0256 Injection, alpha 1 – proteinase inhibitor – human, 10 mg N K2
Aralast, Prolastin
Pub 100-02, 15, 50; 100-4, 17, 10

Ⓘ J0270 Injection, alprostadil, 1.25 mcg (code may be used for Medicare when drug administered under the direct supervision of a physician, not for use when drug is self-administered) ♂ B
Caverject, Edex, Prostin VR Pediatric
Pub 100-02, 15, 50; 100-4, 17, 10

Ⓘ J0275 Alprostadil urethral suppository (code may be used for Medicare when drug administered under the direct supervision of a physician, not for use when drug is self-administered) ♂ B
Muse
Pub 100-02, 15, 50; 100-4, 17, 10

J0278 Injection, amikacin sulfate, 100 mg N N1
Amikin

Ⓘ J0280 Injection, aminophylline, up to 250 mg N N1
Phyllocontin, Theophylline ethylenadiamine, Truphylline
Pub 100-02, 15, 50; 100-4, 17, 10

Ⓘ J0282 Injection, amiodarone hydrochloride, 30 mg N N1
Pub 100-02, 15, 50; 100-4, 17, 10
Cordarone

Ⓘ J0285 Injection, amphotericin B, 50 mg N N1
ABLC, Amphocin, Fungizone
Pub 100-02, 15, 50; 100-4, 17, 10

Ⓘ J0287 Injection, amphotericin B lipid complex, 10 mg K K2
Abelcet
Pub 100-02, 15, 50; 100-4, 17, 10

Ⓘ J0288 Injection, amphotericin B cholesteryl sulfate complex, 10 mg K K2
Amphotec
Pub 100-02, 15, 50; 100-4, 17, 10

Ⓘ J0289 Injection, amphotericin B liposome, 10 mg K K2
AmBisome
Pub 100-02, 15, 50; 100-4, 17, 10

Ⓘ J0290 Injection, ampicillin sodium, 500 mg N N1
Omnipen-N, Polycillin-N, Principen, Totacillin-N
Pub 100-02, 15, 50; 100-4, 17, 10

Ⓘ J0295 Injection, ampicillin sodium/sulbactam sodium, per 1.5 gm N N1
Unasyn
Pub 100-02, 15, 50; 100-4, 17, 10

Ⓘ J0300 Injection, amobarbital, up to 125 mg N N1
Amytal
Pub 100-02, 15, 50; 100-4, 17, 10

Ⓘ J0330 Injection, succinylcholine chloride, up to 20 mg N N1
Anectine, Anectine Flo-Pack, Sucostrin, Quelicin
Pub 100-02, 15, 50; 100-4, 17, 10

J0348 Injection, anidulafungin, 1 mg K K2
Eraxis

Ⓘ J0350 Injection, anistreplase, per 30 units N K2
Eminase
Pub 100-02, 15, 50; 100-4, 17, 10

Ⓘ J0360 Injection, hydralazine HCl, up to 20 mg N N1
Pub 100-02, 15, 50; 100-4, 17, 10

J0364 Injection, apomorphine hydrochloride, 1 mg K N1
Apokyn

Ⓘ J0365 Injection, aprotinin, 10,000 KIU K K2
Trasylol
Pub 100-02, 15, 50; 100-4, 17, 10

Ⓘ J0380 Injection, metaraminol bitartrate, per 10 mg K N1
Aramine
Pub 100-02, 15, 50; 100-4, 17, 10

Ⓘ J0390 Injection, chloroquine hydrochloride, up to 250 mg N N1
Aralen HCl
Pub 100-02, 15, 50; 100-4, 17, 10

Ⓘ J0395 Injection, arbutamine HCl, 1 mg K N1
GenESA
Pub 100-02, 15, 50; 100-4, 17, 10

J0400 Injection, aripiprazole intramuscular, 0.25 mg N K2
Abilify
AHA: 1Q 2008, 7

Ⓘ J0456 Injection, azithromycin, 500 mg N N1
Zithromax
Pub 100-02, 15, 50.5; 100-2, 15, 50.5.2.1; 100-4, 17, 80.3-80.3.2

Ⓘ J0461 Injection, atropine sulfate, 0.01 mg N N1
AtroPen®; Atropine-Care®; Isopto® Atropine; Sal-Tropine™

Ⓘ J0470 Injection, dimercaprol, per 100 mg K N1
BAL in oil
Pub 100-02, 15, 50; 100-4, 17, 10

Ⓘ J0475 Injection, baclofen, 10 mg K K2
Pub 100-02, 15, 50; 100-4, 17, 10
Lioresal

Ⓘ J0476 Injection, baclofen, 50 mcg for intrathecal trial K K2
Pub 100-02, 15, 50; 100-4, 17, 10
Lioresal

Ⓘ J0480 Injection, basiliximab, 20 mg K K2
Simulect
Pub 100-02, 15, 50; 100-4, 17, 10

Ⓘ J0500 Injection, dicyclomine HCl, up to 20 mg N N1
Antispas, A-Spas, Bentyl, Byclomine, Dibent, Dilomine, Di-Spaz, Or-Tyl, Spasmoject
Pub 100-02, 15, 50; 100-4, 17, 10

Ⓘ J0515 Injection, benztropine mesylate, per 1 mg N N1
Cogentin
Pub 100-02, 15, 50; 100-4, 17, 10

Ⓘ J0520 Injection, bethanechol chloride, myotonachol or urecholine, up to 5 mg N N1
Duvoid, Mytonachol, Urabeth, Urecholine
Pub 100-02, 15, 50; 100-4, 17, 10

● J0558 Injection, penicillin G benzathine and penicillin G procaine, 100,000 units N N1
This code is effective January 1, 2011

✖ ~~J0559 Injection, penicillin G benzathine and penicillin G procaine, 2500 units~~
This code is deleted as of December 31, 2010
See code(s) J0558

✖ ~~J0560 Injection, penicillin G benzathine, up to 600,000 units~~
This code is deleted as of December 31, 2010
See code(s) J0561

● Ⓘ J0561 Injection, penicillin G benzathine, 100,000 units N N1
This code is effective January 1, 2011

✖ ~~J0570 Injection, penicillin G benzathine, up to 1,200,000 units~~
This code is deleted as of December 31, 2010
See code(s) J0561

✖ ~~J0580 Injection, penicillin G benzathine, up to 2,400,000 units~~
This code is deleted as of December 31, 2010
See code(s) J0561

J0583 Injection, bivalirudin, 1 mg K K2
Angiomax, Angiox

ⓘ J0585 Injection, onabotulinumtoxinA, 1 unit K K2
Botox, Oculinum
Pub 100-02, 15, 50; 100-4, 17, 10

J0586 Injection, abobotulinumtoxinA, 5 units K K2
Dysport

ⓘ J0587 Injection, rimabotulinumtoxinB, 100 units K K2
Myobloc
Pub 100-02, 15, 50; 100-4, 17, 10

ⓘ J0592 Injection, buprenorphine hydrochloride, 0.1 mg N N1
Buprenex
Pub 100-02, 15, 50; 100-4, 17, 10

J0594 Injection, busulfan, 1 mg K K2
Busulfex

J0595 Injection, butorphanol tartrate, 1 mg N N1
StadoG

● J0597 Injection, C-1 esterase inhibitor (human), Berinert, 10 units N K2
This code is effective January 1, 2011

▲ J0598 Injection, C-1 esterase inhibitor (human), Cinryze, 10 units N K2

ⓘ J0600 Injection, edetate calcium disodium, up to 1000 mg K K2
Calcium disodium versenate, Calcium EDTA
Pub 100-02, 15, 50; 100-4, 17, 10

ⓘ J0610 Injection, calcium gluconate, per 10 ml N N1
Kaleinate
Pub 100-02, 15, 50; 100-4, 17, 10

ⓘ J0620 Injection, calcium glycerophosphate and calcium lactate, per 10 ml N N1
Calphosan
Pub 100-02, 15, 50; 100-4, 17, 10

ⓘ J0630 Injection, calcitonin-salmon, up to 400 units K N1
Calcimar, Miacalcin
Pub 100-02, 15, 50; 100-4, 17, 10

ⓘ J0636 Injection, calcitriol, 0.1 mcg N N1
Calcijex, Rocaltrol
Pub 100-02, 15, 50; 100-4, 17, 10

J0637 Injection, caspofungin acetate, 5 mg K K2
Cancidas

● J0638 Injection, canakinumab, 1 mg K K2
Ilaris
This code is effective January 1, 2011

ⓘ J0640 Injection, leucovorin calcium, per 50 mg N N1
Wellcovorin
Pub 100-02, 15, 50; 100-4, 17, 10

ⓘ J0641 Injection, levoleucovorin calcium, 0.5 mg K K2
Fusilev

ⓘ J0670 Injection, mepivacaine hydrochloride, per 10 ml N N1
Carbocaine, Polocaine, Isocaine
Pub 100-02, 15, 50; 100-4, 17, 10

ⓘ J0690 Injection, cefazolin sodium, 500 mg N N1
Ancef, Kefzol, Zolicef
Pub 100-02, 15, 50; 100-4, 17, 10

J0692 Injection, cefepime hydrochloride, 500 mg N N1
Maxiprime

ⓘ J0694 Injection, cefoxitin sodium, 1 gm N N1
Mefoxin
Pub 100-02, 15, 50; 100-4, 17, 10

ⓘ J0696 Injection, ceftriaxone sodium, per 250 mg N N1
Rocephin
Pub 100-02, 15, 50; 100-4, 17, 10

ⓘ J0697 Injection, sterile cefuroxime sodium, per 750 mg N N1
Zinacef
Pub 100-02, 15, 50; 100-4, 17, 10

ⓘ J0698 Injection, cefotaxime sodium, per gm N N1
Claforan
Pub 100-02, 15, 50; 100-4, 17, 10

ⓘ J0702 Injection, betamethasone acetate 3 mg and betamethasone sodium phosphate, 3 mg N N1
Celestone soluspan
Pub 100-02, 15, 50; 100-4, 17, 10

✕ ~~J0704 Injection, betamethasone sodium phosphate, per 4 mg~~
This code is deleted as of December 31, 2010
See code(s) J0702

J0706 Injection, caffeine citrate, 5mg K N1
Cafcit

ⓘ J0710 Injection, cephapirin sodium, up to 1 gm N N1
Cefadyl
Pub 100-02, 15, 50; 100-4, 17, 10

ⓘ J0713 Injection, ceftazidime, per 500 mg N N1
Ceptaz, Fortaz, Tazicef, Tazidime
Pub 100-02, 15, 50; 100-4, 17, 10

ⓘ J0715 Injection, ceftizoxime sodium, per 500 mg N N1
Cefizox
Pub 100-02, 15, 50; 100-4, 17, 10

J0718 Injection, certolizumab pegol, 1 mg G K2
Cimzia

ⓘ J0720 Injection, chloramphenicol sodium succinate, up to 1 gm N N1
Chloromycetin
Pub 100-02, 15, 50; 100-4, 17, 10

ⓘ J0725 Injection, chorionic gonadotropin, per 1,000 USP units N N1
A.P.L., Chorex-5, Chorex-10, Chorignon, Choron 10, Corgonject-5, Follutein, Gonic, Novarel, Pregnyl, Profas
Pub 100-02, 15, 50; 100-4, 17, 10

ⓘ J0735 Injection, clonidine hydrochloride, 1 mg K K2
Catapres, Duracion, Duraclon
Pub 100-02, 15, 50; 100-4, 17, 10

ⓘ J0740 Injection, cidofovir, 375 mg K K2
Vistide
Pub 100-02, 15, 50; 100-4, 17, 10

ⓘ J0743 Injection, cilastatin sodium; imipenem, per 250 mg N N1
Primaxin IM, Primaxin IV
Pub 100-02, 15, 50; 100-4, 17, 10

J0744 Injection, ciprofloxacin for intravenous infusion, 200 mg N N1
Cipro IV

ⓘ J0745 Injection, codeine phosphate, per 30 mg N N1
Pub 100-02, 15, 50; 100-4, 17, 10

ⓘ J0760 Injection, colchicine, per 1 mg N N1
Pub 100-02, 15, 50; 100-4, 17, 10

ⓘ J0770 Injection, colistimethate sodium, up to 150 mg N N1
Coly-Mycin M
Pub 100-02, 15, 50; 100-4, 17, 10

● J0775 Injection, collagenase, clostridium histolyticum, 0.01 mg N N1
Xiaflex
This code is effective January 1, 2011

ⓘ J0780 Injection, prochlorperazine, up to 10 mg N N1
Compa-Z, Compazine, Cotranzine, Ultrazine-10
Pub 100-02, 15, 50; 100-4, 17, 10

Ⓘ J0795 Injection, corticorelin ovine triflutate, 1 microgram K K2
Acthrel
Pub 100-02, 15, 50; 100-4, 17, 10

Ⓘ J0800 Injection, corticotropin, up to 40 units K K2
Acthar, ACTH
Pub 100-02, 15, 50; 100-4, 17, 10

J0833 Injection, cosyntropin, not otherwise specified, 0.25 mg K K2
Cortrosyn

J0834 Injection, cosyntropin (Cortrosyn), 0.25 mg K K2

Ⓘ J0850 Injection, cytomegalovirus immune globulin intravenous (human), per vial K K2
CytoGam
Pub 100-02, 15, 50; 100-4, 17, 10

J0878 Injection, daptomycin, 1 mg K K2
Cubicin

Ⓘ J0881 Injection, darbepoetin alfa, 1 microgram (non-ESRD use) K K2
Aranesp

Ⓘ J0882 Injection, darbepoetin alfa, 1 microgram (for ESRD on dialysis) A
Aranesp

Ⓘ J0885 Injection, epoetin alfa, (for non-ESRD use), 1000 units K K2
Epogen, Procrit
Pub 100-02, 15, 50; 100-4, 17, 10
AHA: 2Q 2006, 5

Ⓘ J0886 Injection, epoetin alfa, 1000 units (for ESRD on dialysis) A
Epogen, Procrit
AHA: 2Q 2006, 5

J0894 Injection, decitabine, 1 mg K K2
Dacogen

Ⓘ J0895 Injection, deferoxamine mesylate, 500 mg N N1
Desferal
Pub 100-02, 15, 50; 100-4, 17, 10

Ⓘ J0900 Injection, testosterone enanthate and estradiol valerate, up to 1 cc N N1
Andrest 90-4, Andro-Estro 90-4, Androgyn L.A., Deladumone, Deladumone OB, Delatestadiol, Ditate-DS, Dua-Gen L.A., Duoval P.A., Estra-Testrin, TEEV, Testadiate, Testradiol 90/4, Valertest No. 1, Valertest No. 2
Pub 100-02, 15, 50; 100-4, 17, 10

Ⓘ J0945 Injection, brompheniramine maleate, per 10 mg N K2
Codimal-A, Cophene B, Dehist, Histaject, Nasahist B, ND Stat, Oraminic II, Sinusol-B
Pub 100-02, 15, 50; 100-4, 17, 10

✖ ~~J0970 Injection, estradiol valerate, up to 40 mg~~
This code is deleted as of December 31, 2010
See code(s) J1380

Ⓘ J1000 Injection, depo-estradiol cypionate, up to 5 mg ♀ N N1
Estra-D, Estradiol cypionate, Estro-Cyp, Estroject L.A
Pub 100-02, 15, 50; 100-4, 17, 10

Ⓘ J1020 Injection, methylprednisolone acetate, 20 mg N N1
Depo-Medrol, depMedalone 40, depMedalone 80, Depoject, Depopred-40, Depopred-80, D-Med 80, Duralone-40, Duralone-80, Medralone 40, Medralone 80, M-Prednisol-40, M-Prednisol-80, Rep-Pred 40, Rep-Pred 80
Pub 100-02, 15, 50; 100-4, 17, 10

Ⓘ J1030 Injection, methylprednisolone acetate, 40 mg N N1
Depo-Medrol, depMedalone 40, depMedalone 80, Depoject, Depopred-40, Depopred-80, D-Med 80, Duralone-40, Duralone-80, Medralone 40, Medralone 80, M-Prednisol-40, M-Prednisol-80, Rep-Pred 40, Rep-Pred 80
Pub 100-02, 15, 50; 100-4, 17, 10

Ⓘ J1040 Injection, methylprednisolone acetate, 80 mg N N1
Depo-Medrol, depMedalone 40, depMedalone 80, Depoject, Depopred-40, Depopred-80, D-Med 80, Duralone-40, Duralone-80, Medralone 40, Medralone 80, M-Prednisol-40, M-Prednisol-80, Rep-Pred 40, Rep-Pred 80
Pub 100-02, 15, 50; 100-4, 17, 10

Ⓘ J1051 Injection, medroxyprogesterone acetate, 50 mg ♀ N N1
Amen, Cycrin, Depo-Provera, Provera
Pub 100-02, 15, 50; 100-4, 17, 10

⊘ J1055 Injection, medroxyprogesterone acetate for contraceptive use, 150 mg ♀ E
Amen, Cycrin, Depo-Provera, Provera
Medicare Statute 1862(a)(1)

J1056 Injection, medroxyprogesterone acetate/estradiol cypionate, 5mg/25mg ♀ E
Lunelle

Ⓘ J1060 Injection, testosterone cypionate and estradiol cypionate, up to 1 ml N N1
Depo-Testadiol, Andro/Fem, De-Comberol, depAndrogyn, Depotestogen, Duo-Cyp, Duratestrin, Menoject LA, Test-Estro-C, Test-Estro Cypionate
Pub 100-02, 15, 50; 100-4, 17, 10

Ⓘ J1070 Injection, testosterone cypionate, up to 100 mg N N1
Depo-Testosterone, Duratest-100, Andro-Cyp, Andronaq-LA, Andronate-100, depAndro 100, Depotest, Testoject-LA
Pub 100-02, 15, 50; 100-4, 17, 10

Ⓘ J1080 Injection, testosterone cypionate, 1 cc, 200 mg N N1
Depo-Testosterone, Andro-Cyp 200, Andronate-200, depAndro 200, Depotest, Duratest-200, Testa-C, Testadiate-Depo, Testoject-LA
Pub 100-02, 15, 50; 100-4, 17, 10

Ⓘ J1094 Injection, dexamethasone acetate, 1 mg N N1
Cortastat L.A., Dalalone D.P., Dalalone L.A., Decadron - L.A., Decaject - L.A., Dexacen LA-8, Dexasone L.A., Dexone L.A., Solurex L.A.
Pub 100-02, 15, 50; 100-4, 17, 10

Ⓘ J1100 Injection, dexamethasone sodium phosphate, 1 mg N N1
Cortastat, Dalalone, Decadron Phosphate, Decaject, Dexacen-4, Dexasone, Hexadrol Phosphate, Solurex
Pub 100-02, 15, 50; 100-4, 17, 10

Ⓘ J1110 Injection, dihydroergotamine mesylate, per 1 mg N N1
D.H.E. 45, Migranal
Pub 100-02, 15, 50; 100-4, 17, 10

Ⓘ J1120 Injection, acetazolamide sodium, up to 500 mg N N1
Ak-Zol, Dazamide, Diamox, Storzolamide
Pub 100-02, 15, 50; 100-4, 17, 10

Ⓘ J1160 Injection, digoxin, up to 0.5 mg N N1
Lanoxin
Pub 100-02, 15, 50; 100-4, 17, 10

Ⓘ J1162 Injection, digoxin immune fab (ovine), per vial K K2
Digibind, DigiFab
Pub 100-02, 15, 50; 100-4, 17, 10

Ⓘ J1165 Injection, phenytoin sodium, per 50 mg N N1
Dilantin, Phenytek
Pub 100-02, 15, 50; 100-4, 17, 10

Ⓘ J1170 Injection, hydromorphone, up to 4 mg N N1
Dilaudid
Pub 100-02, 15, 50; 100-4, 17, 10

Ⓘ J1180 Injection, dyphylline, up to 500 mg N N1
Dilor, Lufyllin
Pub 100-02, 15, 50; 100-4, 17, 10

ⓘ **J1190** Injection, dexrazoxane hydrochloride, per 250 mg K K2
Zinecard
Pub 100-02, 15, 50; 100-4, 17, 10

ⓘ **J1200** Injection, diphenhydramine HCl, up to 50 mg N N1
Aller-med Banophen, Bena-D 10, Bena-D 50, Benadryl, Benadryl Allergy, Benahist 10, Benahist 50, Ben-Allergin-50, Benoject-10, Benoject-50, Compoz, Dihydrex, Diphenacen-50, Diphenadryl, Diphenhist, Dormarex, Genahist, Hydramine, Hyrexin-50, Siladryl, Wehdryl
Pub 100-02, 15, 50; 100-4, 17, 10

ⓘ **J1205** Injection, chlorothiazide sodium, per 500 mg K K2
Diuril Sodium
Pub 100-02, 15, 50; 100-4, 17, 10

ⓘ **J1212** Injection, DMSO, dimethyl sulfoxide, 50%, 50 ml K N1
Rimso
NCD 230.12; Pub 100-02, 15, 50; 100-4, 17, 10

ⓘ **J1230** Injection, methadone HCl, up to 10 mg N N1
Dolophine, Methadose
Pub 100-02, 15, 50; 100-4, 17, 10

ⓘ **J1240** Injection, dimenhydrinate, up to 50 mg N N1
Dinate, Dramamine, Dramanate, Dramilin, Dramocen, Dramoject, Dymenate, Hydrate, Marmine, Wehamine
Pub 100-02, 15, 50; 100-4, 17, 10

ⓘ **J1245** Injection, dipyridamole, per 10 mg N N1
Persantine
Pub 100-04, 13, 50.2,100-2, 15, 50; 100-4, 17, 10

ⓘ **J1250** Injection, dobutamine hydrochloride, per 250 mg N N1
Dobutrex
Pub 100-02, 15, 50; 100-4, 17, 10

ⓘ **J1260** Injection, dolasetron mesylate, 10 mg K N1
Anzemet
Pub 100-02, 15, 50; 100-4, 17, 10

J1265 Injection, dopamine HCl, 40 mg N N1
Dopastat, Intropin

J1267 Injection, doripenem, 10 mg G K2
Doribax
AHA: 2Q 2008, 8

J1270 Injection, doxercalciferol, 1 mcg N N1
Hectorol

● **J1290** Injection, ecallantide, 1 mg N K2
Kalbitor
This code is effective January 1, 2011

J1300 Injection, eculizumab, 10 mg G K2
Soliris
AHA: 1Q 2008, 7

ⓘ **J1320** Injection, amitriptyline HCl, up to 20 mg N N1
Elavil, Endep, Enovil
Pub 100-02, 15, 50; 100-4, 17, 10

J1324 Injection, enfuvirtide, 1 mg N K2
Fuzeon

ⓘ **J1325** Injection, epoprostenol, 0.5 mg N N1
Flolan
Pub 100-02, 15, 50; 100-4, 17, 10

ⓘ **J1327** Injection, eptifibatide, 5 mg K K2
Integrilin
Pub 100-02, 15, 50; 100-4, 17, 10

ⓘ **J1330** Injection, ergonovine maleate, up to 0.2 mg K N1
Ergotrate
Pub 100-02, 15, 50; 100-4, 17, 10

J1335 Injection, ertapenem sodium, 500 mg N N1
Invanz

ⓘ **J1364** Injection, erythromycin lactobionate, per 500 mg N N1
Erythrocin
Pub 100-02, 15, 50; 100-4, 17, 10

ⓘ **J1380** Injection, estradiol valerate, up to 10 mg N N1
Dioval, Dioval XX, Delestrogen, Duragen-10, Valergen 10
Pub 100-02, 15, 50; 100-4, 17, 10

✖ ~~J1390 Injection, estradiol valerate, up to 20 mg~~
This code is deleted as of December 31, 2010
See code(s) J1380

ⓘ **J1410** Injection, estrogen conjugated, per 25 mg K K2
Cenestin, Premarin
Pub 100-02, 15, 50; 100-4, 17, 10

ⓘ **J1430** Injection, ethanolamine oleate, 100 mg K K2
Ethamolin
Pub 100-02, 15, 50; 100-4, 17, 10

ⓘ **J1435** Injection, estrone, per 1 mg N N1
Estragyn 5, Estrone Aqueous, Estrone 5, Estronol, Kestrone 5, Theelin Aqueous
Pub 100-02, 15, 50; 100-4, 17, 10

ⓘ **J1436** Injection, etidronate disodium, per 300 mg K K2
Didronel
Pub 100-02, 15, 50; 100-4, 17, 10

ⓘ **J1438** Injection, etanercept, 25 mg (code may be used for Medicare when drug administered under the direct supervision of a physician, not for use when drug is self-administered) K K2
Enbrel
Pub 100-02, 15, 50; 100-4, 17, 10

ⓘ **J1440** Injection, filgrastim (G-CSF), 300 mcg K K2
Neupogen
Pub 100-02, 15, 50; 100-4, 17, 10

ⓘ **J1441** Injection, filgrastim (G-CSF), 480 mcg K K2
Neupogen
Pub 100-02, 15, 50; 100-4, 17, 10

ⓘ **J1450** Injection fluconazole, 200 mg N N1
Diflucan
Pub 100-02, 15, 50.5; 100-2, 15, 50.5.2.1; 100-4, 17, 80.3-80.3.2

ⓘ **J1451** Injection, fomepizole, 15 mg K K2
Antizol
Pub 100-02, 15, 50; 100-4, 17, 10

ⓘ **J1452** Injection, fomivirsen sodium, intraocular, 1.65 mg K N1
Vitravene
Pub 100-02, 15, 50.3

J1453 Injection, fosaprepitant, 1 mg G K2
Emend
AHA: 3Q 2008, 6

ⓘ **J1455** Injection, foscarnet sodium, per 1,000 mg K N1
Foscavir
Pub 100-02, 15, 50; 100-4, 17, 10

J1457 Injection, gallium nitrate, 1 mg K K2
Ganite

J1458 Injection, galsulfase, 1 mg K K2
Naglazyme

J1459 Injection, immune globulin (privigen), intravenous, non-lyophilized (e.g. liquid), 500 mg G K2
Privigen
AHA: 2Q 2008, 8, 10

ⓘ **J1460** Injection, gamma globulin, intramuscular, 1 cc K K2
BayGam, Gamastan, Gammar
Pub 100-02, 15, 50; 100-4, 17, 10

× ~~J1470 Injection, gamma globulin, intramuscular, 2 cc~~
This code is deleted as of December 31, 2010
See code(s) J1560

× ~~J1480 Injection, gamma globulin, intramuscular, 3 cc~~
This code is deleted as of December 31, 2010
See code(s) J1560

× ~~J1490 Injection, gamma globulin, intramuscular, 4 cc~~
This code is deleted as of December 31, 2010
See code(s) J1560

× ~~J1500 Injection, gamma globulin, intramuscular, 5 cc~~
This code is deleted as of December 31, 2010
See code(s) J1560

× ~~J1510 Injection, gamma globulin, intramuscular, 6 cc~~
This code is deleted as of December 31, 2010
See code(s) J1560

× ~~J1520 Injection, gamma globulin, intramuscular, 7 cc~~
This code is deleted as of December 31, 2010
See code(s) J1560

× ~~J1530 Injection, gamma globulin, intramuscular, 8 cc~~
This code is deleted as of December 31, 2010
See code(s) J1560

× ~~J1540 Injection, gamma globulin, intramuscular, 9 cc~~
This code is deleted as of December 31, 2010
See code(s) J1560

× ~~J1550 Injection, gamma globulin, intramuscular, 10 cc~~
This code is deleted as of December 31, 2010
See code(s) J1560

● J1559 Injection, immune globulin (Hizentra), 100 mg B K2

J1560 Injection, gamma globulin, intramuscular, over 10 cc B K2
BayGam, Gamastan, Gammar
This code is effective January 1, 2011
Pub 100-02, 15, 50; 100-4, 17, 10

J1561 Injection, immune globulin, (Gamunex), intravenous, non-lyophilized (e.g. liquid), 500 mg K K2
Pub 100-02, 15, 50; 100-4, 17, 10)
AHA: 1Q 2008, 7

J1562 Injection, immune globulin (Vivaglobin), 100 mg K K2
Pub 100-04, 17, 80.6

J1566 Injection, immune globulin, intravenous, lyophilized (e.g. powder), not otherwise specified, 500 mg K K2
Gamimune-N, Gammagard S/D, Gammar-P I.V., Iveegam, Polygam S/D, Sandoglobulin, Venoglobulin-I, Venoglobulin-S
Pub 100-02, 15, 50; 100-4, 17, 10)

J1568 Injection, immune globulin, (Octagam), intravenous, non-lyophilized (e.g. liquid), 500 mg K K2
Pub 100-04, 17, 80.6
AHA: 1Q 2008, 7

J1569 Injection, immune globulin, (Gammagard liquid), intravenous, non-lyophilized (e.g. liquid), 500 mg K K2
Pub 100-02, 15, 50; 100-4, 17, 10)v
AHA: 1Q 2008, 7

J1570 Injection, ganciclovir sodium, 500 mg N N1
Cytovene IV
Pub 100-02, 15, 50; 100-4, 17, 10

J1571 Injection, hepatitis B immune globulin (HepaGam B), intramuscular, 0.5 ml K K2
Pub 100-02, 15, 50; 100-4, 17, 10
AHA: 1Q 2008, 7, 3Q 2008, 7

J1572 Injection, immune globulin, (Flebogamma/Flebogamma DIF), intravenous, non-lyophilized (e.g. liquid), 500 mg K K2
Pub 100-02, 15, 50; 100-4, 17, 10)
AHA: 1Q 2008, 7

J1573 Injection, hepatitis B immune globulin (HepaGam B), intravenous, 0.5 ml K K2
AHA: 1Q 2008, 7, 3Q 2008, 8

J1580 Injection, garamycin, gentamicin, up to 80 mg N N1
G-Mycin, Jenamicin
Pub 100-02, 15, 50; 100-4, 17, 10

J1590 Injection, gatifloxacin, 10 mg N N1
Tequin

J1595 Injection, glatiramer acetate, 20 mg N K2
Copaxone
Pub 100-02, 15, 50; 100-4, 17, 10

● J1599 Injection, immune globulin, intravenous, non-lyophilized (e.g. liquid), not otherwise specified, 500 mg B N1
Hepagram B, Fleogamma, Gammaguard, Gamunex, Octogam, Privigen
This code is effective January 1, 2011

J1600 Injection, gold sodium thiomalate, up to 50 mg N N1
Myochoysine
Pub 100-02, 15, 50; 100-4, 17, 10

J1610 Injection, glucagon hydrochloride, per 1 mg K K2
GlucaGen diagnostic kit, Glucagon diagnostic kit
Pub 100-02, 15, 50; 100-4, 17, 10

J1620 Injection, gonadorelin hydrochloride, per 100 mcg K K2
Factrel
Pub 100-02, 15, 50; 100-4, 17, 10

J1626 Injection, granisetron hydrochloride, 100 mcg K N1
Kytril
Pub 100-02, 15, 50; 100-4, 17, 10

J1630 Injection, haloperidol, up to 5 mg N N1
Haldol
Pub 100-02, 15, 50; 100-4, 17, 10

J1631 Injection, haloperidol decanoate, per 50 mg N N1
Haldol deconoate
Pub 100-02, 15, 50; 100-4, 17, 10

J1640 Injection, hemin, 1 mg K K2
Panhematin
Pub 100-02, 15, 50; 100-4, 17, 10

J1642 Injection, heparin sodium, (heparin lock flush), per 10 units N N1
Hep-Lock, Hep-Lock U/P, Hep-Pak
Pub 100-02, 15, 50; 100-4, 17, 10

J1644 Injection, heparin sodium, per 1,000 units N N1
Calciparine, Liquaemin
Pub 100-02, 15, 50; 100-4, 17, 10

J1645 Injection, dalteparin sodium, per 2500 IU N N1
Fragmin
Pub 100-02, 15, 50; 100-4, 17, 10

J1650 Injection, enoxaparin sodium, 10 mg N N1
Lovenox
Pub 100-02, 15, 50; 100-4, 17, 10

J1652 Injection, fondaparinux sodium, 0.5 mg K K2
Arixtra
Pub 100-02, 15, 50; 100-4, 17, 10

J1655 Injection, tinzaparin sodium, 1,000 IU N N1
Innohep

J1670 Injection, tetanus immune globulin, human, up to 250 units K K2
BayTet, Hyper-Tet
Pub 100-02, 15, 50; 100-4, 17, 10

Medicare Non-Coverage | Special Coverage Instructions | Coverage Carrier Determined | A – Y APC Status Indicators | ● New Code | ▲ Revised Code | × Deleted Code
AHA AHA Coding Clinic for HCPCS | A2 – Z3 ASC Payment Indicators | DMEPOS | ♂ Male | ♀ Female | PQRI PQRI

Ⓘ J1675 Injection, histrelin acetate, 10 micrograms B
Supprelin
Pub 100-02, 15, 50; 100-4, 17, 10

J1680 Injection, human fibrinogen concentrate, 100 mg G K2

Ⓘ J1700 Injection, hydrocortisone acetate, up to 25 mg N N1
Anucort-HC, Anusol-HC, Cortifoam, Hydrocortone Acetate, Proctocort
Pub 100-02, 15, 50; 100-4, 17, 10

Ⓘ J1710 Injection, hydrocortisone sodium phosphate, up to 50 mg N N1
Hydrocortone phosphate
Pub 100-02, 15, 50; 100-4, 17, 10

Ⓘ J1720 Injection, hydrocortisone sodium succinate, up to 100 mg N N1
A-HydroCort, Solu-Cortef
Pub 100-02, 15, 50; 100-4, 17, 10

Ⓘ J1730 Injection, diazoxide, up to 300 mg K K2
Hyperstat IV
Pub 100-02, 15, 50; 100-4, 17, 10

J1740 Injection, ibandronate sodium, 1 mg K K2
Boniva

Ⓘ J1742 Injection, ibutilide fumarate, 1 mg K K2
Corvert
Pub 100-02, 15, 50; 100-4, 17, 10

J1743 Injection, idursulfase, 1 mg K K2
Elaprase
AHA: 1Q 2008, 7

Ⓘ J1745 Injection infliximab, 10 mg K K2
Remicade
Pub 100-02, 15, 50; 100-4, 17, 10

J1750 Injection, iron dextran, 50 mg K K2
AHA: 2Q 2008, 8, 10

J1756 Injection, iron sucrose, 1 mg K K2
Venofer
Pub 100-04, 8, 60.2.4-60.2.4.2

✖ ~~J1785 Injection, imiglucerase, per unit~~
This code is deleted as of December 31, 2010
See code(s) J1786

● Ⓘ J1786 Injection, imiglucerase, 10 units N K2
Cerezym
This code is effective January 1, 2011

Ⓘ J1790 Injection, droperidol, up to 5 mg N N1
Inapsine
Pub 100-02, 15, 50; 100-4, 17, 10

Ⓘ J1800 Injection, propranolol HCl, up to 1 mg N N1
Inderal
Pub 100-02, 15, 50; 100-4, 17, 10

Ⓘ J1810 Injection, droperidol and fentanyl citrate, up to 2 ml ampule E
Innovar
Pub 100-02, 15, 50; 100-4, 17, 10

Ⓘ J1815 Injection, insulin, per 5 units N N1
Humulin-R, Iletin, Novolin-R, NPH, Regular, Velosulin
NCD 40.2; Pub 100-02, 15, 50; 100-4, 17, 10

J1817 Insulin for administration through DME (i.e., insulin pump) per 50 units N K2
Humalog, Lispro

✖ ~~J1825 Injection, interferon beta-1a, 33 mcg~~
This code is deleted as of December 31, 2010
See code(s) J1825, Q3025, Q3026

● J1826 Injection, interferon beta-1A, 30 mcg N
Avonex
This code is effective January 1, 2011

Ⓘ J1830 Injection interferon beta-1b, 0.25 mg (code may be used for Medicare when drug administered under the direct supervision of a physician, not for use when drug is self-administered) K K2
Betaseron
Pub 100-02, 15, 50; 100-4, 17, 10

J1835 Injection, itraconazole, 50 mg K N1
Sporonox

Ⓘ J1840 Injection, kanamycin sulfate, up to 500 mg N N1
Kantrex, Klebcil
Pub 100-02, 15, 50; 100-4, 17, 10

Ⓘ J1850 Injection, kanamycin sulfate, up to 75 mg N N1
Kantrex, Klebcil
Pub 100-02, 15, 50; 100-4, 17, 10

Ⓘ J1885 Injection, ketorolac tromethamine, per 15 mg N N1
Toradol
Pub 100-02, 15, 50; 100-4, 17, 10

Ⓘ J1890 Injection, cephalothin sodium, up to 1 gram N N1
Keflin
Pub 100-02, 15, 50; 100-4, 17, 10

J1930 Injection, lanreotide, 1 mg K K2
Somatuline Depot

J1931 Injection, laronidase, 0.1 mg K K2
Aldurazyme

Ⓘ J1940 Injection, furosemide, up to 20 mg N N1
Furomide M.D., Lasix
Pub 100-02, 15, 50; 100-4, 17, 10

Ⓘ J1945 Injection, lepirudin, 50 mg K K2
Refludan
Pub 100-02, 15, 50; 100-4, 17, 10

Ⓘ J1950 Injection, leuprolide acetate (for depot suspension), per 3.75 mg K K2
Eligard, Lupron, Lupron Depot, Lupron Depot-PED
Pub 100-02, 15, 50; 100-4, 17, 10

J1953 Injection, levetiracetam, 10 mg G K2
Keppra

Ⓘ J1955 Injection, levocarnitine, per 1 gm B
Carnitor
Pub 100-02, 15, 50; 100-4, 17, 10

Ⓘ J1956 Injection, levofloxacin, 250 mg N N1
Levaquin
Pub 100-02, 15, 50; 100-4, 17, 10

Ⓘ J1960 Injection, levorphanol tartrate, up to 2 mg N N1
Levo-Dromoran
Pub 100-02, 15, 50; 100-4, 17, 10

Ⓘ J1980 Injection, hyoscyamine sulfate, up to 0.25 mg N N1
Anaspaz, Cystospaz, Cystospaz-M, Gastrosed, Levbid, Levsin, Levsin Drops, Levsin SL, Levsinex Timecaps, Neoquess
Pub 100-02, 15, 50; 100-4, 17, 10

Ⓘ J1990 Injection, chlordiazepoxide HCl, up to 100 mg N N1
Librax, Librium, Limbitrol
Pub 100-02, 15, 50; 100-4, 17, 10

Ⓘ J2001 Injection, lidocaine HCl for intravenous infusion, 10 mg N N1
Caine-1, Caine-2, Dalcaine, Lidoject-1, Lidoject-2, Dilocaine, L-Caine, Nervocaine 1%, Nervocaine 2%, Nulicaine, Octocaine, Xylocaine
Pub 100-02, 15, 50; 100-4, 17, 10

ⓘ J2010 Injection, lincomycin HCl, up to 300 mg N N1
Lincocin, Lincorex
Pub 100-02, 15, 50; 100-4, 17, 10

J2020 Injection, linezolid, 200 mg K K2
Zyvox

ⓘ J2060 Injection, lorazepam, 2 mg N N1
Ativan
Pub 100-02, 15, 50; 100-4, 17, 10

ⓘ J2150 Injection, mannitol, 25% in 50 ml N N1
Osmitrol
Pub 100-02, 15, 50; 100-4, 17, 10

J2170 Injection, mecasermin, 1 mg N K2
Increlex, Iplex

ⓘ J2175 Injection, meperidine hydrochloride, per 100 mg N N1
Demerol
Pub 100-02, 15, 50; 100-4, 17, 10

ⓘ J2180 Injection, meperidine and promethazine HCl, up to 50 mg N N1
Mepergan
Pub 100-02, 15, 50; 100-4, 17, 10

J2185 Injection, meropenem, 100 mg N N1
Merrem IV

ⓘ J2210 Injection, methylergonovine maleate, up to 0.2 mg N N1
Methergine, Methylergometrine
Pub 100-02, 15, 50; 100-4, 17, 10

J2248 Injection, micafungin sodium, 1 mg K K2
Mycamine

ⓘ J2250 Injection, midazolam hydrochloride, per 1 mg N N1
Versed
Pub 100-02, 15, 50; 100-4, 17, 10

ⓘ J2260 Injection, milrinone lactate, 5 mg N N1
Primacor
Pub 100-02, 15, 50; 100-4, 17, 10

ⓘ J2270 Injection, morphine sulfate, up to 10 mg N N1
Pub 100-02, 15, 50; 100-4, 17, 10
Duramorph, Infumorph

ⓘ J2271 Injection, morphine sulfate, 100 mg N N1
NCD 280.14; Pub 100-02, 15, 50; 100-4, 17, 10
Duramorph, Infumorph

ⓘ J2275 Injection, morphine sulfate (preservative-free sterile solution), per 10 mg N N1
NCD 280.14; Pub 100-02, 15, 50; 100-4, 17, 10
Astramorph PF

ⓘ J2278 Injection, ziconotide, 1 microgram G K2
Prialt

J2280 Injection, moxifloxacin, 100 mg N N1
Avelox

ⓘ J2300 Injection, nalbuphine hydrochloride, per 10 mg N N1
Nubain
Pub 100-02, 15, 50; 100-4, 17, 10

ⓘ J2310 Injection, naloxone hydrochloride, per 1 mg N N1
Narcan
Pub 100-02, 15, 50; 100-4, 17, 10

J2315 Injection, naltrexone, depot form, 1 mg K K2
Vivitrol

ⓘ J2320 Injection, nandrolone decanoate, up to 50 mg N K2
Deca-Durabolin, Decolone-50, Hybolin Decanoate, Kabolin, Nandrobolic L.A., Neo-Durabolic
Pub 100-02, 15, 50; 100-4, 17, 10

✖ ~~J2321 Injection, nandrolone decanoate, up to 100 mg~~
This code is deleted as of December 31, 2010
See code(s) J2320

✖ ~~J2322 Injection, nandrolone decanoate, up to 200 mg~~
This code is deleted as of December 31, 2010
See code(s) J2320

J2323 Injection, natalizumab, 1 mg K K2
Tysabri
AHA: 1Q 2008, 7

ⓘ J2325 Injection, nesiritide, 0.1 mg K K2
Natrecor
Pub 100-02, 15, 50; 100-4, 17, 10

J2353 Injection, octreotide, depot form for intramuscular injection, 1 mg K K2
Sandostatin Lar Depot

J2354 Injection, octreotide, non-depot form for subcutaneous or intravenous injection, 25 mcg N N1
Sandostatin

ⓘ J2355 Injection, oprelvekin, 5 mg K K2
Neumega
Pub 100-02, 15, 50; 100-4, 17, 10

J2357 Injection, omalizumab, 5 mg K K2
Xolair

● J2358 Injection, olanzapine, long-acting, 1 mg K K2
Zyprexa Relprevv
This code is effective January 1, 2011

ⓘ J2360 Injection, orphenadrine citrate, up to 60 mg N N1
Antiflex, Banflex, Flexoject, Flexon, K-Flex, Myolin, Neocyten, Norflex, O-Flex, Orphenate
Pub 100-02, 15, 50; 100-4, 17, 10

ⓘ J2370 Injection, phenylephrine HCl, up to 1 ml N N1
Neo-synephrine
Pub 100-02, 15, 50; 100-4, 17, 10

ⓘ J2400 Injection, chloroprocaine hydrochloride, per 30 ml N N1
Nesacaine, Nesacaine-MPF
Pub 100-02, 15, 50; 100-4, 17, 10

ⓘ J2405 Injection, ondansetron hydrochloride, per 1 mg K N1
Zofran, Zofran ODT
Pub 100-02, 15, 50; 100-4, 17, 10

ⓘ J2410 Injection, oxymorphone HCl, up to 1 mg N N1
Numorphan, Numorphan H.P.
Pub 100-02, 15, 50; 100-4, 17, 10

J2425 Injection, palifermin, 50 micrograms K K2
Kepivance

● J2426 Injection, paliperidone palmitate extended release, 1 mg K K2
Invega Sustenna
This code is effective January 1, 2011

ⓘ J2430 Injection, pamidronate disodium, per 30 mg K K2
Aredia
Pub 100-02, 15, 50; 100-4, 17, 10

ⓘ J2440 Injection, papaverine HCl, up to 60 mg N N1
Cerespan, Genabid, Pavagen
Pub 100-02, 15, 50; 100-4, 17, 10

ⓘ J2460 Injection, oxytetracycline HCl, up to 50 mg K N1
Terramycin
Pub 100-02, 15, 50; 100-4, 17, 10

J2469 Injection, palonosetron HCl, 25 mcg K K2
Aloxi

ⓘ J2501 Injection, paricalcitol, 1 mcg N N1
Zemplar
Pub 100-02, 15, 50; 100-4, 17, 10

J2503 Injection, pegaptanib sodium, 0.3 mg G K2
Macugen

J2504 Injection, pegademase bovine, 25 IU K K2
Adagen
Pub 100-02, 15, 50; 100-4, 17, 10

J2505 Injection, pegfilgrastim, 6 mg K K2
Neulasta

J2510 Injection, penicillin G procaine, aqueous, up to 600,000 units N N1
Wycillin, Duracillin A.S., Crysticillin 300 A.S., Crysticillin 600 A.S., Pfizerpen A.S
Pub 100-02, 15, 50; 100-4, 17, 10

J2513 Injection, pentastarch, 10% solution, 100 ml K K2
Pentaspan
Pub 100-02, 15, 50; 100-4, 17, 10

J2515 Injection, pentobarbital sodium, per 50 mg K N1
Nembutol sodium
Pub 100-02, 15, 50; 100-4, 17, 10

J2540 Injection, penicillin G potassium, up to 600,000 units N N1
Pfizerpen
Pub 100-02, 15, 50; 100-4, 17, 10

J2543 Injection, piperacillin sodium/tazobactam sodium, 1 gram/0.125 grams (1.125 grams) N N1
Zosyn
Pub 100-02, 15, 50; 100-4, 17, 10

J2545 Pentamidine isethionate, inhalation solution, FDA-approved final product, non-compounded, administered through DME, unit dose form, per 300 mg B
NebuPent, Pentacarinat, Pentam 300
Pub 100-02, 15, 50; 100-4, 17, 10

J2550 Injection, promethazine HCl, up to 50 mg N N1
Anergan 50, Phenazine 25, Phenazine 50, Phenergan, Prorex-25, Prorex-50, Prothazine, V-Gan 25, V-Gan 50
Pub 100-02, 15, 50; 100-4, 17, 10

J2560 Injection, phenobarbital sodium, up to 120 mg N N1
Luminal sodium
Pub 100-02, 15, 50; 100-4, 17, 10

J2562 Injection, plerixafor, 1 mg G K2
Mozobil

J2590 Injection, oxytocin, up to 10 units N N1
Pitocin, Syntocinon
Pub 100-02, 15, 50; 100-4, 17, 10

J2597 Injection, desmopressin acetate, per 1 mcg N N1
DDAVP
Pub 100-02, 15, 50; 100-4, 17, 10

J2650 Injection, prednisolone acetate, up to 1 ml N N1
Key-Pred 25, Key-Pred 50, Predcor-25, Predcor-50, Predoject 50, Predalone-50, Predicort-50
Pub 100-02, 15, 50; 100-4, 17, 10

J2670 Injection, tolazoline HCl, up to 25 mg N N1
Priscoline HCl
Pub 100-02, 15, 50; 100-4, 17, 10

J2675 Injection, progesterone, per 50 mg N N1
Gesterol 50
Pub 100-02, 15, 50; 100-4, 17, 10

J2680 Injection, fluphenazine decanoate, up to 25 mg N N1
Prolixin deconoate
Pub 100-02, 15, 50; 100-4, 17, 10

J2690 Injection, procainamide HCl, up to 1 gm ♀ N N1
Procan, Pronestyl, Promine
Pub 100-02, 15, 50; 100-4, 17, 10

J2700 Injection, oxacillin sodium, up to 250 mg N N1
Bactocill, Prostaphlin
Pub 100-02, 15, 50; 100-4, 17, 10

J2710 Injection, neostigmine methylsulfate, up to 0.5 mg N N1
Prostigmin
Pub 100-02, 15, 50; 100-4, 17, 10

J2720 Injection, protamine sulfate, per 10 mg N N1
Pub 100-02, 15, 50; 100-4, 17, 10

J2724 Injection, protein C concentrate, intravenous, human, 10 IU K K2
Ceprotin
AHA: 1Q 2008, 7

J2725 Injection, protirelin, per 250 mcg N N1
Relefact TRH, Thypinone
Pub 100-02, 15, 50; 100-4, 17, 10

J2730 Injection, pralidoxime chloride, up to 1 gm K K2
Protopam chloride
Pub 100-02, 15, 50; 100-4, 17, 10

J2760 Injection, phentolamine mesylate, up to 5 mg N N1
Regitine
Pub 100-02, 15, 50; 100-4, 17, 10

J2765 Injection, metoclopramide HCl, up to 10 mg N N1
Reglan
Pub 100-02, 15, 50; 100-4, 17, 10

J2770 Injection, quinupristin/dalfopristin, 500 mg (150/350) K K2
Synercid
Pub 100-02, 15, 50; 100-4, 17, 10

J2778 Injection, ranibizumab, 0.1 mg K K2
Lucentis
AHA: 1Q 2008, 7

J2780 Injection, ranitidine hydrochloride, 25 mg N N1
Tritec, Zantac
Pub 100-02, 15, 50; 100-4, 17, 10

J2783 Injection, rasburicase, 0.5 mg K K2
Elitek

J2785 Injection, regadenoson, 0.1 mg G K2
Lexiscan

J2788 Injection, Rho (D) immune globulin, human, minidose, 50 micrograms (250 I.U.) K K2
Gamulin RH, HypRho-D, MICRhoGAM, Rhesonativ, RhoGAM
Pub 100-02, 15, 50; 100-4, 17, 10

J2790 Injection, Rho (D) immune globulin, human, full dose, 300 micrograms (1500 I.U.) K K2
Gamulin RH, HypRho-D, MICRhoGAM, Rhesonativ, RhoGAM
Pub 100-02, 15, 50; 100-4, 17, 10

J2791 Injection, Rho (D) immune globulin (human), (Rhophylac), intramuscular or intravenous, 100 IU K K2
Pub 100-02, 15, 50; 100-4, 17, 10
AHA: 1Q 2008, 7

J2792 Injection, Rho (D) immune globulin, intravenous, human, solvent detergent, 100 IU K K2
Win Rho SDF
Pub 100-02, 15, 50; 100-4, 17, 10

J2793 Injection, rilonacept, 1 mg K K2
Arcalyst

J2794 Injection, risperidone, long acting, 0.5 mg K K2
Risperdal, Risperdal M-Tab

J2795 Injection, ropivacaine hydrochloride, 1 mg N N1
Naropin

J2796 Injection, romiplostim, 10 micrograms G K2
Nplate

J2800 Injection, methocarbamol, up to 10 ml N N1
Pub 100-02, 15, 50; 100-4, 17, 10
Robaxin

J2805 Injection, sincalide, 5 micrograms N N1
Kinevac

J2810 Injection, theophylline, per 40 mg K N1
Lanophyllin, Respbid
Pub 100-02, 15, 50; 100-4, 17, 10

J2820 Injection, sargramostim (GM-CSF), 50 mcg K K2
Leukine, Prokine
Pub 100-02, 15, 50; 100-4, 17, 10

J2850 Injection, secretin, synthetic, human, 1 microgram K K2
Secretin
Pub 100-02, 15, 50; 100-4, 17, 10

J2910 Injection, aurothioglucose, up to 50 mg N N1
Solganal
Pub 100-02, 15, 50; 100-4, 17, 10

J2916 Injection, sodium ferric gluconate complex in sucrose injection, 12.5 mg N N1
Ferrlecit
Pub 100-02, 15, 50.4-50.4.1, 100-2, 15, 50.4.3-50.4.4.2; 100-4, 8, 60.2.4-60.2.4.2

J2920 Injection, methylprednisolone sodium succinate, up to 40 mg N N1
A-methaPred, Solu-Medrol
Pub 100-02, 15, 50; 100-4, 17, 10

J2930 Injection, methylprednisolone sodium succinate, up to 125 mg N N1
A-methaPred, Solu-Medrol
Pub 100-02, 15, 50; 100-4, 17, 10

J2940 Injection, somatrem, 1 mg K K2
Protropin
Medicare Statute 1861s2b
Pub 100-02, 15, 50; 100-4, 17, 10

J2941 Injection, somatropin, 1 mg K K2
Genotropin, Humatrope, Nutropin, Nutropin AQ, Norditropin, Saizen, Serostim
Medicare Statute 1861s2b
Pub 100-02, 15, 50; 100-4, 17, 10

J2950 Injection, promazine HCl, up to 25 mg N N1
Sparine, Prozine-50
Pub 100-02, 15, 50; 100-4, 17, 10

J2993 Injection, reteplase, 18.1 mg K K2
Retavase
Pub 100-02, 15, 50; 100-4, 17, 10

J2995 Injection, streptokinase, per 250,000 IU K K2
Kabikinase, Streptase
Pub 100-02, 15, 50; 100-4, 17, 10

J2997 Injection, alteplase recombinant, 1 mg K K2
Activase
Pub 100-02, 15, 50; 100-4, 17, 10

J3000 Injection, streptomycin, up to 1 gm N N1
Pub 100-02, 15, 50; 100-4, 17, 10

J3010 Injection, fentanyl citrate, 0.1 mg N N1
Sublimaze
Pub 100-02, 15, 50; 100-4, 17, 10

J3030 Injection, sumatriptan succinate, 6 mg (code may be used for Medicare when drug administered under the direct supervision of a physician, not for use when drug is self administered) K K2
Imitrex
Pub 100-02, 15, 50; 100-4, 17, 10

J3070 Injection, pentazocine, 30 mg N N1
Talwin
Pub 100-02, 15, 50; 100-4, 17, 10

● J3095 Injection, televancin, 10 mg K K2
Vibativ
This code is effective January 1, 2011

J3101 Injection, tenecteplase, 1 mg K K2
TNKase

J3105 Injection, terbutaline sulfate, up to 1 mg N N1
Brethaire, Brethine, Bricanyl
Pub 100-02, 15, 50; 100-4, 17, 10

J3110 Injection, teriparatide, 10 mcg B
Forteo

J3120 Injection, testosterone enanthate, up to 100 mg N N1
Andropository 100, Delatest, Everone, Testone LA 100
Pub 100-02, 15, 50; 100-4, 17, 10

J3130 Injection, testosterone enanthate, up to 200 mg N N1
Andro L.A. 200, Andryl 200, Delatestryl, Durathate-200, Testone LA 200, Testrin PA
Pub 100-02, 15, 50; 100-4, 17, 10

J3140 Injection, testosterone suspension, up to 50 mg N N1
Andronaq 50, Testosterone Aqueous, Testaqua, Testoject-50, Histerone 50, Histerone 100
Pub 100-02, 15, 50; 100-4, 17, 10

J3150 Injection, testosterone propionate, up to 100 mg N N1
Testex
Pub 100-02, 15, 50; 100-4, 17, 10

J3230 Injection, chlorpromazine HCl, up to 50 mg N N1
Pub 100-02, 15, 50; 100-4, 17, 10
Chlorpromazine, Fluphenazine, Mesoridazine, Perphenazine, Prochlorperazine, Trifluoperazine, Triflupromazine

J3240 Injection, thyrotropin alpha, 0.9 mg, provided in 1.1 mg vial K K2
Thyrogen
Pub 100-02, 15, 50; 100-4, 17, 10

J3243 Injection, tigecycline, 1 mg K K2
Tygacil

J3246 Injection, tirofiban HCl, 0.25mg K K2
Aggrastat

J3250 Injection, trimethobenzamide HCl, up to 200 mg N N1
Arrestin, Tebamide, T-Gen, Ticon, Tigan, Tiject-20, Triban Trimazide
Pub 100-02, 15, 50; 100-4, 17, 10

J3260 Injection, tobramycin sulfate, up to 80 mg N N1
Nebcin
Pub 100-02, 15, 50; 100-4, 17, 10

● J3262 Injection, tocilizumab, 1 mg K K2
Actemra
This code is effective January 1, 2011

J3265 Injection, torsemide, 10 mg/ml N N1
Demadex
Pub 100-02, 15, 50; 100-4, 17, 10

J3280 Injection, thiethylperazine maleate, up to 10 mg N N1
Pub 100-02, 15, 50; 100-4, 17, 10

J3285 Injection, treprostinil, 1 mg K K2
Remodulin

J2795 – J3285

J3300 Injection, triamcinolone acetonide, preservative free, 1 mg N N1
Triesence

ⓘ J3301 Injection, triamcinolone acetonide, not otherwise specified, 10 mg N N1
Cenacort A-40, Kenalog-10, Kenalog-40, Tri-Kort, Kenaject-40, Triam-A, Trilog
Pub 100-02, 15, 50; 100-4, 17, 10

ⓘ J3302 Injection, triamcinolone diacetate, per 5 mg N N1
Aristocort Intralesional, Aristocort Forte, Amcort, Cenacort Forte, Trilone
Pub 100-02, 15, 50; 100-4, 17, 10

ⓘ J3303 Injection, triamcinolone hexacetonide, per 5 mg N N1
Aristospan Intralesional, Aristospan Intra-Articular
Pub 100-02, 15, 50; 100-4, 17, 10

ⓘ J3305 Injection, trimetrexate glucuronate, per 25 mg K K2
Neutrexin
Pub 100-02, 15, 50; 100-4, 17, 10

ⓘ J3310 Injection, perphenazine, up to 5 mg N N1
Trilafon
Pub 100-02, 15, 50; 100-4, 17, 10

ⓘ J3315 Injection, triptorelin pamoate, 3.75 mg K K2
Trelstar Depot
Pub 100-02, 15, 50; 100-4, 17, 10

ⓘ J3320 Injection, spectinomycin dihydrochloride, up to 2 gm N N1
Trobicin
Pub 100-02, 15, 50; 100-4, 17, 10

ⓘ J3350 Injection, urea, up to 40 gm K N1
Ureaphil
Pub 100-02, 15, 50; 100-4, 17, 10

ⓘ J3355 Injection, urofollitropin, 75 IU K K2
Bravelle, Fertinex, Metrodin
Pub 100-02, 15, 50; 100-4, 17, 10

● J3357 Injection, ustekinumab, 1 mg K K2
Stelara
This code is effective January 1, 2011

ⓘ J3360 Injection, diazepam, up to 5 mg N N1
Diastat, Diazepam Intensol, Valium, Zetran
Pub 100-02, 15, 50; 100-4, 17, 10
AHA: 2Q 2007, 6

ⓘ J3364 Injection, urokinase, 5000 IU vial N N1
Abbokinase, Open Cath
Pub 100-02, 15, 50; 100-4, 17, 10

ⓘ J3365 Injection, IV, urokinase, 250,000 IU vial K K2
Abbokinase
Pub 100-02, 15, 50; 100-4, 17, 10

ⓘ J3370 Injection, vancomycin HCl, 500 mg N N1
Vancocin, Vancoled
NCD 40.2; Pub 100-02, 15, 50; 100-4, 17, 10

● J3385 Injection, velaglucerase alfa, 100 units K K2
VPRIV
This code is effective January 1, 2011

ⓘ J3396 Injection, verteporfin, 0.1 mg K K2
Visudyne
NCD 20.290, NCD 80.3

ⓘ J3400 Injection, triflupromazine HCl, up to 20 mg K N1
Vesprin
Pub 100-02, 15, 50; 100-4, 17, 10

ⓘ J3410 Injection, hydroxyzine HCl, up to 25 mg N N1
Atarax, Hyzine-50, Vistaject-50, Vistaril
Pub 100-02, 15, 50; 100-4, 17, 10

J3411 Injection, thiamine HCl, 100 mg N N1
Vitamin B-1

J3415 Injection, pyridoxine HCl, 100 mg N N1
Nestrex, Rodex

ⓘ J3420 Injection, vitamin B-12 cyanocobalamin, up to 1,000 mcg N N1
Berubigen, Betalin 12, Cobex, Crystamine, Cyanoject, Cyomin, Redisol, Rubramin PC, Sytobex
NCD 150.6; Pub 100-02, 15, 50; 100-4, 17, 10

ⓘ J3430 Injection, phytonadione (vitamin K), per 1 mg N N1
AquaMEPHYTON, Konakion, Mephyton
Pub 100-02, 15, 50; 100-4, 17, 10

ⓘ J3465 Injection, voriconazole, 10 mg K K2
Vfend
Pub 100-02, 15, 50; 100-4, 17, 10

ⓘ J3470 Injection, hyaluronidase, up to 150 units N N1
Amphadase, Vitrase, Wydase
Pub 100-02, 15, 50; 100-4, 17, 10

ⓘ J3471 Injection, hyaluronidase, ovine, preservative free, per 1 USP unit (up to 999 USP units) N N1
Vitrase
Pub 100-02, 15, 50; 100-4, 17, 10

ⓘ J3472 Injection, hyaluronidase, ovine, preservative free, per 1000 USP units K N1
Vitrase
Pub 100-02, 15, 50; 100-4, 17, 10

ⓘ J3473 Injection, hyaluronidase, recombinant, 1 usp unit K N1
Hylenex Recombinant
Pub 100-02, 15, 50; 100-4, 17, 10

ⓘ J3475 Injection, magnesium sulfate, per 500 mg N N1
Pub 100-02, 15, 50; 100-4, 17, 10

ⓘ J3480 Injection, potassium chloride, per 2 meq N N1
Pub 100-02, 15, 50; 100-4, 17, 10

ⓘ J3485 Injection, zidovudine, 10 mg N N1
Retrovir
Pub 100-02, 15, 50; 100-4, 17, 10

J3486 Injection, ziprasidone mesylate, 10 mg N N1
Geodon

J3487 Injection, zoledronic acid (Zometa), 1 mg K K2

ⓘ J3488 Injection, zoledronic acid (Reclast), 1 mg G K2
AHA: 1Q 2008, 7

ⓘ J3490 Unclassified drugs N N1
Pub 100-02, 15, 50; 100-4, 17, 10

⊘ J3520 Edetate disodium, per 150 mg E
Chealamide, Disodium EDTA, Disotate, Endrate, Endrate ethylenediamine-tetra-acetic acid
NCD 20.21, NCD 20.22

ⓘ J3530 Nasal vaccine inhalation N N1
Pub 100-02, 15, 50; 100-4, 17, 10

⊘ J3535 Drug administered through a metered dose inhaler E
Pub 100-02, 15, 50

⊘ J3570 Laetrile, amygdalin, vitamin B-17 E
NCD 30.7

J3590 Unclassified biologics N N1

Miscellaneous Drugs and Solutions

ⓘ J7030 Infusion, normal saline solution, 1,000 cc N N1
Pub 100-02, 15, 50; 100-4, 17, 10

ⓘ J7040 Infusion, normal saline solution, sterile (500 ml = 1 unit) N N1
Pub 100-02, 15, 50; 100-4, 17, 10

ⓘ J7042 5% dextrose/normal saline (500 ml = 1 unit) N N1
Pub 100-02, 15, 50; 100-4, 17, 10

ⓘ J7050 Infusion, normal saline solution, 250 cc N N1
Pub 100-02, 15, 50; 100-4, 17, 10

ⓘ J7060 5% dextrose/water (500 ml = 1 unit) N N1
Pub 100-02, 15, 50; 100-4, 17, 10

ⓘ J7070 Infusion, D-5-W, 1000 cc N N1
Dextrose 5% in water
Pub 100-02, 15, 50; 100-4, 17, 10

ⓘ J7100 Infusion, dextran 40, 500 ml N N1
Gentran 40, 10% LMD, Rheomacrodex
Pub 100-02, 15, 50; 100-4, 17, 10

ⓘ J7110 Infusion, dextran 75, 500 ml N N1
Gentran 75
Pub 100-02, 15, 50; 100-4, 17, 10

ⓘ J7120 Ringers lactate infusion, up to 1000 cc N N1
Pub 100-02, 15, 50; 100-4, 17, 10

ⓘ J7130 Hypertonic saline solution, 50 or 100 meq, 20 cc vial N N1
Pub 100-02, 15, 50; 100-4, 17, 10

● ⓘ J7184 Injection, von Willebrand factor complex (human), Wilate, per 100 IU VWF:RCO K K2
This code is effective January 1, 2011

J7185 Injection, factor VIII (antihemophilic factor, recombinant) (Xyntha), per I.U. K K2

ⓘ J7186 Injection, antihemophilic factor VIII/von Willebrand factor complex (human), per factor VIII I.U. K K2
Humate-P
AHA: 2Q 2008, 8, 10

ⓘ J7187 Injection, von Willebrand factor complex (Humate-P), per IU vWF:RCo K K2
Humate-P
Pub 100-02, 15, 50; 100-4, 17, 10

ⓘ J7189 Factor VIIa (antihemophilic factor, recombinant), per 1 microgram K K2
Kogenate FS, NovoSeven
Pub 100-02, 15, 50; 100-4, 17, 10

ⓘ J7190 Factor VIII (antihemophilic factor, human) per IU K K2
Alphanate, Hemofil M, Humate-P, Koate-HP, Monarc-M, Monoclate-P
Pub 100-02, 15, 50; 100-4, 17, 10

ⓘ J7191 Factor VIII (antihemophilic factor (porcine), per IU K N1
Hyate: C
Pub 100-02, 15, 50; 100-4, 17, 10

ⓘ J7192 Factor VIII (antihemophilic factor, recombinant) per I.U., not otherwise specified K K2
Bioclate, Helixate FS, Kogenate, Kogenate FS, Recombinate, ReFacto
Pub 100-02, 15, 50; 100-4, 17, 10

ⓘ J7193 Factor IX (antihemophilic factor, purified, non-recombinant) per IU K K2
Alpha-Nine SD, Bebulin VH, Benefix, Konyne 80, Mononine, Profilnine SD, Proplex SX-T, Proplex T
Pub 100-02, 15, 50; 100-4, 17, 10

ⓘ J7194 Factor IX, complex, per IU K K2
Alpha-Nine SD, Bebulin VH, Benefix, Konyne 80, Mononine, Profilnine SD, Proplex SX-T, Proplex T
Pub 100-02, 15, 50; 100-4, 17, 10

ⓘ J7195 Factor IX (antihemophilic factor, recombinant) per IU K K2
Alpha-Nine SD, Bebulin VH, Benefix, Konyne 80, Mononine, Profilnine SD, Proplex SX-T, Proplex T
Pub 100-02, 15, 50; 100-4, 17, 10

● J7196 Injection, antithrombin recombinant, 50 IU K K2
ATryn
This code is effective January 1, 2011

ⓘ J7197 Antithrombin III (human), per IU N K2
Thrombate III
Pub 100-02, 15, 50; 100-4, 17, 10

ⓘ J7198 Anti-inhibitor, per IU K K2
Autoplex T, Feiba VH Immuno
NCD 110.3,100-2, 15, 50; 100-4, 17, 10; 100-4, 17, 80.4

ⓘ J7199 Hemophilia clotting factor, not otherwise classified B
NCD 110.3,100-2, 15, 50; 100-4, 17, 10; 100-4, 17, 80.4

⊘ J7300 Intrauterine copper contraceptive ♀ E
ParaGard, Paragarel T380A
Medicare Statute 1862(a)(1)

⊘ J7302 Levonorgestrel-releasing intrauterine contraceptive system, 52 mg ♀ E
Mirena
Medicare Statute 1862(a)(1)

⊘ J7303 Contraceptive supply, hormone containing vaginal ring, each ♀ E
NuvaRing
Medicare Statute 1862(a)(1)

⊘ J7304 Contraceptive supply, hormone containing patch, each ♀ E
ORTHO EVRA
Medicare Statute 1862(a)(1)

⊘ J7306 Levonorgestrel (contraceptive) implant system, including implants and supplies ♀ E
Norplant

⊘ J7307 Etonogestrel (contraceptive) implant system, including implant and supplies ♀ E
Implanon

Insertion of implantable contraceptive capsules

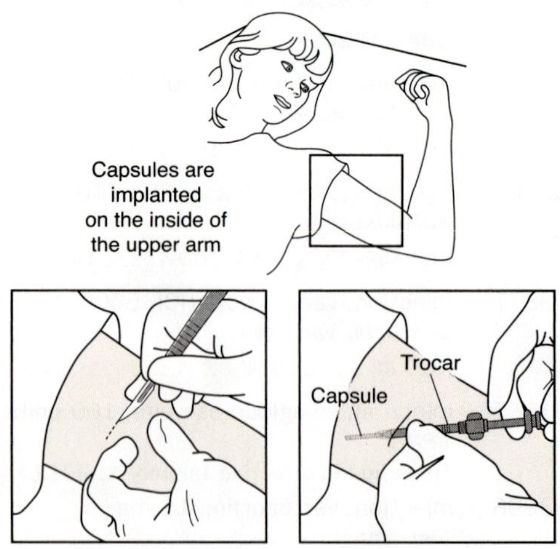

Small incision is made
Capsules are inserted using a trocar

J7308 Aminolevulinic acid HCl for topical administration, 20%, single unit dosage form (354 mg) K K2
Levulan Kerastick for topical solution

● ⓘ J7309 Methyl aminolevulinate (MAL) for topical administration, 16.8%, 1 gram K K2
Metvixia
This code is effective January 1, 2011

ⓘ J7310 Ganciclovir, 4.5 mg, long-acting implant K K2
Vitrasert
Pub 100-02, 15, 50; 100-4, 17, 10

J7311 Fluocinolone acetonide, intravitreal implant G K2
Retisert

● J7312 Injection, dexamethasone, intravitreal implant, 0.1 mg K K2
Ozurdex
This code is effective January 1, 2011

J7321 Hyaluronan or derivative, Hyalgan or Supartz, for intra-articular injection, per dose K K2
AHA: 1Q 2008, 7

J7323 Hyaluronan or derivative, Euflexxa, for intra-articular injection, per dose K K2
AHA: 1Q 2008, 7

J7324 Hyaluronan or derivative, Orthovisc, for intra-articular injection, per dose K K2
AHA: 1Q 2008, 8

J7325 Hyaluronan or derivative, Synvisc or Synvisc-one, for intra-articular injection, 1 mg K K2

J7330 Autologous cultured chondrocytes, implant B
Carticel

● J7335 Capsaicin 8% patch, per 10 square centimeters K K2
Qutenza
This code is effective January 1, 2011

Immunosuppressive Drugs

ⓘ J7500 Azathioprine, oral, 50 mg N N1
Azasan, Imuran
Pub 100-02, 15, 50.5; 100-2, 15, 50.5.2.1; 100-4, 17, 80.3-80.3.2

ⓘ J7501 Azathioprine, parenteral, 100 mg K K2
Azasan, Imuran
Pub 100-02, 15, 50; 100-4, 17, 10

ⓘ J7502 Cyclosporine, oral, 100 mg K K2
Gengraf, Neoral, Sandimmune, SangCya
Pub 100-02, 15, 50.5; 100-2, 15, 50.5.2.1; 100-4, 17, 80.3-80.3.2

ⓘ J7504 Lymphocyte immune globulin, antithymocyte globulin, equine, parenteral, 250 mg K K2
Atgam
NCD 260.7; Pub 100-02, 15, 50; 100-4, 17, 10

ⓘ J7505 Muromonab-CD3, parenteral, 5 mg K K2
Orthoclone OKT3
Pub 100-02, 15, 50; 100-4, 17, 10

ⓘ J7506 Prednisone, oral, per 5 mg N N1
Deltasone, Meticorten, Orasone
Pub 100-02, 15, 50.5; 100-2, 15, 50.5.2.1; 100-4, 17, 80.3-80.3.2

ⓘ J7507 Tacrolimus, oral, per 1 mg K K2
Prograf
Pub 100-02, 15, 50.5; 100-2, 15, 50.5.2.1; 100-4, 17, 80.3-80.3.2

ⓘ J7509 Methylprednisolone oral, per 4 mg N N1
Medrol, Meprolone
Pub 100-02, 15, 50.5; 100-2, 15, 50.5.2.1; 100-4, 17, 80.3-80.3.2

ⓘ J7510 Prednisolone oral, per 5 mg N N1
Delta Cortef
Pub 100-02, 15, 50.5; 100-2, 15, 50.5.2.1; 100-4, 17, 80.3-80.3.2

J7511 Lymphocyte immune globulin, antithymocyte globulin, rabbit, parenteral, 25 mg K K2
Thymoglobulin

ⓘ J7513 Daclizumab, parenteral, 25 mg K K2
Pub 100-02, 15, 50.5; 100-2, 15, 50.5.2.1; 100-4, 17, 80.3-80.3.2
Zenapax

J7515 Cyclosporine, oral, 25 mg N K2
Gengraf, Neoral, Sandimmune, SangCya

J7516 Cyclosporine, parenteral, 250 mg K N1
Gengraf, Neoral, Sandimmune, SangCya

J7517 Mycophenolate mofetil, oral, 250 mg K K2
CellCept

ⓘ J7518 Mycophenolic acid, oral, 180 mg K N1
Myfortic
Pub 100-04, 8, 120.1; 100-4, 17, 80.3

ⓘ J7520 Sirolimus, oral, 1 mg K K2
Rapamune
Pub 100-02, 15, 50.5; 100-2, 15, 50.5.2.1; 100-4, 17, 80.3-80.3.2

ⓘ J7525 Tacrolimus, parenteral, 5 mg K K2
Prograf
Pub 100-02, 15, 50.5; 100-2, 15, 50.5.2.1; 100-4, 17, 80.3-80.3.2

ⓘ J7599 Immunosuppressive drug, not otherwise classified N N1
Pub 100-02, 15, 50.5; 100-2, 15, 50.5.2.1; 100-4, 17, 80.3-80.3.2

Inhalation Solutions

J7604 Acetylcysteine, inhalation solution, compounded product, administered through DME, unit dose form, per gram M

J7605 Arformoterol, inhalation solution, FDA approved final product, non-compounded, administered through DME, unit dose form, 15 micrograms M
Brovana

J7606 Formoterol fumarate, inhalation solution, FDA approved final product, non-compounded, administered through DME, unit dose form, 20 micrograms M

J7607 Levalbuterol, inhalation solution, compounded product, administered through DME, concentrated form, 0.5 mg M
Xopenex HFA

ⓘ J7608 Acetylcysteine, inhalation solution, FDA-approved final product, non-compounded, administered through DME, unit dose form, per gram M
Brovana
Pub 100-02, 15, 110.3

J7609 Albuterol, inhalation solution, compounded product, administered through DME, unit dose, 1 mg M
Ventolin, Proventil

J7610 Albuterol, inhalation solution, compounded product, administered through DME, concentrated form, 1 mg M
Ventolin, Proventil

ⓘ J7611 Albuterol, inhalation solution, FDA-approved final product, non-compounded, administered through DME, concentrated form, 1 mg M
Proventil, Proventil HFA, Proventil Repetabs, Ventolin, Volmax
AHA: 2Q 2008, 10

J7309 – J7611

ⓘ J7612 Levalbuterol, inhalation solution, FDA-approved final product, non-compounded, administered through DME, concentrated form, 0.5 mg M
Xopenex
AHA: 2Q 2008, 10

ⓘ J7613 Albuterol, inhalation solution, FDA-approved final product, non-compounded, administered through DME, unit dose, 1 mg M
Proventil, Proventil HFA, Proventil Repetabs, Ventolin, Volmax
AHA: 2Q 2008, 10

ⓘ J7614 Levalbuterol, inhalation solution, FDA-approved final product, non-compounded, administered through DME, unit dose, 0.5 mg M
Xopenex
AHA: 2Q 2008, 10

J7615 Levalbuterol, inhalation solution, compounded product, administered through DME, unit dose, 0.5 mg M
Xopenex HFA

ⓘ J7617 Levalbuterol, up to 2.5 mg and ipratropium bromide, up to 1 mg, compounded inhalation solution, administered through DME M
Pub 100-02, 15, 110.3

ⓘ J7620 Albuterol, up to 2.5 mg and ipratropium bromide, up to 0.5 mg, FDA-approved final product, non-compounded, administered through DME M
Combivent, DuoNeb
Pub 100-02, 15, 110.3

J7622 Beclomethasone, inhalation solution, compounded product, administered through DME, unit dose form, per milligram M
Beclovent, Beconase, Vanceril, Qvar, Vancenase

J7624 Betamethasone, inhalation solution, compounded product, administered through DME, unit dose form, per milligram M

J7626 Budesonide, inhalation solution, FDA-approved final product, non-compounded, administered through DME, unit dose form, up to 0.5 mg M
Pulmicort Respules, Pulmicort Turbuhaler, Rhinocort Aqua

J7627 Budesonide, inhalation solution, compounded product, administered through DME, unit dose form, up to 0.5 mg M
Pulmicort Respules, Pulmicort Turbuhaler, Rhinocort Aqua

ⓘ J7628 Bitolterol mesylate, inhalation solution, compounded product, administered through DME, concentrated form, per milligram M
Tornalate
Pub 100-02, 15, 110.3

ⓘ J7629 Bitolterol mesylate, inhalation solution, compounded product, administered through DME, unit dose form, per milligram M
Tornalate
Pub 100-02, 15, 110.3

ⓘ J7631 Cromolyn sodium, inhalation solution, FDA-approved final product, non-compounded, administered through DME, unit dose form, per 10 milligrams M
Gastrocrom, Intal inhaler, Intal nebulizer solution, Nasalcrom
Pub 100-02, 15, 110.3

J7632 Cromolyn sodium, inhalation solution, compounded product, administered through DME, unit dose form, per 10 milligrams M
Gastrocrom, Intal inhaler, Intal nebulizer solution, Nasalcrom

J7633 Budesonide, inhalation solution, FDA-approved final product, non-compounded, administered through DME, concentrated form, per 0.25 milligram M
Pulmicort Respules, Pulmicort Turbuhaler, Rhinocort Aqua

J7634 Budesonide, inhalation solution, compounded product, administered through DME, concentrated form, per 0.25 milligram M
Pulmicort Respules

ⓘ J7635 Atropine, inhalation solution, compounded product, administered through DME, concentrated form, per milligram M
Pub 100-02, 15, 110.3

ⓘ J7636 Atropine, inhalation solution, compounded product, administered through DME, unit dose form, per milligram M
Pub 100-02, 15, 110.3

ⓘ J7637 Dexamethasone, inhalation solution, compounded product, administered through DME, concentrated form, per milligram M
Pub 100-02, 15, 110.3
Dexacort Turbinaire

ⓘ J7638 Dexamethasone, inhalation solution, compounded product, administered through DME, unit dose form, per milligram M
Pub 100-02, 15, 110.3
Dexacort Turbinaire

ⓘ J7639 Dornase alfa, inhalation solution, FDA-approved final product, non-compounded, administered through DME, unit dose form, per milligram M
Pulmozyme
Pub 100-02, 15, 110.3

J7640 Formoterol, inhalation solution, compounded product, administered through DME, unit dose form, 12 micrograms E
Foradil

J7641 Flunisolide, inhalation solution, compounded product, administered through DME, unit dose, per milligram M
AeroBid, AeroBid-M, Nasalide, Nasarel

ⓘ J7642 Glycopyrrolate, inhalation solution, compounded product, administered through DME, concentrated form, per milligram M
Pub 100-02, 15, 110.3

ⓘ J7643 Glycopyrrolate, inhalation solution, compounded product, administered through DME, unit dose form, per milligram M
Pub 100-02, 15, 110.3

ⓘ J7644 Ipratropium bromide, inhalation solution, FDA-approved final product, non-compounded, administered through DME, unit dose form, per milligram M
Atrivent
Pub 100-02, 15, 110.3

J7645 Ipratropium bromide, inhalation solution, compounded product, administered through DME, unit dose form, per milligram M
Atrivent

J7647 Isoetharine HCl, inhalation solution, compounded product, administered through DME, concentrated form, per milligram M
Beta-2

ⓘ J7648 Isoetharine HCl, inhalation solution, FDA-approved final product, non-compounded, administered through DME, concentrated form, per milligram M
Arm-a-Med, Beta-2, Bronkometer, Bronkosol, Dey-Lute
Pub 100-02, 15, 110.3

J7649 Isoetharine HCl, inhalation solution, FDA-approved final product, non-compounded, administered through DME, unit dose form, per milligram M
Arm-a-Med, Beta-2, Bronkometer, Bronkosol, Dey-Lute
Pub 100-02, 15, 110.3

J7650 Isoetharine HCl, inhalation solution, compounded product, administered through DME, unit dose form, per milligram M
Beta-2

J7657 Isoproterenol HCl, inhalation solution, compounded product, administered through DME, concentrated form, per milligram M
Isuprel HCl

J7658 Isoproterenol HCl, inhalation solution, FDA-approved final product, non-compounded, administered through DME, concentrated form, per milligram M
Isuprel, Medihaler-ISO
Pub 100-02, 15, 110.3

J7659 Isoproterenol HCl, inhalation solution, FDA-approved final product, non-compounded, administered through DME, unit dose form, per milligram M
Isuprel, Medihaler-ISO
Pub 100-02, 15, 110.3

J7660 Isoproterenol HCl, inhalation solution, compounded product, administered through DME, unit dose form, per milligram M
Isuprel HCl

J7667 Metaproterenol sulfate, inhalation solution, compounded product, concentrated form, per 10 milligrams M
Alupent

J7668 Metaproterenol sulfate, inhalation solution, FDA-approved final product, non-compounded, administered through DME, concentrated form, per 10 milligrams M
Alupent, Metaprel
Pub 100-02, 15, 110.3

J7669 Metaproterenol sulfate, inhalation solution, FDA-approved final product, non-compounded, administered through DME, unit dose form, per 10 milligrams M
Alupent, Metaprel
Pub 100-02, 15, 110.3

J7670 Metaproterenol sulfate, inhalation solution, compounded product, administered through DME, unit dose form, per 10 milligrams M
Alupent

J7674 Methacholine chloride administered as inhalation solution through a nebulizer, per 1 mg N N1
Provocholine

J7676 Pentamidine isethionate, inhalation solution, compounded product, administered through DME, unit dose form, per 300 mg M
Nebupent, Pentam 300

J7680 Terbutaline sulfate, inhalation solution, compounded product, administered through DME, concentrated form, per milligram M
Pub 100-02, 15, 110.3
Brethaire, Bricanyl Turbohaler

J7681 Terbutaline sulfate, inhalation solution, compounded product, administered through DME, unit dose form, per milligram M
Pub 100-02, 15, 110.3
Brethaire, Bricanyl Turbohaler

J7682 Tobramycin, inhalation solution, FDA-approved final product, non-compounded, unit dose form, administered through DME, per 300 milligrams M
TOBI
Pub 100-02, 15, 110.3

J7683 Triamcinolone, inhalation solution, compounded product, administered through DME, concentrated form, per milligram B
Pub 100-02, 15, 110.3
Azmacort

J7684 Triamcinolone, inhalation solution, compounded product, administered through DME, unit dose form, per milligram B
Azmacort
Pub 100-02, 15, 110.3

J7685 Tobramycin, inhalation solution, compounded product, administered through DME, unit dose form, per 300 milligrams B
TOBI

● J7686 Treprostinil, inhalation solution, FDA-approved final product, non-compounded, administered through DME, unit dose form, 1.74 mg K K2
This code is effective January 1, 2011

J7699 NOC drugs, inhalation solution administered through DME Y
Pub 100-02, 15, 110.3

J7799 NOC drugs, other than inhalation drugs, administered through DME N N1
Pub 100-02, 15, 110.3

J8498 Antiemetic drug, rectal/suppository, not otherwise specified B
Medicare Statute 1861(s)(2)(T)

J8499 Prescription drug, oral, non-chemotherapeutic, NOS E
Pub 100-02, 15, 50; 100-4, 17, 10

J8501 Aprepitant, oral, 5 mg G K2
Emend
Pub 100-02, 15, 50.5; 100-2, 15, 50.5.2.1; 100-4, 17, 80.1-80.1.4

J8510 Busulfan; oral, 2 mg K N1
Pub 100-02, 15, 50.5; 100-2, 15, 50.5.2.1; 100-4, 17, 80.1-80.1.4
Busulfex, Myleran

J8515 Cabergoline, oral, 0.25 mg E
Dostinex
Pub 100-02, 15, 50.5; 100-2, 15, 50.5.2.1; 100-4, 17, 80.1-80.1.4

J8520 Capecitabine, oral, 150 mg K K2
Xeloda
Pub 100-02, 15, 50.5; 100-2, 15, 50.5.2.1; 100-4, 17, 80.1-80.1.4

J8521 Capecitabine, oral, 500 mg B K2
Xeloda
Pub 100-02, 15, 50.5; 100-2, 15, 50.5.2.1; 100-4, 17, 80.1-80.1.4

J8530 Cyclophosphamide; oral, 25 mg N N1
Cytoxan
Pub 100-02, 15, 50.5; 100-2, 15, 50.5.2.1; 100-4, 17, 80.1-80.1.4

J8540 Dexamethasone, oral, 0.25 mg N N1
Decadron, Dexameth, Dexacort Turbinaire, Dexone, Hexadrol
Medicare Statute 1861(s)(2)(T)

J8560 Etoposide; oral, 50 mg K K2
Pub 100-02, 15, 50.5; 100-2, 15, 50.5.2.1; 100-4, 17, 80.1-80.1.4
Toposar, VePesid

● J8562 Fludarabine phosphate, oral, 10 mg K K2
Oforta
This code is effective January 1, 2011

⊘ J8565 Gefitinib, oral, 250 mg E
Iressa

ⓘ J8597 Antiemetic drug, oral, not otherwise specified N N1
Medicare Statute 1861(s)(2)(T)

ⓘ J8600 Melphalan; oral, 2 mg N K2
Alkeran
Pub 100-02, 15, 50.5; 100-2, 15, 50.5.2.1; 100-4, 17, 80.1-80.1.4

ⓘ J8610 Methotrexate; oral, 2.5 mg N N1
Rheumatrex
Pub 100-02, 15, 50.5; 100-2, 15, 50.5.2.1; 100-4, 17, 80.1-80.1.4

J8650 Nabilone, oral, 1 mg K N1
Cesamet

ⓘ J8700 Temozolomide, oral, 5 mg K K2
Temodar
Pub 100-02, 15, 50.5.4

J8705 Topotecan, oral, 0.25 mg K K2

ⓘ J8999 Prescription drug, oral, chemotherapeutic, NOS B
Pub 100-02, 15, 50.5; 100-2, 15, 50.5.2.1; 100-4, 17, 80.1-80.1.4

Chemotherapy Drugs J9000–J9999

Note: The code reflects the supply of the chemotherapy drug only, it does not include the administration

ⓘ J9000 Injection, doxorubicin HCl, 10 mg K N1
Adriamycin PFS or RDF, Rubex
Pub 100-02, 15, 50; 100-4, 17, 10

ⓘ J9001 Injection, doxorubicin hydrochloride, all lipid formulations, 10 mg K K2
Doxil
Pub 100-02, 15, 50; 100-4, 17, 10

ⓘ J9010 Injection, alemtuzumab, 10 mg K K2
Campath
Medicare Statute 1833(t)

ⓘ J9015 Injection, aldesleukin, per single use vial K K2
Proleukin
Pub 100-02, 15, 50; 100-4, 17, 10

J9017 Injection, arsenic trioxide, 1 mg K K2
Trisenox

ⓘ J9020 Injection, asparaginase, 10,000 units K K2
Elspar
Pub 100-02, 15, 50; 100-4, 17, 10

J9025 Injection, azacitidine, 1 mg K K2
Vidaza

J9027 Injection, clofarabine, 1 mg G K2
Clolar

ⓘ J9031 BCG (intravesical) per instillation K K2
TheraCys, TICE BCG
Pub 100-02, 15, 50; 100-4, 17, 10

J9033 Injection, bendamustine HCl, 1 mg G K2

J9035 Injection, bevacizumab, 10 mg K K2
Avastin

ⓘ J9040 Injection, bleomycin sulfate, 15 units N K2
Blenoxane
Pub 100-02, 15, 50; 100-4, 17, 10

J9041 Injection, bortezomib, 0.1 mg K K2
Velcade

ⓘ J9045 Injection, carboplatin, 50 mg N K2
Paraplatin
Pub 100-02, 15, 50; 100-4, 17, 10

ⓘ J9050 Injection, carmustine, 100 mg K K2
BiCNU
Pub 100-02, 15, 50; 100-4, 17, 10

J9055 Injection, cetuximab, 10 mg K K2
Erbitux

▲ ⓘ J9060 Injection, cisplatin, powder or solution, 10 mg K K2

✖ ~~J9062 Cisplatin, 50 mg~~
This code is deleted as of December 31, 2010
See code(s) J9060

ⓘ J9065 Injection, cladribine, per 1 mg K K2

ⓘ J9070 Cyclophosphamide, 100 mg N N1

✖ ~~J9080 Cyclophosphamide, 200 mg~~
This code is deleted as of December 31, 2010
See code(s) J9070

✖ ~~J9090 Cyclophosphamide, 500 mg~~
This code is deleted as of December 31, 2010
See code(s) J9070

✖ ~~J9091 Cyclophosphamide, 1.0 gram~~
This code is deleted as of December 31, 2010
See code(s) J9070

✖ ~~J9092 Cyclophosphamide, 2.0 gram~~
This code is deleted as of December 31, 2010
See code(s) J9070

✖ ~~J9093 Cyclophosphamide, lyophilized, 100 mg~~
This code is deleted as of December 31, 2010
See code(s) J9070

✖ ~~J9094 Cyclophosphamide, lyophilized, 200 mg~~
This code is deleted as of December 31, 2010
See code(s) J9070

✖ ~~J9095 Cyclophosphamide, lyophilized, 500 mg~~
This code is deleted as of December 31, 2010
See code(s) J9070

✖ ~~J9096 Cyclophosphamide, lyophilized, 1.0 gram~~
This code is deleted as of December 31, 2010
See code(s) J9070

✖ ~~J9097 Cyclophosphamide, lyophilized, 2.0 gram~~
This code is deleted as of December 31, 2010
See code(s) J9070

J9098 Injection, cytarabine liposome, 10 mg K K2

ⓘ J9100 Injection, cytarabine, 100 mg N N1
Cytosar-U
Pub 100-02, 15, 50; 100-4, 17, 10

✖ ~~J9110 Injection, cytarabine, 500 mg~~
This code is deleted as of December 31, 2010
See code(s) J9100

ⓘ J9120 Injection, dactinomycin, 0.5 mg K K2
Cosmegen
Pub 100-02, 15, 50; 100-4, 17, 10

ⓘ J9130 Dacarbazine, 100 mg K N1
DTIC-Dome
Pub 100-02, 15, 50; 100-4, 17, 10

✖ ~~J9140 Dacarbazine, 200 mg~~
This code is deleted as of December 31, 2010
See code(s) J9130

ⓘ J9150 Injection, daunorubicin, 10 mg K K2
Cerubidine
Pub 100-02, 15, 50; 100-4, 17, 10

ⓘ J9151 Injection, daunorubicin citrate, liposomal formulation, 10 mg K K2
DaunoXome
Pub 100-02, 15, 50; 100-4, 17, 10

J9155 Injection, degarelix, 1 mg ♂ G K2
Firmagon

J9160 Injection, denileukin diftitox, 300 micrograms K K2

ⓘ J9165 Injection, diethylstilbestrol diphosphate, 250 mg K N1
Stilphostrol
Pub 100-02, 15, 50; 100-4, 17, 10

ⓘ J9171 Injection, docetaxel, 1 mg K K2
Taxotere

ⓘ J9175 Injection, Elliotts' B solution, 1 ml N N1
Pub 100-02, 15, 50; 100-4, 17, 10

J9178 Injection, epirubicin HCl, 2 mg K K2
Ellence

ⓘ J9181 Injection, etoposide, 10 mg N N1
Etopophos, Toposar, VePesid
Pub 100-02, 15, 50; 100-4, 17, 10

ⓘ J9185 Injection, fludarabine phosphate, 50 mg K K2
Fludara
Pub 100-02, 15, 50; 100-4, 17, 10

ⓘ J9190 Injection, fluorouracil, 500 mg N N1
Adrucil
Pub 100-02, 15, 50; 100-4, 17, 10

ⓘ J9200 Injection, floxuridine, 500 mg K K2
FUDR
Pub 100-02, 15, 50; 100-4, 17, 10

ⓘ J9201 Injection, gemcitabine hydrochloride, 200 mg K K2
Gemzar
Pub 100-02, 15, 50; 100-4, 17, 10

ⓘ J9202 Goserelin acetate implant, per 3.6 mg K K2
Zoladex
Pub 100-02, 15, 50; 100-4, 17, 10

ⓘ J9206 Injection, irinotecan, 20 mg K K2
Camptosar
Pub 100-02, 15, 50; 100-4, 17, 10

J9207 Injection, ixabepilone, 1 mg G K2

ⓘ J9208 Injection, ifosfamide, 1 gram K K2
Ifex
Pub 100-02, 15, 50; 100-4, 17, 10

ⓘ J9209 Injection, mesna, 200 mg K K2
Mesnex
Pub 100-02, 15, 50; 100-4, 17, 10

ⓘ J9211 Injection, idarubicin hydrochloride, 5 mg K K2
Idamycin, Idamycin PFS
Pub 100-02, 15, 50; 100-4, 17, 10

ⓘ J9212 Injection, interferon Alfacon-1, recombinant, 1 microgram N K2
Amgen, Infergen
Pub 100-02, 15, 50; 100-4, 17, 10

ⓘ J9213 Injection, interferon, alfa-2a, recombinant, 3 million units K K2
Roferon-A
Pub 100-02, 15, 50; 100-4, 17, 10

ⓘ J9214 Injection, interferon, alfa-2b, recombinant, 1 million units K K2
Intron-A
Pub 100-02, 15, 50; 100-4, 17, 10

ⓘ J9215 Injection, interferon, alfa-n3, (human leukocyte derived), 250,000 IU K K2
Alferon N
Pub 100-02, 15, 50; 100-4, 17, 10

ⓘ J9216 Injection, interferon, gamma 1-b, 3 million units K K2
Actimmune
Pub 100-02, 15, 50; 100-4, 17, 10

ⓘ J9217 Leuprolide acetate (for depot suspension), 7.5 mg K K2
Pub 100-02, 15, 50; 100-4, 17, 10
Eligard, Lupron Depot, Lupron Depot-Ped

ⓘ J9218 Leuprolide acetate, per 1 mg K K2
Pub 100-02, 15, 50; 100-4, 17, 10
Eligard, Lupron

ⓘ J9219 Leuprolide acetate implant, 65 mg K K2
Viadur
Pub 100-02, 15, 50; 100-4, 17, 10

ⓘ J9225 Histrelin implant (Vantas), 50 mg K K2
Pub 100-02, 15, 50; 100-4, 17, 10

ⓘ J9226 Histrelin implant (Supprelin LA), 50 mg K K2
Pub 100-02, 15, 50; 100-4, 17, 10
AHA: 1Q 2008, 8

ⓘ J9230 Injection, mechlorethamine hydrochloride, (nitrogen mustard), 10 mg K K2
Mustargen
Pub 100-02, 15, 50; 100-4, 17, 10

ⓘ J9245 Injection, melphalan hydrochloride, 50 mg K K2
Alkeran
Pub 100-02, 15, 50; 100-4, 17, 10

ⓘ J9250 Methotrexate sodium, 5 mg N N1
Folex, Folex PFS, Methotrexate LPF, Rheumatrex
Pub 100-02, 15, 50; 100-4, 17, 10

ⓘ J9260 Methotrexate sodium, 50 mg B N1
Folex, Folex PFS, Methotrexate LPF, Rheumatrex
Pub 100-02, 15, 50; 100-4, 17, 10

J9261 Injection, nelarabine, 50 mg K K2
Arranon

J9263 Injection, oxaliplatin, 0.5 mg K K2
Eloxatin

J9264 Injection, paclitaxel protein-bound particles, 1 mg K K2
Abraxane

ⓘ J9265 Injection, paclitaxel, 30 mg K N1
Onxol, Taxol
Pub 100-02, 15, 50; 100-4, 17, 10

ⓘ J9266 Injection, pegaspargase, per single dose vial K K2
Oncaspar
Pub 100-02, 15, 50; 100-4, 17, 10

ⓘ J9268 Injection, pentostatin, 10 mg K K2
Nipent
Pub 100-02, 15, 50; 100-4, 17, 10

ⓘ J9270 Injection, plicamycin, 2.5 mg K N1
Mithracin
Pub 100-02, 15, 50; 100-4, 17, 10

ⓘ J9280 Mitomycin, 5 mg K K2
Mutamycin
Pub 100-02, 15, 50; 100-4, 17, 10

✖ ~~J9290 Mitomycin, 20 mg~~
This code is deleted as of December 31, 2010
See code(s) J9280

✖ ~~J9291 Mitomycin, 40 mg~~
This code is deleted as of December 31, 2010
See code(s) J9280

ⓘ J9293 Injection, mitoxantrone hydrochloride, per 5 mg K K2
Novantrone
Pub 100-02, 15, 50; 100-4, 17, 10

J9300 Injection, gemtuzumab ozogamicin, 5 mg K K2
Mylotarg

J9165 – J9300

● J9302 Injection, ofatumumab, 10 mg K K2
Arzerra
This code is effective January 1, 2011

J9303 Injection, panitumumab, 10 mg K K2
Vectibix
AHA: 1Q 2008, 8

J9305 Injection, pemetrexed, 10 mg K K2
Alimta

● J9307 Injection, pralatrexate, 1 mg K K2
Folotun
This code is effective January 1, 2011

J9310 Injection, rituximab, 100 mg K K2
Rituxan
Pub 100-02, 15, 50; 100-4, 17, 10

● J9315 Injection, romidepsin, 1 mg K K2
Istodax
This code is effective January 1, 2011

J9320 Injection, streptozocin, 1 gram K K2
Zanosar
Pub 100-02, 15, 50; 100-4, 17, 10

J9328 Injection, temozolomide, 1 mg G K2
Temodar, Temodal

J9330 Injection, temsirolimus, 1 mg G K2
Torisel

J9340 Injection, thiotepa, 15 mg K K2
Thioplex
Pub 100-02, 15, 50; 100-4, 17, 10

× ~~J9350 Injection, topotecan, 4 mg~~
This code is deleted as of December 31, 2010
See code(s) J9351

● J9351 Injection, topotecan, 0.1 mg K K2
Hycamtin
This code is effective January 1, 2011

J9355 Injection, trastuzumab, 10 mg K K2
Herceptin

J9357 Injection, valrubicin, intravesical, 200 mg K K2
Valstar
Pub 100-02, 15, 50; 100-4, 17, 10

J9360 Injection, vinblastine sulfate, 1 mg N N1
Alkaban-AQ, Velban, Velsar
Pub 100-02, 15, 50; 100-4, 17, 10

J9370 Vincristine sulfate, 1 mg N N1
Oncovin, Vincasar PFS, Vincrex
Pub 100-02, 15, 50; 100-4, 17, 10

× ~~J9375 Vincristine sulfate, 2 mg~~
This code is deleted as of December 31, 2010
See code(s) J9370

× ~~J9380 Vincristine sulfate, 5 mg~~
This code is deleted as of December 31, 2010
See code(s) J9370

J9390 Injection, vinorelbine tartrate, 10 mg K N1
Navelbine
Pub 100-02, 15, 50; 100-4, 17, 10

J9395 Injection, fulvestrant, 25 mg K K2
Faslodex

J9600 Injection, porfimer sodium, 75 mg K K2
Photofrin
Pub 100-02, 15, 50; 100-4, 17, 10

J9999 Not otherwise classified, antineoplastic drugs N N1
NCD 110.2; Pub 100-02, 15, 50; 100-4, 17, 10

DME Supplies K0001–K0899

Claims for durable medical equipment (DME) must be filed with the DME Medicare Administrative Contractor (DME MAC).

Wheelchairs

K0001 Standard wheelchair Y
K0002 Standard hemi (low seat) wheelchair Y
K0003 Lightweight wheelchair Y
K0004 High strength, lightweight wheelchair Y
K0005 Ultralightweight wheelchair Y
K0006 Heavy-duty wheelchair Y
K0007 Extra heavy-duty wheelchair Y
K0009 Other manual wheelchair/base Y
K0010 Standard – weight frame motorized/power wheelchair Y
K0011 Standard – weight frame motorized/power wheelchair with programmable control parameters for speed adjustment, tremor dampening, acceleration control and braking Y
K0012 Lightweight portable motorized/power wheelchair Y
K0014 Other motorized/power wheelchair base Y

Wheelchair Accessories

Armrests

K0015 Detachable, non-adjustable height armrest, each Y
K0017 Detachable, adjustable height armrest, base, each Y
K0018 Detachable, adjustable height armrest, upper portion, each Y
K0019 Arm pad, each Y
K0020 Fixed, adjustable height armrest, pair Y

Foot and Leg Rests

K0037 High mount flip-up footrest, each Y
K0038 Leg strap, each Y
K0039 Leg strap, H style, each Y
K0040 Adjustable angle footplate, each Y
K0041 Large size footplate, each Y
K0042 Standard size footplate, each Y
K0043 Footrest, lower extension tube, each Y
K0044 Footrest, upper hanger bracket, each Y
K0045 Footrest, complete assembly Y
K0046 Elevating legrest, lower extension tube, each Y
K0047 Elevating legrest, upper hanger bracket, each Y
K0050 Ratchet assembly Y
K0051 Cam release assembly, footrest or legrest, each Y
K0052 Swingaway, detachable footrests, each Y
K0053 Elevating footrests, articulating (telescoping), each Y

Special Sizes

K0056 Seat height less than 17" or equal to or greater than 21" for a high-strength, lightweight, or ultralightweight wheelchair Y

Wheels for Manual Wheelchairs

K0065 Spoke protectors, each Y
K0069 Rear wheel assembly, complete, with solid tire, spokes or molded, each Y

Medicare Non-Coverage | Special Coverage Instructions | Coverage Carrier Determined | A – Y APC Status Indicators | ● New Code | ▲ Revised Code | × Deleted Code
AHA *AHA Coding Clinic for HCPCS* | A2 – Z3 ASC Payment Indicators | DMEPOS | ♂ Male | ♀ Female | PQRI PQRI

K0070 Rear wheel assembly, complete, with pneumatic tire, spokes or molded, each Y

K0071 Front caster assembly, complete, with pneumatic tire, each Y

K0072 Front caster assembly, complete, with semi-pneumatic tire, each Y

K0073 Caster pin lock, each Y

K0077 Front caster assembly, complete, with solid tire, each Y

Power Wheelchair Parts

K0098 Drive belt for power wheelchair Y

Miscellaneous Wheelchair Accessories

K0105 IV hanger, each Y

K0108 Wheelchair component or accessory, not otherwise specified Y

K0195 Elevating leg rests, pair (for use with capped rental wheelchair base) Y
NCD 280.1

Other Miscellaneous DME Supplies

K0455 Infusion pump used for uninterrupted parenteral administration of medication, (e.g., epoprostenol or treprostinol) Y
NCD 40.2

K0462 Temporary replacement for patient owned equipment being repaired, any type Y
Pub 100-04, 20, 40.1

K0552 Supplies for external drug infusion pump, syringe type cartridge, sterile, each Y
NCD 40.2

K0601 Replacement battery for external infusion pump owned by patient, silver oxide, 1.5 volt, each Y

K0602 Replacement battery for external infusion pump owned by patient, silver oxide, 3 volt, each Y

K0603 Replacement battery for external infusion pump owned by patient, alkaline, 1.5 volt, each Y

K0604 Replacement battery for external infusion pump owned by patient, lithium, 3.6 volt, each Y

K0605 Replacement battery for external infusion pump owned by patient, lithium, 4.5 volt, each Y

K0606 Automatic external defibrillator, with integrated electrocardiogram analysis, garment type Y

K0607 Replacement battery for automated external defibrillator, garment type only, each Y

Defibrillator

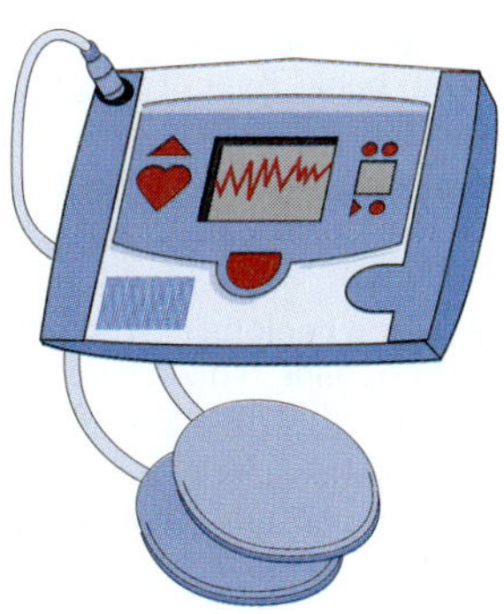

K0608 Replacement garment for use with automated external defibrillator, each Y

K0609 Replacement electrodes for use with automated external defibrillator, garment type only, each Y

K0669 Wheelchair accessory, wheelchair seat or back cushion, does not meet specific code criteria or no written coding verification from DME PDAC Y

K0670 Addition to lower extremity prosthesis, endoskeletal knee shin system, microprocessor control feature, stance phase only, includes electronic sensor(s), any type Y

K0671 Portable oxygen concentrator, rental Y

K0672 Addition to lower extremity orthosis, removable soft interface, all components, replacement only, each A

K0730 Controlled dose inhalation drug delivery system Y

K0733 Power wheelchair accessory, 12 to 24 amp hour sealed lead acid battery, each (e.g., gel cell, absorbed glassmat) Y

✖ ~~K0734 Skin protection wheelchair seat cushion, adjustable, width less than 22 inches, any depth~~
This code is deleted as of December 31, 2010
See code(s) E2603

✖ ~~K0735 Skin protection wheelchair seat cushion, adjustable, width 22 inches or greater, any depth~~
This code is deleted as of December 31, 2010
See code(s) E2604

✖ ~~K0736 Skin protection and positioning wheelchair seat cushion, adjustable, width less than 22 inches, any depth~~
This code is deleted as of December 31, 2010
See code(s) E2607

✖ ~~K0737 Skin protection and positioning wheelchair seat cushion, adjustable, width 22 inches or greater, any depth~~
This code is deleted as of December 31, 2010
See code(s) E2608

K0738 Portable gaseous oxygen system, rental; home compressor used to fill portable oxygen cylinders; includes portable containers, regulator, flowmeter, humidifier, cannula or mask, and tubing Y

K0739 Repair or nonroutine service for durable medical equipment other than oxygen equipment requiring the skill of a technician, labor component, per 15 minutes Y

K0740 Repair or nonroutine service for oxygen equipment requiring the skill of a technician, labor component, per 15 minutes E

K0800 Power operated vehicle, group 1 standard, patient weight capacity up to and including 300 pounds Y

K0801 Power operated vehicle, group 1 heavy duty, patient weight capacity 301 to 450 pounds Y

K0802 Power operated vehicle, group 1 very heavy duty, patient weight capacity 451 to 600 pounds Y

K0806 Power operated vehicle, group 2 standard, patient weight capacity up to and including 300 pounds Y

K0807 Power operated vehicle, group 2 heavy duty, patient weight capacity 301 to 450 pounds Y

K0808 Power operated vehicle, group 2 very heavy duty, patient weight capacity 451 to 600 pounds Y

K0812 Power operated vehicle, not otherwise classified Y

K0813 Power wheelchair, group 1 standard, portable, sling/solid seat and back, patient weight capacity up to and including 300 pounds Y

K0814 Power wheelchair, group 1 standard, portable, captains chair, patient weight capacity up to and including 300 pounds Y

K0815 Power wheelchair, group 1 standard, sling/solid seat and back, patient weight capacity up to and including 300 pounds Y

K0816 Power wheelchair, group 1 standard, captains chair, patient weight capacity up to and including 300 pounds

K0820 Power wheelchair, group 2 standard, portable, sling/solid seat/back, patient weight capacity up to and including 300 pounds

K0821 Power wheelchair, group 2 standard, portable, captains chair, patient weight capacity up to and including 300 pounds

K0822 Power wheelchair, group 2 standard, sling/solid seat/back, patient weight capacity up to and including 300 pounds

K0823 Power wheelchair, group 2 standard, captains chair, patient weight capacity up to and including 300 pounds

K0824 Power wheelchair, group 2 heavy duty, sling/solid seat/ back, patient weight capacity 301 to 450 pounds

K0825 Power wheelchair, group 2 heavy duty, captains chair, patient weight capacity 301 to 450 pounds

K0826 Power wheelchair, group 2 very heavy duty, sling/solid seat/back, patient weight capacity 451 to 600 pounds

K0827 Power wheelchair, group 2 very heavy duty, captains chair, patient weight capacity 451 to 600 pounds

K0828 Power wheelchair, group 2 extra heavy duty, sling/solid seat/back, patient weight capacity 601 pounds or more

K0829 Power wheelchair, group 2 extra heavy duty, captains chair, patient weight 601 pounds or more

K0830 Power wheelchair, group 2 standard, seat elevator, sling/solid seat/back, patient weight capacity up to and including 300 pounds

K0831 Power wheelchair, group 2 standard, seat elevator, captains chair, patient weight capacity up to and including 300 pounds

K0835 Power wheelchair, group 2 standard, single power option, sling/solid seat/back, patient weight capacity up to and including 300 pounds

K0836 Power wheelchair, group 2 standard, single power option, captains chair, patient weight capacity up to and including 300 pounds

K0837 Power wheelchair, group 2 heavy duty, single power option, sling/solid seat/back, patient weight capacity 301 to 450 pounds

K0838 Power wheelchair, group 2 heavy duty, single power option, captains chair, patient weight capacity 301 to 450 pounds

K0839 Power wheelchair, group 2 very heavy duty, single power option sling/solid seat/back, patient weight capacity 451 to 600 pounds

K0840 Power wheelchair, group 2 extra heavy duty, single power option, sling/solid seat/back, patient weight capacity 601 pounds or more

K0841 Power wheelchair, group 2 standard, multiple power option, sling/solid seat/back, patient weight capacity up to and including 300 pounds

K0842 Power wheelchair, group 2 standard, multiple power option, captains chair, patient weight capacity up to and including 300 pounds

K0843 Power wheelchair, group 2 heavy duty, multiple power option, sling/solid seat/back, patient weight capacity 301 to 450 pounds

K0848 Power wheelchair, group 3 standard, sling/solid seat/back, patient weight capacity up to and including 300 pounds

K0849 Power wheelchair, group 3 standard, captains chair, patient weight capacity up to and including 300 pounds

K0850 Power wheelchair, group 3 heavy duty, sling/solid seat/ back, patient weight capacity 301 to 450 pounds

K0851 Power wheelchair, group 3 heavy duty, captains chair, patient weight capacity 301 to 450 pounds

K0852 Power wheelchair, group 3 very heavy duty, sling/solid seat/back, patient weight capacity 451 to 600 pounds

K0853 Power wheelchair, group 3 very heavy duty, captains chair, patient weight capacity 451 to 600 pounds

K0854 Power wheelchair, group 3 extra heavy duty, sling/solid seat/back, patient weight capacity 601 pounds or more

K0855 Power wheelchair, group 3 extra heavy duty, captains chair, patient weight capacity 601 pounds or more

K0856 Power wheelchair, group 3 standard, single power option, sling/solid seat/back, patient weight capacity up to and including 300 pounds

K0857 Power wheelchair, group 3 standard, single power option, captains chair, patient weight capacity up to and including 300 pounds

K0858 Power wheelchair, group 3 heavy duty, single power option, sling/solid seat/back, patient weight 301 to 450 pounds

K0859 Power wheelchair, group 3 heavy duty, single power option, captains chair, patient weight capacity 301 to 450 pounds

K0860 Power wheelchair, group 3 very heavy duty, single power option, sling/solid seat/back, patient weight capacity 451 to 600 pounds

K0861 Power wheelchair, group 3 standard, multiple power option, sling/solid seat/back, patient weight capacity up to and including 300 pounds

K0862 Power wheelchair, group 3 heavy duty, multiple power option, sling/solid seat/back, patient weight capacity 301 to 450 pounds

K0863 Power wheelchair, group 3 very heavy duty, multiple power option, sling/solid seat/back, patient weight capacity 451 to 600 pounds

K0864 Power wheelchair, group 3 extra heavy duty, multiple power option, sling/solid seat/back, patient weight capacity 601 pounds or more

K0868 Power wheelchair, group 4 standard, sling/solid seat/back, patient weight capacity up to and including 300 pounds

K0869 Power wheelchair, group 4 standard, captains chair, patient weight capacity up to and including 300 pounds

K0870 Power wheelchair, group 4 heavy duty, sling/solid seat/back, patient weight capacity 301 to 450 pounds

K0871 Power wheelchair, group 4 very heavy duty, sling/solid seat/ back, patient weight capacity 451 to 600 pounds

K0877 Power wheelchair, group 4 standard, single power option, sling/solid seat/back, patient weight capacity up to and including 300 pounds

K0878 Power wheelchair, group 4 standard, single power option, captains chair, patient weight capacity up to and including 300 pounds

K0879 Power wheelchair, group 4 heavy duty, single power option, sling/solid seat/back, patient weight capacity 301 to 450 pounds

K0880 Power wheelchair, group 4 very heavy duty, single power option, sling/solid seat/back, patient weight 451 to 600 pounds

K0884 Power wheelchair, group 4 standard, multiple power option, sling/solid seat/back, patient weight capacity up to and including 300 pounds

K0885 Power wheelchair, group 4 standard, multiple power option, captains chair, patient weight capacity up to and including 300 pounds

K0886 Power wheelchair, group 4 heavy duty, multiple power option, sling/solid seat/back, patient weight capacity 301 to 450 pounds

K0890 Power wheelchair, group 5 pediatric, single power option, sling/solid seat/back, patient weight capacity up to and including 125 pounds

K0891 Power wheelchair, group 5 pediatric, multiple power option, sling/solid seat/back, patient weight capacity up to and including 125 pounds

K0898 Power wheelchair, not otherwise classified

K0899 Power mobility device, not coded by DME PDAC or does not meet criteria

Orthotic Procedures L0112–L4631

Orthotic Devices – Spinal

Cervical

L0112 Cranial cervical orthosis, congenital torticollis type, with or without soft interface material, adjustable range of motion joint, custom fabricated

L0113 Cranial cervical orthosis, torticollis type, with or without joint, with or without soft interface material, prefabricated, includes fitting and adjustment

L0120 Cervical, flexible, non-adjustable (foam collar)

L0130 Cervical, flexible, thermoplastic collar, molded to patient

L0140 Cervical, semi-rigid, adjustable (plastic collar)

L0150 Cervical, semi-rigid, adjustable molded chin cup (plastic collar with mandibular/occipital piece)

L0160 Cervical, semi-rigid, wire frame occipital/mandibular support

L0170 Cervical, collar, molded to patient model

L0172 Cervical, collar, semi-rigid thermoplastic foam, two-piece

L0174 Cervical, collar, semi-rigid, thermoplastic foam, two-piece with thoracic extension

Multiple Post Collar

L0180 Cervical, multiple post collar, occipital/mandibular supports, adjustable

L0190 Cervical, multiple post collar, occipital/mandibular supports, adjustable cervical bars (SOMI, Guilford, Taylor types)

L0200 Cervical, multiple post collar, occipital/mandibular supports, adjustable cervical bars, and thoracic extension

Thoracic

L0220 Thoracic, rib belt, custom fabricated

Thoracic – Lumbar – Sacral

Flexible Anterior-Posterior-Lateral-Rotary Control

L0430 Spinal orthosis, anterior-posterior-lateral control, with interface material, custom fitted (Dewall posture protector only)

L0450 TLSO, flexible, provides trunk support, upper thoracic region, produces intracavitary pressure to reduce load on the intevertebral disks with rigid stays or panel(s), includes shoulder straps and closures, prefabricated, includes fitting and adjustment

TLSO, flexible upper thoracic trunk support

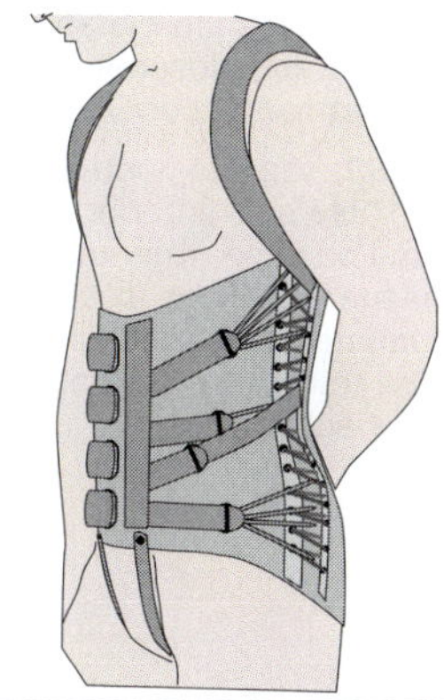

L0452 TLSO, flexible, provides trunk support, upper thoracic region, produces intracavitary pressure to reduce load on the intervertebral disks with rigid stays or panel(s), includes shoulder straps and closures, custom fabricated A

L0454 TLSO flexible, provides trunk support, extends from sacrococcygeal junction to above T9 vertebra, restricts gross trunk motion in the sagittal plane, produces intracavitary pressure to reduce load on the intervertebral disks with rigid stays or panel(s), includes shoulder straps and closures, prefabricated, includes fitting and adjustment A

L0456 TLSO, flexible, provides trunk support, thoracic region, rigid posterior panel and soft anterior apron, extends from the sacrococcygeal junction and terminates just inferior to the scapular spine, restricts gross trunk motion in the sagittal plane, produces intracavitary pressure to reduce load on the intervertebral disks, includes straps and closures, prefabricated, includes fitting and adjustment A

L0458 TLSO, triplanar control, modular segmented spinal system, two rigid plastic shells, posterior extends from the sacrococcygeal junction and terminates just inferior to the scapular spine, anterior extends from the symphysis pubis to the xiphoid, soft liner, restricts gross trunk motion in the sagittal, coronal, and tranverse planes, lateral strength is provided by overlapping plastic and stabilizing closures, includes straps and closures, prefabricated, includes fitting and adjustment A

L0460 TLSO, triplanar control, modular segmented spinal system, two rigid plastic shells, posterior extends from the sacrococcygeal junction and terminates just inferior to the scapular spine, anterior extends from the symphysis pubis to the sternal notch, soft liner, restricts gross trunk motion in the sagittal, coronal, and tranverse planes, lateral strength is provided by overlapping plastic and stabilizing closures, includes straps and closures, prefabricated, includes fitting and adjustment A

L0462 TLSO, triplanar control, modular segmented spinal system, three rigid plastic shells, posterior extends from the sacrococcygeal junction and terminates just inferior to the scapular spine, anterior extends from the symphysis pubis to the sternal notch, soft liner, restricts gross trunk motion in the sagittal, coronal, and transverse planes, lateral strength is provided by overlapping plastic and stabilizing closures, includes straps and closures, prefabricated, includes fitting and adjustment A

L0464 TLSO, triplanar control, modular segmented spinal system, four rigid plastic shells, posterior extends from sacrococcygeal junction and terminates just inferior to scapular spine, anterior extends from symphysis pubis to the sternal notch, soft liner, restricts gross trunk motion in sagittal, coronal, and tranverse planes, lateral strength is provided by overlapping plastic and stabilizing closures, includes straps and closures, prefabricated, includes fitting and adjustment A

L0466 TLSO, sagittal control, rigid posterior frame and flexible soft anterior apron with straps, closures and padding, restricts gross trunk motion in sagittal plane, produces intracavitary pressure to reduce load on intervertebral disks, includes fitting and shaping the frame, prefabricated, includes fitting and adjustment A

L0468 TLSO, sagittal-coronal control, rigid posterior frame and flexible soft anterior apron with straps, closures and padding, extends from sacrococcygeal junction over scapulae, lateral strength provided by pelvic, thoracic, and lateral frame pieces, restricts gross trunk motion in sagittal, and coronal planes, produces intracavitary pressure to reduce load on intervertebral disks, includes fitting and shaping the frame, prefabricated, includes fitting and adjustment A

L0470 TLSO, triplanar control, rigid posterior frame and flexible soft anterior apron with straps, closures and padding, extends from sacrococcygeal junction to scapula, lateral strength provided by pelvic, thoracic, and lateral frame pieces, rotational strength provided by subclavicular extensions, restricts gross trunk motion in sagittal, coronal, and tranverse planes, produces intracavitary pressure to reduce load on the intervertebral disks, includes fitting and shaping the frame, prefabricated, includes fitting and adjustment A

L0472 TLSO, triplanar control, hyperextension, rigid anterior and lateral frame extends from symphysis pubis to sternal notch with two anterior components (one pubic and one sternal), posterior and lateral pads with straps and closures, limits spinal flexion, restricts gross trunk motion in sagittal, coronal, and transverse planes, includes fitting and shaping the frame, prefabricated, includes fitting and adjustment A

L0480 TLSO, triplanar control, one piece rigid plastic shell without interface liner, with multiple straps and closures, posterior extends from sacrococcygeal junction and terminates just inferior to scapular spine, anterior extends from symphysis pubis to sternal notch, anterior or posterior opening, restricts gross trunk motion in sagittal, coronal, and transverse planes, includes a carved plaster or CAD-CAM model, custom fabricated A

L0482 TLSO, triplanar control, one piece rigid plastic shell with interface liner, multiple straps and closures, posterior extends from sacrococcygeal junction and terminates just inferior to scapular spine, anterior extends from symphysis pubis to sternal notch, anterior or posterior opening, restricts gross trunk motion in sagittal, coronal, and transverse planes, includes a carved plaster or CAD-CAM model, custom fabricated A

L0484 TLSO, triplanar control, two piece rigid plastic shell without interface liner, with multiple straps and closures, posterior extends from sacrococcygeal junction and terminates just inferior to scapular spine, anterior extends from symphysis pubis to sternal notch, lateral strength is enhanced by overlapping plastic, restricts gross trunk motion in the sagittal, coronal, and transverse planes, includes a carved plaster or CAD-CAM model, custom fabricated A

L0486 TLSO, triplanar control, two piece rigid plastic shell with interface liner, multiple straps and closures, posterior extends from sacrococcygeal junction and terminates just inferior to scapular spine, anterior extends from symphysis pubis to sternal notch, lateral strength is enhanced by overlapping plastic, restricts gross trunk motion in the sagittal, coronal, and transverse planes, includes a carved plaster or CAD-CAM model, custom fabricated A

L0488 TLSO, triplanar control, one piece rigid plastic shell with interface liner, multiple straps and closures, posterior extends from sacrococcygeal junction and terminates just inferior to scapular spine, anterior extends from symphysis pubis to sternal notch, anterior or posterior opening, restricts gross trunk motion in sagittal, coronal, and transverse planes, prefabricated, includes fitting and adjustment A

L0490 TLSO, sagittal-coronal control, one piece rigid plastic shell, with overlapping reinforced anterior, with multiple straps and closures, posterior extends from sacrococcygeal junction and terminates at or before the T-9 vertebra, anterior extends from symphysis pubis to xiphoid, anterior opening, restricts gross trunk motion in sagittal and coronal planes, prefabricated, includes fitting and adjustment A

L0491 TLSO, sagittal-coronal control, modular segmented spinal system, two rigid plastic shells, posterior extends from the sacrococcygeal junction and terminates just inferior to the scapular spine, anterior extends from the symphysis pubis to the xiphoid, soft liner, restricts gross trunk motion in the sagittal and coronal planes, lateral strength is provided by overlapping plastic and stabilizing closures, includes straps and closures, prefabricated, includes fitting and adjustment A

L0492 TLSO, sagittal-coronal control, modular segmented spinal system, three rigid plastic shells, posterior extends from the sacrococcygeal junction and terminates just inferior to the scapular spine, anterior extends from the symphysis pubis to the xiphoid, soft liner, restricts gross trunk motion in the sagittal and coronal planes, lateral strength is provided by overlapping plastic and stabilizing closures, includes straps and closures, prefabricated, includes fitting and adjustment A

Spinal-Cervical-Thoracic-Lumbar-Sacral-Halo

L0621 Sacroiliac orthosis, flexible, provides pelvic-sacral support, reduces motion about the sacroiliac joint, includes straps, closures, may include pendulous abdomen design, prefabricated, includes fitting and adjustment A

L0622 Sacroiliac orthosis, flexible, provides pelvic-sacral support, reduces motion about the sacroiliac joint, includes straps, closures, may include pendulous abdomen design, custom fabricated A

L0623 Sacroiliac orthosis, provides pelvic-sacral support, with rigid or semi-rigid panels over the sacrum and abdomen, reduces motion about the sacroiliac joint, includes straps, closures, may include pendulous abdomen design, prefabricated, includes fitting and adjustment A

L0624 Sacroiliac orthosis, provides pelvic-sacral support, with rigid or semi-rigid panels placed over the sacrum and abdomen, reduces motion about the sacroiliac joint, includes straps, closures, may include pendulous abdomen design, custom fabricated A

L0625 Lumbar orthosis, flexible, provides lumbar support, posterior extends from L1 to below L5 vertebra, produces intracavitary pressure to reduce load on the intervertebral discs, includes straps, closures, may include pendulous abdomen design, shoulder straps, stays, prefabricated, includes fitting and adjustment A

L0626 Lumbar orthosis, sagittal control, with rigid posterior panel(s), posterior extends from L1 to below L5 vertebra, produces intracavitary pressure to reduce load on the intervertebral discs, includes straps, closures, may include padding, stays, shoulder straps, pendulous abdomen design, prefabricated, includes fitting and adjustment A

L0627 Lumbar orthosis, sagittal control, with rigid anterior and posterior panels, posterior extends from L1 to below L5 vertebra, produces intracavitary pressure to reduce load on the intervertebral discs, includes straps, closures, may include padding, shoulder straps, pendulous abdomen design, prefabricated, includes fitting andadjustment A

L0628 Lumbar-sacral orthosis, flexible, provides lumbo-sacral support, posterior extends from sacrococcygeal junction to T9 vertebra, produces intracavitary pressure to reduce load on the intervertebral discs, includes straps, closures, may include stays, shoulder straps, pendulous abdomen design, prefabricated, includes fitting and adjustment A

L0629 Lumbar-sacral orthosis, flexible, provides lumbo-sacral support, posterior extends from sacrococcygeal junction to T9 vertebra, produces intracavitary pressure to reduce load on the intervertebral discs, includes straps, closures, may include stays, shoulder straps, pendulous abdomen design, custom fabricated A

L0630 Lumbar-sacral orthosis, sagittal control, with rigid posterior panel(s), posterior extends from sacrococcygeal junction to T9 vertebra, produces intracavitary pressure to reduce load on the intervertebral discs, includes straps, closures, may include padding, stays, shoulder straps, pendulous abdomen design, prefabricated, includes fitting and adjustment A

L0631 Lumbar-sacral orthosis, sagittal control, with rigid anterior and posterior panels, posterior extends from sacrococcygeal junction to T9 vertebra, produces intracavitary pressure to reduce load on the intervertebral discs, includes straps, closures, may include padding, shoulder straps, pendulous abdomen design, prefabricated, includes fitting and adjustment A

L0632 Lumbar-sacral orthosis, sagittal control, with rigid anterior and posterior panels, posterior extends from sacrococcygeal junction to T9 vertebra, produces intracavitary pressure to reduce load on the intervertebral discs, includes straps, closures, may include padding, shoulder straps, pendulous abdomen design, custom fabricated A

L0633 Lumbar-sacral orthosis, sagittal-coronal control, with rigid posterior frame/panel(s), posterior extends from sacrococcygeal junction to T9 vertebra, lateral strength provided by rigid lateral frame/panels, produces intracavitary pressure to reduce load on intervertebral discs, includes straps, closures, may include padding, stays, shoulder straps, pendulous abdomen design, prefabricated, includes fitting and adjustment A

L0634 Lumbar-sacral orthosis, sagittal-coronal control, with rigid posterior frame/panel(s), posterior extends from sacrococcygeal junction to T9 vertebra, lateral strength provided by rigid lateral frame/panel(s), produces intracavitary pressure to reduce load on intervertebral discs, includes straps, closures, may include padding, stays, shoulder straps, pendulous abdomen design, custom fabricated A

L0635 Lumbar-sacral orthosis, sagittal-coronal control, lumbar flexion, rigid posterior frame/panel(s), lateral articulating design to flex the lumbar spine, posterior extends from sacrococcygeal junction to T9 vertebra, lateral strength provided by rigid lateral frame/panel(s), produces intracavitary pressure to reduce load on intervertebral discs, includes straps, closures, may include padding, anterior panel, pendulous abdomen design, prefabricated, includes fitting and adjustment A

L0636 Lumbar sacral orthosis, sagittal-coronal control, lumbar flexion, rigid posterior frame/panels, lateral articulating design to flex the lumbar spine, posterior extends from sacrococcygeal junction to T9 vertebra, lateral strength provided by rigid lateral frame/panels, produces intracavitary pressure to reduce load on intervertebral discs, includes straps, closures, may include padding, anterior panel, pendulous abdomen design, custom fabricated A

L0637 Lumbar-sacral orthosis, sagittal-coronal control, with rigid anterior and posterior frame/panels, posterior extends from sacrococcygeal junction to T9 vertebra, lateral strength provided by rigid lateral frame/panels, produces intracavitary pressure to reduce load on intervertebral discs, includes straps, closures, may include padding, shoulder straps, pendulous abdomen design, prefabricated, includes fitting and adjustment

L0638 Lumbar-sacral orthosis, sagittal-coronal control, with rigid anterior and posterior frame/panels, posterior extends from sacrococcygeal junction to T9 vertebra, lateral strength provided by rigid lateral frame/panels, produces intracavitary pressure to reduce load on intervertebral discs, includes straps, closures, may include padding, shoulder straps, pendulous abdomen design, custom fabricated

L0639 Lumbar-sacral orthosis, sagittal-coronal control, rigid shell(s)/panel(s), posterior extends from sacrococcygeal junction to T9 vertebra, anterior extends from symphysis pubis to xyphoid, produces intracavitary pressure to reduce load on the intervertebral discs, overall strength is provided by overlapping rigid material and stabilizing closures, includes straps, closures, may include soft interface, pendulous abdomen design, prefabricated, includes fitting and adjustment

L0640 Lumbar-sacral orthosis, sagittal-coronal control, rigid shell(s)/panel(s), posterior extends from sacrococcygeal junction to T9 vertebra, anterior extends from symphysis pubis to xyphoid, produces intracavitary pressure to reduce load on the intervertebral discs, overall strength is provided by overlapping rigid material and stabilizing closures, includes straps, closures, may include soft interface, pendulous abdomen design, custom fabricated

Anterior-Posterior-Lateral Control

L0700 Cervical-thoracic-lumbar-sacral-orthoses (CTLSO), anterior-posterior-lateral control, molded to patient model, (Minerva type)

L0710 CTLSO, anterior-posterior-lateral-control, molded to patient model, with interface material, (Minerva type)

Halo Procedure

L0810 Halo procedure, cervical halo incorporated into jacket vest

L0820 Halo procedure, cervical halo incorporated into plaster body jacket

L0830 Halo procedure, cervical halo incorporated into Milwaukee type orthosis

L0859 Addition to halo procedure, magnetic resonance image compatible systems, rings and pins, any material

L0861 Addition to halo procedure, replacement liner/interface material

Torso Supports

Additions to Spinal Orthoses

L0970 TLSO, corset front

Spinal orthosis corset

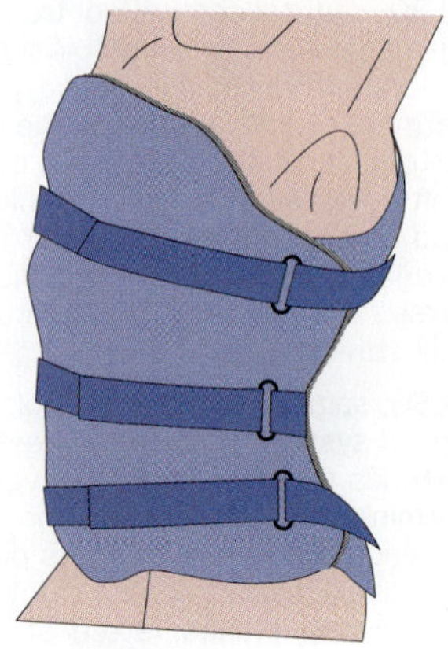

L0972 LSO, corset front

L0974 TLSO, full corset

L0976 LSO, full corset

L0978 Axillary crutch extension

L0980 Peroneal straps, pair

L0982 Stocking supporter grips, set of four (4)

L0984 Protective body sock, each

L0999 Addition to spinal orthosis, not otherwise specified

Orthotic Devices – Scoliosis Procedures

Note: Scoliosis Procedures. The orthotic care of scoliosis differs from other orthotic care in that the treatment is more dynamic in nature and utilizes ongoing, continual modification to the patient's changing condition. This coding structure uses the proper names (or eponyms) of the procedures because they have historic and universal acceptance in the medical profession. It should be recognized that variations to the basic procedures described by the founders/developers are accepted in various medical and orthotic practices throughout the country. All procedures include model of patent when indicated.

Cervical – Thoracic – Lumbar – Sacral (Milwaukee)

L1000 Cervical-thoracic-lumbar-sacral orthosis (CTLSO) (Milwaukee), inclusive of furnishing initial orthosis, including model

L1001 Cervical thoracic lumbar sacral orthosis, immobilizer, infant size, prefabricated, includes fitting and adjustment

L1005 Tension based scoliosis orthosis and accessory pads, includes fitting and adjustment

L1010 Addition to cervical-thoracic-lumbar-sacral orthosis (CTLSO) or scoliosis orthosis, axilla sling

L1020 Addition to CTLSO or scoliosis orthosis, kyphosis pad

L1025 Addition to CTLSO or scoliosis orthosis, kyphosis pad, floating

L1030 Addition to CTLSO or scoliosis orthosis, lumbar bolster pad

L1040 Addition to CTLSO or scoliosis orthosis, lumbar or lumbar rib pad

L1050 Addition to CTLSO or scoliosis orthosis, sternal pad

L1060 Addition to CTLSO or scoliosis orthosis, thoracic pad A

L1070 Addition to CTLSO or scoliosis orthosis, trapezius sling A

L1080 Addition to CTLSO or scoliosis orthosis, outrigger A

L1085 Addition to CTLSO or scoliosis orthosis, outrigger, bilateral with vertical extensions A

L1090 Addition to CTLSO or scoliosis orthosis, lumbar sling A

L1100 Addition to CTLSO or scoliosis orthosis, ring flange, plastic or leather A

L1110 Addition to CTLSO or scoliosis orthosis, ring flange, plastic or leather, molded to patient model A

L1120 Addition to CTLSO, scoliosis orthosis, cover for upright, each A

Thoracic – Lumbar – Sacral (Low Profile)

L1200 Thoracic-lumbar-sacral-orthosis (TLSO), inclusive of furnishing initial orthosis only A

L1210 Addition to TLSO, (low profile), lateral thoracic extension A

L1220 Addition to TLSO, (low profile), anterior thoracic extension A

L1230 Addition to TLSO, (low profile), Milwaukee type superstructure A

L1240 Addition to TLSO, (low profile), lumbar derotation pad A

L1250 Addition to TLSO, (low profile), anterior asis pad A

L1260 Addition to TLSO, (low profile), anterior thoracic derotation pad A

L1270 Addition to TLSO, (low profile), abdominal pad A

L1280 Addition to TLSO, (low profile), rib gusset (elastic), each A

L1290 Addition to TLSO, (low profile), lateral trochanteric pad A

Other Scoliosis Procedures

L1300 Other scoliosis procedure, body jacket molded to patient model A

L1310 Other scoliosis procedure, post-operative body jacket A

L1499 Spinal orthosis, not otherwise specified A

Thoracic – Hip – Knee – Ankle

L1500 Thoracic-hip-knee-ankle orthosis (THKAO), mobility frame (Newington, Parapodium types) A

L1510 THKAO, standing frame, with or without tray and accessories A

L1520 THKAO, swivel walker A

Orthotic Devices – Lower Limb

Hip

L1600 Hip orthosis, abduction control of hip joints, flexible, Frejka type with cover, prefabricated, includes fitting and adjustment A

L1610 Hip orthosis, abduction control of hip joints, flexible, (Frejka cover only), prefabricated, includes fitting and adjustment A

L1620 Hip orthosis, abduction control of hip joints, flexible, (Pavlik harness), prefabricated, includes fitting and adjustment A

L1630 Hip orthosis, abduction control of hip joints, semi-flexible (Von Rosen type), custom-fabricated A

L1640 Hip orthosis, abduction control of hip joints, static, pelvic band or spreader bar, thigh cuffs, custom-fabricated A

L1650 Hip orthosis, abduction control of hip joints, static, adjustable, (Ilfled type), prefabricated, includes fitting and adjustment A

L1652 Hip orthosis, bilateral thigh cuffs with adjustable abductor spreader bar, adult size, prefabricated, includes fitting and adjustment, any type A

L1660 Hip orthosis, abduction control of hip joints, static, plastic, prefabricated, includes fitting and adjustment A

L1680 Hip orthosis, abduction control of hip joints, dynamic, pelvic control, adjustable hip motion control, thigh cuffs (Rancho hip action type), custom fabricated A

L1685 Hip orthosis, abduction control of hip joint, post-operative hip abduction type, custom fabricated A

L1686 Hip orthosis, abduction control of hip joint, postoperative hip abduction type, prefabricated, includes fitting and adjustment A

L1690 Combination, bilateral, lumbo-sacral, hip, femur orthosis providing adduction and internal rotation control, prefabricated, includes fitting and adjustment A

Legg Perthes

L1700 Legg Perthes orthosis, (Toronto type), custom-fabricated A

L1710 Legg Perthes orthosis, (Newington type), custom fabricated A

L1720 Legg Perthes orthosis, trilateral, (Tachdijan type), custom-fabricated A

L1730 Legg Perthes orthosis, (Scottish Rite type), custom-fabricated A

L1755 Legg Perthes orthosis, (Patten bottom type), custom-fabricated A

L1810 Knee orthosis, elastic with joints, prefabricated, includes fitting and adjustment A

L1820 Knee orthosis, elastic with condylar pads and joints, with or without patellar control, prefabricated, includes fitting and adjustment A

L1830 Knee orthosis, immobilizer, canvas longitudinal, prefabricated, includes fitting and adjustment A

L1831 Knee orthosis, locking knee joint(s), positional orthosis, prefabricated, includes fitting and adjustment A

L1832 Knee orthosis, adjustable knee joints (unicentric or polycentric), positional orthosis, rigid support, prefabricated, includes fitting and adjustment A

L1834 Knee orthosis, without knee joint, rigid, custom-fabricated A

L1836 Knee orthosis, rigid, without joint(s), includes soft interface material, prefabricated, includes fitting and adjustment A

L1840 Knee orthosis, derotation, medial-lateral, anterior cruciate ligament, custom fabricated A

L1843 Knee orthosis, single upright, thigh and calf, with adjustable flexion and extension joint (unicentric or polycentric), medial-lateral and rotation control, with or without varus/valgus adjustment, prefabricated, includes fitting and adjustment A

L1844 Knee orthosis, single upright, thigh and calf, with adjustable flexion and extension joint (unicentric or polycentric), medial-lateral and rotation control, with or without varus/valgus adjustment, custom fabricated A

L1845 Knee orthosis, double upright, thigh and calf, with adjustable flexion and extension joint (unicentric or polycentric), medial-lateral and rotation control, with or without varus/valgus adjustment, prefabricated, includes fitting and adjustment

L1846 Knee orthosis, double upright, thigh and calf, with adjustable flexion and extension joint (unicentric or polycentric), medial-lateral and rotation control, with or without varus/valgus adjustment, custom fabricated

L1847 Knee orthosis, double upright with adjustable joint, with inflatable air support chamber(s), prefabricated, includes fitting and adjustment

L1850 Knee orthosis, Swedish type, prefabricated, includes fitting and adjustment

L1860 Knee orthosis, modification of supracondylar prosthetic socket, custom-fabricated (SK)

Ankle – Foot

L1900 Ankle foot orthosis, spring wire, dorsiflexion assist calf band, custom-fabricated

L1902 Ankle foot orthosis, ankle gauntlet, prefabricated, includes fitting and adjustment

L1904 Ankle foot orthosis, molded ankle gauntlet, custom-fabricated

L1906 Ankle foot orthosis, multiligamentus ankle support, prefabricated, includes fitting and adjustment

L1907 AFO, supramalleolar with straps, with or without interface/pads, custom fabricated

L1910 Ankle foot orthosis, posterior, single bar, clasp attachment to shoe counter, prefabricated, includes fitting and adjustment

L1920 Ankle foot orthosis, single upright with static or adjustable stop (Phelps or Perlstein type), custom-fabricated

L1930 Ankle foot orthosis, plastic or other material, prefabricated, includes fitting and adjustment

L1932 AFO, rigid anterior tibial section, total carbon fiber or equal material, prefabricated, includes fitting and adjustment

L1940 Ankle foot orthosis, plastic or other material, custom-fabricated

L1945 Ankle foot orthosis, plastic, rigid anterior tibial section (floor reaction), custom-fabricated

L1950 Ankle foot orthosis, spiral, (institute of rehabilitative medicine type), plastic, custom-fabricated

L1951 Ankle foot orthosis, spiral, (institute of rehabilitative medicine type), plastic or other material, prefabricated, includes fitting and adjustment

L1960 Ankle foot orthosis, posterior solid ankle, plastic, custom-fabricated

L1970 Ankle foot orthosis, plastic, with ankle joint, custom-fabricated

Richie brace

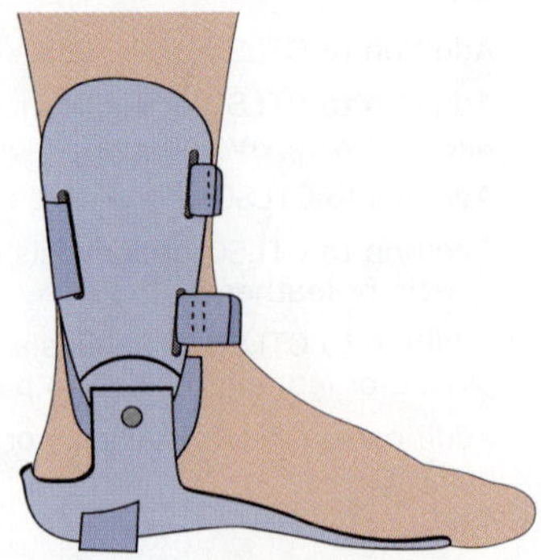

L1971 Ankle foot orthosis, plastic or other material with ankle joint, prefabricated, includes fitting and adjustment

L1980 Ankle foot orthosis, single upright free plantar dorsiflexion, solid stirrup, calf band/cuff (single bar 'BK' orthosis), custom-fabricated

L1990 Ankle foot orthosis, double upright free plantar dorsiflexion, solid stirrup, calf band/cuff (double bar 'BK' orthosis), custom-fabricated

Hip – Knee – Ankle – Foot (or Any Combination)

Note: L2000, L2020, and L2036 are base procedures to be used with any knee joint. L2010 and L2030 are to be used only without knee joint.

L2000 Knee ankle foot orthosis, single upright, free knee, free ankle, solid stirrup, thigh and calf bands/cuffs (single bar 'AK' orthosis), custom-fabricated

L2005 Knee ankle foot orthosis, any material, single or double upright, stance control, automatic lock and swing phase release, mechanical activation, includes ankle joint, any type, custom fabricated

L2010 Knee ankle foot orthosis, single upright, free ankle, solid stirrup, thigh and calf bands/cuffs (single bar 'AK' orthosis), without knee joint, custom-fabricated

L2020 Knee ankle foot orthosis, double upright, free ankle, solid stirrup, thigh and calf bands/cuffs (double bar 'AK' orthosis), custom-fabricated

L2030 Knee ankle foot orthosis, double upright, free ankle, solid stirrup, thigh and calf bands/cuffs, (double bar 'AK' orthosis), without knee joint, custom fabricated

L2034 Knee ankle foot orthosis, full plastic, single upright, with or without free motion knee, medial lateral rotation control, with or without free motion ankle, custom fabricated

L2035 Knee ankle foot orthosis, full plastic, static (pediatric size), without free motion ankle, prefabricated, includes fitting and adjustment

L2036 Knee ankle foot orthosis, full plastic, double upright, with or without free motion knee, with or without free motion ankle, custom fabricated

L2037 Knee ankle foot orthosis, full plastic, single upright, with or without free motion knee, with or without free motion ankle, custom fabricated

L2038 Knee ankle foot orthosis, full plastic, with or without free motion knee, multi-axis ankle, custom fabricated

Torsion Control

L2040 Hip knee ankle foot orthosis, torsion control, bilateral rotation straps, pelvic band/belt, custom fabricated

L2050 Hip knee ankle foot orthosis, torsion control, bilateral torsion cables, hip joint, pelvic band/belt, custom-fabricated

L2060 Hip knee ankle foot orthosis, torsion control, bilateral torsion cables, ball bearing hip joint, pelvic band/ belt, custom-fabricated

L2070 Hip knee ankle foot orthosis, torsion control, unilateral rotation straps, pelvic band/belt, custom fabricated

L2080 Hip knee ankle foot orthosis, torsion control, unilateral torsion cable, hip joint, pelvic band/belt, custom-fabricated

L2090 Hip knee ankle foot orthosis, torsion control, unilateral torsion cable, ball bearing hip joint, pelvic band/ belt, custom-fabricated

Fracture Orthoses

L2106 Ankle foot orthosis, fracture orthosis, tibial fracture cast orthosis, thermoplastic type casting material, custom-fabricated

L2108 Ankle foot orthosis, fracture orthosis, tibial fracture cast orthosis, custom-fabricated

L2112 Ankle foot orthosis, fracture orthosis, tibial fracture orthosis, soft, prefabricated, includes fitting and adjustment

L2114 Ankle foot orthosis, fracture orthosis, tibial fracture orthosis, semi-rigid, prefabricated, includes fitting and adjustment

L2116 Ankle foot orthosis, fracture orthosis, tibial fracture orthosis, rigid, prefabricated, includes fitting and adjustment

L2126 Knee ankle foot orthosis, fracture orthosis, femoral fracture cast orthosis, thermoplastic type casting material, custom-fabricated

L2128 Knee ankle foot orthosis, fracture orthosis, femoral fracture cast orthosis, custom-fabricated

L2132 KAFO, fracture orthosis, femoral fracture cast orthosis, soft, prefabricated, includes fitting and adjustment

L2134 KAFO, fracture orthosis, femoral fracture cast orthosis, semi-rigid, prefabricated, includes fitting and adjustment

L2136 KAFO, fracture orthosis, femoral fracture cast orthosis, rigid, prefabricated, includes fitting and adjustment

Additions to Fracture Orthosis

L2180 Addition to lower extremity fracture orthosis, plastic shoe insert with ankle joints

L2182 Addition to lower extremity fracture orthosis, drop lock knee joint

L2184 Addition to lower extremity fracture orthosis, limited motion knee joint

L2186 Addition to lower extremity fracture orthosis, adjustable motion knee joint, lerman type

L2188 Addition to lower extremity fracture orthosis, quadrilateral brim

L2190 Addition to lower extremity fracture orthosis, waist belt

L2192 Addition to lower extremity fracture orthosis, hip joint, pelvic band, thigh flange, and pelvic belt

Additions to Lower Extremity Orthosis

Additions – Shoe – Ankle – Shin – Knee

L2200 Addition to lower extremity, limited ankle motion, each joint

L2210 Addition to lower extremity, dorsiflexion assist (plantar flexion resist), each joint

L2220 Addition to lower extremity, dorsiflexion and plantar flexion assist/resist, each joint

L2230 Addition to lower extremity, split flat caliper stirrups and plate attachment

L2232 Addition to lower extremity orthosis, rocker bottom for total contact ankle foot orthosis, for custom fabricated orthosis only

L2240 Addition to lower extremity, round caliper and plate attachment

L2250 Addition to lower extremity, foot plate, molded to patient model, stirrup attachment

L2260 Addition to lower extremity, reinforced solid stirrup (Scott-Craig type)

L2265 Addition to lower extremity, long tongue stirrup

L2270 Addition to lower extremity, varus/valgus correction ('T') strap, padded/lined or malleolus pad

L2275 Addition to lower extremity, varus/valgus correction, plastic modification, padded/lined

L2280 Addition to lower extremity, molded inner boot

L2300 Addition to lower extremity, abduction bar (bilateral hip involvement), jointed, adjustable

L2310 Addition to lower extremity, abduction bar, straight

L2320 Addition to lower extremity, non-molded lacer, for custom fabricated orthosis only

L2330 Addition to lower extremity, lacer molded to patient model, for custom fabricated orthosis only

L2335 Addition to lower extremity, anterior swing band

L2340 Addition to lower extremity, pre-tibial shell, molded to patient model

L2350 Addition to lower extremity, prosthetic type, (BK) socket, molded to patient model, (used for 'PTB', 'AFO' orthoses)

L2360 Addition to lower extremity, extended steel shank

L2370 Addition to lower extremity, patten bottom

L2375 Addition to lower extremity, torsion control, ankle joint and half solid stirrup

L2380 Addition to lower extremity, torsion control, straight knee joint, each joint

L2385 Addition to lower extremity, straight knee joint, heavy duty, each joint

L2387 Addition to lower extremity, polycentric knee joint, for custom fabricated knee ankle foot orthosis, each joint

L2390 Addition to lower extremity, offset knee joint, each joint

L2395 Addition to lower extremity, offset knee joint, heavy duty, each joint

L2397 Addition to lower extremity orthosis, suspension sleeve

Additions to Straight Knee or Offset Knee Joints

L2405 Addition to knee joint, drop lock, each

L2415 Addition to knee lock with integrated release mechanism (bail, cable, or equal), any material, each joint

L2425 Addition to knee joint, disc or dial lock for adjustable knee flexion, each joint A

L2430 Addition to knee joint, ratchet lock for active and progressive knee extension, each joint A

L2492 Addition to knee joint, lift loop for drop lock ring A

Additions – Thigh/Weight Bearing

L2500 Addition to lower extremity, thigh/weight bearing, gluteal/ ischial weight bearing, ring A

L2510 Addition to lower extremity, thigh/weight bearing, quadri- lateral brim, molded to patient model A

L2520 Addition to lower extremity, thigh/weight bearing, quadri- lateral brim, custom fitted A

L2525 Addition to lower extremity, thigh/weight bearing, ischial containment/narrow M-L brim molded to patient model A

L2526 Addition to lower extremity, thigh/weight bearing, ischial containment/narrow M-L brim, custom fitted A

L2530 Addition to lower extremity, thigh-weight bearing, lacer, non-molded A

L2540 Addition to lower extremity, thigh/weight bearing, lacer, molded to patient model A

L2550 Addition to lower extremity, thigh/weight bearing, high roll cuff A

Additions – Pelvic and Thoracic Control

L2570 Addition to lower extremity, pelvic control, hip joint, clevis type, two position joint, each A

L2580 Addition to lower extremity, pelvic control, pelvic sling A

L2600 Addition to lower extremity, pelvic control, hip joint, clevis type, or thrust bearing, free, each A

L2610 Addition to lower extremity, pelvic control, hip joint, clevis or thrust bearing, lock, each A

L2620 Addition to lower extremity, pelvic control, hip joint, heavy-duty, each A

L2622 Addition to lower extremity, pelvic control, hip joint, adjustable flexion, each A

L2624 Addition to lower extremity, pelvic control, hip joint, adjustable flexion, extension, abduction control, each A

L2627 Addition to lower extremity, pelvic control, plastic, molded to patient model, reciprocating hip joint and cables A

L2628 Addition to lower extremity, pelvic control, metal frame, reciprocating hip joint and cables A

L2630 Addition to lower extremity, pelvic control, band and belt, unilateral A

L2640 Addition to lower extremity, pelvic control, band and belt, bilateral A

L2650 Addition to lower extremity, pelvic and thoracic control, gluteal pad, each A

L2660 Addition to lower extremity, thoracic control, thoracic band A

L2670 Addition to lower extremity, thoracic control, paraspinal uprights A

L2680 Addition to lower extremity, thoracic control, lateral support uprights A

Additions – General

L2750 Addition to lower extremity orthosis, plating chrome or nickel, per bar A

L2755 Addition to lower extremity orthosis, high strength, lightweight material, all hybrid lamination/prepreg composite, per segment, for custom fabricated orthosis only A

L2760 Addition to lower extremity orthosis, extension, per extension, per bar (for lineal adjustment for growth) A

L2768 Orthotic side bar disconnect device, per bar A

L2780 Addition to lower extremity orthosis, non-corrosive finish, per bar A

L2785 Addition to lower extremity orthosis, drop lock retainer, each A

L2795 Addition to lower extremity orthosis, knee control, full kneecap A

L2800 Addition to lower extremity orthosis, knee control, knee cap, medial or lateral pull, for use with custom fabricated orthosis only A

L2810 Addition to lower extremity orthosis, knee control, condylar pad A

L2820 Addition to lower extremity orthosis, soft interface for molded plastic, below knee section A

L2830 Addition to lower extremity orthosis, soft interface for molded plastic, above knee section A

L2840 Addition to lower extremity orthosis, tibial length sock, fracture or equal, each A

L2850 Addition to lower extremity orthosis, femoral length sock, fracture or equal, each A

L2861 Addition to lower extremity joint, knee or ankle, concentric adjustable torsion style mechanism for custom fabricated orthotics only, each E

L2999 Lower extremity orthoses, not otherwise specified A

Foot Orthopedic Shoes/Shoe Modifications

Transfers/Foot /Insert, Removable, Molded to Patient Model

L3000 Foot, insert, removable, molded to patient model, 'UCB' type, Berkeley shell, each A
Pub 100-02, 15, 290

L3001 Foot, insert, removable, molded to patient model, Spenco, each A
Pub 100-02, 15, 290

L3002 Foot, insert, removable, molded to patient model, Plastazote or equal, each A
Pub 100-02, 15, 290

L3003 Foot, insert, removable, molded to patient model, silicone gel, each A
Pub 100-02, 15, 290

L3010 Foot, insert, removable, molded to patient model, longitudinal arch support, each A
Pub 100-02, 15, 290

L3020 Foot, insert, removable, molded to patient model, longitudinal/ metatarsal support, each A
Pub 100-02, 15, 290

L3030 Foot, insert, removable, formed to patient foot, each A
Pub 100-02, 15, 290

L3031 Foot, insert/plate, removable, addition to lower extremity orthosis, high strength, lightweight material, all hybrid lamination/prepreg composite, each A

Arch Support, Removable, Premolded

L3040 Foot, arch support, removable, premolded, longitudinal, each A
Pub 100-02, 15, 290

ⓘ L3050 Foot, arch support, removable, premolded, metatarsal, each A
Pub 100-02, 15, 290

ⓘ L3060 Foot, arch support, removable, premolded, longitudinal/ metatarsal, each A
Pub 100-02, 15, 290

Arch Support, Non-Removable, Attached to Shoe

ⓘ L3070 Foot, arch support, non-removable attached to shoe, longitudinal, each A
Pub 100-02, 15, 290

ⓘ L3080 Foot, arch support, non-removable attached to shoe, metatarsal, each A
Pub 100-02, 15, 290

ⓘ L3090 Foot, arch support, non-removable attached to shoe, longitudinal/metatarsal, each A
Pub 100-02, 15, 290

ⓘ L3100 Hallus-Valgus night dynamic splint A
Pub 100-02, 15, 290

Abduction and Rotation Bars

ⓘ L3140 Foot, abduction rotation bar, including shoes A
Pub 100-02, 15, 290

ⓘ L3150 Foot, abduction rotatation bar, without shoes A
Pub 100-02, 15, 290

L3160 Foot, adjustable shoe-styled positioning device A

ⓘ L3170 Foot, plastic, silicone or equal, heel stabilizer, each A
Pub 100-02, 15, 290

Orthopedic Footwear

ⓘ L3201 Orthopedic shoe, Oxford with supinator or pronator, infant A
Pub 100-02, 15, 290

ⓘ L3202 Orthopedic shoe, Oxford with supinator or pronator, child A
Pub 100-02, 15, 290

ⓘ L3203 Orthopedic shoe, Oxford with supinator or pronator, junior A
Pub 100-02, 15, 290

ⓘ L3204 Orthopedic shoe, hightop with supinator or pronator, infant A
Pub 100-02, 15, 290

ⓘ L3206 Orthopedic shoe, hightop with supinator or pronator, child A
Pub 100-02, 15, 290

ⓘ L3207 Orthopedic shoe, hightop with supinator or pronator, junior A
Pub 100-02, 15, 290

ⓘ L3208 Surgical boot, each, infant A
Pub 100-02, 15, 100

ⓘ L3209 Surgical boot, each, child A
Pub 100-02, 15, 100

ⓘ L3211 Surgical boot, each, junior A
Pub 100-02, 15, 100

ⓘ L3212 Benesch boot, pair, infant A
Pub 100-02, 15, 100

ⓘ L3213 Benesch boot, pair, child A
Pub 100-02, 15, 100

ⓘ L3214 Benesch boot, pair, junior A
Pub 100-02, 15, 100

⊘ L3215 Orthopedic footwear, ladies shoe, Oxford, each E
Medicare Statute 1862(a)(8)

⊘ L3216 Orthopedic footwear, ladies shoe, depth inlay, each E
Medicare Statute 1862(a)(8)

⊘ L3217 Orthopedic footwear, ladies shoe, hightop, depth inlay, each E
Medicare Statute 1862(a)(8)

⊘ L3219 Orthopedic footwear, mens shoe, Oxford, each E
Medicare Statute 1862(a)(8)

⊘ L3221 Orthopedic footwear, mens shoe, depth inlay, each E
Medicare Statute 1862(a)(8)

⊘ L3222 Orthopedic footwear, mens shoe, hightop, depth inlay, each E
Medicare Statute 1862(a)(8)

ⓘ L3224 Orthopedic footwear, woman's shoe, Oxford, used as an integral part of a brace (orthosis) A
Pub 100-02, 15, 290

ⓘ L3225 Orthopedic footwear, man's shoe, Oxford, used as an integral part of a brace (orthosis) A
Pub 100-02, 15, 290

ⓘ L3230 Orthopedic footwear, custom shoe, depth inlay, each A
Pub 100-02, 15, 290

ⓘ L3250 Orthopedic footwear, custom molded shoe, removable inner mold, prosthetic shoe, each A
Pub 100-02, 15, 290

ⓘ L3251 Foot, shoe molded to patient model, silicone shoe, each A
Pub 100-02, 15, 290

ⓘ L3252 Foot, shoe molded to patient model, Plastazote (or similar), custom fabricated, each A
Pub 100-02, 15, 290

ⓘ L3253 Foot, molded shoe Plastazote (or similar) custom fitted, each A
Pub 100-02, 15, 290

ⓘ L3254 Non-standard size or width A
Pub 100-02, 15, 290

ⓘ L3255 Non-standard size or length A
Pub 100-02, 15, 290

ⓘ L3257 Orthopedic footwear, additional charge for split size A
Pub 100-02, 15, 290

ⓘ L3260 Surgical boot/shoe, each E
Pub 100-02, 15, 100

L3265 Plastazote sandal, each A

Shoe Modification

Lifts

ⓘ L3300 Lift, elevation, heel, tapered to metatarsals, per inch A
Pub 100-02, 15, 290

ⓘ L3310 Lift, elevation, heel and sole, neoprene, per inch A
Pub 100-02, 15, 290

ⓘ L3320 Lift, elevation, heel and sole, cork, per inch A
Pub 100-02, 15, 290

ⓘ L3330 Lift, elevation, metal extension (skate) A
Pub 100-02, 15, 290

⊘ Medicare Non-Coverage ⓘ Special Coverage Instructions Coverage Carrier Determined A – Y APC Status Indicators ● New Code ▲ Revised Code ✖ Deleted Code
AHA AHA Coding Clinic for HCPCS A2 – Z3 ASC Payment Indicators DMEPOS ♂ Male ♀ Female PQR PQRI

ⓘ L3332 Lift, elevation, inside shoe, tapered, up to one-half inch A
Pub 100-02, 15, 290

ⓘ L3334 Lift, elevation, heel, per inch A
Pub 100-02, 15, 290

Wedges

ⓘ L3340 Heel wedge, SACH A
Pub 100-02, 15, 290

ⓘ L3350 Heel wedge A
Pub 100-02, 15, 290

ⓘ L3360 Sole wedge, outside sole A
Pub 100-02, 15, 290

ⓘ L3370 Sole wedge, between sole A
Pub 100-02, 15, 290

ⓘ L3380 Clubfoot wedge A
Pub 100-02, 15, 290

ⓘ L3390 Outflare wedge A
Pub 100-02, 15, 290

ⓘ L3400 Metatarsal bar wedge, rocker A
Pub 100-02, 15, 290

ⓘ L3410 Metatarsal bar wedge, between sole A
Pub 100-02, 15, 290

ⓘ L3420 Full sole and heel wedge, between sole A
Pub 100-02, 15, 290

Heels

ⓘ L3430 Heel, counter, plastic reinforced A
Pub 100-02, 15, 290

ⓘ L3440 Heel, counter, leather reinforced A
Pub 100-02, 15, 290

ⓘ L3450 Heel, SACH cushion type A
Pub 100-02, 15, 290

ⓘ L3455 Heel, new leather, standard A
Pub 100-02, 15, 290

ⓘ L3460 Heel, new rubber, standard A
Pub 100-02, 15, 290

ⓘ L3465 Heel, Thomas with wedge A
Pub 100-02, 15, 290

ⓘ L3470 Heel, Thomas extended to ball A
Pub 100-02, 15, 290

ⓘ L3480 Heel, pad and depression for spur A
Pub 100-02, 15, 290

ⓘ L3485 Heel, pad, removable for spur A
Pub 100-02, 15, 290

Miscellaneous Shoe Additions

ⓘ L3500 Orthopedic shoe addition, insole, leather A
Pub 100-02, 15, 290

ⓘ L3510 Orthopedic shoe addition, insole, rubber A
Pub 100-02, 15, 290

ⓘ L3520 Orthopedic shoe addition, insole, felt covered with leather A
Pub 100-02, 15, 290

ⓘ L3530 Orthopedic shoe addition, sole, half A
Pub 100-02, 15, 290

ⓘ L3540 Orthopedic shoe addition, sole, full A
Pub 100-02, 15, 290

ⓘ L3550 Orthopedic shoe addition, toe tap standard A
Pub 100-02, 15, 290

ⓘ L3560 Orthopedic shoe addition, toe tap, horseshoe A
Pub 100-02, 15, 290

ⓘ L3570 Orthopedic shoe addition, special extension to instep (leather with eyelets) A
Pub 100-02, 15, 290

ⓘ L3580 Orthopedic shoe addition, convert instep to Velcro closure A
Pub 100-02, 15, 290

ⓘ L3590 Orthopedic shoe addition, convert firm shoe counter to soft counter A
Pub 100-02, 15, 290

ⓘ L3595 Orthopedic shoe addition, March bar A
Pub 100-02, 15, 290

Transfer or Replacement

ⓘ L3600 Transfer of an orthosis from one shoe to another, caliper plate, existing A
Pub 100-02, 15, 290

ⓘ L3610 Transfer of an orthosis from one shoe to another, caliper plate, new A
Pub 100-02, 15, 290

ⓘ L3620 Transfer of an orthosis from one shoe to another, solid stirrup, existing A
Pub 100-02, 15, 290

ⓘ L3630 Transfer of an orthosis from one shoe to another, solid stirrup, new A
Pub 100-02, 15, 290

ⓘ L3640 Transfer of an orthosis from one shoe to another, Dennis Browne splint (Riveton), both shoes A
Pub 100-02, 15, 290

ⓘ L3649 Orthopedic shoe, modification, addition or transfer, not otherwise specified A
Pub 100-02, 15, 290

Orthotic Devices – Upper Limb

Upper Limb – Shoulder

L3650 Shoulder orthosis, figure of eight design abduction restrainer, prefabricated, includes fitting and adjustment A

✖ ~~L3660 Shoulder orthosis, figure of eight design abduction restrainer, canvas and webbing, prefabricated, includes fitting and adjustment~~
This code is deleted as of December 31, 2010
See code(s) L3650

✖ ~~L3670 Shoulder orthosis, acromio/clavicular (canvas and webbing type), prefabricated, includes fitting and adjustment~~
This code is deleted as of December 31, 2010
See code(s) L3671, L3677

▲ L3671 Shoulder orthosis, shoulder joint design, without joints, may include soft interface, straps, custom fabricated, includes fitting and adjustment A

✖ ~~L3672 Shoulder orthosis, abduction positioning (airplane design), thoracic component and support bar, without joints, may inlcude soft interface, straps, custom fabricated, includes fitting and adjustment~~
This code is deleted as of December 31, 2010
See code(s) L3674

✖ ~~L3673 Shoulder orthosis, abduction positioning (airplane design), thoracic component and support bar, includes nontorsion joint/turnbuckle, may include soft interface, straps, custom fabricated, includes fitting and adjustment~~

This code is deleted as of December 31, 2010

See code(s) L3674

● L3674 Shoulder orthosis, abduction positioning (airplane design), thoracic component and support bar, with or without nontorsion joint/turnbuckle, may include soft interface, straps, custom fabricated, includes fitting and adjustment A

This code is effective January 1, 2011

✖ ~~L3675 Shoulder orthosis, vest type abduction restrainer, canvas webbing type, or equal, prefabricated, includes fitting and adjustment~~

This code is deleted as of December 31, 2010

▲ ⓘ L3677 Shoulder orthosis, shoulder joint design, without joints, may include soft interface, straps, prefabricated, includes fitting and adjustment E

Pub 100-02, 15, 120

Upper Limb – Elbow

L3702 Elbow orthosis, without joints, may include soft interface, straps, custom fabricated, includes fitting and adjustment A

L3710 Elbow orthosis, elastic with metal joints, prefabricated, includes fitting and adjustment A

L3720 Elbow orthosis, double upright with forearm/arm cuffs, free motion, custom-fabricated A

L3730 Elbow orthosis, double upright with forearm/arm cuffs, extension/ flexion assist, custom-fabricated A

L3740 Elbow orthosis, double upright with forearm/arm cuffs, adjustable position lock with active control, custom-fabricated A

L3760 Elbow orthosis, with adjustable position locking joint(s), prefabricated, includes fitting and adjustments, any type A

L3762 Elbow orthosis, rigid, without joints, includes soft interface material, prefabricated, includes fitting and adjustment A

L3763 Elbow wrist hand orthosis, rigid, without joints, may include soft interface, straps, custom fabricated, includes fitting and adjustment A

L3764 Elbow wrist hand orthosis, includes one or more nontorsion joints, elastic bands, turnbuckles, may include soft interface, straps, custom fabricated, includes fitting and adjustment A

L3765 Elbow wrist hand finger orthosis, rigid, without joints, may include soft interface, straps, custom fabricated, includes fitting and adjustment A

L3766 Elbow wrist hand finger orthosis, includes one or more nontorsion joints, elastic bands, turnbuckles, may include soft interface, straps, custom fabricated, includes fitting and adjustment A

Upper Limb – Wrist – Hand – Finger

L3806 Wrist hand finger orthosis, includes one or more nontorsion joint(s), turnbuckles, elastic bands/ springs, may include soft interface material, straps, custom fabricated, includes fitting and adjustment A

L3807 Wrist hand finger orthosis, without joint(s), prefabricated, includes fitting and adjustments, any type A

L3808 Wrist hand finger orthosis, rigid without joints, may include soft interface material; straps, custom fabricated, includes fitting and adjustment A

⊘ L3891 Addition to upper extremity joint, wrist or elbow, concentric adjustable torsion style mechanism for custom fabricated orthotics only, each E

Dynamic Flexor Hinge, Reciprocal Wrist Extension/ Flexion, Finger Flexion/Extension

L3900 Wrist hand finger orthosis, dynamic flexor hinge, reciprocal wrist extension/ flexion, finger flexion/ extension, wrist or finger driven, custom-fabricated A

L3901 Wrist hand finger orthosis, dynamic flexor hinge, reciprocal wrist extension/ flexion, finger flexion/ extension, cable driven, custom-fabricated A

External Power

⊘ L3902 Wrist hand finger orthosis, external powered, compressed gas, custom-fabricated D

L3904 Wrist hand finger orthosis, external powered, electric, custom-fabricated A

Other Wrist-Hand-Finger Orthoses-Custom Fitted

L3905 Wrist hand orthosis, includes one or more nontorsion joints, elastic bands, turnbuckles, may include soft interface, straps, custom fabricated, includes fitting and adjustment A

L3906 Wrist hand orthosis, without joints, may include soft interface, straps, custom fabricated, includes fitting and adjustment A

L3908 Wrist hand orthosis, wrist extension control cock-up, non molded, prefabricated, includes fitting and adjustment A

L3912 Hand finger orthosis, flexion glove with elastic finger control, prefabricated, includes fitting and adjustment A

L3913 Hand finger orthosis, without joints, may include soft interface, straps, custom fabricated, includes fitting and adjustment A

L3915 Wrist hand orthosis, includes one or more nontorsion joint(s), elastic bands, turnbuckles, may include soft interface, straps, prefabricated, includes fitting and adjustment A

L3917 Hand orthosis, metacarpal fracture orthosis, prefabricated, includes fitting and adjustment A

L3919 Hand orthosis, without joints, may include soft interface, straps, custom fabricated, includes fitting and adjustment A

L3921 Hand finger orthosis, includes one or more nontorsion joints, elastic bands, turnbuckles, may include soft interface, straps, custom fabricated, includes fitting and adjustment A

L3923 Hand finger orthosis, without joints, may include soft interface, straps, prefabricated, includes fitting and adjustment A

L3925 Finger orthosis, proximal interphalangeal (PIP)/ distal interphalangeal (DIP), non torsion joint/spring, extension/flexion, may include soft interface material, prefabricated, includes fitting and adjustment A

L3927 Finger orthosis, proximal interphalangeal (PIP)/distal interphalangeal (DIP), without joint/spring, extension/ flexion (e.g. static or ring type), may include soft interface material, prefabricated, includes fitting and adjustment A

L3929 Hand finger orthosis, includes one or more nontorsion joint(s), turnbuckles, elastic bands/springs, may include soft interface material, straps, prefabricated, includes fitting and adjustment A

L3931 Wrist hand finger orthosis, includes one or more nontorsion joint(s), turnbuckles, elastic bands/springs, may include soft interface material, straps, prefabricated, includes fitting and adjustment A

L3933 Finger orthosis, without joints, may include soft interface, custom fabricated, includes fitting and adjustment A

L3935 Finger orthosis, nontorsion joint, may include soft interface, custom fabricated, includes fitting and adjustment A

L3956 Addition of joint to upper extremity orthosis, any material; per joint A

Upper Limb – Shoulder – Elbow – Wrist – Hand

Abduction Positioning, Custom Fitted

L3960 Shoulder elbow wrist hand orthosis, abduction positioning, airplane design, prefabricated, includes fitting and adjustment A

L3961 Shoulder elbow wrist hand orthosis, shoulder cap design, without joints, may include soft interface, straps, custom fabricated, includes fitting and adjustment A

L3962 Shoulder elbow wrist hand orthosis, abduction positioning, Erbs Palsey design, prefabricated, includes fitting and adjustment A

L3964 Shoulder elbow orthosis, mobile arm support attached to wheelchair, balanced, adjustable, prefabricated, includes fitting and adjustment Y

L3965 Shoulder elbow orthosis, mobile arm support attached to wheelchair, balanced, adjustable Rancho type, prefabricated, includes fitting and adjustment Y

L3966 Shoulder elbow orthosis, mobile arm support attached to wheelchair, balanced, reclining, prefabricated, includes fitting and adjustment Y

L3967 Shoulder elbow wrist hand orthosis, abduction positioning (airplane design), thoracic component and support bar, without joints, may include soft interface, straps, custom fabricated, includes fitting and adjustment A

L3968 Shoulder elbow orthosis, mobile arm support attached to wheelchair, balanced, friction arm support (friction dampening to proximal and distal joints), prefabricated, includes fitting and adjustment Y

L3969 Shoulder elbow orthosis, mobile arm support, monosuspension arm and hand support, overhead elbow forearm hand sling support, yoke type arm suspension support, prefabricated, includes fitting and adjustment Y

Additions to Mobile Arm Supports

L3970 SEO, addition to mobile arm support, elevating proximal arm Y

L3971 Shoulder elbow wrist hand orthosis, shoulder cap design, includes one or more nontorsion joints, elastic bands, turnbuckles, may include soft interface, straps, custom fabricated, includes fitting and adjustment A

L3972 SEO, addition to mobile arm support, offset or lateral rocker arm with elastic balance control Y

L3973 Shoulder elbow wrist hand orthosis, abduction positioning (airplane design), thoracic component and support bar, includes one or more nontorsion joints, elastic bands, turnbuckles, may include soft interface, straps, custom fabricated, includes fitting and adjustment A

L3974 SEO, addition to mobile arm support, supinator Y

L3975 Shoulder elbow wrist hand finger orthosis, shoulder cap design, without joints, may include soft interface, straps, custom fabricated, includes fitting and adjustment A

L3976 Shoulder elbow wrist hand finger orthosis, abduction positioning (airplane design), thoracic component and support bar, without joints, may include soft interface, straps, custom fabricated, includes fitting and adjustment A

Orthosis

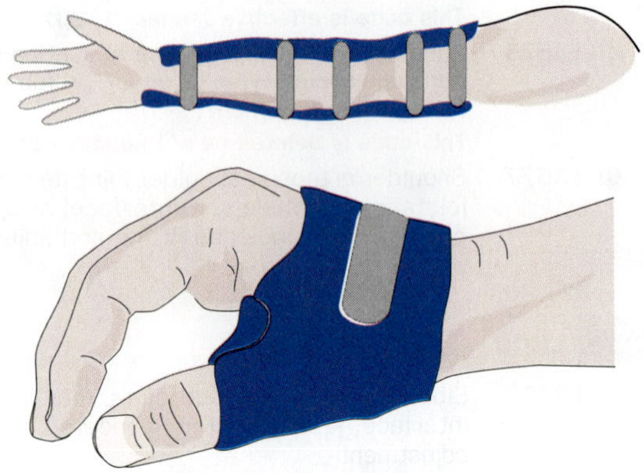

L3977 Shoulder elbow wrist hand finger orthosis, shoulder cap design, includes one or more nontorsion joints, elastic bands, turnbuckles, may include soft interface, straps, custom fabricated, includes fitting and adjustment A

L3978 Shoulder elbow wrist hand finger orthosis, abduction positioning (airplane design), thoracic component and support bar, includes one or more nontorsion joints, elastic bands, turnbuckles, may include soft interface, straps, custom fabricated, includes fitting and adjustment A

Fracture Orthoses

L3980 Upper extremity fracture orthosis, humeral, prefabricated, includes fitting and adjustment A

L3982 Upper extremity fracture orthosis, radius/ulnar, prefabricated, includes fitting and adjustment A

L3984 Upper extremity fracture orthosis, wrist, prefabricated, includes fitting and adjustment

L3995 Addition to upper extremity orthosis, sock, fracture or equal, each A

L3999 Upper limb orthosis, not otherwise specified A

Specific Repair

L4000 Replace girdle for spinal orthosis (CTLSO or SO) A

L4002 Replacement strap, any orthosis, includes all components, any length, any type A

L4010 Replace trilateral socket brim A

L4020 Replace quadrilateral socket brim, molded to patient model A

L4030 Replace quadrilateral socket brim, custom fitted A

L4040 Replace molded thigh lacer, for custom fabricated orthosis only A

L4045 Replace non-molded thigh lacer, for custom fabricated orthosis only A

L4050 Replace molded calf lacer, for custom fabricated orthosis only A

L4055 Replace non-molded calf lacer, for custom fabricated orthosis only

L4060 Replace high roll cuff

L4070 Replace proximal and distal upright for KAFO

L4080 Replace metal bands KAFO, proximal thigh

L4090 Replace metal bands KAFO-AFO, calf or distal thigh

L4100 Replace leather cuff KAFO, proximal thigh

L4110 Replace leather cuff KAFO-AFO, calf or distal thigh

L4130 Replace pretibial shell

Repairs

L4205 Repair of orthotic device, labor component, per 15 minutes

Pub 100-02, 15, 110.2

L4210 Repair of orthotic device, repair or replace minor parts

Pub 100-02, 15, 110.2; 100-2, 15, 130; 100-4, 32, 100-100.4

Ancillary Orthotic Services

L4350 Ankle control orthosis, stirrup style, rigid, includes any type interface (e.g., pneumatic, gel), prefabricated, includes fitting and adjustment

L4360 Walking boot, pneumatic and/or vacuum, with or without joints, with or without interface material, prefabricated, includes fitting and adjustment

L4370 Pneumatic full leg splint, prefabricated, includes fitting and adjustment

L4380 Pneumatic knee splint, prefabricated, includes fitting and adjustment

L4386 Walking boot, non-pneumatic, with or without joints, with or without interface material, prefabricated, includes fitting and adjustment

L4392 Replacement, soft interface material, static AFO

L4394 Replace soft interface material, foot drop splint

L4396 Static or dynamic ankle foot orthosis, including soft interface material, adjustable for fit, for positioning, may be used for minimal ambulation, prefabricated, includes fitting and adjustment

L4398 Foot drop splint, recumbent positioning device, prefabricated, includes fitting and adjustment

● L4631 Ankle foot orthosis, walking boot type, varus/valgus correction, rocker bottom, anterior tibial shell, soft interface, custom arch support, plastic or other material, includes straps and closures, custom fabricated

This code is effective January 1, 2011

Prosthetic Procedures L5000–L9900

Lower Limb

Partial Foot

L5000 Partial foot, shoe insert with longitudinal arch, toe filler

Pub 100-02, 15, 290

L5010 Partial foot, molded socket, ankle height, with toe filler

Pub 100-02, 15, 290

L5020 Partial foot, molded socket, tibial tubercle height, with toe filler

Pub 100-02, 15, 290

Ankle

L5050 Ankle, Symes, molded socket, SACH foot

L5060 Ankle, Symes, metal frame, molded leather socket, articulated ankle/foot

Below Knee

L5100 Below knee, molded socket, shin, SACH foot

Below knee prosthetic

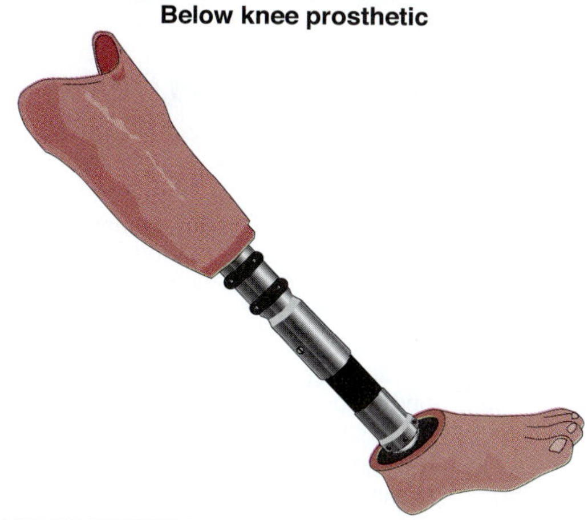

L5105 Below knee, plastic socket, joints and thigh lacer, SACH foot

Knee Disarticulation

L5150 Knee disarticulation (or through knee), molded socket, external knee joints, shin, SACH foot

L5160 Knee disarticulation (or through knee), molded socket, bent knee configuration, external knee joints, shin, SACH foot

Above Knee

L5200 Above knee, molded socket, single axis constant friction knee, shin, SACH foot

L5210 Above knee, short prosthesis, no knee joint ('stubbies'), with foot blocks, no ankle joints, each

L5220 Above knee, short prosthesis, no knee joint ('stubbies'), with articulated ankle/foot, dynamically aligned, each

L5230 Above knee, for proximal femoral focal deficiency, constant friction knee, shin, SACH foot

Hip Disarticulation

L5250 Hip disarticulation, Canadian type; molded socket, hip joint, single axis constant friction knee, shin, SACH foot

L5270 Hip disarticulation, tilt table type; molded socket, locking hip joint, single axis constant friction knee, shin, SACH foot

Hemipelvectomy

L5280 Hemipelvectomy, Canadian type; molded socket, hip joint, single axis constant friction knee, shin, SACH foot

Endoskeletal

L5301 Below knee, molded socket, shin, SACH foot, endoskeletal system

L5311 Knee disarticulation (or through knee), molded socket, external knee joints, shin, SACH foot, endoskeletal system A

L5321 Above knee, molded socket, open end, SACH foot, endoskeletal system, single axis knee A

L5331 Hip disarticulation, Canadian type, molded socket, endoskeletal system, hip joint, single axis knee, SACH foot A

L5341 Hemipelvectomy, Canadian type, molded socket, endoskeletal system, hip joint, single axis knee, SACH foot A

Immediate Post Surgical or Early Fitting Procedures

L5400 Immediate post surgical or early fitting, application of initial rigid dressing, including fitting, alignment, suspension, and one cast change, below knee A

L5410 Immediate post surgical or early fitting, application of initial rigid dressing, including fitting, alignment and suspension, below knee, each additional cast change and realignment A

L5420 Immediate post surgical or early fitting, application of initial rigid dressing, including fitting, alignment and suspension and one cast change 'AK' or knee disarticulation A

L5430 Immediate post surgical or early fitting, application of initial rigid dressing, including fitting, alignment and suspension, 'AK' or knee disarticulation, each additional cast change and realignment A

L5450 Immediate post surgical or early fitting, application of non-weight bearing rigid dressing, below knee A

L5460 Immediate post surgical or early fitting, application of non-weight bearing rigid dressing, above knee A

Initial Prosthesis

L5500 Initial, below knee 'PTB" type socket, non-alignable system, pylon, no cover, SACH foot, plaster socket, direct formed A

L5505 Initial, above knee – knee disarticulation, ischial level socket, non-alignable system, pylon, no cover, SACH foot, plaster socket, direct formed A

Preparatory Prosthesis

L5510 Preparatory, below knee 'PTB" type socket, non-alignable system, pylon, no cover, SACH foot, plaster socket, molded to model A

L5520 Preparatory, below knee 'PTB" type socket, non-alignable system, pylon, no cover, SACH foot, thermoplastic or equal, direct formed A

L5530 Preparatory, below knee 'PTB" type socket, non-alignable system, pylon, no cover, SACH foot, thermoplastic or equal, molded to model A

L5535 Preparatory, below knee 'PTB" type socket, non-alignable system, pylon, no cover, SACH foot, prefabricated, adjustable open end socket A

L5540 Preparatory, below knee 'PTB" type socket, non-alignable system, pylon, no cover, SACH foot, laminated socket, molded to model A

L5560 Preparatory, above knee- knee disarticulation, ischial level socket, non-alignable system, pylon, no cover, SACH foot, plaster socket, molded to model A

L5570 Preparatory, above knee – knee disarticulation, ischial level socket, non-alignable system, pylon, no cover, SACH foot, thermoplastic or equal, direct formed A

L5580 Preparatory, above knee – knee disarticulation, ischial level socket, non-alignable system, pylon, no cover, SACH foot, thermoplastic or equal, molded to model A

L5585 Preparatory, above knee – knee disarticulation, ischial level socket, non-alignable system, pylon, no cover, SACH foot, prefabricated adjustable open end socket A

L5590 Preparatory, above knee – knee disarticulation, ischial level socket, non-alignable system, pylon, no cover, SACH foot, laminated socket, molded to model A

L5595 Preparatory, hip disarticulation-hemipelvectomy, pylon, no cover, SACH foot, thermoplastic or equal, molded to patient model A

L5600 Preparatory, hip disarticulation-hemipelvectomy, pylon, no cover, SACH foot, laminated socket, molded to patient model A

Additions – Lower Extremity

L5610 Addition to lower extremity, endoskeletal system, above knee, hydracadence system A

L5611 Addition to lower extremity, endoskeletal system, above knee – knee disarticulation, 4-bar linkage, with friction swing phase control A

L5613 Addition to lower extremity, endoskeletal system, above knee-knee disarticulation, 4-bar linkage, with hydraulic swing phase control A

L5614 Addition to lower extremity, exoskeletal system, above knee-knee disarticulation, 4-bar linkage, with pneumatic swing phase control A

L5616 Addition to lower extremity, endoskeletal system, above knee, universal multiplex system, friction swing phase control A

L5617 Addition to lower extremity, quick change self-aligning unit, above knee or below knee, each A

L5618 Addition to lower extremity, test socket, Symes A

L5620 Addition to lower extremity, test socket, below knee A

L5622 Addition to lower extremity, test socket, knee disarticulation A

L5624 Addition to lower extremity, test socket, above knee A

L5626 Addition to lower extremity, test socket, hip disarticulation A

L5628 Addition to lower extremity, test socket, hemipelvectomy A

L5629 Addition to lower extremity, below knee, acrylic socket A

Additions – Socket Variations

L5630 Addition to lower extremity, Symes type, expandable wall socket A

L5631 Addition to lower extremity, above knee or knee disarticulation, acrylic socket A

L5632 Addition to lower extremity, Symes type, 'PTB" brim design socket A

L5634 Addition to lower extremity, Symes type, posterior opening (Canadian) socket A

L5636 Addition to lower extremity, Symes type, medial opening socket A

L5637 Addition to lower extremity, below knee, total contact A

L5638 Addition to lower extremity, below knee, leather socket A

L5639 Addition to lower extremity, below knee, wood socket A

L5640 Addition to lower extremity, knee disarticulation, leather socket A

L5642 Addition to lower extremity, above knee, leather socket A

L5643 Addition to lower extremity, hip disarticulation, flexible inner socket, external frame A

L5644 Addition to lower extremity, above knee, wood socket A

L5645 Addition to lower extremity, below knee, flexible inner socket, external frame A

L5646 Addition to lower extremity, below knee, air, fluid, gel or equal, cushion socket A

L5647 Addition to lower extremity, below knee suction socket A

L5648 Addition to lower extremity, above knee, air, fluid, gel or equal, cushion socket A

L5649 Addition to lower extremity, ischial containment/narrow M-L socket A

L5650 Additions to lower extremity, total contact, above knee or knee disarticulation socket A

L5651 Addition to lower extremity, above knee, flexible inner socket, external frame A

L5652 Addition to lower extremity, suction suspension, above knee or knee disarticulation socket A

L5653 Addition to lower extremity, knee disarticulation, expandable wall socket A

Additions – Socket Insert and Suspension

L5654 Addition to lower extremity, socket insert, Symes, (Kemblo, Pelite, Aliplast, Plastazote or equal) A

L5655 Addition to lower extremity, socket insert, below knee (Kemblo, Pelite, Aliplast, Plastazote or equal) A

L5656 Addition to lower extremity, socket insert, knee disarticulation (Kemblo, Pelite, Aliplast, Plastazote or equal) A

L5658 Addition to lower extremity, socket insert, above knee (Kemblo, Pelite, Aliplast, Plastazote or equal) A

L5661 Addition to lower extremity, socket insert, multi-durometer Symes A

L5665 Addition to lower extremity, socket insert, multi-durometer, below knee A

L5666 Addition to lower extremity, below knee, cuff suspension A

L5668 Addition to lower extremity, below knee, molded distal cushion A

L5670 Addition to lower extremity, below knee, molded supracondylar suspension ('PTS" or similar) A

L5671 Addition to lower extremity, below knee / above knee suspension locking mechanism (shuttle, lanyard or equal), excludes socket insert A

L5672 Addition to lower extremity, below knee, removable medial brim suspension A

L5673 Addition to lower extremity, below knee/above knee, custom fabricated from existing mold or prefabricated, socket insert, silicone gel, elastomeric or equal, for use with locking mechanism A

L5676 Additions to lower extremity, below knee, knee joints, single axis, pair A

L5677 Additions to lower extremity, below knee, knee joints, polycentric, pair A

L5678 Additions to lower extremity, below knee, joint covers, pair A

L5679 Addition to lower extremity, below knee/above knee, custom fabricated from existing mold or prefabricated, socket insert, silicone gel, elastomeric or equal, not for use with locking mechanism A

L5680 Addition to lower extremity, below knee, thigh lacer, nonmolded A

L5681 Addition to lower extremity, below knee/above knee, custom fabricated socket insert for congenital or atypical traumatic amputee, silicone gel, elastomeric or equal, for use with or without locking mechanism, initial only (for other than initial, use code L5673 or L5679) A

L5682 Addition to lower extremity, below knee, thigh lacer, gluteal/ischial, molded A

L5683 Addition to lower extremity, below knee/above knee, custom fabricated socket insert for other than congenital or atypical traumatic amputee, silicone gel, elastomeric or equal, for use with or without locking mechanism, initial only (for other than initial, use code L5673 or L5679) A

L5684 Addition to lower extremity, below knee, fork strap A

L5685 Addition to lower extremity prosthesis, below knee, suspension/sealing sleeve, with or without valve, any material, each A

L5686 Addition to lower extremity, below knee, back check (extension control) A

L5688 Addition to lower extremity, below knee, waist belt, webbing A

L5690 Addition to lower extremity, below knee, waist belt, padded and lined A

L5692 Addition to lower extremity, above knee, pelvic control belt, light A

L5694 Addition to lower extremity, above knee, pelvic control belt, padded and lined A

L5695 Addition to lower extremity, above knee, pelvic control, sleeve suspension, neoprene or equal, each A

L5696 Addition to lower extremity, above knee or knee disarticulation, pelvic joint A

L5697 Addition to lower extremity, above knee or knee disarticulation, pelvic band A

L5698 Addition to lower extremity, above knee or knee disarticulation, Silesian bandage A

L5699 All lower extremity prostheses, shoulder harness A

Replacements – Lower Limb

L5700 Replacement, socket, below knee, molded to patient model A

L5701 Replacement, socket, above knee/knee disarticulation, including attachment plate, molded to patient model A

L5702 Replacement, socket, hip disarticulation, including hip joint, molded to patient model A

L5703 Ankle, Symes, molded to patient model, socket without solid ankle cushion heel (SACH) foot, replacement only A

L5704 Custom shaped protective cover, below knee A

L5705 Custom shaped protective cover, above knee A

L5706 Custom shaped protective cover, knee disarticulation A

L5707 Custom shaped protective cover, hip disarticulation A

Additions – Knee – Shin System

Exoskeletal

L5710 Addition, exoskeletal knee-shin system, single axis, manual lock A

L5711 Additions exoskeletal knee-shin system, single axis, manual lock, ultra-light material A

L5712 Addition, exoskeletal knee-shin system, single axis, friction swing and stance phase control (safety knee) A

L5714 Addition, exoskeletal knee-shin system, single axis, variable friction swing phase control A

L5716 Addition, exoskeletal knee-shin system, polycentric, mechanical stance phase lock A

L5718 Addition, exoskeletal knee-shin system, polycentric, friction swing and stance phase control A

L5722 Addition, exoskeletal knee-shin system, single axis, pneumatic swing, friction stance phase control A

L5724 Addition, exoskeletal knee-shin system, single axis, fluid swing phase control A

L5726 Addition, exoskeletal knee-shin system, single axis, external joints fluid swing phase control A

L5728 Addition, exoskeletal knee-shin system, single axis, fluid swing and stance phase control A

L5780 Addition, exoskeletal knee-shin system, single axis, pneumatic/hydra pneumatic swing phase control A

L5781 Addition to lower limb prosthesis, vacuum pump, residual limb volume management and moisture evacuation system A

L5782 Addition to lower limb prosthesis, vacuum pump, residual limb volume management and moisture evacuation system, heavy duty A

L5785 Addition, exoskeletal system, below knee, ultra-light material (titanium, carbon fiber or equal) A

L5790 Addition, exoskeletal system, above knee, ultra-light material (titanium, carbon fiber or equal) A

L5795 Addition, exoskeletal system, hip disarticulation, ultra-light material (titanium, carbon fiber or equal) A

Endoskeletal

L5810 Addition, endoskeletal knee-shin system, single axis, manual lock A

L5811 Addition, endoskeletal knee-shin system, single axis, manual lock, ultra-light material A

L5812 Addition, endoskeletal knee-shin system, single axis, friction swing and stance phase control (safety knee) A

L5814 Addition, endoskeletal knee-shin system, polycentric, hydraulic swing phase control, mechanical stance phase lock A

L5816 Addition, endoskeletal knee-shin system, polycentric, mechanical stance phase lock A

L5818 Addition, endoskeletal knee-shin system, polycentric, friction swing, and stance phase control A

L5822 Addition, endoskeletal knee-shin system, single axis, pneumatic swing, friction stance phase control A

L5824 Addition, endoskeletal knee-shin system, single axis, fluid swing phase control A

L5826 Addition, endoskeletal knee-shin system, single axis, hydraulic swing phase control, with miniature high activity frame A

L5828 Addition, endoskeletal knee-shin system, single axis, fluid swing and stance phase control A

L5830 Addition, endoskeletal knee-shin system, single axis, pneumatic/ swing phase control A

L5840 Addition, endoskeletal knee/shin system, 4-bar linkage or multiaxial, pneumatic swing phase control A

L5845 Addition, endoskeletal, knee-shin system, stance flexion feature, adjustable A

L5848 Addition to endoskeletal knee-shin system, fluid stance extension, dampening feature, with or without adjustability A

L5850 Addition, endoskeletal system, above knee or hip disarticulation, knee extension assist A

L5855 Addition, endoskeletal system, hip disarticulation, mechanical hip extension assist A

L5856 Addition to lower extremity prosthesis, endoskeletal knee-shin system, microprocessor control feature, swing and stance phase, includes electronic sensor(s), any type A

L5857 Addition to lower extremity prosthesis, endoskeletal knee-shin system, microprocessor control feature, swing phase only, includes electronic sensor(s), any type A

L5858 Addition to lower extremity prosthesis, endoskeletal knee shin system, microprocessor control feature, stance phase only, includes electronic sensor(s), any type A

L5910 Addition, endoskeletal system, below knee, alignable system A

L5920 Addition, endoskeletal system, above knee or hip disarticulation, alignable system A

L5925 Addition, endoskeletal system, above knee, knee disarticulation or hip disarticulation, manual lock A

L5930 Addition, endoskeletal system, high activity knee control frame A

L5940 Addition, endoskeletal system, below knee, ultra-light material (titanium, carbon fiber or equal) A

L5950 Addition, endoskeletal system, above knee, ultra-light material (titanium, carbon fiber or equal) A

L5960 Addition, endoskeletal system, hip disarticulation, ultra-light material (titanium, carbon fiber or equal) A

● L5961 Addition, endoskeletal system, polycentric hip joint, pneumatic or hydraulic control, rotation control, with or without flexion and/or extension control A
This code is effective January 1, 2011

L5962 Addition, endoskeletal system, below knee, flexible protective outer surface covering system A

L5964 Addition, endoskeletal system, above knee, flexible protective outer surface covering system A

L5966 Addition, endoskeletal system, hip disarticulation, flexible protective outer surface covering system A

L5968 Addition to lower limb prosthesis, multiaxial ankle with swing phase active dorsiflexion feature A

L5970 All lower extremity prostheses, foot, external keel, SACH foot A

L5971 All lower extremity prosthesis, solid ankle cushion heel (SACH) foot, replacement only A

L5972 All lower extremity prostheses, flexible keel foot (safe, sten, Bock dynamic or equal) A

L5974 All lower extremity prostheses, foot, single axis ankle/
foot A

L5973 Endoskeletal ankle foot system, microprocessor controlled feature, dorsiflexion and/or plantar flexion control, includes power source A

L5975 All lower extremity prosthesis, combination single axis ankle and flexible keel foot A

L5976 All lower extremity prostheses, energy storing foot (Seattle Carbon Copy II or equal) A

L5978 All lower extremity prostheses, foot, multi-axial ankle/ foot A

L5979 All lower extremity prosthesis, multi-axial ankle, dynamic response foot, one piece system A

L5980 All lower extremity prostheses, flex foot system A

L5981 All lower extremity prostheses, flex-walk system or equal A

L5982 All exoskeletal lower extremity prostheses, axial rotation unit

L5984 All endoskeletal lower extremity prosthesis, axial rotation unit, with or without adjustability

L5985 All endoskeletal lower extremity prostheses, dynamic prosthetic pylon

L5986 All lower extremity prostheses, multi-axial rotation unit ("MCP" or equal)

L5987 All lower extremity prosthesis, shank foot system with vertical loading pylon

L5988 Addition to lower limb prosthesis, vertical shock reducing pylon feature

L5990 Addition to lower extremity prosthesis, user adjustable heel height

L5999 Lower extremity prosthesis, not otherwise specified

Upper Limb

Partial Hand

L6000 Partial hand, Robin-Aids, thumb remaining (or equal)

L6010 Partial hand, Robin-Aids, little and/or ring finger remaining (or equal)

L6020 Partial hand, Robin-Aids, no finger remaining (or equal)

L6025 Transcarpal/metacarpal or partial hand disarticulation prosthesis, external power, self-suspended, inner socket with removable forearm section, electrodes and cables, two batteries, charger, myoelectric control of terminal device

Wrist Disarticulation

L6050 Wrist disarticulation, molded socket, flexible elbow hinges, triceps pad

L6055 Wrist disarticulation, molded socket with expandable interface, flexible elbow hinges, triceps pad

Below Elbow

L6100 Below elbow, molded socket, flexible elbow hinge, triceps pad

L6110 Below elbow, molded socket, (Muenster or Northwestern suspension types)

L6120 Below elbow, molded double wall split socket, step-up hinges, half cuff

L6130 Below elbow, molded double wall split socket, stump activated locking hinge, half cuff

Elbow Disarticulation

L6200 Elbow disarticulation, molded socket, outside locking hinge, forearm

L6205 Elbow disarticulation, molded socket with expandable interface, outside locking hinges, forearm

Above Elbow

L6250 Above elbow, molded double wall socket, internal locking elbow, forearm

Shoulder Disarticulation

L6300 Shoulder disarticulation, molded socket, shoulder bulkhead, humeral section, internal locking elbow, forearm

L6310 Shoulder disarticulation, passive restoration (complete prosthesis)

L6320 Shoulder disarticulation, passive restoration (shoulder cap only)

Interscapular Thoracic

L6350 Interscapular thoracic, molded socket, shoulder bulkhead, humeral section, internal locking elbow, forearm

L6360 Interscapular thoracic, passive restoration (complete prosthesis)

L6370 Interscapular thoracic, passive restoration (shoulder cap only)

Immediate and Early Post Surgical Procedures

L6380 Immediate post surgical or early fitting, application of initial rigid dressing, including fitting alignment and suspension of components, and one cast change, wrist disarticulation or below elbow

L6382 Immediate post surgical or early fitting, application of initial rigid dressing including fitting alignment and suspension of components, and one cast change, elbow disarticulation or above elbow

L6384 Immediate post surgical or early fitting, application of initial rigid dressing including fitting alignment and suspension of components, and one cast change, shoulder disarticulation or interscapular thoracic

L6386 Immediate post surgical or early fitting, each additional cast change and realignment

L6388 Immediate post surgical or early fitting, application of rigid dressing only

Upper Limb – Endoskeletal

L6400 Below elbow, molded socket, endoskeletal system, including soft prosthetic tissue shaping

L6450 Elbow disarticulation, molded socket, endoskeletal system, including soft prosthetic tissue shaping

L6500 Above elbow, molded socket, endoskeletal system, including soft prosthetic tissue shaping

L6550 houlder disarticulation, molded socket, endoskeletal system, including soft prosthetic tissue shaping

L6570 Interscapular thoracic, molded socket, endoskeletal system, including soft prosthetic tissue shaping

Preparatory Prosthesis

L6580 Preparatory, wrist disarticulation or below elbow, single wall plastic socket, friction wrist, flexible elbow hinges, figure of eight harness, humeral cuff, Bowden cable control, USMC or equal pylon, no cover, molded to patient model

L6582 Preparatory, wrist disarticulation or below elbow, single wall socket, friction wrist, flexible elbow hinges, figure of eight harness, humeral cuff, Bowden cable control, USMC or equal pylon, no cover, direct formed

L6584 Preparatory, elbow disarticulation or above elbow, single wall plastic socket, friction wrist, locking elbow, figure of eight harness, fair lead cable control, USMC or equal pylon, no cover, molded to patient model

L6586 Preparatory, elbow disarticulation or above elbow, single wall socket, friction wrist, locking elbow, figure of eight harness, fair lead cable control, USMC or equal pylon, no cover, direct formed

L6588 Preparatory, shoulder disarticulation or interscapular thoracic, single wall plastic socket, shoulder joint, locking elbow, friction wrist, chest strap, fair lead cable control, USMC or equal pylon, no cover, molded to patient model

L6590 Preparatory, shoulder disarticulation or interscapular thoracic, single wall socket, shoulder joint, locking elbow, friction wrist, chest strap, fair lead cable control, USMC or equal pylon, no cover, direct formed A

Additions – Upper Limb

L6600 Upper extremity additions, polycentric hinge, pair A

L6605 Upper extremity additions, single pivot hinge, pair A

L6610 Upper extremity additions, flexible metal hinge, pair A

L6611 Addition to upper extremity prosthesis, external powered, additional switch, any type A

L6615 Upper extremity addition, disconnect locking wrist unit A

L6616 Upper extremity addition, additional disconnect insert for locking wrist unit, each A

L6620 Upper extremity addition, flexion/extension wrist unit, with or without friction A

L6621 Upper extremity prosthesis addition, flexion/extension wrist with or without friction, for use with external powered terminal device A

L6623 Upper extremity addition, spring assisted rotational wrist unit with latch release A

L6624 Upper extremity addition, flexion/extension and rotation wrist unit A

L6625 Upper extremity addition, rotation wrist unit with cable lock A

L6628 Upper extremity addition, quick disconnect hook adapter, Otto Bock or equal A

L6629 Upper extremity addition, quick disconnect lamination collar with coupling piece, Otto Bock or equal A

L6630 Upper extremity addition, stainless steel, any wrist A

L6632 Upper extremity addition, latex suspension sleeve, each A

L6635 Upper extremity addition, lift assist for elbow A

L6637 Upper extremity addition, nudge control elbow lock A

L6638 Upper extremity addition to prosthesis, electric locking feature, only for use with manually powered elbow A

L6640 Upper extremity additions, shoulder abduction joint, pair A

L6641 Upper extremity addition, excursion amplifier, pulley type A

L6642 Upper extremity addition, excursion amplifier, lever type A

L6645 Upper extremity addition, shoulder flexion-abduction joint, each A

L6646 Upper extremity addition, shoulder joint, multipositional locking, flexion, adjustable abduction friction control, for use with body powered or external powered system A

L6647 Upper extremity addition, shoulder lock mechanism, body powered actuator A

L6648 Upper extremity addition, shoulder lock mechanism, external powered actuator A

L6650 Upper extremity addition, shoulder universal joint, each A

L6655 Upper extremity addition, standard control cable, extra A

L6660 Upper extremity addition, heavy duty control cable A

L6665 Upper extremity addition, Teflon, or equal, cable lining A

L6670 Upper extremity addition, hook to hand, cable adapter A

L6672 Upper extremity addition, harness, chest or shoulder, saddle type A

L6675 Upper extremity addition, harness, (e.g. figure of eight type), single cable design A

L6676 Upper extremity addition, harness, (e.g. figure of eight type), dual cable design A

L6677 Upper extremity addition, harness, triple control, simultaneous operation of terminal device and elbow A

L6680 Upper extremity addition, test socket, wrist disarticulation or below elbow A

L6682 Upper extremity addition, test socket, elbow disarticulation or above elbow A

L6684 Upper extremity addition, test socket, shoulder disarticulation or interscapular thoracic A

L6686 Upper extremity addition, suction socket A

L6687 Upper extremity addition, frame type socket, below elbow or wrist disarticulation A

L6688 Upper extremity addition, frame type socket, above elbow or elbow disarticulation A

L6689 Upper extremity addition, frame type socket, shoulder disarticulation A

L6690 Upper extremity addition, frame type socket, interscapular-thoracic A

L6691 Upper extremity addition, removable insert, each A

L6692 Upper extremity addition, silicone gel insert or equal, each A

L6693 Upper extremity addition, locking elbow, forearm counterbalance A

L6694 Addition to upper extremity prosthesis, below elbow/above elbow, custom fabricated from existing mold or prefabricated, socket insert, silicone gel, elastomeric or equal, for use with locking mechanism A

L6695 Addition to upper extremity prosthesis, below elbow/above elbow, custom fabricated from existing mold or prefabricated, socket insert, silicone gel, elastomeric or equal, not for use with locking mechanism A

L6696 Addition to upper extremity prosthesis, below elbow/above elbow, custom fabricated socket insert for congenital or atypical traumatic amputee, silicone gel, elastomeric or equal, for use with or without locking mechanism, initial only (for other than initial, use code L6694 or L6695) A

L6697 Addition to upper extremity prosthesis, below elbow/above elbow, custom fabricated socket insert for other than congenital or atypical traumatic amputee, silicone gel, elastomeric or equal, for use with or without locking mechanism, initial only (for other than initial, use code L6694 or L6695) A

L6698 Addition to upper extremity prosthesis, below elbow/above elbow, lock mechanism, excludes socket insert A

Terminal Devices

Hooks and Hands

L6703 Terminal device, passive hand/mitt, any material, any size A

L6704 Terminal device, sport/recreational/work attachment, any material, any size A

L6706 Terminal device, hook, mechanical, voluntary opening, any material, any size, lined or unlined A

L6707 Terminal device, hook, mechanical, voluntary closing, any material, any size, lined or unlined A

L6708 Terminal device, hand, mechanical, voluntary opening, any material, any size A

L6709 Terminal device, hand, mechanical, voluntary closing, any material, any size A

L6711 Terminal device, hook, mechanical, voluntary opening, any material, any size, lined or unlined, pediatric A

L6712 Terminal device, hook, mechanical, voluntary closing, any material, any size, lined or unlined, pediatric A

L6713 Terminal device, hand, mechanical, voluntary opening, any material, any size, pediatric A

L6714 Terminal device, hand, mechanical, voluntary closing, any material, any size, pediatric A

L6721 Terminal device, hook or hand, heavy duty, mechanical, voluntary opening, any material, any size, lined or unlined A

L6722 Terminal device, hook or hand, heavy duty, mechanical, voluntary closing, any material, any size, lined or unlined

L6805 Addition to terminal device, modifier wrist unit A

Pub 100-02, 15, 130

L6810 Addition to terminal device, precision pinch device A

Pub 100-02, 15, 130

L6881 Automatic grasp feature, addition to upper limb electric prosthetic terminal device A

L6882 Microprocessor control feature, addition to upper limb prosthetic terminal device A

Pub 100-02, 15, 130

Replacement Sockets

L6883 Replacement socket, below elbow/wrist disarticulation, molded to patient model, for use with or without external power A

L6884 Replacement socket, above elbow/elbow disarticulation, molded to patient model, for use with or without external power A

L6885 Replacement socket, shoulder disarticulation/ interscapular thoracic, molded to patient model, for use with or without external power A

Gloves for Above Hands

L6890 Addition to upper extremity prosthesis, glove for terminal device, any material, prefabricated, includes fitting and adjustment A

L6895 Addition to upper extremity prosthesis, glove for terminal device, any material, custom fabricated A

Hand Restoration

L6900 Hand restoration (casts, shading and measurements included), partial hand, with glove, thumb or one finger remaining A

L6905 Hand restoration (casts, shading and measurements included), partial hand, with glove, multiple fingers remaining A

L6910 Hand restoration (casts, shading and measurements included), partial hand, with glove, no fingers remaining A

L6915 Hand restoration (shading, and measurements included), replacement glove for above A

External Power – Base Devices

L6920 Wrist disarticulation, external power, self-suspended inner socket, removable forearm shell, Otto Bock or equal, switch, cables, two batteries and one charger, switch control of terminal device A

L6925 Wrist disarticulation, external power, self-suspended inner socket, removable forearm shell, Otto Bock or equal electrodes, cables, two batteries and one charger, myoelectronic control of terminal device A

L6930 Below elbow, external power, self-suspended inner socket, removable forearm shell, Otto Bock or equal switch, cables, two batteries and one charger, switch control of terminal device A

L6935 Below elbow, external power, self-suspended inner socket, removable forearm shell, Otto Bock or equal electrodes, cables, two batteries and one charger, myoelectronic control of terminal device A

L6940 Elbow disarticulation, external power, molded inner socket, removable humeral shell, outside locking hinges, forearm, Otto Bock or equal switch, cables, two batteries and one charger, switch control of terminal device A

L6945 Elbow disarticulation, external power, molded inner socket, removable humeral shell, outside locking hinges, forearm, Otto Bock or equal electrodes, cables, two batteries and one charger, myoelectronic control of terminal device A

L6950 Above elbow, external power, molded inner socket, removable humeral shell, internal locking elbow, forearm, Otto Bock or equal switch, cables, two batteries and one charger, switch control of terminal device A

L6955 Above elbow, external power, molded inner socket, removable humeral shell, internal locking elbow, forearm, Otto Bock or equal electrodes, cables, two batteries and one charger, myoelectronic control of terminal device A

L6960 Shoulder disarticulation, external power, molded inner socket, removable shoulder shell, shoulder bulkhead, humeral section, mechanical elbow, forearm, Otto Bock or equal switch, cables, two batteries and one charger, switch control of terminal device A

L6965 Shoulder disarticulation, external power, molded inner socket, removable shoulder shell, shoulder bulkhead, humeral section, mechanical elbow, forearm, Otto Bock or equal electrodes, cables, two batteries and one charger, myoelectronic control of terminal device A

L6970 Interscapular-thoracic, external power, molded inner socket, removable shoulder shell, shoulder bulkhead, humeral section, mechanical elbow, forearm, Otto Bock or equal switch, cables, two batteries and one charger, switch control of terminal device A

L6975 Interscapular-thoracic, external power, molded inner socket, removable shoulder shell, shoulder bulkhead, humeral section, mechanical elbow, forearm, Otto Bock or equal electrodes, cables, two batteries and one charger, myoelectronic control of terminal device A

External Power – Terminal Devices

L7007 Electric hand, switch or myoelectric controlled, adult A

L7008 Electric hand, switch or myoelectric, controlled, pediatric A

L7009 Electric hook, switch or myoelectric controlled, adult A

L7040 Prehensile actuator, switch controlled A

L7045 Electric hook, switch or myoelectric controlled, pediatric A

External Power – Elbow

L7170 Electronic elbow, Hosmer or equal, switch controlled A

L7180 Electronic elbow, microprocessor sequential control of elbow and terminal device A

L7181 Electronic elbow, microprocessor simultaneous control of elbow and terminal device A

L7185 Electronic elbow, adolescent, Variety Village or equal, switch controlled A

L7186 Electronic elbow, child, Variety Village or equal, switch controlled

L7190 Electronic elbow, adolescent, Variety Village or equal, myoelectronically controlled

L7191 Electronic elbow, child, Variety Village or equal, myoelectronically controlled

External Power – Control Modules

L7260 Electronic wrist rotator, Otto Bock or equal

L7261 Electronic wrist rotator, for Utah arm

L7266 Servo control, steeper or equal

L7272 Analogue control, unb or equal

L7274 Proportional control, 6-12 volt, Liberty, Utah or equal

External Power – Battery Components

L7360 Six volt battery, each

L7362 Battery charger, six volt, each

L7364 Twelve volt battery, each

L7366 Battery charger, twelve volt, each

L7367 Lithium ion battery, replacement

L7368 Lithium ion battery charger

Upper Extremity Prosthesis

L7400 Addition to upper extremity prosthesis, below elbow/wrist disarticulation, ultralight material (titanium, carbon fiber or equal)

L7401 Addition to upper extremity prosthesis, above elbow disarticulation, ultralight material (titanium, carbon fiber or equal)

L7402 Addition to upper extremity prosthesis, shoulder disarticulation/interscapular thoracic, ultralight material (titanium, carbon fiber or equal)

L7403 Addition to upper extremity prosthesis, below elbow/wrist disarticulation, acrylic material

L7404 Addition to upper extremity prosthesis, above elbow disarticulation, acrylic material

L7405 Addition to upper extremity prosthesis, shoulder disarticulation/interscapular thoracic, acrylic material

L7499 Upper extremity prosthesis, not otherwise specified

Repairs, Supplies

L7500 Repair of prosthetic device, hourly rate (excludes V5335 repair of oral or laryngeal prosthesis or artificial larynx)
Pub 100-02, 15, 110.2; 100-4, 32, 100-100.4; 100-2, 15, 130

L7510 Repair of prosthetic device, repair or replace minor parts
Pub 100-02, 15, 110.2; 100-4, 32, 100-100.4; 100-2, 15, 130

L7520 Repair prosthetic device, labor component, per 15 minutes

L7600 Prosthetic donning sleeve, any material, each
Medicare Statute 1862(1)(a)

General

L7900 Male vacuum erection system ♂

General – Breast Prostheses

L8000 Breast prosthesis, mastectomy bra ♀
Pub 100-02, 15, 120

Mastectomy bra

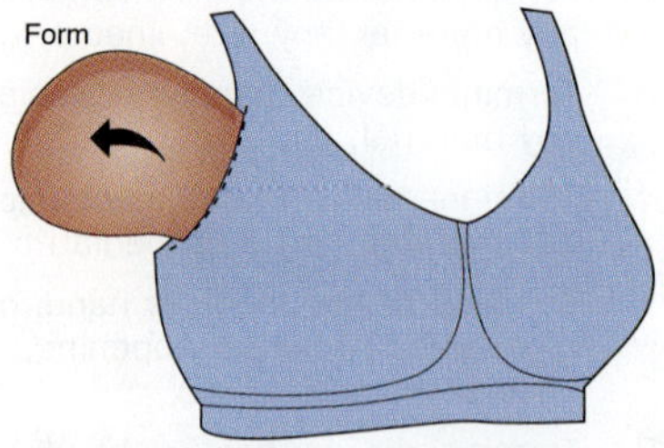

L8001 Breast prosthesis, mastectomy bra, with integrated breast prosthesis form, unilateral ♀
Pub 100-02, 15, 120

L8002 Breast prosthesis, mastectomy bra, with integrated breast prosthesis form, bilateral ♀
Pub 100-02, 15, 120

L8010 Breast prosthesis, mastectomy sleeve ♀
Pub 100-02, 15, 120

L8015 External breast prosthesis garment, with mastectomy form, post mastectomy ♀
Pub 100-02, 15, 120

L8020 Breast prosthesis, mastectomy form ♀
Pub 100-02, 15, 120

L8030 Breast prosthesis, silicone or equal, without integral adhesive ♀
Pub 100-02, 15, 120

L8031 Breast prosthesis, silicone or equal, with integral adhesive

L8032 Nipple prosthesis, reusable, any type, each

L8035 Custom breast prosthesis, post mastectomy, molded to patient model ♀
Pub 100-02, 15, 120

L8039 Breast prosthesis, not otherwise specified ♀

General – Nasal/Face Prostheses

L8040 Nasal prosthesis, provided by a non-physician

L8041 Midfacial prosthesis, provided by a non-physician

L8042 Orbital prosthesis, provided by a non-physician

L8043 Upper facial prosthesis, provided by a non-physician

L8044 Hemi-facial prosthesis, provided by a non-physician

L8045 Auricular prosthesis, provided by a non-physician

L8046 Partial facial prosthesis, provided by a non-physician

L8047 Nasal septal prosthesis, provided by a non-physician

L8048 Unspecified maxillofacial prosthesis, by report, provided by a non-physician

L8049 Repair or modification of maxillofacial prosthesis, labor component, 15 minute increments, provided by a non-physician

General – Trusses

L8300 Truss, single with standard pad
NCD 280.11, 280.12; Pub 100-02, 15, 130

L8310 Truss, double with standard pads
NCD 280.11, 280.12; Pub 100-02, 15, 130

L8320 Truss, addition to standard pad, water pad
NCD 280.11, 280.12; Pub 100-02, 15, 130

ⓘ L8330 Truss, addition to standard pad, scrotal pad A
NCD 280.11, 280.12; Pub 100-02, 15, 130

Prosthetic Socks

ⓘ L8400 Prosthetic sheath, below knee, each A
Pub 100-02, 15, 130

ⓘ L8410 Prosthetic sheath, above knee, each A
Pub 100-02, 15, 130

ⓘ L8415 Prosthetic sheath, upper limb, each A
Pub 100-02, 15, 130

L8417 Prosthetic sheath/sock, including a gel cushion layer, below knee or above knee, each A

ⓘ L8420 Prosthetic sock, multiple ply, below knee, each A
Pub 100-02, 15, 130

ⓘ L8430 Prosthetic sock, multiple ply, above knee, each A
Pub 100-02, 15, 130

ⓘ L8435 Prosthetic sock, multiple ply, upper limb, each A
Pub 100-02, 15, 130

ⓘ L8440 Prosthetic shrinker, below knee, each A
Pub 100-02, 15, 130

ⓘ L8460 Prosthetic shrinker, above knee, each A
Pub 100-02, 15, 130

ⓘ L8465 Prosthetic shrinker, upper limb, each A
Pub 100-02, 15, 130

ⓘ L8470 Prosthetic sock, single ply, fitting, below knee, each A
Pub 100-02, 15, 130

ⓘ L8480 Prosthetic sock, single ply, fitting, above knee, each A
Pub 100-02, 15, 130

ⓘ L8485 Prosthetic sock, single ply, fitting, upper limb, each A
Pub 100-02, 15, 130

L8499 Unlisted procedure for miscellaneous prosthetic services A

Prosthetic Implants

Integumentary System

ⓘ L8500 Artificial larynx, any type A
NCD 50.2; Pub 100-02, 15, 120

ⓘ L8501 Tracheostomy speaking valve A
NCD 20.9

L8505 Artificial larynx replacement battery/ accessory, any type A

L8507 Tracheo-esophageal voice prosthesis, patient inserted, any type, each A

L8509 Tracheo-esophageal voice prosthesis, inserted by a licensed health care provider, any type A

ⓘ L8510 Voice amplifier A
NCD 50.2

L8511 Insert for indwelling tracheoesophageal prosthesis, with or without valve, replacement only, each A

L8512 Gelatin capsules or equivalent, for use with tracheoesophageal voice prosthesis, replacement only, per 10 A

L8513 Cleaning device used with tracheoesophageal voice prosthesis, pipet, brush, or equal, replacement only, each A

L8514 Tracheoesophageal puncture dilator, replacement only, each A

L8515 Gelatin capsule, application device for use with tracheoesophageal voice prosthesis, each A

ⓘ L8600 Implantable breast prosthesis, silicone or equal N N1
NCD 140.2; Pub 100-02, 15, 120

ⓘ L8603 Injectable bulking agent, collagen implant, urinary tract, 2.5 ml syringe, includes shipping and necessary supplies N N1
NCD 230.10

L8604 Injectable bulking agent, dextranomer/hyaluronic acid copolymer implant, urinary tract, 1 ml, includes shipping and necessary supplies N N1

ⓘ L8606 Injectable bulking agent, synthetic implant, urinary tract, 1 ml syringe, includes shipping and necessary supplies N N1
NCD 230.10

Head: Skull, Facial Bones, and Temporomandibular Joint

L8609 Artificial cornea N N1

ⓘ L8610 Ocular implant N N1
Pub 100-02, 15, 120

ⓘ L8612 Aqueous shunt N N1
Pub 100-02, 15, 120

ⓘ L8613 Ossicula implant N N1
Pub 100-02, 15, 120

ⓘ L8614 Cochlear device, includes all internal and external components N N1
NCD 50.3; Pub 100-02, 15, 120; 100-4, 32, 100-100.4

Cochlear device

A device to aid hearing is inserted into the cochlea of the inner ear

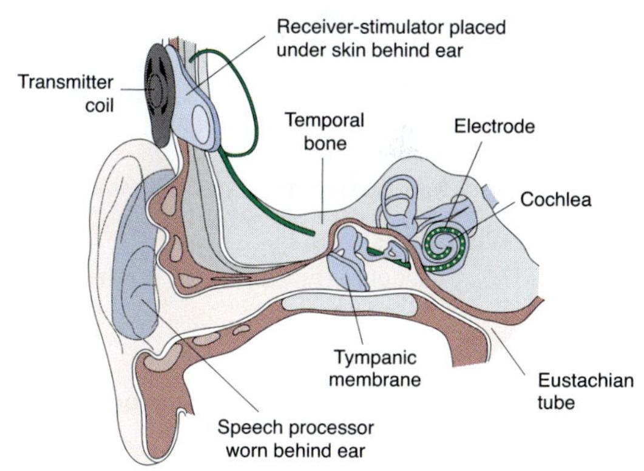

ⓘ L8615 Headset/headpiece for use with cochlear implant device, replacement A
NCD 50.3

ⓘ L8616 Microphone for use with cochlear implant device, replacement A
NCD 50.3

ⓘ L8617 Transmitting coil for use with cochlear implant device, replacement A
NCD 50.3

ⓘ L8618 Transmitter cable for use with cochlear implant device, replacement A
NCD 50.3

ⓘ L8619 Cochlear implant, external speech processor and controller, integrated system, replacementt A
NCD 50.3; Pub 100-02, 15, 120; 100-4, 32, 100-100.4

L8330 – L8619

L8621 Zinc air battery for use with cochlear implant device, replacement, each A

L8622 Alkaline battery for use with cochlear implant device, any size, replacement, each A

L8623 Lithium ion battery for use with cochlear implant device speech processor, other than ear level, replacement, each A

L8624 Lithium ion battery for use with cochlear implant device speech processor, ear level, replacement, each A

L8627 Cochlear implant, external speech processor, component, replacement A

L8628 Cochlear implant, external controller component, replacement A

L8629 Transmitting coil and cable, integrated, for use with cochlear implant device, replacement A

Upper Extremity

L8630 Metacarpophalangeal joint implant N N1

Pub 100-02, 15, 120

L8631 Metacarpal phalangeal joint replacement, two or more pieces, metal (e.g., stainless steel or cobalt chrome), ceramic-like material (e.g., pyrocarbon), for surgical implantation (all sizes, includes entire system) N N1

Pub 100-02, 15, 120

Lower Extremity – Joint: Knee, Ankle, Toe

L8641 Metatarsal joint implant N N1

Pub 100-02, 15, 120

L8642 Hallux implant N N1

Pub 100-02, 15, 120

Miscellaneous Muscular – Skeletal

L8658 Interphalangeal joint spacer, silicone or equal, each N N1

Pub 100-02, 15, 120

L8659 Interphalangeal finger joint replacement, 2 or more pieces, metal (e.g., stainless steel or cobalt chrome), ceramic-like material (e.g., pyrocarbon) for surgical implantation, any size N N1

Pub 100-02, 15, 120

Cardiovascular System

L8670 Vascular graft material, synthetic, implant N N1

Pub 100-02, 15, 120

Neurostimulator

L8680 Implantable neurostimulator electrode (with any number of contact points), each B

NCD 160.7

L8681 Patient programmer (external) for use with implantable programmable neurostimulator pulse generator, replacement only A

NCD 160.7

L8682 Implantable neurostimulator radiofrequency receiver N N1

NCD 160.7

L8683 Radiofrequency transmitter (external) for use with implantable neurostimulator radiofrequency receiver A

NCD 160.7

L8684 Radiofrequency transmitter (external) for use with implantable sacral root neurostimulator receiver for bowel and bladder management, replacement A

NCD 160.7

L8685 Implantable neurostimulator pulse generator, single array, rechargeable, includes extension N

NCD 160.7

L8686 Implantable neurostimulator pulse generator, single array, non-rechargeable, includes extension N

NCD 160.7

L8687 Implantable neurostimulator pulse generator, dual array, rechargeable, includes extension N

NCD 160.7

L8688 Implantable neurostimulator pulse generator, dual array, non-rechargeable, includes extension N

NCD 160.7

L8689 External recharging system for battery (internal) for use with implantable neurostimulator, replacement only A

NCD 160.7

L8690 Auditory osseointegrated device, includes all internal and external components N J7

L8691 Auditory osseointegrated device, external sound processor, replacement A

● L8693 Auditory osseointegrated device abutment, any length, replacement only A

This code is effective January 1, 2011

L8692 Auditory osseointegrated device, external sound processor, used without attachment E

L8695 External recharging system for battery (external) for use with implantable neurostimulator, replacement only A

NCD 160.7

General

L8699 Prosthetic implant, not otherwise specified N N1

L9900 Orthotic and prosthetic supply, accessory, and/or service component of another HCPCS L code N

Medical Services M0064–M0301

Note: Periodic, routine or annual type examinations are preventive type services. The following procedure codes should be used when services rendered fall into this category.

CMS Designation of Office Services

ⓘ M0064 Brief office visit for the sole purpose of monitoring or changing drug prescriptions used in the treatment of mental psychoneurotic and personality disorders Q3

CMS Designation of Other Medical Services

⊘ M0075 Cellular therapy E
NCD 30.8

⊘ M0076 Prolotherapy E
NCD 150.7

⊘ M0100 Intragastric hypothermia using gastric freezing E
NCD 100.6

CMS Designation of Cardiovascular Services

⊘ M0300 IV chelation therapy (chemical endarterectomy) E
NCD 20.21

⊘ M0301 Fabric wrapping of abdominal aneurysm E
NCD 20.23

Laboratory and Pathology P2028–P9615

Chemistry and Toxicology Tests

ⓘ P2028 Cephalin floculation, blood A
NCD 300.1

ⓘ P2029 Congo red, blood A
NCD 300.1

⊘ P2031 Hair analysis (excluding arsenic) A
NCD 190.6

ⓘ P2033 Thymol turbidity, blood A
NCD 300.1

ⓘ P2038 Mucoprotein, blood (seromucoid) (medical necessity procedure) A
NCD 300.1

Pathology Screening Tests

ⓘ P3000 Screening Papanicolaou smear, cervical or vaginal, up to three smears, by technician under physician supervision ♀ A
NCD 190.2

ⓘ P3001 Screening Papanicolaou smear, cervical or vaginal, up to three smears, requiring interpretation by physician ♀ B
NCD 190.2; Pub 100-04, 18, 30-30.9

Microbiology Tests

⊘ P7001 Culture, bacterial, urine; quantitative, sensitivity study E

Miscellaneous Pathology and Lab Tests

ⓘ P9010 Blood (whole), for transfusion, per unit R
Pub 100-1, 3, 20-20.4A

ⓘ P9011 Blood, split unit R
Pub 100-1, 3, 20-20.4

ⓘ P9012 Cryoprecipitate, each unit R
Pub 100-1, 3, 20-20.4

ⓘ P9016 Red blood cells, leukocytes reduced, each unit R
Pub 100-1, 3, 20-20.4

ⓘ P9017 Fresh frozen plasma (single donor), frozen within 8 hours of collection, each unit R
Pub 100-1, 3, 20-20.4

ⓘ P9019 Platelets, each unit R
Pub 100-1, 3, 20-20.4

ⓘ P9020 Platelet rich plasma, each unit R
Pub 100-1, 3, 20-20.4

ⓘ P9021 Red blood cells, each unit R
Pub 100-1, 3, 20-20.4

ⓘ P9022 Red blood cells, washed, each unit R
Pub 100-1, 3, 20-20.4

ⓘ P9023 Plasma, pooled multiple donor, solvent/detergent treated, frozen, each unit R
Pub 100-1, 3, 20-20.4

ⓘ P9031 Platelets, leukocytes reduced, each unit R
Pub 100-1, 3, 20-20.4

ⓘ P9032 Platelets, irradiated, each unit R
Pub 100-1, 3, 20-20.4

ⓘ P9033 Platelets, leukocytes reduced, irradiated, each unit R
Pub 100-1, 3, 20-20.4

ⓘ P9034 Platelets, pheresis, each unit R
Pub 100-1, 3, 20-20.4

ⓘ P9035 Platelets, pheresis, leukocytes reduced, each unit R
Pub 100-1, 3, 20-20.4

ⓘ P9036 Platelets, pheresis, irradiated, each unit R
Pub 100-1, 3, 20-20.4

ⓘ P9037 Platelets, pheresis, leukocytes reduced, irradiated, each unit R
Pub 100-1, 3, 20-20.4

ⓘ P9038 Red blood cells, irradiated, each unit R
Pub 100-1, 3, 20-20.4

ⓘ P9039 Red blood cells, deglycerolized, each unit R
Pub 100-1, 3, 20-20.4

ⓘ P9040 Red blood cells, leukocytes reduced, irradiated, each unit R
Pub 100-1, 3, 20-20.4

P9041 Infusion, albumin (human), 5%, 50 ml K K2

ⓘ P9043 Infusion, plasma protein fraction (human), 5%, 50 ml R
Pub 100-1, 3, 20-20.4

ⓘ P9044 Plasma, cryoprecipitate reduced, each unit R
Pub 100-1, 3, 20-20.4

P9045 Infusion, albumin (human), 5%, 250 ml K K2

P9046 Infusion, albumin (human), 25%, 20 ml K K2

P9047 Infusion, albumin (human), 25%, 50 ml K K2

P9048 Infusion, plasma protein fraction (human), 5%, 250 ml R

P9050 Granulocytes, pheresis, each unit R

ⓘ P9051 Whole blood or red blood cells, leukocytes reduced, CMV-negative, each unit R
Medicare Statute 1833(t)

ⓘ P9052 Platelets, HLA-matched leukocytes reduced, apheresis/pheresis, each unit R
Medicare Statute 1833(t)

ⓘ P9053 Platelets, pheresis, leukocytes reduced, CMV-negative, irradiated, each unit R
Medicare Statute 1833(t)

ⓘ P9054 Whole blood or red blood cells, leukocytes reduced, frozen, deglycerol, washed, each unit R
Medicare Statute 1833(t)

ⓘ P9055 Platelets, leukocytes reduced, CMV-negative, apheresis/pheresis, each unit R
Medicare Statute 1833(t)

ⓘ P9056 Whole blood, leukocytes reduced, irradiated, each unit R
Medicare Statute 1833(t)

ⓘ P9057 Red blood cells, frozen/deglycerolized/washed, leukocytes reduced, irradiated, each unit R
Medicare Statute 1833(t)

ⓘ P9058 Red blood cells, leukocytes reduced, CMV-negative, irradiated, each unit R
Medicare Statute 1833(t)

ⓘ P9059 Fresh frozen plasma between 8-24 hours of collection, each unit R
Medicare Statute 1833(t)

ⓘ P9060 Fresh frozen plasma, donor retested, each unit R
Medicare Statute 1833(t)

ⓘ P9603 Travel allowance one way in connection with medically necessary laboratory specimen collection drawn from home bound or nursing home bound patient; prorated miles actually travelled A
Pub 100-04, 16, 60-60.1.1, 60.2

ⓘ P9604 Travel allowance one way in connection with medically necessary laboratory specimen collection drawn from home bound or nursing home bound patient; prorated trip charge period A
Pub 100-04, 16, 60-60.1.1, 60.2

ⓘ P9612 Catheterization for collection of specimen, single patient, all places of service A
Pub 100-04, 16, 60-60.1.1, 60.2

ⓘ P9615 Catheterization for collection of specimen(s) (multiple patients) N
Pub 100-04, 16, 60-60.1.1, 60.2

Temporary Codes Q0035–Q9967

This section reflects the national codes designated by CMS on a temporary basis.

Q0035 Cardiokymography X
NCD 20.24

Q0081 Infusion therapy, using other than chemotherapeutic drugs, per visit B
NCD 40.2
AHA: 2Q 2004, 11; 1Q 2004, 5, 8; 2Q 2002, 10

Infusion therapy

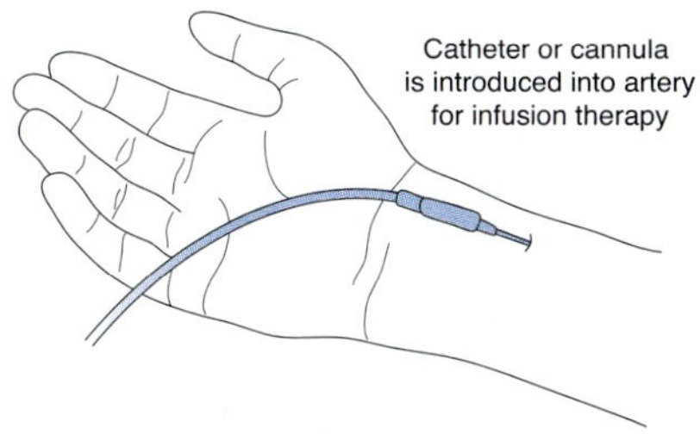

Q0083 Chemotherapy administration by other than infusion technique only (e.g. subcutaneous, intramuscular, push) per visit B
Pub 100-02 , 15, 50.4.5-50.4.5.1

Q0084 Chemotherapy administration by infusion technique only, per visit B
NCD 40.2; Pub 100-02 , 15, 50.4.5-50.4.5.1
AHA: 2Q 2004, 11

Q0085 Chemotherapy administration by both infusion technique and other technique(s) (e.g., subcutaneous, intramuscular, push), per visit B
Pub 100-02 , 15, 50.4.5-50.4.5.1

Q0091 Screening papanicolaou smear; obtaining, preparing and conveyance of cervical or vaginal smear to laboratory ♀ T
Pub 100-04, 18, 30-30.9
AHA: 4Q 2002, 8

Q0092 Set-up portable x-ray equipment N
Pub 100-02, 15, 80.4; 100-4, 13, 90.4

Q0111 Wet mounts, including preparations of vaginal, cervical or skin specimens A
Pub 100-04, 16, 70.6

Q0112 All potassium hydroxide (KOH) preparations A
Pub 100-04, 16, 70.6

Q0113 Pinworm examinations A
Pub 100-04, 16, 70.6

Q0114 Fern test A
Pub 100-04, 16, 70.6

Q0115 Post-coital direct, qualitative examinations of vaginal or cervical mucous ♀ A
Pub 100-04, 16, 70.6

Q0138 Injection, ferumoxytol, for treatment of iron deficiency anemia, 1 mg (non-ESRD use) G K2
Feraheme

Q0139 Injection, ferumoxytol, for treatment of iron deficiency anemia, 1 mg (for ESRD on dialysis) A
Feraheme

Q0144 Azithromycin dihydrate, oral, capsules/powder, 1 gram E
Zithromax

Q0163 Diphenhydramine hydrochloride, 50 mg, oral, FDA approved prescription anti-emetic, for use as a complete therapeutic substitute for an IV anti-emetic at time of chemotherapy treatment not to exceed a 48-hour dosage regimen N N1
Medicare Statute 1861(s)(2)(T)
Pub 100-04, 8, 120.1; 100-4, 17, 80.3.4

Q0164 Prochlorperazine maleate, 5 mg, oral, FDA approved prescription anti-emetic, for use as a complete therapeutic substitute for an IV anti-emetic at the time of chemotherapy treatment, not to exceed a 48-hour dosage regimen N N1
Compazine
Medicare Statute 1861(s)(2)(T)
Pub 100-04, 8, 120.1; 100-4, 17, 80.3.4

Q0165 Prochlorperazine maleate, 10 mg, oral, FDA approved prescription anti-emetic, for use as a complete therapeutic substitute for an IV anti-emetic at the time of chemotherapy treatment, not to exceed a 48-hour dosage regimen N N1
Compazine
Medicare Statute 1861(s)(2)(T)
Pub 100-04, 8, 120.1; 100-4, 17, 80.3.4

Q0166 Granisetron hydrochloride, 1 mg, oral, FDA approved prescription anti-emetic, for use as a complete therapeutic substitute for an IV anti-emetic at the time of chemotherapy treatment, not to exceed a 24-hour dosage regimen K N1
Kytril
Medicare Statute 1861(s)(2)(T)
Pub 100-04, 8, 120.1; 100-4, 17, 80.3.4

Q0167 Dronabinol, 2.5 mg, oral, FDA approved prescription anti-emetic, for use as a complete therapeutic substitute for an IV anti-emetic at the time of chemotherapy treatment, not to exceed a 48-hour dosage regimen N N1
Marinol
Medicare Statute 1861(s)(2)(T)
Pub 100-04, 8, 120.1; 100-4, 17, 80.3.4

Q0168 Dronabinol, 5 mg, oral, FDA approved prescription anti-emetic, for use as a complete therapeutic substitute for an IV anti-emetic at the time of chemotherapy treatment, not to exceed a 48-hour dosage regimen N N1
Marinol
Medicare Statute 1861(s)(2)(T)
Pub 100-04, 8, 120.1; 100-4, 17, 80.3.4

Q0169 Promethazine hydrochloride, 12.5 mg, oral, FDA approved prescription anti-emetic, for use as a complete therapeutic substitute for an IV anti-emetic at the time of chemotherapy treatment, not to exceed a 48-hour dosage regimen N N1
Anergan 50, Phenazine 25, Phenazine 50, Phenergan, Prorex-25, Prorex-50, Prothazine, V-Gan 25, V-Gan 50
Medicare Statute 1861(s)(2)(T)
Pub 100-04, 8, 120.1; 100-4, 17, 80.3.4

Q0170 Promethazine hydrochloride, 25 mg, oral, FDA approved prescription anti-emetic, for use as a complete therapeutic substitute for an IV anti-emetic at the time of chemotherapy treatment, not to exceed a 48-hour dosage regimen N
Anergan 50, Phenazine 25, Phenazine 50, Phenergan, Prorex-25, Prorex-50, Prothazine, V-Gan 25, V-Gan 50
Medicare Statute 1861(s)(2)(T)
Pub 100-04, 8, 120.1; 100-4, 17, 80.3.4

Ⓘ Q0171 Chlorpromazine hydrochloride, 10 mg, oral, FDA approved prescription anti-emetic, for use as a complete therapeutic substitute for an IV anti-emetic at the time of chemotherapy treatment, not to exceed a 48-hour dosage regimen N N1
Thorazine
Medicare Statute 1861(s)(2)(T)
Pub 100-04, 8, 120.1; 100-4, 17, 80.3.4

Ⓘ Q0172 Chlorpromazine hydrochloride, 25 mg, oral, FDA approved prescription anti-emetic, for use as a complete therapeutic substitute for an IV anti-emetic at the time of chemotherapy treatment, not to exceed a 48-hour dosage regimen N
Thorazine
Medicare Statute 1861(s)(2)(T)
Pub 100-04, 8, 120.1; 100-4, 17, 80.3.4

Ⓘ Q0173 Trimethobenzamide hydrochloride, 250 mg, oral, FDA approved prescription anti-emetic, for use as a complete therapeutic substitute for an IV anti-emetic at the time of chemotherapy treatment, not to exceed a 48-hour dosage regimen N N1
Tigan
Medicare Statute 1861(s)(2)(T)
Pub 100-04, 8, 120.1; 100-4, 17, 80.3.4

Ⓘ Q0174 Thiethylperazine maleate, 10 mg, oral, FDA approved prescription anti-emetic, for use as a complete therapeutic substitute for an IV anti-emetic at the time of chemotherapy treatment, not to exceed a 48-hour dosage regimen N
Torecan
Medicare Statute 1861(s)(2)(T)
Pub 100-04, 8, 120.1; 100-4, 17, 80.3.4

Ⓘ Q0175 Perphenazine, 4 mg, oral, FDA approved prescription anti-emetic, for use as a complete therapeutic substitute for an IV anti-emetic at the time of chemotherapy treatment, not to exceed a 48-hour dosage regimen N N1
Trilafon
Medicare Statute 1861(s)(2)(T)
Pub 100-04, 8, 120.1; 100-4, 17, 80.3.4

Ⓘ Q0176 Perphenazine, 8 mg, oral, FDA approved prescription anti-emetic, for use as a complete therapeutic substitute for an IV anti-emetic at the time of chemotherapy treatment, not to exceed a 48-hour dosage regimen N
Trilafon
Medicare Statute 1861(s)(2)(T)
Pub 100-04, 8, 120.1; 100-4, 17, 80.3.4

Ⓘ Q0177 Hydroxyzine pamoate, 25 mg, oral, FDA approved prescription anti-emetic, for use as a complete therapeutic substitute for an IV anti-emetic at the time of chemotherapy treatment, not to exceed a 48-hour dosage regimen N N1
Vistaril
Medicare Statute 1861(s)(2)(T)
Pub 100-04, 8, 120.1; 100-4, 17, 80.3.4

Ⓘ Q0178 Hydroxyzine pamoate, 50 mg, oral, FDA approved prescription anti-emetic, for use as a complete therapeutic substitute for an IV anti-emetic at the time of chemotherapy treatment, not to exceed a 48-hour dosage regimen N
Vistaril
Medicare Statute 1861(s)(2)(T)
Pub 100-04, 8, 120.1; 100-4, 17, 80.3.4

Ⓘ Q0179 Ondansetron hydrochloride 8 mg, oral, FDA approved prescription anti-emetic, for use as a complete therapeutic substitute for an IV anti-emetic at the time of chemotherapy treatment, not to exceed a 48-hour dosage regimen K K1
Zofran, Zofram ODT
Medicare Statute 1861(s)(2)(T)
Pub 100-04, 8, 120.1; 100-4, 17, 80.3.4

Ⓘ Q0180 Dolasetron mesylate, 100 mg, oral, FDA approved prescription anti-emetic, for use as a complete therapeutic substitute for an IV anti-emetic at the time of chemotherapy treatment, not to exceed a 24-hour dosage regimen K K1
Anzemet
Medicare Statute 1861(s)(2)(T)
Pub 100-04, 8, 120.1; 100-4, 17, 80.3.4

Ⓘ Q0181 Unspecified oral dosage form, FDA approved prescription anti-emetic, for use as a complete therapeutic substitute for a IV anti-emetic at the time of chemotherapy treatment, not to exceed a 48-hour dosage regimen E
Medicare Statute 1861(s)(2)(T)
Pub 100-04, 8, 120.1; 100-4, 17, 80.3.4

● Ⓘ Q0478 Power adapter for use with electric or electric/pneumatic ventricular assist device, vehicle type A
This code is effective January 1, 2011

● Ⓘ Q0479 Power module for use with electric or electric/pneumatic ventricular assist device, replacement only A
This code is effective January 1, 2011

Ⓘ Q0480 Driver for use with pneumatic ventricular assist device, replacement only A
NCD 20.9

Ⓘ Q0481 Microprocessor control unit for use with electric ventricular assist device, replacement only A
NCD 20.9

Ⓘ Q0482 Microprocessor control unit for use with electric/pneumatic combination ventricular assist device, replacement only A
NCD 20.9

Ⓘ Q0483 Monitor/display module for use with electric ventricular assist device, replacement only A
NCD 20.9

Ⓘ Q0484 Monitor/display module for use with electric or electric/pneumatic ventricular assist device, replacement only A
NCD 20.9

Ⓘ Q0485 Monitor control cable for use with electric ventricular assist device, replacement only A
NCD 20.9

Ⓘ Q0486 Monitor control cable for use with electric/pneumatic ventricular assist device, replacement only A
NCD 20.9

Ⓘ Q0487 Leads (pneumatic/electrical) for use with any type electric/pneumatic ventricular assist device, replacement only A
NCD 20.9

Ⓘ Q0488 Power pack base for use with electric ventricular assist device, replacement only A
NCD 20.9

Ⓘ Q0489 Power pack base for use with electric/pneumatic ventricular assist device, replacement only A
NCD 20.9

Ⓘ Q0490 Emergency power source for use with electric ventricular assist device, replacement only A
NCD 20.9

Ⓘ Q0491 Emergency power source for use with electric/pneumatic ventricular assist device, replacement only A
NCD 20.9

Ⓘ Q0492 Emergency power supply cable for use with electric ventricular assist device, replacement only A
NCD 20.9

Ⓘ Q0493 Emergency power supply cable for use with electric/pneumatic ventricular assist device, replacement only A
NCD 20.9

Ⓘ Q0494 Emergency hand pump for use with electric or electric/pneumatic ventricular assist device, replacement only A
NCD 20.9

Ⓘ Q0495 Battery/power pack charger for use with electric or electric/ pneumatic ventricular assist device, replacement only A
NCD 20.9

Ⓘ Q0496 Battery, other than lithium-ion, for use with electric or electric/pneumatic ventricular assist device, replacement only A
NCD 20.9

Ⓘ Q0497 Battery clips for use with electric or electric/pneumatic ventricular assist device, replacement only A
NCD 20.9

Ⓘ Q0498 Holster for use with electric or electric/pneumatic ventricular assist device, replacement only A
NCD 20.9

▲ Ⓘ Q0499 Belt/vest/bag for use to carry external peripheral components of any type ventricular assist device, replacement only A

Ⓘ Q0500 Filters for use with electric or electric/pneumatic ventricular assist device, replacement only A
NCD 20.9

Ⓘ Q0501 Shower cover for use with electric or electric/pneumatic ventricular assist device, replacement only A
NCD 20.9

Ⓘ Q0502 Mobility cart for pneumatic ventricular assist device, replacement only A
NCD 20.9

Ⓘ Q0503 Battery for pneumatic ventricular assist device, replacement only, each A
NCD 20.9

Ⓘ Q0504 Power adapter for pneumatic ventricular assist device, replacement only, vehicle type A
NCD 20.9

Ⓘ Q0505 Miscellaneous supply or accessory for use with ventricular assist device A
NCD 20.9

Ⓘ Q0506 Battery, lithium-ion, for use with electric or electric/pneumatic ventricular assist device, replacement only A

Ⓘ Q0510 Pharmacy supply fee for initial immunosuppressive drug(s), first month following transplant B
Medicare Statute 1842(o)(6)
Pub 100-04, 17, 80.7

Ⓘ Q0511 Pharmacy supply fee for oral anti-cancer, oral anti-emetic or immunosuppressive drug(s); for the first prescription in a 30-day period B
Medicare Statute 1842(o)(6)
Pub 100-04, 17, 80.7

Ⓘ Q0512 Pharmacy supply fee for oral anti-cancer, oral anti-emetic or immunosuppressive drug(s); for a subsequent prescription in a 30-day period B
Medicare Statute 1842(o)(6)
Pub 100-04, 17, 80.7

Ⓘ Q0513 Pharmacy dispensing fee for inhalation drug(s); per 30 days B
Medicare Statute 1842(o)(6)
Pub 100-04, 17, 80.7

Ⓘ Q0514 Pharmacy dispensing fee for inhalation drug(s); per 90 days B
Medicare Statute 1842(o)(6)
Pub 100-04, 17, 80.7

Ⓘ Q0515 Injection, sermorelin acetate, 1 microgram K K2
Pub 100-02, 15, 50; 100-4, 17, 10
Geref

Q1003 New technology intraocular lens category 3 (reduced spherical aberration) N L6

Ⓘ Q1004 New technology intraocular lens category 4 as defined in Federal Register notice E

Ⓘ Q1005 New technology intraocular lens category 5 as defined in Federal Register notice E

Ⓘ Q2004 Irrigation solution for treatment of bladder calculi, for example renacidin, per 500 ml N K2
Medicare Statute 1861(s)(2)(B)
Pub 100-02, 15, 50; 100-4, 17, 10

Ⓘ Q2009 Injection, fosphenytoin, 50 mg phenytoin equivalent N N1
Medicare Statute 1861(s)(2)(B)
Pub 100-02, 15, 50; 100-4, 17, 10
Cerebyx

Ⓘ Q2017 Injection, teniposide, 50 mg K K2
Medicare Statute 1861(s)(2)(B)
Pub 100-02, 15, 50; 100-4, 17, 10
Vumon

✖ ~~Q2025 Fludarabine phosphate, oral, 1 mg~~
This code was effective July 1, 2010
This code is deleted as of December 31, 2010

● Ⓘ Q2026 Injection, radiesse, 0.1 ml D
Radiesse
This code was effective July 1, 2010

● Ⓘ Q2027 Injection, sculptra, 0.1 ml D
Sculptra
This code was effective July 1, 2010

● Ⓘ Q2035 Influenza virus vaccine, split virus, when administered to individuals 3 years of age and older, for intramuscular use (afluria) D L1
This code is effective January 1, 2011

● Ⓘ Q2036 Influenza virus vaccine, split virus, when administered to individuals 3 years of age and older, for intramuscular use (flulaval) D L1
This code is effective January 1, 2011

● Ⓘ Q2037 Influenza virus vaccine, split virus, when administered to individuals 3 years of age and older, for intramuscular use (fluvirin) D L1
This code is effective January 1, 2011

Q0490 – Q2037

● ⓘ Q2038 Influenza virus vaccine, split virus, when administered to individuals 3 years of age and older, for intramuscular use (fluzone) D L I
This code is effective January 1, 2011

● ⓘ Q2039 Influenza virus vaccine, split virus, when administered to individuals 3 years of age and older, for intramuscular use (not otherwise specified) D L I
This code is effective January 1, 2011

ⓘ Q3001 Radioelements for brachytherapy, any type, each B
Pub 100-04, 13, 20; 100-4, 13, 90

Q3014 Telehealth originating site facility fee A

ⓘ Q3025 Injection, interferon beta-1a, 11 mcg for intramuscular use K K2
Pub 100-02, 15, 50; 100-4, 17, 10
Avonex

⊘ Q3026 Injection, interferon beta-1a, 11 mcg for subcutaneous use E
Rebif

ⓘ Q3031 Collagen skin test N
NCD 230.10

Casting Supplies

Q4001 Casting supplies, body cast adult, with or without head, plaster B

Q4002 Cast supplies, body cast adult, with or without head, fiberglass B

Q4003 Cast supplies, shoulder cast, adult (11 years +), plaster B

Q4004 Cast supplies, shoulder cast, adult (11 years +), fiberglass B

Q4005 Cast supplies, long arm cast, adult (11 years +), plaster B

Q4006 Cast supplies, long arm cast, adult (11 years +), fiberglass B

Q4007 Cast supplies, long arm cast, pediatric (0-10 years), plaster B

Q4008 Cast supplies, long arm cast, pediatric (0-10 years), fiberglass B

Q4009 Cast supplies, short arm cast, adult (11 years +), plaster B

Q4010 Cast supplies, short arm cast, adult (11 years +), fiberglass B

Q4011 Cast supplies, short arm cast, pediatric (0-10 years), plaster B

Q4012 Cast supplies, short arm cast, pediatric (0-10 years), fiberglass B

Q4013 Cast supplies, gauntlet cast (includes lower forearm and hand), adult (11 years +), plaster B

Cast; hand and lower forearm (gauntlet)

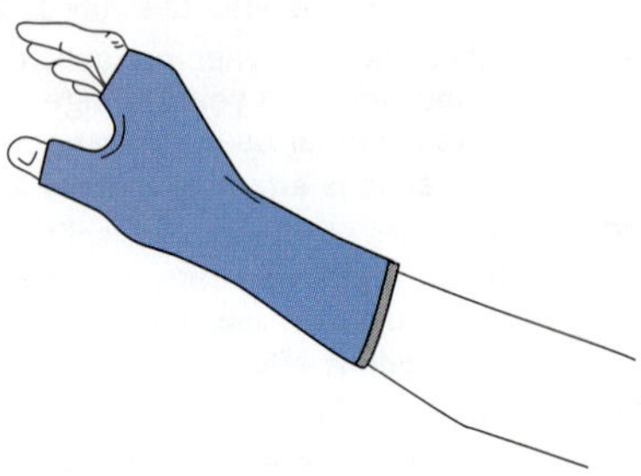

Q4014 Cast supplies, gauntlet cast (includes lower forearm and hand), adult (11 years +), fiberglass B

Q4015 Cast supplies, gauntlet cast (includes lower forearm and hand), pediatric (0-10 years), plaster B

Q4016 Cast supplies, gauntlet cast (includes lower forearm and hand), pediatric (0-10 years), fiberglass B

Q4017 Cast supplies, long arm splint, adult (11 years +), plaster B

Q4018 Cast supplies, long arm splint, adult (11 years +), fiberglass B

Q4019 Cast supplies, long arm splint, pediatric (0-10 years), plaster B

Q4020 Cast supplies, long arm splint, pediatric (0-10 years), fiberglass B

Q4021 Cast supplies, short arm splint, adult (11 years +), plaster B

Q4022 Cast supplies, short arm splint, adult (11 years +), fiberglass B

Q4023 Cast supplies, short arm splint, pediatric (0-10 years), plaster B

Q4024 Cast supplies, short arm splint, pediatric (0-10 years), fiberglass B

Q4025 Cast supplies, hip spica (one or both legs), adult (11 years +), plaster B

Q4026 Cast supplies, hip spica (one or both legs), adult (11 years +), fiberglass B

Q4027 Cast supplies, hip spica (one or both legs), pediatric (0-10 years), plaster B

Q4028 Cast supplies, hip spica (one or both legs), pediatric (0-10 years), fiberglass B

Q4029 Cast supplies, long leg cast, adult (11 years +), plaster B

Q4030 Cast supplies, long leg cast, adult (11 years +), fiberglass B

Q4031 Cast supplies, long leg cast, pediatric (0-10 years), plaster B

Q4032 Cast supplies, long leg cast, pediatric (0-10 years), fiberglass B

Q4033 Cast supplies, long leg cylinder cast, adult (11 years +), plaster B

Q4034 Cast supplies, long leg cylinder cast, adult (11 years +), fiberglass B

Q4035 Cast supplies, long leg cylinder cast, pediatric (0-10 years), plaster B

Q4036 Cast supplies, long leg cylinder cast, pediatric (0-10 years), fiberglass B

Q4037 Cast supplies, short leg cast, adult (11 years +), plaster B

Q4038 Cast supplies, short leg cast, adult (11 years +), fiberglass B

Q4039 Cast supplies, short leg cast, pediatric (0-10 years), plaster B

Q4040 Cast supplies, short leg cast, pediatric (0-10 years), fiberglass B

Q4041 Cast supplies, long leg splint, adult (11 years +), plaster B

Q4042 Cast supplies, long leg splint, adult (11 years +), fiberglass B

Q4043 Cast supplies, long leg splint, pediatric (0-10 years), plaster B

Q4044 Cast supplies, long leg splint, pediatric (0-10 years), fiberglass B

Q4045 Cast supplies, short leg splint, adult (11 years +), plaster B

Q4046 Cast supplies, short leg splint, adult (11 years +), fiberglass B

Q4047 Cast supplies, short leg splint, pediatric (0-10 years), plaster B

Q4048 Cast supplies, short leg splint, pediatric (0-10 years), fiberglass B

Q4049 Finger splint, static B

Q4050 Cast supplies, for unlisted types and materials of casts B

Q4051 Splint supplies, miscellaneous (includes thermoplastics, strapping, fasteners, padding and other supplies) B

Injections and Inhalation Solutions

Q4074 Iloprost, inhalation solution, FDA-approved final product, non-compounded, administered through DME, unit dose form, up to 20 micrograms Y
Ventavis

Q4081 Injection, epoetin alfa, 100 units (for ESRD on dialysis) A
Pub 100-04, 8, 60.4.2-60.4.2.1
Epogen, Procrit

Q4082 Drug or biological, not otherwise classified, part B drug competitive acquisition program (CAP) B

Q4100 Skin substitute, not otherwise specified N NI

▲ Q4101 Apligraf, per square centimeter K K2

▲ Q4102 Oasis Wound Matrix, per square centimeter K K2

▲ Q4103 Oasis Burn Matrix, per square centimeter K K2

▲ Q4104 Integra Bilayer Matrix wound dressing (BMWD), per square centimeter K K2

▲ Q4105 Integra Dermal Regeneration Template (DRT), per square centimeter K K2

▲ Q4106 Dermagraft, per square centimeter K K2

▲ Q4107 Graftjacket, per square centimeter K K2

▲ Q4108 Integra Matrix, per square centimeter K K2

× ~~Q4109 Skin substitute, Tissuemend, per square centimeter~~
This code is deleted as of December 31, 2010

▲ Q4110 Primatrix, per square centimeter K K2

▲ Q4111 Gammagraft, per square centimeter K K2

▲ Q4112 Cymetra, injectable, 1cc K K2

▲ Q4113 Graftjacket Xpress, injectable, 1cc K K2

Q4114 Integra Flowable Wound Matrix, injectable, 1cc G K2

▲ Q4115 Alloskin, per square centimeter K

▲ Q4116 Alloderm, per square centimeter K

● Q4117 Hyalomatrix, per square centimeter K

● Q4118 Matristem Micromatrix, 1 mg K
This code is effective January 1, 2011

● Q4119 Matristem Wound Matrix, per square centimeter K
This code is effective January 1, 2011

● Q4120 Matristem Burn Matrix, per square centimeter K
This code is effective January 1, 2011

● Q4121 Theraskin, per square centimeter K
This code is effective January 1, 2011

Hospice Care

Q5001 Hospice care provided in patient's home/residence B

Q5002 Hospice care provided in assisted living facility B

Q5003 Hospice care provided in nursing long term care facility (LTC) or non-skilled nursing facility (NF) B

Q5004 Hospice care provided in skilled nursing facility (SNF) B

Q5005 Hospice care provided in inpatient hospital B

Q5006 Hospice care provided in inpatient hospice facility B

Q5007 Hospice care provided in long term care facility B

Q5008 Hospice care provided in inpatient psychiatric facility B

Q5009 Hospice care provided in place not otherwise specified (NOS) B

● Q5010 Hospice home care provided in a hospice facility D
This code was effective October 1, 2010

Contrast agents

Q9951 Low osmolar contrast material, 400 or greater mg/ml iodine concentration, per ml N NI
Pub 100-04, 13, 20; 100-4, 13, 90

Q9953 Injection, iron-based magnetic resonance contrast agent, per ml N NI
Pub 100-04, 13, 20; 100-4, 13, 90

Q9954 Oral magnetic resonance contrast agent, per 100 ml N NI
Pub 100-04, 13, 20; 100-4, 13, 90

Q9955 Injection, perflexane lipid microspheres, per ml N NI

Q9956 Injection, octafluoropropane microspheres, per ml N NI

Q9957 Injection, perflutren lipid microspheres, per ml N NI

Q9958 High osmolar contrast material, up to 149 mg/ml iodine concentration, per ml N NI
Pub 100-04, 13, 20; 100-4, 13, 90
AHA: 1Q 2007, 6

Q9959 High osmolar contrast material, 150-199 mg/ml iodine concentration, per ml N NI
Pub 100-04, 13, 20; 100-4, 13, 90
AHA: 1Q 2007, 6

Q9960 High osmolar contrast material, 200-249 mg/ml iodine concentration, per ml N NI
Pub 100-04, 13, 20; 100-4, 13, 90
AHA: 1Q 2007, 6

Q9961 High osmolar contrast material, 250-299 mg/ml iodine concentration, per ml N NI
Pub 100-04, 13, 20; 100-4, 13, 90
AHA: 1Q 2007, 6

Q9962 High osmolar contrast material, 300-349 mg/ml iodine concentration, per ml N NI
Pub 100-04, 13, 20; 100-4, 13, 90
AHA: 1Q 2007, 6

Q9963 High osmolar contrast material, 350-399 mg/ml iodine concentration, per ml N NI
Pub 100-04, 13, 20; 100-4, 13, 90
AHA: 1Q 2007, 6

Q9964 High osmolar contrast material, 400 or greater mg/ml iodine concentration, per ml N NI
Pub 100-04, 13, 20; 100-4, 13, 90
AHA: 1Q 2007, 6

Q9965 Low osmolar contrast material, 100-199 mg/ml iodine concentration, per ml N NI
Pub 100-04, 13, 20; 100-4, 13, 90

Q9966 Low osmolar contrast material, 200-299 mg/ml iodine concentration, per ml N NI
Pub 100-04, 13, 20; 100-4, 13, 90
AHA: 1Q 2008, 8

Q9967 Low osmolar contrast material, 300-399 mg/ml iodine concentration, per ml N NI
Pub 100-04, 13, 20; 100-4, 13, 90
AHA: 1Q 2008, 8

Q9968 Injection, non-radioactive, non-contrast, visualization adjunct (e.g., methylene blue, isosulfan blue), 1 mg K K2

Diagnostic Radiology Services R0070–R0076

ⓘ R0070 Transportation of portable x-ray equipment and personnel to home or nursing home, per trip to facility or location, one patient seen B
Pub 100-02, 15, 80.4; 100-4, 13, 90.4; 100-4, 13, 90.3

ⓘ R0075 Transportation of portable x-ray equipment and personnel to home or nursing home, per trip to facility or location, more than one patient seen, per patient B
Pub 100-02, 15, 80.4; 100-4, 13, 90.4; 100-4, 13, 90.3

ⓘ R0076 Transportation of portable EKG to facility or location, per patient B
NCD 20.15; Pub 100-1, 5, 90.2; 100-2, 15, 80.1; 100-2, 15, 80.4; 100-4, 13, 90.4; 100-4, 16, 10-10.1

Temporary National Codes (Non-Medicare) S0012–S9999

Note: These codes are not covered and are not valid for Medicare. The submission of these codes to the Medicare program will result in non-payment of services.

⊘ S0012 Butorphanol tartrate, nasal spray, 25 mg
Stadol NS

⊘ S0014 Tacrine hydrochloride, 10 mg
Cognex

⊘ S0017 Injection, aminocaproic acid, 5 grams
Amicar

⊘ S0020 Injection, bupivicaine hydrochloride, 30 ml
Marcaine, Sensorcaine, Bupivacaine

⊘ S0021 Injection, cefoperazone sodium, 1 gram

⊘ S0023 Injection, cimetidine hydrochloride, 300 mg

⊘ S0028 Injection, famotidine, 20 mg
Pepcid

⊘ S0030 Injection, metronidazole, 500 mg
Flagyl, METROnidazole

⊘ S0032 Injection, nafcillin sodium, 2 grams
Flexyx

⊘ S0034 Injection, ofloxacin, 400 mg
Floxin

⊘ S0039 Injection, sulfamethoxazole and trimethoprim, 10 ml
Bactrim, Septra

⊘ S0040 Injection, ticarcillin disodium and clavulanate potassium, 3.1 grams
Timentin

⊘ S0073 Injection, aztreonam, 500 mg
Azactam

⊘ S0074 Injection, cefotetan disodium, 500 mg
Cefotan

⊘ S0077 Injection, clindamycin phosphate, 300 mg
Cleocin, Dalacin C

⊘ S0078 Injection, fosphenytoin sodium, 750 mg
Cerebyx

⊘ S0080 Injection, pentamidine isethionate, 300 mg
Pentam 300, Pentacarinat

⊘ S0081 Injection, piperacillin sodium, 500 mg
Pipracil, Zosyn

⊘ S0088 Imatinib, 100 mg
Gleevec

⊘ S0090 Sildenafil citrate, 25 mg
Viagra

⊘ S0091 Granisetron hydrochloride, 1 mg (for circumstances falling under the Medicare Statute, use Q0166)
Kytril

⊘ S0092 Injection, hydromorphone hydrochloride, 250 mg (loading dose for infusion pump)
Dilaudid-HP

⊘ S0093 Injection, morphine sulfate, 500 mg (loading dose for infusion pump)
Astramorph

⊘ S0104 Zidovudine, oral, 100 mg
Retrovir

⊘ S0106 Bupropion HCl sustained release tablet, 150 mg, per bottle of 60 tablets
Wellbutrin SR

⊘ S0108 Mercaptopurine, oral, 50 mg
Purinethol

⊘ S0109 Methadone, oral, 5 mg
Dolophine

⊘ S0117 Tretinoin, topical, 5 grams
Renova

⊘ S0122 Injection, menotropins, 75 IU
Menopur, Repronex

⊘ S0126 Injection, follitropin alfa, 75 IU
Gonal-f RFF

⊘ S0128 Injection, follitropin beta, 75 IU
Follistim AQ

⊘ S0132 Injection, ganirelix acetate, 250 mcg

⊘ S0136 Clozapine, 25 mg

⊘ S0137 Didanosine (ddI), 25 mg

⊘ S0138 Finasteride, 5 mg

⊘ S0139 Minoxidil, 10 mg

⊘ S0140 Saquinavir, 200 mg

⊘ S0142 Colistimethate sodium, inhalation solution administered through DME, concentrated form, per mg

⊘ S0145 Injection, pegylated interferon Alfa-2A, 180 mcg per ml

✖ ~~S0146 Injection, pegylated interferon Alfa-2B, 10 mcg per 0.5 ml~~
This code's delete date: September 30, 2010
See code(s) S0148

● ⊘ S0148 Injection, pegylated interferon Alfa-2B, 10 mcg
This code was effective October 1, 2010

⊘ S0155 Sterile dilutant for epoprostenol, 50 ml

⊘ S0156 Exemestane, 25 mg

⊘ S0157 Becaplermin gel 0.01%, 0.5 gm

⊘ S0160 Dextroamphetamine sulfate, 5 mg

✖ ~~S0161 Calcitrol, 0.25 mg~~
This code's delete date: September 30, 2010
See code(s) S0169

⊘ S0164 Injection, pantoprazole sodium, 40 mg

⊘ S0166 Injection, olanzapine, 2.5 mg

● ⊘ S0169 Calcitrol, 0.25 microgram
This code was effective October 1, 2010

⊘ S0170 Anastrozole, oral, 1 mg

⊘ S0171 Injection, bumetanide, 0.5 mg

⊘ S0172 Chlorambucil, oral, 2 mg

⊘ S0174 Dolasetron mesylate, oral 50 mg (for circumstances falling under the Medicare Statute, use Q0180)

⊘ S0175 Flutamide, oral, 125 mg

⊘ S0176 Hydroxyurea, oral, 500 mg

⊘ S0177 Levamisole hydrochloride, oral, 50 mg

⊘ S0178 Lomustine, oral, 10 mg

⊘ S0179 Megestrol acetate, oral, 20 mg

⊘ S0181 Ondansetron hydrochloride, oral, 4 mg (for circumstances falling under the Medicare Statute, use Q0179)

⊘ S0182 Procarbazine hydrochloride, oral, 50 mg

⊘ S0183 Prochlorperazine maleate, oral, 5 mg (for circumstances falling under the Medicare Statute, use Q0164 – Q0165)

⊘ S0187 Tamoxifen citrate, oral, 10 mg

⊘ S0189 Testosterone pellet, 75 mg

⊘ S0190 Mifepristone, oral, 200 mg

⊘ S0191 Misoprostol, oral, 200 mcg

⊘ S0194 Dialysis/stress vitamin supplement, oral, 100 capsules

⊘ S0195 Pneumococcal conjugate vaccine, polyvalent, intramuscular, for children from five years to nine years of age who have not previously received the vaccine

✖ ~~S0196 Injectable poly-L-lactic acid, restorative implant, 1 ml, face (deep dermis, subcutaneous layers)~~
This code's delete date: September 30, 2010
See code(s) C9800, Q2027

⊘ S0197 Prenatal vitamins, 30-day supply ♀

⊘ S0199 Medically induced abortion by oral ingestion of medication including all associated services and supplies (e.g., patient counseling, office visits, confirmation of pregnancy by HCG, ultrasound to confirm duration of pregnancy, ultrasound to confirm completion of abortion) except drugs ♀

⊘ S0201 Partial hospitalization services, less than 24 hours, per diem

⊘ S0207 Paramedic Intercept, non-hospital-based ALS service (non-voluntary), non-transport

⊘ S0208 Paramedic intercept, hospital-based ALS service (non-voluntary), non-transport

⊘ S0209 Wheelchair van, mileage, per mile

⊘ S0215 Non-emergency transportation; mileage, per mile

⊘ S0220 Medical conference by a physician with interdisciplinary team of health professionals or representatives of community agencies to coordinate activities of patient care (patient is present); approximately 30 minutes

⊘ S0221 Medical conference by a physician with interdisciplinary team of health professionals or representatives of community agencies to coordinate activities of patient care (patient is present); approximately 60 minutes

⊘ S0250 Comprehensive geriatric assessment and treatment planning performed by assessment team

⊘ S0255 Hospice referral visit (advising patient and family of care options) performed by nurse, social worker, or other designated staff

⊘ S0257 Counseling and discussion regarding advance directives or end of life care planning and decisions, with patient and/or surrogate (list separately in addition to code for appropriate evaluation and management service)

⊘ S0260 History and physical (outpatient or office) related to surgical procedure (list separately in addition to code for appropriate evaluation and management service)

⊘ S0265 Genetic counseling, under physician supervision, each 15 minutes

⊘ S0270 Physician management of patient home care, standard monthly case rate (per 30 days)

⊘ S0271 Physician management of patient home care, hospice monthly case rate (per 30 days)

⊘ S0272 Physician management of patient home care, episodic care monthly case rate (per 30 days)

⊘ S0273 Physician visit at member's home, outside of a capitation arrangement

⊘ S0274 Nurse practitioner visit at member's home, outside of a capitation arrangement

⊘ S0280 Medical home program, comprehensive care coordination and planning, initial plan

⊘ S0281 Medical home program, comprehensive care coordination and planning, maintenance of plan

⊘ S0302 Completed early periodic screening diagnosis and treatment (EPSDT) service (list in addition to code for appropriate evaluation and management service)

⊘ Medicare Non-Coverage ⓘ Special Coverage Instructions Coverage Carrier Determined A – Y APC Status Indicators ● New Code ▲ Revised Code ✖ Deleted Code
AHA AHA Coding Clinic for HCPCS A2 – Z3 ASC Payment Indicators DMEPOS ♂ Male ♀ Female PQR PQRI

⊘ S0310 Hospitalist services (list separately in addition to code for appropriate evaluation and management service)

⊘ S0315 Disease management program; initial assessment and initiation of the program

⊘ S0316 Disease management program, follow-up/ reassessment

⊘ S0317 Disease management program; per diem

⊘ S0320 Telephone calls by a registered nurse to a disease management program member for monitoring purposes; per month

⊘ S0340 Lifestyle modification program for management of coronary artery disease, including all supportive services; first quarte/stage

⊘ S0341 Lifestyle modification program for management of coronary artery disease, including all supportive services; second or third quarter/stage

⊘ S0342 Lifestyle modification program for management of coronary artery disease, including all supportive services; fourth quarter/stage

⊘ S0390 Routine foot care; removal and/or trimming of corns, calluses and/or nails and preventive maintenance in specific medical conditions (e.g. diabetes), per visit

⊘ S0395 Impression casting of a foot performed by a practitioner other than the manufacturer of the orthotic

⊘ S0400 Global fee for extracorporeal shock wave lithotripsy treatment of kidney stone(s)

⊘ S0500 Disposable contact lens, per lens

⊘ S0504 Single vision prescription lens (safety, athletic, or sunglass), per lens

⊘ S0506 Bifocal vision prescription lens (safety, athletic, or sunglass), per lens

⊘ S0508 Trifocal vision prescription lens (safety, athletic, or sunglass), per lens

⊘ S0510 Non-prescription lens (safety, athletic, or sunglass), per lens

⊘ S0512 Daily wear specialty contact lens, per lens

⊘ S0514 Color contact lens, per lens

⊘ S0515 Scleral lens, liquid bandage device, per lens

⊘ S0516 Safety eyeglass frames

⊘ S0518 Sunglasses frames

⊘ S0580 Polycarbonate lens (list this code in addition to the basic code for the lens)

⊘ S0581 Nonstandard lens (list this code in addition to the basic code for the lens)

⊘ S0590 Integral lens service, miscellaneous services reported separately

⊘ S0592 Comprehensive contact lens evaluation

⊘ S0595 Dispensing new spectacle lenses for patient supplied frame

⊘ S0601 Screening proctoscopy

⊘ S0610 Annual gynecological examination, new patient ♀

⊘ S0612 Annual gynecological examination, established patient ♀

⊘ S0613 Annual gynecological examination; clinical breast ♀ examination without pelvic evaluation

⊘ S0618 Audiometry for hearing aid evaluation to determine the level and degree of hearing loss

⊘ S0620 Routine ophthalmological examination including refraction; new patient

⊘ S0621 Routine ophthalmological examination including refraction; established patient

⊘ S0622 Physical exam for college, new or established patient (list separately in addition to appropriate evaluation and management code)

⊘ S0625 Retinal telescreening by digital imaging of multiple different fundus areas to screen for vision-threatening conditions, including imaging, interpretation and report

⊘ S0630 Removal of sutures; by a physician other than the physician who originally closed the wound

Treatment of superficial dehiscence

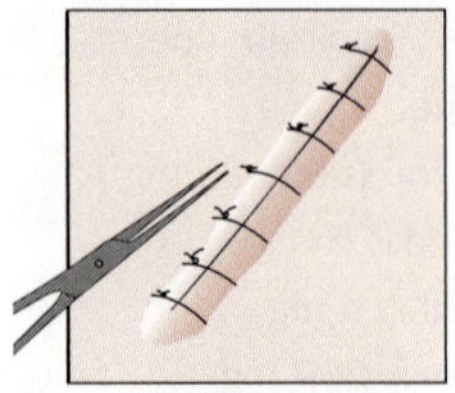

Wound sutures are removed

⊘ S0800 Laser in situ keratomileusis (LASIK)

⊘ S0810 Photorefractive keratectomy (PRK)

⊘ S0812 Phototherapeutic keratectomy (PTK)

⊘ S1001 Deluxe item, patient aware (list in addition to code for basic item)

⊘ S1002 Customized item (list in addition to code for basic item)

⊘ S1015 IV tubing extension set

⊘ S1016 Non-PVC (polyvinyl chloride) intravenous administration set, for use with drugs that are not stable in PVC e.g. paclitaxel

⊘ S1030 Continuous noninvasive glucose monitoring device, purchase (for physician interpretation of data, use CPT code)

⊘ S1031 Continuous noninvasive glucose monitoring device, rental, including sensor, sensor replacement, and download to monitor (for physician interpretation of data, use CPT code)

⊘ S1040 Cranial remolding orthosis, pediatric, rigid, with soft interface material, custom fabricated, includes fitting and adjustment(s)

⊘ S2053 Transplantation of small intestine and liver allografts

⊘ S2054 Transplantation of multivisceral organs

⊘ S2055 Harvesting of donor multivisceral organs, with preparation and maintenance of allografts; from cadaver donor

⊘ S2060 Lobar lung transplantation

⊘ S2061 Donor lobectomy (lung) for transplantation, living donor

⊘ S2065 Simultaneous pancreas kidney transplantation

⊘ S2066 Breast reconstruction with gluteal artery perforator (GAP) flap, including harvesting of the flap, microvascular transfer, closure of donor site and shaping the flap into a breast, unilateral

⊘ S2067 Breast reconstruction of a single breast with "stacked" deep inferior epigastric perforator (DIEP) flap(s) and/or gluteal artery perforator (GAP) flap(s), including harvesting of the flap(s), microvascular transfer, closure of donor site(s) and shaping the flap into a breast, unilateral

⊘ S2068 Breast reconstruction with deep inferior epigastric perforator (DIEP) flap or superficial inferior epigastric artery (SIEA) flap, including harvest of the flap, microvascular transfer, closure of donor site and shaping the flap into a breast, unilateral

⊘ S2070 Cystourethroscopy, with ureteroscopy and/or pyeloscopy; with endoscopic laser treatment of ureteral calculi (includes ureteral catheterization)

⊘ S2079 Laparoscopic esophagomyotomy (Heller type)

⊘ S2080 Laser-assisted uvulopalatoplasty (LAUP)

⊘ S2083 Adjustment of gastric band diameter via subcutaneous port by injection or aspiration of saline

⊘ S2095 Transcatheter occlusion or embolization for tumor destruction, percutaneous, any method, using yttrium-90 microspheres

⊘ S2102 Islet cell tissue transplant from pancreas; allogeneic

⊘ S2103 Adrenal tissue transplant to brain

⊘ S2107 Adoptive immunotherapy i.e. development of specific anti-tumor reactivity (e.g. tumor-infiltrating lymphocyte therapy) per course of treatment

⊘ S2112 Arthroscopy, knee, surgical for harvesting of cartilage (chondrocyte cells)

⊘ S2115 Osteotomy, periacetabular, with internal fixation

⊘ S2117 Arthroereisis, subtalar

⊘ S2118 Metal-on-metal total hip resurfacing, including acetabular and femoral components

⊘ S2120 Low density lipoprotein (LDL) apheresis using Heparin-induced extracorporeal LDL precipitation

⊘ S2140 Cord blood harvesting for transplantation, allogeneic

⊘ S2142 Cord blood-derived stem-cell transplantation, allogeneic

⊘ S2150 Bone marrow or blood-derived stem cells (peripheral or umbilical), allogeneic or autologous, harvesting, transplantation, and related complications; including: pheresis and cell preparation/storage; marrow ablative therapy; drugs, supplies, hospitalization with outpatient follow-up; medical/surgical, diagnostic, emergency, and rehabilitative services; and the number of days of pre- and post-transplant care in the global definition

Bone marrow or blood-derived stem cells

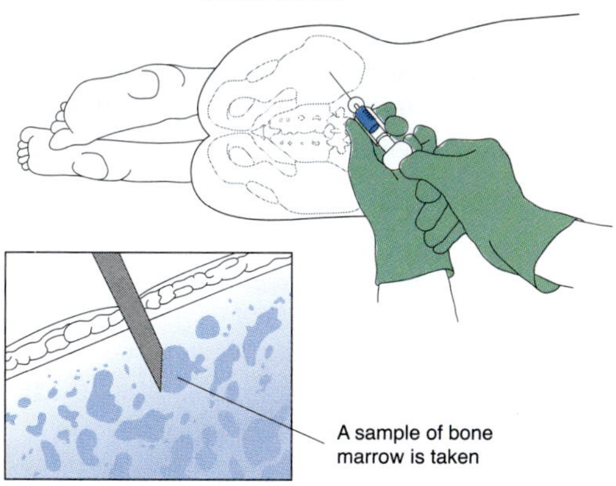

⊘ S2152 Solid organ(s), complete or segmental, single organ or combination of organs; deceased or living donor(s), procurement, transplantation, and related complications; including: drugs; supplies; hospitalization with outpatient follow-up; medical/surgical, diagnostic, emergency, and rehabilitative services, and the number of days of pre- and post-transplant care in the global definition

⊘ S2202 Echosclerotherapy

⊘ S2205 Minimally invasive direct coronary artery bypass surgery involving mini-thoracotomy or mini-sternotomy surgery, performed under direct vision; using arterial graft(s), single coronary arterial graft

⊘ S2206 Minimally invasive direct coronary artery bypass surgery involving mini-thoracotomy or mini-sternotomy surgery, performed under direct vision; using arterial graft(s), two coronary arterial grafts

⊘ S2207 Minimally invasive direct coronary artery bypass surgery involving mini-thoracotomy or mini-sternotomy surgery, performed under direct vision; using venous graft only, single coronary venous graft

⊘ S2208 Minimally invasive direct coronary artery bypass surgery involving mini-thoracotomy or mini-sternotomy surgery, performed under direct vision; using single arterial and venous graft(s), single venous graft

⊘ S2209 Minimally invasive direct coronary artery bypass surgery involving mini-thoracotomy or mini-sternotomy surgery, performed under direct vision; using two arterial grafts and single venous graft

⊘ S2225 Myringotomy, laser-assisted

⊘ S2230 Implantation of magnetic component of semi-implantable hearing device on ossicles in middle ear

⊘ S2235 Implantation of auditory brain stem implant

⊘ S2260 Induced abortion, 17 to 24 weeks ♀

⊘ S2265 Induced abortion, 25 to 28 weeks ♀

⊘ S2266 Induced abortion, 29 to 31 weeks ♀

⊘ S2267 Induced abortion, 32 weeks or greater ♀

⊘ S2270 Insertion of vaginal cylinder for application of radiation source or clinical brachytherapy (report separately in addition to radiation source delivery) ♀

⊘ S2300 Arthroscopy, shoulder, surgical; with thermally-induced capsulorrhaphy

⊘ S2325 Hip core decompression

⊘ S2340 Chemodenervation of abductor muscle(s) of vocal cord

⊘ S2341 Chemodenervation of adductor muscle(s) of vocal cord

⊘ S2342 Nasal endoscopy for post-operative debridement following functional endoscopic sinus surgery, nasal and/or sinus cavity(s), unilateral or bilateral

⊘ S2344 Nasal/sinus endoscopy, surgical; with enlargement of sinus ostium opening using inflatable device (i.e., balloon sinuplasty)

⊘ S2348 Decompression procedure, percutaneous, of nucleus pulposus of intervertebral disc, using radiofrequency energy, single or multiple levels, lumbar

⊘ S2350 Diskectomy, anterior, with decompression of spinal cord and/or nerve root(s), including osteophytectomy; lumbar, single interspace

⊘ S2351 Diskectomy, anterior, with decompression of spinal cord and/or nerve root(s), including osteophytectomy; lumbar, each additional interspace (list separately in addition to code for primary procedure)

⊘ S2360 Percutaneous vertebroplasty, one vertebral body, unilateral or bilateral injection; cervical

⊘ S2361 Each additional cervical vertebral body (list separately in addition to code for primary procedure)

⊘ S2400 Repair, congenital diaphragmatic hernia in the fetus using temporary tracheal occlusion, procedure performed in utero ♀

⊘ S2401 Repair, urinary tract obstruction in the fetus, procedure performed in utero ♀

⊘ S2402 Repair, congenital cystic adenomatoid malformation in the fetus, procedure performed in utero ♀

⊘ S2403 Repair, extralobar pulmonary sequestration in the fetus, procedure performed in utero ♀

⊘ S2404 Repair, myelomeningocele in the fetus, procedure performed in utero ♀

⊘ S2405 Repair of sacrococcygeal teratoma in the fetus, procedure performed in utero ♀

⊘ S2409 Repair, congenital malformation of fetus, procedure performed in utero, not otherwise classified ♀

⊘ S2411 Fetoscopic laser therapy for treatment of twin-to-twin transfusion syndrome ♀

⊘ S2900 Surgical techniques requiring use of robotic surgical system (list separately in addition to code for primary procedure)

⊘ S3000 Diabetic indicator; retinal eye exam, dilated, bilateral

⊘ S3005 Performance measurement, evaluation of patient self assessment, depression

⊘ S3600 Stat laboratory request (situations other than S3601)

⊘ S3601 Emergency stat laboratory charge for patient who is homebound or residing in a nursing facility

⊘ S3620 Newborn metabolic screening panel, includes test kit, postage and the laboratory tests specified by the state for inclusion in this panel (e.g., galactose; hemoglobin, electrophoresis; hydroxyprogesterone, 17-D; phenylanine (PKU); and thyroxine, total)

⊘ S3625 Maternal serum triple marker screen including alpha-fetoprotein (AFP), estriol, and human chorionic gonadotropin (HCG) ♀

⊘ S3626 Maternal serum quadruple marker screen including alpha-fetoprotein (AFP), estriol, human chorionic gonadotropin (HCG) and inhibin A ♀

⊘ S3628 Placental alpha microglobulin-1 rapid immunoassay for detection of rupture of fetal membranes ♀

⊘ S3630 Eosinophil count, blood, direct

⊘ S3645 HIV-1 antibody testing of oral mucosal transudate

Pub 100-03, 1, 190.14, 210.7

⊘ S3650 Saliva test, hormone level; during menopause ♀

⊘ S3652 Saliva test, hormone level; to assess preterm labor risk ♀

⊘ S3655 Antisperm antibodies test (immunobead)

⊘ S3708 Gastrointestinal fat absorption study

⊘ S3711 Circulating tumor cell test

⊘ S3713 KRAS mutation analysis testing

⊘ S3800 Genetic testing for amyotrophic lateral sclerosis (ALS)

⊘ S3818 Complete gene sequence analysis; BRCA1 gene

⊘ S3819 Complete gene sequence analysis; BRCA2 gene

⊘ S3820 Complete BRCA1 and BRCA2 gene sequence analysis for susceptibility to breast and ovarian cancer

⊘ S3822 Single mutation analysis (in individual with a known BRCA1 or BRCA2 mutation in the family) for susceptibility to breast and ovarian cancer

⊘ S3823 Three-mutation BRCA1 and BRCA2 analysis for susceptibility to breast and ovarian cancer in Ashkenazi individuals

⊘ S3828 Complete gene sequence analysis; MLH1 gene

⊘ S3829 Complete gene sequence analysis; MLH2 gene

⊘ S3830 Complete MLH1 and MLH2 gene sequence analysis for hereditary nonpolyposis colorectal cancer (HNPCC) genetic testing

⊘ S3831 Single-mutation analysis (in individual with a known MLH1 and MLH2 mutation in the family) for hereditary nonpolyposis colorectal cancer (HNPCC) genetic testing

⊘ S3833 Complete APC gene sequence analysis for susceptibility to familial adenomatous polyposis (FAP) and attenuated FAP

⊘ S3834 Single-mutation analysis (in individual with a known APC mutation in the family) for susceptibility to familial adenomatous polyposis (FAP) and attenuated FAP

⊘ S3835 Complete gene sequence analysis for cystic fibrosis genetic testing

⊘ S3837 Complete gene sequence analysis for hemochromatosis genetic testing

⊘ S3840 DNA analysis for germline mutations of the ret proto-oncogene for susceptibility to multiple endocrine neoplasia type 2

⊘ S3841 Genetic testing for retinoblastoma

⊘ S3842 Genetic testing for Von Hippel-Lindau disease

⊘ S3843 DNA analysis of the F5 gene for susceptibility to Factor V Leiden thrombophilia

⊘ S3844 DNA analysis of the connexin 26 gene (GJB2) for susceptibility to congenital, profound deafness

⊘ S3845 Genetic testing for alpha-thalassemia

⊘ S3846 Genetic testing for hemoglobin E beta-thalassemia

⊘ S3847 Genetic testing for Tay-Sachs disease

⊘ S3848 Genetic testing for Gaucher disease

⊘ S3849 Genetic testing for Niemann-Pick disease

⊘ S3850 Genetic testing for sickle cell anemia

⊘ S3851 Genetic testing for Canavan disease

⊘ S3852 DNA analysis for APOE epsilon 4 allele for susceptibility to Alzheimer's disease

⊘ S3853 Genetic testing for myotonic muscular dystrophy

⊘ S3854 Gene expression profiling panel for use in the management of breast cancer treatment

⊘ S3855 Genetic testing for detection of mutations in the presenilin – 1 gene

⊘ S3860 Genetic testing, comprehensive cardiac ion channel analysis, for variants in 5 major cardiac ION channel genes for individuals with high index of suspicion for familial long qt syndrome (LQTS) or related syndromes

⊘ S3861 Genetic testing, sodium channel, voltage-gated, type V, alpha subunit (SCN5a) and variants for suspected Brugada syndrome

⊘ S3862 Genetic testing, family-specific ion channel analysis, for blood-relatives of individuals (index case) who have previously tested positive for a genetic variant of a cardiac ion channel syndrome using either one of the above test configurations or confirmed results from another laboratory

⊘ S3865 Comprehensive gene sequence analysis for hypertrophic cardiomyopathy

⊘ S3866 Genetic analysis for a specific gene mutation for hypertrophic cardiomyopathy (HCM) in an individual with a known HCM mutation in the family

⊘ S3870 Comparative genomic hybrization (CGH) microarray testing for developmental delay, autism spectrum disorder and/or mental retardation

⊘ S3890 DNA analysis, fecal, for colorectal cancer screening

⊘ S3900 Surface electromyography (EMG)

⊘ S3902 Ballistocardiogram

⊘ S3904 Masters two step

⊘ S3905 Non-invasive electrodiagnostic testing with automatic computerized hand-held device to stimulate and measure neuromuscular signals in diagnosing and evaluating systemic and entrapment neuropathies

⊘ S4005 Interim labor facility global (labor occurring but not resulting in delivery) ♀

⊘ S4011 In vitro fertilization; including but not limited to identification and incubation of mature oocytes, fertilization with sperm, incubation of embryo(s), and subsequent visualization for determination of development ♀

⊘ S4013 Complete cycle, gamete intrafallopian transfer (GIFT), case rate ♀

⊘ S4014 Complete cycle, zygote intrafallopian transfer (ZIFT), case rate ♀
⊘ S4015 Complete in vitro fertilization cycle, not otherwise specified, case rate ♀
⊘ S4016 Frozen in vitro fertilization cycle, case rate ♀
⊘ S4017 Incomplete cycle, treatment cancelled prior to stimulation, case rate ♀
⊘ S4018 Frozen embryo transfer procedure cancelled before transfer, case rate ♀
⊘ S4020 In vitro fertilization procedure cancelled before aspiration, case rate ♀
⊘ S4021 In vitro fertilization procedure cancelled after aspiration, case rate
⊘ S4022 Assisted oocyte fertilization, case rate ♀
⊘ S4023 Donor egg cycle, incomplete, case rate ♀
⊘ S4025 Donor services for in vitro fertilization (sperm or embryo), case rate
⊘ S4026 Procurement of donor sperm from sperm bank ♂
⊘ S4027 Storage of previously frozen embryos ♀
⊘ S4028 Microsurgical epididymal sperm aspiration (MESA)
⊘ S4030 Sperm procurement and cryopreservation services; initial visit ♂
⊘ S4031 Sperm procurement and cryopreservation services; subsequent visit ♂
⊘ S4035 Stimulated intrauterine insemination (IUI), case rate ♀
⊘ S4037 Cryopreserved embryo transfer, case rate ♀
⊘ S4040 Monitoring and storage of cryopreserved embryos, per 30 days ♀
⊘ S4042 Management of ovulation induction (interpretation of diagnostic tests and studies, non-face-to-face medical management of the patient), per cycle ♀
⊘ S4981 Insertion of levonorgestrel-releasing intrauterine system ♀
⊘ S4989 Contraceptive intrauterine device (e.g. Progestacert IUD), including implants and supplies ♀
⊘ S4990 Nicotine patches, legend
⊘ S4991 Nicotine patches, non-legend
⊘ S4993 Contraceptive pills for birth control
⊘ S4995 Smoking cessation gum
⊘ S5000 Prescription drug, generic
⊘ S5001 Prescription drug, brand name
⊘ S5010 5% dextrose and 0.45% normal saline, 1000 ml
⊘ S5011 5% dextrose in lactated Ringer's, 1000 ml
⊘ S5012 5% dextrose with potassium chloride, 1000 ml
⊘ S5013 5% dextrose/0.45% normal saline with potassium chloride and magnesium sulfate, 1000 ml
⊘ S5014 5% dextrose/0.45% normal saline with potassium chloride and magnesium sulfate, 1500 ml
⊘ S5035 Home infusion therapy, routine service of infusion device (e.g. pump maintenance)
⊘ S5036 Home infusion therapy, repair of infusion device (e.g. pump repair)
⊘ S5100 Day care services, adult; per 15 minutes
⊘ S5101 Day care services, adult; per half day
⊘ S5102 Day care services, adult; per diem
⊘ S5105 Day care services, center-based; services not included in program fee, per diem
⊘ S5108 Home care training to home care client, per 15 minutes
⊘ S5109 Home care training to home care client, per session
⊘ S5110 Home care training, family; per 15 minutes
⊘ S5111 Home care training, family; per session
⊘ S5115 Home care training, non-family; per 15 minutes
⊘ S5116 Home care training, non-family; per session
⊘ S5120 Chore services; per 15 minutes
⊘ S5121 Chore services; per diem
⊘ S5125 Attendant care services; per 15 minutes
⊘ S5126 Attendant care services; per diem
⊘ S5130 Homemaker service, NOS; per 15 minutes
⊘ S5131 Homemaker service, NOS; per diem
⊘ S5135 Companion care, adult (e.g. IADL/ADL); per 15 minutes
⊘ S5136 Companion care, adult (e.g. IADL/ADL); per diem
⊘ S5140 Foster care, adult; per diem
⊘ S5141 Foster care, adult; per month
⊘ S5145 Foster care, therapeutic, child; per diem
⊘ S5146 Foster care, therapeutic, child; per month
⊘ S5150 Unskilled respite care, not hospice; per 15 minutes
⊘ S5151 Unskilled respite care, not hospice; per diem
⊘ S5160 Emergency response system; installation and testing
⊘ S5161 Emergency response system; service fee, per month (excludes installation and testing)
⊘ S5162 Emergency response system; purchase only
⊘ S5165 Home modifications; per service
⊘ S5170 Home delivered meals, including preparation; per meal
⊘ S5175 Laundry service, external, professional; per order
⊘ S5180 Home health respiratory therapy, initial evaluation
⊘ S5181 Home health respiratory therapy, NOS, per diem
⊘ S5185 Medication reminder service, non-face-to-face; per month
⊘ S5190 Wellness assessment, performed by non-physician
⊘ S5199 Personal care item, NOS, each
⊘ S5497 Home infusion therapy, catheter care/maintenance, not otherwise classified; includes administrative services, professional pharmacy services, care coordination, and all necessary supplies and equipment (drugs and nursing visits coded separately), per diem
⊘ S5498 Home infusion therapy, catheter care/maintenance, simple (single lumen), includes administrative services, professional pharmacy services, care coordination and all necessary supplies and equipment, (drugs and nursing visits coded separately), per diem
⊘ S5501 Home infusion therapy, catheter care/maintenance, complex (more than one lumen), includes administrative services, professional pharmacy services, care coordination, and all necessary supplies and equipment (drugs and nursing visits coded separately), per diem
⊘ S5502 Home infusion therapy, catheter care/maintenance, implanted access device, includes administrative services, professional pharmacy services, care coordination and all necessary supplies and equipment, (drugs and nursing visits coded separately), per diem (use this code for interim maintenance of vascular access not currently in use)
⊘ S5517 Home infusion therapy, all supplies necessary for restoration of catheter patency or declotting
⊘ S5518 Home infusion therapy, all supplies necessary for catheter repair
⊘ S5520 Home infusion therapy, all supplies (including catheter) necessary for a peripherally inserted central venous catheter (PICC) line insertion

⊘ S5521 Home infusion therapy, all supplies (including catheter) necessary for a midline catheter insertion

⊘ S5522 Home infusion therapy, insertion of peripherally inserted central venous catheter (PICC), nursing services only (no supplies or catheter included)

⊘ S5523 Home infusion therapy, insertion of midline venous catheter, nursing services only (no supplies or catheter included)

⊘ S5550 Insulin, rapid onset, 5 units

⊘ S5551 Insulin, most rapid onset (Lispro or Aspart); 5 units

⊘ S5552 Insulin, intermediate acting (NPH or Lente); 5 units

⊘ S5553 Insulin, long acting; 5 units

⊘ S5560 Insulin delivery device, reusable pen; 1.5 ml size

⊘ S5561 Insulin delivery device, reusable pen; 3 ml size

⊘ S5565 Insulin cartridge for use in insulin delivery device other than pump; 150 units

⊘ S5566 Insulin cartridge for use in insulin delivery device other than pump; 300 units

⊘ S5570 Insulin delivery device, disposable pen (including insulin); 1.5 ml size

⊘ S5571 Insulin delivery device, disposable pen (including insulin); 3 ml size

⊘ S8030 Scleral application of tantalum ring(s) for localization of lesions for proton beam therapy

⊘ S8035 Magnetic source imaging

Pub 100-03, 1, 220.2

⊘ S8037 Magnetic resonance cholangiopancreatography (MRCP)

Pub 100-03, 1, 220.2

⊘ S8040 Topographic brain mapping

⊘ S8042 Magnetic resonance imaging (MRI), low-field

Pub 100-03, 1, 220.2

⊘ S8049 Intraoperative radiation therapy (single administration)

⊘ S8055 Ultrasound guidance for multifetal pregnancy reduction(s), technical component (only to be used when the physician doing the reduction procedure does not perform the ultrasound, guidance is included in the CPT code for multifetal pregnancy reduction – 59866) ♀

⊘ S8080 Scintimammography (radioimmunoscintigraphy of the breast), unilateral, including supply of radiopharmaceutical

⊘ S8085 Fluorine-18 fluorodeoxyglucose (F-18 FDG) imaging using dual-head coincidence detection system (non-dedicated PET scan)

⊘ S8092 Electron beam computed tomography (also known as ultrafast CT, cine CT)

⊘ S8096 Portable peak flow meter

⊘ S8097 Asthma kit (including but not limited to portable peak expiratory flow meter, instructional video, brochure, and/or spacer)

⊘ S8100 Holding chamber or spacer for use with an inhaler or nebulizer; without mask

⊘ S8101 Holding chamber or spacer for use with an inhaler or nebulizer; with mask

⊘ S8110 Peak expiratory flow rate (physician services)

⊘ S8120 Oxygen contents, gaseous, 1 unit equals 1 cubic foot

⊘ S8121 Oxygen contents, liquid, 1 unit equals 1 pound

⊘ S8185 Flutter device

⊘ S8186 Swivel adaptor

⊘ S8189 Tracheostomy supply, not otherwise classified

⊘ S8210 Mucus trap

⊘ S8262 Mandibular orthopedic repositioning device, each

⊘ S8265 Haberman feeder for cleft lip/palate

⊘ S8270 Enuresis alarm, using auditory buzzer and/or vibration device

⊘ S8301 Infection control supplies, not otherwise specified

⊘ S8415 Supplies for home delivery of infant

⊘ S8420 Gradient pressure aid (sleeve and glove combination), custom made

⊘ S8421 Gradient pressure aid (sleeve and glove combination), ready made

⊘ S8422 Gradient pressure aid (sleeve), custom made, medium weight

⊘ S8423 Gradient pressure aid (sleeve), custom made, heavy weight

⊘ S8424 Gradient pressure aid (sleeve), ready made

⊘ S8425 Gradient pressure aid (glove), custom made, medium weight

⊘ S8426 Gradient pressure aid (glove), custom made, heavy weight

⊘ S8427 Gradient pressure aid (glove), ready made

⊘ S8428 Gradient pressure aid (gauntlet), ready made

⊘ S8429 Gradient pressure exterior wrap

⊘ S8430 Padding for compression bandage, roll

⊘ S8431 Compression bandage, roll

⊘ S8450 Splint, prefabricated, digit (specify digit by use of modifier)

⊘ S8451 Splint, prefabricated, wrist or ankle

Wrist splint

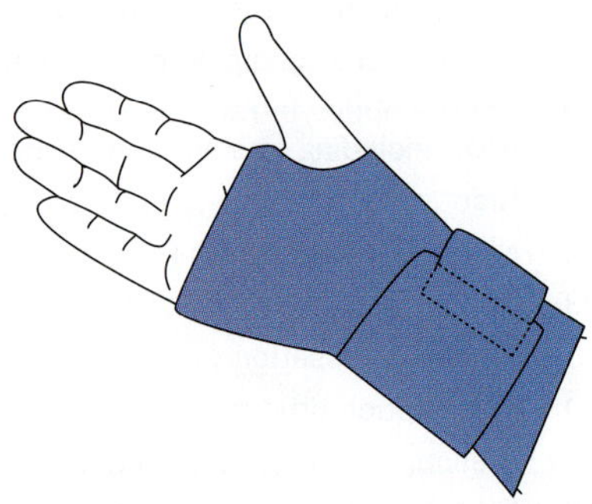

⊘ S8452 Splint, prefabricated, elbow

⊘ S8460 Camisole, post-mastectomy

⊘ S8490 Insulin syringes (100 syringes, any size)

⊘ S8940 Equestrian/hippotherapy, per session

⊘ S8948 Application of a modality (requiring constant provider attendance) to one or more areas; low-level laser; each 15 minutes

⊘ S8950 Complex lymphedema therapy, each 15 minutes

⊘ S8990 Physical or manipulative therapy performed for maintenance rather than restoration

⊘ S8999 Resuscitation bag (for use by patient on artificial respiration during power failure or other catastrophic event)

⊘ S9001 Home uterine monitor with or without associated nursing services

⊘ S9007 Ultrafiltration monitor

⊘ S9015 Automated EEG monitoring

⊘ S9024 Paranasal sinus ultrasound

⊘ S9025 Omnicardiogram/cardiointegram

⊘ S9034 Extracorporeal shockwave lithotripsy for gall stones (if performed with ERCP, use CPT 43265)

⊘ S9055 Procuren or other growth factor preparation to promote wound healing

⊘ S9056 Coma stimulation per diem

⊘ S9061 Home administration of aerosolized drug therapy (e.g., pentamidine); administrative services, professional pharmacy services, care coordination, all necessary supplies and equipment (drugs and nursing visits coded separately), per diem

⊘ S9075 Smoking cessation treatment

⊘ S9083 Global fee urgent care centers

⊘ S9088 Services provided in an urgent care center (list in addition to code for service)

⊘ S9090 Vertebral axial decompression, per session

⊘ S9097 Home visit for wound care

⊘ S9098 Home visit, phototherapy services (e.g. Bili-lite), including equipment rental, nursing services, blood draw, supplies, and other services, per diem

⊘ S9109 Congestive heart failure telemonitoring, equipment rental, including telescale, computer system and software, telephone connections, and maintenance, per month

⊘ S9117 Back school, per visit

⊘ S9122 Home health aide or certified nurse assistant, providing care in the home; per hour

⊘ S9123 Nursing care, in the home; by registered nurse, per hour (use for general nursing care only, not to be used when CPT codes 99500-99602 can be used)

⊘ S9124 Nursing care, in the home; by licensed practical nurse, per hour

⊘ S9125 Respite care, in the home, per diem

⊘ S9126 Hospice care, in the home, per diem

⊘ S9127 Social work visit, in the home, per diem

⊘ S9128 Speech therapy, in the home, per diem

⊘ S9129 Occupational therapy, in the home, per diem

⊘ S9131 Physical therapy; in the home, per diem

⊘ S9140 Diabetic management program, follow-up visit to non-MD provider

⊘ S9141 Diabetic management program, follow-up visit to MD provider

⊘ S9145 Insulin pump initiation, instruction in initial use of pump (pump not included)

⊘ S9150 Evaluation by ocularist

⊘ S9152 Speech therapy, re-evaluation

⊘ S9208 Home management of preterm labor, including administrative services, professional pharmacy services, care coordination, and all necessary supplies or equipment (drugs and nursing visits coded separately), per diem (do not use this code with any home infusion per diem code) ♀

⊘ S9209 Home management of preterm premature rupture of membranes (PPROM), including administrative services, professional pharmacy services, care coordination, and all necessary supplies or equipment (drugs and nursing visits coded separately), per diem (do not use this code with any home infusion per diem code) ♀

⊘ S9211 Home management of gestational hypertension, includes administrative services, professional pharmacy services, care coordination and all necessary supplies and equipment (drugs and nursing visits coded separately); per diem (do not use this code with any home infusion per diem code) ♀

⊘ S9212 Home management of postpartum hypertension, includes administrative services, professional pharmacy services, care coordination, and all necessary supplies and equipment (drugs and nursing visits coded separately), per diem (do not use this code with any home infusion per diem code) ♀

⊘ S9213 Home management of preeclampsia, includes administrative services, professional pharmacy services, care coordination, and all necessary supplies and equipment (drugs and nursing services coded separately); per diem (do not use this code with any home infusion per diem code) ♀

⊘ S9214 Home management of gestational diabetes, includes administrative services, professional pharmacy services, care coordination, and all necessary supplies and equipment (drugs and nursing visits coded separately); per diem (do not use this code with any home infusion per diem code) ♀

⊘ S9325 Home infusion therapy, pain management infusion; administrative services, professional pharmacy services, care coordination, and all necessary supplies and equipment, (drugs and nursing visits coded separately), per diem (do not use this code with S9326, S9327 or S9328)

⊘ S9326 Home infusion therapy, continuous (twenty-four hours or more) pain management infusion; administrative services, professional pharmacy services, care coordination and all necessary supplies and equipment (drugs and nursing visits coded separately), per diem

⊘ S9327 Home infusion therapy, intermittent (less than twenty-four hours) pain management infusion; administrative services, professional pharmacy services, care coordination, and all necessary supplies and equipment (drugs and nursing visits coded separately), per diem

⊘ S9328 Home infusion therapy, implanted pump pain management infusion; administrative services, professional pharmacy services, care coordination, and all necessary supplies and equipment (drugs and nursing visits coded separately), per diem

⊘ S9329 Home infusion therapy, chemotherapy infusion; administrative services, professional pharmacy services, care coordination, and all necessary supplies and equipment (drugs and nursing visits coded separately), per diem (do not use this code with S9330 or S9331)

⊘ S9330 Home infusion therapy, continuous (twenty-four hours or more) chemotherapy infusion; administrative services, professional pharmacy services, care coordination, and all necessary supplies and equipment (drugs and nursing visits coded separately), per diem

⊘ S9331 Home infusion therapy, intermittent (less than twenty-four hours) chemotherapy infusion; administrative services, professional pharmacy services, care coordination, and all necessary supplies and equipment (drugs and nursing visits coded separately), per diem

⊘ S9335 Home therapy, hemodialysis; administrative services, professional pharmacy services, care coordination, and all necessary supplies and equipment (drugs and nursing services coded separately), per diem

⊘ S9336 Home infusion therapy, continuous anticoagulant infusion therapy (e.g. Heparin), administrative services, professional pharmacy services, care coordination and all necessary supplies and equipment (drugs and nursing visits coded separately), per diem

⊘ S9338 Home infusion therapy, immunotherapy; administrative services, professional pharmacy services, care coordination, and all necessary supplies and equipment (drug and nursing visits coded separately), per diem

⊘ S9339 Home therapy; peritoneal dialysis, administrative services, professional pharmacy services, care coordination and all necessary supplies and equipment (drugs and nursing visits coded separately), per diem

⊘ S9340 Home therapy; enteral nutrition; administrative services, professional pharmacy services, care coordination, and all necessary supplies and equipment (enteral formula and nursing visits coded separately), per diem

⊘ S9341 Home therapy; enteral nutrition via gravity; administrative services, professional pharmacy services, care coordination, and all necessary supplies and equipment (enteral formula and nursing visits coded separately), per diem

⊘ S9342 Home therapy; enteral nutrition via pump; administrative services, professional pharmacy services, care coordination, and all necessary supplies and equipment (enteral formula and nursing visits coded separately), per diem

⊘ S9343 Home therapy; enteral nutrition via bolus; administrative services, professional pharmacy services, care coordination, and all necessary supplies and equipment (enteral formula and nursing visits coded separately), per diem

⊘ S9345 Home infusion therapy, anti-hemophilic agent infusion therapy (e.g. factor VIII); administrative services, professional pharmacy services, care coordination, and all necessary supplies and equipment (drugs and nursing visits coded separately), per diem

Home infusion therapy

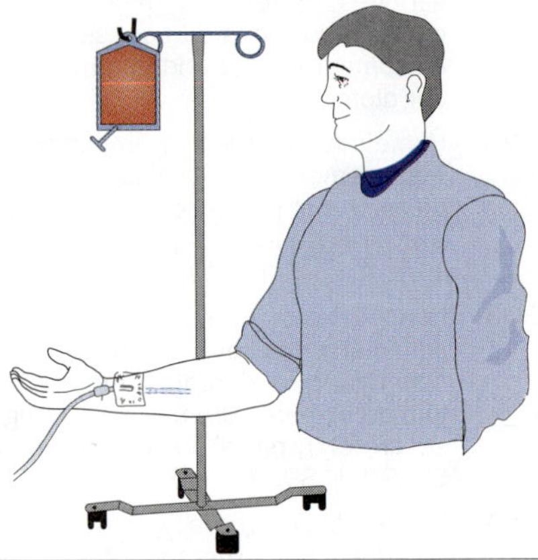

⊘ S9346 Home infusion therapy, alpha-1-proteinase inhibitor (e.g., Prolastin); administrative services, professional pharmacy services, care coordination, and all necessary supplies and equipment (drugs and nursing visits coded separately), per diem

⊘ S9347 Home infusion therapy, uninterrupted, long-term, controlled rate intravenous or subcutaneous infusion therapy (e.g. epoprostenol); administrative services, professional pharmacy services, care coordination, and all necessary supplies and equipment (drugs and nursing visits coded separately), per diem

⊘ S9348 Home infusion therapy, sympathomimetic/ inotropic agent infusion therapy (e.g., Dobutamine); administrative services, professional pharmacy services, care coordination, all necessary supplies and equipment (drugs and nursing visits coded separately), per diem

⊘ S9349 Home infusion therapy, tocolytic infusion therapy; administrative services, professional pharmacy services, care coordination, and all necessary supplies and equipment (drugs and nursing visits coded separately), per diem

⊘ S9351 Home infusion therapy, continuous or intermittent anti-emetic infusion therapy; administrative services, professional pharmacy services, care coordination, and all necessary supplies and equipment (drugs and visits coded separately), per diem

⊘ S9353 Home infusion therapy, continuous insulin infusion therapy; administrative services, professional pharmacy services, care coordination, and all necessary supplies and equipment (drugs and nursing visits coded separately), per diem

⊘ S9355 Home infusion therapy, chelation therapy; administrative services, professional pharmacy services, care coordination, and all necessary supplies and equipment (drugs and nursing visits coded separately), per diem

⊘ S9357 Home infusion therapy, enzyme replacement intravenous therapy; (e.g. Imiglucerase); administrative services, professional pharmacy services, care coordination, and all necessary supplies and equipment (drugs and nursing visits coded separately), per diem

⊘ S9359 Home infusion therapy, anti-tumor necrosis factor intravenous therapy; (e.g. Infliximab); administrative services, professional pharmacy services, care coordination, and all necessary supplies and equipment (drugs and nursing visits coded separately), per diem

⊘ S9361 Home infusion therapy, diuretic intravenous therapy; administrative services, professional pharmacy services, care coordination, and all necessary supplies and equipment (drugs and nursing visits coded separately), per diem

⊘ S9363 Home infusion therapy, anti-spasmotic therapy; administrative services, professional pharmacy services, care coordination, and all necessary supplies and equipment (drugs and nursing visits coded separately), per diem

⊘ S9364 Home infusion therapy, total parenteral nutrition (TPN); administrative services, professional pharmacy services, care coordination, and all necessary supplies and equipment including standard TPN formula (lipids, specialty amino acid formulas, drugs other than in standard formula and nursing visits coded separately), per diem (do not use with home infusion codes S9365-S9368 using daily volume scales)

⊘ S9365 Home infusion therapy, total parenteral nutrition (TPN); one liter per day, administrative services, professional pharmacy services, care coordination, and all necessary supplies and equipment including standard TPN formula (lipids, specialty amino acid formulas, drugs other than in standard formula and nursing visits coded separately), per diem

⊘ S9366 Home infusion therapy, total parenteral nutrition (TPN); more than one liter but no more than two liters per day, administrative services, professional pharmacy services, care coordination, and all necessary supplies and equipment including standard tpn formula (lipids, specialty amino acid formulas, drugs other than in standard formula and nursing visits coded separately), per diem

⊘ S9367 Home infusion therapy, total parenteral nutrition (TPN); more than two liters but no more than three liters per day, administrative services, professional pharmacy services, care coordination, and all necessary supplies and equipment including standard TPN formula (lipids, specialty amino acid formulas, drugs other than in standard formula and nursing visits coded separately), per diem

⊘ S9368 Home infusion therapy, total parenteral nutrition (TPN); more than three liters per day, administrative services, professional pharmacy services, care coordination, and all necessary supplies and equipment including standard TPN formula (lipids, specialty amino acid formulas, drugs other than in standard formula and nursing visits coded separately), per diem

⊘ S9370 Home therapy, intermittent anti-emetic injection therapy; administrative services, professional pharmacy services, care coordination, and all necessary supplies and equipment (drugs and nursing visits coded separately), per diem

⊘ S9372 Home therapy; intermittent anticoagulant injection therapy (e.g. Heparin); administrative services, professional pharmacy services, care coordination, and all necessary supplies and equipment (drugs and nursing visits coded separately), per diem (do not use this code for flushing of infusion devices with Heparin to maintain patency)

⊘ S9373 Home infusion therapy, hydration therapy; administrative services, professional pharmacy services, care coordination, and all necessary supplies and equipment (drugs and nursing visits coded separately), per diem (do not use with hydration therapy codes S9374-S9377 using daily volume scales)

⊘ S9374 Home infusion therapy, hydration therapy; one liter per day, administrative services, professional pharmacy services, care coordination, and all necessary supplies and equipment (drugs and nursing visits coded separately), per diem

⊘ S9375 Home infusion therapy, hydration therapy; more than one liter but no more than two liters per day, administrative services, professional pharmacy services, care coordination, and all necessary supplies and equipment (drugs and nursing visits coded separately), per diem

⊘ S9376 Home infusion therapy, hydration therapy; more than two liters but no more than three liters per day, administrative services, professional pharmacy services, care coordination, and all necessary supplies and equipment (drugs and nursing visits coded separately), per diem

⊘ S9377 Home infusion therapy, hydration therapy; more than three liters per day, administrative services, professional pharmacy services, care coordination, and all necessary supplies (drugs and nursing visits coded separately), per diem

⊘ S9379 Home infusion therapy, infusion therapy, not otherwise classified; administrative services, professional pharmacy services, care coordination, and all necessary supplies and equipment (drugs and nursing visits coded separately), per diem

⊘ S9381 Delivery or service to high risk areas requiring escort or extra protection, per visit

⊘ S9401 Anticoagulation clinic, inclusive of all services except laboratory tests, per session

⊘ S9430 Pharmacy compounding and dispensing services

⊘ S9433 Medical food nutritionally complete, administered orally, providing 100% of nutritional intake

⊘ S9434 Modified solid food supplements for inborn errors of metabolism

⊘ S9435 Medical foods for inborn errors of metabolism

⊘ S9436 Childbirth preparation/lamaze classes, non-physician provider, per session

⊘ S9437 Childbirth refresher classes, non-physician provider, per session

⊘ S9438 Cesarean birth classes, non-physician provider, per session

⊘ S9439 VBAC (vaginal birth after Cesarean) classes, non-physician provider, per session

⊘ S9441 Asthma education, non-physician provider, per session

⊘ S9442 Birthing classes, non-physician provider, per session

⊘ S9443 Lactation classes, non-physician provider, per session

⊘ S9444 Parenting classes, non-physician provider, per session

⊘ S9445 Patient education, not otherwise classified, non-physician provider, individual, per session

⊘ S9446 Patient education, not otherwise classified, non-physician provider, group, per session

⊘ S9447 Infant safety (including CPR) classes, non-physician provider, per session

⊘ S9449 Weight management classes, non-physician provider, per session

⊘ S9451 Exercise classes, non-physician provider, per session

⊘ S9452 Nutrition classes, non-physician provider, per session

⊘ S9453 Smoking cessation classes, non-physician provider, per session

⊘ S9454 Stress management classes, non-physician provider, per session

⊘ S9455 Diabetic management program, group session

⊘ S9460 Diabetic management program, nurse visit

⊘ S9465 Diabetic management program, dietitian visit

⊘ S9470 Nutritional counseling, dietitian visit

⊘ S9472 Cardiac rehabilitation program, non-physician provider, per diem

⊘ S9473 Pulmonary rehabilitation program, non-physician provider, per diem

⊘ S9474 Enterostomal therapy by a registered nurse certified in enterostomal therapy, per diem

⊘ S9475 Ambulatory setting substance abuse treatment or detoxification services, per diem

⊘ S9476 Vestibular rehabilitation program, non-physician provider, per diem

⊘ S9480 Intensive outpatient psychiatric services, per diem

⊘ S9482 Family stabilization services, per 15 minutes

⊘ S9484 Crisis intervention mental health services, per hour

⊘ S9485 Crisis intervention mental health services, per diem

⊘ S9490 Home infusion therapy, corticosteroid infusion; administrative services, professional pharmacy services, care coordination, and all necessary supplies and equipment (drugs and nursing visits coded separately), per diem

⊘ S9494 Home infusion therapy, antibiotic, antiviral, or antifungal therapy; administrative services, professional pharmacy services, care coordination, and all necessary supplies and equipment (drugs and nursing visits coded separately, per diem) (do not use this code with home infusion codes for hourly dosing schedules S9497-S9504)

⊘ S9497 Home infusion therapy, antibiotic, antiviral, or antifungal therapy; once every 3 hours; administrative services, professional pharmacy services, care coordination, and all necessary supplies and equipment (drugs and nursing visits coded separately), per diem

⊘ S9500 Home infusion therapy, antibiotic, antiviral, or antifungal therapy; once every 24 hours; administrative services, professional pharmacy services, care coordination, and all necessary supplies and equipment (drugs and nursing visits coded separately), per diem

⊘ S9501 Home infusion therapy, antibiotic, antiviral, or antifungal therapy; once every 12 hours; administrative services, professional pharmacy services, care coordination, and all necessary supplies and equipment (drugs and nursing visits coded separately), per diem

⊘ S9502 Home infusion therapy, antibiotic, antiviral, or antifungal therapy; once every 8 hours, administrative services, professional pharmacy services, care coordination, and all necessary supplies and equipment (drugs and nursing visits coded separately), per diem

⊘ S9503 Home infusion therapy, antibiotic, antiviral, or antifungal; once every 6 hours; administrative services, professional pharmacy services, care coordination, and all necessary supplies and equipment (drugs and nursing visits coded separately), per diem

⊘ S9504 Home infusion therapy, antibiotic, antiviral, or antifungal; once every 4 hours; administrative services, professional pharmacy services, care coordination, and all necessary supplies and equipment (drugs and nursing visits coded separately), per diem

⊘ S9529 Routine venipuncture for collection of specimen(s), single home bound, nursing home, or skilled nursing facility patient

⊘ S9537 Home therapy; hematopoietic hormone injection therapy (e.g., erythropoietin, G-CSF, GM-CSF); administrative services, professional pharmacy services, care coordination, and all necessary supplies and equipment (drugs and nursing visits coded separately), per diem

⊘ S9538 Home transfusion of blood product(s); administrative services, professional pharmacy services, care coordination and all necessary supplies and equipment (blood products, drugs, and nursing visits coded separately), per diem

⊘ S9542 Home injectable therapy, not otherwise classified, including administrative services, professional pharmacy services, care coordination, and all necessary supplies and equipment (drugs and nursing visits coded separately), per diem

⊘ S9558 Home injectable therapy; growth hormone, including administrative services, professional pharmacy services, care coordination, and all necessary supplies and equipment (drugs and nursing visits coded separately), per diem

⊘ S9559 Home injectable therapy, interferon, including administrative services, professional pharmacy services, care coordination, and all necessary supplies and equipment (drugs and nursing visits coded separately), per diem

⊘ S9560 Home injectable therapy; hormonal therapy (e.g.; leuprolide, goserelin), including administrative services, professional pharmacy services, care coordination, and all necessary supplies and equipment (drugs and nursing visits coded separately), per diem

⊘ S9562 Home injectable therapy, palivizumab, including administrative services, professional pharmacy services, care coordination, and all necessary supplies and equipment (drugs and nursing visits coded separately), per diem

⊘ S9590 Home therapy, irrigation therapy (e.g. sterile irrigation of an organ or anatomical cavity); including administrative services, professional pharmacy services, care coordination, and all necessary supplies and equipment (drugs and nursing visits coded separately), per diem

⊘ S9810 Home therapy; professional pharmacy services for provision of infusion, specialty drug administration, and/or disease state management, not otherwise classified, per hour (do not use this code with any per diem code)

⊘ S9900 Services by authorized Christian Science Practitioner for the process of healing, per diem; not to be used for rest or study; excludes in-patient services

⊘ S9970 Health club membership, annual

⊘ S9975 Transplant related lodging, meals and transportation, per diem

⊘ S9976 Lodging, per diem, not otherwise classified

⊘ S9977 Meals, per diem, not otherwise specified

⊘ S9981 Medical records copying fee, administrative

⊘ S9982 Medical records copying fee, per page

⊘ S9986 Not medically necessary service (patient is aware that service not medically necessary)

⊘ S9988 Services provided as part of a phase I clinical trial

⊘ S9989 Services provided outside of the United States of America (list in addition to code(s) for services(s))

⊘ S9990 Services provided as part of a phase II clinical trial

⊘ S9991 Services provided as part of a phase III clinical trial

⊘ S9992 Transportation costs to and from trial location and local transportation costs (e.g., fares for taxicab or bus) for clinical trial participant and one caregiver/companion

⊘ S9994 Lodging costs (e.g., hotel charges) for clinical trial participant and one caregiver/companion

⊘ S9996 Meals for clinical trial participant and one caregiver/companion

⊘ S9999 Sales tax

National Codes Established for State Medicaid Agencies T1000–T5999

⊘ T1000 Private duty/independent nursing service(s) – licensed, up to 15 minutes

⊘ T1001 Nursing assessment / evaluation

⊘ T1002 RN services, up to 15 minutes

⊘ T1003 LPN/LVN services, up to 15 minutes

⊘ T1004 Services of a qualified nursing aide, up to 15 minutes

⊘ T1005 Respite care services, up to 15 minutes

⊘ T1006 Alcohol and/or substance abuse services, family/couple counseling

⊘ T1007 Alcohol and/or substance abuse services, treatment plan development and/or modification

⊘ T1009 Child sitting services for children of the individual receiving alcohol and/or substance abuse services

⊘ T1010 Meals for individuals receiving alcohol and/or substance abuse services (when meals not included in the program)

⊘ T1012 Alcohol and/or substance abuse services, skills development

⊘ T1013 Sign language or oral interpretive services, per 15 minutes

⊘ T1014 Telehealth transmission, per minute, professional services bill separately

⊘ T1015 Clinic visit/encounter, all-inclusive

⊘ T1016 Case management, each 15 minutes

⊘ T1017 Targeted case management, each 15 minutes

⊘ T1018 School-based individualized education program (IEP) services, bundled

⊘ T1019 Personal care services, per 15 minutes, not for an inpatient or resident of a hospital, nursing facility, ICF/MR or IMD, part of the individualized plan of treatment (code may not be used to identify services provided by home health aide or certified nurse assistant)

⊘ T1020 Personal care services, per diem, not for an inpatient or resident of a hospital, nursing facility, ICF/MR or IMD, part of the individualized plan of treatment (code may not be used to identify services provided by home health aide or certified nurse assistant)

⊘ T1021 Home health aide or certified nurse assistant, per visit

⊘ T1022 Contracted home health agency services, all services provided under contract, per day

⊘ T1023 Screening to determine the appropriateness of consideration of an individual for participation in a specified program, project or treatment protocol, per encounter

⊘ T1024 Evaluation and treatment by an integrated, specialty team contracted to provide coordinated care to multiple or severely handicapped children, per encounter

⊘ T1025 Intensive, extended multidisciplinary services provided in a clinic setting to children with complex medical, physical, mental and psychosocial impairments, per diem

⊘ T1026 Intensive, extended multidisciplinary services provided in a clinic setting to children with complex medical, physical, medical and psychosocial impairments, per hour

⊘ T1027 Family training and counseling for child development, per 15 minutes

⊘ T1028 Assessment of home, physical and family environment, to determine suitability to meet patient's medical needs

⊘ T1029 Comprehensive environmental lead investigation, not including laboratory analysis, per dwelling

⊘ T1030 Nursing care, in the home, by registered nurse, per diem

⊘ T1031 Nursing care, in the home, by licensed practical nurse, per diem

⊘ T1502 Administration of oral, intramuscular and/or subcutaneous medication by health care agency/professional, per visit

⊘ T1503 Administration of medication, other than oral and/or injectable, by a health care agency/professional, per visit

● ⊘ T1505 Electronic medication compliance management device, includes all components and accessories, not otherwise classified

This code is effective January 1, 2011

⊘ T1999 Miscellaneous therapeutic items and supplies, retail purchases, not otherwise classified; identify product in "remarks"

⊘ T2001 Non-emergency transportation; patient attendant/escort

⊘ T2002 Non-emergency transportation; per diem

⊘ T2003 Non-emergency transportation; encounter/ trip

⊘ T2004 Non-emergency transport; commercial carrier, multi-pass

⊘ T2005 Non-emergency transportation; stretcher van

⊘ T2007 Transportation waiting time, air ambulance and non-emergency vehicle, one-half (1/2) hour increments

⊘ T2010 Preadmission screening and resident review (PASRR) level I identification screening, per screen

⊘ T2011 Preadmission screening and resident review (PASRR) level II evaluation, per evaluation

⊘ T2012 Habilitation, educational; waiver, per diem

⊘ T2013 Habilitation, educational, waiver; per hour

⊘ T2014 Habilitation, prevocational, waiver; per diem

⊘ T2015 Habilitation, prevocational, waiver; per hour

⊘ T2016 Habilitation, residential, waiver; per diem

⊘ T2017 Habilitation, residential, waiver; 15 minutes

⊘ T2018 Habilitation, supported employment, waiver; per diem

⊘ T2019 Habilitation, supported employment, waiver; per 15 minutes

⊘ T2020 Day habilitation, waiver; per diem

⊘ T2021 Day habilitation, waiver; per 15 minutes

⊘ T2022 Case management, per month

⊘ T2023 Targeted case management; per month

⊘ T2024 Service assessment/plan of care development, waiver

⊘ T2025 Waiver services; not otherwise specified (NOS)

⊘ T2026 Specialized childcare, waiver; per diem

⊘ T2027 Specialized childcare, waiver; per 15 minutes

⊘ T2028 Specialized supply, not otherwise specified, waiver

⊘ T2029 Specialized medical equipment, not otherwise specified, waiver

⊘ T2030 Assisted living, waiver; per month

⊘ T2031 Assisted living; waiver, per diem

⊘ T2032 Residential care, not otherwise specified (NOS), waiver; per month

⊘ T2033 Residential care, not otherwise specified (NOS), waiver; per diem

⊘ T2034 Crisis intervention, waiver; per diem

⊘ T2035 Utility services to support medical equipment and assistive technology/devices, waiver

⊘ T2036 Therapeutic camping, overnight, waiver; each session

⊘ T2037 Therapeutic camping, day, waiver; each session

⊘ T2038 Community transition, waiver; per service

⊘ T2039 Vehicle modifications, waiver; per service

⊘ T2040 Financial management, self-directed, waiver; per 15 minutes

⊘ T2041 Supports brokerage, self-directed, waiver; per 15 minutes

⊘ T2042 Hospice routine home care; per diem

⊘ T2043 Hospice continuous home care; per hour

⊘ T2044 Hospice inpatient respite care; per diem

⊘ T2045 Hospice general inpatient care; per diem

⊘ T2046 Hospice long term care, room and board only; per diem

⊘ T2048 Behavioral health; long-term care residential (non-acute care in a residential treatment program where stay is typically longer than 30 days), with room and board, per diem

⊘ T2049 Non-emergency transportation; stretcher van, mileage; per mile

⊘ T2101 Human breast milk processing, storage and distribution only

⊘ T4521 Adult sized disposable incontinence product, brief/diaper, small, each
NCD 280.1

⊘ T4522 Adult sized disposable incontinence product, brief/diaper, medium, each
NCD 280.1

⊘ T4523 Adult sized disposable incontinence product, brief/diaper, large, each
NCD 280.1

⊘ T4524 Adult sized disposable incontinence product, brief/diaper, extra large, each
NCD 280.1

⊘ T4525 Adult sized disposable incontinence product, protective underwear/pull-on, small size, each
NCD 280.1

⊘ T4526 Adult sized disposable incontinence product, protective underwear/pull-on, medium size, each
NCD 280.1

⊘ T4527 Adult sized disposable incontinence product, protective underwear/pull-on, large size, each
NCD 280.1

⊘ T4528 Adult sized disposable incontinence product, protective underwear/pull-on, extra large size, each
NCD 280.1

⊘ T4529 Pediatric sized disposable incontinence product, brief/diaper, small/medium size, each
NCD 280.1

⊘ T4530 Pediatric sized disposable incontinence product, brief/diaper, large size, each
NCD 280.1

⊘ T4531 Pediatric sized disposable incontinence product, protective underwear/pull-on, small/medium size, each
NCD 280.1

⊘ T4532 Pediatric sized disposable incontinence product, protective underwear/pull-on, large size, each
NCD 280.1

⊘ T4533 Youth sized disposable incontinence product, brief/diaper, each
NCD 280.1

⊘ T4534 Youth sized disposable incontinence product, protective underwear/pull-on, each
NCD 280.1

⊘ T4535 Disposable liner/ shield/ guard/ pad/ undergarment, for incontinence, each
NCD 280.1

⊘ T4536 Incontinence product, protective underwear/pull-on, reusable, any size, each
NCD 280.1

⊘ T4537 Incontinence product, protective underpad, reusable, bed size, each
NCD 280.1

⊘ T4538 Diaper service, reusable diaper, each diaper
NCD 280.1

⊘ T4539 Incontinence product, diaper/brief, reusable, any size, each
NCD 280.1

⊘ T4540 Incontinence product, protective underpad, reusable, chair size, each
NCD 280.1

⊘ T4541 Incontinence product, disposable underpad, large, each

⊘ T4542 Incontinence product, disposable underpad, small size, each

⊘ T4543 Disposable incontinence product, brief/diaper, bariatric, each
NCD 280.1

⊘ T5001 Positioning seat for persons with special orthopedic needs

⊘ T5999 Supply, not otherwise specified

Vision and Hearing Services V2020–V5364

Frames

- V2020 Frames, purchases
  Pub 100-02, 15, 120
- V2025 Deluxe frame
  Pub 100-04, 1, 30.3.5

Spectacle Lenses

Report with the specific lens type supply codes listed below. For aphakic temporary spectacle correction, see CPT® 92358

Single Vision, Glass or Plastic

- V2100 Sphere, single vision, plano to plus or minus 4.00, per lens
- V2101 Sphere, single vision, plus or minus 4.12 to plus or minus 7.00d, per lens
- V2102 Sphere, single vision, plus or minus 7.12 to plus or minus 20.00d, per lens
- V2103 Spherocylinder, single vision, plano to plus or minus 4.00d sphere, 0.12 to 2.00d cylinder, per lens
- V2104 Spherocylinder, single vision, plano to plus or minus 4.00d sphere, 2.12 to 4.00d cylinder, per lens
- V2105 Spherocylinder, single vision, plano to plus or minus 4.00d sphere, 4.25 to 6.00d cylinder, per lens
- V2106 Spherocylinder, single vision, plano to plus or minus 4.00d sphere, over 6.00d cylinder, per lens
- V2107 Spherocylinder, single vision, plus or minus 4.25 to plus or minus 7.00 sphere, 0.12 to 2.00d cylinder, per lens
- V2108 Spherocylinder, single vision, plus or minus 4.25d to plus or minus 7.00d sphere, 2.12 to 4.00d cylinder, per lens
- V2109 Spherocylinder, single vision, plus or minus 4.25 to plus or minus 7.00d sphere, 4.25 to 6.00d cylinder, per lens
- V2110 Spherocylinder, single vision, plus or minus 4.25 to 7.00d sphere, over 6.00d cylinder, per lens
- V2111 Spherocylinder, single vision, plus or minus 7.25 to plus or minus 12.00d sphere, 0.25 to 2.25d cylinder, per lens
- V2112 Spherocylinder, single vision, plus or minus 7.25 to plus or minus 12.00d sphere, 2.25d to 4.00d cylinder, per lens
- V2113 Spherocylinder, single vision, plus or minus 7.25 to plus or minus 12.00d sphere, 4.25 to 6.00d cylinder, per lens
- V2114 Spherocylinder, single vision, sphere over plus or minus 12.00d, per lens
- V2115 Lenticular, (myodisc), per lens, single vision
- V2118 Aniseikonic lens, single vision
- V2121 Lenticular lens, per lens, single
  Pub 100-02, 15, 120
- V2199 Not otherwise classified, single vision lens

Bifocal, Glass, or Plastic

- V2200 Sphere, bifocal, plano to plus or minus 4.00d, per lens
- V2201 Sphere, bifocal, plus or minus 4.12 to plus or minus 7.00d, per lens
- V2202 Sphere, bifocal, plus or minus 7.12 to plus or minus 20.00d, per lens
- V2203 Spherocylinder, bifocal, plano to plus or minus 4.00d sphere, 0.12 to 2.00d cylinder, per lens
- V2204 Spherocylinder, bifocal, plano to plus or minus 4.00d sphere, 2.12 to 4.00d cylinder, per lens
- V2205 Spherocylinder, bifocal, plano to plus or minus 4.00d sphere, 4.25 to 6.00d cylinder, per lens
- V2206 Spherocylinder, bifocal, plano to plus or minus 4.00d sphere, over 6.00d cylinder, per lens
- V2207 Spherocylinder, bifocal, plus or minus 4.25 to plus or minus 7.00d sphere, 0.12 to 2.00d cylinder, per lens
- V2208 Spherocylinder, bifocal, plus or minus 4.25 to plus or minus 7.00d sphere, 2.12 to 4.00d cylinder, per lens
- V2209 Spherocylinder, bifocal, plus or minus 4.25 to plus or minus 7.00d sphere, 4.25 to 6.00d cylinder, per lens
- V2210 Spherocylinder, bifocal, plus or minus 4.25 to plus or minus 7.00d sphere, over 6.00d cylinder, per lens
- V2211 Spherocylinder, bifocal, plus or minus 7.25 to plus or minus 12.00d sphere, 0.25 to 2.25d cylinder, per lens
- V2212 Spherocylinder, bifocal, plus or minus 7.25 to plus or minus 12.00d sphere, 2.25 to 4.00d cylinder, per lens
- V2213 Spherocylinder, bifocal, plus or minus 7.25 to plus or minus 12.00d sphere, 4.25 to 6.00d cylinder, per l ens
- V2214 Spherocylinder, bifocal, sphere over plus or minus 12.00d, per lens
- V2215 Lenticular (myodisc), per lens, bifocal
- V2218 Aniseikonic, per lens, bifocal
- V2219 Bifocal seg width over 28mm
- V2220 Bifocal add over 3.25d
- V2221 Lenticular lens, per lens, bifocal
  Pub 100-02, 15, 120
- V2299 Specialty bifocal (by report)

Trifocal, Glass or Plastic

- V2300 Sphere, trifocal, plano to plus or minus 4.00d, per lens
- V2301 Sphere, trifocal, plus or minus 4.12 to plus or minus 7.00d, per lens
- V2302 Sphere, trifocal, plus or minus 7.12 to plus or minus 20.00, per lens
- V2303 Spherocylinder, trifocal, plano to plus or minus 4.00d sphere, 0.12 to 2.00d cylinder, per lens
- V2304 Spherocylinder, trifocal, plano to plus or minus 4.00d sphere, 2.25 to 4.00d cylinder, per lens
- V2305 Spherocylinder, trifocal, plano to plus or minus 4.00d sphere, 4.25 to 6.00 cylinder, per lens
- V2306 Spherocylinder, trifocal, plano to plus or minus 4.00d sphere, over 6.00d cylinder, per lens
- V2307 Spherocylinder, trifocal, plus or minus 4.25 to plus or minus 7.00d sphere, 0.12 to 2.00d cylinder, per lens
- V2308 Spherocylinder, trifocal, plus or minus 4.25 to plus or minus 7.00d sphere, 2.12 to 4.00d cylinder, per lens
- V2309 Spherocylinder, trifocal, plus or minus 4.25 to plus or minus 7.00d sphere, 4.25 to 6.00d cylinder, per lens
- V2310 Spherocylinder, trifocal, plus or minus 4.25 to plus or minus 7.00d sphere, over 6.00d cylinder, per lens
- V2311 Spherocylinder, trifocal, plus or minus 7.25 to plus or minus 12.00d sphere, 0.25 to 2.25d cylinder, per lens
- V2312 Spherocylinder, trifocal, plus or minus 7.25 to plus or minus 12.00d sphere, 2.25 to 4.00d cylinder, per lens

V2313 Spherocylinder, trifocal, plus or minus 7.25 to plus or minus 12.00d sphere, 4.25 to 6.00d cylinder, per lens

V2314 Spherocylinder, trifocal, sphere over plus or minus 12 .00d, per lens

V2315 Lenticular, (myodisc), per lens, trifocal

V2318 Aniseikonic lens, trifocal

V2319 Trifocal seg width over 28 mm

V2320 Trifocal add over 3.25d

V2321 Lenticular lens, per lens, trifocal
Pub 100-02, 15, 120

V2399 Specialty trifocal (by report)

Variable Asphericity Lens, Glass, or Plastic

V2410 Variable asphericity lens, single vision, full field, glass or plastic, per lens

V2430 Variable asphericity lens, bifocal, full field, glass or plastic, per lens

V2499 Variable sphericity lens, other type

Contact Lens

Note: Record with specific lens type listed below [per lens]

V2500 Contact lens, PMMA, spherical, per lens

V2501 Contact lens, PMMA, toric or prism ballast, per lens

V2502 Contact lens PMMA, bifocal, per lens

V2503 Contact lens, PMMA, color vision deficiency, per lens

V2510 Contact lens, gas permeable, spherical, per lens

V2511 Contact lens, gas permeable, toric, prism ballast, per lens

V2512 Contact lens, gas permeable, bifocal, per lens

V2513 Contact lens, gas permeable, extended wear, per lens

V2520 Contact lens, hydrophilic, spherical, per lens
NCD 80.1, 80.4

V2521 Contact lens, hydrophilic, toric, or prism ballast, per lens
NCD 80.1, 80.4

V2522 Contact lens, hydrophillic, bifocal, per lens
NCD 80.1, 80.4

V2523 Contact lens, hydrophilic, extended wear, per lens
NCD 80.1, 80.4

V2530 Contact lens, scleral, gas impermeable, per lens (for contact lens modification, see CPT 92325)

V2531 Contact lens, scleral, gas permeable, per lens (for contact lens modification, see CPT 92325)
NCD 80.5

V2599 Contact lens, other type

Vision Aids

Note: Report with specific systems listed below

V2600 Hand held low vision aids and other nonspectacle mounted aids

V2610 Single lens spectacle mounted low vision aids

V2615 Telescopic and other compound lens system, including distance vision telescopic, near vision telescopes and compound microscopic lens system

Prosthetic Eye

V2623 Prosthetic eye, plastic, custom
Pub 100-02, 15, 130

Prosthetic eye

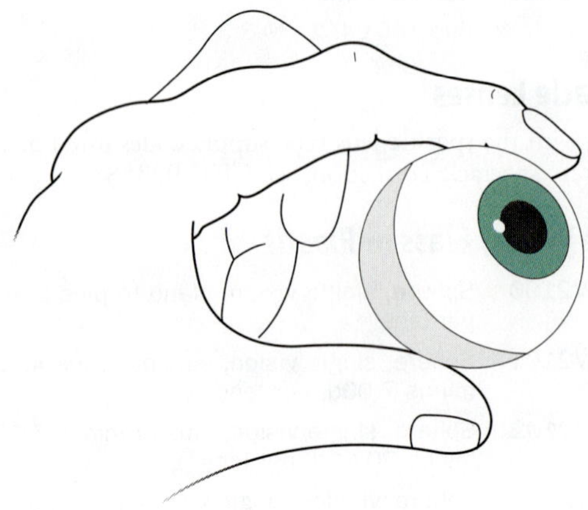

V2624 Polishing/resurfacing of ocular prosthesis

V2625 Enlargement of ocular prosthesis

V2626 Reduction of ocular prosthesis

V2627 Scleral cover shell
NCD 80.5

V2628 Fabrication and fitting of ocular conformer

V2629 Prosthetic eye, other type

Intraocular Lenses

V2630 Anterior chamber intraocular lens
Pub 100-02, 15, 120

Intraocular lens

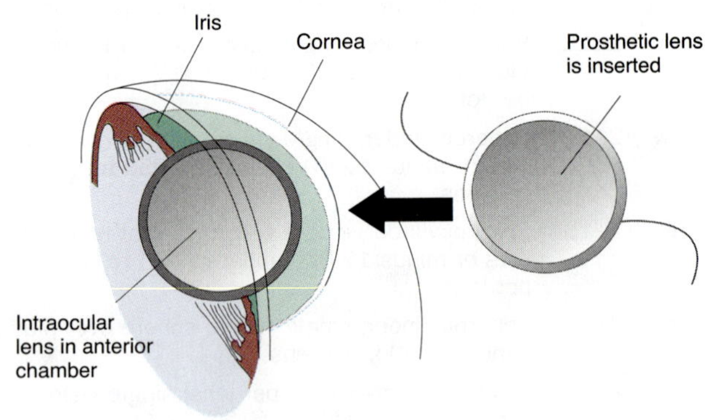

V2631 Iris supported intraocular lens
Pub 100-02, 15, 120

V2632 Posterior chamber intraocular lens
Pub 100-02, 15, 120

Miscellaneous

V2700 Balance lens, per lens

V2702 Deluxe lens feature
Pub 100-02, 15, 120

V2710 Slab off prism, glass or plastic, per lens

V2715 Prism, per lens A

V2718 Press-on lens, Fresnell prism, per lens A

V2730 Special base curve, glass or plastic, per lens A

V2744 Tint, photochromatic, per lens A
Pub 100-02, 15, 120

V2745 Addition to lens; tint, any color, solid, gradient or equal, excludes photochromatic, any lens material, per lens A
Pub 100-02, 15, 120

V2750 Anti-reflective coating, per lens A
Pub 100-02, 15, 120

V2755 UV lens, per lens A
Pub 100-02, 15, 120

V2756 Eye glass case E

V2760 Scratch resistant coating, per lens A

V2761 Mirror coating, any type, solid, gradient or equal, any lens material, per lens B
Pub 100-02, 15, 120

V2762 Polarization, any lens material, per lens A
Pub 100-02, 15, 120

V2770 Occluder lens, per lens A

V2780 Oversize lens, per lens A

V2781 Progressive lens, per lens B

V2782 Lens, index 1.54 to 1.65 plastic or 1.60 to 1.79 glass, excludes polycarbonate, per lens A
Pub 100-02, 15, 120

V2783 Lens, index greater than or equal to 1.66 plastic or greater than or equal to 1.80 glass, excludes polycarbonate, per lens A
Pub 100-02, 15, 120

V2784 Lens, polycarbonate or equal, any index, per lens A
Pub 100-02, 15, 120

V2785 Processing, preserving and transporting corneal tissue F F4

V2786 Specialty occupational multifocal lens, per lens A
Pub 100-02, 15, 120

V2787 Astigmatism correcting function of intraocular lens E
Medicare statute 1862(a)(7)

V2788 Presbyopia correcting function of intraocular lens E
Medicare Statute 1862(a)(7)

V2790 Amniotic membrane for surgical reconstruction, per procedure N N1

V2797 Vision supply, accessory and/or service component of another HCPCS vision code A

V2799 Vision service, miscellaneous A

Hearing Services

Note: These codes are not covered by Medicare. Submission of these codes to the Medicare program will result in non-payment.

V5008 Hearing screening E
Pub 100-02, 15, 80.3; Pub 100-04, 12, 30.3

V5010 Assessment for hearing aid E
Pub 100-02, 15, 80.3; Pub 100-04, 12, 30.3
Medicare Statute 1862(a)(7)

V5011 Fitting/orientation/checking of hearing aid E
Pub 100-02, 15, 80.3; Pub 100-04, 12, 30.3
Medicare Statute 1862(a)(7)

V5014 Repair/modification of a hearing aid E
Pub 100-02, 15, 80.3; Pub 100-04, 12, 30.3
Medicare Statute 1862(a)(7)

V5020 Conformity evaluation E
Pub 100-02, 15, 80.3; Pub 100-04, 12, 30.3
Medicare Statute 1862(a)(7)

V5030 Hearing aid, monaural, body worn, air conduction E
Medicare Statute 1862(a)(7)

V5040 Hearing aid, monaural, body worn, bone conduction E
Medicare Statute 1862(a)(7)

V5050 Hearing aid, monaural, in the ear E
Medicare Statute 1862(a)(7)

V5060 Hearing aid, monaural, behind the ear E
Medicare Statute 1862(a)(7)

V5070 Glasses, air conduction E
Medicare Statute 1862(a)(7)

V5080 Glasses, bone conduction E
Medicare Statute 1862(a)(7)

V5090 Dispensing fee, unspecified hearing aid E
Medicare Statute 1862(a)(7)

V5095 Semi-implantable middle ear hearing prosthesis E
Medicare Statute 1862(a)(7)

V5100 Hearing aid, bilateral, body worn E
Medicare Statute 1862(a)(7)

V5110 Dispensing fee, bilateral E
Medicare Statute 1862(a)(7)

V5120 Binaural, body E
Medicare Statute 1862(a)(7)

V5130 Binaural, in the ear E
Medicare Statute 1862(a)(7)

V5140 Binaural, behind the ear E
Medicare Statute 1862(a)(7)

V5150 Binaural, glasses E
Medicare Statute 1862(a)(7)

V5160 Dispensing fee, binaural E
Medicare Statute 1862(a)(7)

V5170 Hearing aid, CROS, in the ear E
Medicare Statute 1862(a)(7)

V5180 Hearing aid, CROS, behind the ear E
Medicare Statute 1862(a)(7)

V5190 Hearing aid, CROS, glasses E
Medicare Statute 1862(a)(7)

V5200 Dispensing fee, CROS E
Medicare Statute 1862(a)(7)

V5210 Hearing aid, BICROS, in the ear E
Medicare Statute 1862(a)(7)

V5220 Hearing aid, BICROS, behind the ear E
Medicare Statute 1862(a)(7)

V5230 Hearing aid, BICROS, glasses E
Medicare Statute 1862(a)(7)

V5240 Dispensing fee, BICROS E
Medicare Statute 1862(a)(7)

V5241 Dispensing fee, monaural hearing aid, any type E
Medicare Statute 1862(a)(7)

⊘ V5242 Hearing aid, analog, monaural, CIC (completely in the ear canal) E
Medicare Statute 1862(a)(7)

⊘ V5243 Hearing aid, analog, monaural, ITC (in the canal) E
Medicare Statute 1862(a)(7)

⊘ V5244 Hearing aid, digitally programmable analog, monaural, CIC E
Medicare Statute 1862(a)(7)

(CIC) Hearing aid

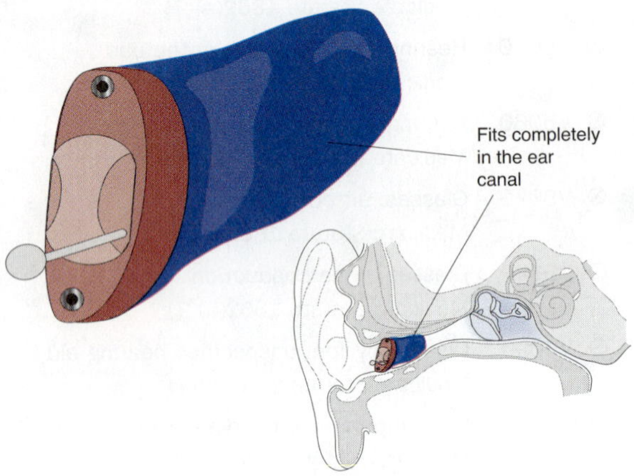

⊘ V5245 Hearing aid, digitally programmable, analog, monaural, ITC E
Medicare Statute 1862(a)(7)

⊘ V5246 Hearing aid, digitally programmable analog, monaural, ITE (in the ear) E
Medicare Statute 1862(a)(7)

⊘ V5247 Hearing aid, digitally programmable analog, monaural, BTE (behind the ear) E
Medicare Statute 1862(a)(7)

⊘ V5248 Hearing aid, analog, binaural, CIC E
Medicare Statute 1862(a)(7)

⊘ V5249 Hearing aid, analog, binaural, ITC E
Medicare Statute 1862(a)(7)

⊘ V5250 Hearing aid, digitally programmable analog, binaural, CIC E
Medicare Statute 1862(a)(7)

⊘ V5251 Hearing aid, digitally programmable analog, binaural, ITC E
Medicare Statute 1862(a)(7)

⊘ V5252 Hearing aid, digitally programmable, binaural, ITE E
Medicare Statute 1862(a)(7)

⊘ V5253 Hearing aid, digitally programmable, binaural, BTE E
Medicare Statute 1862(a)(7)

⊘ V5254 Hearing aid, digital, monaural, CIC E
Medicare Statute 1862(a)(7)

⊘ V5255 Hearing aid, digital, monaural, ITC E
Medicare Statute 1862(a)(7)

⊘ V5256 Hearing aid, digital, monaural, ITE E
Medicare Statute 1862(a)(7)

⊘ V5257 Hearing aid, digital, monaural, BTE E
Medicare Statute 1862(a)(7)

⊘ V5258 Hearing aid, digital, binaural, CIC E
Medicare Statute 1862(a)(7)

⊘ V5259 Hearing aid, digital, binaural, ITC E
Medicare Statute 1862(a)(7)

⊘ V5260 Hearing aid, digital, binaural, ITE E
Medicare Statute 1862(a)(7)

⊘ V5261 Hearing aid, digital, binaural, BTE E
Medicare Statute 1862(a)(7)

⊘ V5262 Hearing aid, disposable, any type, monaural E
Medicare Statute 1862(a)(7)

⊘ V5263 Hearing aid, disposable, any type, binaural E
Medicare Statute 1862(a)(7)

⊘ V5264 Ear mold/insert, not disposable, any type E
Medicare Statute 1862(a)(7)

⊘ V5265 Ear mold/insert, disposable, any type E
Medicare Statute 1862(a)(7)

⊘ V5266 Battery for use in hearing device E
Medicare Statute 1862(a)(7)

⊘ V5267 Hearing aid supplies / accessories E
Medicare Statute 1862(a)(7)

⊘ V5268 Assistive listening device, telephone amplifier, any type E
Medicare Statute 1862(a)(7)

⊘ V5269 Assistive listening device, alerting, any type E
Medicare Statute 1862(a)(7)

⊘ V5270 Assistive listening device, television amplifier, any type E
Medicare Statute 1862(a)(7)

⊘ V5271 Assistive listening device, television caption decoder E
Medicare Statute 1862(a)(7)

⊘ V5272 Assistive listening device, TDD E
Medicare Statute 1862(a)(7)

⊘ V5273 Assistive listening device, for use with cochlear implant E
Medicare Statute 1862(a)(7)

⊘ V5274 Assistive listening device, not otherwise specified E
Medicare Statute 1862(a)(7)

⊘ V5275 Ear impression, each E
Medicare Statute 1862(a)(7)

⊘ V5298 Hearing aid, not otherwise classified E
Medicare Statute 1862(a)(7)

ⓘ V5299 Hearing service, miscellaneous B
2320; 100-4, 12, 30.3

Speech-Language Pathology Services

⊘ V5336 Repair/modification of augmentative communicative system or device (excludes adaptive hearing aid) E
Medicare Statute 1862(a)(7)

⊘ V5362 Speech screening E
Medicare Statute 1862(a)(7)
Pub 100-04, 12, 30.3

⊘ V5363 Language screening E
Medicare Statute 1862(a)(7)
Pub 100-04, 12, 30.3

⊘ V5364 Dysphagia screening E
CFR 42CFR410.62
Pub 100-04, 12, 30.3

⊘ Medicare Non-Coverage ⓘ Special Coverage Instructions Coverage Carrier Determined A – Y APC Status Indicators ● New Code ▲ Revised Code ✖ Deleted Code
AHA AHA Coding Clinic for HCPCS A2 – Z3 ASC Payment Indicators DMEPOS ♂ Male ♀ Female PQRI PQRI

Appendix A

HCPCS Level II Modifiers

A1 Dressing for one wound
A2 Dressing for two wounds
A3 Dressing for three wounds
A4 Dressing for four wounds
A5 Dressing for five wounds
A6 Dressing for six wounds
A7 Dressing for seven wounds
A8 Dressing for eight wounds
A9 Dressing for nine or more wounds
AA Anesthesia services performed personally by anesthesiologist
AD Medical supervision by a physician: more than four concurrent anesthesia procedures
AE Registered dietician
AF Specialty physician
AG Primary physician
AH Clinical psychologist
AI Principal physician of record
AJ Clinical social worker
AK Non participating physician
AM Physician, team member service
AP Determination of refractive state was not performed in the course of diagnostic ophthalmological examination
AQ Physician providing a service in an unlisted health professional shortage area (HPSA)
AR Physician provider services in a physician scarcity area
AS Physician assistant, nurse practitioner, or clinical nurse specialist services for assistant at surgery
AT Acute treatment (this modifier should be used when reporting service CPT® 98940, 98941, 98942)
AU Item furnished in conjunction with a urological, ostomy, or tracheostomy supply
AV Item furnished in conjunction with a prosthetic device, prosthetic or orthotic
AW Item furnished in conjunction with a surgical dressing
AX Item furnished in conjunction with dialysis services
● AY Item or service furnished to an esrd patient that is not for the treatment of ESRD
● AZ Physician providing a service in a dental health professional shortage area for the purpose of an electronic health record incentive payment
BA Item furnished in conjunction with parenteral enteral nutrition (PEN) services
BL Special acquisition of blood and blood products
BO Orally administered nutrition, not by feeding tube
BP The beneficiary has been informed of the purchase and rental options and has elected to purchase the item
BR The beneficiary has been informed of the purchase and rental options and has elected to rent the item
BU The beneficiary has been informed of the purchase and rental options and after 30 days has not informed the supplier of his/her decision
CA Procedure payable only in the inpatient setting when performed emergently on an outpatient who expires prior to admission.
CB Service ordered by a renal dialysis facility (RDF) physician as part of the beneficiary's benefit, is not part of the composite rate, and is seperately reimbursable.
CC Procedure code change (use -CC when the procedure code submitted was changed either for administrative reasons or because an incorrect code was filed)
CD AMCC test has been ordered by an ESRD facility or MCP physician that is part of the composite rate and is not separately billable
CE AMCC test has been ordered by an ESRD facility or MCP physician that is a part of the composite rate, but is beyond the normal frequency covered under the rate, and is separately reimbursable based on medical necessity
CF AMCC test has been ordered by an ESRD facility or MCP physician that is not part of the composite rate and is separately billable
CG Policy criteria applied
CR Catastrophe/disaster related
● CS Item or service related, in whole or in part, to an illness, injury, or condition that was caused by or exacerbated by the effects, direct or indirect, of the 2010 oil spill in the Gulf of Mexico, including but not limited to subsequent clean-up activities
● DA Oral health assessment by a licensed health professional other than a dentist
E1 Upper left, eyelid
E2 Lower left, eyelid
E3 Upper right, eyelid
E4 Lower right, eyelid
EA Erythropoetic stimulating agent (ESA) administered to treat anemia due to anti-cancer chemotherapy
EB Erythropoetic stimulating agent (ESA) administered to treat anemia due to anti-cancer radiotherapy
EC Erythropoetic stimulating agent (ESA) administered to treat anemia not due to anti-cancer radiotherapy or anti-cancer chemotherapy
ED Hematocrit level has exceeded 39% (or hemoglobin level has exceeded 13.0 g/dL) for 3 or more consecutive billing cycles immediately prior to and including the current cycle
EE Hematocrit level has not exceeded 39% (or hemoglobin level has not exceeded 13.0 g/dL) for 3 or more consecutive billing cycles immediately prior to and including the current cycle
EJ Subsequent claims for a defined course of therapy, e.g., EPO, sodium hyaluronate, infliximab
EM Emergency reserve supply (for ESRD benefit only)
EP Service provided as part of medicaid early periodic screening diagnosis and treatment (EPSDT) program
ET Emergency services
EY No physician or other licensed health care provider order for this item or service
F1 Left hand, second digit
F2 Left hand, third digit
F3 Left hand, fourth digit
F4 Left hand, fifth digit
F5 Right hand, thumb
F6 Right hand, second digit
F7 Right hand, third digit
F8 Right hand, fourth digit

● New Modifier ▲ Revised Modifier ✖ Deleted Modifier

F9 Right hand, fifth digit
FA Left hand, thumb
FB Item provided without cost to provider, supplier or practitioner, or full credit received for replaced device (examples, but not limited to, covered under warranty, replaced due to defect, free samples)
FC Partial credit received for replaced device
FP Service provided as part of family planning program
G1 Most recent URR reading of less than 60
G2 Most recent URR reading of 60 to 64.9
G3 Most recent URR reading of 65 to 69.9
G4 Most recent URR reading of 70 to 74.9
G5 Most recent URR reading of 75 or greater
G6 ESRD patient for whom less than six dialysis sessions have been provided in a month
G7 Pregnancy resulted from rape or incest or pregnancy certified by physician as life threatening
G8 Monitored anesthesia care (MAC) for deep complex, complicated, or markedly invasive surgical procedure
G9 Monitored anesthesia care for patient who has history of severe cardio-pulmonary condition
▲ GA Waiver of liability statement issued as required by payer policy, individual case
GB Claim being re-submitted for payment because it is no longer covered under a global payment demonstration
GC This service has been performed in part by a resident under the direction of a teaching physician
GD Units of service exceeds medically unlikely edit value and represents reasonable and necessary services
GE This service has been performed by a resident without the presence of a teaching physician under the primary care exception
GF Non-physician (e.g. nurse practitioner (NP), certified registered nurse anaesthetist (CRNA), certified registered nurse (CRN), clinical nurse anaesthetist (CRNA), certified registered nurse (CRN), CLI
GG Performance and payment of a screening mammogram and diagnostic mammogram on the same patient, same day
GH Diagnostic mammogram converted from screening mammogram on same day
GJ "Opt out" physician or practitioner emergency or urgent service
GK Reasonable and necessary item/service associated with a GA or GZ modifier
GL Medically unnecessary upgrade provided instead of non-upgraded item, no charge, no advance beneficiary notice (ABN)
GM Multiple patients on one ambulance trip
GN Services delivered under an outpatient speech language pathology plan of care
GO Services delivered under an outpatient occupational therapy plan of care
GP Services delivered under an outpatient physical therapy plan of care
GQ Via asynchronous telecommunications system
GR This service was performed in whole or in part by a resident in a Department of Veterans Affairs medical center or clinic, supervised in accordance with VA policy
GS Dosage of EPO or darbepoetin alfa has been reduced and maintained in response to hematocrit or hemoglobin level
GT Via interactive audio and video telecommunication systems
● GU Waiver of liability statement issued as required by payer policy, routine notice
GV Attending physician not employed or paid under arrangement by the patient's hospice provider
GW Service not related to the hospice patient's terminal condition
● GX Notice of liability issued, voluntary under payer policy
GY Item or service statutorily excluded, does not meet the definition of any Medicare benefit or, for non-Medicare insurers, is not a contract benefit
GZ Item or service expected to be denied as not reasonable and necessary
H9 Court-ordered
HA Child/adolescent program
HB Adult program, non geriatric
HC Adult program, geriatric
HD Pregnant/parenting women's program
HE Mental health program
HF Substance abuse program
HG Opioid addiction treatment program
HH Integrated mental health/substance abuse program
HI Integrated mental health and mental retardation/developmental disabilities program
HJ Employee assistance program
HK Specialized mental health programs for high-risk populations
HL Intern
HM Less than bachelor degree level
HN Bachelors degree level
HO Masters degree level
HP Doctoral level
HQ Group setting
HR Family/couple with client present
HS Family/couple without client present
HT Multi-disciplinary team
HU Funded by child welfare agency
HV Funded state addictions agency
HW Funded by state mental health agency
HX Funded by county/local agency
HY Funded by juvenile justice agency
HZ Funded by criminal justice agency
J1 Competitive acquisition program no-pay submission for a prescription number
J2 Competitive acquisition program, restocking of emergency drugs after emergency administration
J3 Competitive acquisition program (CAP), drug not available through CAP as written, reimbursed under average sales price methodology
J4 DMEPOS item subject to DMEPOS competitive bidding program that is furnished by a hospital upon discharge
JA Administered intravenously
JB Administered subcutaneously
JC Skin substitute used as a graft
JD Skin substitute not used as a graft
JW Drug amount discarded/not administered to any patient
K0 Lower extremity prosthesis functional level 0 – does not have the ability or potential to ambulate or transfer safely with or without assistance and a prosthesis does not enhance their quality of life or mobility
K1 Lower extremity prosthesis functional level 1 – has the ability or potential to use a prosthesis for transfers or ambulation on level surfaces at fixed cadence. Typical of the limited and unlimited household ambulator.
K2 Lower extremity prosthesis functional level 2 – has the ability or potential for ambulation with the ability to traverse low level environmental barriers such as curbs, stairs or uneven surfaces. Typical of the limited community ambulator.
K3 Lower extremity prosthesis functional level 3 – has the ability or potential for ambulation with variable

cadence. Typical of the community ambulator who has the ability to transverse most environmental barriers and may have vocational, therapeutic, or exercise activity that demands prosthetic utilization beyond simple locomotion.

K4 Lower extremity prosthesis functional level 4 – has the ability or potential for prosthetic ambulation that exceeds the basic ambulation skills, exhibiting high impact, stress, or energy levels, typical of the prosthetic demands of the child, active adult, or athlete

KA Add on option/accessory for wheelchair

KB Beneficiary requested upgrade for ABN, more than 4 modifiers identified on claim

KC Replacement of special power wheelchair interface

KD Drug or biological infused through DME

KE Bid under round one of the DMEPOS competitive bidding program for use with non-competitive bid base equipment

KF Item designated by FDA as class III device

KG DMEPOS item subject to DMEPOS competitive bidding program number 1

KH DMEPOS item, initial claim, purchase or first month rental

KI DMEPOS item, second or third month rental

KJ DMEPOS item, parenteral enteral nutrition (PEN) pump or capped rental, months four to fifteen

KK DMEPOS item subject to DMEPOS competitive bidding program number 2

KL DMEPOS item delivered via mail

KM Replacement of facial prosthesis including new impression/moulage

KN Replacement of facial prosthesis using previous master model

KO Single drug unit dose formulation

KP First drug of a multiple drug unit dose formulation

KQ Second or subsequent drug of a multiple drug unit dose formulation

KR Rental item, billing for partial month

KS Glucose monitor supply for diabetic beneficiary not treated with insulin

KT Beneficiary resides in a ~~non~~competitive bidding area and travels outside that competitive bidding area and receives a competitive bid item

KU DMEPOS item subject to DMEPOS competitive bidding program number 3

KV DMEPOS item subject to DMEPOS competitive bidding program that is furnished as part of a professional service

KW DMEPOS item subject to DMEPOS competitive bidding program number 4

KX Specific required documentation on file

KY DMEPOS item subject to DMEPOS competitive bidding program number 5

KZ New coverage not implemented by managed care

LC Left circumflex coronary artery

LD Left anterior descending coronary artery

LL Lease/rental (use the -LL modifier when DME equipment rental is to be applied against the purchase price)

LR Laboratory round trip

LS FDA-monitored intraocular lens implant

LT Left side (used to identify procedures performed on the left side of the body)

M2 Medicare secondary payer (MSP)

MS Six month maintenance and servicing fee for reasonable and necessary parts and labor which are not covered under any manufacturer or supplier warranty

● NB Nebulizer system, any type, FDA-cleared for use with specific drug

NR New when rented (use the -NR modifier when DME which was new at the time of rental is subsequently purchased)

NU New equipment

P1 A normal healthy patient

P2 A patient with mild systemic disease

P3 A patient with severe systemic disease

P4 A patient with severe systemic disease that is a constant threat to life

P5 A moribund patient who is not expected to survive without the operation

P6 A declared brain-dead patient whose organs are being removed for donor purposes

PA Surgical or other invasive procedure on wrong body part

PB Surgical or other invasive procedure on wrong patient

PC Wrong surgery or other invasive procedure on patient

PI Positron emission tomography (PET) or PET/computed tomography (CT) to inform the initial treatment strategy of tumors that are biopsy proven or strongly suspected of being cancerous based on other diagnostic testing

PL Progressive addition lenses

PS Positron emission tomography (PET) or PET/computed tomography (CT) to inform the subsequent treatment strategy of cancerous tumors when the beneficiary's treating physician determines that the PET study is needed to inform subsequent anti-tumor strategy

● PT Colorectal cancer screening test; converted to diagnostic test or other procedure

Q0 Investigational clinical service provided in a clinical research study that is in an approved clinical research study

Q1 Routine clinical service provided in a clinical research study that is in an approved clinical research study

Q2 CMS/ORD demonstration project procedure/service

Q3 Live kidney donor surgery and related services

Q4 Service for ordering/referring physician qualifies as a service exemption

Q5 Service furnished by a substitute physician under a reciprocal billing arrangement

Q6 Service furnished by a locum tenens physician

Q7 One class A finding

Q8 Two class B findings

Q9 One class B and two class C findings

QC Single channel monitoring

QD Recording and storage in solid state memory by a digital recorder

QE Prescribed amount of oxygen is less than 1 liter per minute (LPM)

QF Prescribed amount of oxygen exceeds 4 liters per minute (LPM) and portable oxygen is prescribed

QG Prescribed amount of oxygen is greater than 4 liters per minute (LPM)

QH Oxygen conserving device is being used with an oxygen delivery system

QJ Services/items provided to a prisoner or patient in state or local custody, however the state or local government, as applicable, meets the requirements in 42 CFR 411.4 (B)

QK Medical direction of two, three, or four concurrent anesthesia procedures involving qualified individuals

QL Patient pronounced dead after ambulance called

QM Ambulance service provided under arrangement by a provider of services

QN Ambulance service furnished directly by a provider of services

QP Documentation is on file showing that the laboratory test(s) was ordered individually or ordered as a CPT®-recognized panel other than automated profile codes 80002-80019, G0058, G0059, and G0060.
QS Monitored anesthesia care service
QT Recording and storage on tape by an analog tape recorder
QW CLIA waived test
QX CRNA service: with medical direction by a physician
QY Medical direction of one certified registered nurse anesthetist (CRNA) by an anesthesiologist
QZ CRNA service: without medical direction by a physician
▲ RA Replacement of a DME, orthotic or prosthetic item
▲ RB Replacement of a part of a DME, orthotic or prosthetic item furnished as part of a repair
RC Right coronary artery
RD Drug provided to beneficiary, but not administered "incident-to"
RE Furnished in full compliance with FDA-mandated risk evaluation and mitigation strategy (REMS)
RR Rental (use the -RR modifier when DME is to be rented)
RT Right side (used to identify procedures performed on the right side of the body)
SA Nurse practitioner rendering service in collaboration with a physician
SB Nurse midwife
SC Medically necessary service or supply
SD Services provided by registered nurse with specialized, highly technical home infusion training
SE State and/or Federally-funded programs/services
SF Second opinion ordered by a Professional Review Organization (PRO) per Section 9401, P.l. 99-272 (100% reimbursement - no Medicare deductible or coinsurance)
SG Ambulatory Surgical Center (ASC) facility service
SH Second concurrently administered infusion therapy
SJ Third or more concurrently administered infusion therapy
SK Member of high risk population (use only with codes for immunization)
SL State supplied vaccine
SM Second surgical opinion
SN Third surgical opinion
SQ Item ordered by home health
SS Home infusion services provided in the infusion suite of the IV therapy provider
ST Related to trauma or injury
SU Procedure performed in physician's office (to denote use of facility and equipment)
SV Pharmaceuticals delivered to patient's home but not utilized
SW Services provided by a certified diabetic educator
SY Persons who are in close contact with member of high-risk population (use only with codes for immunization)
T1 Left foot, second digit
T2 Left foot, third digit
T3 Left foot, fourth digit
T4 Left foot, fifth digit
T5 Right foot, great toe
T6 Right foot, second digit
T7 Right foot, third digit
T8 Right foot, fourth digit
T9 Right foot, fifth digit
TA Left foot, great toe
TC Technical component. Under certain circumstances, a charge may be made for the technical component alone. Under those circumstances the technical component charge is identified by adding modifier TC to the usual procedure number. Technical component charges are institutional charges and not billed separately by physicians. However, portable X-ray suppliers only bill for technical component and should utilize modifier TC. The charge data from portable X-ray suppliers will then be used to build customary and prevailing profiles.
TD RN
TE LPN/LVN
TF Intermediate level of care
TG Complex/high tech level of care
TH Obstetrical treatment/services, prenatal or postpartum
TJ Program group, child and/or adolescent
TK Extra patient or passenger, non-ambulance
TL Early intervention/individualized family service plan (IFSP)
TM Individualized education program (IEP)
TN Rural/outside providers' customary service area
TP Medical transport, unloaded vehicle
TQ Basic life support transport by a volunteer ambulance provider
TR School-based individualized education program (IEP) services provided outside the public school district responsible for the student
TS Follow-up service
TT Individualized service provided to more than one patient in same setting
TU Special payment rate, overtime
TV Special payment rates, holidays/weekends
TW Back-up equipment
U1 Medicaid level of care 1, as defined by each state
U2 Medicaid level of care 2, as defined by each state
U3 Medicaid level of care 3, as defined by each state
U4 Medicaid level of care 4, as defined by each state
U5 Medicaid level of care 5, as defined by each state
U6 Medicaid level of care 6, as defined by each state
U7 Medicaid level of care 7, as defined by each state
U8 Medicaid level of care 8, as defined by each state
U9 Medicaid level of care 9, as defined by each state
UA Medicaid level of care 10, as defined by each state
UB Medicaid level of care 11, as defined by each state
UC Medicaid level of care 12, as defined by each state
UD Medicaid level of care 13, as defined by each state
UE Used durable medical equipment
UF Services provided in the morning
UG Services provided in the afternoon
UH Services provided in the evening
UJ Services provided at night
UK Services provided on behalf of the client to someone other than the client (collateral relationship)
UN Two patients served
UP Three patients served
UQ Four patients served
UR Five patients served
US Six or more patients served
▲ V5 Vascular catheter (alone or with any other vascular access)
▲ V6 Arteriovenous graft (or other vascular access not including a vascular catheter)
▲ V7 Arteriovenous fistula only (in use with two needles)
V8 Infection present
V9 No infection present
VP Aphakic patient

Appendix B

Table of Drugs

Drug Name	Additional Name(s)	Dosage	Delivery Method	HCPCS Code
A				
Abatacept	Orencia	10 mg	IM	J0129
Abbokinase	Urokinase	250,000 IU vial	IV	J3365
Abbokinase, Open Cath	Urokinase	5,000 IU vial	IV	J3364
Abciximab	ReoPro	10 mg	IV	J0130
Abelcet	Amphotericin B, lipid complex	10 mg	IV	J0287
ABLC	Amphotericin B	50 mg	IV	J0285
Abilify	Aripiprazole	0.25 mg	IM	J0400
AbobotulinumtoxinA	Dysport	5 units	IM	J0586
Abraxane	Paclitaxel protein-bound particles	1 mg	IV	J9264
Acetadote	Acetylcysteine	100 mg	IV	J0132
Acetazolamide sodium	Ak-Zol, Dazamide, Diamox, Storzolamide	up to 500 mg	IM, IV	J1120
Acetylcysteine	Acetadote, Mucomyst, Mucosil-10, Mucosil-20	100 mg per gram, unit dose form	IV INH	J0132 J7604, J7608
Achromycin	Tetracycline	up to 250 mg	IM, IV	J0120
Actemra	Tocilizumab	1mg	IV	J3262
ACTH	Corticotropin	up to 40 units	IV, IM, SC	J0800
Acthar	Corticotropin	up to 40 units	IV, IM, SC	J0800
Acthrel	Corticorelin ovine triflutate	1 mcg	IV	J0795
Actimmune	Interferon gamma 1-B	3 million units	SC	J9216
Activase	Alteplase recombinant	1 mg	IV	J2997
Acyclovir	Zovirax	5 mg	IV	J0133
Adagen	Pegademase bovine	25 IU	IM	J2504
Adalimumab	Humira	20 mg	SC	J0135
Adenocard	Adenosine	6 mg 30 mg	IV IV	J0150 J0152
Adenoscan	Adenosine	6 mg 30 mg	IV IV	J0150 J0152
Adenosine	Adenocard, Adenoscan	6 mg 30 mg	IV IV	J0150 J0152
Adrenalin chloride	Adrenalin, epinephrine	up to 1 ml ampule	IV, IM, SC	J0170
Adrenalin, epinephrine	Adrenalin chloride, Bronkaid Mist, EpiPen, Primatene Mist, Sus-Phrine	up to 1 ml ampule	IV, IM, SC	J0171
Adriamycin PFS	Doxorubicin HCl	10 mg	IV	J9000
Adriamycin RDF	Doxorubicin HCl	10 mg	IV	J9000
Adrucil	Fluorouracil	500 mg	IV	J9190
Advate	Factor VIII (antihemophiliac factor, recombinant)	per IU	IV	J7192
AeroBid	Flunisolide	per mg	INH	J7641
AeroBid-M	Flunisolide	per mg	INH	J7641
Agalsidase beta	Fabrazyme	1 mg	IV	J0180
Aggrastat	Tirofiban hydrochloride	0.25 mg	IM, IV	J3246
A-hydroCort	Hydrocortisone sodium succinate	up to 50 mg	IV, IM, SC	J1710
Ak-Zol	Acetazolamide sodium	up to 500 mg	IM, IV	J1120
Akineton	Biperiden lactate	per 5 mg	IM, IV	J0190
Alatrofloxacin mesylate	Trovan IV	100 mg	IV	J0200
Albuterol, compounded	Proventil, Ventolin	1 mg, concentrated dose, via DME 1 mg, unit dose, via DME	INH INH	J7609 J7610
Albuterol, all formulations including separated isomers, non-compounded	Proventil, Ventolin	1 mg, concentrated dose, via DME 1 mg, unit dose, via DME	INH INH	J7611 J7613
Albuterol, ipratropium bromide	Combivent, DuoNeb	up to 2.5 mg (albuterol) and up to 0.5 mg (ipratropium bromide)	INH	J7620
Aldesleukin	Proleukin	per single use vial	IM, IV	J9015
Aldomet	Methyldopate HCl	up to 250 mg	IV	J0210
Aldurazyme	Laronidase	0.1 mg	IV	J1931
Alefacept	Amevive	.5 mg	IM	J0215
Alemtuzumab	Campath	10 mg	IV	J9010
Alferon N	Interferon alfa-N3 (human leukocyte derived)	250,000 IU	IM	J9215
Alglucerase	Ceredase	per 10 units	IV	J0205
Alglucosidase alfa	Myozyme Lumizyme	10 mg 1 mg	IV IM	J0220 C9277
Alimta	Pemetrexed	10 mg	IV	J9305
Alkaban-AQ	Vinblastine sulfate	1 mg	IV	J9360
Alkeran	Melphalan, oral	2 mg	ORAL	J8600
Alkeran	Melphalan HCl	50 mg	IV	J9245
AllerMax Caplets	Diphenhydramine HCl	50 mg	ORAL	Q0163
Aller-med	Diphenhydramine HCl	50 mg	ORAL	Q0163
Aloxi	Palonosetron HCl	25 mcg	IV	J2469
Alpha 1-proteinase inhibitor, human	Aralast, Prolastin	10 mg	IV	J0256
Alphanate	Factor VIII (antihemophilic factor, human)	per IU	IV	J7190
AlphanNine SD	Factor IX	per IU	IV	J7193-J7195
Alprostadil	Caverject, Edex, Prostin VR Pediatric	1.25 mcg	IV	J0270
Alprostadil, urethral suppository	Muse	per dose	OTH	J0275

IA – intraarterial IM – intramuscular INH – inhalation IT – intrathecal IV – intravenous OTH – other SC – subcutaneous VAR – various administration methods

Table of Drugs

Drug Name	Additional Name(s)	Dosage	Delivery Method	HCPCS Code
Alteplase recombinant	Activase	1 mg	IV	J2997
Alupent	Metaproterenol sulfate	per 10 mg, concentrated form per 10 mg, unit dose form	INH INH	J7667, J7668 J7669, J7670
AmBisome	Amphotericin B, liposomal	10 mg	IV	J0289
Amcort	Triamcinolone diacetate	per 5 mg	IM	J3302
Amen	Medroxyprogesterone acetate	50 mg 150 mg, for contraceptive use	IM IM	J1051 J1055
A-methaPred	Methylprednisolone sodium phosphate	up to 40 mg up to 125 mg	IM, IV IM, IV	J2920 J2930
Amevive	Alefacept	.5 mg	IM	J0215
Amgen	Interferon alphacon-1, recombinant	1 mcg	IM	J9212
Amicar	Aminocaproic acid	5 g	IV	S0017
Amifostine	Ethyol, Ethiofos, Gammaphos, WR-2721	500 mg	IV	J0207
Amikacin sulfate	Amikin	100 mg	IM, IV	J0278
Amikin	Amikacin sulfate	100 mg	IM, IV	J0278
Aminocaproic acid	Amicar	5 g	IV	S0017
Aminolevalinic acid HCl	Levulan Kerastick	20%, single unit dosage form (354 mg)	OTH (TOPICAL)	J7308
Aminophylline	Phyllocontin, Theophylline ethylenadiamine, Truphylline	up to 250 mg	IV	J0280
Amiodarone HCl	Cordarone	30 mg	IV	J0282
Amitriptyline HCl	Elavil, Endep, Enovil	up to 20 mg	IM	J1320
Amobarbital	Amytal	up to 125 mg	IM, IV	J0300
Amphadase	Hyaluronidase	up to 150 units	IV, SC	J3470
Amphocin	Amphotericin B	50 mg	IV	J0285
Amphotec	Amphotericin B, cholesteryl sulfate complex	10 mg	IV	J0288
Amphotericin B	ABLC, Amphocin, Fungizone	50 mg	IV	J0285
Amphotericin B, cholesteryl sulfate complex	Amphotec	10 mg	IV	J0288
Amphotericin B, lipid complex	Abelcet	10 mg	IV	J0287
Amphotericin B, liposomal	AmBisome	10 mg	IV	J0289
Ampicillin sodium	Omnipen-N, Polycillin-N, Principen, Totacillin-N	500 mg	IM, IV	J0290
Ampicillin sodium/ sulbactam sodium	Unasyn	per 1.5 gm	IM, IV	J0295
Amygdalin, vitamin B-17	Laetrile		VAR	J3570
Amytal	Amobarbital	up to 125 mg	IM, IV	J0300
Anabolin LA 100	Nandrolone decanoate	up to 50 mg	IM	J2320
Anaspaz	Hyoscyamine sulfate	up to 0.25 mg	SC, IM, IV	J1980
Anastrozole	Arimidex	1 mg	ORAL	S0170
Ancef	Cefazolin sodium	500 mg	IV, IM	J0690
Andrest 90-4	Testosterone enanthate and estradiol valerate	up to 1 cc	IM	J0900
Andro-Cyp	Testosterone cypionate	up to 100 mg	IM	J1070
Andro-Cyp 200	Testosterone cypionate	1 cc, 200 mg	IM	J1080
Andro L.A. 200	Testosterone enanthate	up to 200 mg	IM	J3130
Andro-Estro 90-4	Testosterone enanthate and estradiol valerate	up to 1 cc	IM	J0900
Andro/Fem	Testosterone cypionate and estradiol cypionate	up to 1 ml	IM	J1060
Androgyn L.A.	Testosterone enanthate and estradiol valerate	up to 1 cc	IM	J0900
Androlone-D 100	Nandrolone decanoate	up to 50 mg	IM	J2320
Andronaq-50	Testosterone suspension	up to 50 mg	IM	J3140
Andronaq-LA	Testosterone cypionate	up to 100 mg	IM	J1070
Andronate-100	Testosterone cypionate	up to 100 mg	IM	J1070
Andronate-200	Testosterone cypionate	1 cc, 200 mg	IM	J1080
Andropository 100	Testosterone enanthate	up to 100 mg	IM	J3120
Andryl 200	Testosterone enanthate	up to 200 mg	IM	J3130
AN-DTPA	Technetium Tc-99m pentetate	up to 25 mCi	IV	A9539
Anectine	Succinylcholine chloride	up to 20 mg	IV, IM	J0330
Anectine Flo-Pack	Succinylcholine chloride	up to 20 mg	IV, IM	J0330
Anergan 50	Promethazine HCl	up to 50 mg 12.5 mg 25 mg	IM, IV ORAL ORAL	J2550 Q0169 Q0170
Angiomax	Bivalirudin	1 mg	IV	J0583
Angiox	Bivalirudin	1 mg	IV	J0583
Anidulafungin	Eraxis	1 mg	IM	J0348
Anistreplase	Eminase	per 30 units	IV	J0350
Antiemetic drug		per dose	ORAL	J8597
Antiemetic drug, rectal/suppository		per dose	OTH	J8498
Antiflex	Orphenadrine citrate	up to 60 mg	IV, IM	J2360
Anti-Inhibitor coagulant complex	Autoplex T, Feiba VH Immuno	per IU	IV	J7198
Antispas	Dicyclomine HCl	up to 20 mg	IM	J0500
Antithrombin III (human)	Thrombate III	per IU	IV	J7197
Antithrombin recombinant	ATryn	50 IU	IV	J7196
Antizol	Fomepizole	15 mg	IV	J1451
Anucort-HC	Hydrocortisone acetate	up to 25 mg	IV, IM, SC	J1700
Anusol-HC	Hydrocortisone acetate	up to 25 mg	IV, IM, SC	J1700

IA – intraarterial IM – intramuscular INH – inhalation IT – intrathecal IV – intravenous OTH – other SC – subcutaneous VAR – various administration methods

Drug Name	Additional Name(s)	Dosage	Delivery Method	HCPCS Code
Anzemet	Dolasetron mesylate	10 mg 50 mg 100 mg	IV ORAL ORAL	J1260 S0174 Q0180
A.P.L.	Chorionic gonadotropin	per 1,000 USP units	IM	J0725
Apokyn	Apomorphine HCl	1 mg	IM	J0364
Apomorphine HCl	Apokyn	1 mg	IM	J0364
Aprepitant	Emend	5 mg	ORAL	J8501
Apresoline	Hydralazine HCl	up to 20 mg	IV, IM	J0360
Aprotinin	Trasylol	10,000 KIU	IV	J0365
AquaMEPHYTON	Phytonadione (Vitamin K)	per 1 mg	IM, SC, IV	J3430
Aralast	Alpha 1-proteinase inhibitor, human	10 mg	IV	J0256
Aralen HCl	Chloroquine HCl	up to 250 mg	IM	J0390
Aramine	Metaraminol bitartrate	per 10 mg	IV, IM, SC	J0380
Aranesp	Darbepoetin alfa	1 mcg	IV, SC	J0881-J0882
Arbutamine HCl	GenESA	1 mg	IV	J0395
Arcalyst	rilonacept	1 mg	SC	J2793
Aredia	Pamidronate disodium	per 30 mg	IV	J2430
Arformoterol tartrate	Brovana	15 mcg	INH	J7605
Arimidex	Anastrozole	1 mg	ORAL	S0170
Aripiprazole	Abilify	0.25 mg	IM	J0400
Aristocort Forte	Triamcinolone diacetate	per 5 mg	IM	J3302
Aristocort Intralesional	Triamcinolone diacetate	per 5 mg	IM	J3302
Aristospan Intra-Articular	Triamcinolone hexacetonide	per 5 mg	VAR	J3303
Aristospan Intralesional	Triamcinolone hexacetonide	per 5 mg	VAR	J3303
Arixtra	Fondaparinux sodium	0.5 mg	SC	J1652
Arm-a-Med	Isoetharine HCl	per mg, concentrated form per mg, unit dose form	INH INH	J7647-J7648 J7649-J7650
Arranon	Nelarabine	50 mg	IM	J9261
Arrestin	Trimethobenzamide HCl	up to 200 mg 250 mg	IM ORAL	J3250 Q0173
Arsenic trioxide	Trisenox	1 mg	IV	J9017
Aromasin	Exemestane	25 mg	ORAL	S0156
Arzerra	Ofatumumab	10 mg	IV	J9302
Asparaginase	Elspar	10,000 units	IM, IV	J9020
A-Spas	Dicyclomine HCl	up to 20 mg	IM	J0500
Astramorph PF	Morphine sulfate	per 10 mg	IM, IV, SC	J7725
Atarax	Hydroxyzine HCl	up to 25 mg	IM	J3410
Atgam	Lymphocyte immune globulin, anti-thymocyte globulin, equine, parenteral	250 mg	IV	J7504
Ativan	Lorazepam	2 mg	IM, IV	J2060
Atropine		per mg, concentrated form per mg, unit dose form	INH INH	J7635 J7636
Atropine sulfate	Sabex, Hospira	.01 mg	IV, IM, SC	J0461
Atrovent	Ipratropium bromide	per mg, unit dose form	INH	J7644, J7645
ATryn	Antithrombin recombitant	50 IU	IV	J7196
Aurothioglucose	Solganal	up to 50 mg	IM	J2910
Autologous cultured chondrocytes, implant	Carticel		OTH	J7330
Autoplex T	Anti-inhibitor coagulant complex	per IU	IV	J7198
Avastin	Bevacizumab	10 mg	IV	J9035
Avelox	Moxifloxacin	100 mg	IV	J2280
Avonex	Interferon beta-1a	11 mcg 11 mcg 33 mcg	IM SC IM	Q3025 Q3026 J1825
Azacitidine	Vidaza	1 mg	SC	J9025
Azactam	Aztreonam	500 mg per gram	IM, IV INH	S0073 S0143
Azasan	Azathioprine	50 mg 100 mg	ORAL IV	J7500 J7501
Azathioprine	Azasan, Imuran	50 mg 100 mg	ORAL IV	J7500 J7501
Azithromycin	Zithromax	500 mg	IV	J0456
Azithromycin dihydrate	Zithromax	1 gm	ORAL	Q0144
Azmacort	Triamcinolone	per 1 mg, concentrated form per 1 mg, unit dose form	INH INH	J7683 J7684
Aztreonam	Azactam	500 mg per gram	IM, IV INH	S0073 S0143
B				
Baclofen	Lioresal	10 mg 50 mcg, for intrathecal trial	IT IT	J0475 J0476
Baclofen Intrathecal Refill Kit		10 mg	IT	J0475
Baclofen Intrathecal Screening Kit		50 mcg	IT	J0476
Bactocill	Oxacillin sodium	up to 250 mg	IM, IV	J2700
Bactrim IV	Sulfamethoxazole and trimethoprim	10 ml	IV	S0039
BAL in oil	Dimercaprol	per 100 mg	IM	J0470
Banflex	Orphenadrine citrate	up to 60 mg	IV, IM	J2360
Banophen	Diphenhydramine HCl	up to 50 mg 50 mg	IV, IM ORAL	J1200 Q0163
Basiliximab	Simulect	20 mg	IV	J0480
BayTet	Tetanus immune globulin, human	up to 250 units	IM	J1670
Bebulin VH	Factor IX	per IU	IV	J7193-J7195
BCG (Bacillus Calmette and Guérin), live	TheraCys, TICE BCG	per vial	INTRAVESICAL INSTILLATION	J9031
Becaplermin gel, 0.01%	Regranex Gel	0.5 gm	OTH	S0157
Beclomethasone	Beclovent, Beconase, Qvar, Vanceril, Vancenase	per mg, unit dose form	INH	J7622
Beclovent	Beclomethasone	per mg, unit dose form	INH	J7622

Table of Drugs

IA – intraarterial IM – intramuscular INH – inhalation IT – intrathecal IV – intravenous OTH – other SC – subcutaneous VAR – various administration methods

Drug Name	Additional Name(s)	Dosage	Delivery Method	HCPCS Code
Beconase	Beclomethasone	per mg, unit dose form	INH	J7622
Bena-D 10	Diphenhydramine HCl	up to 50 mg 50 mg	IV, IM ORAL	J1200 Q0163
Bena-D 50	Diphenhydramine HCl	up to 50 mg 50 mg	IV, IM ORAL	J1200 Q0163
Benadryl	Diphenhydramine HCl	up to 50 mg 50 mg	IV, IM ORAL	J1200 Q0163
Benadryl Allergy	Diphenhydramine HCl	up to 50 mg 50 mg	IV, IM ORAL	J1200 Q0163
Benahist 10	Diphenhydramine HCl	up to 50 mg 50 mg	IV, IM ORAL	J1200 Q0163
Benahist 50	Diphenhydramine HCl	up to 50 mg 50 mg	IV, IM ORAL	J1200 Q0163
Ben-Allergin-50	Diphenhydramine HCl	up to 50 mg 50 mg	IV, IM ORAL	J1200 Q0163
Bendamustine	Treanda, Ribomustin	1 mg	IV	J9033
Benefix	Factor IX, recombinant	per IU	IV	J7193-J7195
Benoject-10	Diphenhydramine HCl	up to 50 mg 50 mg	IV, IM ORAL	J1200 Q0163
Benoject-50	Diphenhydramine HCl	up to 50 mg 50 mg	IV, IM ORAL	J1200 Q0163
Bentyl	Dicyclomine HCl	up to 20 mg	IM	J0500
Benztropine mesylate	Cogentin	per 1 mg	IM, IV	J0515
Benylin Cough	Diphenhydramine HCl	up to 50 mg 50 mg	IV, IM ORAL	J1200 Q0163
Berinert	C-1 esterase inhibitor (human)	10 units	IV	J0597
Berubigen	Vitamin B-12 cyanocobalamin	up to 1,000 mcg	IM, SC	J3420
Beta-2	Isoetharine HCl	per mg, concentrated form per mg, unit dose form	INH INH	J7647, J7648 J7649, J7650
Betalin 12	Vitamin B-12 cyanocobalamin	up to 1,000 mcg	IM, SC	J3420
Betamethasone		per mg, unit dose form	INH	J7624
Betamethasone acetate & betamethasone sodium phosphate	Celestone soluspan	3 mg	IM	J0702
Betaseron	Interferon beta-1B, recombinant	0.25 mg	SC	J1830
Bethanechol chloride	Duvoid, Mytonachol, Urabeth, Urecholine	up to 5 mg	SC	J0520
Bexxar	Iodine I-131 tositumomab	per treatment dose	IV	A9545
Bevacizumab	Avastin	10 mg	IV	J9035
Bicillin C-R 900/300	Penicillin G benzathine and penicillin G procaine	2,500 units	IM	J0559
Bicillin L-A	Penicillin G benzathine	up to 600,000 units up to 1,200,000 units up to 2,400,000 units	IM IM IM	J0560 J0570 J0580
BiCNU	Carmustine	100 mg	IV	J9050
Bioclate	Factor VIII (antihemophilic factor, recombinant)	per IU	IV	J7192
Biperiden lactate	Akineton	per 5 mg	IM, IV	J0190
Bitolterol mesylate	Tornalate	per mg, concentrated form per mg, unit dose form	INH INH	J7628 J7629
Bivalirudin	Angiomax, Angiox	1 mg	IV	J0583
Blenoxane	Bleomycin sulfate	15 units	IM, IV, SC	J9040
Bleomycin sulfate	Blenoxane	15 units	IM, IV, SC	J9040
Boniva	Ibandronate sodium	1 mg	IM	J1740
Bortezomib	Velcade	0.1 mg	IV	J9041
Botox /Botox cosmetic	onabotulimtoxinA	per unit	IM	J0585
Botulinum toxin type B	Myobloc	per 100 units	IM	J0587
Bravelle	Urofollitropin	75 IU	IM, SC	J3355
Brethaire	Terbutaline sulfate	per 1 mg, concentrated form per 1 mg, unit dose form	INH INH	J7680 J7681
Brethine	Terbutaline sulfate	up to 1 mg	SC, IV	J3105
Bricanyl	Terbutaline sulfate	up to 1 mg	SC, IV	J3105
Bricanyl Turbuhaler	Terbutaline sulfate	per 1 mg, concentrated form per 1 mg, unit dose form	INH INH	J7680 J7681
Brodspec	Tetracycline	up to 250 mg	IM, IV	J0120
Brompheniramine maleate	Codimal-A, Cophene B, Dehist, Histaject, Nasahist B, ND Stat, Oraminic II, Sinusol-B	per 10 mg	IM, SC, IV	J0945
Bronkaid Mist	Epinephrine, adrenaline	up to 1 ml ampule	IV, IM, SC	J0170
Bronkometer	Isoetharine HCl	per mg, concentrated form per mg, unit dose form	INH INH	J7647, J7648 J7649, J7650
Bronkosol	Isoetharine HCl	per mg, concentrated form per mg, unit dose form	INH INH	J7647, J7648 J7649, J7650
Brovana	Arformoterol tartrate	15 mcg	INH	J7605
Budesonide, compounded	Pulmicort Respules, Pulmicort Turbuhaler, Rhinocort Aqua	up to 0.5 mg unit dose form per 0.25 mg	INH INH	J7626, J7627 J7633, J7634
Budesonide, non-compounded	Pulmicort Respules, Pulmicort Turbuhaler, Rhinocort Aqua	up to 0.5 mg unit dose form	INH	J7626
Bumetanide	Bumex	0.5 mg	IV, IM	S0171
Bumex	Bumetanide	0.5 mg	IV, IM	S0171
Bupivicaine HCl	Marcaine, Sensorcaine	30 ml	IV	S0020
Buprenex	Buprenorphine hydrochloride	0.1 mg	IM, IV	J0592
Buprenorphine hydrochloride	Buprenex	0.1 mg	IM, IV	J0592

IA – intraarterial IM – intramuscular INH – inhalation IT – intrathecal IV – intravenous OTH – other SC – subcutaneous VAR – various administration methods

Drug Name	Additional Name(s)	Dosage	Delivery Method	HCPCS Code
Busulfan	Busulfex, Myleran	1 mg 2 mg	IV ORAL	J0594 J8510
Busulfex	Busulfan	1 mg 2 mg	IV ORAL	J0594 J8510
Butorphanol tartrate, injection	Stadol	1 mg	IM	J0595
Butorphanol tartrate, nasal spray	Stadol NS	25 mg	NASAL SPRAY	S0012
Byclomine	Dicyclomine HCl	up to 20 mg	IM	J0500
C				
C1 esterase inhibitor	Berinert Cinryze	10 units	IV, IM, SC	J0597 J0598
Cabazitaxel	Jevtana	1 mg	IM	C9276
Cabergoline	Dostinex	0.25 mg	ORAL	J8515
Cafcit	Caffeine citrate	5 mg	IV	J0706
Caffeine citrate	Cafcit	5 mg	IV	J0706
Caine-1	Lidocaine HCl	10 mg	IV	J2001
Caine-2	Lidocaine HCl	10 mg	IV	J2001
Calcijex	Calcitriol	0.1 mcg	IM	J0636
Calcimar	Calcitonin-salmon	up to 400 units	SC, IM	J0630
Calciparine	Heparin sodium	per 1,000 units	IV, SC	J1644
Calcitonin-salmon	Calcimar, Miacalcin	up to 400 units	SC, IM	J0630
Calcitriol	Calcijex, Rocaltrol	0.1 mcg	IM	J0636
Calcium disodium versenate	Edetate calcium disodium	up to 1,000 mg	IV, SC, IM	J0600
Calcium EDTA	Edetate calcium disodium	up to 1,000 mg	IV, SC, IM	J0600
Calcium gluconate	Kaleinate	per 10 ml	IV	J0610
Calcium glycerophosphate & calcium lactate	Calphosan	per 10 ml	IM, SC	J0620
Calcium lactate & calcium glycerophosphate	Calphosan	per 10 ml	IM, SC	J0620
Caldor	Ibuprofen	100 mg	IM	C9279
Calphosan	Calcium glycerophosphate and calcium lactate	per 10 ml	IM, SC	J0620
Campath	Alemtuzumab	10 mg	IV	J9010
Camptosar	Irinotecan HCl	20 mg	IV	J9206
Cancidas	Caspofungin acetate	5 mg	IV	J0637
Canakinumab	Ilaris	1 mg	IM	J0638
Capecitabine	Xeloda	150 mg 500 mg	ORAL ORAL	J8520 J8521
Capsaicin patch	Qutenza	per 10 sq cm	OTH	J7335
Carbocaine	Mepivacaine HCl	per 10 ml	VAR	J0670
Carboplatin	Paraplatin	50 mg	IV	J9045
Cardiogen-82	Rubidium Rb-82	up to 60 mCi	IV	A9555
Cardiolite	Technetium Tc-99m sestamibi	up to 40 millicuries	IV	A9500
Carmustine	BiCNU	100 mg	IV	J9050
Carnitor	Levocarnitine	per 1 gm	IV	J1955
Carticel	Autologous cultured chondrocytes, implant		OTH	J7330
Caspofungin acetate	Cancidas	5 mg	IV	J0637
Catapres	Clonidine HCl	1 mg	IT	J0735
Caverject	Alprostadil	1.25 mcg	IV	J0270
CeeNu	Lomustine	10 mg	ORAL	S0178
Cefadyl	Cephapirin Sodium	up to 1 g	IV, IM	J0710
Cefazolin sodium	Ancef, Kefzol, Zolicef	500 mg	IV, IM	J0690
Cefepime hydrochloride	Maxiprime	500 mg	IV	J0692
Cefizox	Ceftizoxime sodium	per 500 mg	IV, IM	J0715
Cefobid	Cefoperazone sodium	1 g	IV, IM	S0021
Cefoperazone sodium	Cefobid	1 g	IV, IM	S0021
Cefotan	Cefotetan disodium	500 mg	IV, IM	S0074
Cefotaxime sodium	Claforan	per 1 g	IV, IM	J0698
Cefotetan disodium	Cefotan	500 mg	IV, IM	S0074
Cefoxitin sodium	Mefoxin	1 g	IV, IM	J0694
Ceftazidime	Ceptaz, Fortaz, Tazicef, Tazidime	per 500 mg	IM, IV	J0713
Ceftin	Cefuroxime sodium, sterile	per 750 mg	IM, IV	J0697
Ceftizoxime sodium	Cefizox	per 500 mg	IV, IM	J0715
Ceftriaxone sodium	Rocephin	per 250 mg	IV, IM	J0696
Cefuroxime sodium, sterile	Ceftin, Kefurox, Zinacef	per 750 mg	IM, IV	J0697
Celestone soluspan	Betamethasone acetate and betamethasone sodium phosphate	3 mg	IM	J0702
CellCept	Mycophenolate mofetil	250 mg	ORAL	J7517
Cenacort A-40	Triamcinolone acetonide	per 10 mg	IM	J3301
Cenacort Forte	Triamcinolone diacetate	per 5 mg	IM	J3302
Cenestin	Estrogen, conjugated	per 25 mg	IV, IM	J1410
Cephalothin sodium	Keflin	up to 1 g	IM, IV	J1890
Cephapirin sodium	Cefadyl	up to 1 g	IV, IM	J0710
Ceprotin	Protein C concentrate, human	10 iu	IV	J2724
Ceptaz	Ceftazidime	per 500 mg	IM, IV	J0713
Cerebyx	Fosphenytoin sodium	750 mg	IV, IM	S0078
Cerebyx	Fosphenytoin	50 mg	IV, IM	Q2009
Ceredase	Alglucerase	per 10 units	IV	J0205
Cerespan	Papaverine HCl	up to 60 mg	IV, IM	J2440
Ceretec	Technetium Tc-99m exametazime	up to 25 millicuries	IV	A9521
Cerezyme	Imiglucerase	per unit	IV	J1785
Certolizumab pegol	Cimzia	1 mg	SC	J0718
Cerubidine	Daunorubicin HCl	10 mg	IV	J9150
Cesamet	Nabilone	1 mg	ORAL	J8650
Cetuximab	Erbitux	10 mg	IV	J9055
Chealamide	Endrate ethylenediamine-tetra-acetic acid	per 150 mg	IV	J3520
Chlorambucil	Leukeran	2 mg	ORAL	S0172
Chloramphenicol sodium succinate	Chloromycetin	up to 1 g	IV	J0720
Chlordiazepoxide HCl	Librax, Librium, Limbitrol	up to 100 mg	IM, IV	J1990
Chloromycetin	Chloramphenicol sodium succinate	up to 1 g	IV	J0720
Chloroprocaine HCl	Nesacaine, Nesacaine-MPF	per 30 ml	VAR	J2400
Chloroquine HCl	Aralen HCl	up to 250 mg	IM	J0390
Chlorothiazide sodium	Diuril Sodium	per 500 mg	IV	J1205

Table of Drugs

IA – intraarterial IM – intramuscular INH – inhalation IT – intrathecal IV – intravenous OTH – other SC – subcutaneous VAR – various administration methods

Drug Name	Additional Name(s)	Dosage	Delivery Method	HCPCS Code
Chlorpromazine HCl	Ormazine, Thorazine	10 mg 25 mg up to 50 mg	ORAL ORAL IM, IV	Q0171 Q0172 J3230
Choletec	Technetium Tc-99m mebrofenin	up to 15 mCi	IV	A9537
Chorex-5	Chorionic gonadotropin	per 1,000 USP units	IM	J0725
Chorex-10	Chorionic gonadotropin	per 1,000 USP units	IM	J0725
Chorignon	Chorionic gonadotropin	per 1,000 USP units	IM	J0725
Chorionic gonadotropin	A.P.L., Chorex-5, Chorex-10, Chorignon, Choron 10, Corgonject-5, Follutein, Gonic, Novarel, Pregnyl, Profasi	per 1,000 USP units	IM	J0725
Choron 10	Chorionic gonadotropin	per 1,000 USP units	IM	J0725
Chromic phosphate P-32	Phosphocol P 32	per mCi	OTH	A9564
Chromitope	Chromium Cr-51 sodium chromate	up to 250 μCi	IV	A9553
Chromium Cr-51 sodium chromate	Chromitope	up to 250 μCi	IV	A9553
Cidofovir	Vistide	375 mg	IV	J0740
Cilastatin sodium, imipenem	Primaxin IM, Primaxin IV	per 250 mg	IV, IM	J0743
Cimetidine hydrochloride	Tagamet	300 mg	IV, IM	S0023
Cimzia	Certolizumab pegol	1 mg	SC	J0718
Cinryze	C1 esterase inhibitor	10 units	IV, IM, SC	J0598
Cipro IV	Ciprofloxacin	200 mg	IV	J0744
Ciprofloxacin	Cipro IV	200 mg	IV	J0744
CIS-MDP	Technetium Tc-99m medronate	up to 30 millicuries	IV	A9503
Cisplatin	Platinol AQ	per 10 mg	IV	J9060
Cladribine	Leustatin	per 1 mg	IV	J9065
Claforan	Cefotaxime sodium	per g	IV, IM	J0698
Cleocin phosphate	Clindamycin phosphate	300 mg	IM, IV	S0077
Clindamycin phosphate	Cleocin phosphate	300 mg	IM, IV	S0077
Clofarabine	Clolar	1 mg	IV	J9027
Clolar	Clofarabine	1 mg	IV	J9027
Clonidine hydrochloride	Catapres, Duracion, Duraclon	1 mg	IT	J0735
Cobalt Co-57 cyanocobalamin	Rubratope-57	up to 1 μCi	ORAL	A9559
Cobex	Vitamin B-12 cyanocobalamin	up to 1,000 mcg	IM, SC	J3420
Codeine phosphate		per 30 mg	IM, IV, SC	J0745
Codimal-A	Brompheniramine maleate	per 10 mg	IM, SC, IV	J0945
Cofatrim Forte	Sulfamethoxazole and trimethoprim	10 ml	IV	S0039
Cogentin	Benztropine mesylate	per 1 mg	IM, IV	J0515
Cognex	Tacrine hydrochloride	10 mg	ORAL	S0014
Colchicine		per 1 mg	IV	J0760
Colistimethate sodium	Coly-Mycin M	up to 150 mg per mg	IM, IV INH	J0770 S0142

Drug Name	Additional Name(s)	Dosage	Delivery Method	HCPCS Code
Collagenase, clostridium histolyticum	Xiaflex	0.01 mg	IM	J0775
Coly-Mycin M	Colistimethate sodium	up to 150 per mg	IM, IV INH	J0770 S0142
Combivent	Albuterol, ipratropium bromide	up to 2.5 mg (albuterol) and up to 0.5 mg (ipratropium bromide)	INH	J7620
Compa-Z	Prochlorperazine	up to 10 mg	IM, IV	J0780
Compazine	Prochlorperazine	up to 10 mg	IM, IV	J0780
Compazine	Prochlorperazine maleate	5 mg 10 mg	ORAL ORAL	Q0164 Q0165
Compoz	Diphenhydramine HCl	50 mg	ORAL	Q0163
Copaxone	Glatiramer acetate	20 mg	SC	J1595
Cophene-B	Brompheniramine maleate	per 10 mg	IM, SC, IV	J0945
Copper contraceptive, intrauterine	ParaGard, Paragarel T380A		OTH	J7300
Cordarone	Amiodarone HCl	30 mg	IV	J0282
Corgonject-5	Chorionic gonadotropin	per 1,000 USP units	IM	J0725
Cortastat	Dexamethasone sodium phosphate	1 mg	IM, IV, OTH	J1100
Cortastat L.A.	Dexamethasone acetate	1 mg	IM	J1094
Corticorelin ovine triflutate	Acthrel	1 mcg	IV	J0795
Corticotropin	Acthar, ACTH	up to 40 units	IV, IM, SC	J0800
Cortifoam	Hydrocortisone acetate	up to 25 mg	IV, IM, SC	J1700
Cortrosyn	Cosyntropin	per 0.25 mg	IM, IV	J0833, J0834
Corvert	Ibutilide fumarate	1 mg	IV	J1742
Cosmegen	Dactinomycin	0.5 mg	IV	J9120
Cosyntropin	Cortrosyn	per 0.25 mg	IM, IV	J0833, J0834
Cotranzine	Prochlorperazine	up to 10 mg	IM, IV	J0780
Cotrim	Sulfamethoxazole and trimethoprim	10 ml	IV	S0039
Cromolyn sodium	Gastrocrom, Intal inhaler, Intal nebulizer solution, Nasalcrom	per 10 mg, unit dose form	INH	J7631- J7632
Crystamine	Vitamin B-12 cyanocobalamin	up to 1,000 mcg	IM, SC	J3420
Crysticillin 300 A.S.	Penicillin G procaine, aqueous	up to 600,000 units	IM, IV	J2510
Crysticillin 600 A.S.	Penicillin G procaine, aqueous	up to 600,000 units	IM, IV	J2510
Cubicin	Daptomycin	1 mg	IV	J0878
Cyanoject	Vitamin B-12 cyanocobalamin	up to 1,000 mcg	IM, SC	J3420
Cyclophosphamide	Cytoxan, Neosar	25 mg 100 mg	ORAL IV	J8530 J9070
Cyclophosphamide, oral	Cytoxan	25 mg	ORAL	J8530
Cyclosporine	Gengraf, Neoral, Sandimmune, SangCya	25 mg 100 mg 250 mg	ORAL ORAL IV	J7515 J7502 J7516

IA – intraarterial IM – intramuscular INH – inhalation IT – intrathecal IV – intravenous OTH – other SC – subcutaneous VAR – various administration methods

Drug Name	Additional Name(s)	Dosage	Delivery Method	HCPCS Code
Cycrin	Medroxyprogesterone acetate	50 mg 150 mg, for contraceptive use	IM IM	J1051 J1055
Cyomin	Vitamin B-12 cyanocobalamin	up to 1,000 mcg	IM, SC	J3420
Cysview	hexaminolevulinate hydrochloride	100 mg	OTH	C9275
Cystospaz	Hyoscyamine sulfate	up to 0.25 mg	SC, IM, IV	J1980
Cystospaz-M	Hyoscyamine sulfate	up to 0.25 mg	SC, IM, IV	J1980
Cytarabine	Cytosar-U	100 mg	SC, IV	J9100
Cytarabine liposome	DepoCyt	10 mg		J9098
CytoGam	Cytomegalovirus immune globulin intravenous (human)	per vial	IV	J0850
Cytomegalovirus immune globulin intravenous (human)	CytoGam	per vial	IV	J0850
Cytosar-U	Cytarabine	100 mg	SC, IV	J9100
Cytotec	Misoprostol	200 mcg	ORAL	S0191
Cytovene IV	Ganciclovir sodium	500 mg	IV	J1570
Cytoxan	Cyclophosphamide	25 mg 100 mg	ORAL IV	J8530 J9070
D				
D.H.E. 45	Dihydroergotamine mesylate	per 1 mg	IM, IV	J1110
D-5-W, Dextrose 5% in water, infusion		1,000 cc	IV	J7070
Dacarbazine	DTIC-Dome	100 mg	IV	J9130
Daclizumab	Zenapax	25 mg	IV	J7513
Dacogen	Decitabine	1 mg	IM	J0894
Dactinomycin	Cosmegen	0.5 mg	IV	J9120
Dalalone	Dexamethasone sodium phosphate	1 mg	IM, IV, OTH	J1100
Dalalone D.P.	Dexamethasone acetate	1 mg	IM	J1094
Dalalone L.A.	Dexamethasone acetate	1 mg	IM	J1094
Dalcaine	Lidocaine HCl	10 mg	IV	J2001
Dalteparin sodium	Fragmin	per 2,500 IU	SC	J1645
Daptomycin	Cubicin	1 mg	IV	J0878
Darbepoetin alfa, for ESRD on dialysis	Aranesp	1 mcg	IV, SC	J0882
Darbepoetin alfa, non-ESRD use	Aranesp	1 mcg	IV, SC	J0881
Daunorubicin citrate, liposomal formulation	DaunoXome	10 mg	IV	J9151
Daunorubicin HCl	Cerubidine	10 mg	IV	J9150
DaunoXome	Daunorubicin citrate, liposome formula	10 mg	IV	J9151
Dazamide	Acetazolamide sodium	up to 500 mg	IM, IV	J1120
DDAVP	Desmopressin acetate	1 mcg	IV, SC	J2597
Decadron	Dexamethasone	0.25 mg per mg, concentrated form per mg, unit dose form	ORAL INH INH	J8540 J7637 J7638
Decadron-LA	Dexamethasone acetate	1 mg	IM	J1094
Decadron phosphate	Dexamethasone sodium phosphate	1 mg	IM, IV, OTH	J1100
Deca-Durabolin	Nandrolone decanoate	up to 50 mg	IM	J2320
Decaject	Dexamethasone sodium phosphate	1 mg	IM, IV, OTH	J1100
Decaject-L.A.	Dexamethasone acetate	1 mg	IM	J1094
Decitabine	Dacogen	1 mg	IM	J0894
Decolone-50	Nandrolone decanoate	up to 50 mg	IM	J2320
Decolone-100	Nandrolone decanoate	up to 50 mg	IM	J2320
De-Comberol	Testosterone cypionate and estradiol cypionate	up to 1 ml	IM	J1060
Deferoxamine mesylate	Desferal	500 mg	IM, SC, IV	J0895
Definity	Perflutren lipid microsphere	per ml	IV	Q9957
Degarelix	Firmagon	1 mg	SC	J9155
Dehist	Brompheniramine maleate	per 10 mg	IM, SC, IV	J0945
Deladumone	Testosterone enanthate and estradiol valerate	up to 1 cc	IM	J0900
Deladumone OB	Testosterone enanthate and estradiol valerate	up to 1 cc	IM	J0900
Delatest	Testosterone enanthate	up to 100 mg	IM	J3120
Delatestadiol	Testosterone enanthate and estradiol valerate	up to 1 cc	IM	J0900
Delatestryl	Testosterone enanthate	up to 200 mg	IM	J3130
Delestrogen	Estradiol valerate	up to 10 mg up to 20 mg up to 40 mg	IM IM IM	J1380 J1390 J0970
Delta-Cortef	Prednisolone	per 5 mg	ORAL	J7510
Deltasone	Prednisone	per 5 mg	ORAL	J7506
Demadex	Torsemide	10 mg/ml	IV	J3265
Demerol	Meperidine HCl	per 100 mg	IM, IV, SC	J2175
Denileukin diftitox	Ontak	300 mcg		J9160
Denosumab	Prolia	1 mg	IM	C9272
DepAndro 100	Testosterone cypionate	up to 100 mg	IM	J1070
DepAndro 200	Testosterone cypionate	1 cc, 200 mg	IM	J1080
DepAndrogyn	Testosterone cypionate and estradiol cypionate	up to 1 ml	IM	J1060
DepGynogen	Estradiol cypionate	up to 5 mg	IM	J1000
DepMedalone 40	Methylprednisolone acetate	40 mg	IM	J1030
DepMedalone 80	Methylprednisolone acetate	80 mg	IM	J1040
DepoCyt	Cytarabine liposome	10 mg		J9098
Depo-estradiol cypionate	Estra-D, Estradiol cypionate, Estro-Cyp, Estroject L.A.	up to 5 mg	IM	J1000
Depogen	Estradiol cypionate	up to 5 mg	IM	J1000

IA – intraarterial IM – intramuscular INH – inhalation IT – intrathecal IV – intravenous OTH – other SC – subcutaneous VAR – various administration methods

Drug Name	Additional Name(s)	Dosage	Delivery Method	HCPCS Code
Depoject	Methyprednisolone acetate	20 mg 40 mg 80 mg	IM IM IM	J1020 J1030 J1040
Depo-Medrol	Methylprednisolone acetate	20 mg 40 mg 80 mg	IM IM IM	J1020 J1030 J1040
Depopred-40	Methylprednisolone acetate	20 mg 40 mg 80 mg	IM IM IM	J1020 J1030 J1040
Depopred-80	Methylprednisolone acetate	20 mg 40 mg 80 mg	IM IM IM	J1020 J1030 J1040
Depo-Provera	Medroxyprogesterone acetate	50 mg 150 mg, for contraceptive use	IM IM	J1051 J1055
Depotest	Testosterone cypionate	up to 100 mg 1 cc, 200 mcg	IM IM	J1070 J1080
Depo-Testadiol	Testosterone cypionate and estradiol cypionate	up to 1 ml	IM	J1060
Depotestogen	Testosterone cypionate and estradiol cypionate	up to 1 ml	IM	J1060
Depo-Testosterone	Testosterone cypionate	up to 100 mg 1 cc, 200 mg	IM IM	J1070 J1080
Desferal	Deferoxamine mesylate	500 mg	IM, SC, IV	J0895
Desmopressin acetate	DDAVP	1 mcg	IV, SC	J2597
Dexacen-4	Dexamethasone sodium phosphate	1 mg	IM, IV, OTH	J1100
Dexacen LA-8	Dexamethasone acetate	1 mg	IM	J1094
Dexacort Turbinaire	Dexamethasone	per mg, unit dose form	INH	J7638
Dexameth	Dexamethasone	0.25 mg per mg, concentrated form per mg, unit dose form	ORAL INH INH	J8540 J7637 J7638
Dexamethasone	Decadron, Dexameth, Dexacort Turbinaire, Dexone, Hexadrol	0.25 mg per mg, concentrated form per mg, unit dose form	ORAL INH INH	J8540 J7637 J7638
Dexamethasone acetate	Cortastat L.A., Dalalone D.P., Dalalone L.A., Decadron - L.A., Decaject - L.A., Dexacen LA-8, Dexasone L.A., Dexone L.A., Solurex L.A.	1 mg	IM	J1094
Dexamethasone intravitreal implant	Ozurdex	0.1 mg	OTH	J7312
Dexamethasone sodium phosphate	Cortastat, Dalalone, Decadron Phosphate, Decaject, Dexacen-4, Dexasone, Hexadrol Phosphate, Solurex	1 mg	IM, IV, OTH	J1100
Dexasone	Dexamethasone sodium phosphate	1 mg	IM, IV, OTH	J1100
Dexasone L.A.	Dexamethasone acetate	1 mg	IM	J1094
Dexone	Dexamethasone	0.25 mg per mg, concentrated form per mg, unit dose form	ORAL INH INH	J8540 J7637 J7638
Dexone L.A.	Dexamethasone acetate	1 mg	IM	J1094
Dexrazoxane hydrochloride	Zinecard	per 250 mg	IV	J1190
Dextran 40	Gentran 40, 10% LMD, Rheomacrodex	500 ml	IV	J7100
Dextran 75	Gentran 75	500 ml	IV	J7110
Dextrose 5%/45% normal saline with potassium chloride & magnesium sulfate		1,000 ml 1,500 ml	IV IV	S5013 S5014
Dextrose 5% and normal saline 45%		1,000 ml	IV	S5010
Dextrose 5% in lactated ringer's		1,000 ml	IV	S5011
Dextrose 5% with potassium chloride		1,000 ml	IV	S5012
Dextrose 5%/normal saline solution		500 ml = 1 unit	IV	J7042
Dextrose/water 5%		500 ml = 1 unit	IV	J7060
Dey-Lute	Isoetharine HCl	per mg, concentrated form per mg, unit dose form	INH INH	J7647, J7648 J7649, J7650
Diamox	Acetazolamide sodium	up to 500 mg	IM, IV	J1120
Diastat	Diazepam	up to 5 mg	IM, IV	J3360
Diazepam	Diastat, Diazepam Intensol, Valium, Zetran	up to 5 mg	IM, IV	J3360
Diazepam Intensol	Diazepam	up to 5 mg	IM, IV	J3360
Diazoxide	Hyperstat IV	up to 300 mg	IV	J1730
Dibent	Dicyclomine HCl	up to 20 mg	IM	J0500
Dicyclomine HCl	Antispas, A-Spas, Bentyl, Byclomine, Dibent, Dilomine, Di-Spaz, Or-Tyl, Spasmoject	up to 20 mg	IM	J0500
Didronel	Etidronate disodium	per 300 mg	IV	J1436
Diethylstilbestrol diphosphate	Stilphostrol	250 mg	IV	J9165
Diflucan	Fluconazole	200 mg	IV	J1450
Digibind	Digoxin immune fab (ovine)	per vial	IV	J1162
DigiFab	Digoxin immune fab (ovine)	per vial	IV	J1162
Digoxin	Lanoxin	up to 0.5 mg	IM, IV	J1160
Digoxin immune fab (ovine)	Digibind, DigiFab	per vial	IV	J1162
Dihydrex	Diphenhydramine HCl	up to 50 mg 50 mg	IV, IM ORAL	J1200 Q0163
Dihydroergotamine mesylate	D.H.E. 45, Migranal	per 1 mg	IM, IV	J1110
Dilantin	Phenytoin sodium	per 50 mg	IM, IV	J1165

IA – intraarterial IM – intramuscular INH – inhalation IT – intrathecal IV – intravenous OTH – other SC – subcutaneous VAR – various administration methods

Drug Name	Additional Name(s)	Dosage	Delivery Method	HCPCS Code
Dilaudid	Hydromorphone	up to 4 mg	IM, IV, SC	J1170
Dilaudid	Hydromorphone HCl	250 mg	LOADING DOSE FOR INFUSION PUMP	S0092
Dilaudid-5	Hydromorphone HCl	250 mg	LOADING DOSE FOR INFUSION PUMP	S0092
Dilaudid-HP	Hydromorphone HCl	250 mg	LOADING DOSE FOR INFUSION PUMP	S0092
Dilocaine	Lidocaine HCl	10 mg	IV	J2001
Dilomine	Dicyclomine HCl	up to 20 mg	IM	J0500
Dilor	Dyphylline	up to 500 mg	IM	J1180
Dimenhydrinate	Dinate, Dramamine, Dramanate, Dramilin, Dramocen, Dramoject, Dymenate, Hydrate, Marmine, Wehamine	up to 50 mg	IM, IV	J1240
Dimercaprol	BAL in oil	per 100 mg	IM	J0470
Dimethyl sulfoxide, DMSO, 50%	Rimso	50 ml	OTH	J1212
Dinate	Dimenhydrinate	up to 50 mg	IM, IV	J1240
Dioval	Estradiol valerate	up to 10 mg up to 20 mg up to 40 mg	IM IM IM	J1380 J1390 J0970
Dioval 40	Estradiol valerate	up to 10 mg up to 20 mg up to 40 mg	IM IM IM	J1380 J1390 J0970
Dioval XX	Estradiol valerate	up to 10 mg up to 20 mg up to 40 mg	IM IM IM	J1380 J1390 J0970
Diphenacen-50	Diphenhydramine HCl	up to 50 mg 50 mg	IV, IM ORAL	J1200 Q0163
Diphenadryl	Diphenhydramine HCl	up to 50 mg 50 mg	IV, IM ORAL	J1200 Q0163
Diphen Cough	Diphenhydramine HCl	50 mg	ORAL	Q0163
Diphenhist	Diphenhydramine HCl	up to 50 mg 50 mg	IV, IM ORAL	J1200 Q0163
Diphenhydramine HCl	AllerMax Caplets, Aller-med Banophen, Bena-D 10, Bena-D 50, Benadryl, Benadryl Allergy, Benahist 10, Benahist 50, Ben-Allergin-50, Benoject-10, Benoject-50, Benylin Cough, Compoz, Dihydrex, Diphenacen-50, Diphenadryl, Diphen Cough, Diphenhist, Dormarex, Genahist, Hydramine, Hyrexin-50, Nervine Nighttime Sleep-Aid, Nordryl Cough, Nytol, Siladryl, Sleep-Eze D, Sominex, Twilite Caplets, Unisom SleepGels, Wehdryl	up to 50 mg 50 mg	IV, IM ORAL	J1200 Q0163
Dipyridamole	Persantine	per 10 mg	IV	J1245
Disodium EDTA	Edetate disodium	per 150 mg	IV	J3520
Disotate	Endrate ethylenediamine-tetra-acetic acid	per 150 mg	IV	J3520
Di-Spaz	Dicyclomine HCl	up to 20 mg	IM	J0500
Ditate-DS	Testosterone enanthate and estradiol valerate	up to 1 cc	IM	J0900
Diuril sodium	Chlorothiazide sodium	per 500 mg	IV	J1205
D-Med 80	Methylprednisolone acetate	20 mg 40 mg 80 mg	IM IM IM	J1020 J1030 J1040
DMSO, Dimethyl sulfoxide, 50%	Rimso 50	50%, 50 ml	OTH	J1212
Dobutamine HCl	Dobutrex	per 250 mg	IV	J1250
Dobutrex	Dobutamine HCl	per 250 mg	IV	J1250
Docetaxel	Taxotere	1 mg	IV	J9171
Dolasetron mesylate	Anzemet	10 mg 50 mg 100 mg	IV ORAL ORAL	J1260 S0174 Q0180
Dolophine	Methadone HCl	up to 10 mg	IM, SC	J1230
Dormarex	Diphenhydramine HCl	50 mg	ORAL	Q0163
Dopamine HCl	Dopastat, Intropin	40 mg	IV	J1265
Dopastat	Dopamine HCl	40 mg	IV	J1265
Doribax	Doripenem	10 mg	IM	J1267
Doripenem	Doribax	10 mg	IM	J1267
Dornase alpha	Pulmozyme	per mg, unit dose form	INH	J7639
Dostinex	Cabergoline	0.25 mg	ORAL	J8515
Doxercalciferol	Hectorol	1 mcg	IV	J1270
Doxil	Doxorubicin HCl, all lipid formulations	10 mg	IV	J9001
Doxorubicin HCl	Adriamycin PFS or RDF, Rubex	10 mg	IV	J9000
Doxorubicin HCl, all lipid formulations	Doxil	10 mg	IV	J9001
Dramamine	Dimenhydrinate	up to 50 mg	IM, IV	J1240
Dramanate	Dimenhydrinate	up to 50 mg	IM, IV	J1240
Dramilin	Dimenhydrinate	up to 50 mg	IM, IV	J1240
Dramocen	Dimenhydrinate	up to 50 mg	IM, IV	J1240
Dramoject	Dimenhydrinate	up to 50 mg	IM, IV	J1240
Dronabinol	Marinol	2.5 mg 5 mg	ORAL ORAL	Q0167 Q0168
Droperidol	Inapsine	up to 5 mg	IM, IV	J1790
Droperidol and fentanyl citrate	Innovar	up to 2 ml ampule	IM, IV	J1810
Droxia	Hydroxyurea	500 mg	ORAL	S0176
Drug administered through a metered dose inhaler			INH	J3535
DTIC-Dome	Dacarbazine	100 mg	IV	J9130
Dua-Gen L.A.	Testosterone enanthate and estradiol valerate cypionate	up to 1 cc	IM	J0900
Duo-Cyp	Testosterone cypionate and estradiol cypionate	up to 1 ml	IM	J1060
DuoNeb	Albuterol, ipratropium bromide	up to 2.5 mg (albuterol) and up to 0.5 mg (ipratropium bromide)	INH	J7620

IA – intraarterial IM – intramuscular INH – inhalation IT – intrathecal IV – intravenous OTH – other SC – subcutaneous VAR – various administration methods

Drug Name	Additional Name(s)	Dosage	Delivery Method	HCPCS Code
Duoval P.A.	Testosterone enanthate and estradiol valerate	up to 1 cc	IM	J0900
Duracion	Clonidine hydrochloride	1 mg	IT	J0735
Duraclon	Clonidine hydrochloride	1 mg	IT	J0735
Duracillin A.S.	Penicillin G procaine, aqueous	up to 600,000 units	IM, IV	J2510
Dura-Estrin	Testosterone cypionate and estradiol cypionate	up to 1 ml	IM	J1060
Duragen-10	Estradiol valerate	up to 10 mg up to 20 mg up to 40 mg	IM IM IM	J1380 J1390 J0970
Duragen-20	Estradiol valerate	up to 10 mg up to 20 mg up to 40 mg	IM IM IM	J1380 J1390 J0970
Duragen-40	Estradiol valerate	up to 10 mg up to 20 mg up to 40 mg	IM IM IM	J1380 J1390 J0970
Duralone-40	Methylprednisolone acetate	40 mg	IM	J1030
Duralone-80	Methylprednisolone acetate	80 mg	IM	J1040
Duramorph	Morphine sulfate	500 mg up to 10 mg 100 mg	LOADING DOSE FOR INFUSION PUMP IM, IV, SC IM, IV, SC	S0093 J2270 J2271
Duratest-100	Testosterone cypionate	up to 100 mg	IM	J1070
Duratest-200	Testosterone cypionate	1 cc, 200 mg	IM	J1080
Duratestrin	Testosterone cypionate and estradiol cypionate	up to 1 ml	IM	J1060
Durathate-200	Testosterone enanthate	up to 200 mg	IM	J3130
Duvoid	Bethanechol chloride	up to 5 mg	SC	J0520
Dymenate	Dimenhydrinate	up to 50 mg	IM, IV	J1240
Dyphylline	Lufyllin, Dilor	up to 500 mg	IM	J1180
Dysport	AbobotulinumtoxinA	5 units	IM	J0586
E				
Ecallantide	Kalbitor	1 mg	SC	J1290
Eculizumab	Soliris	10 mg	IV	J1300
Edetate calcium disodium	Calcium disodium versenate, Calcium EDTA	up to 1,000 mg	IV, SC, IM	J0600
Edetate disodium	Chealamide, Endrate ethylenediamine-tetra-acetic acid, Disodium EDTA, Disotate, Endrate	per 150 mg	IV	J3520
Edex	Alprostadil	1.25 mcg	IV	J0270
Elaprase	Idursulfase	1 mg	IV	J1743
Elavil	Amitriptyline HCl	up to 20 mg	IM	J1320
Eligard	Leuprolide acetate	1 mg 3.75 mg 7.5 mg	SC, IV IM, IV IM, IV	J9218 J1950 J9217
Elitek	Rasburicase	0.5 mg	IV	J2783
Ellence	Epirubicin HCl	2 mg	IV	J9178
Elliotts' B solution		1 ml	INTRATHECAL	J9175
Eloxatin	Oxaliplatin	0.5 mg	IV	J9263
Elspar	Asparaginase	10,000 units	IV, IM	J9020
Emend	Aprepitant Fosaprepitant	5 mg 1 mg	ORAL IM	J8501 J1453
Eminase	Anistreplase	per 30 units	IV	J0350
Enbrel	Etanercept	25 mg	IM, IV	J1438
Endep	Amitriptyline HCl	up to 20 mg	IM	J1320
Endrate	Edetate disodium	per 150 mg	IV	J3520
Endrate ethylenediamine-tetra-acetic acid	Chealamide, Disotate, Edetate disodium	per 150 mg	IV	J3520
Enfuvirtide	Fuzeon	1 mg	IM	J1324
Enovil	Amitriptyline HCl	up to 20 mg	IM	J1320
Enoxaparin sodium	Lovenox	10 mg	SC	J1650
Epinephrine, adrenalin	Bronkaid Mist, Primatene Mist	up to 1 ml ampule	SC, IM, IV	J0170
EpiPen	Adrenalin, epinephrine	up to 1 ml ampule	IV, IM, SC	J0170
Epirubicin hydrochloride	Ellence	2 mg	IV	J9178
Epoetin alfa, for ESRD on dialysis	Epogen, Procrit	100 units 1,000 units	IV, SC IV, SC	Q4081 J0886
Epoetin alfa, for non-ESRD use	Epogen, Procrit	1,000 units	IV, SC	J0885
Epogen	Epoetin alfa	100 units 1,000 units	IV, SC IV, SC	Q4081 J0885-J0886
Epoprostenol	Flolan	0.5 mg	IV	J1325
Eptifibatide	Integrilin	5 mg	IM, IV	J1327
Eraxis	Anidulafungin	1 mg	IM	J0348
Erbitux	Cetuximab	10 mg	IV	J9055
Ergamisol	Levamisole hydrochloride	50 mg	ORAL	S0177
Ergonovine maleate	Ergotrate	up to 0.2 mg	IM, IV	J1330
Ergotrate	Ergonovine maleate	up to 0.2 mg	IM, IV	J1330
Ertapenem sodium	Invanz	500 mg	IV, IM	J1335
Erythrocin	Erythromycin lactobionate	per 500 mg	IV	J1364
Erythromycin lactobionate	Erythrocin	per 500 mg	IV	J1364
Estra-D	Depo-estradiol cypionate	up to 5 mg	IM	J1000
Estra-L 20	Estradiol valerate	up to 10 mg up to 20 mg up to 40 mg	IM IM IM	J1380 J1390 J0970
Estra-L 40	Estradiol valerate	up to 10 mg up to 20 mg up to 40 mg	IM IM IM	J1380 J1390 J0970
Estra-Testrin	Testosterone enanthate and estradiol valerate	up to 1 cc	IM	J0900
Estradiol cypionate	Depo-estradiol cypionate, DepGynogen, Depogen	up to 5 mg	IM	J1000
Estradiol L.A.	Estradiol valerate	up to 10 mg up to 20 mg up to 40 mg	IM IM IM	J1380 J1390 J0970
Estradiol L.A. 20	Estradiol valerate	up to 10 mg up to 20 mg up to 40 mg	IM IM IM	J1380 J1390 J0970
Estradiol L.A. 40	Estradiol valerate	up to 10 mg up to 20 mg up to 40 mg	IM IM IM	J1380 J1390 J0970

IA – intraarterial IM – intramuscular INH – inhalation IT – intrathecal IV – intravenous OTH – other SC – subcutaneous VAR – various administration methods

Drug Name	Additional Name(s)	Dosage	Delivery Method	HCPCS Code
Estradiol valerate	Dioval, Dioval 40, Dioval XX, Delestrogen, Duragen-10, Duragen-20, Duragen-40, Estra-L 20, Estra-L 40, Estradiol L.A., Estradiol L.A. 20, Estradiol L.A. 40, Gynogen L.A., L.A.E. 20, Valergen 10, Valergen 20, Valergen 40	up to 10 mg	IM	J1380
Estragyn 5	Estrone	per 1 mg	IM	J1435
Estro-Cyp	Depo-estradiol cypionate	up to 5 mg	IM	J1000
Estrogen, conjugated	Cenestin, Premarin	per 25 mg	IV, IM	J1410
Estroject L.A.	Depo-estradiol cypionate	up to 5 mg	IM	J1000
Estrone	Estragyn 5, Estrone Aqueous, Estrone 5, Estronol, Kestrone 5, Theelin Aqueous	per 1 mg	IM	J1435
Estrone 5	Estrone	per 1 mg	IM	J1435
Estrone Aqueous	Estrone	per 1 mg	IM	J1435
Estronol	Estrone	per 1 mg	IM	J1435
Etanercept	Enbrel	25 mg	IM, IV	J1438
Ethamolin	Ethanolamine oleate	100 mg	IV	J1430
Ethanolamine oleate	Ethamolin	100 mg	IV	J1430
Ethiofos	Amifostine	500 mg	IV	J0207
Ethyol	Amifostine	500 mg	IV	J0207
Etidronate disodium	Didronel	per 300 mg	IV	J1436
Etonogestrel implant system	Implanon	1 implant system	OTH	J7307
Etopophos	Etoposide	10 mg 50 mg	IV ORAL	J9181 J8560
Etoposide	Etopophos, Toposar, VePesid	10 mg 50 mg	IV ORAL	J9181 J8560
Eulexin	Flutamide	125 mg	ORAL	S0175
Euflexxa	Hyaluronan (sodium hyaluronate or derivative)	per dose	INTRA-ARTICULAR	J7323
Everone	Testosterone Enanthate	up to 100 mg	IM	J3120
Exemestane	Aromasin	25 mg	ORAL	S0156
F				
Fabrazyme	Agalsidase beta	1 mg	IV	J0180
Factor, hemophilia clotting, not otherwise specified				J7199
Factor VIIa (antihemophilic factor, recombinant)	Kogenate FS, NovoSeven	per 1 mcg	IV	J7189
Factor VIII (antihemophilic factor, human)	Alphanate, Monarc-M, Hemofil M, Humate-P, Koate-HP, Monoclate-P	per IU	IV	J7190
Factor VIII (antihemophilic factor, porcine)	Hyate: C	per IU	IV	J7191
Factor VIII (antihemophilic factor, recombinant)	Bioclate, Kogenate, Recombinate, ReFacto, Xyntha	per IU	IV	J7185, J7192
Factor IX (antihemophilic factor, purified, non-recombinant)	Alpha-Nine SD, Bebulin VH, Benefix, Konyne 80, Mononine, Profilnine SD, Proplex SX-T, Proplex T	per IU	IV	J7193
Factor IX, complex	Alpha-Nine SD, Bebulin VH, Benefix, Konyne 80, Mononine, Profilnine SD, Proplex SX-T, Proplex T	per IU	IV	J7194
Factor IX antihemophilic factor, purified, non-recombinant (human)	Alpha-Nine SD, Bebulin VH, Benefix, Konyne 80, Mononine, Profilnine SD, Proplex SX-T, Proplex T	per IU	IV	J7193
Factor IX, antihemophilic factor, recombinant (Human Complex)	Alpha-Nine SD, Bebulin VH, Benefix, Konyne 80, Mononine, Profilnine SD, Proplex SX-T, Proplex T	per IU	IV	J7195
Factrel	Gonadorelin HCl	per 100 mcg	SC, IV	J1620
Famotidine	Pepcid	20 mg	IV	S0028
Faslodex	Fulvestrant	25 mg	IM	J9395
Feiba VH Immuno	Hemophilia clotting factor	per IU	IV	J7198
Fentanyl citrate	Sublimaze	0.1 mg	IM, IV	J3010
Ferrlecit	Sodium ferric gluconate complex in sucrose	12.5 mg	IV	J2916
Fertinex	Urofollitropin	75 IU	IM, SC	J3355
Ferumoxytol	Feraheme	1 mg	IV	Q0138 Q0139
Filgrastim (G-CSF)	Neupogen	300 mcg 480 mcg	SC, IV SC, IV	J1440 J1441
Firmagon	Degarelix	1 mg	SC	J9155
Flagyl	Metronidazole	500 mg	IV	S0030
Flebogamma	Immune globulin, non-lyophilized (e.g. liquid)	500 mg	IV	J1572
Flexoject	Orphenadrine citrate	up to 60 mg	IV, IM	J2360
Flexon	Orphenadrine citrate	up to 60 mg	IV, IM	J2360
Floxin	Ofloxacin	400 mg	IV	S0034
Floxin IV	Ofloxacin	400 mg	IV	S0034
Flolan	Epoprostenol	0.5 mg	IV	J1325
Flolan	Sterile dilutant for Epoprostenol	50 ml	IV	S0155
Floxuridine	FUDR	500 mg	IV	J9200
Fluconazole	Diflucan	200 mg	IV	J1450
Fludara	Fludarabine phosphate	50 mg	IV	J9185
Fludarabine phosphate	Fludara Oforta	50 mg 10 mg	IV ORAL	J9185 J8562
Flunisolide	AeroBid, AeroBid-M, Nasalide, Nasarel	per mg	INH	J7641
Fluocinolone acetonide	Retisert	.59 mg	INTRAVITREAL	J7311
Fluorouracil	Adrucil	500 mg	IV	J9190

Table of Drugs

IA – intraarterial IM – intramuscular INH – inhalation IT – intrathecal IV – intravenous OTH – other SC – subcutaneous VAR – various administration methods

Drug Name	Additional Name(s)	Dosage	Delivery Method	HCPCS Code
Fluphenazine decanoate	Prolixin deconoate	up to 25 mg	IM, SC	J2680
Flutamide	Eulexin	125 mg	ORAL	S0175
Folex	Methotrexate sodium	5 mg 50 mg	IV, IM, IT, IA IV, IM, IT, IA	J9250 J9260
Folex PFS	Methotrexate sodium	5 mg 50 mg	IV, IM, IT, IA IV, IM, IT, IA	J9250 J9260
Follutein	Chorionic gonadotropin	per 1,000 USP units	IM	J0725
Folotyn	Pralatrexate	1 mg	IV	J9307
Fomepizole	Antizol	15 mg	IV	J1451
Fomivirsen sodium	Vitravene	1.65 mg	INTRAOCULAR	J1452
Fondaparinux sodium	Arixtra	0.5 mg	SC	J1652
Foradil	Formoterol	12 mcg, unit dose form	INH	J7640
Formoterol	Foradil, Perforomist	12 mcg, unit dose form	INH	J7640 J7606
Fortaz	Ceftazidime	per 500 mg	IM, IV	J0713
Forteo	Teriparatide	10 mcg	SC	J3110
Fosaprepitant	Emend	1 mg	IM	J1453
Foscarnet sodium	Foscavir	per 1,000 mg	IV	J1455
Foscavir	Foscarnet sodium	per 1,000 mg	IV	J1455
Fosphenytoin	Cerebyx	50 mg	IV, IM	Q2009
Fosphenytoin Sodium	Cerebyx	750 mg	IV, IM	S0078
Fragmin	Dalteparin sodium	per 2,500 IU	SC	J1645
FUDR	Floxuridine	500 mg	IV	J9200
Fulvestrant	Faslodex	25 mg	IM	J9395
Fungizone	Amphotericin B	50 mg	IV	J0285
Furomide M.D.	Furosemide	up to 20 mg	IM, IV	J1940
Furosemide	Furomide M.D., Lasix	up to 20 mg	IM, IV	J1940
Fusilev	Levoleucovorin calcium	.5 mg	IM	J0641
Fuzeon	Enfuvirtide	1 mg	IM	J1324
G				
Gadobenate dimeglumine	MultiHance, MultiHance multipack	per ml	IV	A9577-A9578
Gadoteridol	ProHance	per ml	IV	A9576
Gallium nitrate	Ganite	1 mg	IV	J1457
Galsulfase	Naglazyme	1 mg	IM	J1458
Gamastan	Gamma globulin and Immune globulin	1 cc 2 cc 3 cc 4 cc 5 cc 6 cc 7 cc 8 cc 9 cc 10 cc over 10 cc	IM IM IM IM IM IM IM IM IM IM IM	J1460 J1470 J1480 J1490 J1500 J1510 J1520 J1530 J1540 J1550 J1560
Gamimune N	Immune globulin, lyophilized (e.g. powder)	500 mg	IV	J1566
Gammagard	Immune globulin, non-lyophilized (e.g. liquid)	500 mg	IV	J1569
Gammagard S/D	Immune globulin, lyophilized (e.g. powder)	500 mg	IV	J1566
Gamma globulin	Gamastan, Gammar	1 cc over 10 cc	IM IM	J1460 J1560
Gammaphos	Amifostine	500 mg	IV	J0207
Gammar	Gamma globulin and Immune globulin	1 cc over 10 cc	IM IM	J1460 J1560
Gammar-P I.V.	Immune globulin, lyophilized (e.g. powder)	500 mg	IV	J1566
Gamulin RH	Rho(D) immune globulin, human	minidose, 50 mcg full dose, 300 mcg	IM IM	J2788 J2790
Gamunex	Immune globulin, non-lyophilized (e.g. liquid)	500 mg	IV	J1561
Ganciclovir, long-acting implant	Vitrasert	4.5 mg	OTH	J7310
Ganciclovir sodium	Cytovene IV	500 mg	IV	J1570
Ganite	Gallium nitrate	1 mg	IV	J1457
Garamycin	Gentamicin sulfate	up to 80 mg	IM, IV	J1580
Garamycin, gentamicin	G-Mycin, Jenamicin	up to 80 mg	IM, IV	J1580
Gastrocrom	Cromolyn sodium	per 10 mg, unit dose form	INH	J7631-J7632
Gastrosed	Hyoscyamine sulfate	up to 0.25 mg	SC, IM, IV	J1980
Gatifloxacin	Tequin	10 mg	IV	J1590
Gefitinib	Iressa	250 mg	ORAL	J8565
Gemcitabine HCl	Gemzar	200 mg	IV	J9201
Gemtuzumab ozogamicin	Mylotarg	5 mg	IV	J9300
Gemzar	Gemcitabine HCl	200 mg	IV	J9201
Genabid	Papaverine HCl	up to 60 mg	IV, IM	J2440
Genahist	Diphenhydramine HCl	50 mg	ORAL	Q0163
GenESA	Arbutamine HCl	1 mg	IV	J0395
Gengraf	Cyclosporine	25 mg 100 mg	ORAL ORAL	J7515 J7502
Genotropin	Somatropin	1 mg	IM, SC	J2941
Gentamicin sulfate	Garamycin	up to 80 mg	IM, IV	J1580
Gentran 40	Dextran 40	500 ml	IV	J7100
Gentran 75	Dextran 75	500 ml	IV	J7110
Geodon	Ziprasidone mesylate	10 mg	IM	J3486
Geref	Sermorelin acetate	1 mcg 0.5 mg	SC IV	Q0515 Q2014
Gesterol 50	Progesterone	per 50 mg	IM	J2675
Glatiramer acetate	Copaxone	20 mg	SC	J1595
Glofil-125	Iodine I-125 sodium iothalamate	up to 10 µCi	IV	A9554
GlucaGen diagnostic kit	Glucagon HCl	per 1 mg	SC, IM, IV	J1610
Glucagon diagnostic kit	Glucagon HCl	per 1 mg	SC, IM, IV	J1610
Glucagon HCl	GlucaGen diagnostic kit, Glucagon diagnostic kit	per 1 mg	SC, IM, IV	J1610
Glukor	Chorionic gonadotropin	per 1,000 USP units	IM	J0725
Glycopyrrolate		per 1 mg, concentrated form per 1 mg, unit dose form	INH INH	J7642 J7643
G-Mycin	Garamycin, gentamicin	up to 80 mg	IM, IV	J1580
Gold sodium thiomalate	Myochoysine	up to 50 mg	IM	J1600

IA – intraarterial IM – intramuscular INH – inhalation IT – intrathecal IV – intravenous OTH – other SC – subcutaneous VAR – various administration methods

Drug Name	Additional Name(s)	Dosage	Delivery Method	HCPCS Code
Gonadorelin HCl	Factrel	per 100 mcg	SC, IV	J1620
Gonic	Chorionic gonadotropin	per 1,000 USP units	IM	J0725
Goserelin acetate implant	Zoladex	per 3.6 mg	SC	J9202
Granisetron HCl	Kytril	100 mcg 1 mg 1 mg	IV ORAL IV	J1626 Q0166 S0091
Gynogen L.A.	Estradiol valerate	up to 10 mg up to 20 mg up to 40 mg	IM IM IM	J1380 J1390 J0970
H				
Habitrol	Nicotine patches, non-legend		OTH	S4991
Haldol	Haloperidol	up to 5 mg	IM, IV	J1630
Haloperidol	Haldol	up to 5 mg	IM, IV	J1630
Haloperidol decanoate	Haldol deconoate	per 50 mg	IM	J1631
Hectorol	Doxercalciferol	1 mcg	IV	J1270
Helixate FS	Factor VIII (antihemophilic factor, recombinant)	per IU	IV	J7192
Hemin	Panhematin	1 mg	IV	J1640
Hemofil M	Factor VIII (antihemophilic factor, human)	per IU	IV	J7190
Hemophilia clotting factors	Feiba VH Immuno	per IU	IV	J7198
Hemophilia clotting factors, NOC		per IU	IV	J7199
Hep-Lock	Heparin sodium (heparin lock flush)	per 10 units	IV	J1642
Hep-Lock U/P	Heparin sodium (heparin lock flush)	per 10 units	IV	J1642
Hep-Pak	Heparin sodium (heparin lock flush)	per 10 units	IV	J1642
HepaGam B	Hepatitis B immune globulin	0.5 ml 0.5 ml	IM IV	J1571 J1573
Heparin sodium	Calciparine, Liquaemin	per 1,000 units	IV, SC	J1644
Heparin sodium (heparin lock flush)	Hep-Lock, Hep-Lock U/P, Hep-Pak	per 10 units	IV	J1642
Hepatitis B immune globulin	HepaGam B	0.5 ml 0.5 ml	IM IV	J1571 J1573
Herceptin	Trastuzumab	10 mg	IV	J9355
Hexadrol	Dexamethasone	0.25 mg per mg, concentrated form per mg, unit dose form	ORAL INH INH	J8540 J7637 J7638
Hexadrol phosphate	Dexamethasone sodium phosphate	1 mg	IM, IV, OTH	J1100
Hexaminolevulinate hydrochloride	Cysview	100 mg	OTH	C9275
Histaject	Brompheniramine maleate	per 10 mg	IM, SC, IV	J0945
Histerone 50	Testosterone suspension	up to 50 mg	IM	J3140
Histerone 100	Testosterone suspension	up to 50 mg	IM	J3140
Histrelin acetate	Supprelin	10 mcg	SC	J1675
Histrelin implant	Supprelin LA, Vantas	50 mg	SC implant	J9225, J9226
Hizentra immune globulin		100 mg	IV, SC	J1559
Hospira	atropine sulfate Sabex	.01 mg	IV, IM, SC	J0461
Humalog	Insulin (Lispro)	per 50 units	INJ	J1817
Human Fibrinogen Concentrate	RiaSTAP	100 mg	IV	J1680
Humate-P	antihemophilic factor, human	per IU	IV	J7186, J7187, J7190
Humatrope	Somatropin	1 mg	IM, SC	J2941
Humira	Adalimumab	20 mg	SC	J0135
Humulin-R	Insulin	per 5 units	SC	J1815
Hyalgan	Hyaluronan (sodium hyaluronate or derivative)	per dose	INTRA-ARTICULAR	J7321
Hyaluronan (sodium hyaluronate) or derivative	Euflexxa, Hyalgan, Orthovisc, Supartz, Synvisc	per dose	INTRA-ARTICULAR	J7321-J7325
Hyaluronidase	Amphadase, Vitrase, Wydase	up to 150 units	IV, SC	J3470
Hyaluronidase, ovine, preservative free	Vitrase	1 USP unit up to 999 units per 1,000 USP units	IM, IV, SC IM, IV, SC	J3471 J3472
Hyaluronidase, recombinant	Hylenex, recombinant	1 USP unit	IM	J3473
Hyate: C	Factor VIII (antihemophilic factor (porcine))	per IU	IV	J7191
Hybolin decanoate	Nandrolone decanoate	up to 50 mg	IM	J2320
Hycamtin	Topotecan hydrochloride	.1 mg	IV	J9351
Hydralazine HCl	Apresoline	up to 20 mg	IV, IM	J0360
Hydramine	Diphenhydramine HCl	up to 50 mg 50 mg	IV, IM ORAL	J1200 Q0163
Hydrate	Dimenhydrinate	up to 50 mg	IV, IM	J1240
Hydrea	Hydroxyurea	500 mg	ORAL	S0176
Hydrocortisone acetate	Anucort-HC, Anusol-HC, Cortifoam, Hydrocortone acetate, Proctocort	up to 25 mg	IV, IM, SC	J1700
Hydrocortisone sodium phosphate	A-HydroCort, Hydrocortone phosphate	up to 50 mg	IV, IM, SC	J1710
Hydrocortisone sodium succinate	Solu-Cortef	up to 100 mg	IV, IM, SC	J1720
Hydrocortone acetate	Hydrocortisone acetate	up to 25 mg	IV, IM, SC	J1700
Hydrocortone phosphate	Hydrocortisone sodium phosphate	up to 50 mg	IV, IM, SC	J1710
Hydromorphone	Dilaudid	up to 4 mg	IV, IM, SC	J1170
Hydromorphone HCl	Dilaudid, Dilaudid-5, Dilaudid-HP	250 mg	LOADING DOSE FOR INFUSION PUMP	S0092
Hydroxyurea	Droxia, Hydrea	500 mg	ORAL	S0176
Hydroxyzine HCl	Atarax, Hyzine-50, Vistaject-50, Vistaril	up to 25 mg	IM	J3410
Hydroxyzine pamoate	Vistaril	25 mg 50 mg	ORAL ORAL	Q0177 Q0178
Hylan G-F 20	Synvisc	per dose	INTRA-ARTICULAR	J7325

Table of Drugs

IA – intraarterial IM – intramuscular INH – inhalation IT – intrathecal IV – intravenous OTH – other SC – subcutaneous VAR – various administration methods

Drug Name	Additional Name(s)	Dosage	Delivery Method	HCPCS Code
Hylenex, recombinant	Hyaluronidase, recombinant	1 USP unit	IM	J3473
Hyoscyamine sulfate	Anaspaz, Cystospaz, Cystospaz-M, Gastrosed, Levbid, Levsin, Levsin Drops, Levsin SL, Levsinex Timecaps, Neoquess	up to 0.25 mg	SC, IM, IV	J1980
Hyperstat IV	Diazoxide	up to 300 mg	IV	J1730
Hyper-Tet	Tetanus immune globulin, human	up to 250 units	IM	J1670
HypRho-D	Rho(D) immune globulin, human	minidose, 50 mcg full dose, 300 mg	IM IM	J2788 J2790
Hyrexin-50	Diphenhydramine HCl	up to 50 mg 50 mg	IV, IM ORAL	J1200 Q0163
Hyzine-50	Hydroxyzine HCl	up to 25 mg	IM	J3410
I				
Ibandronate sodium	Boniva	1 mg	IM	J1740
Ibuprofen	Caldolox, NeoProfen	100 mg	IM	C9279
Ibutilide fumarate	Corvert	1 mg	IV	J1742
Idamycin	Idarubicin HCl	5 mg	IV	J9211
Idamycin PFS	Idarubicin HCl	5 mg	IV	J9211
Idarubicin HCl	Idamycin, Idamycin PFS	5 mg	IV	J9211
Idursulfase	Elaprase	1 mg	IV	J1743
Ifex	Ifosfamide	1 g	IV	J9208
Ifosfamide	Ifex	1 g	IV	J9208
Ilaris	Canakinumab	1 mg	IM	J0638
Iletin	Insulin	per 5 units	SC	J1815
Iloprost	Ventavis	up to 20 mcg	INH	Q4074
Imagent	Perflexane lipid microspheres	per ml	IV	Q9955
Imiglucerase	Cerezyme	10 units	IV	J1786
Imitrex	Sumatriptan succinate	6 mg	SC	J3030
Immune globulin, lyophilized (e.g. powder)	Gamimune-N, Gammagard S/D, Gammar-P I.V., Iveegam, Polygam S/D, Sandoglobulin, Venoglobulin-I, Venoglobulin-S	500 mg	IV	J1566
Immune globulin, non-lyophilized (e.g. liquid)	Flebogamma, Gammagard, Gamunex, Hepagam B, Hizentra, Octagam, Privigen	500 mg .5 ml 100 mg	IV IM	J1459, J1559, J1561, J1568, J1569, J1571, J1572, J1599
Immune globulin, subcutaneous	Vivaglobin	100 mg	SC	J1562
Immunosuppressive drug, not otherwise classified				J7599
Implanon	Etonogestrel implant system	1 implant system	OTH	J7307
Imuran	Azathioprine	50 mg 100 mg	ORAL IV	J7500 J7501
In-111 Zevalin	Indium In-111 ibritumomab tiuxetan	up to 5 mCi	IV	A9542
Inapsine	Droperidol	up to 5 mg	IM, IV	J1790
Incobotulinumtoxin	Xeomin	1 unit	IM	C9278
Increlex	Mecasermin	1 mg	IM	J2170
Inderal	Propranolol HCl	up to 1 mg	IV	J1800
Indium DTPA	Indium In-111 pentetate	per 0.5 mCi	IT	A9548
Indium In-111 capromab pendetide	ProstaScint	up to 10 millicuries	IV	A9507
Indium In-111 ibritumomab tiuxetan	Zevalin	up to 5 mCi	IV	A9542
Indium In-111 pentetate	Indium DTPA	per 0.5 mCi	IT	A9548
Indium In-111 pentetreotide	OctreoScan	up to 6 millicuries	IV	A9572
Infergen	Interferon Alfacon-1, recombinant	1 mcg	IM	J9212
Infliximab	Remicade	10 mg	IM, IV	J1745
Infumorph	Morphine sulfate	500 mg up to 10 mg 100 mg	LOADING DOSE FOR INFUSION PUMP IM, IV, SC IM, IV, SC	S0093 J2270 J2271
Innohep	Tinzarparin sodium	1,000 IU	SC	J1655
Innovar	Droperidol and fentanyl citrate	up to 2 ml ampule	IM, IV	J1810
Insulin	Humulin-R, Iletin, Novolin-R, NPH, Regular, Velosulin	per 5 units	SC	J1815
Insulin (lispro)	Humalog	per 50 units	SC	J1817
Intal Inhaler	Cromolyn sodium	per 10 mg, unit dose form	INH	J7631-J7632
Intal Nebulizer Solution	Cromolyn sodium	per 10 mg, unit dose form	INH	J7631-J7632
Integrilin	Eptifibatide	5 mg	IM, IV	J1327
Interferon Alphacon-1, recombinant	Amgen, Infergen	1 mcg	IM	J9212
Interferon alfa-2A, recombinant	Roferon-A	3 million units	SC, IM	J9213
Interferon alfa-2B, recombinant	Intron-A	1 million units	SC, IM	J9214
Interferon alfa-N3 (human leukocyte derived)	Alferon N	250,000 IU	IM	J9215
Interferon beta-1A	Avonex, Rebif	11 mcg 11 mcg 30 mcg	IM SC IM	Q3025 Q3026 J1826
Interferon beta-1B, recombinant	Betaseron	0.25 mg	SC	J1830
Interferon gamma-1B	Actimmune	3 million units	SC	J9216
Intrauterine copper contraceptive	Paragard T 380 A		OTH	J7300
Intron-A	Interferon alfa-2b, recombinant	1 million units	SC, IM	J9214
Intropin	Dopamine HCl	40 mg	IV	J1265
Invanz	Ertapenem sodium	500 mg	IM, IV	J1335
Invega sustenna	Paliperidon palmitate	1 mg	IM	J2426
Iodine I-125 sodium iothalamate	Glofil-125	up to 10 µCi	IV	A9554
Iodine I-131 tositumomab	Bexxar	per treatment dose	IV	A9545
Ipratropium bromide, compounded	Atrovent	per mg, unit dose form	INH	J7645

IA – intraarterial IM – intramuscular INH – inhalation IT – intrathecal IV – intravenous OTH – other SC – subcutaneous VAR – various administration methods

Drug Name	Additional Name(s)	Dosage	Delivery Method	HCPCS Code
Ipratropium bromide, non-compounded	Atrovent	per mg, unit dose form	INH	J7644
Iressa	Gefitinib	250 mg	ORAL	J8565
Irinotecan HCl	Camptosar	20 mg	IV	J9206
Iron sucrose	Venofer	1 mg	IV	J1756
Irrigation solution for treatment of bladder calculi	Renacidin	per 500 ml	OTH	Q2004
Isocaine	Mepivacaine HCl	per 10 ml	VAR	J0670
Isoetharine HCl	Arm-a-Med, Beta-2, Bronkometer, Bronkosol, Dey-Lute	per mg, concentrated form per mg, unit dose form	INH INH	J7647, J7648 J7649, J7650
Isoproterenol HCl	Isuprel, Medihaler-ISO	per mg, concentrated form per mg, unit dose form	INH INH	J7657, J7658 J7659, J7660
Istodax	Romidepsin	1 mg	IV	J9315
Isuprel	Isoproterenol HCl	per mg, concentrated form per mg, unit dose form	INH INH	J7657, J7658 J7659, J7660
Itraconazole	Sporonox	50 mg	IV	J1835
Iveegam	Immune globulin, lyophilized (e.g. powder)	500 mg	IV	J1566
Ixabepilone	Ixempra	1 mg	IV	J9207
Ixempra	Ixabepilone	1 mg	IV	J9207
J				
Jenamicin	Garamycin, Gentamicin	up to 80 mg	IM, IV	J1580
Jevtana	Cabazitaxel	1 mg	IM	C9276
K				
Kabikinase	Streptokinase	per 250,000 IU	IV	J2995
Kabolin	Nandrolone decanoate	up to 50 mg	IM	J2320
Kaleinate	Calcium gluconate	per 10 ml	IV	J0610
Kanamycin sulfate	Kantrex, Klebcil	up to 75 mg up to 500 mg	IM, IV IM, IV	J1850 J1840
Kantrex	Kanamycin sulfate	up to 75 mg up to 500 mg	IM, IV IM, IV	J1850 J1840
Keflin	Cephalothin sodium	up to 1 g	IM, IV	J1890
Kefurox	Cefuroxime sodium, sterile	per 750 mg	IM, IV	J0697
Kefzol	Cefazolin sodium	500 mg	IV, IM	J0690
Kenaject-40	Triamcinolone acetonide	per 10 mg	IM	J3301
Kenalog-10	Triamcinolone acetonide	per 10 mg	IM	J3301
Kenalog-40	Triamcinolone acetonide	per 10 mg	IM	J3301
Kepivance	Palifermin	50 mcg	IV	J2425
Keppra	Levetiracetam	10 mg	IV	J1953
Kestrone 5	Estrone	per 1 mg	IM	J1435
Ketorolac tromethamine	Toradol	per 15 mg	IM, IV	J1885
Key-Pred 25	Prednisolone acetate	up to 1 ml	IM	J2650
Key-Pred 50	Prednisolone acetate	up to 1 ml	IM	J2650
K-Flex	Orphenadrine citrate	up to 60 mg	IV, IM	J2360
Kinevac	Sincalide	5 mcg	IM, IV, SC	J2805
Klebcil	Kanamycin sulfate	up to 75 mg up to 500 mg	IM, IV IM, IV	J1850 J1840
Koate-HP	Factor VIII (antihemophilic factor, human)	per IU	IV	J7190
Kogenate	Factor VIII (antihemophilic factor, recombinant)	per IU	IV	J7192
Kogenate FS	Factor VIIa (antihemophilic factor, recombinant)	per 1 mcg	IV	J7189
Kogenate FS	Factor VIII (antihemophilic factor, recombinant)	per IU	IV	J7192
Konakion	Phytonadione (Vitamin K)	per 1 mg	IM, SC, IV	J3430
Konyne-80	Factor IX	per IU		J7193-J7195
Kytril	Granisetron HCl	100 mcg 1 mg 1 mg	IV ORAL IV	J1626 Q0166 S0091
L				
Lacomaside	Vimpat	1 mg	IM	C9254
L.A.E. 20	Estradiol valerate	up to 10 mg up to 20 mg up to 40 mg	IM IM IM	J1380 J1390 J0970
Laetrile	Amygdalin, vitamin B-17		VAR	J3570
Lanophyllin	Theophylline	per 40 mg	IV	J2810
Lanoxin	Digoxin	up to 0.5 mg	IM, IV	J1160
Lanreotide	Somatuline Depot	1 mg	SC, IM	J1930
Laronidase	Aldurazyme	0.1 mg	IV	J1931
Lasix	Furosemide	up to 20 mg	IM, IV	J1940
L-Caine	Lidocaine HCl	10 mg	IV	J2001
Lepirudin	Refludan	50 mg	IV	J1945
Leucovorin calcium	Wellcovorin	per 50 mg	IM, IV	J0640
Leukeran	Chlorambucil	2 mg	ORAL	S0172
Leukine	Sargramostim (GM-CSF)	50 mcg	IV	J2820
Leuprolide acetate	Eligard, Lupron	per 1 mg	SC, IM	J9218
Leuprolide acetate (for depot suspension)	Eligard, Lupron Depot, Lupron Depot-Ped	3.75 mg 7.5 mg	IM IM	J1950 J9217
Leuprolide acetate implant	Viadur	65 mg	SC, IM	J9219
Leustatin	Cladribine	per 1 mg	IV	J9065
Levalbuterol HCl, compounded	Xopenex	0.5 mg, concentrated form 0.5 mg, unit dose form	INH INH	J7607 J7615
Levalbuterol HCl, non-compounded	Xopenex	0.5 mg, concentrated form 0.5 mg, unit dose form	INH INH	J7612 J7614
Levamisole hydrochloride	Ergamisol	50 mg	ORAL	S0177
Levaquin	Levofloxacin	250 mg	IV	J1956
Levbid	Hyoscyamine sulfate	up to 0.25 mg	SC, IM, IV	J1980
Levetiracetam	Keppra	10 mg	IV	J1953
Levocarnitine	Carnitor	per 1 gm	IV	J1955

IA – intraarterial IM – intramuscular INH – inhalation IT – intrathecal IV – intravenous OTH – other SC – subcutaneous VAR – various administration methods

Table of Drugs

Drug Name	Additional Name(s)	Dosage	Delivery Method	HCPCS Code
Levo-Dromoran	Levorphanol tartrate	up to 2 mg	SC, IV	J1960
Levofloxacin	Levaquin	250 mg	IV	J1956
Levoleucovorin calcium	Fusilev	.5 mg	IM	J0641
Levonorgestrel (contraceptive) implant system, including implants and supplies	Norplant	Kit	OTH	J7306
Levonorgestrel-releasing intrauterine contraceptive	Mirena	52 mg	OTH	J7302
Levorphanol tartrate	Levo-Dromoran	up to 2 mg	SC, IV	J1960
Levsin	Hyoscyamine sulfate	up to 0.25 mg	SC, IM, IV	J1980
Levsin Drops	Hyoscyamine sulfate	up to 0.25 mg	SC, IM, IV	J1980
Levsin SL	Hyoscyamine sulfate	up to 0.25 mg	SC, IM, IV	J1980
Levsinex Timecaps	Hyoscyamine sulfate	up to 0.25 mg	SC, IM, IV	J1980
Levulan Kerastick	Aminolevulinic acid HCl	20%, single unit dosage form (354 mg)	OTH (TOPICAL)	J7308
Lexiscan	Regadenoson	.1 mg	IM	J2785
Librax	Chlordiazepoxide HCl	up to 100 mg	IM, IV	J1990
Librium	Chlordiazepoxide HCl	up to 100 mg	IM, IV	J1990
Lidocaine HCl	Caine-1, Caine-2, Dalcaine, Lidoject-1, Lidoject-2, Dilocaine, L-Caine, Nervocaine 1%, Nervocaine 2%, Nulicaine, Octocaine, Xylocaine	10 mg	IV	J2001
Lidoject-1	Lidocaine HCl	10 mg	IV	J2001
Lidoject-2	Lidocaine HCl	10 mg	IV	J2001
Limbitrol	Chlordiazepoxide HCl	up to 100 mg	IM, IV	J1990
Lincocin	Lincomycin HCl	up to 300 mg	IV	J2010
Lincomycin HCl	Lincocin, Lincorex	up to 300 mg	IV	J2010
Lincorex	Lincomycin HCl	up to 300 mg	IV	J2010
Linezolid	Zyvox	200 mg	IV	J2020
Lioresal	Baclofen	10 mg 50 mcg, for intrathecal trial	IT IT	J0475 J0476
Liquaemin	Heparin sodium	per 1,000 units	IV, SC	J1644
LMD 10%	Dextran 40	500 ml	IV	J7100
Lomustine	CeeNu	10 mg	ORAL	S0178
Lovenox	Enoxaparin sodium	10 mg	SC	J1650
Lorazepam	Ativan	2 mg	IM, IV	J2060
Lucentis	Ranibizumab	0.5 mg	IV	J2778
Lufyllin	Dyphylline	up to 500 mg	IM	J1180
Luminal Sodium	Phenobarbitol sodium	up to 120 mg	IM, IV	J2560
Lumizyme	Alglucosidase alfa	1 mg	IM	C9277
Lunelle	Medroxyprogesterone acetate/estradiol cypionate	5 mg/25 mg	IM	J1056
Lupron	Leuprolide acetate	1 mg	SC, IV	J9218
Lupron Depot	Leuprolide acetate (for depot suspension)	3.75 mg 7.5 mg	IM, IV IM, IV	J1950 J9217
Lupron Depot-PED	Leuprolide acetate (for depot suspension)	3.75 mg 7.5 mg	IM, IV IM, IV	J1950 J9217
Lymphocyte immune globulin, anti-thymocyte globulin, equine	Atgam	250 mg	IV	J7504
Lymphocyte immune globulin, anti-thymocyte globulin, rabbit	Thymoglobulin	25 mg	IV	J7511
M				
Macugen	Pegaptanib sodium	0.3 mg 0.3 mg	INTRAVITREOUS INTRAVITREOUS	C9128 J2503
Magnesium sulfate		per 500 mg	IM, IV	J3475
Mannitol	Osmitrol	25% in 50 ml	IV	J2150
Marcaine	Bupivicaine HCl	30 ml	IV	S0020
Marinol	Dronabinol	2.5 mg 5 mg	ORAL ORAL	Q0167 Q0168
Marmine	Dimenhydrinate	up to 50 mg	IM, IV	J1240
Matulane	Procarbazine hydrochloride	50 mg	ORAL	S0182
Maxipime	Cefepime hydrochloride	500 mg	IV	J0692
Mecasermin	Increlex	1 mg	IM	J2170
Mechlorethamine HCl (nitrogen mustard), HN_2	Mustargen	10 mg	IV	J9230
Medihaler-ISO	Isoproterenol HCl	per mg, concentrated form per mg, unit dose form	INH INH	J7657, J7658 J7659, J7660
Medralone 40	Methylprednisolone acetate	20 mg 40 mg 80 mg	IM IM IM	J1020 J1030 J1040
Medralone 80	Methylprednisolone acetate	20 mg 40 mg 80 mg	IM IM IM	J1020 J1030 J1040
Medrol	Methylprednisolone	per 4 mg	ORAL	J7509
Medroxyprogesterone acetate	Amen, Cycrin, Depo-Provera, Provera	50 mg 150 mg, for contraceptive use	IM IM	J1051 J1055
Medroxyprogesterone acetate/estradiol cypionate	Lunelle	5 mg/25 mg	IM	J1056
Mefoxin	Cefoxitin sodium	1 g	IV, IM	J0694
Megace	Megestrol acetate	20 mg	ORAL	S0179
Megestrol acetate	Megace	20 mg	ORAL	S0179
Melphalan HCl	Alkeran	50 mg	IV	J9245
Melphalan, oral	Alkeran	2 mg	ORAL	J8600
Menoject LA	Testosterone cypionate and estradiol cypionate	up to 1 ml	IM	J1060
Mepergan	Meperdine and promethazine HCl	up to 50 mg	IM, IV	J2180
Meperidine HCl	Demerol	per 100 mg	IM, IV, SC	J2175
Meperidine and promethazine HCl	Mepergan	up to 50 mg	IM, IV	J2180
Mephyton	Phytonadione (Vitamin K)	per 1 mg	IM, SC, IV	J3430
Mepivacaine HCl	Carbocaine, Polocaine, Isocaine	per 10 ml	VAR	J0670
Meprolone	Methylprednisolone	per 4 mg	ORAL	J7509

IA – intraarterial IM – intramuscular INH – inhalation IT – intrathecal IV – intravenous OTH – other SC – subcutaneous VAR – various administration methods

Drug Name	Additional Name(s)	Dosage	Delivery Method	HCPCS Code
Meropenem	Merrem IV	100 mg	IV	J2185
Merrem IV	Meropenem	100 mg	IV	J2185
Mesna	Mesnex	200 mg	IV	J9209
Mesnex	Mesna	200 mg	IV	J9209
Metaprel	Metaproterenol sulfate	per 10 mg, concentrated form per 10 mg, unit dose form	INH INH	J7667, J7668 J7669, J7670
Metaproterenol sulfate	Alupent, Metaprel	per 10 mg, concentrated form per 10 mg, unit dose form	INH INH	J7667, J7668 J7669, J7670
Metaraminol bitartrate	Aramine	per 10 mg	IV, IM, SC	J0380
Metastron	Strontium-89 chloride	per mCi	IV	A9600
Methacholine chloride	Provocholine	1 mg	INH	J7674
Methadone HCl	Dolophine, Methadose	up to 10 mg	IM, SC	J1230
Methadose	Methadone HCl	up to 10 mg	IM, SC	J1230
Methergine	Methylergonovine maleate	up to 0.2 mg	IM, IV	J2210
Methocarbamol	Robaxin	up to 10 ml	IV, IM	J2800
Methotrexate	Rheumatrex	2.5 mg	ORAL	J8610
Methotrexate LPF	Methotrexate sodium	5 mg 50 mg	IV, IM, IT, IA IV, IM, IT, IA	J9250 J9260
Methotrexate sodium	Folex, Folex PFS, Methotrexate LPF, Rheumatrex	5 mg 50 mg	IV, IM, IT, IA IV, IM, IT, IA	J9250 J9260
Methylaminolevulinate	Metvixia	1 gram	OTH	J7309
Methyldopate HCl	Aldomet	up to 250 mg	IV	J0210
Methylene blue	Urolene Blue	1 mg	IV	Q9968
Methylergometrine	Methylergonovine maleate	up to 0.2 mg	IM, IV	J2210
Methylergonovine maleate	Methergine, Methylergometrine	up to 0.2 mg	IM, IV	J2210
Methylprednisolone	Medrol, Meprolone	per 4 mg	ORAL	J7509
Methylprednisolone acetate	Depo-Medrol, depMedalone 40, depMedalone 80, Depoject, Depopred-40, Depopred-80, D-Med 80, Duralone-40, Duralone-80, Medralone 40, Medralone 80, M-Prednisol-40, M-Prednisol-80, Rep-Pred 40, Rep-Pred 80	20 mg 40 mg 80 mg	IM IM IM	J1020 J1030 J1040
Methylprednisolone sodium succinate	A-methaPred, Solu-Medrol	up to 40 mg up to 125 mg	IM, IV IM, IV	J2920 J2930
Meticorten	Prednisone	per 5 mg	ORAL	J7506
Metoclopramide HCl	Reglan	up to 10 mg	IV	J2765
Metric 21	Metronidazole	500 mg	IV	S0030
Metrodin	Urofollitropin	75 IU	IM, SC	J3355
Metro IV	Metronidazole	500 mg	IV	S0030
Metronidazole	Flagyl, Metric 21, Metro IV, Protostat	500 mg	IV	S0030
Metvixia	Methylaminolevulinate	1 gram	OTH	J7309
Miacalcin	Calcitonin-salmon	up to 400 units	SC, IM	J0630
Micafungin sodium	Mycamine	1 mg	IM	J2248
MICRhoGAM	Rho(D) immune globulin, human	minidose, 50 mcg full dose, 300 mg	IM IM	J2788 J2790
Midazolam HCl	Versed	per 1 mg	IM, IV	J2250
Mifeprex	Mifepristone	200 mg	ORAL	S0190
Mifepristone	Mifeprex	200 mg	ORAL	S0190
Migranal	Dihydroergotamine mesylate	per 1 mg	IM, IV	J1110
Milrinone lactate	Primacor	5 mg	IV	J2260
Mirena	Levonorgestrel releasing intrauterine contraceptive	52 mg	OTH	J7302
Misoprostol	Cytotec	200 mcg	ORAL	S0191
Mithracin	Plicamycin	2.5 mg	IV	J9270
Mitomycin	Mutamycin	5 mg	IV	J9280
Mitoxantrone HCl	Novantrone	per 5 mg	IV	J9293
Monarc-M	Factor VIII (antihemophilic factor, human)	per IU	IV	J7190
Monoclate-P	Factor VIII (antihemophilic factor, human)	per IU	IV	J7190
Monoclonal antibodies, parenteral		5 mg	IV	J7505
Mononine	Factor IX	per IU	IV	J7193-J7195
Morphine sulfate	Duramorph, Infumorph	500 mg up to 10 mg 100 mg	LOADING DOSE FOR INFUSION PUMP IM, IV, SC IM, IV, SC	S0093 J2270 J2271
Morphine sulfate (preservative-free sterile solution)	Astramorph PF	per 10 mg	IM, IV, SC	J2275
Moxifloxacin	Avelox	100 mg	IV	J2280
Mozobil	Plerixafor	1 mg	SC	J2562
M-Prednisol-40	Methylprednisolone acetate	20 mg 40 mg 80 mg	IM IM IM	J1020 J1030 J1040
M-Prednisol-80	Methylprednisolone acetate	20 mg 40 mg 80 mg	IM IM IM	J1020 J1030 J1040
Mucomyst	Acetylcysteine	per gram, unit dose form	INH	J7604, J7608
Mucosil-10	Acetylcysteine	per gram, unit dose form	INH	J7604, J7608
Mucosil-20	Acetylcysteine	per gram, unit dose form	INH	J7604, J7608
MultiHance	Gadobenate dimeglumine	per mg	IV	A9577
MultiHance multipack	Gadobenate dimeglumine	per mg	IV	A9578
Muromonab-CD3	Orthoclone OKT3	5 mg	IV	J7505
Muse	Alprostadil, urethral suppository	per dose	OTH	J0275
Mustargen	Mechlorethamine HCl (Nitrogen mustard) HN2	10 mg	IV	J9230
Mutamycin	Mitomycin	5 mg	IV	J9280
Mycamine	Micafungin sodium	1 mg	IM	J2248

IA – intraarterial IM – intramuscular INH – inhalation IT – intrathecal IV – intravenous OTH – other SC – subcutaneous VAR – various administration methods

Table of Drugs

Drug Name	Additional Name(s)	Dosage	Delivery Method	HCPCS Code
Mycophenolate mofetil	CellCept	250 mg	ORAL	J7517
Mycophenolic acid	Myfortic	180 mg	ORAL	J7518
Myfortic	Mycophenolic acid	180 mg	ORAL	J7518
Myleran	Busulfan	1 mg 2 mg	IM ORAL	J0594 J8510
Mylotarg	Gemtuzumab ozogamicin	5 mg	IV	J9300
Myobloc	Botulinum toxin type B rimabotulinumtoxinB	per 100 units 100 units	IM IM	J0587 J0587
Myochrysine	Gold sodium thiomalate	up to 50 mg	IM	J1600
Myolin	Orphenadrine citrate	up to 60 mg	IV, IM	J2360
Myozyme	Alglucosidase alfa	10 mg	IV	J0220
Mytonachol	Bethanechol chloride	up to 5 mg	SC	J0520
N				
Nabilone	Cesamet	1 mg	ORAL	J8650
Nafcil	Nafcillin sodium	2 g	IV, IM	S0032
Nafcillin Sodium	Nafcil, Nallpen, Unipen	2 g	IV, IM	S0032
Naglazyme	Galsulfase	1 mg	IM	J1458
Nalbuphine HCl	Nubain	per 10 mg	IM, IV, SC	J2300
Nallpen	Nafcillin sodium	2 g	IV, IM	S0032
Naloxone HCl	Narcan	per 1 mg	IM, IV, SC	J2310
Naltrexone, depot form	Vivatrol	1 mg	IM	J2315
Nandrobolic L.A.	Nandrolone decanoate	up to 50 mg	IM	J2320
Nandrolone decanoate	Anabolin LA 100, Androlone-D 100, Deca-Durabolin, Decolone-50, Decolone-100, Hybolin Decanoate, Kabolin, Nandrobolic L.A., Neo-Durabolic	up to 50 mg	IM	J2320
Narcan	Naloxone HCl	per 1 mg	IM, IV, SC	J2310
Naropin	Ropivacaine HCl	1 mg	OTH	J2795
Nasahist B	Brompheniramine maleate	per 10 mg	IM, SC, IV	J0945
Nasal vaccine inhalation			INH	J3530
Nasalcrom	Cromolyn sodium	per 10 mg, unit dose form	INH	J7631-J7632
Nasalide	Flunisolide	per mg	INH	J7641
Nasarel	Flunisolide	per mg	INH	J7641
Natalizumab	Tysabri	1 mg	IV	J2323
Natrecor	Nesiritide	0.1 mg	IV	J2325
Navelbine	Vinorelbine tartrate	per 10 mg	IV	J9390
ND Stat	Brompheniramine maleate	per 10 mg	IM, SC, IV	J0945
Nebcin	Tobramycin sulfate	up to 80 mg	IM, IV	J3260
NebuPent	Pentamidine isethionate	per 300 mg, unit dose form 300 mg	INH IV, IM	J2545, J7676 S0080
Nelarabine	Arranon	50 mg	IM	J9261
Nembutal Sodium	Pentobarbital sodium	per 50 mg	IM, IV	J2515
Neocyten	Orphenadrine citrate	up to 60 mg	IV, IM	J2360
Neo-Durabolic	Nandrolone decanoate	up to 50 mg	IM	J2320
NeoProfen	Ibuprofen	100 mg	IM	C9279
Neoquess	Hyoscyamine sulfate	up to 0.25 mg	SC, IM, IV	J1980
Neoral	Cyclosporine	25 mg 100 mg 250 mg	ORAL ORAL IV	J7515 J7502 J7516
Neosar	Cyclophosphamide	25 mg 100 mg	ORAL IV	J8530 J9070
Neostigmine methylsulfate	Prostigmin	up to 0.5 mg	IM, IV, SC	J2710
Neo-Synephrine	Phenylephrine HCl	up to 1 ml	SC, IM, IV	J2370
Nervine Nighttime Sleep-Aid	Diphenhydramine HCl	50 mg	ORAL	Q0163
Nervocaine 1%	Lidocaine HCl	10 mg	IV	J2001
Nervocaine 2%	Lidocaine HCl	10 mg	IV	J2001
Nesacaine	Chloroprocaine HCl	per 30 ml	VAR	J2400
Nesacaine-MPF	Chloroprocaine HCl	per 30 ml	VAR	J2400
Nesiritide	Natrecor	0.1 mg	IV	J2325
Nestrex	Pyridoxine HCl	100 mg	IM, IV	J3415
Neulasta	Pegfilgrastim	6 mg	SC	J2505
Neumega	Oprelvekin	5 mg	SC	J2355
Neupogen	Filgrastim (G-CSF)	300 mcg 480 mcg	SC, IV SC, IV	J1440 J1441
Neutrexin	Trimetrexate glucuronate	per 25 mg	IV	J3305
NeutroSpec	Technetium Tc-99m fanolesomab	up to 25 mCi	IV	A9566
Nicoderm	Nicotine patches, legend		OTH	S4990
Nicotine patches, legend	ProStep, Nicoderm		OTH	S4990
Nicotine patches, non-legend	Habitrol, Nicotrol		OTH	S4991
Nicotrol	Nicotine patches, non-legend		OTH	S4991
Nipent	Pentostatin	per 10 mg	IV	J9268
Norditropin	Somatropin	1 mg	IM, SC	J2941
Nordryl Cough	Diphenhydramine HCl	up to 50 mg 50 mg	IV, IM ORAL	J1200 Q0163
Norflex	Orphenadrine citrate	up to 60 mg	IV, IM	J2360
Norplant	Levonorgestrel (contraceptive implants system, including implants and supplies)	Kit	OTH	J7306
Norzine	Thiethylperazine maleate	10 mg up to 10 mg	ORAL IM	Q0174 J3280
Not otherwise classified drugs	Unclassified drugs		VAR INH ADMIN. THRU DME OTHER THAN INH ADMIN. THRU DME	J3490 J7699 J7799
Not otherwise classified drugs, anti-emetic			ORAL	Q0181
Not otherwise classified drugs, anti-neoplastic			IV	J9999
Not otherwise classified drugs, chemotherapeutic			ORAL	J8999
Not otherwise classified drugs, immunosuppressive				J7599

IA – intraarterial IM – intramuscular INH – inhalation IT – intrathecal IV – intravenous OTH – other SC – subcutaneous VAR – various administration methods

Drug Name	Additional Name(s)	Dosage	Delivery Method	HCPCS Code
Not otherwise classified drugs, nonchemotherapeutic			ORAL	J8499
Novantrone	Mitoxantrone HCl	per 5 mg	IV	J9293
Novarel	Chorionic gonadotropin	per 1,000 USP units	IM	J0725
Novolin-R	Insulin	per 5 units	SC	J1815
NovoSeven	Factor VIIa (antihemophilic factor, recombinant)	per 1 mcg	IV	J7189
NPH	Insulin	per 5 units	SC	J1815
Nplate	Romiplostim	10 mcg	SC	J2795
Nubain	Nalbuphine HCl	per 10 mg	IM, IV, SC	J2300
Nulicaine	Lidocaine HCl	10 mg	IV	J2001
Numorphan	Oxymorphone HCl	up to 1 mg	IV, SC, IM	J2410
Numorphan H.P.	Oxymorphone HCl	up to 1 mg	IV, SC, IM	J2410
Nutropin	Somatropin	1 mg	IM, SC	J2941
Nutropin AQ	Somatropin	1 mg	IM, SC	J2941
Nytol	Diphenhydramine HCl	50 mg	ORAL	Q0163
O				
Octafluoropropane microspheres		per ml	IV	Q9956
Octagam	Immune globulin, non-lyophilized (e.g. liquid)	500 mg	IV	J1568
Octocaine	Lidocaine HCl	10 mg	IV	J2001
OctreoScan	Indium In-111 pentetreotide	up to 6 millicuries	IV	A9572
Octreotide acetate	Sandostatin, Sandostatin Lar Depot	1 mg 25 mcg	IM IV, SC	J2353 J2354
Oculinum	Botulinum toxin type A	per unit	IM	J0585
Ofatumumab	Arzerra	10 mg	IV	J9302
O-Flex	Orphenadrine citrate	up to 60 mg	IM, IV	J2360
Ofloxacin	Floxin, Floxin IV	400 mg	IV	S0034
Oforta	Fludarabine phosphate	10 mg	ORAL	J8562
Olanzapine	Zyprexa RelPrevv	1 mg	IM	J2358
Omalizumab	Xolair	5 mg	SC	J2357
Omnipen-N	Ampicillin sodium	500 mg	IM, IV	J0290
OnabotulinumtoxinA	Botox	1 unit	IV, IM, SC	J0585
Oncaspar	Pegaspargase	per single dose vial	IM, IV	J9266
Oncovin	Vincristine sulfate	1 mg	IV	J9370
Ondansetron HCl	Zofran, Zofran ODT	per 1 mg 8 mg	IV ORAL	J2405 Q0179
Ontak	Denileukin diftitox	300 mcg	IV	J9160
Onxol	Paclitaxel	30 mg	IV	J9265
Oprelvekin	Neumega	5 mg	SC	J2355
Oraminic II	Brompheniramine maleate	per 10 mg	IM, SC, IV	J0945
Orasone	Prednisone	per 5 mg	ORAL	J7506
Orencia	Abatacept	10 mg	IM	J0129
Ormazine	Chlorpromazine HCl	10 mg 25 mg up to 50 mg	ORAL ORAL IM, IV	Q0171 Q0172 J3230
Orphenadrine citrate	Antiflex, Banflex, Flexoject, Flexon, K-Flex, Myolin, Neocyten, Norflex, O-Flex, Orphenate	up to 60 mg	IV, IM	J2360
Orphenate	Orphenadrine citrate	up to 60 mg	IV, IM	J2360
Orthoclone OKT3	Muromonab-CD3	5 mg	IV	J7505
Orthovisc	Hyaluronan (sodium hyaluronate or derivative)	per dose	INTRA-ARTICULAR	J7324
Or-Tyl	Dicyclomine HCl	up to 20 mg	IM	J0500
Osmitrol	Mannitol	25% in 50 ml	IV	J2150
Oxacillin sodium	Bactocill, Prostaphlin	up to 250 mg	IM, IV	J2700
Oxaliplatin	Eloxatin	0.5 mg	IV	J9263
Oxymorphone HCl	Numorphan, Numorphan H.P.	up to 1 mg	IV, SC, IM	J2410
Oxytetracycline HCl	Terramycin	up to 50 mg	IM	J2460
Oxytocin	Pitocin, Syntocinon	up to 10 units	IV, IM	J2590
Ozurdex	Dexamethasone intravitreal implant	0.1 mg	OTH	J7312
P				
Paclitaxel	Onxol, Taxol	30 mg	IV	J9265
Paclitaxel protein-bound particles	Abraxane	1 mg	IV	J9264
Palifermin	Kepivance	50 mcg	IV	J2425
Paliperidone palmitate	Invega Sustema	1 mg	IM	J2426
Palivizumab-RSV-IGM	Synagis	per 50 mg	IM	C9003
Palonosetron HCl	Aloxi	25 mcg	IV	J2469
Pamidronate disodium	Aredia	per 30 mg	IV	J2430
Panglobulin	Immune globulin, lyophilized (e.g. powder)	500 mg	IV	J1566
Panhematin	Hemin	1 mg	IV	J1640
Panitumumab	Vectibix	10 mg	IV	J9303
Panmycin	Tetracycline	up to 250 mg	IM, IV	J0120
Pantoprazole sodium	Protonix	per vial	IV	C9113
Papaverine HCl	Cerespan, Genabid, Pavagen	up to 60 mg	IV, IM	J2440
ParaGard	Copper contraceptive, intrauterine		OTH	J7300
Paragard T 380 A	Intrauterine copper contraceptive		OTH	J7300
Paraplatin	Carboplatin	50 mg	IV	J9045
Paricalcitol	Zemplar	1 mcg	IV, IM	J2501
Pavagen	Papaverine HCl	up to 60 mg	IV, IM	J2440
Pegademase bovine	Adagen	25 IU	IM	J2504
Pegaptanib sodium	Macugen	0.3 mg 0.3 mg	INTRAVITREOUS INTRAVITREOUS	C9128 J2503
Pegaspargase	Oncaspar	per single dose vial	IM, IV	J9266
Pegasys	Pegylated interferon alfa-2A	180 mcg per ml	SC	S0145
Pegasys	Pegylated interferon alfa-2B	10 mcg per 0.5 ml	SC	S0146
Pegfilgrastim	Neulasta	6 mg	SC	J2505
Pegylated interferon alfa-2A	Pegasys	180 mcg per ml	SC	S0145
Pegylated interferon alfa-2B	Pegasys	10 mcg per 0.5 ml	SC	S0146
Pemetrexed	Alimta	10 mg	IV	J9305
Penicillin G benzathine	Bicillin L.A., Permapen	100,000 units	IM	J0561

Table of Drugs

IA – intraarterial IM – intramuscular INH – inhalation IT – intrathecal IV – intravenous OTH – other SC – subcutaneous VAR – various administration methods

Table of Drugs

Drug Name	Additional Name(s)	Dosage	Delivery Method	HCPCS Code
Penicillin G benzathine and penicillin G procaine	Bicillin C-R 900/300	100,000 units	IM	J0558
Penicillin G potassium	Pfizerpen	up to 600,000 units	IM, IV	J2540
Penicillin G procaine, aqueous	Crysticillin 300 A.S., Crysticillin 600 A.S., Duracillin A.S., Pfizerpen A.S., Wycillin,	up to 600,000 units	IM	J2510
Pentacarinat	Pentamidine isethionate	per 300 mg, unit dose form 300 mg	INH IV, IM	J2545, J7676 S0080
Pentam 300	Pentamidine isethionate	per 300 mg, unit dose form 300 mg	INH IV, IM	J2545, J7676 S0080
Pentamidine isethionate	NebuPent, Pentacarinat, Pentam 300	per 300 mg, unit dose form 300 mg	INH IV, IM	J2545, J7676 S0080
Pentaspan	Pentastarch, 10% solution	100 ml	IV	J2513
Pentastarch, 10% solution	Pentaspan	100 ml	IV	J2513
Pentazocine HCl	Talwin	30 mg	IM, SC, IV	J3070
Pentobarbital sodium	Nembutol Sodium	per 50 mg	IM, IV, OTH	J2515
Pentostatin	Nipent	per 10 mg	IV	J9268
Pepcid	Famotidine	20 mg	IV	S0028
Perflexane lipid microspheres	Imagent	per ml	IV	Q9955
Perflutren lipid microsphere	Definity	per ml	IV	Q9957
Permapen	Penicillin G benzathine	100,000 units	IM	J0561
Perphenazine	Trilafon	up to 5 mg 4 mg 8 mg	IM, IV ORAL ORAL	J3310 Q0175 Q0176
Persantine	Dipyridamole	per 10 mg	IV	J1245
Pfizerpen	Penicillin G potassium	up to 600,000 units	IM, IV	J2540
Pfizerpen A.S.	Penicillin G procaine, aqueous	up to 600,000 units		J2510
Phenazine 25	Promethazine HCl	up to 50 mg 12.5 mg 25 mg	IM, IV ORAL ORAL	J2550 Q0169 Q0170
Phenazine 50	Promethazine HCl	up to 50 mg 12.5 mg 25 mg	IM, IV ORAL ORAL	J2550 Q0169 Q0170
Phenergan	Promethazine HCl	up to 50 mg	IM, IV	J2550
Phenobarbital sodium	Luminal sodium	up to 120 mg	IM, IV	J2560
Phentolamine mesylate	Regitine	up to 5 mg	IM, IV	J2760
Phenylephrine HCl	Neo-synephrine	up to 1 ml	SC, IM, IV	J2370
Phenytek	Phenytoin sodium	per 50 mg	IM, IV	J1165
Phenytoin sodium	Dilantin, Phenytek	per 50 mg	IM, IV	J1165
Phosphocol P 32	Chromic phosphate P-32	per mCi	OTH	A9564
Photofrin	Porfimer sodium	75 mg	IV	J9600
Phyllocontin	Aminophylline	up to 250 mg	IV	J0280
Phytonadione (Vitamin K)	Konakion, AquaMEPHYTON, Mephyton	per 1 mg	IM, SC, IV	J3430
Piperacillin sodium	Pipracil	1.125 g	IV	S0081
Piperacillin/ tazobactam sodium	Zosyn	1 g/0.125 g (1.125 g)	IV	J2543
Pipracil	Piperacillin sodium	1.125 g	IV	S0081
Pitocin	Oxytocin	up to 10 units	IV, IM	J2590
Plas+SD	Plasma, pooled multiple donor, solvent/detergent treated, frozen	each unit	IV	P9023
Plasma, cryoprecipitate reduced		each unit		P9044
Plasma, pooled multiple donor, solvent/detergent treated, frozen	Plas+SD	each unit	IV	P9023
Platinol AQ	Cisplatin	per 10 mg	IV	J9060
Plerixafor	Mozobil	1 mg	SC	J2562
Plicamycin	Mithracin	2.5 mg	IV	J9270
Polocaine	Mepivacaine HCl	per 10 ml	VAR	J0670
Polycillin-N	Ampicillin	500 mg	IM, IV	J0290
Polygram S/D	Immune globulin, lyophilized (e.g. powder)	500 mg	IV	J1566
Porfimer sodium	Photofrin	75 mg	IV	J9600
Potassium chloride		per 2 meq	IV	J3480
Pralidoxime chloride	Protopam chloride	up to 1 g	IV, IM, SC	J2730
Pralatrexate	Folotyn	1 mg	IV	J9307
Predalone-50	Prednisolone acetate	up to 1 ml	IM	J2650
Predcor-25	Prednisolone acetate	up to 1 ml	IM	J2650
Predcor-50	Prednisolone acetate	up to 1 ml	IM	J2650
Predicort-50	Prednisolone acetate	up to 1 ml	IM	J2650
Prednisolone	Delta Cortef	per 5 mg	ORAL	J7510
Prednisolone acetate	Key-Pred 25, Key-Pred 50, Predcor-25, Predcor-50, Predoject 50, Predalone-50, Predicort-50	up to 1 ml	IM	J2650
Prednisone	Deltasone, Meticorten, Orasone	per 5 mg	ORAL	J7506
Predoject-50	Prednisolone acetate	up to 1 ml	IM	J2650
Pregnyl	Chorionic gonadotropin	per 1,000 USP units	IM	J0725
Premarin	Estrogen, conjugated	per 25 mg	IV, IM	J1410
Prescription anti-emetic drug, oral, for use in conjunction with oral anti-cancer drug, not otherwise specified		per dose	ORAL	J8597
Prescription anti-emetic drug, rectal, for use in conjunction with oral anti-cancer drug, not otherwise specified		per dose	OTH	J8498
Prescription, chemotherapeutic, not otherwise specified			ORAL	J8999
Prescription, non-chemotherapeutic, not otherwise specified			ORAL	J8499

IA – intraarterial IM – intramuscular INH – inhalation IT – intrathecal IV – intravenous OTH – other SC – subcutaneous VAR – various administration methods

Drug Name	Additional Name(s)	Dosage	Delivery Method	HCPCS Code
Prescription drug, band name				S5001
Prescription, drug, generic				S5000
Prialt	Ziconotide	1 mcg	IT	J2278
Primacor	Milrinone lactate	5 mg	IV	J2260
Primatene Mist	Epinephrine, adrenaline	up to 1 ml ampule	IV, IM, SC	J0170
Primaxin I.M.	Cilastatin sodium, imipenem	per 250 mg	IM	J0743
Primaxin I.V.	Cilastatin sodium, imipenem	per 250 mg	IV	J0743
Principen	Ampicillin sodium	500 mg	IM, IV	J0290
Priscoline HCl	Tolazoline HCl	up to 25 mg	IV	J2670
Privigen	Immune globulin	500 mg	IV	J1459
Procainamide HCl	Procan, Pronestyl, Promine	up to 1 g	IM, IV	J2690
Procan	Procainamide HCl	up to 1 g	IM, IV	J2690
Procarbazine hydrochloride	Matulane	50 mg	ORAL	S0182
Prochlorperazine	Compa-Z, Compazine, Cotranzine, Ultrazine-10	up to 10 mg	IM, IV	J0780
Prochlorperazine maleate	Compazine	5 mg 10 mg	ORAL ORAL	Q0164 Q0165
Procrit	Epoetin alfa	100 units 1,000 units	IV, SC IV, SC	Q4081 J0885-J0886
Proctocort	Hydrocortisone acetate	up to 25 mg	IV, IM, SC	J1700
Profasi	Chorionic gonadotropin	per 1,000 USP units	IM	J0725
Profilnine SD	Factor IX	per IU	IV	J7193-J7195
Progesterone	Gesterol 50	per 50 mg	IM	J2675
Prograf	Tacrolimus	per 1 mg 5 mg	ORAL IV	J7507 J7525
ProHance	Gadoteridol	per ml	IV	A9576
Prokine	Sargramostim (GM-CSF)	50 mcg	IV	J2820
Prolastin	Alpha 1-proteinase inhibitor, human	10 mg	IV	J0256
Proleukin	Aldesleukin	per single use vial	IM, IV	J9015
Prolia	Denosumab	1 mg	IM	C9272
Prolixin decanoate	Fluphenazine decanoate	up to 25 mg	IM, SC	J2680
Promazine HCl	Sparine, Prozine-50	up to 25 mg	IM	J2950
Promethazine HCl	Anergan 50, Phenazine 25, Phenazine 50, Phenergan, Prorex-25, Prorex-50, Prothazine, V-Gan 25, V-Gan 50	up to 50 mg 12.5 mg 25 mg	IM, IV ORAL ORAL	J2550 Q0169 Q0170
Promine	Procainamide HCl	up to 1 g	IM, IV	J2690
Pronestyl	Procainamide HCl	up to 1 g	IM, IV	J2690
Proplex SX-T	Factor IX	per IU	IV	J7193-J7195
Proplex T	Factor IX	per IU	IV	J7193-J7195
Propranolol HCl	Inderal	up to 1 mg	IV	J1800
Prorex-25	Promethazine HCl	up to 50 mg 12.5 mg 25 mg	IM, IV ORAL ORAL	J2550 Q0169 Q0170
Prorex-50	Promethazine HCl	up to 50 mg 12.5 mg 25 mg	IM, IV ORAL ORAL	J2550 Q0169 Q0170
Prostaphlin	Oxacillin sodium	up to 250 mg	IM, IV	J2700
ProstaScint	Indium In-111 capromab pendetide	up to 10 millicuries	IV	A9507
ProStep	Nicotine patches, legend		OTH	S4990
Prostigmin	Neostigmine methylsulfate	up to 0.5 mg	IM, IV, SC	J2710
Prostin VR Pediatric	Alprostadil	1.25 mcg	IV	J0270
Protamine sulfate		per 10 mg	IV	J2720
Protamine sulfate, for hemodialysis		per 50 mg	IV	A4802
Protein C concentrate, human	Ceprotin	10 iu	IV	J2724
Prothazine	Promethazine HCl	up to 50 mg 12.5 mg 25 mg	IM, IV ORAL ORAL	J2550 Q0169 Q0170
Protirelin	Relefact TRH, Thypinone	per 250 mcg	IV	J2725
Protonix	Pantoprazole sodium	per vial	IV	C9113
Protopam Chloride	Pralidoxime chloride	up to 1 g	IV, IM, SC	J2730
Protostat	Metronidazole	500 mg	IV	S0030
Protropin	Somatrem	1 mg	IM, SC	J2940
Proventil	Albuterol	1 mg, concentrated dose, via DME 1 mg, concentrated dose, via DME	INH INH	J7609 J7610
Provera	Medroxyprogesterone acetate	50 mg 150 mg, for contraceptive use	IM IM	J1051 J1055
Provocholine	Methacholine chloride	1 mg	INH	J7674
Prozine-50	Promazine HCl	up to 25 mg	IM	J2950
Pulmicort Respules	Budesonide, compounded	up to 0.5 mg unit dose form per 0.25 mg	INH INH	J7627 J7633
Pulmicort Respules	Budesonide, non-compounded	up to 0.5 mg unit dose form	INH	J7626
Pulmicort Turbuhaler	Budesonide, compounded	up to 0.5 mg unit dose form per 0.25 mg	INH INH	J7627 J7633
Pulmicort Turbuhaler	Budesonide, non-compounded	up to 0.5 mg unit dose form	INH	J7626
Pulmozyme	Dornase alpha	per mg, unit dose form	INH	J7639
Pyridoxine HCl	Nestrex, Rodex	100 mg	IM, IV	J3415
Q				
Quadramet	Samarium Sm-153 lexidronamm	per 50 millicuries	IV	A9604
Quelicin	Succinylcholine chloride	up to 20 mg	IV, IM	J0330
Quinupristin/ dalfopristin	Synercid	500 mg (150/350)	IV	J2770
Qutenza	Capsaicin patch	per 10 sq cm	OTH	J7335
Qvar	Beclomethasone	per mg, unit dose form	INH	J7622

IA – intraarterial IM – intramuscular INH – inhalation IT – intrathecal IV – intravenous OTH – other SC – subcutaneous VAR – various administration methods

Table of Drugs

Drug Name	Additional Name(s)	Dosage	Delivery Method	HCPCS Code
R				
Ranibizumab	Lucentis	0.5 mg	IV	J2778
Ranitidine HCl	Tritec, Zantac	25 mg	IV, IM	J2780
Rapamune	Sirolimus	1 mg	ORAL	J7520
Rasburicase	Elitek	0.5 mg	IV	J2783
Rebif	Interferon beta-1a	11 mcg 11 mcg 33 mcg	IM SC IM	Q3025 Q3026 J1825
Reclast	Zoledronic acid	1 mg	IV	J3488
Recombinate	Factor VIII (antihemophilic factor, recombinant)	per IU	IV	J7192
Redisol	Vitamin B-12 cyanocobalamin	up to 1,000 mcg	IM, SC	J3420
ReFacto	Factor VIII (antihemophilic factor, recombinant)	per IU	IV	J7192
Refludan	Lepirudin	50 mg	IV	J1945
Regadenoson	Lexiscan	.1 mg	IM	J2785
Regitine	Phentolamine mesylate	up to 5 mg	IM, IV	J2760
Reglan	Metoclopramide HCl	up to 10 mg	IV	J2765
Regranex Gel	Becaplermin gel, 0.01%	0.5 gm	OTH	S0157
Regular	Insulin	per 5 units	SC	J1815
Relefact TRH	Protirelin	per 250 mcg	IV	J2725
Remicade	Infliximab	10 mg	IM, IV	J1745
Remodulin	Treprostinil sodium	1 mg	SC	J3285
Renacidin	Irrigation solution for treatment of bladder calculi	per 500 ml	OTH	Q2004
ReoPro	Abciximab	10 mg	IV	J0130
Rep-Pred 40	Methylprednisolone acetate	20 mg 40 mg 80 mg	IM IM IM	J1020 J1030 J1040
Rep-Pred 80	Methylprednisolone acetate	20 mg 40 mg 80 mg	IM IM IM	J1020 J1030 J1040
Respbid	Theophylline	per 40 mg	IV	J2810
Retavase	Reteplase	18.1 mg	IV	J2993
Reteplase	Retavase	18.1 mg	IV	J2993
Retisert	Fluocinolone acetonide	.59 mg	INTRAVITREAL	J7311
Retrovir	Zidovudine	10 mg	IV	J3485
Rheomacrodex	Dextran 40	500 ml	IV	J7100
Rhesonativ	Rho(D) immune globulin, human	minidose, 50 mcg full dose, 300 mg	IM IM	J2788 J2790
Rheumatrex	Methotrexate	2.5 mg	ORAL	J8610
Rheumatrex	Methotrexate sodium	5 mg 50 mg	IV, IM, IT, IA IV, IM, IT, IA	J9250 J9260
Rhinocort Aqua	Budesonide, compounded	up to 0.5 mg unit dose form per 0.25 mg	INH INH	J7627 J7633
Rhinocort Aqua	Budesonide, non-compounded	up to 0.5 mg unit dose form	INH	J7626
Rho(D) immune globulin, human	Gamulin RH, HypRho-D, MICRhoGAM, Rhesonativ, RhoGAM, Rhophylac	minidose, 50 mcg full dose, 300 mg 100 mg	IM IM IM, IV	J2788 J2790 J2791
Rho(D) immune globulin, human, solvent detergent	Win Rho SDF	100 IU	IV	J2792
RhoGAM	Rho(D) immune globulin, human	minidose, 50 mcg full dose, 300 mg	IM IM	J2788 J2790
Rhophylac	Rho(D) immune globulin, human	100 mg	IM, IV	J2791
RiaSTAP	Human Fibrinogen Concentrate	100 mg	IV	J1680
Rilonacept	Arcalyst	1 mg	SC	J2793
RimabotulinumtoxinB	Myobloc	100 units	IM	J0587
Rimso 50	DMSO, Dimethyl sulfoxide, 50%	50 ml	OTH	J1212
Ringer's lactate infusion		up to 1,000 cc	IV	J7120
Risperdal	Risperidone	0.5 mg	ORAL	J2794
Risperdal M-Tab	Risperidone	0.5 mg	ORAL	J2794
Risperidone	Risperdal, Risperdal M-Tab	0.5 mg	ORAL	J2794
Rituxan	Rituximab	100 mg	IV	J9310
Rituximab	Rituxan	100 mg	IV	J9310
Robaxin	Methocarbamol	up to 10 ml	IV, IM	J2800
Rocaltrol	Calcitriol	0.1 mcg	IM	J0636
Rocephin	Ceftriaxone sodium	per 250 mg	IV, IM	J0696
Rodex	Pyridoxine HCl	100 mg	IM, IV	J3415
Roferon-A	Interferon alfa-2a, recombinant	3 million units	SC, IM	J9213
Romidepsin	Istodax	1 mg	IV	J9315
Romiplostim	Nplate	10 mcg	SC	J2795
Ropivacaine hydrochloride	Naropin	1 mg	OTH	J2795
Rubex	Doxorubicin HCl	10 mg	IV	J9000
Rubidium Rb-82	Cardiogen-82	up to 60 mCi	IV	A9555
Rubramin PC	Vitamin B-12 cyanocobalamin	up to 1,000 mcg	IM, SC	J3420
Rubratope-57	Cobalt Co-57 cyanocobalamin	up to 1 µCi	ORAL	A9559
S				
Sabex	atropine sulfate Hospira	.01 mg	IV, IM, SC	J0461
Saizen	Somatropin	1 mg	IM, SC	J2941
Saline hypertonic solution		50 or 100 meq, 20 cc vial	IV, IM	J7130
Saline solution, normal		5% dextrose/ normal saline (500 ml= 1 unit) infusion, 250 cc infusion, 1,000 cc	IV IV IV	J7042 J7050 J7030
Saline solution, sterile		500 ml = 1 unit 30 cc 10 ml	IV, OTH IV, OTH IV, OTH	J7040 A4214 A4218
Samarium Sm-153 lexidronamm	Quadramet	per 50 millicuries	IV	A9604
Sandimmune	Cyclosporine	25 mg 100 mg 250 mg	ORAL ORAL IV	J7515 J7502 J7516

IA – intraarterial IM – intramuscular INH – inhalation IT – intrathecal IV – intravenous OTH – other SC – subcutaneous VAR – various administration methods

Drug Name	Additional Name(s)	Dosage	Delivery Method	HCPCS Code
Sandoglobulin	Immune globulin, lyophilized (e.g. powder)	500 mg	IV	J1566
Sandostatin	Octreotide acetate	1 mg 25 mcg	IM IV, SC	J2353 J2354
Sandostatin Lar Depot	Octreotide acetate	1 mg 25 mcg	IM IV, SC	J2353 J2354
SangCya	Cyclosporine	25 mg 100 mg	ORAL ORAL	J7515 J7502
Sargramostim	GM-CSF (Leukine, Prokine)	50 mcg	IV	J2820
Secretin	Secretin, synthetic, human	1 mcg	IV	J2850
Secretin, synthetic, human	Secretin	1 mcg	IV	J2850
Sensorcaine	Bupivicaine hydrochloride	30 ml	IV	S0020
Septra IV	Sulfamethoxazole and trimethoprim	10 ml	IV	S0039
Sermorelin acetate	Geref	1 mcg 0.5 mg	SC IV	Q0515 Q2014
Serostim	Somatropin	1 mg	IM, SC	J2941
Siladryl	Diphenhydramine HCl	50 mg	ORAL	Q0163
Sildenafil citrate	Viagra	25 mg	ORAL	S0090
Simulect	Basiliximab	20 mg	IV	J0480
Sincalide	Kinevac	5 mcg	IM, IV, SC	J2805
Sinusol-B	Brompheniramine maleate	per 10 mg	IM, SC, IV	J0945
Sirolimus	Rapamune	1 mg	ORAL	J7520
Sleep-Eze D	Diphenhydramine HCl	50 mg	ORAL	Q0163
SMZ-TMP	Sulfamethoxazole and trimethoprim	10 ml	IV	S0039
Sodium ferric gluconate complex in sucrose, injection	Ferrlecit	12.5 mg	IV	J2916
Sodium hyaluronate (hyaluronan) or derivative	Euflexxa, Hyalgan, Orthovisc, Supartz, Synvisc	per dose	INTRA-ARTICULAR	J7321-J7324
Solganal	Aurothioglucose	up to 50 mg	IM	J2910
Soliris	Eculizumab	10 mg	IV	J1300
Solu-Cortef	Hydrocortisone sodium succinate	up to 100 mg	IV, IM, SC	J1720
Solu-Medrol	Methylprednisolone sodium succinate	up to 40 mg up to 125 mg	IM, IV IM, IV	J2920 J2930
Solurex	Dexamethasone sodium phosphate	1 mg	IM, IV, OTH	J1100
Solurex LA	Dexamethasone acetate	1 mg	IM	J1094
Somatrem	Protropin	1 mg	IM, SC	J2940
Somatropin	Genotropin, Humatrope, Saizen, Serostim, Nutropin, Nutropin AQ, Norditropin	1 mg	IM, SC	J2941
Somatuline depot	Lanreotide	1 mg	SC, IM	J1930
Sominex	Diphenhydramine HCl	up to 50 mg 50 mg	IV, IM ORAL	J1200 Q0163
Sparine	Promazine HCl	up to 25 mg	IM	J2950
Spasmoject	Dicyclomine HCl	up to 20 mg	IM	J0500
Spectinomycin dihydrochloride	Trobicin	up to 2 g	IM	J3320
Sporanox	Itraconazole	50 mg	IV	J1835
Stadol	Butorphanol tartrate, injection	1 mg	IM	J0595
Stadol NS	Butorphanol tartrate, nasal spray	25 mg	NASAL SPRAY	S0012
Stelara	Ustekinumab	1 mg	SC	J3357
Sterile dilutant for Epoprostenol	Flolan	50 ml	IV	S0155
Stilphostrol	Diethylstilbestrol diphosphate	250 mg	IV	J9165
Storzolamide	Acetazolamide sodium	up to 500 mg	IM, IV	J1120
Streptase	Streptokinase	per 250,000 IU	IV	J2995
Streptokinase	Kabikinase, Streptase	per 250,000 IU	IV	J2995
Streptomycin		up to 1 g	IM	J3000
Streptozocin	Zanosar	1 gm	IV	J9320
Strontium-89 chloride	Metastron	per mCi	IV	A9600
Sublimaze	Fentanyl citrate	0.1 mg	IM, IV	J3010
Succinylcholine chloride	Anectine, Anectine Flo-Pack, Sucostrin, Quelicin	up to 20 mg	IV, IM	J0330
Sucostrin	Succinycholine chloride	up to 20 mg	IV, IM	J0330
Sulfamethoxazole and trimethoprim	Bactrim IV, Cofatrim Forte, Cotrim, Septra IV, SMZ-TMP, Sulfatrim	10 ml	IV	S0039
Sulfatrim	Sulfamethoxazole and trimethoprim	10 ml	IV	S0039
Sumatriptan succinate	Imitrex	6 mg	SC	J3030
Sumycin	Tetracycline	up to 250 mg	IM, IV	J0120
Supartz	Hyaluronan (sodium hyaluronate or derivative)	per dose	INTRA-ARTICULAR	J7321
Supprelin	Histrelin acetate	10 mcg	SC	J1675
Supprelin LA	Histrelin implant	50 mg	SC implant	J9226
Sus-Phrine	Adrenalin, epinephrine	up to 1 ml ampule	IV, IM, SC	J0170
Synagis	Palivizumab-RSV-IGM	per 50 mg	IM	C9003
Synercid	Quinupristin/dalfopristin	500 mg (150/350)	IV	J2770
Synkavite	Vitamin K (phytonadione)	per 1 mg	IM, SC, IV	J3430
Syntocinon	Oxytocin	up to 10 units	IV, IM	J2590
Synvisc	Hylan G-F 20	per dose	INTRA-ARTICULAR	J7325
Sytobex	Vitamin B-12 cyanocobalamin	up to 1,000 mcg	IM, SC	J3420
T				
Tacrine hydrochloride	Cognex	10 mg	ORAL	S0014
Tacrolimus	Prograf	per 1 mg 5 mg	ORAL IV	J7507 J7525
Tagamet	Cimetidine hydrochloride	300 mg	IV, IM	S0023
Talwin	Pentazocine HCl	30 mg	IM, SC, IV	J3070
Taxol	Paclitaxel	30 mg	IV	J9265
Taxotere	Docetaxel	20 mg	IV	J9171
Tazicef	Ceftazidime	per 500 mg	IM, IV	J0713
Tazidime	Ceftazidime	per 500 mg	IM, IV	J0713
Tebamide	Trimethobenzamide HCl	up to 200 mg 250 mg	IM ORAL	J3250 Q0173

IA – intraarterial IM – intramuscular INH – inhalation IT – intrathecal IV – intravenous OTH – other SC – subcutaneous VAR – various administration methods

Drug Name	Additional Name(s)	Dosage	Delivery Method	HCPCS Code
TechneScan MAG3	Technetium Tc-99m mertiatide	up to 15 mCi	IV	A9562
TechneScan PYP	Technetium Tc-99m pyrophosphate	up to 25 mCi	IV	A9538
Technetium Tc-99m exametazime	Ceretec	up to 25 millicuries	IV	A9521
Technetium Tc-99m fanolesomab	NeutroSpec	up to 25 mCi	IV	A9566
Technetium Tc-99m mebrofenin	Choletec	up to 15 mCi	IV	A9537
Technetium Tc-99m medronate	CIS-MDP	up to 30 millicuries	IV	A9503
Technetium Tc-99m mertiatide	TechneScan MAG3	up to 15 mCi	IV	A9562
Technetium Tc-99m pentetate	AN-DTPA	up to 25 mCi	IV	A9539
Technetium Tc-99m pyrophosphate	TechneScan PYP	up to 25 mCi	IV	A9538
Technetium Tc-99m sestamibi	Cardiolite	up to 40 millicuries	IV	A9500
TEEV	Testosterone enanthate and estradiol valerate	up to 1 cc	IM	J0900
Televancin	Vibativ	10 mg	IV	J3095
Temodar	Temozolomide	5 mg	ORAL	J8700
Temozolomide	Temodar	5 mg 1 mg	ORAL IV	J8700 J9328
Temsirolimus	Torisel	1 mg	IV	J9330
Tenecteplase	TNKase	1 mg	IM, IV	J3101
Teniposide	Vumon	50 mg	IV	Q2017
Tequin	Gatifloxacin	10 mg	IV	J1590
Terbutaline sulfate	Brethaire, Brethine, Bricanyl, Bricanyl Turbuhaler	up to 1 mg per 1 mg, concentrated form per 1 mg, unit dose form	SC, IV INH INH	J3105 J7680 J7681
Teriparatide	Forteo	10 mcg	SC	J3110
Terramycin	Oxytetracycline HCl	up to 50 mg	IM	J2460
Testa-C	Testosterone cypionate	1 cc, 200 mg	IM	J1080
Testadiate	Testosterone enanthate and estradiol valerate	up to 1 cc	IM	J0900
Testadiate-Depo	Testosterone cypionate	1 cc, 200 mg	IM	J1080
Testaqua	Testosterone suspension	up to 50 mg	IM	J3140
Test-Estro-C	Testosterone cypionate and estradiol cypionate	up to 1 ml	IM	J1060
Test-Estro Cypionate	Testosterone cypionate and estradiol cypionate	up to 1 ml	IM	J1060
Testex	Testosterone propionate	up to 100 mg	IM	J3150
Testoject-50	Testosterone suspension	up to 50 mg	IM	J3140
Testoject-LA	Testosterone cypionate	up to 100 mg 1 cc, 200 mg	IM IM	J1070 J1080
Testone LA 100	Testosterone enanthate	up to 100 mg	IM	J3120
Testone LA 200	Testosterone enanthate	up to 200 mg	IM	J3130

Drug Name	Additional Name(s)	Dosage	Delivery Method	HCPCS Code
Testosterone aqueous	Testosterone suspension	up to 50 mg	IM	J3140
Testosterone cypionate	Andro-Cyp, Andronaq-LA, Andronate-100, depAndro 100, Depotest, Depo-Testosterone, Duratest-100, Testadiate-Depo, Testoject-LA	up to 100 mg	IM	J1070
Testosterone cypionate	Andro-Cyp 200, Andronate-200, depAndro 200, Depotest, Depo-Testosterone, Duratest-200, Testa-C, Testoject-LA	1 cc, 200 mg	IM	J1080
Testosterone cypionate and estradiol cypionate	Depo-Testadiol, Andro/Fem, De-Comberol, depAndrogyn, Depotestogen, Duo-Cyp, Duratestrin, Menoject LA, Test-Estro-C, Test-Estro Cypionate	up to 1 ml	IM	J1060
Testosterone enanthate	Andropository 100, Delatest, Everone, Testone LA 100	up to 100 mg	IM	J3120
Testosterone enanthate	Andro L.A. 200, Andryl 200, Delatestryl, Durathate-200, Testone LA 200, Testrin PA	up to 200 mg	IM	J3130
Testosterone enanthate and estradiol valerate	Deladumone, Andrest 90-4, Andro-Estro 90-4, Androgyn L.A., Delatestadiol, Dua-Gen L.A., Duoval P.A., Estra-Testrin, TEEV, Testadiate, Testradiol 90/4, Valertest No. 1, Valertest No. 2, Deladumone OB, Ditate-DS	up to 1 cc	IM	J0900
Testosterone propionate	Testex	up to 100 mg	IM	J3150
Testosterone suspension	Andronaq 50, Testosterone Aqueous, Testaqua, Testoject-50, Histerone 50, Histerone 100	up to 50 mg	IM	J3140
Testradiol 90/4	Testosterone enanthate and estradiol valerate	up to 1 cc	IM	J0900
Testrin PA	Testosterone enanthate	up to 200 mg	IM	J3130
Tetanus immune globulin, human	BayTet, Hyper-Tet	up to 250 units	IM	J1670
Tetracon	Tetracycline	up to 250 mg	IM, IV	J0120
Tetracycline	Achromycin, Brodspec, Panmycin, Sumycin, Tetracon, Wesmycin	up to 250 mg	IM, IV	J0120

IA – intraarterial IM – intramuscular INH – inhalation IT – intrathecal IV – intravenous OTH – other SC – subcutaneous VAR – various administration methods

Drug Name	Additional Name(s)	Dosage	Delivery Method	HCPCS Code
T-Gen	Trimethobenzamide HCl	up to 200 mg 250 mg	IM ORAL	J3250 Q0173
Thallous chloride (Tl-201)		per mCi	IM	A9505
Theelin aqueous	Estrone	per 1 mg	IM	J1435
Theophylline	Lanophyllin, Respbid	per 40 mg	IV	J2810
Theophylline ethylenadiamine	Aminophylline	up to 250 mg	IV	J0280
TheraCys	BCG, live	per vial	IV	J9031
Thiamine HCl	Vitamin B-1	100 mg	IM, IV	J3411
Thiethylperazine maleate	Norzine, Torecan	10 mg up to 10 mg	ORAL IM	Q0174 J3280
Thioplex	Thiotepa	15 mg	IV	J9340
Thiotepa	Thioplex	15 mg	IV	J9340
Thorazine	Chlorpromazine HCl	up to 50 mg 10 mg 25 mg	IM, IV ORAL ORAL	J3230 Q0171 Q0172
Thrombate III	Antithrombin III (human)	per IU	IV	J7197
Thymoglobulin	Lymphocyte Immune globulin, anti-thymocyte globulin, rabbit, parenteral	25 mg	IV	J7511
Thypinone	Protirelin	per 250 mcg	IV	J2725
Thyrogen	Thyrotropin Alfa	0.9 mg, provided in a 1.1 mg vial	IM, SC	J3240
Thyrotropin Alfa	Thyrogen	0.9 mg, provided in a 1.1 mg vial	IM, SC	J3240
Ticarcillin disodium and clavulanate potassium	Timentin	3.1 g	IV, IM	S0040
TICE BCG	BCG live	per vial	INTRAVESICAL INSTILLATION	J9031
Ticon	Trimethobenzamide HCl	up to 200 mg 250 mg	IM ORAL	J3250 Q0173
Tigan	Trimethobenzamide HCl	up to 200 mg 250 mg	IM ORAL	J3250 Q0173
Tigecycline	Tygacil	1 mg	IM	J3243
Tiject-20	Trimethobenzamide HCl	up to 200 mg 250 mg	IM ORAL	J3250 Q0173
Timentin	Ticarcillin disodium and clavulanate potassium	3.1 g	IV, IM	S0040
Tinzaparin Sodium	Innohep	1000 IU	SC	J1655
Tirofiban hydrochloride	Aggrastat	0.25 mg	IM, IV	J3246
TNKase	Tenecteplase	1 mg	IM, IV	J3101
TOBI	Tobramycin	300 mg, unit dose form	INH	J7682, J7685
Tobramycin	TOBI	300 mg, unit dose form	INH	J7682, J7685
Tobramycin sulfate	Nebcin	up to 80 mg	IM, IV	J3260
Tocilizumab	Actemra	1 mg	IV	J3262
Tolazoline HCl	Priscoline HCl	up to 25 mg	IV	J2670
Toposar	Etoposide	10 mg 50 mg	IV ORAL	J9181 J8560
Topotecan	Hycamtin	.1 mg .25 mg	IV ORAL	J9351 J8705
Toradol	Ketorolac tromethamine	per 15 mg	IM, IV	J1885
Torecan	Thiethylperazine maleate	10 mg up to 10 mg	ORAL IM	Q0174 J3280
Torisel	Temsirolimus	1 mg	IV	J9330
Tornalate	Bitolterol mesylate	per mg, concentrated form per mg, unit dose form	INH INH	J7628 J7629
Torsemide	Demadex	10 mg/ml	IV	J3265
Totacillin-N	Ampicillin sodium	500 mg	IM, IV	J0290
Trastuzumab	Herceptin	10 mg	IV	J9355
Trasylol	Aprotinin	10,000 KIU	IV	J0365
Treanda	Bendamustine	1 mg	IV	J9033
Trelstar Depot	Triptorelin pamoate	3.75 mg	IM	J3315
Treprostinil	Remodulin	1 mg	SC	J3285
Triam-A	Triamcinolone acetonide	per 10 mg	IM	J3301
Triamcinolone	Azmacort	per 1 mg, concentrated form per 1 mg, unit dose form	INH INH	J7683 J7684
Triamcinolone acetonide	Cenacort A-40, Kenalog-10, Kenalog-40, Tri-Kort, Kenaject-40, Triam-A, Trilog	per 10 mg	IM	J3301
Triamcinolone, preservative free	Triesence	1 mg	IM	J3300
Triamcinolone diacetate	Aristocort Intralesional, Aristocort Forte, Amcort, Cenacort Forte, Trilone	per 5 mg	IM	J3302
Triamcinolone hexacetonide	Aristospan Intralesional, Aristospan Intra-Articular	per 5 mg	VAR	J3303
Triban	Trimethobenzamide HCl	up to 200 mg 250 mg	IM ORAL	J3250 Q0173
Triesence	Triamcinolone acetonide	1 mg	IM	J3300
Triflupromazine HCl	Vesprin	up to 20 mg	IM, IV	J3400
Tri-Kort	Triamcinolone acetonide	per 10 mg	IM	J3301
Trilafon	Perphenazine	up to 5 mg 4 mg 8 mg	IM, IV ORAL ORAL	J3310 Q0175 Q0176
Trilog	Triamcinolone acetonide	per 10 mg	IM	J3301
Trilone	Triamcinolone diacetate	per 5 mg	IM	J3302
Trimazide	Trimethobenzamide HCl	up to 200 mg 250 mg	IM ORAL	J3250 Q0173
Trimethobenzamide HCl	Arrestin, Tebamide, T-Gen, Ticon, Tigan, Tiject-20, Triban Trimazide	up to 200 mg 250 mg	IM ORAL	J3250 Q0173
Trimetrexate glucuronate	Neutrexin	per 25 mg	IV	J3305
Triptorelin pamoate	Trelstar Depot	3.75 mg	IM	J3315
Trisenox	Arsenic trioxide	1 mg	IV	J9017
Tritec	Ranitidine HCl	25 mg	IV, IM	J2780
Trobicin	Spectinomycin dihydrochloride	up to 2 g	IM	J3320

Table of Drugs

IA – intraarterial IM – intramuscular INH – inhalation IT – intrathecal IV – intravenous OTH – other SC – subcutaneous VAR – various administration methods

Drug Name	Additional Name(s)	Dosage	Delivery Method	HCPCS Code
Trovan IV	Alatrofloxacin mesylate	100 mg	IV	J0200
Truphylline	Aminophylline	up to 250 mg	IV	J0280
Twilite Caplets	Diphenhydramine HCl	50 mg	ORAL	Q0163
Tygacil	Tigecycline	1 mg	IM	J3243
Tysabri	Natalizumab	1 mg	IV	J2323
U				
Ultrazine-10	Prochlorperazine	up to 10 mg	IM, IV	J0780
Unasyn	Ampicillin sodium/ sulbactam sodium	per 1.5 gm	IM, IV	J0295
Unclassified drugs	Not otherwise classified drugs		VAR	J3490
Unclassified drugs	Not otherwise classified drugs		INH ADMIN. THRU DME	J7699
Unclassified drugs	Not otherwise classified drugs		OTHER THAN INH ADMIN. THRU DME	J7799
Unipen	Nafcillin sodium	2 g	IV, IM	S0032
Unisom SleepGels	Diphenhydramine HCl	50 mg	ORAL	Q0163
Unspecified oral antiemetic			ORAL	Q0181
Urabeth	Bethanechol chloride	up to 5 mg	SC	J0520
Urea	Ureaphil	up to 40 g	IV	J3350
Ureaphil	Urea	up to 40 g	IV	J3350
Urecholine	Bethanechol chloride	up to 5 mg	SC	J0520
Urofollitropin	Bravelle, Fertinex, Metrodin	75 IU	IM, SC	J3355
Urokinase	Abbokinase	250,000 IU vial	IV	J3365
Urokinase	Abbokinase, Open Cath	5,000 IU vial	IV	J3364
Urolene Blue	Methylene blue	1 mg	IV	A9604
Ustenkinumab	Stelara	1 mg	SC	J3357
V				
Valergen 10	Estradiol valerate	up to 10 mg up to 20 mg up to 40 mg	IM IM IM	J1380 J1390 J0970
Valergen 20	Estradiol valerate	up to 10 mg up to 20 mg up to 40 mg	IM IM IM	J1380 J1390 J0970
Valergen 40	Estradiol valerate	up to 10 mg up to 20 mg up to 40 mg	IM IM IM	J1380 J1390 J0970
Valertest No. 1	Testosterone enanthate and estradiol valerate	up to 1 cc	IM	J0900
Valertest No. 2	Testosterone enanthate and estradiol valerate	up to 1 cc	IM	J0900
Valium	Diazepam	up to 5 mg	IM, IV	J3360
Valrubicin	Valstar	200 mg	INTRAVESICAL	J9357
Valstar	Valrubicin	200 mg	INTRAVESICAL	J9357
Vancenase	Beclomethasone	per mg, unit dose form	INH	J7622
Vanceril	Beclomethasone	per mg, unit dose form	INH	J7622
Vancocin	Vancomycin HCl	500 mg	IV, IM	J3370
Vancoled	Vancomycin HCl	500 mg	IV, IM	J3370
Vancomycin HCl	Vancocin, Vancoled	500 mg	IV, IM	J3370
Vantas	Histrelin implant	50 mg	SC implant	J9225
Vectibix	Panitumumab	10 mg	IV	J9303
Velaglucerase alfa	VPRIV	100 units	IV	J3385
Velban	Vinblastine sulfate	1 mg	IV	J9360
Velcade	Bortezomib	0.1 mg	IV	J9041
Velosulin	Insulin	per 5 units	SC	J1815
Velsar	Vinblastine sulfate	1 mg	IV	J9360
Venoglubulin-I	Immune globulin, lyophilized (e.g. powder)	500 mg	IV	J1566
Venoglubulin-S	Immune globulin, lyophilized (e.g. powder)	500 mg	IV	J1566
Venofer	Iron sucrose	1 mg	IV	J1756
Ventavis	Iloprost	up to 20 mcg	INH	Q4074
Ventolin	Albuterol	1 mg, concentrated dose, via DME 1 mg, unit dose, via DME	INH INH	J7609 J7610
VePesid	Etoposide	10 mg 50 mg	IV ORAL	J9181 J8560
Versed	Midazolam HCl	per 1 mg	IM, IV	J2250
Verteporfin	Visudyne	0.1 mg	IV	J3396
Vesprin	Triflupromazine HCl	up to 20 mg	IM, IV	J3400
Vfend	Voriconazole	10 mg	IV	J3465
V-Gan 25	Promethazine HCl	up to 50 mg 12.5 mg 25 mg	IM, IV ORAL ORAL	J2550 Q0169 Q0170
V-Gan 50	Promethazine HCl	up to 50 mg 12.5 mg 25 mg	IM, IV ORAL ORAL	J2550 Q0169 Q0170
Viadur	Leuprolide acetate implant	65 mg	SC, IM	J9219
Viagra	Sildenafil citrate	25 mg	ORAL	S0090
Vibativ	Televancin	10 mg	IV	J3262
Vidaza	Azacitidine	1 mg	SC	J9025
Vimpat	Lacosamide	1 mg	IM	C9257
Vinblastine sulfate	Alkaban-AQ, Velban, Velsar	1 mg	IV	J9360
Vincasar PFS	Vincristine sulfate	1 mg	IV	J9370
Vincrex	Vincristine sulfate	1 mg	IV	J9370
Vincristine sulfate	Oncovin, Vincasar PFS, Vincrex	1 mg	IV	J9370
Vinorelbine tartrate	Navelbine	per 10 mg	IV	J9390
Vistaject-50	Hydroxyzine HCl	up to 25 mg	IM	J3410
Vistaril	Hydroxyzine HCl	up to 25 mg	IM	J3410
Vistaril	Hydroxyzine pamoate	25 mg 50 mg	ORAL ORAL	Q0177 Q0178
Vistide	Cidofovir	375 mg	IV	J0740
Visudyne	Verteporfin	0.1 mg	IV	J3396
Vitamin B-1	Thiamine HCl	100 mg	IM, IV	J3411
Vitamin B-12 cyanocobalamin	Berubigen, Betalin12, Cobex, Crystamine, Cyanoject, Cyomin, Redisol, Rubramin PC, Sytobex	up to 1,000 mcg	IM, SC	J3420
Vitamin B-17, amygdalin	Laetrile		VAR	J3570
Vitamin K	phytonadione (AquaMEPHYTON, Konakion, Mephyton, Synkavite)	per 1 mg	IM, SC, IV	J3430

IA – intraarterial IM – intramuscular INH – inhalation IT – intrathecal IV – intravenous OTH – other SC – subcutaneous VAR – various administration methods

Drug Name	Additional Name(s)	Dosage	Delivery Method	HCPCS Code
Vitrase	Hyaluronidase	1 USP unit up to 999 units per 1,000 USP units	IM, IV, SC IM, IV, SC	J3471 J3472
Vitrasert	Ganciclovir, long-acting implant	4.5 mg	OTH	J7310
Vitravene	Fomivirsen sodium	1.65 mg	INTRAOCULAR	J1452
Vivaglobin	Immune globulin, subcutaneous	100 mg	SC	J1562
Vivatrol	Naltrexone, depot form	1 mg	IM	J2315
Von Willebrand factor complex, vWF:RCo	Humate-P Wilate	per IU per 100 IU	IV IV	J7187 J7184
VPRIV	Velaglucerase	100 units	IV	J3385
Voriconazole	Vfend	10 mg	IV	J3465
Vumon	Teniposide	50 mg	IV	Q2017
W				
Wehamine	Dimenhydrinate	up to 50 mg	IM, IV	J1240
Wehdryl	Diphenhydramine HCl	up to 50 mg 50 mg	IV, IM ORAL	J1200 Q0163
Wellcovorin	Leucovorin calcium	per 50 mg	IM, IV	J0640
Wesmycin	Tetracycline	up to 250 mg	IM, IV	J0120
Wilate	Von Willebrand factor complex, vWF:RCo	per 100 IU	IV	J7184
Win Rho SDF	Rho(D) immune globulin, human, solvent detergent	100 IU	IV	J2792
WR-2721	Amifostine	500 mg	IV	J0207
Wycillin	Penicillin G procaine, aqueous	up to 600,000 units	IM, IV	J2510
Wydase	Hyaluronidase	up to 150 units	SC, IV	J3470
X				
Xeloda	Capecitabine	150 mg 500 mg	ORAL ORAL	J8520 J8521
Xeomin	Incobotulinum toxin A	1 unit	IM	C9278
Xiaflex	Collagenase, clostrodium histolyticum	0.01 mg	IM	J0775
Xolair	Omalizumab	5 mg	SC	J2357
Xopenex	Levalbuterol HCl	0.5 mg, concentrated form 0.5 mg, unit dose form	INH INH	J7607 J7615
Xylocaine	Lidocaine HCl	10 mg	IV	J2001
Xyntha	Factor VIII (antihemophillic factor, recombinant)	per I.U.	IV	J7185, J7192
Y				
Y-90 Zevalin	Yttrium Y-90 ibritumomab tiuxetan	up to 40 mCi	IV	A9543
Yttrium Y-90 ibritumomab tiuxetan	Y-90 Zevalin	up to 40 mCi	IV	A9543
Z				
Zanosar	Streptozocin	1 gm	IV	J9320
Zantac	Ranitidine HCl	25 mg	IV, IM	J2780
Zemplar	Paricalcitol	1 mcg	IV, IM	J2501
Zenapax	Daclizumab	25 mg	IV	J7513
Zetran	Diazepam	up to 5 mg	IM, IV	J3360
Zevalin	Indium In-111 ibritumomab tiuxetan	up to 5 mCi	IV	A9542
Ziconotide	Prialt	1 mcg	IT	J2278
Zidovudine	Retrovir	10 mg	IV	J3485
Zinacef	Cefuroxime sodium, sterile	per 750 mg	IM, IV	J0697
Zinecard	Dexrazoxane hydrochloride	per 250 mg	IV	J1190
Ziprasidone mesylate	Geodon	10 mg	IM	J3486
Zithromax	Azithromycin, Azithromycin dihydrate	500 mg 1 gm	IV ORAL	J0456 Q0144
Zofran	Ondansetron HCl	per 1 mg 8 mg	IV ORAL	J2405 Q0179
Zofran ODT	Ondansetron HCl	per 1 mg 8 mg	IV ORAL	J2405 Q0179
Zoladex	Goserelin acetate implant	per 3.6 mg	SC	J9202
Zoledronic acid	Reclast, Zometa	1 mg	IV	J3487-J3488
Zolicef	Cefazolin sodium	500 mg	IV, IM	J0690
Zometa	Zoledronic acid	1 mg	IV	J3487
Zosyn	Piperacillin/ tazobactam sodium	1 g/ 0.125 g (1.125 g)	IV	J2543
Zovirax	Acyclovir	5 mg	IV	J0133
Zyprexa, Relprevv	Olanzapine	1 mg	IM	J2358
Zyvox	Linezolid	200 mg	IV	J2020

Medicare References

Internet Only Manuals

Pub 100-1: **Medicare General Information, Eligibility and Entitlement Manual**
Pub 100-2: **Medicare Benefit Policy Manual**
Pub 100-3: **National Coverage Decisions (NCD)**
Pub 100-4: **Medicare Claims Processing Manual**
Pub 100-5: **Medicare Secondary Payor Manual**
Pub 100-8: **Medicare Program Integrity Manual**

Pub 100-1: Medicare General Information, Eligibility and Entitlement Manual

Pub 100-1, 3, 20.4 – Exceptions to Annual Deductible and Coinsurance

(Rev. 11, Issued: 10-22-04, Effective: 11-22-04, Implementation: 11-22-04)

There is no deductible for screening mammography effective for services January 1, 1998 and later.

Neither the annual deductible nor the 20 percent coinsurance apply with respect to:

- Parts A and B home health services, except that there is a coinsurance of 20 percent of the payment amount for supplies, drugs, DME and prosthetics /orthotics furnished as a home health benefit;
- Clinical diagnostic laboratory tests (including specimen collection fees) performed or supervised by a physician, laboratory, or other entity paid on an assigned basis;
- Pneumococcal vaccine and its administration;
- Influenza vaccine and its administration; and
- Services or items denied as medically unnecessary.

NOTE: Services which are not subject to the deductible cannot be used to satisfy the deductible.

Pub 100-1, 5, 90.2 – Laboratory Defined

(Rev. 1, 09-11-02)

Laboratory means a facility for the biological, microbiological, serological, chemical, immuno-hematological, hematological, biophysical, cytological, pathological, or other examination of materials derived from the human body for the purpose of providing information for the diagnosis, prevention, or treatment of any disease or impairment of, or the assessment of the health of, human beings. These examinations also include procedures to determine, measure, or otherwise describe the presence or absence of various substances or organisms in the body. Facilities only collecting or preparing specimens (or both) or only serving as a mailing service and not performing testing are not considered laboratories.

Pub 100-2: Medicare Benefit Policy Manual

Pub 100-2, 1, 120 – Services Related to and Required as a Result of Services Which Are Not Covered Under Medicare

(Rev. 1, 10-01-03)

A3-3101.14, HO-210.12, B3-2300.1, A3-3101.14, HO-210.12

Medical and hospital services are sometimes required to treat a condition that arises as a result of services that are not covered because they are determined to be not reasonable and necessary or because they are excluded from coverage for other reasons. Services "related to" noncovered services (e.g., cosmetic surgery, noncovered organ transplants, noncovered artificial organ implants, etc.), including services related to follow-up care and complications of noncovered services which require treatment during a hospital stay in which the noncovered service was performed, are not covered services under Medicare. Services "not related to" noncovered services are covered under Medicare.

Following are examples of services "related to" and "not related to" noncovered services while the beneficiary is an inpatient:

- A beneficiary was hospitalized for a noncovered service and broke a leg while in the hospital. Services related to care of the broken leg during this stay is a clear example of "not related to" services and are covered under Medicare.
- A beneficiary was admitted to the hospital for covered services, but during the course of hospitalization became a candidate for a noncovered transplant or implant and actually received the transplant or implant during that hospital stay. When the original admission was entirely unrelated to the diagnosis that led to a recommendation for a noncovered transplant or implant, the services related to the admitting condition would be covered.
- A beneficiary was admitted to the hospital for covered services related to a condition which ultimately led to identification of a need for transplant and receipt of a transplant during the same hospital stay. If, on the basis of the nature of the services and a comparison of the date they are received with the date on which the beneficiary is identified as a transplant candidate, the services could reasonably be attributed to preparation for the noncovered transplant, the services would be "related to" noncovered services and would also be noncovered.

Following is an example of services received subsequent to a noncovered inpatient stay:

> After a beneficiary has been discharged from the hospital stay in which the beneficiary received noncovered services, medical and hospital services required to treat a condition or complication that arises as a result of the prior noncovered services may be covered when they are reasonable and necessary in all other respects. Thus, coverage could be provided for subsequent inpatient stays or outpatient treatment ordinarily covered by Medicare, even if the need for treatment arose because of a previous noncovered procedure. Some examples of services that may be found to be covered under this policy are the reversal of intestinal bypass surgery for obesity, repair of complications from transsexual surgery or from cosmetic surgery, removal of a noncovered bladder stimulator, or treatment of any infection at the surgical site of a noncovered transplant that occurred following discharge from the hospital.

However, any subsequent services that could be expected to have been incorporated into a global fee are not covered. Thus, where a patient undergoes cosmetic surgery and the treatment regimen calls for a series of postoperative visits to the surgeon for evaluating the patient's progress, these visits are not covered.

Pub 100-2, 10, 10 – Ambulance Service

(Rev. 1, 10-01-03)

B3-2120, A3-3114, HO-236

Ambulance services are separately payable only under Part B. There are certain circumstances in which the service is covered and payable as a beneficiary transportation service under Part A; however in this case the service cannot be classified and paid for as an ambulance service under Part B. (See §10.3.3 for a description of this exception. Also see §10.2.4 for the required documentation for ambulance services.)

Payment may be made for expenses incurred for ambulance service provided the conditions specified in the following subsections are met. (See the Medicare **Claims Processing Manual**, Chapter 15, "Ambulance," for instructions for processing ambulance service claims.)

The Medicare ambulance benefit is a transportation benefit and without a transport there is no payable service. When multiple ground and/or air ambulance providers/suppliers respond, payment may be made only to the ambulance provider/supplier that actually furnishes the transport.

Pub 100-2, 10, 10.1 – Vehicle and Crew Requirement

(Rev. 1, 10-01-03)

B3-2120.1, A3-3114, HO-236.1

Pub 100-2, 10, 10.1.1 – The Vehicle

(Rev. 1, 10-01-03)

B3-2120.1.A, A3-3114.A, HO-236.1.A

Any vehicle used as an ambulance must be designed and equipped to respond to medical emergencies and, in nonemergency situations, be capable of transporting beneficiaries with acute medical conditions. The vehicle must comply with State or local laws governing the licensing and certification of an emergency medical transportation vehicle. At a minimum, the ambulance must contain a stretcher, linens, emergency medical supplies, oxygen equipment, and other lifesaving emergency medical equipment and be equipped with emergency warning lights, sirens, and telecommunications equipment as required by State or local law. This should include, at a minimum, one 2-way voice radio or wireless telephone.

Pub 100-2, 10, 10.1.2 – Vehicle Requirements for Basic Life Support and Advanced Life Support

(Rev. 1, 10-01-03)

A3-3114, B3-2120.1, HO-236.1

Basic Life Support ambulances must be staffed by at least two people, at least one of whom must be certified as an emergency medical technician (EMT) by the State or local authority where the services are being furnished and be legally authorized to operate all lifesaving and life-sustaining equipment on board the vehicle. Advanced Life Support (ALS) vehicles must be staffed by at least two people, at least one of whom must be certified by the State or local authority as an EMT-Intermediate or an EMT-Paramedic.

Pub 100-2, 10, 10.1.3 – Verification of Compliance

(Rev. 1, 10-01-03)

B3-2120.1.C, B3-2120.1.C, HO-236.1

In determining whether the vehicles and personnel of each supplier meet all of the above requirements, carriers may accept the supplier's statement (absent information to the contrary) that its vehicles and personnel meet all of the requirements if:

1. The statement describes the first aid, safety, and other patient care items with which the vehicles are equipped;
2. The statement shows the extent of first aid training acquired by the personnel assigned to those vehicles;
3. The statement contains the supplier's agreement to notify the carrier of any change in operation which could affect the coverage of ambulance services; and
4. The information provided indicates that the requirements are met.

The statement must be accompanied by documentary evidence that the ambulance has the equipment required by State and local authorities. Documentary evidence could include a letter from such authorities, a copy of a license, permit, certificate, etc., issued by the authorities. The carrier will keep the statement and supporting documentation on file.

When a supplier does not submit such a statement or whenever there is a question about a supplier's compliance with any of the above requirements for vehicle and crew (including suppliers who have completed the statement), carriers will take appropriate action including, where necessary, on-site inspection of the vehicles and verification of the qualifications of personnel to determine whether the ambulance service qualifies for reimbursement under Medicare. Since the requirements described above for coverage of ambulance services are applicable to the overall operation of the ambulance supplier's service, information regarding personnel and vehicles need not be obtained on an individual trip basis.

Pub 100-2, 10, 10.1.4 – Ambulance Services Furnished by Providers of Services

(Rev. 1, 10-01-03)

A3-3114, B3-2120.1, HO-236.1

The Part A intermediary is responsible for the processing of claims for ambulance service furnished under arrangements by participating hospitals, skilled nursing facilities, and home health agencies. Since provider ambulance services furnished "under arrangements" with suppliers can be covered only if the supplier meets the above requirements, the Part A intermediary may ask the carrier to identify those suppliers who meet the requirements. Where the "under arrangement" supplier also supplies ambulance services directly to Medicare beneficiaries, i.e., services that are not pursuant to an arrangement with a provider, the intermediary contacts the Part B carrier to ascertain whether it has already determined whether the crew and ambulance requirements are met. In such a situation, the intermediary should accept the carrier's determination without pursuing its own investigation.

Pub 100-2, 10, 10.1.5 – Equipment and Supplies

(Rev. 1, 10-01-03)

A3-3114.A, B3-2120.2.E

As mentioned above, the ambulance must have customary patient care equipment and first aid supplies, including reusable devices and equipment such as backboards, neckboards, and inflatable leg and arm splints. These are all considered part of the general ambulance service and payment for them is included in the payment rate for the transport.

Pub 100-2, 10, 20 – Coverage Guidelines for Ambulance Service Claims

(Rev. 103; Issued: 02-20-09; Effective Date: 01-05-09; Implementation Date: 03- 20-09)

B3-2125

Payment may be made for expenses incurred by a patient for ambulance service provided conditions l, 2, and 3 in the left-hand column have been met. The right-hand column indicates the documentation needed to establish that the condition has been met.

Conditions	Review Action
1. Patient was transported by an approved supplier of ambulance services.	1. Ambulance supplier is listed in the table of approved ambulance companies (§10.1.3)
2. The patient was suffering from an illness or injury, which contraindicated transportation by other means. (§10.2)	2. (a) The contractor presumes the requirement was met if the submitted documentation indicates that the patient:
	• Was transported in an emergency situation, e.g., as a result of an accident, injury or acute illness, or

Conditions	Review Action
	• Needed to be restrained to prevent injury to the beneficiary or others; or
	• Was unconscious or in shock; or
	• Required oxygen or other emergency treatment during transport to the nearest appropriate facility; or
	• Exhibits signs and symptoms of acute respiratory distress or cardiac distress such as shortness of breath or chest pain; or
	• Exhibits signs and symptoms that indicate the possibility of acute stroke; or
	• Had to remain immobile because of a fracture that had not been set or the possibility of a fracture; or
	• Was experiencing severe hemorrhage; or
	• Could be moved only by stretcher; or
	• Was bed-confined before and after the ambulance trip.
	(b) In the absence of any of the conditions listed in (a) above additional documentation should be obtained to establish medical need where the evidence indicates the existence of the circumstances listed below: (i) Patient's condition would not ordinarily require movement by stretcher, or (ii) The individual was not admitted as a hospital inpatient (except in accident cases), or (iii) The ambulance was used solely because other means of transportation were unavailable, or (iv) The individual merely needed assistance in getting from his room or home to a vehicle. (c) Where the information indicates a situation not listed in 2(a) or 2(b) above, refer the case to your supervisor.
3. The patient was transported from and to points listed below. (a) From patient's residence (or other place where need arose) to hospital or skilled nursing facility.	3. Claims should show the ZIP code of the point of pickup (a) i. Condition met if trip began within the institution's service area as shown in the carrier's locality guide ii. Condition met where the trip began outside the institution's service area if the institution was the nearest one with appropriate facilities.
NOTE: A patient's residence is the place where he or she makes his/her home and dwells permanently, or for an extended period of time. A skilled nursing facility is one, which is listed in the Directory of Medical Facilities as a participating SNF or as an institution which meets §1861(j)(1) of the Act. NOTE: A claim for ambulance service to a participating hospital or skilled nursing facility should not be denied on the grounds that there is a nearer nonparticipating institution having appropriate facilities.	
(b) Skilled nursing facility to a hospital or hospital to a skilled nursing facility.	(b) (i) Condition met if the ZIP code of the pickup point is within the service area of the destination as shown in the carrier's locality guide. (ii) Condition met where the ZIP code of the pickup point is outside the service area of the destination if the destination institution was the nearest appropriate facility.
(c) Hospital to hospital or skilled nursing facility to skilled nursing facility.	(c) Condition met if the discharging institution was not an appropriate facility and the admitting institution was the nearest appropriate facility.
(d) From a hospital or skilled nursing facility to patient's residence.	(d) (i) Condition met if patient's residence is within the institution's service area as shown in the carrier's locality guide. (ii) Condition met where the patient's residence is outside the institution's service area if the institution was the nearest appropriate facility.
(e) Round trip for hospital or participating skilled nursing facility inpatients to the nearest hospital or nonhospital treatment facility.	(e) Condition met if the reasonable and necessary diagnostic or therapeutic service required by patient's condition is not available at the institution where the beneficiary is an inpatient.

Conditions	Review Action
NOTE: Ambulance service to a physician's office or a physician-directed clinic is not covered. See §10.3.8 above, where a stop is made at a physician's office en route to a hospital and §10.3.3 for additional exceptions.)	
4. Ambulance services involving hospital admissions in Canada or Mexico are covered (Medicare Claims Processing Manual, Chapter 1, "General Billing Requirements, " §§10.1.3.) if the following conditions are met:	(a) The foreign hospitalization has been determined to be covered; and (b) The ambulance service meets the coverage requirements set forth in §§10-10.3. If the foreign hospitalization has been determined to be covered on the basis of emergency services (See the Medicare Claims Processing Manual, Chapter 1, "General Billing Requirements," §10.1.3), the necessity requirement (§10.2) and the destination requirement (§10.3) are considered met.
5. The carrier will make partial payment for otherwise covered ambulance service, which exceeded limits defined in item 6. The carrier will base the payment on the amount payable had the patient been transported: 6. The carrier will base the payment on the amount payable had the patient been transported:.	(a) From the pickup point to the nearest appropriate facility, or (b) From the nearest appropriate facility to the beneficiary's residence where he or she is being returned home from a distant institution.

Pub 100-2, 11, 10 – Definitions Relating to ESRD

(Rev. 1, 10-01-03)

A3-3165, A3-3166.1, B3-2230.1, PR 1-2703, RDF-245.1, B3-2230.1, B3-2230.2, A3- 3171, HO-238, B3-2231, RDF-240

End Stage Renal Disease (ESRD) occurs from the destruction of normal kidney tissues over a long period of time. Often there are no symptoms until the kidney has lost more than half its function. The loss of kidney function in ESRD is usually irreversible and permanent.

Some services are listed in the definitions shown below. Medicare covers these services unless otherwise noted.

Note that services furnished to hospital inpatients are covered under Part A and paid in accordance with the applicable payment rules for the type of provider. Other dialysis services are payable under Part B.

A. Dialysis

Dialysis is a process by which waste products are removed from the body by diffusion from one fluid compartment to another across a semi-permeable membrane. There are two types of renal dialysis procedures in common clinical usage: hemodialysis and peritoneal dialysis. Both hemodialysis and peritoneal dialysis are acceptable modes of treatment for ESRD under Medicare.

1. Hemodialysis – Blood passes through an artificial kidney machine and the waste products diffuse across a manmade membrane into a bath solution known as dialysate after which the cleansed blood is returned to the patient's body. Hemodialysis is accomplished usually in three to four hour sessions, three times a week.
2. Peritoneal – Waste products pass from the patient's body through the peritoneal membrane into the peritoneal (abdominal) cavity where the bath solution (dialysate) is introduced and removed periodically.

   Peritoneal dialysis is particularly suited for:
   - Patients without family members to assist in self-dialysis;
   - Children;
   - Patients with no peripheral sites available for fistula or cannula placement;
   - Patients who have difficulty learning the more complex hemodialysis technique; and
   - Elderly patients with cardiovascular disease who are unable to tolerate intravascular fluid shifts associated with hemodialysis.

   The three types of peritoneal dialysis are listed below:

   a. Continuous Ambulatory Peritoneal Dialysis (CAPD) – In CAPD, the patient's peritoneal membrane is used as a dialyzer. The patient connects a 2-liter plastic bag of dialysate to a surgically implanted indwelling catheter that allows the dialysate to pour into the beneficiary's peritoneal cavity.

Medicare References

Four to 6 hours later, the patient drains the fluid out into the same bag and replaces the old bag with a new bag of fresh dialysate. This is done three to five times a day, with the first exchange being made when the patient wakes up in the morning, and the last exchange being made at bedtime. Because no machine is used, CAPD frees patients from the confinement of a machine; and because it is continuous, CAPD frees patients from the dietary restrictions associated with intermittent hemodialysis or intermittent peritoneal dialysis. For more information, see §70.

b. Continuous Cycling Peritoneal Dialysis (CCPD) – CCPD is a treatment modality that combines the advantages of the long dwell, continuous steady state dialysis of CAPD, with the advantages of automation inherent in intermittent peritoneal dialysis (IPD). The major difference between CCPD and CAPD is that the solution exchanges, which are performed manually during the day by the patient on CAPD, are moved to nighttime with CCPD and are performed automatically with a peritoneal dialysis cycler. The long nighttime dwell of CCPD is moved to the daytime with CAPD.

At night, the patient connects a surgically implanted catheter to the cycler system, which has four 2-liter containers of dialysate suspended. The cycler automatically empties the patient's peritoneal cavity of the all-day dwell. The cycler then cycles the nocturnal exchanges automatically while the patient sleeps. The number of nocturnal exchanges with CCPD are prescribed by the physician; generally there are three nocturnal exchanges occurring at intervals of 2 1/2 to 3 hours, with the fourth exchange being instilled in the morning upon awakening. The patient then disconnects from the cycler and leaves the last 2-liter fill inside the peritoneum to continue the daytime long dwell dialysis.

c. Intermittent Peritoneal Dialysis (IPD) – Waste products pass from the patient's body through the peritoneal membrane into the peritoneal cavity where the dialysate is introduced and removed periodically by machine. Peritoneal dialysis generally is required for approximately 30 hours a week, either as three 10-hour sessions or less frequent, but longer, sessions.

3. Hemofiltration – Hemofiltration is a safe and effective technique for the treatment of ESRD patients and an alternative to peritoneal dialysis and hemodialysis. Hemofiltration (which is also known as diafiltration) removes fluid, electrolytes, and other low molecular weight toxic substances from the blood by filtration through hollow artificial membranes and may be routinely performed in three weekly sessions. In contrast to both hemodialysis and peritoneal dialysis treatments, which eliminate dissolved substances via diffusion across semipermeable membranes, hemofiltration mimics the filtration process of the normal kidney. The technique requires an arteriovenous access. Hemofiltration may be performed either in facility or at home. (See §100.)

4. Hemoperfusion – Hemoperfusion is a process that removes substances from the blood through the dialysis membrane by using a charcoal or resin artificial kidney. When used in the treatment of a life threatening drug overdose, hemoperfusion is a covered service for patients with or without renal failure. Hemoperfusion is also covered when used in conjunction with DFO to treat aluminum toxicity. (See §110.) However, hemoperfusion is not covered when used to improve the results of hemodialysis or when used in conjunction with deferoxamine (DFO) to remove iron overload.

One or two treatments are usually all that is necessary to remove the toxic compound; additional treatments should be documented. Hemoperfusion may be performed concurrently with dialysis, and in those cases payment for the hemoperfusion should reflect only the additional care rendered over and above the care, which would have been given during the dialysis.

Hemoperfusion generally requires a physician to be present to initiate treatment and to be present in the hospital or an adjacent medical office during the entire procedure, as changes may be sudden. Special staff training and equipment are required.

5. Therapeutic Pheresis (Apheresis) – Apheresis is a medical procedure utilizing specialized equipment to remove selected blood constituents (plasma or cells) from whole blood and return the remaining constituents to the person from whom the blood was taken.

See the **Medicare National Coverage Determinations Manual**, Chapter 1, for the national coverage determination for apheresis.

6. Ultrafiltration – A process of removing excess fluid from the blood through a dialysis membrane by exerting pressure. It is not a substitute for dialysis. Occasionally, medical complications may occur which require that ultrafiltration be performed separately from the dialysis treatment.

B. ESRD Facility

An ESRD facility is a facility which is approved to furnish at least one specific ESRD service. Such facilities are:

1. Renal Transplantation Center – A hospital unit, which is approved to furnish transplantation, and other medical and surgical specialty services required for the care of the ESRD transplant patients, including inpatient dialysis furnished directly or under arrangement. A renal transplantation center may also be a renal dialysis center.
2. Renal Dialysis Center – A hospital unit, which is approved to furnish the full spectrum of diagnostic, therapeutic, and rehabilitative services required for the care of ESRD dialysis patients (including inpatient dialysis furnished directly or under arrangement). A hospital need not provide renal transplantation to qualify as a renal dialysis center.
3. Renal Dialysis Facility – An independent unit that is approved to furnish dialysis service(s) directly to ESRD patients.
4. Self-Dialysis Unit – A unit that is part of an approved renal transplantation center, renal dialysis center, or renal dialysis facility, and furnishes self-dialysis services.
5. Special Purpose Renal Dialysis Facility – A renal dialysis facility that is approved to furnish dialysis at special locations on a short-term basis to a group of dialysis patients otherwise unable to obtain treatment in the geographical area. The special locations must be either special rehabilitative (including vacation) locations serving ESRD patients temporarily residing there, or locations in need of ESRD facilities under emergency circumstances.

C. Dialysis Services

The types of care available are:

1. Transplantation Service – A process by which: (a) a kidney is excised from a live or cadaveric donor, (b) a kidney is implanted in an ESRD patient, and (c) supportive care is furnished to the living donor and to the recipient following implantation.
2. Dialysis Service
   a. Acute Dialysis – Dialysis given to patients who are not ESRD patients, but who require dialysis because of temporary kidney failure due to a sudden trauma; e.g., traffic accident or ingestion of certain drugs.
   b. Back-Up Dialysis – Dialysis given to patients under special circumstances. Examples are: dialysis of a home dialysis patient in a dialysis facility when the patient's equipment fails, inpatient dialysis when a patient's illness requires more comprehensive care on an inpatient basis, and preoperative and postoperative dialysis provided to transplant patients.
   c. Institutional Dialysis Services – Institutional dialysis services include all services, supplies, items, equipment, and ESRD related laboratory tests covered under the composite rate necessary to perform dialysis in an approved renal dialysis facility or center.
   d. Inpatient Dialysis – Dialysis, which, because of medical necessity, is furnished to an ESRD patient on a temporary inpatient basis in a hospital.
   e. Outpatient Dialysis – Dialysis furnished on an outpatient basis at a renal dialysis center or facility. Outpatient dialysis includes:
      - Staff-assisted Dialysis – Dialysis performed by the staff of the center or facility.
      - Self-Dialysis – Dialysis performed by an ESRD patient with little or no professional assistance. The patient must have completed an appropriate course of training.
      - Home Dialysis – Dialysis performed by an appropriately trained patient (and the patient's caregiver) and at home.
      - Infacility Dialysis – Dialysis furnished on an outpatient basis at an approved renal dialysis facility.
      - Self-Dialysis and Home Dialysis Training – A program that trains ESRD patients to perform self-dialysis or home dialysis with little or no professional assistance, and trains other individuals to assist patients in performing self dialysis or home dialysis.

D. Home Dialysis – Supplies, Equipment, and Support Services

1. Home Dialysis Equipment – Home dialysis equipment includes all of the medically necessary equipment prescribed by the attending physician, including (but not limited to) artificial kidney, automated peritoneal dialysis machines, and support equipment. Home dialysis supplies and equipment may be covered if used by an ESRD beneficiary in a nursing home.
2. Installation – Installation includes (but is not limited to): the identification of any minor plumbing and electrical changes required to accommodate the equipment; the ordering and performing of these changes; delivery of the equipment and its actual installation (i.e., hookup), as well as any necessary testing to assure proper installation and function.

   Minor plumbing and electrical changes include those parts and labor required to connect the dialysis equipment to plumbing and electrical lines that already exist in the room where the patient will dialyze. Medicare does not cover wiring or rewiring of the patient's home or installing any plumbing to the patient's home or to the room of the home where the patient will dialyze.
3. Maintenance – Maintenance includes (but is not limited to): travel to the patient's home or, if needed, transportation of the equipment to a repair site; the actual performance of the maintenance or repair; and all necessary parts. Water purification equipment maintenance includes replacing the filter on a reverse osmosis device, regenerating the resin tanks on a deionization device, using chemicals in a water softener, and periodic water testing to assure proper performance. Routine maintenance customarily performed by a patient are not covered services except for the cost of parts involved in this maintenance furnished by the facility to a patient.
4. Supplies – Supplies include all durable and disposable items and medical supplies necessary for the effective performance of a patient's dialysis. Supplies include (but are not limited to): dialyzers, forceps, sphygmomanometer with cuff and stethoscope, scales, scissors, syringes, alcohol wipes, sterile drapes, needles, topical anesthetics, and rubber gloves.
5. Support Services – Support services include (but are not limited to):
   1. Periodic monitoring of a patient's adaptation to home dialysis and performance of dialysis, including provisions for visits to the home or the facility;
   2. Visits by trained personnel for the patient with a qualified social worker and a qualified dietitian, made in accordance with a plan prepared and periodically reviewed by a professional team which includes the physician;
   3. Individual's unscheduled visits to a facility made on an as-needed basis; e.g., assistance with difficult access situations;
   4. ESRD related laboratory tests covered under the composite rate;
   5. Providing, installing, repairing, testing, and maintaining home dialysis equipment, including appropriate water testing and treatment;
   6. Ordering of supplies on an ongoing basis; and
   7. A record keeping system that assures continuity of care. (See §70.3 for CAPD support services.)

      NOTE: The CMS requires that suppliers billing Medicare under Method II must have a written agreement with a certified dialysis facility to provide these services.
   6. Support Equipment – Support equipment is equipment used in conjunction with the basic dialysate delivery system. Such equipment includes (but is not limited to) pumps, such as blood and heparin pumps, alarms, such as bubble detectors, water purification equipment used to improve the quality of the water used for dialysis, and adjustable dialysis chairs.
   7. Method Selection – For home dialysis, a beneficiary selects one of two methods for payment and billing. Under Method I (composite rate), the facility with which the patient is associated assumes responsibility for providing all home dialysis equipment, supplies and support services. Under Method II (direct dealing) the beneficiary deals directly with a single home dialysis supplier to secure the necessary supplies and equipment to dialyze at home.

E. Hospital-Based ESRD Facility

Hospital-based ESRD facility is an integral and subordinate part of a hospital and is operated with other departments of the hospital under common licensure, governance, and professional supervision, with all services of the hospital and facility fully integrated. Specifically, the facility would be hospital-based only if all the following conditions are met:

- The facility and hospital are subject to the bylaws and operating decisions of a common governing board. All authority in management flows from this administrative body which approves all personnel actions, appoints medical staff, and carries out similar management functions;
- The ESRD facility's director or administrator is under the supervision of the hospital's chief executive officer and reports through that officer to the governing board;
- The facility personnel policies and practices conform to those of the hospital;
- The administrative functions of the facility (that is, records, billing, laundry, housekeeping, and purchasing) are integrated with those of the hospital; and
- The dialysis unit and hospital are financially integrated, as evidenced by the cost report, which must reflect allocation of hospital overhead to the facility through the required step-down methodology (see the Medicare Provider Reimbursement Manual (Pub 15-1), §2306). For example, where a single dialysis department in a hospital is responsible for inpatient and outpatient dialysis and the costs are subsequently split between inpatient and outpatient, the outpatient department will normally be classified as hospital-based. In determining compliance with this criterion, the key issue is whether Pub 15-1, §2306, would require the hospital to make this cost allocation, rather than whether the hospital has actually made the allocation. If no allocation is made because the hospital failed to follow Pub 15-1, §2306, the hospital must resubmit a corrected cost report, and the facility will normally be classified as hospital-based.

The existence of an agreement or an arrangement between a facility and a hospital for referral of patients, a shared service arrangement between a facility and a hospital (a common practice recognized by both Medicare and Medicaid), or the physical location of a dialysis unit on the premises of a hospital, does not mean that a facility is hospital-based.

Any facility that does not meet all of the above criteria would be considered an independent facility.

Pub 100-2, 11, 20 – Coverage of Outpatient Maintenance Dialysis

(Rev. 1, 10-01-03)

A3-3167, B3-2230.2, RDF-202, SOM-2272, RDF-317.1, PM AB-03-001

Medicare covers maintenance dialysis treatments when they are provided to ESRD patients by an approved hospital-based dialysis facility, an independent dialysis facility, or a special purpose dialysis facility. Outpatient dialysis treatments are covered in various settings: hospital outpatient facility, independent dialysis facility, or the patient's home. Dialysis treatments at dialysis facilities differ according to the types of patients being treated, the types of equipment and supplies used, the preferences of the treating physician, and the capability and makeup of the staff. Although not all facilities provide an identical range of services, the most common elements of a dialysis treatment are:

a. Personnel services;
b. Equipment and supplies – dialysis machine and its maintenance;
c. Administrative services;
d. Overhead costs;
e. Monitoring access and related declotting the access or referring the patient;
f. ESRD related laboratory tests; and
g. Biologicals.

Direct nursing services include registered nurses, licensed practical nurses, technicians, social workers, and dietitians.

Facilities with self-dialysis units must meet specific health and safety requirements. Certain standards applicable to staff assisted dialysis have been adjusted for self-dialysis units in consideration of the differences in the two modalities. Before participating in self-dialysis, patients must have

Medicare References

completed an appropriate training program in emergency procedures and have a safe storage area for their supplies. Access to the self-dialysis unit is limited to patients for whom the facility maintains patient care plans in order to exclude transient patients who might not be familiar with the facility's equipment or emergency procedures. The self-dialysis unit need not be physically separate from the rest of the facility nor operate on a separate shift.

Pub 100-2, 11, 80 – Physician's Services for Renal Dialysis Patients – General

(Rev. 1, 10-01-03)

B3-2230.3

Payment for physician's services generally is subject to the guidelines in the **Medicare Benefit Policy Manual**, Chapter 15, "Covered Medical and Other Health Services," §30. Medicare pays physician's services furnished in connection with dialysis sessions for outpatients who are on maintenance dialysis in a facility or at home by the monthly capitation payment method or the initial method. (See the Medicare **Claims Processing Manual**, Chapter 8, "Outpatient ESRD Hospital, Independent Facility, and Physician/Supplier Claims," for payment instructions.)

Pub 100-2, 11, 80.1 – Physicians' Services to an ESRD Inpatient

(Rev. 1, 10-01-03)

B3-2230.4

Physicians' services furnished to ESRD patients, who require inpatient hospital care in connection with the renal condition or any other condition, are covered if the carrier determines the services to be reasonable and necessary. Inpatient physician's visits are covered in addition to the composite rate or MCP amount.

Pub 100-2, 11, 80.2 – Physicians' Services – Outpatient Maintenance Dialysis

(Rev. 1, 10-01-03)

B3-2230.5, A3-3172.5, B3-2231.4

A physician's services, furnished to dialysis patients who are treated as outpatients, are divided into two major categories: direct patient care and administrative services. See §80.4 for physician services to a kidney donor. Medicare covers physician services furnished to beneficiaries on CAPD.

A. Direct Patient Care Services

These services are part of the medical treatment furnished to an individual patient that:

1. Are personally furnished by a physician to an individual patient;
2. Contribute directly to the diagnosis or treatment of an individual patient; and
3. A physician must ordinarily perform.

   They include:

   - Visits to the patient during dialysis, in conjunction with review of laboratory test results, nurses' notes, and any other medical documentation, as a basis for adjustment of the patient's medication or diet or the dialysis procedure, prescription of medical supplies, and evaluation of the patient's psychosocial status and the appropriateness of the treatment modality.
   - Medical direction of staff in delivering services to a patient during a dialysis session;
   - Pre- and post-dialysis examinations where medically appropriate;
   - Insertions of a catheter for patients on maintenance peritoneal dialysis who are not provided an indwelling catheter;
   - Services which must be furnished at a time other than during the dialysis procedure; e.g., monthly and semi-annual examinations to review health status and treatment; and
   - Other services furnished during dialysis; e.g., declotting of shunts, needle insertions into fistulae, care during immediately life-threatening complications related to the dialysis procedure, and care of nonrenal conditions.

B. Administrative Services

A component of the facility's cost or charge for dialysis is for "administrative services" furnished by physicians. Administrative services are differentiated from physicians' direct patient care services because they constitute supervision of staff or are not directly related to the care of an individual patient, but benefit all patients and the facility as a whole. The administrative type of physician's service are services that are supportive of the facility as a whole and have benefit to patients in general. Examples of such services include participation in management of the facility, advice on and procurement of facility equipment and supplies, supervision of staff, staff training, and staff conferences. The carrier will disallow all claims for these services with an explanation that such services are paid as part of the dialysis services that are included in the facility charge for dialysis.

Pub 100-2, 11, 80.3 – Physicians' Services During Self-Dialysis Training

(Rev. 1, 10-01-03)

B3-2230.6, A3-3172.5

A. Initial Training

All physicians' services required creating the capacity for self-dialysis are covered. For example:

1. Direction of, and participation in, training of dialysis patients;
2. Review of family and home status, environment, and counseling and training of family members; or
3. Review of training progress.

B. Subsequent Training

Occasionally, it is necessary to furnish additional training to an ESRD self-dialysis beneficiary after the initial training course is completed, e.g., because of a change from hemodialysis to peritoneal dialysis, a change in equipment. The amount of additional training required depends upon the transferability of the skills the patient has already learned. Subsequent training would normally be very limited. Physicians' training services furnished during subsequent training of an ESRD beneficiary are covered and reimbursed in addition to the initial training fee.

The payment for subsequent training sessions should be based on the amount of $20 per training session. The total payment for a course of subsequent training may not be based on an amount that exceeds $500.

Subsequent training sessions that are reimbursable under this rule must be distinguished from the ongoing services for which the original training fee is considered payment in full, e.g., answering the patient's questions arising after home dialysis has begun about the machine the patient has already been trained to use. No additional payment is made after the initial training course unless the subsequent training is required because of a change from the patient's treatment machine to a machine that the patient had not been trained to use in the initial training course, a change in the type of dialysis, or a change in setting or dialysis partner.

Pub 100-2, 15, 50 – Drugs and Biologicals

(Rev. 1, 10-01-03)

B3-2049, A3-3112.4.B, HO-230.4.B

The Medicare program provides limited benefits for outpatient drugs. The program covers drugs that are furnished "incident to" a physician's service provided that the drugs are not usually self-administered by the patients who take them. Generally, drugs and biologicals are covered only if all of the following requirements are met:

- They meet the definition of drugs or biologicals (see 254H§50.1);
- They are of the type that are not usually self-administered. (see 25H§50.2);
- They meet all the general requirements for coverage of items as incident to a physician's services (see §§50.1 and 256H50.3);
- They are reasonable and necessary for the diagnosis or treatment of the illness or injury for which they are administered according to accepted standards of medical practice (see 257H§50.4);
- They are not excluded as noncovered immunizations (see 258H§50.4.4.2); and
- They have not been determined by the FDA to be less than effective. (See 259H§§50.4.4).

Medicare Part B does generally not cover drugs that can be self-administered, such as those in pill form, or are used for self-injection. However, the statute provides for the coverage of some self-administered

Medicare References

drugs. Examples of self-administered drugs that are covered include blood-clotting factors, drugs used in immunosuppressive therapy, erythropoietin for dialysis patients, osteoporosis drugs for certain homebound patients, and certain oral cancer drugs. (See 260H§110.3 for coverage of drugs, which are necessary to the effective use of Durable Medical Equipment (DME) or prosthetic devices.)

Pub 100-2, 15, 50.1 – Definition of Drug or Biological

(Rev. 1, 10-01-03)

B3-2049.1

Drugs and biologicals must be determined to meet the statutory definition. Under the statute 261H§1861(t)(1), payment may be made for a drug or biological only where it is included, or approved for inclusion, in the latest official edition of the United States Pharmacopoeia National Formulary (USP-NF), the United States Pharmacopoeia-Drug Information (USD-DI), or the American Dental Association (AOA) Guide to Dental Therapeutics, except for those drugs and biologicals unfavorably evaluated in the ADA Guide to Dental Therapeutics. The inclusion of an item in the USP DI does not necessarily mean that the item is a drug or biological. The USP DI is a database of drug information developed by the U.S. Pharmacopoeia but maintained by Micromedex, which contains medically accepted uses for generic and brand name drug products.

Inclusion in such reference (or approval by a hospital committee) is a necessary condition for a product to be considered a drug or biological under the Medicare program, however, it is not enough. Rather, the product must also meet all other program requirements to be determined to be a drug or biological. Combination drugs are also included in the definition of drugs if the combination itself or all of the therapeutic ingredients of the combination are included, or approved for inclusion, in any of the above drug compendia.

Drugs and biologicals are considered approved for inclusion in a compendium if approved under the established procedure by the professional organization responsible for revision of the compendium.

Pub 100-2, 15, 50.2 – Determining Self-Administration of Drug or Biological

(Rev. 123, Issued: 04-30-10, Effective: 07-30-10, Implementation: 07-30-10)

The Medicare program provides limited benefits for outpatient prescription drugs. The program covers drugs that are furnished "incident to" a physician's service provided that the drugs are not usually self-administered by the patients who take them. Section 112 of the Benefits, Improvements & Protection Act of 2000 (BIPA) amended sections 1861(s)(2)(A) and 1861(s)(2)(B) of the Act to redefine this exclusion. The prior statutory language referred to those drugs "which cannot be self-administered." Implementation of the BIPA provision requires interpretation of the phrase "not usually self-administered by the patient".

A. Policy

Fiscal intermediaries, carriers and Medicare Administrative Contractors (MACs) are instructed to follow the instructions below when applying the exclusion for drugs that are usually self-administered by the patient. Each individual contractor must make its own individual determination on each drug. Contractors must continue to apply the policy that not only the drug is medically reasonable and necessary for any individual claim, but also that the route of administration is medically reasonable and necessary. That is, if a drug is available in both oral and injectable forms, the injectable form of the drug must be medically reasonable and necessary as compared to using the oral form.

For certain injectable drugs, it will be apparent due to the nature of the condition(s) for which they are administered or the usual course of treatment for those conditions, they are, or are not, usually self-administered. For example, an injectable drug used to treat migraine headaches is usually self-administered. On the other hand, an injectable drug, administered at the same time as chemotherapy, used to treat anemia secondary to chemotherapy is not usually self-administered.

B. Administered

The term "administered" refers only to the physical process by which the drug enters the patient's body. It does not refer to whether the process is supervised by a medical professional (for example, to observe proper technique or side-effects of the drug). Injectable drugs, including intravenously administered drugs, are typically eligible for inclusion under the "incident to" benefit. With limited exceptions, other routes of administration including, but not limited to, oral drugs, suppositories, topical medications are considered to be usually self-administered by the patient.

C. Usually

For the purposes of applying this exclusion, the term "usually" means more than 50 percent of the time for all Medicare beneficiaries who use the drug. Therefore, if a drug is self-administered by more than 50 percent of Medicare beneficiaries, the drug is excluded from coverage and the contractor may not make any Medicare payment for it. In arriving at a single determination as to whether a drug is usually self-administered, contractors should make a separate determination for each indication for a drug as to whether that drug is usually self-administered.

After determining whether a drug is usually self-administered for each indication, contractors should determine the relative contribution of each indication to total use of the drug (i.e., weighted average) in order to make an overall determination as to whether the drug is usually self-administered. For example, if a drug has three indications, is not self-administered for the first indication, but is self administered for the second and third indications, and the first indication makes up 40 percent of total usage, the second indication makes up 30 percent of total usage, and the third indication makes up 30 percent of total usage, then the drug would be considered usually self-administered.

Reliable statistical information on the extent of self-administration by the patient may not always be available. Consequently, CMS offers the following guidance for each contractor's consideration in making this determination in the absence of such data:

1. Absent evidence to the contrary, presume that drugs delivered intravenously are not usually self-administered by the patient.
2. Absent evidence to the contrary, presume that drugs delivered by intramuscular injection are not usually self-administered by the patient. (Avonex, for example, is delivered by intramuscular injection, not usually self-administered by the patient.) The contractor may consider the depth and nature of the particular intramuscular injection in applying this presumption. In applying this presumption, contractors should examine the use of the particular drug and consider the following factors:
   A. **Acute Condition**—Is the condition for which the drug is used an acute condition? If so, it is less likely that a patient would self-administer the drug. If the condition were longer term, it would be more likely that the patient would self-administer the drug.
   B **Frequency of Administration**—How often is the injection given? For example, if the drug is administered once per month, it is less likely to be self-administered by the patient. However, if it is administered once or more per week, it is likely that the drug is self-administered by the patient.
3. Absent evidence to the contrary, presume that drugs delivered by subcutaneous injection are self-administered by the patient. However, contractors should examine the use of the particular drug and consider the following factors:
   A. **Acute Condition**—Is the condition for which the drug is used an acute condition? If so, it is less likely that a patient would self-administer the drug. If the condition were longer term, it would be more likely that the patient would self-administer the drug.
   B. **Frequency of Administration**—How often is the injection given? For example, if the drug is administered once per month, it is less likely to be self-administered by the patient. However, if it is administered once or more per week, it is likely that the drug is self-administered by the patient.

In some instances, carriers may have provided payment for one or perhaps several doses of a drug that would otherwise not be paid for because the drug is usually self-administered. Carriers may have exercised this discretion for limited coverage, for example, during a brief time when the patient is being trained under the supervision of a physician in the proper technique for self-administration. Medicare will no longer pay for such doses. In addition, contractors may no longer pay for any drug when it is administered on an outpatient emergency basis, if the drug is excluded because it is usually self-administered by the patient.

D. Definition of Acute Condition

For the purposes of determining whether a drug is usually self-administered, an acute condition means a condition that begins over a short time period, is likely to be of short duration and/or the expected course of treatment is for a short, finite interval. A course of treatment consisting of scheduled injections lasting less than 2 weeks, regardless of frequency or route of administration, is considered acute. Evidence to support this may include Food and Drug administration (FDA) approval language, package inserts, drug compendia, and other information.

E. By the Patient

The term "by the patient" means Medicare beneficiaries as a collective whole. The carrier includes only the patients themselves and not other individuals (that is, spouses, friends, or other care-givers are not considered the patient). The determination is based on whether the drug is self-administered by the patient a majority of the time that the drug is used on an outpatient basis by Medicare beneficiaries for medically necessary indications. The carrier ignores all instances when the drug is administered on an inpatient basis.

The carrier makes this determination on a drug-by-drug basis, not on a beneficiary-by-beneficiary basis. In evaluating whether beneficiaries as a collective whole self-administer, individual beneficiaries who do not have the capacity to self-administer any drug due to a condition other than the condition for which they are taking the drug in question are not considered. For example, an individual afflicted with paraplegia or advanced dementia would not have the capacity to self-administer any injectable drug, so such individuals would not be included in the population upon which the determination for self-administration by the patient was based. Note that some individuals afflicted with a less severe stage of an otherwise debilitating condition would be included in the population upon which the determination for "self-administered by the patient" was based; for example, an early onset of dementia.

F. Evidentiary Criteria

Contractors are only required to consider the following types of evidence: peer reviewed medical literature, standards of medical practice, evidence-based practice guidelines, FDA approved label, and package inserts. Contractors may also consider other evidence submitted by interested individuals or groups subject to their judgment.

Contractors should also use these evidentiary criteria when reviewing requests for making a determination as to whether a drug is usually self-administered, and requests for reconsideration of a pending or published determination.

Note that prior to August 1, 2002, one of the principal factors used to determine whether a drug was subject to the self-administered exclusion was whether the FDA label contained instructions for self-administration. However, CMS notes that under the new standard, the fact that the FDA label includes instructions for self-administration is not, by itself, a determining factor that a drug is subject to this exclusion.

G. Provider Notice of Noncovered Drugs

Contractors must describe on their Web site the process they will use to determine whether a drug is usually self-administered and thus does not meet the "incident to" benefit category. Contractors must publish a list of the injectable drugs that are subject to the self-administered exclusion on their Web site, including the data and rationale that led to the determination. Contractors will report the workload associated with developing new coverage statements in CAFM 21208.

Contractors must provide notice 45 days prior to the date that these drugs will not be covered. During the 45-day time period, contractors will maintain existing medical review and payment procedures. After the 45-day notice, contractors may deny payment for the drugs subject to the notice.

Contractors must not develop local coverage determinations (LCDs) for this purpose because further elaboration to describe drugs that do not meet the 'incident to' and the 'not usually self-administered' provisions of the statute are unnecessary. Current LCDs based solely on these provisions must be withdrawn. LCDs that address the self-administered exclusion and other information may be reissued absent the self-administered drug exclusion material. Contractors will report this workload in CAFM 21206. However, contractors may continue to use and write LCDs to describe reasonable and necessary uses of drugs that are not usually self-administered.

H. Conferences Between Contractors

Contractors' Medical Directors may meet and discuss whether a drug is usually self-administered without reaching a formal consensus. Each contractor uses its discretion as to whether or not it will participate in such discussions. Each contractor must make its own individual determinations, except that fiscal intermediaries may, at their discretion, follow the determinations of the local carrier with respect to the self-administered exclusion.

I. Beneficiary Appeals

If a beneficiary's claim for a particular drug is denied because the drug is subject to the "self-administered drug" exclusion, the beneficiary may appeal the denial. Because it is a "benefit category" denial and not a denial based on medical necessity, an Advance Beneficiary Notice (ABN) is not required. A "benefit category" denial (i.e., a denial based on the fact that there is no benefit category under which the drug may be covered) does not trigger the financial liability protection provisions of Limitation On Liability (under §1879 of the Act). Therefore, physicians or providers may charge the beneficiary for an excluded drug.

J. Provider and Physician Appeals

A physician accepting assignment may appeal a denial under the provisions found in Chapter 29 of the ***Medicare Claims Processing Manual.***

K. Reasonable and Necessary

Contractors will make the determination of reasonable and necessary with respect to the medical appropriateness of a drug to treat the patient's condition. Contractors will continue to make the determination of whether the intravenous or injection form of a drug is appropriate as opposed to the oral form. Contractors will also continue to make the determination as to whether a physician's office visit was reasonable and necessary. However, contractors should not make a determination of whether it was reasonable and necessary for the patient to choose to have his or her drug administered in the physician's office or outpatient hospital setting. That is, while a physician's office visit may not be reasonable and necessary in a specific situation, in such a case an injection service would be payable.

L. Reporting Requirements

Each carrier, intermediary and Medicare Administrative Contractor (MAC) must report to CMS its complete list of injectable drugs that the contractor has determined are excluded when furnished incident to a physician's service on the basis that the drug is usually self-administered. The CMS expects that contractors will review injectable drugs on a rolling basis and update their list of excluded drugs as it is developed and no less frequently than annually. For example, contractors should not wait to publish this list until every drug has been reviewed. Contractors must enter their self-administered drug exclusion list to the Medicare Coverage Database (MCD). This database can be accessed at www.cms.hhs.gov/mcd. See Pub.100-08, Medicare Program Integrity Manual, Chapter 3, Section 3.3, "Articles", for instructions on submitting these lists to the MCD.

Pub 100-2, 15, 50.3 – Incident-to Requirements

(Rev. 1, 10-01-03)

B3-2049.3

In order to meet all the general requirements for coverage under the incident-to provision, an FDA approved drug or biological must:

- Be of a form that is not usually self-administered;
- Must be furnished by a physician; and
- Must be administered by the physician, or by auxiliary personnel employed by the physician and under the physician's personal supervision.

The charge, if any, for the drug or biological must be included in the physician's bill, and the cost of the drug or biological must represent an expense to the physician. Drugs and biologicals furnished by other health professionals may also meet these requirements. (See 26H§§170, 267H180, 268H190 and 269H200 for specific instructions.)

Whole blood is a biological, which cannot be self-administered and is covered when furnished incident to a physician's services. Payment may also be made for blood fractions if all coverage requirements are satisfied and the blood deductible has been met.

Pub 100-2, 15, 50.4 – Reasonableness and Necessity

(Rev. 1, 10-01-03)

B3-2049.4

Pub 100-2, 15, 50.4.1 – Approved Use of Drug

(Rev. 1, 10-01-03)

B3-2049.4

Use of the drug or biological must be safe and effective and otherwise reasonable and necessary. (See the **Medicare Benefit Policy Manual**, Chapter 16, "General Exclusions from Coverage," §20.) Drugs or biologicals approved for marketing by the Food and Drug Administration (FDA) are considered safe and effective for purposes of this requirement when used for indications specified on the labeling. Therefore, the program may pay for the use of an FDA approved drug or biological, if:

- It was injected on or after the date of the FDA's approval;
- It is reasonable and necessary for the individual patient; and
- All other applicable coverage requirements are met.

The carrier, DMERC, or intermediary will deny coverage for drugs and biologicals, which have not received final marketing approval by the FDA unless it receives instructions from CMS to the contrary. For specific guidelines on coverage of Group C cancer drugs, see the **Medicare National Coverage Determinations Manual**.

If there is reason to question whether the FDA has approved a drug or biological for marketing, the carrier or intermediary must obtain satisfactory evidence of FDA's approval. Acceptable evidence includes:

- A copy of the FDA's letter to the drug's manufacturer approving the new drug application (NDA);
- A listing of the drug or biological in the FDA's "Approved Drug Products" or "FDA Drug and Device Product Approvals";
- A copy of the manufacturer's package insert, approved by the FDA as part of the labeling of the drug, containing its recommended uses and dosage, as well as possible adverse reactions and recommended precautions in using it; or
- Information from the FDA's Web site. When necessary, the regional office (RO) may be able to help in obtaining information.

Pub 100-2, 15, 50.4.2 – Unlabeled Use of Drug

(Rev. 1, 10-01-03)

B3-2049.3

An unlabeled use of a drug is a use that is not included as an indication on the drug's label as approved by the FDA. FDA approved drugs used for indications other than what is indicated on the official label may be covered under Medicare if the carrier determines the use to be medically accepted, taking into consideration the major drug compendia, authoritative medical literature and/or accepted standards of medical practice. In the case of drugs used in an anti-cancer chemotherapeutic regimen, unlabeled uses are covered for a medically accepted indication as defined in §50.5.

These decisions are made by the contractor on a case-by-case basis.

Pub 100-2, 15, 50.4.3 – Examples of Not Reasonable and Necessary

(Rev. 1, 10-01-03)

B3-2049.4

Determinations as to whether medication is reasonable and necessary for an individual patient should be made on the same basis as all other such determinations (i.e., with the advice of medical consultants and with reference to accepted standards of medical practice and the medical circumstances of the individual case). The following guidelines identify three categories with specific examples of situations in which medications would not be reasonable and necessary according to accepted standards of medical practice:

1. Not for Particular Illness

   Medications given for a purpose other than the treatment of a particular condition, illness, or injury are not covered (except for certain immunizations). Charges for medications, e.g., vitamins, given simply for the general good and welfare of the patient and not as accepted therapies for a particular illness are excluded from coverage.

2. Injection Method Not Indicated

   Medication given by injection (parenterally) is not covered if standard medical practice indicates that the administration of the medication by mouth (orally) is effective and is an accepted or preferred method of administration. For example, the accepted standard of medical practice for the treatment of certain diseases is to initiate therapy with parenteral penicillin and to complete therapy with oral penicillin. Carriers exclude the entire charge for penicillin injections given after the initiation of therapy if oral penicillin is indicated unless there are special medical circumstances that justify additional injections.

3. Excessive Medications

   Medications administered for treatment of a disease and which exceed the frequency or duration of injections indicated by accepted standards of medical practice are not covered. For example, the accepted standard of medical practice in the maintenance treatment of pernicious anemia is one vitamin B-12 injection per month. Carriers exclude the entire charge for injections given in excess of this frequency unless there are special medical circumstances that justify additional injections.

Carriers will supplement the guidelines as necessary with guidelines concerning appropriate use of specific injections in other situations. They will use the guidelines to screen out questionable cases for special review, further development, or denial when the injection billed for would not be reasonable and necessary. They will coordinate any type of drug treatment review with the Quality Improvement Organization (QIO). If a medication is determined not to be reasonable and necessary for diagnosis or treatment of an illness or injury according to these guidelines, the carrier excludes the entire charge (i.e., for both the drug and its administration). Also, carriers exclude from payment any charges for other services (such as office visits) which were primarily for the purpose of administering a noncovered injection (i.e., an injection that is not reasonable and necessary for the diagnosis or treatment of an illness or injury).

Pub 100-2, 15, 50.4.4 – Payment for Antigens and Immunizations

(Rev. 1, 10-01-03)

Pub 100-2, 15, 50.4.4.1 – Antigens

(Rev. 1, 10-01-03)

B3-2049.4

Payment may be made for a reasonable supply of antigens that have been prepared for a particular patient if: (1) the antigens are prepared by a physician who is a doctor of medicine or osteopathy, and (2) the physician who prepared the antigens has examined the patient and has determined a plan of treatment and a dosage regimen. Antigens must be administered in accordance with the plan of treatment and by a doctor of medicine or osteopathy or by a properly instructed person (who could be the patient) under the supervision of the doctor. The associations of allergists that CMS consulted advised that a reasonable supply of antigens is considered to be not more than a 12-month supply of antigens that has been prepared for a particular patient at any one time. The purpose of the reasonable supply limitation is to assure that the antigens retain their potency and effectiveness over the period in which they are to be administered to the patient. (See 270H§§20.2 and 271H50.2.)

Pub 100-2, 15, 50.4.4.2 – Immunizations

(Rev. 1, 10-01-03)

A3-3157.A, B3-2049.4, HO-230.4.C

Vaccinations or inoculations are excluded as immunizations unless they are directly related to the treatment of an injury or direct exposure to a disease or condition, such as anti-rabies treatment, tetanus antitoxin or booster vaccine, botulin antitoxin, antivenin sera, or immune globulin. In the absence of injury or direct exposure, preventive immunization (vaccination or inoculation) against such diseases as smallpox, polio, diphtheria, etc., is not covered. However, pneumococcal, hepatitis B, and influenza virus vaccines are exceptions to this rule. (See items A, B, and C below.) In cases where a vaccination or inoculation is excluded from coverage, related charges are also not covered.

A. Pneumococcal Pneumonia Vaccinations

Effective for services furnished on or after May 1, 1981, the Medicare Part B program covers pneumococcal pneumonia vaccine and its administration when furnished in compliance with any applicable State law by any provider of services or any entity or individual with a supplier number. This includes revaccination of patients at highest risk of pneumococcal infection. Typically, these vaccines are administered once in a lifetime except for persons at highest risk. Effective July 1, 2000, Medicare does not require for coverage purposes that a doctor of medicine or osteopathy order the vaccine. Therefore, the beneficiary may receive the vaccine upon request without a physician's order and without physician supervision.

An initial vaccine may be administered only to persons at high risk (see below) of pneumococcal disease. Revaccination may be administered only to persons at highest risk of serious pneumococcal infection and those likely to have a rapid decline in pneumococcal antibody levels, provided that at least five years have [passed since the previous doe of pneumococcal vaccine.

Persons at high risk for whom an initial vaccine may be administered include all people age 65 and older; immunocompetent adults who are at increased risk of pneumococcal disease or its complications because of chronic illness (e.g., cardiovascular disease, pulmonary disease, diabetes mellitus, alcoholism, cirrhosis, or cerebrospinal fluid leaks); and individuals with compromised immune systems (e.g., splenic dysfunction or anatomic asplenia, Hodgkin's disease, lymphoma, multiple myeloma, chronic renal failure, HIV infection, nephrotic syndrome, sickle cell disease, or organ transplantation).

Persons at highest risk and those most likely to have rapid declines in antibody levels are those for whom revaccination may be appropriate. This group includes persons with functional or anatomic asplenia (e.g., sickle cell disease, splenectomy), HIV infection, leukemia, lymphoma, Hodgkin's disease, multiple myeloma, generalized malignancy, chronic renal failure, nephrotic syndrome, or other conditions associated with immunosuppression such as organ or bone marrow transplantation, and those receiving immunosuppressive chemotherapy. It is not appropriate for routine revaccination of people age 65 or older that are not at highest risk.

Those administering the vaccine should not require the patient to present an immunization record prior to administering the pneumococcal vaccine, nor should they feel compelled to review the patient's complete medical record if it is not available. Instead, provided that the patient is competent, it is acceptable to rely on the patient's verbal history to determine prior vaccination status. If the patient is uncertain about his or her vaccination history in the past five years, the vaccine should be given. However, if the patient is certain he/she was were vaccinated in the last five years, the vaccine should not be given. If the patient is certain that the vaccine was given more than five years ago, revaccination is covered only if the patient is at high risk.

B. Hepatitis B Vaccine

Effective for services furnished on or after September 1, 1984, P.L. 98-369 provides coverage under Part B for hepatitis B vaccine and its administration, furnished to a Medicare beneficiary who is at high or intermediate risk of contracting hepatitis B. This coverage is effective for services furnished on or after September 1, 1984. High-risk groups currently identified include (see exception below):

- ESRD patients;
- Hemophiliacs who receive Factor VIII or IX concentrates;
- Clients of institutions for the mentally retarded;
- Persons who live in the same household as an Hepatitis B Virus (HBV) carrier;
- Homosexual men; and
- Illicit injectable drug abusers.

Intermediate risk groups currently identified include:

- Staff in institutions for the mentally retarded; and
- Workers in health care professions who have frequent contact with blood or blood-derived body fluids during routine work.

EXCEPTION: Persons in both of the above-listed groups in paragraph B, would not be considered at high or intermediate risk of contracting hepatitis B, however, if there were laboratory evidence positive for antibodies to hepatitis B. (ESRD patients are routinely tested for hepatitis B antibodies as part of their continuing monitoring and therapy.) For Medicare program purposes, the vaccine may be administered upon the order of a doctor of medicine or osteopathy, by a doctor of medicine or osteopathy, or by home health agencies, skilled nursing facilities, ESRD facilities, hospital outpatient departments, and persons recognized under the incident to physicians' services provision of law.

A charge separate from the ESRD composite rate will be recognized and paid for administration of the vaccine to ESRD patients.

C. Influenza Virus Vaccine

Effective for services furnished on or after May 1, 1993, the Medicare Part B program covers influenza virus vaccine and its administration when furnished in compliance with any applicable State law by any provider of services or any entity or individual with a supplier number. Typically, these vaccines are administered once a year in the fall or winter. Medicare does not require, for coverage purposes, that a doctor of medicine or osteopathy order the vaccine. Therefore, the beneficiary may receive the vaccine upon request without a physician's order and without physician supervision.

Pub 100-2, 15, 50.4.5 – Off-Label Use of Drugs and Biologicals in an Anti-Cancer Chemotherapeutic Regimen

(Rev. 96, Issued: 10-24-08, Effective: 06-05-08 NCCN / 06-10-08 Thomson Micromedex / 07-02-08 Clinical Pharmacology, Implementation: 11-25-08)

A. Overview

Effective January 1, 1994, off-label, medically accepted indications of Food and Drug Administration-(FDA) approved drugs and biologicals used in an anti-cancer chemotherapeutic regimen are identified under the conditions described below. A regimen is a combination of anti-cancer agents clinically recognized for the treatment of a specific type of cancer. Off-label, medically accepted indications are supported in either one or more of the compendia or in peer-reviewed medical literature. The contractor may maintain its own subscriptions to the listed compendia or peer-reviewed publications to determine the medically accepted indication of drugs or biologicals used off-label in an anti-cancer chemotherapeutic regimen. Compendia documentation or peer-reviewed literature supporting off-label use by the treating physician may also be requested of the physician by the contractor.

B. Recent Revisions to the Compendia List

Do not deny coverage based solely on the absence of FDA-approved labeling for the use, if the use is supported by any of the following compendia and the use is not listed as unsupported, not indicated, not recommended, or equivalent terms, in any of the following compendia:

Existing – American Hospital Formulary Service-Drug Information (AHFS-DI)

Effective June 5, 2008 – National Comprehensive Cancer Network (NCCN) Drugs and Biologics Compendium

Effective June 10, 2008 – Thomson Micromedex DrugDex

Effective July 2, 2008 – Clinical Pharmacology

The listed compendia employ various rating and recommendation systems that may not be readily cross-walked from compendium to compendium. In general, a use is identified by a compendium as medically accepted if the:

1. indication is a Category 1 or 2A in NCCN, or Class I, Class IIa, or Class IIb in DrugDex; or,
2. narrative text in AHFS-DI or Clinical Pharmacology is supportive. A use is not medically accepted by a compendium if the:
   a. indication is a Category 3 in NCCN or a Class III in DrugDex; or,
   b. narrative text in AHFS or Clinical Pharmacology is "not supportive."

The complete absence of narrative text on a use is considered neither supportive nor non-supportive.

C. Use Supported by Clinical Research That Appears in Peer-Reviewed Medical Literature

Contractors may also identify off-label uses that are supported by clinical research under the conditions identified in this section. Peer-reviewed medical literature may appear in scientific, medical, and pharmaceutical publications in which original manuscripts are

Medicare References

published, only after having been critically reviewed for scientific accuracy, validity, and reliability by unbiased, independent experts prior to publication. In-house publications of entities whose business relates to the manufacture, sale, or distribution of pharmaceutical products are excluded from consideration. Abstracts (including meeting abstracts) are excluded from consideration.

In determining whether an off-label use is supported, the contractors will evaluate the evidence in published, peer-reviewed medical literature listed below. When evaluating this literature, they will consider (among other things) the following:

- Whether the clinical characteristics of the beneficiary and the cancer are adequately represented in the published evidence
- Whether the administered chemotherapy regimen is adequately represented in the published evidence.
- Whether the reported study outcomes represent clinically meaningful outcomes experienced by patients.
- Whether the study is appropriate to address the clinical question. The contractor will consider:
    1. whether the experimental design, in light of the drugs and conditions under investigation, is appropriate to address the investigative question. (For example, in some clinical studies, it may be unnecessary or not feasible to use randomization, double blind trials, placebos, or crossover.);
    2. that non-randomized clinical trials with a significant number of subjects may be a basis for supportive clinical evidence for determining accepted uses of drugs; and,
    3. that case reports are generally considered uncontrolled and anecdotal information and do not provide adequate supportive clinical evidence for determining accepted uses of drugs.

The contractor will use peer-reviewed medical literature appearing in the regular editions of the following publications, not to include supplement editions privately funded by parties with a vested interest in the recommendations of the authors:

- American Journal of Medicine;
- Annals of Internal Medicine;
- Annals of Oncology;
- Annals of Surgical Oncology;
- Biology of Blood and Marrow Transplantation;
- Blood;
- Bone Marrow Transplantation;
- British Journal of Cancer;
- British Journal of Hematology;
- British Medical Journal;
- Cancer;
- Clinical Cancer Research;
- Drugs;
- European Journal of Cancer (formerly the European Journal of Cancer and Clinical Oncology);
- Gynecologic Oncology;
- International Journal of Radiation, Oncology, Biology, and Physics;
- The Journal of the American Medical Association;
- Journal of Clinical Oncology;
- Journal of the National Cancer Institute;
- Journal of the National Comprehensive Cancer Network (NCCN);
- Journal of Urology;
- Lancet;
- Lancet Oncology;
- Leukemia;
- The New England Journal of Medicine; or
- Radiation Oncology

D. Generally

FDA-approved drugs and biologicals may also be considered for use in the determination of medically accepted indications for off-label use if determined by the contractor to be reasonable and necessary.

If a use is identified as not indicated by the Centers for Medicare and Medicaid Services (CMS) or the FDA, or if a use is specifically identified as not indicated in one or more of the compendia listed, or if the contractor determines, based on peer-reviewed medical literature, that a particular use of a drug is not safe and effective, the off-label usage is not supported and, therefore, the drug is not covered.

Pub 100-2, 15, 50.4.5.1 – Process for Amending the List of Compendia for Determination of Medically-Accepted Indications for Off-Label Uses of Drugs and Biologicals in an Anti-Cancer Chemotherapeutic Regimen

(Rev. 120, Issued: 01-29-10, Effective:01-01-10, Implementation: 03-01-10)

A. Background

In the Physician Fee Schedule final rule for calendar year (CY) 2008, the CMS established a process for revising the list of compendia, as authorized under section 1861(t)(2) of the Social Security Act, and also established a definition for "compendium." At 42 CFR 414.930(a), a compendium is defined "as a comprehensive listing of FDA-approved drugs and biologicals or a comprehensive listing of a specific subset of drugs and biologicals in a specialty compendium, for example, a compendium of anti-cancer treatment." A compendium: (1) includes a summary of the pharmacologic characteristics of each drug or biological and may include information on dosage, as well as recommended or endorsed uses in specific diseases; (2) is indexed by drug or biological, and, (3) effective January 1, 2010, pursuant to section 182(b) of the Medicare Improvements for Patients and Providers Act (MIPPA), has a publicly transparent process for evaluating therapies and for identifying potential conflicts of interests. See 42 CFR 414.930(a); 72 FR 66222, 66404, and 74 FR 61901.

B. Desirable Characteristics of Compendia

CMS increased the transparency of the process by incorporating a list of desirable compendium characteristics outlined by the Medicare Evidence Development and

Coverage Advisory Committee (MedCAC) as criteria for decision-making. The list of desirable compendium characteristics was developed by the MedCAC during a public session on March 30, 2006. T he goal of this session was to review the evidence and advise CMS on the desirable characteristics of compendia for use in the determination of medically accepted indications of drugs and biologicals in anti-cancer therapy. As a result of this meeting, the MedCAC generated the following list of desirable characteristics:

- Extensive breadth of listings,
- Quick processing from application for inclusion to listing,
- Detailed description of the evidence reviewed for every individual listing,
- Use of pre-specified published criteria for weighing evidence,
- Use of prescribed published process for making recommendations,
- Publicly transparent process for evaluating therapies,
- Explicit "Not Recommended" listing when validated evidence is appropriate,
- Explicit listing and recommendations regarding therapies, including sequential use or combination in relation to other therapies,
- Explicit "Equivocal" listing when validated evidence is equivocal, and,
- Process for public identification and notification of potential conflicts of interest of the compendias' parent and sibling organizations, reviewers, and committee members, with an established procedure to manage recognized conflicts.

Furthermore, the provisions discussed in section 182(b) of MIPPA bring more uniformity in compendia conflict of interest disclosure practices and allow the public the ability to monitor how these policies impact compendia off-label recommendations.

C. Process for Changing List of Compendia

CMS will provide an annual 30-day open request period starting January 15 for the public to submit requests for additions or deletions to the compendia list contained on the CMS Web site at http://www.cms.hhs.gov/CoverageGenInfo/02_compendia.asp.

Complete requests as defined in section 50.4.5.1.D will be posted to the Web site annually by March 15 for public notice and comment. The request will identify the requestor and the requested action CMS is being asked to make to the list. Public comments will be accepted for a 30-day period beginning on the day the request is posted on the Web site. In addition to the annual process, CMS may generate a request for changes to the list at any time an urgent action is needed to protect the interests of the Medicare program and its beneficiaries.

D. Content of Requests

For a request to be considered complete, and therefore accepted for review, it must include the following information:

- The full name and contact information (including the mailing address, e-mail address, and telephone number) of the requestor. If the requestor is not an individual person, the information shall identify the officer or other representative who is authorized to act for the requestor on all matters related to the request.
- Full identification of the compendium that is the subject of the request, including name, publisher, edition if applicable, date of publication, and any other information needed for the accurate and precise identification of the specific compendium.
- A complete, written copy of the compendium that is the subject of the request. If the complete compendium is available electronically, it may be submitted electronically in place of hard copy. If the compendium is available online, the requestor may provide CMS with electronic access by furnishing at no cost to the Federal Government sufficient accounts for the purposes and duration of the review of the application in place of hard copy.
- The specific action that the requestor wishes CMS to take, for example to add or delete a specific compendium.
- Detailed, specific documentation that the compendium that is the subject of the request does or does not comply with the conditions of this rule. Broad, nonspecific claims without supporting documentation cannot be efficiently reviewed; therefore, they will not be accepted.
- A publicly transparent process for evaluating therapies, which includes the following: (1) internal or external request for listing of a therapy recommendation, including criteria used to evaluate the request (the complete application), (2) listing of all the evidentiary materials reviewed or considered for inclusion in the compendium (3) listing of all individuals who substantively participated in the review and development of the request, and (4) minutes and voting records of meetings for the review and disposition of the request. The information from an internal or external request for inclusion of a therapy in a compendium are available to the public for a period of not less than 5 years, which includes availability on the compendium's Web site for a period of not less than 3 years, coincident with the compendium's publication.
- A publicly transparent process for identifying potential conflicts of interests that provides: (1) direct or indirect financial relationships, and (2) ownership or investment interests that exist between individuals or the spouse or minor child of individuals who have substantively participated in the development or disposition of compendia recommendations, and the manufacturer or seller of the drug or biological being reviewed by the compendium. This information shall be identified and made timely available in response to a public request for a period of not less than 5 years, which includes availability on the compendium's Web site for a period of not less than 3 years, coincident with the compendium's publication.

A request may have only a single compendium as its subject. This will provide greater clarity to the scope of the Agency's review of a given request. A requestor may submit multiple requests, each requesting a different action.

E. Submission of Requests

Requests must be in writing and submitted in one of the following two ways (no duplicates please):

1. Electronic requests are encouraged to facilitate administrative efficiency. Each solicitation will include the electronic address for submissions.
2. Hard copy requests can be sent to:

   Centers for Medicare & Medicaid Services Coverage and Analysis Group
   Mailstop C1–09–06
   7500 Security Boulevard
   Baltimore, MD 21244

Allow sufficient time for hard copies to be received prior to the close of the open request period.

F. Review of Requests

CMS will consider a compendium's attainment of the desirable characteristics specified in 50.4.5.1.B when reviewing requests. CMS may consider additional, reasonable factors in making a determination. For example, CMS may consider factors that are likely to impact the compendium's suitability for this use, such as a change in the compendium's ownership or affiliation, and the standards applicable to the evidence considered by the compendium. CMS may consider that broad accessibility by the general public to the information contained in the compendium may assist beneficiaries, their treating physicians, or both, in choosing among treatment options. CMS will also consider a compendium's grading of evidence used in making recommendations regarding off-label uses, and the process by which the compendium grades the evidence. CMS may, at its discretion, combine and consider multiple requests that refer to the same compendium, even if those requests are for different actions. This facilitates administrative efficiency in the review of requests.

G. Publishing Review Results

CMS will publish decisions on the CMS Web site within 90 days after the close of the public comment period. (This instruction was last reviewed by CMS in December 2009.)

Pub 100-2, 15, 50.4.6 – Less Than Effective Drug

(Rev. 1, 10-01-03)

B3-2049.4.C.5

This is a drug that has been determined by the Food and Drug Administration (FDA) to lack substantial evidence of effectiveness for all labeled indications. Also, a drug that has been the subject of a Notice of an Opportunity for a Hearing (NOOH) published in the "Federal Register" before being withdrawn from the market, and for which the Secretary has not determined there is a compelling justification for its medical need, is considered less than effective. This includes any other drug product that is identical, similar, or related. Payment may not be made for a less than effective drug.

Because the FDA has not yet completed its identification of drug products that are still on the market, existing FDA efficacy decisions must be applied to all similar products once they are identified.

Pub 100-2, 15, 50.4.7 – Denial of Medicare Payment for Compounded Drugs Produced in Violation of Federal Food, Drug, and Cosmetic Act

(Rev. 1, 10-01-03)

B3-2049.4.C.6

The Food and Drug Administration (FDA) has found that, from time to time, firms established as retail pharmacies engage in mass production of compounded drugs, beyond the normal scope of pharmaceutical practice, in violation of the Federal Food, Drug, and Cosmetic Act (FFDCA). By compounding drugs on a large scale, a company may be operating as a drug manufacturer within the meaning of the FFDCA, without complying with requirements of that law. Such companies may be manufacturing drugs, which are subject to the new drug application (NDA) requirements of the FFDCA, but for which FDA has not approved an NDA or which are misbranded or adulterated. If the FDA has not approved the manufacturing and processing procedures used by these facilities, the FDA has no assurance that the drugs these companies are producing are safe and effective. The safety and effectiveness issues pertain to such factors as chemical stability, purity, strength, bioequivalency, and biovailability.

272HSection 1862(a)(1)(A) of the Act requires that drugs must be reasonable and necessary in order to by covered under Medicare. This means, in the case of drugs, the FDA must approve them for marketing. Section 273H50.4.1 instructs carriers and intermediaries to deny coverage for drugs that have not received final marketing approval by the FDA, unless instructed otherwise by CMS. The **Medicare Benefit Policy Manual**, Chapter 16, "General Exclusions from Coverage," §180, instructs carriers to deny coverage of services related to the use of noncovered drugs as well. Hence, if DME or a prosthetic device is used to administer a noncovered drug, coverage is denied for both the nonapproved drug and the DME or prosthetic device.

In those cases in which the FDA has determined that a company is producing compounded drugs in violation of the FFDCA, Medicare does not pay for the drugs because they do not meet the FDA approval requirements of the Medicare program. In addition, Medicare does not pay for the DME or prosthetic device used to administer such a drug if FDA determines that a required NDA has not been approved or that the drug is misbranded or adulterated.

The CMS will notify the carrier when the FDA has determined that compounded drugs are being produced in violation of the FFDCA. The carrier does not stop Medicare payment for such a drug unless it is notified that it is appropriate to do so through a subsequent instruction. In addition, if the carrier or Regional Offices (ROs) become aware that other companies are possibly operating in violation of the FFDCA, the carrier or RO notifies:

Centers for Medicare & Medicaid Services
Center for Medicare Management
7500 Security Blvd.
Baltimore, MD 21244-1850

Pub 100-2, 15, 50.5 – Self-Administered Drugs and Biologicals

(Rev. 1, 10-01-03)

B3-2049.5

Medicare Part B does not cover drugs that are usually self-administered by the patient unless the statute provides for such coverage. The statute explicitly provides coverage, for blood clotting factors, drugs used in immunosuppressive therapy, erythropoietin for dialysis patients, certain oral anti-cancer drugs and anti-emetics used in certain situations.

Pub 100-2, 15, 50.5.1 – Immunosuppressive Drugs

(Rev. 1, 10-01-03)

A3-3112.4.B.3, HO-230.4.B.3, AB-01-10

Until January 1, 1995, immunosuppressive drugs were covered under Part B for a period of one year following discharge from a hospital for a Medicare covered organ transplant. The CMS interpreted the 1-year period after the date of the transplant procedure to mean 365 days from the day on which an inpatient is discharged from the hospital.

Beneficiaries are eligible to receive additional Part B coverage within 18 months after the discharge date for drugs furnished in 1995; within 24 months for drugs furnished in 1996; within 30 months for drugs furnished in 1997; and within 36 months for drugs furnished after 1997.

For immunosuppressive drugs furnished on or after December 21, 2000, this time limit for coverage is eliminated.

Covered drugs include those immunosuppressive drugs that have been specifically labeled as such and approved for marketing by the FDA. (This is an exception to the standing drug policy which permits coverage of FDA approved drugs for nonlabeled uses, where such uses are found to be reasonable and necessary in an individual case.)

Covered drugs also include those prescription drugs, such as prednisone, that are used in conjunction with immunosuppressive drugs as part of a therapeutic regimen reflected in FDA approved labeling for immunosuppressive drugs. Therefore, antibiotics, hypertensives, and other drugs that are not directly related to rejection are not covered.

The FDA has identified and approved for marketing the following specifically labeled immunosuppressive drugs. They are:

- Sandimmune (cyclosporine), Sandoz Pharmaceutical;
- Imuran (azathioprine), Burroughs Wellcome;
- Atgam (antithymocyte globulin), Upjohn;
- Orthoclone OKT3 (Muromonab-CD3), Ortho Pharmaceutical;
- Prograf (tacrolimus), Fujisawa USA, Inc;
- Celicept (mycophenolate mefetil, Roche Laboratories;
- Daclizumab (Zenapax);
- Cyclophosphamide (Cytoxan);
- Prednisone; and
- Prednosolone.

The CMS expects contractors to keep informed of FDA additions to the list of the immunosuppressive drugs.

Pub 100-2, 15, 50.5.2 – Erythropoietin (EPO)

(Rev. 1, 10-01-03)

A3-3112.4.B.4, HO-230.4.B.4

The statute provides that EPO is covered for the treatment of anemia for patients with chronic renal failure who are on dialysis. Coverage is available regardless of whether the drug is administered by the patient or the patient's caregiver. EPO is a biologically engineered protein which stimulates the bone marrow to make new red blood cells.

NOTE: Non-ESRD patients who are receiving EPO to treat anemia induced by other conditions such as chemotherapy or the drug zidovudine (commonly called AZT) must meet the coverage requirements in 274H§50.

EPO is covered for the treatment of anemia for patients with chronic renal failure who are on dialysis when:

- It is administered in the renal dialysis facility; or
- It is self-administered in the home by any dialysis patient (or patient caregiver) who is determined competent to use the drug and meets the other conditions detailed below.

NOTE: Payment may not be made for EPO under the incident to provision when EPO is administered in the renal dialysis facility.

Also, in the office setting, reimbursement will be made for the administration charge only for non-ESRD patients receiving EPO.

Pub 100-2, 15, 50.5.2.1 – Requirements for Medicare Coverage for EPO

(Rev. 1, 10-01-03)

B3-2049.5

Medicare covers EPO and items related to its administration for dialysis patients who use EPO in the home when the following conditions are met:

A. Patient Care Plan

A dialysis patient who uses EPO in the home must have a current care plan (a copy of which must be maintained by the designated backup facility for Method II patients) for monitoring home use of EPO that includes the following:

1. Review of diet and fluid intake for aberrations as indicated by hyperkalemia and elevated blood pressure secondary to volume overload;
2. Review of medications to ensure adequate provision of supplemental iron;
3. Ongoing evaluations of hematocrit and iron stores;
4. Reevaluation of the dialysis prescription taking into account the patient's increased appetite and red blood cell volume;
5. Method for physician and facility (including backup facility for Method II patients) follow-up on blood tests and a mechanism (such as a patient log) for keeping the physician informed of the results;
6. Training of the patient to identify the signs and symptoms of hypotension and hypertension; and
7. The decrease or discontinuance of EPO if hypertension is uncontrollable.

B. Patient Selection

The dialysis facility, or the physician responsible for all dialysis-related services furnished to the patient, must make a comprehensive assessment that includes the following:

1. Preselection Monitoring

   The patient's hematocrit (or hemoglobin), serum iron, transferrin saturation, serum ferritin, and blood pressure must be measured.
2. Conditions the Patient Must Meet

   The assessment must find that the patient meets the following conditions:

Medicare References

a. Is a dialysis patient;

b. Has a hematocrit (or comparable hemoglobin level) that is as follows:

- For a patient who is initiating EPO treatment, no higher than 30 percent unless there is medical documentation showing the need for EPO despite a hematocrit (or comparable hemoglobin level) higher than 30 percent. Patients with severe angina, severe pulmonary distress, or severe hypotension may require EPO to prevent adverse symptoms even if they have higher hematocrit or hemoglobin levels.
- For a patient who has been receiving EPO from the facility or the physician, between 30 and 36 percent.

c. Is under the care of:

- A physician who is responsible for all dialysis-related services and who prescribes the EPO and follows the drug labeling instructions when monitoring the EPO home therapy; and
- A renal dialysis facility that establishes the plan of care and monitors the progress of the home EPO therapy.

3. The assessment must find that the patient or a caregiver meets the following conditions:
   - Is trained by the facility to inject EPO and is capable of carrying out the procedure;
   - Is capable of reading and understanding the drug labeling; and
   - Is trained in, and capable of observing, aseptic techniques.
4. Care and Storage of Drug

   The assessment must find that EPO can be stored in the patient's residence under refrigeration and that the patient is aware of the potential hazard of a child's having access to the drug and syringes.

C. Responsibilities of Physician or Dialysis Facility

The patient's physician or dialysis facility must:

- Develop a protocol that follows the drug label instructions;
- Make the protocol available to the patient to ensure safe and effective home use of EPO;
- Through the amounts prescribed, ensure that the drug on hand at any time does not exceed a 2-month supply;
- Maintain adequate records to allow quality assurance for review by the Network and State Survey Agencies. For Method II patients, current records must be provided to and maintained by the designated backup facility; and
- The dialysis facility must submit claims for EPO, if the facility provides it.

See the Medicare **Claims Processing Manual**, Chapter 11, "End Stage Renal Disease," for instructions for billing and processing claims for EPO under Method 1 and Method 2. Note that hematocrit readings are required on claims. It is expected that the ESRD facility or hospital outpatient department will maintain the following information in each patient's medical record to permit the review of the medical necessity of EPO.

1. Diagnostic coding;
2. Most recent creatinine prior to initiation of EPO therapy;
3. Date of most recent creatinine prior to initiation of EPO therapy;
4. Most recent hematocrit (HCT) prior to initiation of EPO therapy;
5. Date of most recent hematocrit (HCT) prior to initiation of EPO therapy;
6. Dosage in units/kg;
7. Weight in kgs; and
8. Number of units administered.

Pub 100-2, 15, 50.5.2.2 – Medicare Coverage of Epoetin Alfa (Procrit) for Preoperative Use

(Rev. 1, 10-01-03)

PM-AB-99-59, Dated 8/1/99

This instruction pertains exclusively to the preoperative surgical indication of the drug Procrit, in which it is administered to specific patients prior to surgery to reduce risk of transfusion. It does not affect Medicare policies related to other Food and Drug Administration (FDA) approved uses of Procrit. It is not a national coverage decision.

Procrit as Preventive Service

The carrier may determine that Procrit is covered for individuals who:

1. Are undergoing hip or knee surgery
2. Have an anemia with a hemoglobin between 10 and 13 mg/dL;
3. Are not a candidate for autologous blood transfusion;
4. Are expected to lose more than 2 units of blood; and
5. Have had a workup so that their anemia appears to be that of chronic disease.

The preoperative use of Procrit may be afforded to these individuals when carriers, exercising their discretion, determine that this treatment is reasonable and necessary. In other cases, Procrit is considered a preventive service and therefore not covered.

Pub 100-2, 15, 50.5.3 – Oral Anti-Cancer Drugs

(Rev. 1, 10-01-03)

A3-3112.4.B.5, HO-230.4.B.5

Effective January 1, 1994, Medicare Part B coverage is extended to include oral anticancer drugs that are prescribed as anti-cancer chemotherapeutic agents providing they have the same active ingredients and are used for the same indications as anti-cancer chemotherapeutic agents which would be covered if they were not self-administered and they were furnished incident to a physician's service as drugs and biologicals.

For an oral anti-cancer drug to be covered under Part B, it must:

- Be prescribed by a physician or other practitioner licensed under State law to prescribe such drugs as anti-cancer chemotherapeutic agents;
- Be a drug or biological that has been approved by the Food and Drug Administration (FDA);
- Have the same active ingredients as a non-self-administrable anti-cancer chemotherapeutic drug or biological that is covered when furnished incident to a physician's service. The oral anti-cancer drug and the non-self-administrable drug must have the same chemical/generic name as indicated by the FDA's "Approved Drug Products" (Orange Book), "Physician's Desk Reference" (PDR), or an authoritative drug compendium;
- Be used for the same indications, including unlabeled uses, as the non-self-administrable version of the drug; and
- Be reasonable and necessary for the individual patient.

Pub 100-2, 15, 50.5.4 – Oral Anti-Nausea (Anti-Emetic) Drugs

(Rev. 1, 10-01-03)

PM AB-97-26

Effective January 1, 1998, Medicare also covers self-administered anti-emetics, which are necessary for the administration and absorption of the anti-neoplastic chemotherapeutic agents when a high likelihood of vomiting exists. The anti-emetic drug is covered as a necessary means for administration of the antineoplastic chemotherapeutic agents. Oral drugs prescribed for use with the primary drug, which enhance the antineoplastic effect of the primary drug or permit the patient to tolerate the primary antineoplastic drug in higher doses for longer periods are not covered. Self-administered anti-emetics to reduce the side effects of nausea and vomiting brought on by the primary drug are not included beyond the administration necessary to achieve drug absorption.

275HSection 1861(s)(2) of the Act extends coverage to oral anti-emetic drugs that are used as full replacement for intravenous dosage forms of a cancer regimen under the following conditions:

- Coverage is provided only for oral drugs approved by the Food and Drug Administration (FDA) for use as anti-emetics;
- The oral anti-emetic must either be administered by the treating physician or in accordance with a written order from the physician as part of a cancer chemotherapy regimen;
- Oral anti-emetic drugs administered with a particular chemotherapy treatment must be initiated within two hours of the administration of the chemotherapeutic agent and may be continued for a period not to exceed 48 hours from that time;
- The oral anti-emetic drugs provided must be used as a full therapeutic replacement for the intravenous anti-emetic drugs

that would have otherwise been administered at the time of the chemotherapy treatment.

Only drugs pursuant to a physician's order at the time of the chemotherapy treatment qualify for this benefit. The dispensed number of dosage units may not exceed a loading dose administered within two hours of the treatment, plus a supply of additional dosage units not to exceed 48 hours of therapy.

Oral drugs that are not approved by the FDA for use as anti-emetics and which are used by treating physicians adjunctively in a manner incidental to cancer chemotherapy are not covered by this benefit and are not reimbursable within the scope of this benefit.

It is recognized that a limited number of patients will fail on oral anti-emetic drugs. Intravenous anti-emetics may be covered (subject to the rules of medical necessity) when furnished to patients who fail on oral anti-emetic therapy. More than one oral anti emetic drug may be prescribed and may be covered for concurrent use if needed to fully replace the intravenous drugs that otherwise would be given.

Pub 100-2, 15, 50.5.5 – Hemophilia Clotting Factors

(Rev. 1, 10-01-03)

A3-3112.4.B.2, HO-230.4.B.2

276HSection 1861(s)(2)(I) of the Act provides Medicare coverage of blood clotting factors for hemophilia patients competent to use such factors to control bleeding without medical supervision, and items related to the administration of such factors. Hemophilia, a blood disorder characterized by prolonged coagulation time, is caused by deficiency of a factor in plasma necessary for blood to clot. For purposes of Medicare Part B coverage, hemophilia encompasses the following conditions:

- Factor VIII deficiency (classic hemophilia);
- Factor IX deficiency (also termed plasma thromboplastin component (PTC) or Christmas factor deficiency); and
- Von Willebrand's disease.

Claims for blood clotting factors for hemophilia patients with these diagnoses may be covered if the patient is competent to use such factors without medical supervision. The amount of clotting factors determined to be necessary to have on hand and thus covered under this provision is based on the historical utilization pattern or profile developed by the contractor for each patient. It is expected that the treating source, e.g., a family physician or comprehensive hemophilia diagnostic and treatment center, have such information. From this data, the contractor is able to anticipate and make reasonable projections concerning the quantity of clotting factors the patient will need over a specific period of time. Unanticipated occurrences involving extraordinary events, such as automobile accidents or inpatient hospital stays, will change this base line data and should be appropriately considered. In addition, changes in a patient's medical needs over a period of time require adjustments in the profile.

Pub 100-2, 15, 50.6 – Coverage of Intravenous Immune Globulin for Treatment of Primary Immune Deficiency Diseases in the Home

(Rev. 6, 01-23-04)

Beginning for dates of service on or after January 1, 2004, The Medicare Prescription Drug, Improvement, and Modernization Act of 2003 provides coverage of intravenous immune globulin (IVIG) for the treatment of primary immune deficiency diseases (ICD-9 diagnosis codes 279.04, 279.05, 279.06, 279.12, and 279.2) in the home. The corresponding HCPCS codes are J1563 and J1564. The Act defines "intravenous immune globulin" as an approved pooled plasma derivative for the treatment of primary immune deficiency disease. It is covered under this benefit when the patient has a diagnosed primary immune deficiency disease, it is administered in the home of a patient with a diagnosed primary immune deficiency disease, and the physician determines that administration of the derivative in the patient's home is medically appropriate. The benefit does not include coverage for items or services related to the administration of the derivative. For coverage of IVIG under this benefit, it is not necessary for the derivative to be administered through a piece of durable medical equipment.

Pub 100-2, 15, 80.1 – Clinical Laboratory Services

(Rev. 79; Issued: 10-19-07; Effective: 01-01-03; Implementation: 11-19-07)

Section 1833 and 1861 of the Act provides for payment of clinical laboratory services under Medicare Part B. Clinical laboratory services involve the biological, microbiological, serological, chemical, immunohematological, hematological, biophysical, cytological, pathological, or other examination of materials derived from the human body for the diagnosis, prevention, or treatment of a disease or assessment of a medical condition. Laboratory services must meet all applicable requirements of the Clinical Laboratory Improvement Amendments of 1988 (CLIA), as set forth at 42 CFR part 493. Section 1862(a)(1)(A) of the Act provides that Medicare payment may not be made for services that are not reasonable and necessary. Clinical laboratory services must be ordered and used promptly by the physician who is treating the beneficiary as described in 42 CFR 410.32(a), or by a qualified nonphysician practitioner, as described in 42 CFR 410.32(a)(3).

See section 80.6 of this manual for related physician ordering instructions.

Pub 100-2, 15, 80.1.1 – Certification Changes

(Rev. 1, 10-01-03)

B3-2070.1.E

Each page of the lists of approved specialties also includes a column "Certification Changed" in which the following codes are used:

"C" indicates a change in the laboratory's approved certification since the preceding listing.

"A" discloses an accretion.

"TERM" – Laboratory not approved for payment after the indicated date which follows the code. The reason for termination also is given in the following codes:

1. Involuntary termination – no longer meets requirements
2. Voluntary withdrawal
3. Laboratory closed, merged with other interests, or organizational change
4. Ownership change with new ownership participating under different name
5. Ownership change with new owner not participating
6. Change in ownership – new provider number assigned
7. Involuntary termination – failure to abide by agreement
8. Former "emergency" hospital now fully participating

Pub 100-2, 15, 80.1.2 – Carrier Contacts With Independent Clinical Laboratories

(Rev. 1, 10-01-03)

B3-2070.1.F

An important role of the carrier is as a communicant of necessary information to independent clinical laboratories. Experience has shown that the failure to inform laboratories of Medicare regulations and claims processing procedures may have an adverse effect on prosecution of laboratories suspected of fraudulent activities with respect to tests performed by, or billed on behalf of, independent laboratories. United States Attorneys often have to prosecute under a handicap or may simply refuse to prosecute cases where there is no evidence that a laboratory has been specifically informed of Medicare regulations and claims processing procedures.

Carriers must follow the Provider Education and Training (PET) guidelines to assure that laboratories are aware of Medicare regulations and the carrier's policy when any changes are made in coverage policy or claims processing procedures. The PET guidelines require carriers to use various methods of communication (such as print, Internet, face-toface instruction). Newsletters/bulletins that contain program and billing information must be produced at least quarterly and posted on the carrier Web site where duplicate copies may be obtained.

Some items which should be communicated to laboratories and responsibilities that laboratories are required to perform are:

- The requirements to have the same fee schedule for Medicare and private patients;

Medicare References

- To specify whether the tests are manual or automated;
- To document fully the medical necessity for pickup of specimens from a skilled nursing facility or a beneficiary's home, and
- In cases when a laboratory service is referred from one independent laboratory to another independent laboratory, to identify the laboratory actually performing the test.

Additionally, when carrier professional relations representatives make personal contacts with particular laboratories, the representative should prepare and retain reports of contact indicating dates, persons present, and issues discussed. Finally, carriers should inform independent laboratories that the **Medicare National Coverage Determinations Manual** as well as other guidelines contained in the manual for determining medical necessity are on the Web site. Carriers should also publish local guidelines on its Web site; the carrier should not duplicate national instructions here. Timely paper or electronic communications concerning the Internet publications to independent laboratories new to the carrier's service area are essential.

Pub 100-2, 15, 80.1.3 – Independent Laboratory Service to a Patient in the Patient's Home or an Institution

(Rev. 1, 10-01-03)

B3-2070.1.G

Where it is medically necessary for an independent laboratory to visit a patient to obtain a specimen, the service would be covered in the following circumstances:

1. Patient Confined to Home

   If a patient is confined to the home or other place of residence used as his or her home (see 303H§60.4.1 for the definition of a "homebound patient"), medical necessity would exist (e.g., where a laboratory technician draws a blood specimen). However, where the specimen is a type which would require only the services of a messenger and would not require the skills of a laboratory technician, e.g., urine or sputum, a specimen pickup service would not be considered medically necessary.

2. Place of Residence is an Institution

   Medical necessity could also exist where the patient's place of residence is an institution, including a skilled nursing facility that does not perform venipunctures. This would apply even though the institution meets the basic definition of a skilled nursing facility and would not ordinarily be considered a beneficiary's home. (This policy is intended for independent laboratories only and does not expand the range of coverage of services to homebound patients under the incident to provision.) A trip by an independent laboratory technician to a facility (other than a hospital) for the purpose of performing a venipuncture is considered medically necessary only if:

   a. The patient was confined to the facility; and

   b. The facility did not have on duty personnel qualified to perform this service.

When facility personnel actually obtained and prepared the specimens for the independent laboratory to pick them up, the laboratory provides this pickup service as a service to the facility in the same manner as it does for physicians.

Pub 100-2, 15, 100 – Surgical Dressings, Splints, Casts, and Other Devices Used for Reductions of Fractures and Dislocations

(Rev. 1, 10-01-03)

B3-2079, A3-3110.3, HO-228.3,

Surgical dressings are limited to primary and secondary dressings required for the treatment of a wound caused by, or treated by, a surgical procedure that has been performed by a physician or other health care professional to the extent permissible under State law. In addition, surgical dressings required after debridement of a wound are also covered, irrespective of the type of debridement, as long as the debridement was reasonable and necessary and was performed by a health care professional acting within the scope of his/her legal authority when performing this function. Surgical dressings are covered for as long as they are medically necessary.

Primary dressings are therapeutic or protective coverings applied directly to wounds or lesions either on the skin or caused by an opening to the skin. Secondary dressing materials that serve a therapeutic or protective function and that are needed to secure a primary dressing are also covered. Items such as adhesive tape, roll gauze, bandages, and disposable compression material are examples of secondary dressings. Elastic stockings, support hose, foot coverings, leotards, knee supports, surgical leggings, gauntlets, and pressure garments for the arms and hands are examples of items that are not ordinarily covered as surgical dressings. Some items, such as transparent film, may be used as a primary or secondary dressing.

If a physician, certified nurse midwife, physician assistant, nurse practitioner, or clinical nurse specialist applies surgical dressings as part of a professional service that is billed to Medicare, the surgical dressings are considered incident to the professional services of the health care practitioner. (See 31H§§60.1, 312H180, 313H190, 314H200, and 315H210.) When surgical dressings are not covered incident to the services of a health care practitioner and are obtained by the patient from a supplier (e.g., a drugstore, physician, or other health care practitioner that qualifies as a supplier) on an order from a physician or other health care professional authorized under State law or regulation to make such an order, the surgical dressings are covered separately under Part B.

Splints and casts, and other devices used for reductions of fractures and dislocations are covered under Part B of Medicare. This includes dental splints.

Pub 100-2, 15, 110 – Durable Medical Equipment – General

(Rev. 1, 10-01-03)

B3-2100, A3-3113, HO-235, HHA-220

Expenses incurred by a beneficiary for the rental or purchases of durable medical equipment (DME) are reimbursable if the following three requirements are met:

- The equipment meets the definition of DME 316H(§110.1);
- The equipment is necessary and reasonable for the treatment of the patient's illness or injury or to improve the functioning of his or her malformed body member (§110.1); and
- The equipment is used in the patient's home.

The decision whether to rent or purchase an item of equipment generally resides with the beneficiary, but the decision on how to pay rests with CMS. For some DME, program payment policy calls for lump sum payments and in others for periodic payment. Where covered DME is furnished to a beneficiary by a supplier of services other than a provider of services, the DMERC makes the reimbursement. If a provider of services furnishes the equipment, the intermediary makes the reimbursement. The payment method is identified in the annual fee schedule update furnished by CMS.

The CMS issues quarterly updates to a fee schedule file that contains rates by HCPCS code and also identifies the classification of the HCPCS code within the following categories.

Category	Code Definition
IN	Inexpensive and Other Routinely Purchased Items
FS	Frequently Serviced Items
CR	Capped Rental Items
OX	Oxygen and Oxygen Equipment
OS	Ostomy, Tracheostomy & Urological Items
SD	Surgical Dressings
PO	Prosthetics & Orthotics
SU	Supplies
TE	Transcutaneous Electrical Nerve Stimulators

The DMERCs, carriers, and intermediaries, where appropriate, use the CMS files to determine payment rules. See the Medicare **Claims Processing Manual**, Chapter 20, "Durable Medical Equipment, Surgical Dressings and Casts, Orthotics and Artificial Limbs, and Prosthetic Devices," for a detailed description of payment rules for each classification.

Payment may also be made for repairs, maintenance, and delivery of equipment and for expendable and nonreusable items essential to the effective use of the equipment subject to the conditions in 317H§110.2.

See the **Medicare Benefit Policy Manual**, Chapter 11, "End Stage Renal Disease," for hemodialysis equipment and supplies.

Pub 100-2, 15, 110.1 – Definition of Durable Medical Equipment

(Rev. 1, 10-01-03)

B3-2100.1, A3-3113.1, HO-235.1, HHA-220.1, B3-2100.2, A3-3113.2, HO-235.2, HHA-220.2

Durable medical equipment is equipment which:

- Can withstand repeated use;
- Is primarily and customarily used to serve a medical purpose;
- Generally is not useful to a person in the absence of an illness or injury; and
- Is appropriate for use in the home.

All requirements of the definition must be met before an item can be considered to be durable medical equipment.

The following describes the underlying policies for determining whether an item meets the definition of DME and may be covered.

A. Durability

An item is considered durable if it can withstand repeated use, i.e., the type of item that could normally be rented. Medical supplies of an expendable nature, such as incontinent pads, lambs wool pads, catheters, ace bandages, elastic stockings, surgical facemasks, irrigating kits, sheets, and bags are not considered "durable" within the meaning of the definition. There are other items that, although durable in nature, may fall into other coverage categories such as supplies, braces, prosthetic devices, artificial arms, legs, and eyes.

B. Medical Equipment

Medical equipment is equipment primarily and customarily used for medical purposes and is not generally useful in the absence of illness or injury. In most instances, no development will be needed to determine whether a specific item of equipment is medical in nature. However, some cases will require development to determine whether the item constitutes medical equipment. This development would include the advice of local medical organizations (hospitals, medical schools, medical societies) and specialists in the field of physical medicine and rehabilitation. If the equipment is new on the market, it may be necessary, prior to seeking professional advice, to obtain information from the supplier or manufacturer explaining the design, purpose, effectiveness and method of using the equipment in the home as well as the results of any tests or clinical studies that have been conducted.

1. Equipment Presumptively Medical

   Items such as hospital beds, wheelchairs, hemodialysis equipment, iron lungs, respirators, intermittent positive pressure breathing machines, medical regulators, oxygen tents, crutches, canes, trapeze bars, walkers, inhalators, nebulizers, commodes, suction machines, and traction equipment presumptively constitute medical equipment. (Although hemodialysis equipment is covered as a prosthetic device (§120), it also meets the definition of DME, and reimbursement for the rental or purchase of such equipment for use in the beneficiary's home will be made only under the provisions for payment applicable to DME. See the **Medicare Benefit Policy Manual**, Chapter 11, "End Stage Renal Disease," §30.1, for coverage of home use of hemodialysis.) NOTE: There is a wide variety in types of respirators and suction machines. The DMERC's medical staff should determine whether the apparatus specified in the claim is appropriate for home use.

2. Equipment Presumptively Nonmedical

   Equipment which is primarily and customarily used for a nonmedical purpose may not be considered "medical" equipment for which payment can be made under the medical insurance program. This is true even though the item has some remote medically related use. For example, in the case of a cardiac patient, an air conditioner might possibly be used to lower room temperature to reduce fluid loss in the patient and to restore an environment conducive to maintenance of the proper fluid balance. Nevertheless, because the primary and customary use of an air conditioner is a nonmedical one, the air conditioner cannot be deemed to be medical equipment for which payment can be made. Other devices and equipment used for environmental control or to enhance the environmental setting in which the beneficiary is placed are not considered covered DME. These include, for example, room heaters, humidifiers, dehumidifiers, and electric air cleaners. Equipment which basically serves comfort or convenience functions or is primarily for the convenience of a person caring for the patient, such as elevators, stairway elevators, and posture chairs, do not constitute medical equipment. Similarly, physical fitness equipment (such as an exercycle), first-aid or precautionary-type equipment (such as preset portable oxygen units), self-help devices (such as safety grab bars), and training equipment (such as Braille training texts) are considered nonmedical in nature.

3. Special Exception Items

   Specified items of equipment may be covered under certain conditions even though they do not meet the definition of DME because they are not primarily and customarily used to serve a medical purpose and/or are generally useful in the absence of illness or injury. These items would be covered when it is clearly established that they serve a therapeutic purpose in an individual case and would include:

   a. Gel pads and pressure and water mattresses (which generally serve a preventive purpose) when prescribed for a patient who had bed sores or there is medical evidence indicating that they are highly susceptible to such ulceration; and

   b. Heat lamps for a medical rather than a soothing or cosmetic purpose, e.g., where the need for heat therapy has been established.

In establishing medical necessity for the above items, the evidence must show that the item is included in the physician's course of treatment and a physician is supervising its use.

NOTE: The above items represent special exceptions and no extension of coverage to other items should be inferred

C. Necessary and Reasonable

Although an item may be classified as DME, it may not be covered in every instance. Coverage in a particular case is subject to the requirement that the equipment be necessary and reasonable for treatment of an illness or injury, or to improve the functioning of a malformed body member. These considerations will bar payment for equipment which cannot reasonably be expected to perform a therapeutic function in an individual case or will permit only partial therapeutic function in an individual case or will permit only partial payment when the type of equipment furnished substantially exceeds that required for the treatment of the illness or injury involved.

See the Medicare **Claims Processing Manual**, Chapter 1, "General Billing Requirements;" §60, regarding the rules for providing advance beneficiary notices (ABNs) that advise beneficiaries, before items or services actually are furnished, when Medicare is likely to deny payment for them. ABNs allow beneficiaries to make an informed consumer decision about receiving items or services for which they may have to pay out-of-pocket and to be more active participants in their own health care treatment decisions.

1. Necessity for the Equipment

   Equipment is necessary when it can be expected to make a meaningful contribution to the treatment of the patient's illness or injury or to the improvement of his or her malformed body member. In most cases the physician's prescription for the equipment and other medical information available to the DMERC will be sufficient to establish that the equipment serves this purpose.

2. Reasonableness of the Equipment

   Even though an item of DME may serve a useful medical purpose, the DMERC or intermediary must also consider to what extent, if any, it would be reasonable for the Medicare program to pay for the item prescribed. The following considerations should enter into the determination of reasonableness:

   1. Would the expense of the item to the program be clearly disproportionate to the therapeutic benefits which could ordinarily be derived from use of the equipment?
   2. Is the item substantially more costly than a medically appropriate and realistically feasible alternative pattern of care?

3. Does the item serve essentially the same purpose as equipment already available to the beneficiary?

3. Payment Consistent With What is Necessary and Reasonable

   Where a claim is filed for equipment containing features of an aesthetic nature or features of a medical nature which are not required by the patient's condition or where there exists a reasonably feasible and medically appropriate alternative pattern of care which is less costly than the equipment furnished, the amount payable is based on the rate for the equipment or alternative treatment which meets the patient's medical needs.

   The acceptance of an assignment binds the supplier-assignee to accept the payment for the medically required equipment or service as the full charge and the supplier-assignee cannot charge the beneficiary the differential attributable to the equipment actually furnished.

4. Establishing the Period of Medical Necessity

   Generally, the period of time an item of durable medical equipment will be considered to be medically necessary is based on the physician's estimate of the time that his or her patient will need the equipment. See the **Medicare Program Integrity Manual**, Chapters 5 and 6, for medical review guidelines.

D. Definition of a Beneficiary's Home

For purposes of rental and purchase of DME a beneficiary's home may be his/her own dwelling, an apartment, a relative's home, a home for the aged, or some other type of institution. However, an institution may not be considered a beneficiary's home if it:

- Meets at least the basic requirement in the definition of a hospital, i.e., it is primarily engaged in providing by or under the supervision of physicians, to inpatients, diagnostic and therapeutic services for medical diagnosis, treatment, and care of injured, disabled, and sick persons, or rehabilitation services for the rehabilitation of injured, disabled, or sick persons; or
- Meets at least the basic requirement in the definition of a skilled nursing facility, i.e., it is primarily engaged in providing to inpatients skilled nursing care and related services for patients who require medical or nursing care, or rehabilitation services for the rehabilitation of injured, disabled, or sick persons.

Thus, if an individual is a patient in an institution or distinct part of an institution which provides the services described in the bullets above, the individual is not entitled to have separate Part B payment made for rental or purchase of DME. This is because such an institution may not be considered the individual's home. The same concept applies even if the patient resides in a bed or portion of the institution not certified for Medicare. If the patient is at home for part of a month and, for part of the same month is in an institution that cannot qualify as his or her home, or is outside the U.S., monthly payments may be made for the entire month. Similarly, if DME is returned to the provider before the end of a payment month because the beneficiary died in that month or because the equipment became unnecessary in that month, payment may be made for the entire month.

Pub 100-2, 15, 110.2 – Repairs, Maintenance, Replacement, and Delivery

(Rev. 30, Issued 02-18-05, Effective/Implementation: Not Applicable)

Under the circumstances specified below, payment may be made for repair, maintenance, and replacement of medically required DME, including equipment which had been in use before the user enrolled in Part B of the program. However, do not pay for repair, maintenance, or replacement of equipment in the frequent and substantial servicing or oxygen equipment payment categories. In addition, payments for repair and maintenance may not include payment for parts and labor covered under a manufacturer's or supplier's warranty.

A. Repairs

To repair means to fix or mend and to put the equipment back in good condition after damage or wear. Repairs to equipment which a beneficiary owns are covered when necessary to make the equipment serviceable. However, do not pay for repair of previously denied equipment or equipment in the frequent and substantial servicing or oxygen equipment payment categories. If the expense for repairs exceeds the estimated expense of purchasing or renting another item of equipment for the remaining period of medical need, no payment can be made for the amount of the excess. (See 318Hsubsection C where claims for repairs suggest malicious damage or culpable neglect.)

Since renters of equipment recover from the rental charge the expenses they incur in maintaining in working order the equipment they rent out, separately itemized charges for repair of rented equipment are not covered. This includes items in the frequent and substantial servicing, oxygen equipment, capped rental, and inexpensive or routinely purchased payment categories which are being rented.

A new Certificate of Medical Necessity (CMN) and/or physician's order is not needed for repairs.

For replacement items, see Subsection C below.

B. Maintenance

Routine periodic servicing, such as testing, cleaning, regulating, and checking of the beneficiary's equipment, is not covered. The owner is expected to perform such routine maintenance rather than a retailer or some other person who charges the beneficiary. Normally, purchasers of DME are given operating manuals which describe the type of servicing an owner may perform to properly maintain the equipment. It is reasonable to expect that beneficiaries will perform this maintenance. Thus, hiring a third party to do such work is for the convenience of the beneficiary and is not covered. However, more extensive maintenance which, based on the manufacturers' recommendations, is to be performed by authorized technicians, is covered as repairs for medically necessary equipment which a beneficiary owns. This might include, for example, breaking down sealed components and performing tests which require specialized testing equipment not available to the beneficiary. Do not pay for maintenance of purchased items that require frequent and substantial servicing or oxygen equipment.

Since renters of equipment recover from the rental charge the expenses they incur in maintaining in working order the equipment they rent out, separately itemized charges for maintenance of rented equipment are generally not covered. Payment may not be made for maintenance of rented equipment other than the maintenance and servicing fee established for capped rental items. For capped rental items which have reached the 15- month rental cap, contractors pay claims for maintenance and servicing fees after 6 months have passed from the end of the final paid rental month or from the end of the period the item is no longer covered under the supplier's or manufacturer's warranty, whichever is later. See the Medicare **Claims Processing Manual**, Chapter 20, "Durable Medical Equipment, Prosthetics and Orthotics, and Supplies (DMEPOS)," for additional instruction and an example.

A new CMN and/or physician's order is not needed for covered maintenance.

C. Replacement

Replacement refers to the provision of an identical or nearly identical item. Situations involving the provision of a different item because of a change in medical condition are not addressed in this section.

Equipment which the beneficiary owns or is a capped rental item may be replaced in cases of loss or irreparable damage. Irreparable damage refers to a specific accident or to a natural disaster (e.g., fire, flood). A physician's order and/or new Certificate of Medical Necessity (CMN), when required, is needed to reaffirm the medical necessity of the item.

Irreparable wear refers to deterioration sustained from day-to-day usage over time and a specific event cannot be identified. Replacement of equipment due to irreparable wear takes into consideration the reasonable useful lifetime of the equipment. If the item of equipment has been in continuous use by the patient on either a rental or purchase basis for the equipment's useful lifetime, the beneficiary may elect to obtain a new piece of equipment. Replacement may be reimbursed when a new physician order and/or new CMN, when required, is needed to reaffirm the medical necessity of the item.

The reasonable useful lifetime of durable medical equipment is determined through program instructions. In the absence of program instructions, carriers may determine the reasonable useful lifetime of equipment, but in no case can it be less than 5 years. Computation of the useful lifetime is based on when the equipment is delivered to the beneficiary, not the age of the equipment. Replacement due to wear is not covered during the reasonable useful lifetime of the equipment. During the reasonable useful lifetime, Medicare does cover repair up to the cost of replacement (but not actual replacement) for medically necessary equipment owned by the beneficiary. (See subsection A.)

Charges for the replacement of oxygen equipment, items that require frequent and substantial servicing or inexpensive or routinely purchased items which are being rented are not covered.

Cases suggesting malicious damage, culpable neglect, or wrongful disposition of equipment should be investigated and denied where the DMERC determines that it is unreasonable to make program payment under the circumstances. DMERCs refer such cases to the program integrity specialist in the RO.

D. Delivery

Payment for delivery of DME whether rented or purchased is generally included in the fee schedule allowance for the item. See Pub. 100-04, Medicare **Claims Processing Manual**, Chapter 20, "Durable Medical Equipment, Prosthetics and Orthotics, and Supplies (DMEPOS)," for the rules that apply to making reimbursement for exceptional cases.

Pub 100-2, 15, 110.3 – Coverage of Supplies and Accessories

(Rev. 1, 10-01-03)

B3-2100.5, A3-3113.4, HO-235.4, HHA-220.5

Payment may be made for supplies, e.g., oxygen, that are necessary for the effective use of durable medical equipment. Such supplies include those drugs and biologicals which must be put directly into the equipment in order to achieve the therapeutic benefit of the durable medical equipment or to assure the proper functioning of the equipment, e.g., tumor chemotherapy agents used with an infusion pump or heparin used with a home dialysis system. However, the coverage of such drugs or biologicals does not preclude the need for a determination that the drug or biological itself is reasonable and necessary for treatment of the illness or injury or to improve the functioning of a malformed body member.

In the case of prescription drugs, other than oxygen, used in conjunction with durable medical equipment, prosthetic, orthotics, and supplies (DMEPOS) or prosthetic devices, the entity that dispenses the drug must furnish it directly to the patient for whom a prescription is written. The entity that dispenses the drugs must have a Medicare supplier number, must possess a current license to dispense prescription drugs in the State in which the drug is dispensed, and must bill and receive payment in its own name. A supplier that is not the entity that dispenses the drugs cannot purchase the drugs used in conjunction with DME for resale to the beneficiary. Reimbursement may be made for replacement of essential accessories such as hoses, tubes, mouthpieces, etc., for necessary DME, only if the beneficiary owns or is purchasing the equipment.

Pub 100-2, 15, 110.4 – Miscellaneous Issues Included in the Coverage of Equipment

(Rev. 1, 10-01-03)

B3-2100.6, A3-3113.5, HO-235.5, HHA-220.6

Payment can be made for the purchase of DME even though rental payments may have been made for prior months. This could occur where, because of a change in his/her condition, the beneficiary feels that it would be to his/her advantage to purchase the equipment rather than to continue to rent it.

A beneficiary may sell or otherwise dispose of equipment for which they have no further use, for example, because of recovery from the illness or injury that gave rise to the need for the equipment. (There is no authority for the program to repossess the equipment.) If after such disposal there is again medical need for similar equipment, payment can be made for the rental or purchase of that equipment.

However, where an arrangement is motivated solely by a desire to create artificial expenses to be met by the program and to realize a profit thereby, such expenses would not be covered under the program. The resolution of questions involving the disposition and subsequent acquisition of durable medical equipment must be made on a case-by-case basis.

Cases where it appears that there has been an attempt to create an artificial expense and realize a profit thereby should be developed and when appropriate denied. After adjudication the DMERC would refer such cases to the program integrity specialist in the RO.

When payments stop because the beneficiary's condition has changed and the equipment is no longer medically necessary, the beneficiary is responsible for the remaining noncovered charges. Similarly, when payments stop because the beneficiary dies, the beneficiary's estate is responsible for the remaining noncovered charges.

Contractors do not get involved in issues relating to ownership or title of property.

Pub 100-2, 15, 110.5 – Incurred Expense Dates for Durable Medical Equipment

(Rev. 1, 10-01-03)

A3-3113.7.B, HO-235.7.B, B3-3011

The date of service on the claim must be the date that the beneficiary or authorized representative received the DMEPOS item. If the date of delivery is not specified on the bill, the contractor should assume, in the absence of evidence to the contrary, that the date of purchase was the date of delivery.

For mail order DMEPOS items, the date of service on the claim must be the shipping date.

The date of service on the claim must be the date that the DMEPOS item(s) was received by the nursing facility if the supplier delivered it or the shipping date if the supplier utilized a delivery/shipping service.

An exception to the preceding statements concerning the date of service on the claim occurs when items are provided in anticipation of discharge from a hospital or nursing facility. If a DMEPOS item is delivered to a patient in a hospital up to two days prior to discharge to home and it is for the benefit of the patient for purposes of fitting or training of the patient on its use, the supplier should bill the date of service on the claim as the date of discharge to home and should use POS=12.

See the **Medicare Program Integrity Manual**, Chapter 5, "Items and Services Having Special DMERC Review Considerations," for additional information pertaining to the date of service on the claim. Also see the Medicare **Claims Processing Manual**, Chapter 20, "Durable Medical Equipment, Surgical dressings and Casts, Orthotics and Artificial Limbs, and Prosthetic Devices," for additional DME billing and claims processing information.

Pub 100-2, 15, 110.6 – Determining Months for Which Periodic Payments May Be Made for Equipment Used in an Institution

(Rev. 1, 10-01-03)

A3-3113.7.D, HO-235.7.C

If a patient uses equipment subject to the monthly payment rule in an institution, which does not qualify as his or her home, the used months during which the beneficiary was institutionalized are not covered.

Pub 100-2, 15, 110.7 – No Payment for Purchased Equipment Delivered Outside the United States or Before Beneficiary's Coverage Began

(Rev. 1, 10-01-03)

A3-3113.7.C

In the case of equipment subject to the lump sum payment rules, the beneficiary must have been in the United States and must have had Medicare coverage at the time the item was delivered. Therefore, where an item of durable medical equipment paid for as a lump sum was delivered to an individual outside the United States or before his or her coverage period began, the entire expense of the item would be excluded from coverage. Payment cannot be made in such cases even though the individual later uses the item inside the United States or after his or her coverage begins.

If the individual is outside the U.S. for more than 30 days and then returns to the U.S., the DMERC determines medical necessity as in an initial case before resuming payments.

Pub 100-2, 15, 120 – Prosthetic Devices

(Rev. 1, 10-01-03)

B3-2130, A3-3110.4, HO-228.4, A3-3111, HO-229

A. General

Prosthetic devices (other than dental) which replace all or part of an internal body organ (including contiguous tissue), or replace all or part of the function of a permanently inoperative or malfunctioning internal body organ are covered when furnished on a physician's order. This does not require a determination that there is no possibility that the patient's condition may improve sometime in the future. If the medical record, including the judgment of the attending physician, indicates the condition is of long and indefinite duration, the test of permanence is considered met. (Such a device may also be covered under 319H§60.1 as a supply when furnished incident to a physician's service.) Examples of prosthetic devices include artificial limbs, parenteral and enteral (PEN) nutrition, cardiac pacemakers, prosthetic lenses (see subsection B), breast prostheses (including a surgical brassiere) for postmastectomy patients, maxillofacial devices, and devices which replace all or part of the ear or nose. A urinary collection and retention system with or without a tube is a prosthetic device replacing bladder function in case of permanent urinary incontinence. The foley catheter is also considered a prosthetic device when ordered for a patient with permanent urinary incontinence. However, chucks, diapers, rubber sheets, etc., are supplies that are not covered under this provision. Although hemodialysis equipment is a prosthetic device, payment for the rental or purchase of such equipment in the home is made only for use under the provisions for payment applicable to durable medical equipment.

An exception is that if payment cannot be made on an inpatient's behalf under Part A, hemodialysis equipment, supplies, and services required by such patient could be covered under Part B as a prosthetic device, which replaces the function of a kidney. See the **Medicare Benefit Policy Manual**, Chapter 11, "End Stage Renal Disease," for payment for hemodialysis equipment used in the home. See the **Medicare Benefit Policy Manual**, Chapter 1, "Inpatient Hospital Services," §10, for additional instructions on hospitalization for renal dialysis.

NOTE: Medicare does not cover a prosthetic device dispensed to a patient prior to the time at which the patient undergoes the procedure that makes necessary the use of the device. For example, the carrier does not make a separate Part B payment for an intraocular lens (IOL) or pacemaker that a physician, during an office visit prior to the actual surgery, dispenses to the patient for his or her use. Dispensing a prosthetic device in this manner raises health and safety issues. Moreover, the need for the device cannot be clearly established until the procedure that makes its use possible is successfully performed. Therefore, dispensing a prosthetic device in this manner is not considered reasonable and necessary for the treatment of the patient's condition.

Colostomy (and other ostomy) bags and necessary accouterments required for attachment are covered as prosthetic devices. This coverage also includes irrigation and flushing equipment and other items and supplies directly related to ostomy care, whether the attachment of a bag is required.

Accessories and/or supplies which are used directly with an enteral or parenteral device to achieve the therapeutic benefit of the prosthesis or to assure the proper functioning of the device may also be covered under the prosthetic device benefit subject to the additional guidelines in the **Medicare National Coverage Determinations Manual**.

Covered items include catheters, filters, extension tubing, infusion bottles, pumps (either food or infusion), intravenous (I.V.) pole, needles, syringes, dressings, tape, Heparin Sodium (parenteral only), volumetric monitors (parenteral only), and parenteral and enteral nutrient solutions. Baby food and other regular grocery products that can be blenderized and used with the enteral system are not covered. Note that some of these items, e.g., a food pump and an I.V. pole, qualify as DME. Although coverage of the enteral and parenteral nutritional therapy systems is provided on the basis of the prosthetic device benefit, the payment rules relating to lump sum or monthly payment for DME apply to such items.

The coverage of prosthetic devices includes replacement of and repairs to such devices as explained in subsection D.

Finally, the Benefits Improvement and Protection Act of 2000 amended 320H§1834(h)(1) of the Act by adding a provision (1834 (h)(1)(G)(i)) that requires Medicare payment to be made for the replacement of prosthetic devices which are artificial limbs, or for the replacement of any part of such devices, without regard to continuous use or useful lifetime restrictions if an ordering physician determines that the replacement device, or replacement part of such a device, is necessary.

Payment may be made for the replacement of a prosthetic device that is an artificial limb, or replacement part of a device if the ordering physician determines that the replacement device or part is necessary because of any of the following:

1. A change in the physiological condition of the patient;
2. An irreparable change in the condition of the device, or in a part of the device; or
3. The condition of the device, or the part of the device, requires repairs and the cost of such repairs would be more than 60 percent of the cost of a replacement device, or, as the case may be, of the part being replaced.

This provision is effective for items replaced on or after April 1, 2001. It supersedes any rule that that provided a 5-year or other replacement rule with regard to prosthetic devices.

B. Prosthetic Lenses

The term "internal body organ" includes the lens of an eye. Prostheses replacing the lens of an eye include post-surgical lenses customarily used during convalescence from eye surgery in which the lens of the eye was removed. In addition, permanent lenses are also covered when required by an individual lacking the organic lens of the eye because of surgical removal or congenital absence. Prosthetic lenses obtained on or after the beneficiary's date of entitlement to supplementary medical insurance benefits may be covered even though the surgical removal of the crystalline lens occurred before entitlement.

1. Prosthetic Cataract Lenses

   One of the following prosthetic lenses or combinations of prosthetic lenses furnished by a physician (see 321H§30.4 for coverage of prosthetic lenses prescribed by a doctor of optometry) may be covered when determined to be reasonable and necessary to restore essentially the vision provided by the crystalline lens of the eye:

   - Prosthetic bifocal lenses in frames;
   - Prosthetic lenses in frames for far vision, and prosthetic lenses in frames for near vision; or
   - When a prosthetic contact lens(es) for far vision is prescribed (including cases of binocular and monocular aphakia), make payment for the contact lens(es) and prosthetic lenses in frames for near vision to be worn at the same time as the contact lens(es), and prosthetic lenses in frames to be worn when the contacts have been removed.

   Lenses which have ultraviolet absorbing or reflecting properties may be covered, in lieu of payment for regular (untinted) lenses, if it has been determined that such lenses are medically reasonable and necessary for the individual patient.

   Medicare does not cover cataract sunglasses obtained in addition to the regular (untinted) prosthetic lenses since the sunglasses duplicate the restoration of vision function performed by the regular prosthetic lenses.

2. Payment for Intraocular Lenses (IOLs) Furnished in Ambulatory Surgical Centers (ASCs)

   Effective for services furnished on or after March 12, 1990, payment for intraocular lenses (IOLs) inserted during or subsequent to cataract surgery in a Medicare certified ASC is included with the payment for facility services that are furnished in connection with the covered surgery.

   Refer to the **Medicare Claims Processing Manual**, Chapter 14, "Ambulatory Surgical Centers," for more information.

3. Limitation on Coverage of Conventional Lenses

   One pair of conventional eyeglasses or conventional contact lenses furnished after each cataract surgery with insertion of an IOL is covered.

C. Dentures

Dentures are excluded from coverage. However, when a denture or a portion of the denture is an integral part (built-in) of a covered prosthesis (e.g., an obturator to fill an opening in the palate), it is covered as part of that prosthesis.

D. Supplies, Repairs, Adjustments, and Replacement

Supplies are covered that are necessary for the effective use of a prosthetic device (e.g., the batteries needed to operate an artificial larynx). Adjustment of prosthetic devices required by wear or by a change in the patient's condition is covered when ordered by a physician. General provisions relating to the repair and replacement of durable medical equipment in 32H§110.2 for the repair and replacement of prosthetic devices are applicable. (See the **Medicare Benefit Policy Manual**, Chapter 16, "General Exclusions from Coverage," §40.4, for payment for devices replaced under a warranty.) Replacement of conventional eyeglasses or contact lenses furnished in accordance with §120.B.3 is not covered.

Necessary supplies, adjustments, repairs, and replacements are covered even when the device had been in use before the user enrolled in Part B of the program, so long as the device continues to be medically required.

Pub 100-2, 15, 130 – Leg, Arm, Back, and Neck Braces, Trusses, and Artificial Legs, Arms, and Eyes

(Rev. 1, 10-01-03)

B3-2133, A3-3110.5, HO-228.5, AB-01-06 dated 1/18/01

These appliances are covered under Part B when furnished incident to physicians' services or on a physician's order. A brace includes rigid and semi-rigid devices which are used for the purpose of supporting a weak or deformed body member or restricting or eliminating motion in a diseased or injured part of the body. Elastic stockings, garter belts, and similar devices do not come within the scope of the definition of a brace. Back braces include, but are not limited to, special corsets, e.g., sacroiliac, sacrolumbar, dorsolumbar corsets, and belts. A terminal device (e.g., hand or hook) is covered under this provision whether an artificial limb is required by the patient. Stump stockings and harnesses (including replacements) are also covered when these appliances are essential to the effective use of the artificial limb.

Adjustments to an artificial limb or other appliance required by wear or by a change in the patient's condition are covered when ordered by a physician.

Adjustments, repairs and replacements are covered even when the item had been in use before the user enrolled in Part B of the program so long as the device continues to be medically required.

Pub 100-2, 15, 140 – Therapeutic Shoes for Individuals with Diabetes

(Rev. 1, 10-01-03)

B3-2134

Coverage of therapeutic shoes (depth or custom-molded) along with inserts for individuals with diabetes is available as of May 1, 1993. These diabetic shoes are covered if the requirements as specified in this section concerning certification and prescription are fulfilled. In addition, this benefit provides for a pair of diabetic shoes even if only one foot suffers from diabetic foot disease. Each shoe is equally equipped so that the affected limb, as well as the remaining limb, is protected. Claims for therapeutic shoes for diabetics are processed by the Durable Medical Equipment Regional Carriers (DMERCs).

Therapeutic shoes for diabetics are not DME and are not considered DME nor orthotics, but a separate category of coverage under Medicare Part B. (See 323H§1861(s)(12) and 324H§1833(o) of the Act.)

A. Definitions

The following items may be covered under the diabetic shoe benefit:

1. Custom-Molded Shoes

   Custom-molded shoes are shoes that:

   - Are constructed over a positive model of the patient's foot;
   - Are made from leather or other suitable material of equal quality;
   - Have removable inserts that can be altered or replaced as the patient's condition warrants; and
   - Have some form of shoe closure.

2. Depth Shoes

   Depth shoes are shoes that:

   - Have a full length, heel-to-toe filler that, when removed, provides a minimum of 3/16 inch of additional depth used to accommodate custom-molded or customized inserts;
   - Are made from leather or other suitable material of equal quality;
   - Have some form of shoe closure; and
   - Are available in full and half sizes with a minimum of three widths so that the sole is graded to the size and width of the upper portions of the shoes according to the American standard last sizing schedule or its equivalent. (The American standard last sizing schedule is the numerical shoe sizing system used for shoes sold in the United States.)

3. Inserts

Inserts are total contact, multiple density, removable inlays that are directly molded to the patient's foot or a model of the patient's foot and that are made of a suitable material with regard to the patient's condition.

B. Coverage

1. Limitations

   For each individual, coverage of the footwear and inserts is limited to one of the following within one calendar year:

   - No more than one pair of custom-molded shoes (including inserts provided with such shoes) and two additional pairs of inserts; or
   - No more than one pair of depth shoes and three pairs of inserts (not including the noncustomized removable inserts provided with such shoes).

2. Coverage of Diabetic Shoes and Brace

   Orthopedic shoes, as stated in the Medicare Claims Processing Manual, Chapter 20, "Durable Medical Equipment, Surgical Dressings and Casts, Orthotics and Artificial Limbs, and Prosthetic Devices," generally are not covered. This exclusion does not apply to orthopedic shoes that are an integral part of a leg brace. In situations in which an individual qualifies for both diabetic shoes and a leg brace, these items are covered separately. Thus, the diabetic shoes may be covered if the requirements for this section are met, while the brace may be covered if the requirements of 325H§130 are met.

3. Substitution of Modifications for Inserts

   An individual may substitute modification(s) of custom-molded or depth shoes instead of obtaining a pair(s) of inserts in any combination. Payment for the modification(s) may not exceed the limit set for the inserts for which the individual is entitled. The following is a list of the most common shoe modifications available, but it is not meant as an exhaustive list of the modifications available for diabetic shoes:

   - Rigid Rocker Bottoms – These are exterior elevations with apex positions for 51 percent to 75 percent distance measured from the back end of the heel. The apex is a narrowed or pointed end of an anatomical structure. The apex must be positioned behind the metatarsal heads and tapered off sharply to the front tip of the sole. Apex height helps to eliminate pressure at the metatarsal heads. Rigidity is ensured by the steel in the shoe. The heel of the shoe tapers off in the back in order to cause the heel to strike in the middle of the heel;
   - Roller Bottoms (Sole or Bar) – These are the same as rocker bottoms, but the heel is tapered from the apex to the front tip of the sole;
   - Metatarsal Bars – An exterior bar is placed behind the metatarsal heads in order to remove pressure from the metatarsal heads. The bars are of various shapes, heights, and construction depending on the exact purpose;
   - Wedges (Posting) – Wedges are either of hind foot, fore foot, or both and may be in the middle or to the side. The function is to shift or transfer weight bearing upon standing or during ambulation to the opposite side for added support, stabilization, equalized weight distribution, or balance; and
   - Offset Heels – This is a heel flanged at its base either in the middle, to the side, or a combination, that is then extended upward to the shoe in order to stabilize extreme positions of the hind foot.

   Other modifications to diabetic shoes include, but are not limited to flared heels, Velcro closures, and inserts for missing toes.

4. Separate Inserts

   Inserts may be covered and dispensed independently of diabetic shoes if the supplier of the shoes verifies in writing that the patient has appropriate footwear into which the insert can be placed. This footwear must meet the definitions found above for depth shoes and custom-molded shoes.

C. Certification

The need for diabetic shoes must be certified by a physician who is a doctor of medicine or a doctor of osteopathy and who is responsible for diagnosing and treating the patient's diabetic systemic condition through a comprehensive plan of care. This managing physician must:

- Document in the patient's medical record that the patient has diabetes;
- Certify that the patient is being treated under a comprehensive plan of care for diabetes, and that the patient needs diabetic shoes; and
- Document in the patient's record that the patient has one or more of the following conditions:
  - Peripheral neuropathy with evidence of callus formation;
  - History of pre-ulcerative calluses;
  - History of previous ulceration;
  - Foot deformity;
  - Previous amputation of the foot or part of the foot; or
  - Poor circulation.

D. Prescription

Following certification by the physician managing the patient's systemic diabetic condition, a podiatrist or other qualified physician who is knowledgeable in the fitting of diabetic shoes and inserts may prescribe the particular type of footwear necessary.

E. Furnishing Footwear

The footwear must be fitted and furnished by a podiatrist or other qualified individual such as a pedorthist, an orthotist, or a prosthetist. The certifying physician may not furnish the diabetic shoes unless the certifying physician is the only qualified individual in the area. It is left to the discretion of each carrier to determine the meaning of "in the area."

Pub 100-2, 15, 150 – Dental Services

(Rev. 1, 10-01-03)

B3-2136

As indicated under the general exclusions from coverage, items and services in connection with the care, treatment, filling, removal, or replacement of teeth or structures directly supporting the teeth are not covered. "Structures directly supporting the teeth" means the periodontium, which includes the gingivae, dentogingival junction, periodontal membrane, cementum of the teeth, and alveolar process.

In addition to the following, see Pub 100-01, the Medicare General Information, Eligibility, and Entitlement Manual, Chapter 5, Definitions and Pub 3, the **Medicare National Coverage Determinations Manual** for specific services which may be covered when furnished by a dentist. If an otherwise noncovered procedure or service is performed by a dentist as incident to and as an integral part of a covered procedure or service performed by the dentist, the total service performed by the dentist on such an occasion is covered.

EXAMPLE 1:

The reconstruction of a ridge performed primarily to prepare the mouth for dentures is a noncovered procedure. However, when the reconstruction of a ridge is performed as a result of and at the same time as the surgical removal of a tumor (for other than dental purposes), the totality of surgical procedures is a covered service.

EXAMPLE 2:

Medicare makes payment for the wiring of teeth when this is done in connection with the reduction of a jaw fracture.

The extraction of teeth to prepare the jaw for radiation treatment of neoplastic disease is also covered. This is an exception to the requirement that to be covered, a noncovered procedure or service performed by a dentist must be an incident to and an integral part of a covered procedure or service performed by the dentist. Ordinarily, the dentist extracts the patient's teeth, but another physician, e.g., a radiologist, administers the radiation treatments.

When an excluded service is the primary procedure involved, it is not covered, regardless of its complexity or difficulty. For example, the extraction of an impacted tooth is not covered. Similarly, an alveoplasty (the surgical improvement of the shape and condition of the alveolar process) and a frenectomy are excluded from coverage when either of these procedures is performed in connection with an excluded service, e.g., the preparation of the mouth for dentures. In a like manner, the removal of a torus palatinus (a bony protuberance of the hard palate) may be a covered service. However, with rare exception, this surgery is performed in connection with an excluded service, i.e., the preparation of the mouth for dentures. Under such circumstances, Medicare does not pay for this procedure.

Dental splints used to treat a dental condition are excluded from coverage under 326H1862(a)(12) of the Act. On the other hand, if the treatment is determined to be a covered medical condition (i.e., dislocated upper/lower jaw joints), then the splint can be covered. Whether such services as the administration of anesthesia, diagnostic x-rays, and other related procedures are covered depends upon whether the primary procedure being performed by the dentist is itself covered. Thus, an x-ray taken in connection with the reduction of a fracture of the jaw or facial bone is covered. However, a single x-ray or xray survey taken in connection with the care or treatment of teeth or the periodontium is not covered.

Medicare makes payment for a covered dental procedure no matter where the service is performed. The hospitalization or nonhospitalization of a patient has no direct bearing on the coverage or exclusion of a given dental procedure.

Payment may also be made for services and supplies furnished incident to covered dental services. For example, the services of a dental technician or nurse who is under the direct supervision of the dentist or physician are covered if the services are included in the dentist's or physician's bill.

Pub 100-2, 15, 230 – Practice of Physical Therapy, Occupational Therapy, and Speech-Language Pathology

(Rev. 63, Issued: 12-29-06, Effective: 01-01-07, Implementation: on or before 01-29-07)

A. Group Therapy Services

Contractors pay for outpatient physical therapy services (which includes outpatient speech-language pathology services) and outpatient occupational therapy services provided simultaneously to two or more individuals by a practitioner as group therapy services (97150). The individuals can be, but need not be performing the same activity. The physician or therapist involved in group therapy services must be in constant attendance, but one-on-one patient contact is not required.

B. Therapy Students

1. General

   Only the services of the therapist can be billed and paid under Medicare Part B. The services performed by a student are not reimbursed even if provided under "line of sight" supervision of the therapist; however, the presence of the student "in the room" does not make the service unbillable. Pay for the direct (one-to-one) patient contact services of the physician or therapist provided to Medicare Part B patients. Group therapy services performed by a therapist or physician may be billed when a student is also present "in the room".

   EXAMPLES:

   Therapists may bill and be paid for the provision of services in the following scenarios:

   - The qualified practitioner is present and in the room for the entire session. The student participates in the delivery of services when the qualified practitioner is directing the service, making the skilled judgment, and is responsible for the assessment and treatment.
   - The qualified practitioner is present in the room guiding the student in service delivery when the therapy student and the therapy assistant student are participating in the provision of services, and the practitioner is not engaged in treating another patient or doing other tasks at the same time.
   - The qualified practitioner is responsible for the services and as such, signs all documentation. (A student may, of course, also sign but it is not necessary since the Part B payment is for the clinician's service, not for the student's services).

2. Therapy Assistants as Clinical Instructors

   Physical therapist assistants and occupational therapy assistants are not precluded from serving as clinical instructors for therapy students, while providing services within their scope of work and performed under the direction and supervision of a licensed physical or occupational therapist to a Medicare beneficiary.

3. Services Provided Under Part A and Part B

   The payment methodologies for Part A and B therapy services rendered by a student are different. Under the MPFS (Medicare Part B), Medicare pays for services provided by physicians and practitioners that are specifically authorized by statute. Students do not meet the definition of practitioners under Medicare Part B. Under SNF PPS, payments are based upon the case mix or Resource Utilization Group (RUG) category that describes the patient. In the rehabilitation groups, the number of therapy minutes delivered to the patient determines the RUG category. Payment levels for each category are based upon the costs of caring for patients in each group rather than providing specific payment for each therapy service as is done in Medicare Part B.

Pub 100-2, 15, 230.1 – Practice of Physical Therapy

(Rev. 88, Issued: 05-07-08, Effective: 01-01-08, Implementation: 06-09-08)

A. General

Physical therapy services are those services provided within the scope of practice of physical therapists and necessary for the diagnosis and treatment of impairments, functional limitations, disabilities or changes in physical function and health status. (See Pub. 100-03, the Medicare National Coverage Determinations Manual, for specific conditions or services.) For descriptions of aquatic therapy in a community center pool see section 220C of this chapter.

B. Qualified Physical Therapist Defined

Reference: 42CFR484.4

The new personnel qualifications for physical therapists were discussed in the 2008 Physician Fee Schedule. See the Federal Register of November 27, 2007, for the full text. See also the correction notice for this rule, published in the Federal Register on January 15, 2008.

The regulation provides that a qualified physical therapist (PT) is a person who is licensed, if applicable, as a PT by the state in which he or she is practicing unless licensure does not apply, has graduated from an accredited PT education program and passed a national examination approved by the state in which PT services are provided. The phrase, "by the state in which practicing" includes any authorization to practice provided by the same state in which the service is provided, including temporary licensure, regardless of the location of the entity billing the services. The curriculum accreditation is provided by the Commission on Accreditation in Physical Therapy Education (CAPTE) or, for those who graduated before CAPTE, curriculum approval was provided by the American Physical Therapy Association (APTA). For internationally educated PTs, curricula are approved by a credentials evaluation organization either approved by the APTA or identified in 8 CFR 212.15(e) as it relates to PTs. For example, in 2007, 8 CFR 212.15(e) approved the credentials evaluation provided by the Federation of State Boards of Physical Therapy (FSBPT) and the Foreign Credentialing Commission on Physical Therapy (FCCPT). The requirements above apply to all PTs effective January 1, 2010, if they have not met any of the following requirements prior to January 1, 2010.

Physical therapists whose current license was obtained on or prior to December 31, 2009, qualify to provide PT services to Medicare beneficiaries if they:

- graduated from a CAPTE approved program in PT on or before December 31, 2009 (examination is not required), or
- graduated on or before December 31, 2009, from a PT program outside the U.S. that is determined to be substantially equivalent to a U.S. program by a credentials evaluating organization approved by either the APTA or identified in 8 CFR 212.15(e) and also passed an examination for PTs approved by the state in which practicing

  Or, PTs whose current license was obtained before January 1, 2008, may meet the requirements in place on that date (i.e., graduation from a curriculum approved by either the APTA, the Committee on Allied Health Education and Accreditation of the American Medical Association, or both).

  Or, PTs meet the requirements who are currently licensed and were licensed or qualified as a PT on or before December 31, 1977, and had 2 years appropriate experience as a PT, and passed a proficiency examination conducted, approved, or sponsored by the U.S. Public Health Service.

  Or, PTs meet the requirements if they are currently licensed and before January 1, 1966, they were:

  - admitted to membership by the APTA; or
  - admitted to registration by the American Registry of Physical Therapists; or
  - graduated from a 4-year PT curriculum approved by a State Department of Education; or
  - licensed or registered and prior to January 1, 1970, they had 15 years of full-time experience in PT under the order and direction of attending and referring doctors of medicine or osteopathy.

Or, PTs meet requirements if they are currently licensed and they were trained outside the U.S. before January 1, 2008, and after 1928 graduated from a PT curriculum approved in the country in which the curriculum was located, if that country had an organization that was a member of the World Confederation for Physical Therapy, and that PT qualified as a member of the organization.

For outpatient PT services that are provided incident to the services of physicians/NPPs, the requirement for PT licensure does not apply; all other personnel qualifications do apply. The qualified personnel providing PT services incident to the services of a physician/NPP must be trained in an accredited PT curriculum. For example, a person who, on or before December 31, 2009, graduated from a PT curriculum accredited by CAPTE, but who has not passed the national examination or obtained a license, could provide Medicare outpatient PT therapy services incident to the services of a physician/NPP if the physician assumes responsibility for the services according to the incident to policies. On or after January 1, 2010, although licensure does not apply, both education and examination requirements that are effective January 1, 2010, apply to qualified personnel who provide PT services incident to the services of a physician/NPP.

C. Services of Physical Therapy Support Personnel

Reference: 42CFR 484.4

Personnel Qualifications. The new personnel qualifications for physical therapist assistants (PTA) were discussed in the 2008 Physician Fee Schedule. See the Federal Register of November 27, 2007, for the full text. See also the correction notice for this rule, published in the Federal Register on January 15, 2008.

The regulation provides that a qualified PTA is a person who is licensed as a PTA unless licensure does not apply, is registered or certified, if applicable, as a PTA by the state in which practicing, and graduated from an approved curriculum for PTAs, and passed a national examination for PTAs. The phrase, "by the state in which practicing" includes any authorization to practice provided by the same state in which the service is provided, including temporary licensure, regardless of the location or the entity billing for the services. Approval for the curriculum is provided by CAPTE or, if internationally or military trained PTAs apply, approval will be through a credentialing body for the curriculum for PTAs identified by either the American Physical Therapy Association or identified in 8 CFR 212.15(e). A national examination for PTAs is, for example the one furnished by the Federation of State Boards of Physical Therapy. These requirements above apply to all PTAs effective January 1, 2010, if they have not met any of the following requirements prior to January 1, 2010.

Those PTAs also qualify who, on or before December 31, 2009, are licensed, registered or certified as a PTA and met one of the two following requirements:

1. Is licensed or otherwise regulated in the state in which practicing; or
2. In states that have no licensure or other regulations, or where licensure does not apply, PTAs have:
   - graduated on or before December 31, 2009, from a 2-year college-level program approved by the APTA or CAPTE; and
   - effective January 1, 2010, those PTAs must have both graduated from a CAPTE approved curriculum and passed a national examination for PTAs; or

   PTAs may also qualify if they are licensed, registered or certified as a PTA, if applicable and meet requirements in effect before January 1, 2008, that is:

   - they have graduated before January 1, 2008, from a 2 year college level program approved by the APTA; or

- on or before December 31, 1977, they were licensed or qualified as a PTA and passed a proficiency examination conducted, approved, or sponsored by the **U.S. Public Health Service**.

Services. The services of PTAs used when providing covered therapy benefits are included as part of the covered service. These services are billed by the supervising physical therapist. PTAs may not provide evaluation services, make clinical judgments or decisions or take responsibility for the service. They act at the direction and under the supervision of the treating physical therapist and in accordance with state laws.

A physical therapist must supervise PTAs. The level and frequency of supervision differs by setting (and by state or local law). General supervision is required for PTAs in all settings except private practice (which requires direct supervision) unless state practice requirements are more stringent, in which case state or local requirements must be followed. See specific settings for details. For example, in clinics, rehabilitation agencies, and public health agencies, 42CFR485.713 indicates that when a PTA provides services, either on or off the organization's premises, those services are supervised by a qualified physical therapist who makes an onsite supervisory visit at least once every 30 days or more frequently if required by state or local laws or regulation.

The services of a PTA shall not be billed as services incident to a physician/NPP's service, because they do not meet the qualifications of a therapist.

The cost of supplies (e.g., theraband, hand putty, electrodes) used in furnishing covered therapy care is included in the payment for the HCPCS codes billed by the physical therapist, and are, therefore, not separately billable. Separate coverage and billing provisions apply to items that meet the definition of brace in §130.

Services provided by aides, even if under the supervision of a therapist, are not therapy services and are not covered by Medicare. Although an aide may help the therapist by providing unskilled services, those services that are unskilled are not covered by Medicare and shall be denied as not reasonable and necessary if they are billed as therapy services.

D. Application of Medicare Guidelines to PT Services

This subsection will be used in the future to illustrate the application of the above guidelines to some of the physical therapy modalities and procedures utilized in the treatment of patients.

Pub 100-2, 15, 230.2 – Practice of Occupational Therapy

(Rev. 88, Issued: 05-07-08, Effective: 01-01-08, Implementation: 06-09-08)

A. General

Occupational therapy services are those services provided within the scope of practice of occupational therapists and necessary for the diagnosis and treatment of impairments, functional disabilities or changes in physical function and health status. (See Pub. 10003, the Medicare National Coverage Determinations Manual, for specific conditions or services.)

Occupational therapy is medically prescribed treatment concerned with improving or restoring functions which have been impaired by illness or injury or, where function has been permanently lost or reduced by illness or injury, to improve the individual's ability to perform those tasks required for independent functioning. Such therapy may involve:

- The evaluation, and reevaluation as required, of a patient's level of function by administering diagnostic and prognostic tests;
- The selection and teaching of task-oriented therapeutic activities designed to restore physical function; e.g., use of woodworking activities on an inclined table to restore shoulder, elbow, and wrist range of motion lost as a result of burns;
- The planning, implementing, and supervising of individualized therapeutic activity programs as part of an overall "active treatment" program for a patient with a diagnosed psychiatric illness; e.g., the use of sewing activities which require following a pattern to reduce confusion and restore reality orientation in a schizophrenic patient;
- The planning and implementing of therapeutic tasks and activities to restore sensory-integrative function; e.g., providing motor and tactile activities to increase sensory input and improve response for a stroke patient with functional loss resulting in a distorted body image;
- The teaching of compensatory technique to improve the level of independence in the activities of daily living, for example:
  - Teaching a patient who has lost the use of an arm how to pare potatoes and chop vegetables with one hand;
  - Teaching an upper extremity amputee how to functionally utilize a prosthesis;
  - Teaching a stroke patient new techniques to enable the patient to perform feeding, dressing, and other activities as independently as possible; or
  - Teaching a patient with a hip fracture/hip replacement techniques of standing tolerance and balance to enable the patient to perform such functional activities as dressing and homemaking tasks.

The designing, fabricating, and fitting of orthotics and self-help devices; e.g., making a hand splint for a patient with rheumatoid arthritis to maintain the hand in a functional position or constructing a device which would enable an individual to hold a utensil and feed independently; or Vocational and prevocational assessment and training, subject to the limitations specified in item B below.

Only a qualified occupational therapist has the knowledge, training, and experience required to evaluate and, as necessary, reevaluate a patient's level of function, determine whether an occupational therapy program could reasonably be expected to improve, restore, or compensate for lost function and, where appropriate, recommend to the physician/NPP a plan of treatment.

B. Qualified Occupational Therapist Defined

Reference: 42CFR484.4

The new personnel qualifications for occupational therapists (OT) were discussed in the 2008 Physician Fee Schedule. See the Federal Register of November 27, 2007, for the full text. See also the correction notice for this rule, published in the Federal Register on January 15, 2008.

The regulation provides that a qualified OT is an individual who is licensed, if licensure applies, or otherwise regulated, if applicable, as an OT by the state in which practicing, and graduated from an accredited education program for OTs, and is eligible to take or has passed the examination for OTs administered by the National Board for Certification in Occupational Therapy, Inc. (NBCOT). The phrase, "by the state in which practicing" includes any authorization to practice provided by the same state in which the service is provided, including temporary licensure, regardless of the location of the entity billing the services. The education program for U.S. trained OTs is accredited by the Accreditation Council for Occupational Therapy Education (ACOTE). The requirements above apply to all OTs effective January 1, 2010, if they have not met any of the following requirements prior to January 1, 2010.

The OTs may also qualify if on or before December 31, 2009:

- they are licensed or otherwise regulated as an OT in the state in which practicing (regardless of the qualifications they met to obtain that licensure or regulation); or
- when licensure or other regulation does not apply, OTs have graduated from an OT education program accredited by ACOTE and are eligible to take, or have successfully completed the NBCOT examination for OTs.

Also, those OTs who met the Medicare requirements for OTs that were in 42CFR484.4 prior to January 1, 2008, qualify to provide OT services for Medicare beneficiaries if:

- on or before January 1, 2008, they graduated an OT program approved jointly by the American Medical Association and the AOTA, or
- they are eligible for the National Registration Examination of AOTA or the National Board for Certification in OT

Also, they qualify who on or before December 31, 1977, had 2 years of appropriate experience as an occupational therapist, and had achieved a satisfactory grade on a proficiency examination conducted, approved, or sponsored by the U.S. Public Health Service.

Those educated outside the U.S. may meet the same qualifications for domestic trained OTs. For example, they qualify if they were licensed or otherwise regulated by the state in which practicing on or before December 31, 2009. Or they are qualified if they:

- graduated from an OT education program accredited as substantially equivalent to a U.S. OT education program by ACOTE, the World

Federation of Occupational Therapists, or a credentialing body approved by AOTA
- passed the NBCOT examination for OT
- Effective January 1, 2010, are licensed or otherwise regulated, if applicable as an OT by the state in which practicing

For outpatient OT services that are provided incident to the services of physicians/NPPs, the requirement for OT licensure does not apply; all other personnel qualifications do apply. The qualified personnel providing OT services incident to the services of a physician/NPP must be trained in an accredited OT curriculum. For example, a person who, on or before December 31, 2009, graduated from an OT curriculum accredited by ACOTE and is eligible to take or has successfully completed the entry-level certification examination for OTs developed and administered by NBCOT, could provide Medicare outpatient OT services incident to the services of a physician/NPP if the physician assumes responsibility for the services according to the incident to policies. On or after January 1, 2010, although licensure does not apply, both education and examination requirements that are effective January 1, 2010, apply to qualified personnel who provide OT services incident to the services of a physician/NPP.

C. Services of Occupational Therapy Support Personnel

Reference: 42CFR 484.4

The new personnel qualifications for occupational therapy assistants were discussed in the 2008 Physician Fee Schedule. See the Federal Register of November 27, 2007, for the full text. See also the correction notice for this rule, published in the Federal Register on January 15, 2008.

The regulation provides that an occupational therapy assistant is a person who is licensed, unless licensure does not apply, or otherwise regulated, if applicable, as an OTA by the state in which practicing, and graduated from an OTA education program accredited by ACOTE and is eligible to take or has successfully completed the NBCOT examination for OTAs. The phrase, "by the state in which practicing" includes any authorization to practice provided by the same state in which the service is provided, including temporary licensure, regardless of the location of the entity billing the services.

If the requirements above are not met, an OTA may qualify if, on or before December 31, 2009, the OTA is licensed or otherwise regulated as an OTA, if applicable, by the state in which practicing, or meets any qualifications defined by the state in which practicing.

Or, where licensure or other state regulation does not apply, OTAs may qualify if they have, on or before December 31, 2009:

- completed certification requirements to practice as an OTA established by a credentialing organization approved by AOTA; and
- after January 1, 2010, they have also completed an education program accredited by ACOTE and passed the NBCOT examination for OTAs.

OTAs who qualified under the policies in effect prior to January 1, 2008, continue to qualify to provide OT directed and supervised OTA services to Medicare beneficiaries.

Therefore, OTAs qualify who after December 31, 1977, and on or before December 31, 2007:

- completed certification requirements to practice as an OTA established by a credentialing organization approved by AOTA; or
- completed the requirements to practice as an OTA applicable in the state in which practicing.

Those OTAs who were educated outside the U.S. may meet the same requirements as domestically trained OTAs. Or, if educated outside the U.S. on or after January 1, 2008, they must have graduated from an OTA program accredited as substantially equivalent to OTA entry level education in the U.S. by ACOTE, its successor organization, or the World Federation of Occupational Therapists or a credentialing body approved by AOTA. In addition, they must have passed an exam for OTAs administered by NBCOT.

Services. The services of OTAs used when providing covered therapy benefits are included as part of the covered service. These services are billed by the supervising occupational therapist. OTAs may not provide evaluation services, make clinical judgments or decisions or take responsibility for the service. They act at the direction and under the supervision of the treating occupational therapist and in accordance with state laws.

An occupational therapist must supervise OTAs. The level and frequency of supervision differs by setting (and by state or local law). General supervision is required for OTAs in all settings except private practice (which requires direct supervision) unless state practice requirements are more stringent, in which case state or local requirements must be followed. See specific settings for details. For example, in clinics, rehabilitation agencies, and public health agencies, 42CFR485.713 indicates that when an OTA provides services, either on or off the organization's premises, those services are supervised by a qualified occupational therapist who makes an onsite supervisory visit at least once every 30 days or more frequently if required by state or local laws or regulation.

The services of an OTA shall not be billed as services incident to a physician/NPP's service, because they do not meet the qualifications of a therapist.

The cost of supplies (e.g., looms, ceramic tiles, or leather) used in furnishing covered therapy care is included in the payment for the HCPCS codes billed by the occupational therapist and are, therefore, not separately billable. Separate coverage and billing provisions apply to items that meet the definition of brace in §130 of this manual.

Services provided by aides, even if under the supervision of a therapist, are not therapy services in the outpatient setting and are not covered by Medicare. Although an aide may help the therapist by providing unskilled services, those services that are unskilled are not covered by Medicare and shall be denied as not reasonable and necessary if they are billed as therapy services.

D. Application of Medicare Guidelines to Occupational Therapy Services

Occupational therapy may be required for a patient with a specific diagnosed psychiatric illness. If such services are required, they are covered assuming the coverage criteria are met. However, where an individual's motivational needs are not related to a specific diagnosed psychiatric illness, the meeting of such needs does not usually require an individualized therapeutic program. Such needs can be met through general activity programs or the efforts of other professional personnel involved in the care of the patient. Patient motivation is an appropriate and inherent function of all health disciplines, which is interwoven with other functions performed by such personnel for the patient. Accordingly, since the special skills of an occupational therapist are not required, an occupational therapy program for individuals who do not have a specific diagnosed psychiatric illness is not to be considered reasonable and necessary for the treatment of an illness or injury. Services furnished under such a program are not covered.

Occupational therapy may include vocational and prevocational assessment and training. When services provided by an occupational therapist are related solely to specific employment opportunities, work skills, or work settings, they are not reasonable or necessary for the diagnosis or treatment of an illness or injury and are not covered. However, carriers and intermediaries exercise care in applying this exclusion, because the assessment of level of function and the teaching of compensatory techniques to improve the level of function, especially in activities of daily living, are services which occupational therapists provide for both vocational and nonvocational purposes. For example, an assessment of sitting and standing tolerance might be nonvocational for a mother of young children or a retired individual living alone, but could also be a vocational test for a sales clerk. Training an amputee in the use of prosthesis for telephoning is necessary for everyday activities as well as for employment purposes. Major changes in life style may be mandatory for an individual with a substantial disability. The techniques of adjustment cannot be considered exclusively vocational or nonvocational.

Pub 100-2, 15, 230.3 – Practice of Speech-Language Pathology

(Rev. 106, Issued: 04-24-09, Effective: 07-01-09, Implementation: 07-06-09)

A. General

Speech-language pathology services are those services provided within the scope of practice of speech-language pathologists and necessary for the diagnosis and treatment of speech and language disorders, which result in communication disabilities and for the diagnosis and treatment of swallowing disorders (dysphagia), regardless of the presence of a communication disability. (See Pub. 100-03, chapter 1, §170.3) See section 230.4 of this chapter for benefit policies on speech-language pathologists in private practice (SLPP). See Pub. 100-08, Medicare Program Integrity Manual, chapter 10, section 12.4.14 for policy on enrollment in an SLPP.

B. Qualified Speech-Language Pathologist Defined

A qualified speech-language pathologist for program coverage purposes meets one of the following requirements:

- The education and experience requirements for a Certificate of Clinical Competence in (speech-language pathology) granted by the American Speech-Language Hearing Association; or
- Meets the educational requirements for certification and is in the process of accumulating the supervised experience required for certification.

For outpatient speech-language pathology services that are provided incident to the services of physicians/NPPs, the requirement for speech-language pathology licensure does not apply; all other personnel qualifications do apply. Therefore, qualified personnel providing speech-language pathology services incident to the services of a physician/NPP must meet the above qualifications.

C. Services of Speech-Language Pathology Support Personnel

Services of speech-language pathology assistants are not recognized for Medicare coverage. Services provided by speech-language pathology assistants, even if they are licensed to provide services in their states, will be considered unskilled services and denied as not reasonable and necessary if they are billed as therapy services.

Services provided by aides, even if under the supervision of a therapist, are not therapy services and are not covered by Medicare. Although an aide may help the therapist by providing unskilled services, those services are not covered by Medicare and shall be denied as not reasonable and necessary if they are billed as therapy services.

D. Application of Medicare Guidelines to Speech-Language Pathology Services

1. Evaluation Services

Speech-language pathology evaluation services are covered if they are reasonable and necessary and not excluded as routine screening by §1862(a)(7) of the Act. The speech-language pathologist employs a variety of formal and informal speech, language, and dysphagia assessment tests to ascertain the type, causal factor(s), and severity of the speech and language or swallowing disorders. Reevaluation of patients for whom speech, language and swallowing were previously contraindicated is covered only if the patient exhibits a change in medical condition. However, monthly reevaluations; e.g., a Western Aphasia Battery, for a patient undergoing a rehabilitative speech-language pathology program, are considered a part of the treatment session and shall not be covered as a separate evaluation for billing purposes. Although hearing screening by the speech-language pathologist may be part of an evaluation, it is not billable as a separate service.

2. Therapeutic Services

The following are examples of common medical disorders and resulting communication deficits, which may necessitate active rehabilitative therapy. This list is not all-inclusive:

- Cerebrovascular disease such as cerebral vascular accidents presenting with dysphagia, aphasia/dysphasia, apraxia, and dysarthria
- Neurological disease such as Parkinsonism or Multiple Sclerosis with dysarthria, dysphagia, inadequate respiratory volume/control, or voice disorder
- Laryngeal carcinoma requiring laryngectomy resulting in aphonia

3. Impairments of the Auditory System

The terms, aural rehabilitation, auditory rehabilitation, auditory processing, lipreading and speech reading are among the terms used to describe covered services related to perception and comprehension of sound through the auditory system. See Pub. 100-04, chapter 12, section 30.3 for billing instructions. For example:

- Auditory processing evaluation and treatment may be covered and medically necessary. Examples include but are not limited to services for certain neurological impairments or the absence of natural auditory stimulation that results in impaired ability to process sound. Certain auditory processing disorders require diagnostic audiological tests in addition to speech-language pathology evaluation and treatment.
- Evaluation and treatment for disorders of the auditory system may be covered and medically necessary, for example, when it has been determined by a speech-language pathologist in collaboration with an audiologist that the hearing impaired beneficiary's current amplification options (hearing aid, other amplification device or cochlear implant) will not sufficiently meet the patient's functional communication needs. Audiologists and speech-language pathologists both evaluate beneficiaries for disorders of the auditory system using different skills and techniques, but only speech-language pathologists may provide treatment.

Assessment for the need for rehabilitation of the auditory system (but not the vestibular system) may be done by a speech language pathologist. Examples include but are not limited to: evaluation of comprehension and production of language in oral, signed or written modalities, speech and voice production, listening skills, speech reading, communications strategies, and the impact of the hearing loss on the patient/client and family.

Examples of rehabilitation include but are not limited to treatment that focuses on comprehension, and production of language in oral, signed or written modalities; speech and voice production, auditory training, speech reading, multimodal (e.g., visual, auditory-visual, and tactile) training, communication strategies, education and counseling. In determining the necessity for treatment, the beneficiary's performance in both clinical and natural environment should be considered.

4. Dysphagia

Dysphagia, or difficulty in swallowing, can cause food to enter the airway, resulting in coughing, choking, pulmonary problems, aspiration or inadequate nutrition and hydration with resultant weight loss, failure to thrive, pneumonia and death. It is most often due to complex neurological and/or structural impairments including head and neck trauma, cerebrovascular accident, neuromuscular degenerative diseases, head and neck cancer, dementias, and encephalopathies. For these reasons, it is important that only qualified professionals with specific training and experience in this disorder provide evaluation and treatment.

The speech-language pathologist performs clinical and instrumental assessments and analyzes and integrates the diagnostic information to determine candidacy for intervention as well as appropriate compensations and rehabilitative therapy techniques. The equipment that is used in the examination may be fixed, mobile or portable. Professional guidelines recommend that the service be provided in a team setting with a physician/NPP who provides supervision of the radiological examination and interpretation of medical conditions revealed in it.

Swallowing assessment and rehabilitation are highly specialized services. The professional rendering care must have education, experience and demonstrated competencies. Competencies include but are not limited to: identifying abnormal upper aerodigestive tract structure and function; conducting an oral, pharyngeal, laryngeal and respiratory function examination as it relates to the functional assessment of swallowing; recommending methods of oral intake and risk precautions; and developing a treatment plan employing appropriate compensations and therapy techniques.

Pub 100-2, 15, 230.4 – Services Furnished by a Physical or Occupational Therapist in Private Practice (TPP)

(Rev. 106, Issued: 04-24-09, Effective: 07-01-09, Implementation: 07-06-09)

A. General

See section 220 of this chapter for definitions. Therapist refers only to a qualified physical therapist, occupational therapist or speech-language pathologist. TPP refers to therapists in private practice (qualified physical therapists, occupational therapists and speech-language pathologists).

In order to qualify to bill Medicare directly as a therapist, each individual must be enrolled as a private practitioner and employed in one of the following practice types: an unincorporated solo practice, unincorporated partnership, unincorporated group practice, physician/NPP group or groups that are not professional corporations, if allowed by state and local law. Physician/NPP group practices may employ TPP if state and local law permits this employee relationship.

For purposes of this provision, a physician/NPP group practice is defined as one or more physicians/NPPs enrolled with Medicare who may bill as one entity. For further details on issues concerning enrollment, see the provider enrollment Web site at www.cms.hhs.gov/MedicareProviderSupEnroll and Pub. 100-08, Medicare Program Integrity Manual, chapter10, section 12.4.14.

Private practice also includes therapists who are practicing therapy as employees of another supplier, of a professional corporation or other incorporated therapy practice. Private practice does not include individuals when they are working as employees of an institutional provider.

Services should be furnished in the therapist's or group's office or in the patient's home. The office is defined as the location(s) where the practice is operated, in the state(s) where the therapist (and practice, if applicable) is legally authorized to furnish services, during the hours that the therapist engages in the practice at that location. If services are furnished in a private practice office space, that space shall be owned, leased, or rented by the practice and used for the exclusive purpose of operating the practice. For descriptions of aquatic therapy in a community center pool see section 220C of this chapter.

Therapists in private practice must be approved as meeting certain requirements, but do not execute a formal provider agreement with the Secretary.

If therapists who have their own Medicare National Provider Identifier (NPI) are employed by therapist groups, physician/NPP groups, or groups that are not professional organizations, the requirement that therapy space be owned, leased, or rented may be satisfied by the group that employs the therapist. Each therapist employed by a group should enroll as a TPP.

When therapists with a Medicare NPI provide services in the physician's/NPP's office in which they are employed, and bill using their NPI for each therapy service, then the direct supervision requirement for enrolled staff apply.

When the therapist who has a Medicare NPI is employed in a physician's/NPP's office the services are ordinarily billed as services of the therapist, with the therapist identified on the claim as the supplier of services. However, services of the therapist who has a Medicare NPI may also be billed by the physician/NPP as services incident to the physician's/NPP's service. (See §230.5 for rules related to therapy services incident to a physician.) In that case, the physician/NPP is the supplier of service, the NPI of the supervising physician/NPP is reported on the claim with the service and all the rules for both therapy services and incident to services (§230.5) must be followed.

B. Private Practice Defined

Reference: ***Federal Register*** November, 1998, pages 58863-58869; 42CFR 410.38(b), 42CFR410.59, 42CFR410.60, 42CFR410.62

The contractor considers a therapist to be in private practice if the therapist maintains office space at his or her own expense and furnishes services only in that space or the patient's home. Or, a therapist is employed by another supplier and furnishes services in facilities provided at the expense of that supplier.

The therapist need not be in full-time private practice but must be engaged in private practice on a regular basis; i.e., the therapist is recognized as a private practitioner and for that purpose has access to the necessary equipment to provide an adequate program of therapy.

The therapy services must be provided either by or under the direct supervision of the TPP. Each TPP should be enrolled as a Medicare provider. If a therapist is not enrolled, the services of that therapist must be directly supervised by an enrolled therapist. Direct supervision requires that the supervising private practice therapist be present in the office suite at the time the service is performed. These direct supervision requirements apply only in the private practice setting and only for therapists and their assistants. In other outpatient settings, supervision rules differ. The services of support personnel must be included in the therapist's bill. The supporting personnel, including other therapists, must be W-2 or 1099 employees of the TPP or other qualified employer.

Coverage of outpatient therapy under Part B includes the services of a qualified TPP when furnished in the therapist's office or the beneficiary's home. For this purpose, "home" includes an institution that is used as a home, but not a hospital, CAH or SNF, (***Federal Register*** Nov. 2, 1998, pg 58869). Place of Service (POS) includes:

- 03/School, only if residential
- 04/Homeless Shelter
- 12/Home, other than a facility that is a private residence
- 14/Group Home
- 33/Custodial Care Facility

C. Assignment

Reference: Nov. 2, 1998 ***Federal Register***, pg. 58863 See also Pub. 100-04 chapter 1, §30.2.

When physicians, NPPs, or TPPs obtain provider numbers, they have the option of accepting assignment (participating) or not accepting assignment (nonparticipating). In contrast, providers, such as outpatient hospitals, SNFs, rehabilitation agencies, and CORFs, do not have the option. For these providers, assignment is mandatory.

If physicians/NPPs, or TPPs accept assignment (are participating), they must accept the Medicare Physician Fee Schedule amount as payment. Medicare pays 80% and the patient is responsible for 20%. In contrast, if they do not accept assignment, Medicare will only pay 95% of the fee schedule amount. However, when these services are not furnished on an assignment-related basis, the limiting charge applies. (See §1848(g)(2)(c) of the Act.)

NOTE: Services furnished by a therapist in the therapist's office under arrangements with hospitals in rural communities and public health agencies (or services provided in the beneficiary's home under arrangements with a provider of outpatient physical or occupational therapy services) are not covered under this provision. See section 230.6.

Pub 100-2, 15, 230.5 – Physical Therapy, Occupational Therapy and Speech-Language Pathology Services Provided Incident to the Services of Physicians and Non-Physician Practitioners (NPP)

(Rev. 36, Issued: 06-24-05, Effective: 06-06-05, Implementation: 06-06-05)

References: 460H§1861(s)(2)(A) of the Act

42 CFR 410.10(b)

42 CFR 410.26

Pub. 100-02, 15, §60.

The Benefit. Therapy services have their own benefit under 461H§1861 of the Social Security Act and shall be covered when provided according to the standards and conditions of the benefit described in Medicare manuals. The statute 462H1862(a)(20) requires that payment be made for a therapy service billed by a physician/NPP only if the service meets the standards and conditions--other than licensing--that would apply to a therapist. (For example, see coverage requirements in Pub. 463H100-08, chapter 13, §13.5.1(C), Pub. 464H100-04, chapter 5, and also the requirements of this manual, §465H220 and §46H230.

Incident to a Therapist. There is no coverage for services provided incident to the services of a therapist. Although PTAs and OTAs work under the supervision of a therapist and their services may be billed by the therapist, their services are covered under the benefit for therapy services and not by the benefit for services incident to a physician/NPP. The services furnished by PTAs and OTAs are not incident to the therapist's service.

Qualifications of Auxiliary Personnel. Therapy services appropriately billed incident to a physician's/NPP's service shall be subject to the same requirements as therapy services that would be furnished by a physical therapist, occupational therapist or speech-language pathologist in any other outpatient setting with one exception. When therapy services are performed incident to a physician's/NPP's service, the qualified personnel who perform the service do not need to have a license to practice therapy, unless it is required by state law. The qualified personnel must meet all the other requirements except licensure.

Qualifications for therapists are found in 42CFR484.4 and in section 467H230.1, 468H230.2, and 469H230.3 of this manual. In effect, these rules require that the person who furnishes the service to the patient must, at least, be a graduate of a program of training for one of the therapy services as described above. Regardless of any state licensing that allows other health professionals to provide therapy services, Medicare is authorized to pay only for services provided by those trained specifically in physical therapy, occupational therapy or speech-language pathology. That means that the services of athletic trainers, massage therapists, recreation therapists, kinesiotherapists, low vision specialists or any other profession may not be billed as therapy services.

The services of PTAs and OTAs also may not be billed incident to a physician's/NPP's service. However, if a PT and PTA (or an OT and OTA) are both employed in a physician's office, the services of the PTA, when directly supervised by the PT or the services of the OTA, when directly supervised by the OT may be billed by the physician group as PT or OT services using the PIN/NPI of the enrolled PT (or OT). (See Section 470H230.4 for private practice rules on billing services performed in a physician's office.) If the PT or OT is not enrolled, Medicare shall not pay for the services of a PTA or OTA billed incident to the physician's service, because they do not meet the qualification standards in 471H42CFR484.4.

Therapy services provided and billed incident to the services of a physician/NPP also must meet all incident-to requirements in this manual in 472Hchapter 15, §60. Where the policies have different requirements, the more stringent requirement shall be met.

For example, when therapy services are billed as incident to a physician/NPP services, the requirement for direct supervision by the physician/NPP and other incident to requirements must be met, even though the service is provided by a licensed therapist who may perform the services unsupervised in other settings.

The mandatory assignment provision does not apply to therapy services furnished by a physician/NPP or "incident to" a physician's/NPP's service. However, when these services are not furnished on an assignment-related basis; the limiting charge applies.

For emphasis, following are some of the standards that apply to therapy services billed incident-to the services of a physician/NPP in the physician's/NPP's office or the beneficiary's residence.

A. Therapy services provided to the beneficiary must be covered and payable outpatient rehabilitation services as described, for example, in this section as well as Pub. 473H100-08, chapter 13, §13.5.1.

B. Therapy services must be provided by, or under the direct supervision of a physician (a doctor of medicine or osteopathy) or NPP who is legally authorized to practice therapy services by the state in which he or she performs such function or action. Direct supervision requirements are the same as in 474H42CFR410.32(b)(3).

   The supervisor must be present in the office suite and immediately available to furnish assistance and direction throughout the performance of the procedure. It does not mean that the physician/NPP must be present in the same room in the office where the service is performed.

C. The services must be of a level of complexity that require that they be performed by a therapist or under the direct supervision of the therapist, physician/NPP who is licensed to perform them. Services that do not require the performance or supervision of the therapist, physician/NPP, are not considered reasonable or necessary therapy services even if they are performed or supervised by a physician/NPP or other qualified professional.

D. Services must be furnished under a plan of treatment as in §475H220.1.2 of this chapter. The services provided must relate directly to the physician/NPP service to which it is incident.

Pub 100-2, 15, 230.6 – Therapy Services Furnished Under Arrangements With Providers and Clinics

(Rev. 36, Issued: 06-24-05, Effective: 06-06-05, Implementation: 06-06-05)

References: See also 476HPub. 100-01, chapter 5, §10.3.

A. General

For rules regarding services provided under arrangement, see Pub. 47H100-01, chapter 5, §10.3.

A provider may have others furnish outpatient therapy (physical therapy, occupational therapy, or speech-language pathology) services through arrangements under which receipt of payment by the provider for the services discharges the liability of the beneficiary or any other person to pay for the service.

However, it is not intended that the provider merely serve as a billing mechanism for the other party. For such services to be covered the provider must assume professional responsibility for the services.

The provider's professional supervision over the services requires application of many of the same controls that are applied to services furnished by salaried employees. The provider must:

- Accept the patient for treatment in accordance with its admission policies;
- Maintain a complete and timely clinical record on the patient which includes diagnosis, medical history, orders, and progress notes relating to all services received;
- Maintain liaison with the attending physician/NPP with regard to the progress of the patient and to assure that the required plan of treatment is periodically reviewed by the physician/NPP;
- Secure from the physician/NPP the required certifications and recertifications; and
- Ensure that the medical necessity of such service is reviewed on a sample basis by the agency's staff or an outside review group.

In addition, when a provider provides outpatient services under an arrangement with others, such services must be furnished in accordance with the terms of a written contract, which provides for retention by the provider of responsibility for and control and supervision of such services. The terms of the contract should include at least the following:

- Provide that the therapy services are to be furnished in accordance with the plan of care established according to Medicare policies for therapy plans of care in section 478H220.1.2 of this chapter;
- Specify the geographical areas in which the services are to be furnished;
- Provide that contracted personnel and services meet the same requirements as those which would be applicable if the personnel and services were furnished directly by the provider;
- Provide that the therapist will participate in conferences required to coordinate the care of an individual patient;
- Provide for the preparation of treatment records, with progress notes and observations, and for the prompt incorporation of such into the clinical records of the clinic;
- Specify the financial arrangements. The contracting organization or individual may not bill the patient or the health insurance program; and
- Specify the period of time the contract is to be in effect and the manner of termination or renewal.

B. Special Rules for Hospitals

- A hospital may bill Medicare for outpatient therapy (physical therapy, occupational therapy, or speech-language pathology) services that it furnishes to its outpatients either directly or under arrangements in the hospital's outpatient department. If a hospital furnishes medically necessary therapy services in its outpatient department to individuals who are registered as its outpatients, those services must be billed directly by the hospital using bill type 13X or 85X for critical access hospitals. Note that services provided to residents of a Medicare-certified SNF may not be billed by the hospital as services to its outpatients.
- When a hospital sends its therapists to the home of an individual who is registered as an outpatient of the hospital but who is unable, for medical reasons, to come to the hospital to receive medically necessary therapy services, the services must meet the requirements applicable to outpatient hospital therapy services, as set forth in the regulations and applicable Medicare manuals. The hospital may bill for those services directly using bill type 13X or 85X for critical access hospitals.
- If a hospital sends its therapists to provide therapy services to individuals who are registered as its outpatients and who are residing in the non-certified part of a SNF, or in another residential setting (e.g., a group home, assisted living facility or domiciliary care home), the hospital may bill for the services as hospital outpatient services if the services meet the requirements

Medicare References

applicable to outpatient hospital therapy services, as set forth in the regulations and applicable Medicare manuals.

- A hospital may make an arrangement with another entity such as an Outpatient Rehab Facility (Rehabilitation Agency) or a private practice, to provide therapy services to individuals who are registered as outpatients of the hospital. These services must meet the requirements applicable to services furnished under arrangements and the requirements applicable to the outpatient hospital therapy services as set forth in the regulations and applicable Medicare manuals. The hospital uses bill type 13X or 85X for critical access hospitals to bill for the services that another entity furnishes under arrangement to its outpatients.
- Where the provider is a public health agency or a hospital in a rural community, it may enter into arrangements to have outpatient physical therapy services furnished in the private office of a qualified physical therapist if the agency or hospital does not have the capacity to provide on its premises all of the modalities of treatment, tests, and measurements that are included in an adequate outpatient physical therapy program and the services and modalities which the public health agency or hospital cannot provide on its premises are not available on an outpatient basis in another accessible certified facility.
- In certain settings and under certain circumstances, hospitals may not bill Medicare for therapy services as services of the hospital:
  - If a hospital sends its therapists to provide therapy services to patients of another hospital, including a patient at an inpatient rehabilitation facility or a long term care facility, the services must be furnished under arrangements made with the hospital sending the therapists by the hospital having the patients and billed as hospital services by the facility whose patients are treated. These services would be subject to existing hospital bundling rules and would be paid under the payment method applicable to the hospital at which the individuals are patients.
  - A hospital may not send its therapists to provide therapy services to individuals who are receiving services from an HHA under a home health plan of care and bill for the therapy services as hospital outpatient services. For patients under a home health plan of care, payment for therapy services (unless provided by physicians/NPPs) is included or bundled into Medicare's episodic payment to the HHA, and those services must be billed by the HHA under the HHA consolidated billing rules. For patients receiving HHA services under an HHA plan of care, therapy services must be furnished directly or under arrangements made by the HHA, and only the HHA may bill for those services.

If a hospital sends its therapists to provide services under arrangements made by a SNF to residents of the Medicare-certified part of a SNF, SNF consolidated billing rules apply. For arrangements specific to SNF Part A, see Pub. 479H100-04, chapter 6, §10.4. This means that therapy services furnished to SNF residents in the Medicare-certified part of a SNF cannot be billed by any entity other than the SNF. Therefore, a hospital may not bill Medicare for PT/OT/SLP services furnished to residents of a Medicare-certified part of a SNF by its therapists as services of the hospital.

NOTE: If the SNF resident is in a covered Part A stay, the therapy services would be included in the SNF's global PPS per diem payment for the covered Part A stay itself. If the resident is in a noncovered stay (Part A benefits exhausted, no prior qualifying hospital stay, etc.), but remains in the Medicare-certified part of a SNF, the SNF would submit the Part B therapy bill to its fiscal intermediary.

SNF Setting Applicable Rules

Medicare Part A or B Consolidated Billing Rules Apply?	Hospital May Bill For Outpatient Services?
Part A (Medicare Covered / PPS)	Resident in Medicare-certified part of a SNF
Yes	No
Medicare Part B Resident in Medicare-certified part of a SNF	
Yes	No
Medicare Part B	Not a Resident in Medicare-certified part of a SNF
No	Yes

- A hospital may not send therapy staff to provide therapy services in nonresidential health care settings and bill for the services as if they were provided at the hospital, even if the hospital owns the other facility or entity.

Examples of such non-residential settings include CORFs, rehabilitation agencies, ORFs and offices of physicians/NPPs or other practitioners, such as physical therapists. For example, services furnished to patients of a CORF must be billed as CORF services and not as outpatient hospital services. Even if a CORF contracts with a hospital to furnish services to CORF patients, the hospital may not bill Medicare for the services as hospital outpatient services.

However, the CORF could have the hospital furnish services to its patients under arrangements, in which case the CORF would bill for the services.

Psychiatric hospitals are treated the same as other hospitals for the purpose of therapy billing.

Pub 100-2, 15, 270 – Telehealth Services

(Rev. 97, Issued: 11-14-08, Effective: 01-01-09, Implementation: 01-05-09)

Background

Section 223 of the *Medicare, Medicaid and SCHIP Benefits Improvement and Protection Act of 2000* (BIPA) – Revision of Medicare Reimbursement for Telehealth Services amended §1834 of the Act to provide for an expansion of Medicare payment for telehealth services.

Effective October 1, 2001, coverage and payment for Medicare telehealth includes consultation, office visits, individual psychotherapy, and pharmacologic management delivered via a telecommunications system. Eligible geographic areas include rural health professional shortage areas and counties not classified as a metropolitan statistical area (MSA). Additionally, Federal telemedicine demonstration projects as of December 31, 2000, may serve as the originating site regardless of geographic location.

An interactive telecommunications system is required as a condition of payment; however, BIPA does allow the use of asynchronous "store and forward" technology in delivering these services when the originating site is a Federal telemedicine demonstration program in Alaska or Hawaii. BIPA does not require that a practitioner present the patient for interactive telehealth services.

With regard to payment amount, BIPA specified that payment for the professional service performed by the distant site practitioner (i.e., where the expert physician or practitioner is physically located at time of telemedicine encounter) is equal to what would have been paid without the use of telemedicine. Distant site practitioners include only a physician as described in §1861(r) of the Act and a medical practitioner as described in §1842(b)(18)(C) of the Act. BIPA also expanded payment under Medicare to include a $20 originating site facility fee (location of beneficiary).

Previously, the Balanced Budget Act of 1997 (BBA) limited the scope of Medicare telehealth coverage to consultation services and the implementing regulation prohibited the use of an asynchronous 'store and forward' telecommunications system. The BBA of 1997 also required the professional fee to be shared between the referring and consulting practitioners, and prohibited Medicare payment for facility fees and line charges associated with the telemedicine encounter.

The BIPA required that Medicare Part B (Supplementary Medical Insurance) pay for this expansion of telehealth services beginning with services furnished on October 1, 2001.

Section 149 of the Medicare Improvements for Patients and Providers Act of 2008 (MIPPA) amended §1834(m) of the Act to add certain entities as originating sites for payment of telehealth services. Effective for services furnished on or after January 1, 2009, eligible originating sites include a hospital-based or critical access hospital-based renal dialysis center (including satellites); a skilled nursing facility (as defined in §1819(a) of the Act); and a community mental health center (as defined in §1861(ff)(3)(B) of the Act). MIPPA also amended§1888(e)(2)(A)(ii) of the Act to exclude telehealth services furnished under §1834(m)(4)(C)(ii)(VII) from the consolidated billing provisions of the skilled nursing facility prospective payment system (SNF PPS).

NOTE: MIPPA did not add independent renal dialysis facilities as originating sites for payment of telehealth services.

The telehealth provisions authorized by §1834(m) of the Act are implemented in 42 CFR 410.78 and 414.65.

Pub 100-2, 15, 270.1 – Eligibility Criteria

(Rev. 97, Issued: 11-14-08, Effective: 01-01-09, Implementation: 01-05-09)

Beneficiaries are eligible for telehealth services only if they are presented from an originating site located either in a rural HPSA or in a county outside of an MSA.

Entities participating in a Federal telemedicine demonstration project that were approved by or were receiving funding from the Secretary of Health and Human Services as of December 31, 2000, qualify as originating sites regardless of geographic location. Such entities are not required to be in a rural HPSA or non-MSA.

An originating site is the location of an eligible Medicare beneficiary at the time the service being furnished via telecommunications system occurs. Originating sites authorized by law are listed below.

- The office of a physician or practitioner
- A hospital
- A critical access hospital (CAH)
- A rural health clinic (RHC)
- A federally qualified health center (FQHC)
- A hospital-based or critical access hospital-based renal dialysis center (including satellites) (Effective January 1, 2009)
- A skilled nursing facility (SNF) (Effective January 1, 2009)
- A community mental health center (CMHC) (Effective January 1, 2009)

NOTE: Independent renal dialysis facilities are not eligible originating sites.

Pub 100-2, 15, 270.2 – List of Medicare Telehealth Services

(Rev. 99; Issued: 12-24-08; Effective Date: 01-01-09; Implementation Date: 01-05-09)

Furnished by CMS

The use of a telecommunications system may substitute for a face-to-face, "hands on" encounter for consultations, office visits, individual psychotherapy, pharmacologic management, psychiatric diagnostic interview examination, end stage renal disease related services, and individual medical nutrition therapy. These services are listed below.

- Consultations
- Office or other outpatient visits
- Individual psychotherapy
- Pharmacologic management
- Psychiatric diagnostic interview examination (Effective March 1, 2003)
- End stage renal disease related services (Effective January 1, 2005)
- Individual Medical Nutrition Therapy (Effective January 1, 2006)
- Neurobehavioral status exam (Effective January 1, 2008)
- Follow-up inpatient telehealth consultations (Effective January 1, 2009)

For detailed coding for these services, see Pub.100-04, chapter 12, §190.3.

Pub 100-2, 15, 270.2.1 – Follow-Up Inpatient Telehealth Consultations Defined

(Rev. 99; Issued: 12-24-08; Effective Date: 01-01-09; Implementation Date: 01-05-09)

Follow-up inpatient telehealth consultations are consultative visits furnished via telehealth to follow up on an initial consultation, or subsequent consultative visits requested by the attending physician. The initial inpatient consultation may have been provided in person or via telehealth.

The conditions of payment for follow-up inpatient telehealth consultations, including qualifying originating sites and the types of telecommunications systems recognized by Medicare, are subject to the provisions of 42 CFR 410.78. Payment for these services is subject to the provisions of 42 CFR 414.65.

Follow-up inpatient telehealth consultations include monitoring progress, recommending management modifications, or advising on a new plan of care in response to changes in the patient's status or no changes on the consulted health issue. Counseling and coordination of care with other providers or agencies is included as well, consistent with the nature of the problem(s) and the patient's needs.

The physician or practitioner who furnishes the inpatient follow-up consultation via telehealth cannot be the physician of record or the attending physician, and the follow-up inpatient consultation would be distinct from the follow-up care provided by the physician of record or the attending physician. If a physician consultant has initiated treatment at an initial consultation and participates thereafter in the patient's ongoing care management, such care would not be included in the definition of a follow-up inpatient consultation and is not appropriate for delivery via telehealth. Follow-up inpatient telehealth consultations are subject to the criteria for consultation services, as described in Pub. 100-04, chapter 12, §30.6.10.

Payment for follow-up inpatient telehealth consultations includes all consultation related services furnished before, during, and after communicating with the patient via telehealth. Pre-service activities would include, but would not be limited to, reviewing patient data (for example, diagnostic and imaging studies, interim labwork) and communicating with other professionals or family members. Key elements of the intra-service activities are taking an interval history, conducting an examination, and engaging in medical decision making. Follow-up inpatient telehealth consultations must include at least two of these three key elements, as described in Pub. 100-04, chapter 12, §190.3.1. Post-service activities would include, but would not be limited to, completing medical records or other documentation and communicating results of the consultation and further care plans to other health care professionals. No additional evaluation and management service could be billed for work related to a follow-up inpatient telehealth consultation.

Pub 100-2, 15, 270.4.1 – Payment for ESRD-Related Services as a Telehealth Service

(Rev. 97, Issued: 11-14-08, Effective: 01-01-09, Implementation: 01-05-09)

The ESRD-related services included in the monthly capitation payment (MCP) with 2 or 3 visits per month and ESRD-related services with 4 or more visits per month may be paid as Medicare telehealth services. However, at least 1 visit must be furnished face-toface "hands on" to examine the vascular access site by a physician, clinical nurse specialist, nurse practitioner, or physicians assistant. An interactive audio and video telecommunications system may be used for providing additional visits required under the 2-to-3 visit MCP and the 4-or-more visit MCP. The medical record must indicate that at least one of the visits was furnished face-to-face "hands on" by a physician, clinical nurse specialist, nurse practitioner, or physician assistant.

The MCP physician, for example, the physician or practitioner who is responsible for the complete monthly assessment of the patient and establishes the patient's plan of care, may use other physicians and practitioners to furnish ESRD-related visits through an interactive audio and video telecommunications system. The non-MCP physician or practitioner must have a relationship with the billing physician or practitioner such as a partner, employees of the same group practice or an employee of the MCP physician, for example, the non MCP physician or practitioner is either a W-2 employee or 1099 independent contractor. However, the physician or practitioner who is responsible for the complete monthly assessment and establishes the ESRD beneficiary's plan of care should bill for the MCP in any given month.

Clinical Criteria

The visit including a clinical examination of the vascular access site must be conducted face-to-face "hands on" by a physician, clinical nurse specialist, nurse practitioner or physician's assistant. For additional visits, the physician or practitioner at the distant site is required, at a minimum, to use an interactive audio and video telecommunications system that allows the physician or practitioner to provide medical management services for a maintenance dialysis beneficiary. For example, an ESRD-related visit conducted via telecommunications system must permit the physician or practitioner at the distant site to perform an assessment of whether the dialysis is working effectively and whether the patient is tolerating the procedure well (physiologically and psychologically). During this assessment, the physician or practitioner at the distant site must be able to determine whether alteration in any aspect of the beneficiary's prescription is indicated, due to such changes as the estimate of the patient's dry weight.

Pub 100-2, 15, 280.2 – Colorectal Cancer Screening

Pub 100-2, 15, 280.2.1 – Covered Services and HCPCS Codes

(Rev. 3, 12-19-03)

See *Business Requirements* at http://cms.hhs.gov/manuals/pm_trans/R3BP.pdf

Medicare covers colorectal cancer screening test/procedures for the early detection of colorectal cancer for the HCPCS codes indicated.

A. Effective for Services Furnished On or After January 1, 1998:

G0104 Colorectal cancer screening; flexible sigmoidoscopy

G0105 Colorectal cancer screening; colonoscopy on individual at high risk

G0106 Colorectal cancer screening barium enema; alternative to GO104, screening sigmoidoscopy

G0120 Colorectal cancer screening barium enema; alternative to GO105, screening sigmoidoscopy

B. Effective for Services Furnished On or After July 1, 2001:

G0121 Colorectal Cancer Screening; Colonoscopy on Individual Not Meeting Criteria for High Risk

C. Effective for Services Furnished On or After January 1, 2004:

G0328 Colorectal cancer screening; fecal-occult blood test, immunoassay, 1-3 simultaneous determinations

Pub 100-2, 15, 280.2.2 – Coverage Criteria

(Rev. 3, 12-19-03)

The following are the coverage criteria for these screenings:

A. Screening Fecal-Occult Blood Tests (FOBT) (Codes G0107 and G0328)

Effective for services furnished on or after January 1, 2004, one screening FOBT (code G0107 or G0328) is covered for beneficiaries who have attained age 50, at a frequency of once every 12 months (i.e., at least 11 months have passed following the month in which the last covered screening FOBT was done). Screening FOBT means: (1) a guaiac-based test for peroxidase activity in which the beneficiary completes it by taking samples from two different sites of three consecutive stools **or**, (2) a immunoassay (or immunochemical) test for antibody activity in which the beneficiary completes the test by taking the appropriate number of samples according to the specific manufacturer's instructions. This expanded coverage is in accordance with revised regulations at 42 CFR 410.37(a)(2) that includes " other tests determined by the Secretary through a national coverage determination." This screening requires a written order from the beneficiary's attending physician. (The term "attending physician" is defined to mean a doctor of medicine or osteopathy (as defined in §1861(r)(1) of the Act) who is fully knowledgeable about the beneficiary's medical condition, and who would be responsible for using the results of any examination performed in the overall management of the beneficiary's specific medical problem.)

B. Screening Flexible Sigmoidoscopies (code G0104)

For claims with dates of service on or after January 1, 2002, carriers pay for screening flexible sigmoidoscopies (Code G0104) for beneficiaries who have attained age 50 when these services were performed by a doctor of medicine or osteopathy, or by a physician assistant, nurse practitioner, or clinical nurse specialist (as defined in §1861(aa)(5) of the Act and in the Code of Federal Regulations at 42 CFR 410.74, 410.75, and 410.76) at the frequencies noted below. For claims with dates of service prior to January 1, 2002, pay for these services under the conditions noted only when they are performed by a doctor of medicine or osteopathy.

For services furnished from January 1, 1998, through June 30, 2001, inclusive

Once every 48 months (i.e., at least 47 months have passed following the month in which the last covered screening flexible sigmoidoscopy was done).

For services furnished on or after July 1, 2001

Once every 48 months as calculated above **unless** the beneficiary does not meet the criteria for high risk of developing colorectal cancer (refer to §280.2.3) **and** the beneficiary has had a screening colonoscopy (code G0121) within the preceding 10 years. If such a beneficiary has had a screening colonoscopy within the preceding 10 years, then he or she can have covered a screening flexible sigmoidoscopy only after at least 119 months have passed following the month that he/she received the screening colonoscopy (code G0121).

NOTE: If during the course of a screening flexible sigmoidoscopy a lesion or growth is detected which results in a biopsy or removal of the growth, the appropriate diagnostic procedure classified as a flexible sigmoidoscopy with biopsy or removal should be billed and paid rather than code G0104.

C. Screening Colonoscopies for Beneficiaries at High Risk of Developing Colorectal Cancer (Code G0105)

The carrier must pay for screening colonoscopies (code G0105) when performed by a doctor of medicine or osteopathy at a frequency of once every 24 months for beneficiaries at high risk for developing colorectal cancer (i.e., at least 23 months have passed following the month in which the last covered G0105 screening colonoscopy was performed). Refer to §280.2.3 for the criteria to use in determining whether or not an individual is at high risk for developing colorectal cancer.

NOTE: If during the course of the screening colonoscopy, a lesion or growth is detected which results in a biopsy or removal of the growth, the appropriate diagnostic procedure classified as a colonoscopy with biopsy or removal should be billed and paid rather than code G0105.

D. Screening Colonoscopies Performed on Individuals Not Meeting the Criteria for Being at High-Risk for Developing Colorectal Cancer (Code G0121)

Effective for services furnished on or after July 1, 2001, screening colonoscopies (code G0121) are covered when performed under the following conditions:

1. On individuals not meeting the criteria for being at high risk for developing colorectal cancer (refer to §280.2.3);
2. At a frequency of once every 10 years (i.e., at least 119 months have passed following the month in which the last covered G0121 screening colonoscopy was performed); and
3. If the individual would otherwise qualify to have covered a G0121 screening colonoscopy based on the above (see §§280.2.2.D.1 and 2) **but** has had a covered screening flexible sigmoidoscopy (code G0104), then the individual may have a covered G0121 screening colonoscopy only after at least 47 months have passed following the month in which the last covered G0104 flexible sigmoidoscopy was performed.

NOTE: If during the course of the screening colonoscopy, a lesion or growth is detected which results in a biopsy or removal of the growth, the appropriate diagnostic procedure classified as a colonoscopy with biopsy or removal should be billed and paid rather than code G0121.

E. Screening Barium Enema Examinations (codes G0106 and G0120)

Screening barium enema examinations are covered as an alternative to either a screening sigmoidoscopy (code G0104) or a screening colonoscopy (code G0105) examination. The same frequency parameters for screening sigmoidoscopies and screening colonoscopies above apply.

In the case of an individual aged 50 or over, payment may be made for a screening barium enema examination (code G0106) performed after at least 47 months have passed following the month in which the last screening barium enema or screening flexible sigmoidoscopy was performed. For example, the beneficiary received a screening barium enema examination as an alternative to a screening flexible sigmoidoscopy in January 1999. The count starts beginning February 1999. The beneficiary is eligible for another screening barium enema in January 2003.

Medicare References

In the case of an individual who is at high risk for colorectal cancer, payment may be made for a screening barium enema examination (code G0120) performed after at least 23 months have passed following the month in which the last screening barium enema or the last screening colonoscopy was performed. For example, a beneficiary at high risk for developing colorectal cancer received a screening barium enema examination (code G0120) as an alternative to a screening colonoscopy (code G0105) in January 2000. The count starts beginning February 2000. The beneficiary is eligible for another screening barium enema examination (code G0120) in January 2002.

The screening barium enema must be ordered in writing after a determination that the test is the appropriate screening test. Generally, it is expected that this will be a screening double contrast enema unless the individual is unable to withstand such an exam. This means that in the case of a particular individual, the attending physician must determine that the estimated screening potential for the barium enema is equal to or greater than the screening potential that has been estimated for a screening flexible sigmoidoscopy, or for a screening colonoscopy, as appropriate, for the same individual. The screening single contrast barium enema also requires a written order from the beneficiary's attending physician in the same manner as described above for the screening double contrast barium enema examination.

Pub 100-2, 15, 280.2.3 – Determining Whether or Not the Beneficiary is at High Risk for Developing Colorectal Cancer

(Rev. 1, 10-01-03)

A. Characteristics of the High Risk Individual

An individual at high risk for developing colorectal cancer has one or more of the following:

- A close relative (sibling, parent, or child) who has had colorectal cancer or an adenomatous polyp.
- A family history of familial adenomatous polyposis.
- A family history of hereditary nonpolyposis colorectal cancer.
- A personal history of colorectal cancer.
- A personal history of adenomatous polyps.
- Inflammatory bowel disease, including Crohn's Disease, and ulcerative colitis.

B. Partial List of ICD-9-CM Codes Indicating High Risk

Listed below are some examples of diagnoses that meet the high risk criteria for colorectal cancer. This is not an all-inclusive list. There may be more instances of conditions which may be coded and could be at the medical directors' discretion.

- **Personal History**

  V10.05 Personal history of malignant neoplasm of large intestine

  V10.06 Personal history of malignant neoplasm of rectum, rectosigmoid junction, and anus

- **Chronic Digestive Disease Condition**

  555.0 Regional enteritis of small intestine

  555.1 Regional enteritis of large intestine

  555.2 Regional enteritis of small intestine with large intestine

  555.9 Regional enteritis of unspecified site

  556.0 Ulcerative (chronic) enterocolitis

  556.1 Ulcerative (chronic) ileocolitis

  556.2 Ulcerative (chronic) proctitis

  556.3 Ulcerative (chronic) proctosigmoiditis

  556.8 Other ulcerative colitis

  556.9 Ulcerative colitis, unspecified (nonspecific PDX on the MCE)

- **Inflammatory Bowel**

  558.2 Toxic gastroenteritis and colitis

  558.9 Other and unspecified noninfectious gastroenteritis and colitis

Pub 100-2, 15, 280.2.4 – Determining Frequency Standards

(Rev. 1, 10-01-03)

To determine the 11, 23, 47, and 119-month periods, the count starts beginning with the month after the month in which a previous test/ procedure was performed.

EXAMPLE: The beneficiary received a fecal-occult blood test in January 2000. The carrier starts its count beginning with February 2000. The beneficiary is eligible to receive another blood test in January 2001 (the month after 11 full months have passed).

Pub 100-2, 15, 280.2.5 – Noncovered Services

(Rev. 1, 10-01-03)

The following noncovered HCPCS codes are used to allow claims to be billed and denied for beneficiaries who need a Medicare denial for other insurance purposes for the dates of service indicated:

A. From January 1, 1998 Through June 30, 2001, Inclusive

Code G0121 (colorectal cancer screening; colonoscopy on an individual not meeting criteria for high risk) should be used when this procedure is performed on a beneficiary who does NOT meet the criteria for high risk. This service should be denied as noncovered because it fails to meet the requirements of the benefit for these dates of service. The beneficiary is liable for payment. Note that this code is a covered service for dates of service on or after July 1, 2001.

B. On or After January 1, 1998

Code G0122 (colorectal cancer screening; barium enema) should be used when a screening barium enema is performed NOT as an alternative to either a screening colonoscopy (code G0105) or a screening flexible sigmoidoscopy (code G0104). This service should be denied as noncovered because it fails to meet the requirements of the benefit. The beneficiary is liable for payment.

Pub 100-2, 15, 280.4 – Screening Pap Smears

(Rev. 1, 10-01-03)

Effective, January 1, 1998, §4102 of the Balanced Budget Act (BBA) of 1997 (P.L. 105-33) amended §1861(nn) of the Act (42 USC 1395X(nn)) to include coverage every three years for a screening Pap smear or more frequent coverage for women:

1. At high risk for cervical or vaginal cancer.
2. Of childbearing age who have had a Pap smear during any of the preceding three years indicating the presence of cervical or vaginal cancer or other abnormality.

Effective July 1, 2001, the Consolidated Appropriations Act of 2001 (P.L. 106-554) modifies §1861(nn) to provide Medicare coverage for biennial screening Pap smears. Specifications for frequency limitations are defined below.

For claims with dates of service from January 1, 1998, through June 30, 2001, screening Pap smears are covered when ordered and collected by a doctor of medicine or osteopathy (as defined in §1861(r)(1) of the Act), or other authorized practitioner (e.g., a certified nurse midwife, physician assistant, nurse practitioner, or clinical nurse specialist, who is authorized under State law to perform the examination) under one of the following conditions.

The beneficiary has not had a screening Pap smear test during the preceding three years (i.e., 35 months have passed following the month that the woman had the last covered Pap smear ICD-9-CM code V76.2 is used to indicate special screening for malignant neoplasm, cervix); or

There is evidence (on the basis of her medical history or other findings) that she is of childbearing age and has had an examination that indicated the presence of cervical or vaginal cancer or other abnormalities during any of the preceding three years; and at least 11 months have passed following the month that the last covered Pap smear was performed; or

She is at high risk of developing cervical or vaginal cancer ICD-9-CM code V15.89, other specified personal history presenting hazards to health) and at least 11 months have passed following the month that the last covered screening Pap smear was performed. The high risk factors for cervical and vaginal cancer are:

Cervical Cancer High Risk Factors

- Early onset of sexual activity (under 16 years of age).
- Multiple sexual partners (five or more in a lifetime).
- History of a sexually transmitted disease (including HIV infection).
- Fewer than three negative or any Pap smears within the previous seven years.

Vaginal Cancer High Risk Factors

The DES (diethylstilbestrol)—exposed daughters of women who took DES during pregnancy

The term "woman of childbearing age" means a woman who is premenopausal, and has been determined by a physician, or qualified practitioner, to be of childbearing age, based on her medical history or other findings. Payment is not made for a screening Pap smear for women at high risk or who qualify for coverage under the childbearing provision more frequently than once every 11 months after the month that the last screening Pap smear covered by Medicare was performed.

For Claims with Dates of Service on or After July 1, 2001

When the beneficiary does not qualify for a more frequently performed screening Pap smear as noted in items 1 and 2 above, contractors pay for the screening Pap smear only after at least 23 months have passed following the month during which the beneficiary received her last covered screening Pap smear. All other coverage and payment requirements remain the same.

See the *Medicare Claims Processing Manual*, Chapter 18, "Preventive and Screening Services," for billing procedures.

Pub 100-2, 15, 290 – Foot Care

(Rev. 1, 10-01-03)

A3-3158, B3-2323, HO-260.9, B3-4120.1

A. Treatment of Subluxation of Foot

Subluxations of the foot are defined as partial dislocations or displacements of joint surfaces, tendons ligaments, or muscles of the foot. Surgical or nonsurgical treatments undertaken for the sole purpose of correcting a subluxated structure in the foot as an isolated entity are not covered.

However, medical or surgical treatment of subluxation of the ankle joint (talo-crural joint) is covered. In addition, reasonable and necessary medical or surgical services, diagnosis, or treatment for medical conditions that have resulted from or are associated with partial displacement of structures is covered. For example, if a patient has osteoarthritis that has resulted in a partial displacement of joints in the foot, and the primary treatment is for the osteoarthritis, coverage is provided.

B. Exclusions from Coverage

The following foot care services are generally excluded from coverage under both Part A and Part B. (See 516H§290.F and 517H§290.G for instructions on applying foot care exclusions.)

1. Treatment of Flat Foot

   The term "flat foot" is defined as a condition in which one or more arches of the foot have flattened out. Services or devices directed toward the care or correction of such conditions, including the prescription of supportive devices, are not covered.

2. Routine Foot Care

   Except as provided above, routine foot care is excluded from coverage. Services that normally are considered routine and not covered by Medicare include the following:

   - The cutting or removal of corns and calluses;
   - The trimming, cutting, clipping, or debriding of nails; and
   - Other hygienic and preventive maintenance care, such as cleaning and soaking the feet, the use of skin creams to maintain skin tone of either ambulatory or bedfast patients, and any other service performed in the absence of localized illness, injury, or symptoms involving the foot.

3. Supportive Devices for Feet

   Orthopedic shoes and other supportive devices for the feet generally are not covered. However, this exclusion does not apply to such a shoe if it is an integral part of a leg brace, and its expense is included as part of the cost of the brace. Also, this exclusion does not apply to therapeutic shoes furnished to diabetics.

C. Exceptions to Routine Foot Care Exclusion

1. Necessary and Integral Part of Otherwise Covered Services

   In certain circumstances, services ordinarily considered to be routine may be covered if they are performed as a necessary and integral part of otherwise covered services, such as diagnosis and treatment of ulcers, wounds, or infections.

2. Treatment of Warts on Foot

   The treatment of warts (including plantar warts) on the foot is covered to the same extent as services provided for the treatment of warts located elsewhere on the body.

3. Presence of Systemic Condition

   The presence of a systemic condition such as metabolic, neurologic, or peripheral vascular disease may require scrupulous foot care by a professional that in the absence of such condition(s) would be considered routine (and, therefore, excluded from coverage). Accordingly, foot care that would otherwise be considered routine may be covered when systemic condition(s) result in severe circulatory embarrassment or areas of diminished sensation in the individual's legs or feet. (See 518Hsubsection A.)

   In these instances, certain foot care procedures that otherwise are considered routine (e.g., cutting or removing corns and calluses, or trimming, cutting, clipping, or debriding nails) may pose a hazard when performed by a nonprofessional person on patients with such systemic conditions. (See 519H§290.G for procedural instructions.)

4. Mycotic Nails

   In the absence of a systemic condition, treatment of mycotic nails may be covered. The treatment of mycotic nails for an ambulatory patient is covered only when the physician attending the patient's mycotic condition documents that (1) there is clinical evidence of mycosis of the toenail, and (2) the patient has marked limitation of ambulation, pain, or secondary infection resulting from the thickening and dystrophy of the infected toenail plate.

   The treatment of mycotic nails for a nonambulatory patient is covered only when the physician attending the patient's mycotic condition documents that (1) there is clinical evidence of mycosis of the toenail, and (2) the patient suffers from pain or secondary infection resulting from the thickening and dystrophy of the infected toenail plate. For the purpose of these requirements, documentation means any written information that is required by the carrier in order for services to be covered. Thus, the information submitted with claims must be substantiated by information found in the patient's medical record. Any information, including that contained in a form letter, used for documentation purposes is subject to carrier verification in order to ensure that the information adequately justifies coverage of the treatment of mycotic nails.

D. Systemic Conditions That Might Justify Coverage

Although not intended as a comprehensive list, the following metabolic, neurologic, and peripheral vascular diseases (with synonyms in parentheses) most commonly represent the underlying conditions that might justify coverage for routine foot care.

Diabetes mellitus *

Arteriosclerosis obliterans (A.S.O., arteriosclerosis of the extremities, occlusive peripheral arteriosclerosis)

Buerger's disease (thromboangiitis obliterans)

Chronic thrombophlebitis *

Peripheral neuropathies involving the feet -

Associated with malnutrition and vitamin deficiency *

- Malnutrition (general, pellagra)
- Alcoholism
- Malabsorption (celiac disease, tropical sprue)
- Pernicious anemia

Associated with carcinoma *

Associated with diabetes mellitus *

Associated with drugs and toxins *

Associated with multiple sclerosis *

Associated with uremia (chronic renal disease) *

Medicare References

Associated with traumatic injury

Associated with leprosy or neurosyphilis

Associated with hereditary disorders

- Hereditary sensory radicular neuropathy
- Angiokeratoma corporis diffusum (Fabry's)
- Amyloid neuropathy

When the patient's condition is one of those designated by an asterisk (*), routine procedures are covered only if the patient is under the active care of a doctor of medicine or osteopathy who documents the condition.

E. Supportive Devices for Feet

Orthopedic shoes and other supportive devices for the feet generally are not covered. However, this exclusion does not apply to such a shoe if it is an integral part of a leg brace, and its expense is included as part of the cost of the brace. Also, this exclusion does not apply to therapeutic shoes furnished to diabetics.

F. Presumption of Coverage

In evaluating whether the routine services can be reimbursed, a presumption of coverage may be made where the evidence available discloses certain physical and/or clinical findings consistent with the diagnosis and indicative of severe peripheral involvement. For purposes of applying this presumption the following findings are pertinent:

Class A Findings

Nontraumatic amputation of foot or integral skeletal portion thereof.

Class B Findings

Absent posterior tibial pulse;

Advanced trophic changes as: hair growth (decrease or absence) nail changes (thickening) pigmentary changes (discoloration) skin texture (thin, shiny) skin color (rubor or redness) (Three required); and

Absent dorsalis pedis pulse.

Class C Findings

Claudication;

Temperature changes (e.g., cold feet);

Edema;

Paresthesias (abnormal spontaneous sensations in the feet); and

Burning.

The presumption of coverage may be applied when the physician rendering the routine foot care has identified:

1. A Class A finding;
2. Two of the Class B findings; or
3. One Class B and two Class C findings.

Cases evidencing findings falling short of these alternatives may involve podiatric treatment that may constitute covered care and should be reviewed by the intermediary's medical staff and developed as necessary.

For purposes of applying the coverage presumption where the routine services have been rendered by a podiatrist, the contractor may deem the active care requirement met if the claim or other evidence available discloses that the patient has seen an M.D. or D.O. for treatment and/or evaluation of the complicating disease process during the 6-month period prior to the rendition of the routine-type services. The intermediary may also accept the podiatrist's statement that the diagnosing and treating M.D. or D.O. also concurs with the podiatrist's findings as to the severity of the peripheral involvement indicated.

Services ordinarily considered routine might also be covered if they are performed as a necessary and integral part of otherwise covered services, such as diagnosis and treatment of diabetic ulcers, wounds, and infections.

G. Application of Foot Care Exclusions to Physician's Services

The exclusion of foot care is determined by the nature of the service. Thus, payment for an excluded service should be denied whether performed by a podiatrist, osteopath, or a doctor of medicine, and without regard to the difficulty or complexity of the procedure. When an itemized bill shows both covered services and noncovered services not integrally related to the covered service, the portion of charges attributable to the noncovered services should be denied. (For example, if an itemized bill shows surgery for an ingrown toenail and also removal of calluses not necessary for the performance of toe surgery, any additional charge attributable to removal of the calluses should be denied.)

In reviewing claims involving foot care, the carrier should be alert to the following exceptional situations:

1. Payment may be made for incidental noncovered services performed as a necessary and integral part of, and secondary to, a covered procedure. For example, if trimming of toenails is required for application of a cast to a fractured foot, the carrier need not allocate and deny a portion of the charge for the trimming of the nails. However, a separately itemized charge for such excluded service should be disallowed. When the primary procedure is covered the administration of anesthesia necessary for the performance of such procedure is also covered.
2. Payment may be made for initial diagnostic services performed in connection with a specific symptom or complaint if it seems likely that its treatment would be covered even though the resulting diagnosis may be one requiring only noncovered care.

The name of the M.D. or D.O. who diagnosed the complicating condition must be submitted with the claim. In those cases, where active care is required, the approximate date the beneficiary was last seen by such physician must also be indicated.

NOTE: Section 939 of P.L. 96-499 removed "warts" from the routine foot care exclusion effective July 1, 1981.

Relatively few claims for routine-type care are anticipated considering the severity of conditions contemplated as the basis for this exception. Claims for this type of foot care should not be paid in the absence of convincing evidence that nonprofessional performance of the service would have been hazardous for the beneficiary because of an underlying systemic disease. The mere statement of a diagnosis such as those mentioned in §D above does not of itself indicate the severity of the condition. Where development is indicated to verify diagnosis and/or severity the carrier should follow existing claims processing practices, which may include review of carrier's history and medical consultation as well as physician contacts.

The rules in 520H§290.F concerning presumption of coverage also apply. Codes and policies for routine foot care and supportive devices for the feet are not exclusively for the use of podiatrists. These codes must be used to report foot care services regardless of the specialty of the physician who furnishes the services. Carriers must instruct physicians to use the most appropriate code available when billing for routine foot care.

Pub 100-2, 16, 10 – General Exclusions From Coverage

(Rev. 1, 10-01-03)

A3-3150, HO-260, HHA-232, B3-2300

No payment can be made under either the hospital insurance or supplementary medical insurance program for certain items and services, when the following conditions exist:

- Not reasonable and necessary (§20);
- No legal obligation to pay for or provide (§40);
- Paid for by a governmental entity (§50);
- Not provided within United States (§60);
- Resulting from war (§70);
- Personal comfort (§80);
- Routine services and appliances (§90);
- Custodial care (§110);
- Cosmetic surgery (§120);
- Charges by immediate relatives or members of household (§130);
- Dental services (§140);
- Paid or expected to be paid under workers' compensation (§150);
- Nonphysician services provided to a hospital inpatient that were not provided directly or arranged for by the hospital (§170);
- Services Related to and Required as a Result of Services Which are not Covered Under Medicare (§180);
- Excluded foot care services and supportive devices for feet (§30); or
- Excluded investigational devices (See Chapter 14, §30).

Pub 100-2, 16, 20 – Services Not Reasonable and Necessary

(Rev. 1, 10-01-03)

A3-3151, HO-260.1, B3-2303, AB-00-52 – 6/00

Items and services which are not reasonable and necessary for the diagnosis or treatment of illness or injury or to improve the functioning of a malformed body member are not covered, e.g., payment cannot be made for the rental of a special hospital bed to be used by the patient in their home unless it was a reasonable and necessary part of the patient's treatment. See also §80.

A health care item or service for the purpose of causing, or assisting to cause, the death of any individual (assisted suicide) is not covered. This prohibition does not apply to the provision of an item or service for the purpose of alleviating pain or discomfort, even if such use may increase the risk of death, so long as the item or service is not furnished for the specific purpose of causing death.

Pub 100-2, 16, 90 – Routine Services and Appliances

(Rev. 1, 10-01-03)

A3-3157, HO-260.7, B3-2320, R-1797A3 – 5/00

Routine physical checkups; eyeglasses, contact lenses, and eye examinations for the purpose of prescribing, fitting, or changing eyeglasses; eye refractions by whatever practitioner and for whatever purpose performed; hearing aids and examinations for hearing aids; and immunizations are not covered.

The routine physical checkup exclusion applies to (a) examinations performed without relationship to treatment or diagnosis for a specific illness, symptom, complaint, or injury; and (b) examinations required by third parties such as insurance companies, business establishments, or Government agencies.

If the claim is for a diagnostic test or examination performed solely for the purpose of establishing a claim under title IV of Public Law 91-173, "Black Lung Benefits," the service is not covered under Medicare and the claimant should be advised to contact their Social Security office regarding the filing of a claim for reimbursement under the "Black Lung" program.

The exclusions apply to eyeglasses or contact lenses, and eye examinations for the purpose of prescribing, fitting, or changing eyeglasses or contact lenses for refractive errors. The exclusions do not apply to physicians' services (and services incident to a physicians' service) performed in conjunction with an eye disease, as for example, glaucoma or cataracts, or to post-surgical prosthetic lenses which are customarily used during convalescence from eye surgery in which the lens of the eye was removed, or to permanent prosthetic lenses required by an individual lacking the organic lens of the eye, whether by surgical removal or congenital disease. Such prosthetic lens is a replacement for an internal body organ – the lens of the eye. (See the **Medicare Benefit Policy Manual**, Chapter 15, "Covered Medical and Other Health Services," §120).

Expenses for all refractive procedures, whether performed by an ophthalmologist (or any other physician) or an optometrist and without regard to the reason for performance of the refraction, are excluded from coverage.

A. Immunizations

Vaccinations or inoculations are excluded as immunizations unless they are either

- Directly related to the treatment of an injury or direct exposure to a disease or condition, such as antirabies treatment, tetanus antitoxin or booster vaccine, botulin antitoxin, antivenin sera, or immune globulin.(In the absence of injury or direct exposure, preventive immunization (vaccination or inoculation) against such diseases as smallpox, polio, diphtheria, etc., is not covered.); or
- Specifically covered by statute, as described in the **Medicare Benefit Policy Manual**, Chapter 15, "Covered Medical and Other Health Services," §50.

B. Antigens

Prior to the Omnibus Reconciliation Act of 1980, a physician who prepared an antigen for a patient could not be reimbursed for that service unless the physician also administered the antigen to the patient.

Effective January 1, 1981, payment may be made for a reasonable supply of antigens that have been prepared for a particular patient even though they have not been administered to the patient by the same physician who prepared them if:

- The antigens are prepared by a physician who is a doctor of medicine or osteopathy, and
- The physician who prepared the antigens has examined the patient and has determined a plan of treatment and a dosage regimen.

A reasonable supply of antigens is considered to be not more than a 12-week supply of antigens that has been prepared for a particular patient at any one time. The purpose of the reasonable supply limitation is to assure that the antigens retain their potency and effectiveness over the period in which they are to be administered to the patient. (See the **Medicare Benefit Policy Manual**, Chapter 15, "Covered Medical and Other Health Services," §50.4.4.2)

Pub 100-2, 16, 140 – Dental Services Exclusion

(Rev. 1, 10-01-03)

A3-3162, HO-260.13, B3-2336

Items and services in connection with the care, treatment, filling, removal, or replacement of teeth, or structures directly supporting the teeth are not covered. Structures directly supporting the teeth mean the periodontium, which includes the gingivae, dentogingival junction, periodontal membrane, cementum, and alveolar process. However, payment may be made for certain other services of a dentist. (See the **Medicare Benefit Policy Manual**, Chapter 15, "Covered Medical and Other Health Services," §150.)

The hospitalization or nonhospitalization of a patient has no direct bearing on the coverage or exclusion of a given dental procedure.

When an excluded service is the primary procedure involved, it is not covered regardless of its complexity or difficulty. For example, the extraction of an impacted tooth is not covered. Similarly, an alveoplasty (the surgical improvement of the shape and condition of the alveolar process) and a frenectomy are excluded from coverage when either of these procedures is performed in connection with an excluded service, e.g., the preparation of the mouth for dentures. In like manner, the removal of the torus palatinus (a bony protuberance of the hard palate) could be a covered service. However, with rare exception, this surgery is performed in connection with an excluded service, i.e., the preparation of the mouth for dentures. Under such circumstances, reimbursement is not made for this purpose.

The extraction of teeth to prepare the jaw for radiation treatments of neoplastic disease is also covered. This is an exception to the requirement that to be covered, a noncovered procedure or service performed by a dentist must be an incident to and an integral part of a covered procedure or service performed by the dentist. Ordinarily, the dentist extracts the patient's teeth, but another physician, e.g., a radiologist, administers the radiation treatments.

Whether such services as the administration of anesthesia, diagnostic x-rays, and other related procedures are covered depends upon whether the primary procedure being performed by the dentist is covered. Thus, an x-ray taken in connection with the reduction of a fracture of the jaw or facial bone is covered. However, a single x-ray or xray survey taken in connection with the care or treatment of teeth or the periodontium is not covered.

See also the **Medicare Benefit Policy Manual**, Chapter 1, "Inpatient Hospital Services," §70, and Chapter 15, "Covered Medical and Other Health Services," §150 for additional information on dental services.

Pub 100-3 – National Coverage Decisions (NCD)

The revision numbers on the following National Coverage Decisions (NCDs) refer to the transmittal number. Any quarterly updates of NCDs can always be found on the CMS website at http://www.cms.hhs.gov/mcd/index_list.asp?list_type=ncd.

Pub 100-3, 20.8.1 – Cardiac Pacemaker Evaluation Services

(Rev. 1, 10-03-03)

Medicare covers a variety of services for the post-implant follow-up and evaluation of implanted cardiac pacemakers. The following guidelines are designed to assist contractors in identifying and processing claims for such services. These new guidelines are limited to lithium battery-powered pacemakers, because mercury-zinc battery-powered pacemakers are no longer being manufactured and virtually all have been replaced by lithium units. Contractors still receiving claims for monitoring such units should continue to apply the guidelines published in 1980 to those units until they are replaced.

There are two general types of pacemakers in current use – single-chamber pacemakers which sense and pace the ventricles of the heart, and dual-chamber pacemakers which sense and pace both the atria and the ventricles. These differences require different monitoring patterns over the expected life of the units involved. One fact of which contractors should be aware is that many dual-chamber units may be programmed to pace only the ventricles; this may be done either at the time the pacemaker is implanted or at some time afterward. In such cases, a dual-chamber unit, when programmed or reprogrammed for ventricular pacing, should be treated as a single-chamber pacemaker in applying screening guidelines.

The decision as to how often any patient's pacemaker should be monitored is the responsibility of the patient's physician who is best able to take into account the condition and circumstances of the individual patient. These may vary over time, requiring modifications of the frequency with which the patient should be monitored. In cases where monitoring is done by some entity other than the patient's physician, such as a commercial monitoring service or hospital outpatient department, the physician's prescription for monitoring is required and should be periodically renewed (at least annually) to assure that the frequency of monitoring is proper for the patient. Where a patient is monitored both during clinic visits and transtelephonically, the contractor should be sure to include frequency data on both types of monitoring in evaluating the reasonableness of the frequency of monitoring services received by the patient. Since there are over 200 pacemaker models in service at any given point, and a variety of patient conditions that give rise to the need for pacemakers, the question of the appropriate frequency of monitoring is a complex one. Nevertheless, it is possible to develop guidelines within which the vast majority of pacemaker monitoring will fall and contractors should do this, using their own data and experience, as well as the frequency guidelines which follow, in order to limit extensive claims development to those cases requiring special attention.

Pub 100-3, 20.8.1.1 – Transtelephonic Monitoring of Cardiac Pacemakers

(Rev. 1, 10-03-03)

A. General

Transtelephonic monitoring of pacemakers is furnished by commercial suppliers, hospital outpatient departments and physicians offices. Telephone monitoring of cardiac pacemakers as described below is medically efficacious in identifying early signs of possible pacemaker failure, thus reducing the number of sudden pacemaker failures requiring emergency replacement. All systems that monitor the pacemaker rate (bpm) in both the free-running and/or magnetic mode are effective in detecting subclinical pacemaker failure due to battery depletion. More sophisticated systems are also capable of detecting internal electronic problems within the pulse generator itself and other potential problems. In the case of dual chamber pacemakers in particular, such monitoring may detect failure of synchronization of the atria and ventricles, and the need for adjustment and reprogramming of the device. The transmitting device furnished to the patient is simply one component of the diagnostic system, and is not covered as durable medical equipment. Those engaged in transtelephonic pacemaker monitoring should reflect the costs of the transmitters in setting their charges for monitoring.

B. Definition of Transtelephonic Monitoring

In order for transtelephonic monitoring services to be covered, the services must consist of the following elements:

- A minimum 30-second readable strip of the pacemaker in the free-running mode;
- Unless contraindicated, a minimum 30-second readable strip of the pacemaker in the magnetic mode; and
- A minimum 30 seconds of readable ECG strip.

Pub 100-3, 20.8.2 – Self-Contained Pacemaker Monitors

(Rev. 1, 10-03-03)

Self-contained pacemaker monitors are accepted devices for monitoring cardiac pacemakers. Accordingly, program payment may be made for the rental or purchase of either of the following pacemaker monitors when a physician for a patient prescribes it with a cardiac pacemaker:

A Digital Electronic Pacemaker Monitor

This device provides the patient with an instantaneous digital readout of his pacemaker pulse rate. Use of this device does not involve professional services until there has been a change of five pulses (or more) per minute above or below the initial rate of the pacemaker; when such change occurs, the patient contacts his physician.

B Audible/Visible Signal Pacemaker Monitor

This device produces an audible and visible signal which indicates the pacemaker rate. Use of this device does not involve professional services until a change occurs in these signals; at such time, the patient contacts his physician.

Note: The design of the self-contained pacemaker monitor makes it possible for the patient to monitor his pacemaker periodically and minimizes the need for regular visits to the outpatient department of the provider.

Therefore, documentation of the medical necessity for pacemaker evaluation in the outpatient department of the provider should be obtained where such evaluation is employed in addition to the self-contained pacemaker monitor used by the patient in his home.

C Frequency Guidelines for Transtelephonic Monitoring

The guidelines below constitute a system which contractors should use, in conjunction with their knowledge of local medical practices, to screen claims for transtelephonic monitoring prior to payment. It is important to note that they are not recommendations with respect to a minimum frequency for such monitorings, but rather a maximum frequency (within which payment may be made without further claims development). As with previous guidelines, more frequent monitorings may be covered in cases where contractors are satisfied that such monitorings are medically necessary; e.g., based on the condition of the patient, or with respect to pacemakers exhibiting unexpected defects or premature failure. Contractors should seek written justification for more frequent monitorings from the patient's physician and/or any monitoring service involved.

These guidelines are divided into two broad categories. Guideline I which will apply to the majority of pacemakers now in use, and Guideline II which will apply only to pacemaker systems (pacemaker and leads) for which sufficient long-term clinical information exists to assure that they meet the standards of the Inter-Society Commission for Heart Disease Resources (ICHD) for longevity and end-of-life decay. (The ICHD standards are: (l) 90 percent cumulative survival at 5 years following implant; and (2) an end-of-life decay of less than a 50 percent drop of output voltage and less than 20 percent deviation of magnet rate, or a drop of 5 beats per minute or less, over a period of 3 months or more.) Contractors should consult with their medical advisers and other appropriate individuals and organizations (such as the North American Society of Pacing and Electrophysiology which publishes product reliability information) should questions arise over whether a pacemaker system meets the ICHD standards.

The two groups of guidelines are then further broken down into two general categories – single chamber and dual-chamber pacemakers. Contractors should be aware that the frequency with which a patient is monitored may be changed from time to time for a number of reasons, such as a change in the patient's overall condition, a reprogramming of the patient's pacemaker, the development of better information on the pacemaker's longevity or failure mode, etc. Consequently, changes in the proper set of guidelines may be required. Contractors should inform physicians and monitoring services to alert contractors to any changes in the patient's monitoring prescription that might necessitate changes in the screening guidelines applied to that patient. (Of particular importance is the reprogramming of a dual-chamber pacemaker to a single-chamber mode of operation. Such reprogramming would shift the patient from the appropriate dual-chamber guideline to the appropriate single-chamber guideline.)

Guideline I

1 – Single-chamber pacemakers

1st month – every 2 weeks.
2nd through 36th month – every 8 weeks.
37th month to failure – every 4 weeks.

2 – Dual-chamber pacemaker

1st month – every 2 weeks.
2nd through 6th month – every 4 weeks.
7th through 36th month – every 8 weeks.
37th month to failure – every 4 weeks.

Guideline II

1 – Single-chamber pacemakers

1st month – every 2 weeks.
2nd through 48th month – every 12 weeks.
49th through 72nd month – every 8 weeks.
Thereafter – every 4 weeks.

2 – Dual-chamber pacemaker

1st month – every 2 weeks.
2nd through 30th month – every 12 weeks.
31st through 48th month – every 8 weeks.
Thereafter – every 4 weeks.

D Pacemaker Clinic Services

1 General

Pacemaker monitoring is also covered when done by pacemaker clinics. Clinic visits may be done in conjunction with transtelephonic monitoring or as a separate service; however, the services rendered by a pacemaker clinic are more extensive than those currently possible by telephone. They include, for example, physical examination of patients and reprogramming of pacemakers. Thus, the use of one of these types of monitoring does not preclude concurrent use of the other.

2 Frequency Guidelines

As with transtelephonic pacemaker monitoring, the frequency of clinic visits is the decision of the patient's physician, taking into account, among other things, the medical condition of the patient. However, contractors can develop monitoring guidelines that will prove useful in screening claims. The following are recommendations for monitoring guidelines on lithium-battery pacemakers:

- For single-chamber pacemakers – twice in the first 6 months following implant, then once every 12 months.
- For dual-chamber pacemakers – twice in the first 6 months, then once every 6 months.

Cross-reference: §20.8.1

Pub 100-3, 20.9 – Artificial Hearts and Related Devices

(Rev. 95; Issued: 09-10-08 ; Effective Date: 05-01-08; Implementation Date: 12-01-08)

A.Covered Indications

1. Postcardiotomy (effective for services performed on or after October 18, 1993)

A ventricular assist device (VAD) or left ventricular assist device (LVAD) is surgically attached to one or both intact ventricles and is used to assist a damaged or weakened native heart in pumping blood. Improvement in the performance of the native heart may allow the device to be removed.

An artificial heart is a biventricular replacement device which requires removal of a substantial part of the native heart, including both ventricles. Removal of this device is not compatible with life, unless the patient has a heart transplant.

B. Nationally Covered Indications

1. Postcardiotomy (effective for services performed on or after October 18, 1993)

Post-cardiotomy is the period following open-heart surgery. VADs used for support of blood circulation post-cardiotomy are covered only if they have received approval from the Food and Drug Administration (FDA) for that purpose, and the VADs are used according to the FDA-approved labeling instructions.

2. Bridge-to-Transplant

a. VADs as Bridge-to-Transplant (effective for services performed on or after January 22, 1996)

The VADs used for bridge-to-transplant are covered only if they have received approval from the FDA for that purpose, and the VADs are used according to the FDA-approved labeling instructions. All of the following criteria must be fulfilled in order for Medicare coverage to be provided for a VAD used as a bridge-to-transplant:

a. The patient is approved and listed as a candidate for heart transplantation by a Medicare-approved heart transplant center; and,
b. The implanting site, if different than the Medicare-approved transplant center, must receive written permission from the Medicare-approved heart transplant center under which the patient is listed prior to implantation of the VAD.

The Medicare-approved heart transplant center should make every reasonable effort to transplant patients on such devices as soon as medically reasonable. Ideally, the Medicare-approved heart transplant centers should determine patient-specific timetables for transplantation, and should not maintain such patients on VADs if suitable hearts become available.

b. Artificial Heart as Bridge-to-Transplant (effective for services performed on or after May 1, 2008)

An artificial heart for bridge-to-transplantation is covered when performed under coverage with evidence development (CED) when a clinical study meets all of the criteria listed below.

The clinical study must address at least one of the following questions:

- Were there unique circumstances such as expertise available in a particular facility or an unusual combination of conditions in particular patients that affected their outcomes?
- What will be the average time to device failure when the device is made available to larger numbers of patients?
- Do results adequately give a reasonable indication of the full range of outcomes (both positive and negative) that might be expected from more widespread use?

The clinical study must meet all of the following criteria:

- The study must be reviewed and approved by the FDA.
- The principal purpose of the research study is to test whether a particular intervention potentially improves the participants' health outcomes.
- The research study is well supported by available scientific and medical information, or it is intended to clarify or

Medicare References

establish the health outcomes of interventions already in common clinical use.

- The research study does not unjustifiably duplicate existing studies.
- The research study design is appropriate to answer the research question being asked in the study.
- The research study is sponsored by an organization or individual capable of executing the proposed study successfully.
- The research study is in compliance with all applicable Federal regulations concerning the protection of human subjects found at 45 CFR Part 46. If a study is FDA-regulated it also must be in compliance with 21 CFR Parts 50 and 56.
- All aspects of the research study are conducted according to appropriate standards of scientific integrity (see http://www.icmje.org).
- The research study has a written protocol that clearly addresses, or incorporates by reference, the standards listed here as Medicare requirements for coverage with study participation (CSP) or CED coverage.
- The clinical research study is not designed to exclusively test toxicity or disease pathophysiology in healthy individuals. Trials of all medical technologies measuring therapeutic outcomes as one of the objectives meet this standard only if the disease or condition being studied is life threatening as defined in 21 CFR § 312.81(a) and the patient has no other viable treatment options.
- The clinical research study is registered on the ClinicalTrials.gov website by the principal sponsor/investigator as demonstrated by having a National Clinical Trial control number.
- The research study protocol specifies the method and timing of public release of all pre-specified outcomes to be measured including release of outcomes if outcomes are negative or study is terminated early. The results must be made public within 24 months of the end of data collection. If a report is planned to be published in a peer- reviewed journal, then that initial release may be an abstract that meets the requirements of the International Committee of Medical Journal Editors (http://www.icmje.org). However a full report of the outcomes must be made public no later than three (3) years after the end of data collection.
- The research study protocol must explicitly discuss subpopulations affected by the treatment under investigation, particularly traditionally underrepresented groups in clinical studies, how the inclusion and exclusion criteria effect enrollment of these populations, and a plan for the retention and reporting of said populations in the trial. If the inclusion and exclusion criteria are expected to have a negative effect on the recruitment or retention of underrepresented populations, the protocol must discuss why these criteria are necessary.

The research study protocol explicitly discusses how the results are or are not expected to be generalizable to the Medicare population to infer whether Medicare patients may benefit from the intervention. Separate discussions in the protocol may be necessary for populations eligible for Medicare due to age, disability, or Medicaid eligibility.

Consistent with section 1142 of the Social Security Act (the Act), the Agency for Healthcare Research and Quality (AHRQ) supports clinical research studies that CMS determines meet the above-listed standards and address the above-listed research questions.

The principal investigator of an artificial heart clinical study seeking Medicare payment should submit the following documentation to the Centers for Medicare & Medicaid Services (CMS) and should expect to be notified when the CMS review is complete:

- Complete study protocol (must be dated or identified with a version number);
- Protocol summary;
- Statement that the submitted protocol version has been agreed upon by the FDA;
- Statement that the above study standards are met;
- Statement that the study addresses at least one of the above questions related to artificial hearts;
- Complete contact information (phone number, email address, and mailing address); and,
- Clinicaltrials.gov registration number.

The above information should be mailed to:

Director, Coverage and Analysis Group Centers for Medicare and Medicaid Services Re: Artificial Heart Mailstop C1-09-06 7500 Security Blvd. Baltimore, MD 21244-1850

Clinical studies that are determined by CMS to meet the above requirements will be listed on the CMS Web site at: http://www.cms.hhs.gov/MedicareApprovedFacilitie/06_artificialhearts.asp..

Pub 100-3, 20.15 – Electrocardiographic Services

(Rev. 26, Issued: 12-10-04, Effective: 08-26-04, Implementation: 12-10-04)

A. General

1. An electrocardiogram (EKG) is a graphic representation of electrical activity within the heart. Electrodes placed on the body in predetermined locations sense this electrical activity, which is then recorded by various means for review and interpretation. EKG recordings are used to diagnose a wide range of heart disease and other conditions that manifest themselves by abnormal cardiac electrical activity.

   EKG services are covered diagnostic tests when there are documented signs and symptoms or other clinical indications for providing the service. Coverage includes the review and interpretation of EKGs only by a physician. There is no coverage for EKG services when rendered as a screening test or as part of a routine examination unless performed as part of the one-time, "Welcome to Medicare" preventive physical examination under section 611 of the Medicare Prescription Drug, Improvement, and Modernization Act of 2003.
2. Ambulatory electrocardiography (AECG) refers to services rendered in an outpatient setting over a specified period of time, generally while a patient is engaged in daily activities, including sleep. AECG devices are intended to provide the physician with documented episodes of arrhythmia, which may not be detected using a standard 12-lead EKG. AECG is most typically used to evaluate symptoms that may correlate with intermittent cardiac arrhythmias and/or myocardial ischemia. Such symptoms include syncope, dizziness, chest pain, palpitations, or shortness of breath. Additionally, AECG is used to evaluate patient response to initiation, revision, or discontinuation of arrhythmic drug therapy.
3. The Centers for Medicare & Medicaid Services (CMS), through the national coverage determination (NCD) process, may create new ambulatory EKG monitoring device categories if published, peer-reviewed clinical studies demonstrate evidence of improved clinical utility, or equal utility with additional advantage to the patient, as indicated by improved patient management and/or improved health outcomes in the Medicare population (such as superior ability to detect serious or life-threatening arrhythmias) as compared to devices or services in the currently described categories below.

Descriptions of Ambulatory EKG Monitoring Technologies

1. Dynamic electrocardiography devices that continuously record a real-time EKG, commonly known as Holter™ monitors, typically record over a 24-hour period. The recording is captured either on a magnetic tape or other digital medium. The data is then computer-analyzed at a later time, and a physician interprets the computer-generated report. A 24-hour recording is generally adequate to detect most transient arrhythmias. Documentation of medical necessity is required for monitoring longer than 24 hours. The recording device itself is not covered as durable medical equipment (DME) separate from the total diagnostic service.
2. An event monitor, or event recorder, is a patient-activated or event-activated EKG device that intermittently records cardiac arrhythmic events as they occur. The EKG is recorded on magnetic tape or other digital medium.

   Cardiac event monitor technology varies among different devices. For patient-activated event monitors, the patient initiates recording when symptoms appear or when instructed to do so by a physician (e.g., following exercise). For self-sensing, automatically triggered monitors, an EKG is automatically recorded when the device detects an arrhythmia, without patient intervention. Some devices permit a patient to transmit EKG data trans-telephonically (i.e., via telephone) to a receiving center where the data is reviewed. A technician may be available at these centers to review transmitted data 24-hours per day. In some instances, when the EKG is determined to be outside certain pre-set criteria by a technician or other non-physician, a physician is available 24-hours per day to review the transmitted data and to make clinical decisions regarding the patient. These services are known as "24-hour attended monitoring". In other instances, transmitted EKG data is reviewed at a later time and are, therefore, considered "non-attended."

Cardiac event monitors without trans-telephonic capability must be removed from the patient and taken to a location for review of the stored EKG data. Some devices also permit a "time sampling" mode of operation. The "time sampling" mode is not covered under ambulatory EKG monitoring technology. Some cardiac event monitoring devices with trans-telephonic capabilities require the patient to dial the phone number of a central EKG data reception center and initiate transmission of EKG data. Other devices use Internet-based in-home computers to capture and store EKG data. When such devices detect pre-programmed arrhythmias, data is automatically sent via modem and standard telephone lines to a central receiving center, or independent diagnostic testing facility (IDTF), where the data is reviewed. Internet-based in-home computer systems may also provide the receiving center with a daily computer-generated report that summarizes 24 hours of EKG data.

Certain cardiac event monitors capture electrical activity with a single electrode attached to the skin. Other devices may employ multiple electrodes in order to record more complex EKG tracings. Additionally, devices may be individually programmed to detect patient-specific factors, electrode malfunction, or other factors. Cardiac event monitors can be further categorized as either "pre-event" or "post-event" recorders, based on their memory capabilities:

a. Pre-symptom Memory Loop Recorder (MLR)
   Upon detecting symptoms, the wearer presses a button, which activates the recorder to save (i.e., memorize) an interval of pre-symptom EKG data along with data during and subsequent to the symptomatic event. Self-sensing recorders (also known as event-activated or automatic trigger) do not require patient input to capture these data. Single or multiple events may be recorded. The device is worn at all times, usually for up to 30 days.

   Implantable (or Insertable Loop) Recorder (ILR)

   Another type of pre-symptom MLR, it is implanted subcutaneously in a patient's upper left chest and may remain implanted for many months. An ILR is used when syncope is thought to be cardiac-related, but is too infrequent to be detected by either a Holter™ monitor or a traditional pre-symptom MLR.
b. Post-symptom Recorder
   The patient temporarily places this device against the chest when symptoms occur and activates it by pressing a button. These recorders represent old technology, as they do not include a memory loop. The device transmits EKG data telephonically in real-time and is usually used for up to 30 days.

B. Nationally Covered Indications

The following indications are covered nationally unless otherwise indicated:

1. Computer analysis of EKGs when furnished in a setting and under the circumstances required for coverage of other EKG services.
2. EKG services rendered by an independent diagnostic testing facility (IDTF), including physician review and interpretation. Separate physician services are not covered unless he/she is the patient's attending or consulting physician.
3. Emergency EKGs (i.e., when the patient is or may be experiencing a life-threatening event) performed as a laboratory or diagnostic service by a portable x-ray supplier only when a physician is in attendance at the time the service is performed or immediately thereafter.
4 Home EKG services with documentation of medical necessity.
5. Trans-telephonic EKG transmissions (effective March 1, 1980) as a diagnostic service for the indications described below, when performed with equipment meeting the standards described below, subject to the limitations and conditions specified below. Coverage is further limited to the amounts payable with respect to the physician's service in interpreting the results of such transmissions, including charges for rental of the equipment. The device used by the beneficiary is part of a total diagnostic system and is not considered DME separately. Covered uses are to:
   a. Detect, characterize, and document symptomatic transient arrhythmias;
   b. Initiate, revise, or discontinue arrhythmic drug therapy; or,
   c. Carry out early post-hospital monitoring of patients discharged after myocardial infarction (MI); (only if 24-hour coverage is provided, see C.5. below).

Certain uses other than those specified above may be covered if, in the judgment of the local contractor, such use is medically necessary.

Additionally, the transmitting devices must meet at least the following criteria:

a. They must be capable of transmitting EKG Leads, I, II, or III; and,
b. The tracing must be sufficiently comparable to a conventional EKG.

24-hour attended coverage used as early post-hospital monitoring of patients discharged after MI is only covered if provision is made for such 24-hour attended coverage in the manner described below:

24-hour attended coverage means there must be, at a monitoring site or central data center, an EKG technician or other non-physician, receiving calls and/or EKG data; tape recording devices do not meet this requirement. Further, such technicians should have immediate, 24-hour access to a physician to review transmitted data and make clinical decisions regarding the patient. The technician should also be instructed as to when and how to contact available facilities to assist the patient in case of emergencies.

C. Nationally Non-covered Indications

The following indications are non-covered nationally unless otherwise specified below:

1. The time-sampling mode of operation of ambulatory EKG cardiac event monitoring/recording.
2. Separate physician services other than those rendered by an IDTF unless rendered by the patient's attending or consulting physician.
3. Home EKG services without documentation of medical necessity.
4. Emergency EKG services by a portable x-ray supplier without a physician in attendance at the time of service or immediately thereafter.
5. 24-hour attended coverage used as early post-hospital monitoring of patients discharged after MI unless provision is made for such 24-hour attended coverage in the manner described in section B.5. above.
6. Any marketed Food and Drug Administration (FDA)-approved ambulatory cardiac monitoring device or service that cannot be categorized according to the framework below.

D. Other

Ambulatory cardiac monitoring performed with a marketed, FDA-approved device, is eligible for coverage if it can be categorized according to the framework below. Unless there is a specific NCD for that device or service, determination as to whether a device or service that fits into the framework is reasonable and necessary is according to local contractor discretion.

Electrocardiographic Services Framework

1. Patient/Event-Activated Intermittent Recorders
   A. Pre-symptom memory loop (Insertable or Non-insertable)
      a. Attended
      b. Non-attended
   B. Post-symptom (no memory loop)
      a. Non-attended

Medicare References

2. Non-Activated Continuous Recorders
   A. Dynamic Electrocardiography (e.g., Holter™ Monitor)
      a. Non-attended

(This NCD last reviewed December 2004.)

Pub 100-3, 20.19 – Ambulatory Blood Pressure Monitoring

(Rev. 2, 7-01-03)

Ambulatory blood pressure monitoring (ABPM) involves the use of a noninvasive device whichis used to measure blood pressure in 24-hour cycles. These 24-hour measurements are stored in the device and are later interpreted by the physician. ABPM must be performed for at least 24 hours to meet coverage criteria.

ABPM is only covered for those patients with suspected white coat hypertension. Suspected white coat hypertension is defined as

1. Office blood pressure > 140/90 mm Hg on at least three separate clinic/office visits with two separate measurements made at each visit;
2. At least two documented blood pressure measurements taken outside the office which are < 140/90 mm Hg; and
3. No evidence of end-organ damage.

The information obtained by ABPM is necessary in order to determine the appropriate management of the patient. ABPM is not covered for any other uses. In the rare circumstance that ABPM needs to be performed more than once in a patient, the qualifying criteria described above must be met for each subsequent ABPM test.

For those patients that undergo ABPM and have an ambulatory blood pressure of < 135/85 with no evidence of end-organ damage, it is likely that their cardiovascular risk is similar to that of normotensives. They should be followed over time. Patients for which ABPM demonstrates a blood pressure of > 135/85 may be at increased cardiovascular risk, and a physician may wish to consider antihypertensive therapy.

Pub 100-3, 20.20 – External Counterpulsation (ECP) for Severe Angina

(Rev. 2, 03-20-06)

A. General

External counterpulsation (ECP), commonly referred to as enhanced external counterpulsation, is a noninvasive outpatient treatment for coronary artery disease refractory to medical and/or surgical therapy. Although ECP devices are cleared by the Food and Drug Administration (FDA) for use in treating a variety of cardiac conditions, including stable or unstable angina pectoris, acute myocardial infarction and cardiogenic shock, the use of this device to treat cardiac conditions other than stable angina pectoris is not covered, since only that use has developed sufficient evidence to demonstrate its medical effectiveness. Non-coverage of hydraulic versions of these types of devices remains in force.

Indications and Limitations of Coverage

B. Nationally Covered Indications

Effective for services performed on or after July 1, 1999, coverage is provided for the use of ECP for patients who have been diagnosed with disabling angina (Class III or Class IV, Canadian Cardiovascular Society Classification or equivalent classification) who, in the opinion of a cardiologist or cardiothoracic surgeon, are not readily amenable to surgical intervention, such as PTCA or cardiac bypass, because:

- Their condition is inoperable, or at high risk of operative complications or post-operative failure;
- Their coronary anatomy is not readily amenable to such procedures; or
- They have co-morbid states which create excessive risk.

A full course of therapy usually consists of 35 one-hour treatments, which may be offered once or twice daily, usually 5 days per week. The patient is placed on a treatment table where their lower trunk and lower extremities are wrapped in a series of three compressive air cuffs which inflate and deflate in synchronization with the patient's cardiac cycle.

During diastole the three sets of air cuffs are inflated sequentially (distal to proximal) compressing the vascular beds within the muscles of the calves, lower thighs and upper thighs. This action results in an increase in diastolic pressure, generation of retrograde arterial blood flow and an increase in venous return. The cuffs are deflated simultaneously just prior to systole, which produces a rapid drop in vascular impedance, a decrease in ventricular workload and an increase in cardiac output.

The augmented diastolic pressure and retrograde aortic flow appear to improve myocardial perfusion, while systolic unloading appears to reduce cardiac workload and oxygen requirements. The increased venous return coupled with enhanced systolic flow appears to increase cardiac output. As a result of this treatment, most patients experience increased time until onset of ischemia, increased exercise tolerance, and a reduction in the number and severity of anginal episodes. Evidence was presented that this effect lasted well beyond the immediate post-treatment phase, with patients symptom-free for several months to two years. This procedure must be done under direct supervision of a physician.

C. Nationally Non-Covered Indications

All other cardiac conditions not otherwise specified as nationally covered for the use of ECP remain nationally non-covered. (This NCD last reviewed March 2006.)

Pub 100-3, 20.21 – Chelation Therapy for Treatment of Atherosclerosis

(Rev. 1, 10-03-03)

Chelation therapy is the application of chelation techniques for the therapeutic or preventive effects of removing unwanted metal ions from the body. The application of chelation therapy using ethylenediamine-tetra-acetic acid (EDTA) for the treatment and prevention of atherosclerosis is controversial. There is no widely accepted rationale to explain the beneficial effects attributed to this therapy. Its safety is questioned and its clinical effectiveness has never been established by well-designed, controlled clinical trials. It is not widely accepted and practiced by American physicians. EDTA chelation therapy for atherosclerosis is considered experimental. For these reasons, EDTA chelation therapy for the treatment or prevention of atherosclerosis is not covered.

Some practitioners refer to this therapy as chemoendarterectomy and may also show a diagnosis other than atherosclerosis, such as arteriosclerosis or calcinosis. Claims employing such variant terms should also be denied under this section.

Cross-reference: §20.22.

Pub 100-3, 20.22 – Ethylenediamine-Tetra-Acetic (EDTA) Chelation Therapy for Treatment of Atherosclerosis

(Rev. 1, 10-03-03)

The use of EDTA as a chelating agent to treat atherosclerosis, arteriosclerosis, calcinosis, or similar generalized condition not listed by the FDA as an approved use is not covered. Any such use of EDTA is considered experimental. See §20.21 for an explanation of this conclusion.

Pub 100-3, 20.23 – Fabric Wrapping of Abdominal Aneurysms

(Rev. 1, 10-03-03)

Not Covered

Fabric wrapping of abdominal aneurysms is not a covered Medicare procedure. This is a treatment for abdominal aneurysms which involves wrapping aneurysms with cellophane or fascia lata. This procedure has not been shown to prevent eventual rupture. In extremely rare instances, external wall reinforcement may be indicated when the current accepted treatment (excision of the aneurysm and reconstruction with synthetic materials) is not a viable alternative, but external wall reinforcement is not fabric wrapping. Accordingly, fabric wrapping of abdominal aneurysms is not considered reasonable and necessary within the meaning of §1862(a)(1) of the Act.

Pub 100-3, 20.24 – Displacement Cardiography

(Rev. 1, 10-03-03)

Displacement cardiography, including cardiokymography and photokymography, is a noninvasive diagnostic test used in evaluating coronary artery disease.

A Cardiokymography

Cardiokymography is covered for services rendered on or after October 12, 1988.

Cardiokymography is a covered service only when it is used as an adjunct to electrocardiographic stress testing in evaluating coronary artery disease and only when the following clinical indications are present:

- For male patients, atypical angina pectoris or nonischemic chest pain; or
- For female patients, angina, either typical or atypical.

B Photokymography – Not Covered

Photokymography remains excluded from coverage.

Pub 100-3, 20.29 – Hyperbaric Oxygen Therapy

(Rev. 2, 06-19-06)

Indications and Limitations of Coverage

A. Covered Conditions

Program reimbursement for HBO therapy will be limited to that which is administered in a chamber (including the one man unit) and is limited to the following conditions:

- Acute carbon monoxide intoxication,
- Decompression illness,
- Gas embolism,
- Gas gangrene,
- Acute traumatic peripheral ischemia. HBO therapy is a valuable adjunctive treatment to be used in combination with accepted standard therapeutic measures when loss of function, limb, or life is threatened.
- Crush injuries and suturing of severed limbs. As in the previous conditions, HBO therapy would be an adjunctive treatment when loss of function, limb, or life is threatened.
- Progressive necrotizing infections (necrotizing fasciitis),
- Acute peripheral arterial insufficiency,
- Preparation and preservation of compromised skin grafts (not for primary management of wounds),
- Chronic refractory osteomyelitis, unresponsive to conventional medical and surgical management,
- Osteoradionecrosis as an adjunct to conventional treatment,
- Soft tissue radionecrosis as an adjunct to conventional treatment,
- Cyanide poisoning,
- Actinomycosis, only as an adjunct to conventional therapy when the disease process is refractory to antibiotics and surgical treatment,
- Diabetic wounds of the lower extremities in patients who meet the following three criteria:
  - Patient has type I or type II diabetes and has a lower extremity wound that is due to diabetes;
  - Patient has a wound classified as Wagner grade III or higher; and
  - Patient has failed an adequate course of standard wound therapy.

The use of HBO therapy is covered as adjunctive therapy only after there are no measurable signs of healing for at least 30 –days of treatment with standard wound therapy and must be used in addition to standard wound care. Standard wound care in patients with diabetic wounds includes: assessment of a patient's vascular status and correction of any vascular problems in the affected limb if possible, optimization of nutritional status, optimization of glucose control, debridement by any means to remove devitalized tissue, maintenance of a clean, moist bed of granulation tissue with appropriate moist dressings, appropriate off-loading, and necessary treatment to resolve any infection that might be present. Failure to respond to standard wound care occurs when there are no measurable signs of healing for at least 30 consecutive days. Wounds must be evaluated at least every 30 days during administration of HBO therapy. Continued treatment with HBO therapy is not covered if measurable signs of healing have not been demonstrated within any 30-day period of treatment.

B. Noncovered Conditions

All other indications not specified under §270.4(A) are not covered under the Medicare program. No program payment may be made for any conditions other than those listed in §270.4(A).

No program payment may be made for HBO in the treatment of the following conditions:

- Cutaneous, decubitus, and stasis ulcers.
- Chronic peripheral vascular insufficiency.
- Anaerobic septicemia and infection other than clostridial.
- Skin burns (thermal).
- Senility.
- Myocardial infarction.
- Cardiogenic shock.
- Sickle cell anemia.
- Acute thermal and chemical pulmonary damage, i.e., smoke inhalation with pulmonary insufficiency.
- Acute or chronic cerebral vascular insufficiency.
- Hepatic necrosis.
- Aerobic septicemia.
- Nonvascular causes of chronic brain syndrome (Pick's disease, Alzheimer's disease, Korsakoff's disease).
- Tetanus.
- Systemic aerobic infection.
- Organ transplantation.
- Organ storage
- Pulmonary emphysema.
- Exceptional blood loss anemia.
- Multiple Sclerosis.
- Arthritic Diseases.
- Acute cerebral edema.

C. Topical Application of Oxygen

This method of administering oxygen does not meet the definition of HBO therapy as stated above. Also, its clinical efficacy has not been established. Therefore, no Medicare reimbursement may be made for the topical application of oxygen.

Pub 100-3, 30.1.1 – Biofeedback Therapy for the Treatment of Urinary Incontinence

(Rev. 1, 10-03-03)

Biofeedback Therapy for the Treatment of Urinary Incontinence

This policy applies to biofeedback therapy rendered by a practitioner in an office or other facility setting.

Biofeedback is covered for the treatment of stress and/or urge incontinence in cognitively intact patients who have failed a documented trial of pelvic muscle exercise (PME) training. Biofeedback is not a treatment, per se, but a tool to help patients learn how to perform PME. Biofeedback-assisted PME incorporates the use of an electronic or mechanical device to relay visual and/or auditory evidence of pelvic floor muscle tone, in order to improve awareness of pelvic floor musculature and to assist patients in the performance of PME.

A failed trial of PME training is defined as no clinically significant improvement in urinary incontinence after completing four weeks of an ordered plan of pelvic muscle exercises to increase periurethral muscle strength.

Contractors may decide whether or not to cover biofeedback as an initial treatment modality. Home use of biofeedback therapy is not covered.

Pub 100-3, 30.7 – Laetrile and Related Substances

(Rev. 1, 10-03-03)

Not Covered

Laetrile (and the other drugs called by the various terms mentioned below) have been used primarily in the treatment or control of cancer. Although the terms "Laetrile," "laetrile," "amygdalin," "Sarcarcinase," "vitamin B-17," and "nitriloside" have been used interchangeably, the chemical identity of the substances to which these terms refer has varied.

The FDA has determined that neither Laetrile nor any other drug called by the various terms mentioned above, nor any other product which might be characterized as a "nitriloside" is generally recognized (by experts qualified by scientific training and experience to evaluate the safety and effectiveness of drugs) to be safe and effective for any therapeutic use. Therefore, use of this drug cannot be considered to be reasonable and necessary within the meaning of §1862(a)(1) of the Act and program payment may not be made for its use or any services furnished in connection with its administration.

A hospital stay only for the purpose of having laetrile (or any other drug called by the terms mentioned above) administered is not covered. Also, program payment may not be made for laetrile (or other drug noted above) when it is used during the course of an otherwise covered hospital stay.

Pub 100-3, 30.8 – Cellular Therapy

(Rev. 1, 10-03-03)

Not Covered

Cellular therapy involves the practice of injecting humans with foreign proteins like the placenta or lungs of unborn lambs. Cellular therapy is without scientific or statistical evidence to document its therapeutic efficacy and, in fact, is considered a potentially dangerous practice. Accordingly, cellular therapy is not considered reasonable and necessary within the meaning of §1862 (a) (1) of the Act.

Pub 100-3, 40.2 – Home Blood Glucose Monitors

(Rev. 48, 06-19-06)

There are several different types of blood glucose monitors that use reflectance meters to determine blood glucose levels. Medicare coverage of these devices varies, with respect to both the type of device and the medical condition of the patient for whom the device is prescribed.

Reflectance colorimeter devices used for measuring blood glucose levels in clinical settings are not covered as durable medical equipment for use in the home because their need for frequent professional re-calibration makes them unsuitable for home use. However, some types of blood glucose monitors which use a reflectance meter specifically designed for home use by diabetic patients may be covered as durable medical equipment, subject to the conditions and limitations described below.

Blood glucose monitors are meter devices that read color changes produced on specially treated reagent strips by glucose concentrations in the patient's blood. The patient, using a disposable sterile lancet, draws a drop of blood, places it on a reagent strip and, following instructions which may vary with the device used, inserts it into the device to obtain a reading. Lancets, reagent strips, and other supplies necessary for the proper functioning of the device are also covered for patients for whom the device is indicated. Home blood glucose monitors enable certain patients to better control their blood glucose levels by frequently checking and appropriately contacting their attending physician for advice and treatment. Studies indicate that the patient's ability to carefully follow proper procedures is critical to obtaining satisfactory results with these devices. In addition, the cost of the devices, with their supplies, limits economical use to patients who must make frequent checks of their blood glucose levels. Accordingly, coverage of home blood glucose monitors is limited to patients meeting the following conditions:

1. The patient has been diagnosed as having diabetes;
2. The patient's physician states that the patient is capable of being trained to use the particular device prescribed in an appropriate manner. In some cases, the patient may not be able to perform this function, but a responsible individual can be trained to use the equipment and monitor the patient to assure that the intended effect is achieved. This is permissible if the record is properly documented by the patient's physician; and
3. The device is designed for home rather than clinical use.

There is also a blood glucose monitoring system designed especially for use by those with visual impairments. The monitors used in such systems are identical in terms of reliability and sensitivity to the standard blood glucose monitors described above. They differ by having such features as voice synthesizers, automatic timers, and specially designed arrangements of supplies and materials to enable the visually impaired to use the equipment without assistance.

These special blood glucose monitoring systems are covered under Medicare if the following conditions are met:

- The patient and device meet the three conditions listed above for coverage of standard home blood glucose monitors; and
- The patient's physician certifies that he or she has a visual impairment severe enough to require use of this special monitoring system.

The additional features and equipment of these special systems justify a higher reimbursement amount than allowed for standard blood glucose monitors. Separately identify claims for such devices and establish a separate reimbursement amount for them.

Pub 100-3, 40.5 – Treatment of Obesity

(Rev. 54, Effective: 02-21-06, Implementation: 05-30-06)

A. General

Obesity may be caused by medical conditions such as hypothyroidism, Cushing's disease, and hypothalamic lesions, or can aggravate a number of cardiac and respiratory diseases as well as diabetes and hypertension. Non-surgical services in connection with the treatment of obesity are covered when such services are an integral and necessary part of a course of treatment for one of these medical conditions. Certain designated surgical services for the treatment of obesity are covered for Medicare beneficiaries who have a BMI >35, have at least one co-morbidity related to obesity and have been previously unsuccessful with the medical treatment of obesity.

In addition, supplemented fasting is a type of very low calorie weight reduction regimen used to achieve rapid weight loss. The reduced calorie intake is supplemented by a mixture of protein, carbohydrates, vitamins, and minerals. Serious questions exist about the safety of prolonged adherence for 2 months or more to a very low calorie weight reduction regimen as a general treatment for obesity, because of instances of cardiopathology and sudden death, as well as possible loss of body protein.

Indications and Limitations of Coverage

B. Nationally Covered Indications

Certain designated surgical services for the treatment of obesity are covered for Medicare beneficiaries who have a BMI >35, have at least one co-morbidity related to obesity and have been previously unsuccessful with the medical treatment of obesity. See §100.1.

C. Nationally Noncovered Indications

1. Treatments for obesity alone remain non-covered.
2. Supplemented fasting is not covered under the Medicare program as a general treatment for obesity (see section D. below for discretionary local coverage).

D. Other

Where weight loss is necessary before surgery in order to ameliorate the complications posed by obesity when it coexists with pathological conditions such as cardiac and respiratory diseases, diabetes, or hypertension (and other more conservative techniques to achieve this end are not regarded as appropriate), supplemented fasting with adequate monitoring of the patient is eligible for coverage on a case-by-case basis or pursuant to a local coverage determination. The risks associated with the achievement of rapid weight loss must be carefully balanced against the risk posed by the condition requiring surgical treatment.

(This NCD last reviewed February 2006.)

See §§ 100.1, 100.8, 100.11

Pub 100-3, 50.1 – Speech Generating Devices

(Rev. 1, 10-03-03)

Effective January 1, 2001, augmentative and alternative communication devices or communicators which are hereafter referred to as "speech generating devices" are now considered to fall within the DME benefit category established by §1861(n) of the Social Security Act. They may be covered if the contractor's medical staff determines that the patient suffers from a severe speech impairment and that the medical condition warrants the use of a device based on the following definitions.

Definition of Speech Generating Devices

Speech generating devices are defined as speech aids that provide an individual who has a severe speech impairment with the ability to meet his functional speaking needs. Speech generating are characterized by:

- Being a dedicated speech device, used solely by the individual who has a severe speech impairment;
- May have digitized speech output, using prerecorded messages, less than or equal to 8 minutes recording time;
- May have digitized speech output, using prerecorded messages, greater than 8 minutes recording time;
- May have synthesized speech output which requires message formulation by spelling and device access by physical contact with the device-direct selection techniques;
- May have synthesized speech output which permits multiple methods of message formulation and multiple methods of device access; or
- May be software that allows a laptop computer, desktop computer or personal digital assistant (PDA) to function as a speech generating device.

Devices that would not meet the definition of speech generating devices and therefore, do not fall within the scope of §1861(n) of the Act are characterized by:

- Devices that are not dedicated speech devices, but are devices that are capable of running software for purposes other than for speech generation, e.g., devices that can also run a word processing package, an accounting program, or perform other than non-medical function.
- Laptop computers, desktop computers, or PDA's which may be programmed to perform the same function as a speech generating device, are noncovered since they are not primarily medical in nature and do not meet the definition of DME. For this reason, they cannot be considered speech-generating devices for Medicare coverage purposes.
- A device that is useful to someone without severe speech impairment is not considered a speech-generating device for Medicare coverage purposes.

Pub 100-3, 50.2 – Electronic Speech Aids

(Rev. 1, 10-03-03)

Electronic speech aids are covered under Part B as prosthetic devices when the patient has had a laryngectomy or his larynx is permanently inoperative. There are two types of speech aids. One operates by placing a vibrating head against the throat; the other amplifies sound waves through a tube which is inserted into the user's mouth. A patient who has had radical neck surgery and/or extensive radiation to the anterior part of the neck would generally be able to use only the "oral tube" model or one of the more sensitive and more expensive "throat contact" devices.

Cross-reference:

The **Medicare Benefit Policy Manual**, Chapter 15, "Covered Medical and Other Health Services," §120.

Pub 100-3, 50.3 – Cochlear Implantation

(Rev. 42, Implementation: 07/25/05)

A. General

A cochlear implant device is an electronic instrument, part of which is implanted surgically to stimulate auditory nerve fibers, and part of which is worn or carried by the individual to capture, analyze, and code sound. Cochlear implant devices are available in single-channel and multi-channel models. The purpose of implanting the device is to provide awareness and identification of sounds and to facilitate communication for persons who are moderately to profoundly hearing impaired.

B. Nationally Covered Indications

1. Effective for services performed on or after April 4, 2005, cochlear implantation may be covered for treatment of bilateral pre- or-post-linguistic, sensorineural, moderate-to-profound hearing loss in individuals who demonstrate limited benefit from amplification. Limited benefit from amplification is defined by test scores of less than or equal to 40% correct in the best-aided listening condition on tape-recorded tests of open-set sentence cognition. Medicare coverage is provided only for those patients who meet all of the following selection guidelines.
    - Diagnosis of bilateral moderate-to-profound sensorineural hearing impairment with limited benefit from appropriate hearing (or vibrotactile) aids;
    - Cognitive ability to use auditory clues and a willingness to undergo an extended program of rehabilitation;
    - Freedom from middle ear infection, an accessible cochlear lumen that is structurally suited to implantation, and freedom from lesions in the auditory nerve and acoustic areas of the central nervous system;
    - No contraindications to surgery; and
    - The device must be used in accordance with Food and Drug Administration (FDA)-approved labeling.
2. Effective for services performed on or after April 4, 2005, cochlear implantation may be covered for individuals meeting the selection guidelines above and with hearing test scores of greater than 40% and less than or equal to 60% only when the provider is participating in, and patients are enrolled in, either an FDA-approved category B investigational device exemption clinical trial as defined at 42 CFR 405.201, a trial under the Centers for Medicare & Medicaid (CMS) Clinical Trial Policy as defined at section 310.1 of the National Coverage Determinations Manual, or a prospective, controlled comparative trial approved by CMS as consistent with the evidentiary requirements for National Coverage Analyses and meeting specific quality standards.

C. Nationally Noncovered Indications

Medicare beneficiaries not meeting all of the coverage criteria for cochlear implantation listed are deemed not eligible for Medicare coverage under section 1862(a)(1)(A) of the Social Security Act.

D. Other

All other indications for cochlear implantation not otherwise indicated as nationally covered or non-covered above remain at local contractor discretion.

(This NCD last reviewed May 2005.)

Pub 100-3, 70.2 – Consultation Services Rendered by a Podiatrist in a Skilled Nursing Facility

(Rev. 1, 10-03-03)

Consultation services rendered by a podiatrist in a skilled nursing facility are covered if the services are reasonable and necessary and do not come within any of the specific statutory exclusions. Section 1862(a)(13) of the Act excludes payment for the treatment of flat foot conditions, the treatment of subluxations of the foot, and routine foot care. To determine whether the consultation comes within the foot care exclusions, apply the same rule as for initial diagnostic examinations, i.e., where services are performed in connection with specific symptoms or complaints which suggest the need for, covered services, the services are covered regardless of the resulting diagnosis. The exclusion of routine physician examinations is also pertinent and would generally exclude podiatric consultation performed on all patients in a skilled nursing facility on a routine basis for screening purposes, except in those cases where a specific foot ailment is involved. Section 1862(a)(7) of the Act excludes payment for routine physical checkups. (See the Medicare Benefit Policy Manual, Chapter 16, "General Exclusions from Coverage," §90 and §100.)

Pub 100-3, 80.1 – Hydrophilic Contact Lens for Corneal Bandage

(Rev. 1, 10-03-03)

Some hydrophilic contact lenses are used as moist corneal bandages for the treatment of acute or chronic corneal pathology, such as bulbous keratopathy, dry eyes, corneal ulcers and erosion, keratitis, corneal edema, descemetocele, corneal ectasis, Mooren's ulcer, anterior corneal dystrophy, neurotrophic keratoconjunctivitis, and for other therapeutic reasons.

Payment may be made under §1861(s)(2) of the Act for a hydrophilic contact lens approved by the Food and Drug Administration (FDA) and used as a supply incident to a physician's service. Payment for the lens is included in the payment for the physician's service to which the lens is incident. Contractors are authorized to accept an FDA letter of approval or other FDA published material as evidence of FDA approval. (See §80.4 for coverage of a hydrophilic contact lens as a prosthetic device.) See the Medicare Benefit Policy Manual, Chapter 15, "Covered Medical and Other Health Services," and the Medicare Benefit Policy Manual, Chapter 6, "Hospital Services Covered Under Part B," §20.4.

Pub 100-3, 80.2 – Photodynamic Therapy

(Rev. 9, 04-01-04)

Photodynamic therapy is a medical procedure which involves the infusion of a photosensitive (light-activated) drug with a very specific absorption peak. This drug is chemically designed to have a unique affinity for the diseased tissue intended for treatment. Once introduced to the body, the drug accumulates and is retained in diseased tissue to a greater degree than in normal tissue. Infusion is followed by the targeted irradiation of this tissue with a non-thermal laser, calibrated to emit light at a wavelength that corresponds to the drug's absorption peak. The drug then becomes active and locally treats the diseased tissue.

A. General

OPT is used in the treatment of ophthalmologic diseases; specifically, for age-related macular degeneration (AMD), a common eye disease among the elderly. OPT involves the infusion of an intravenous photosensitizing drug called verteporfin followed by exposure to a laser. OPT is only covered when used in conjunction with verteporfin.

Effective July 1, 2001, OPT with verteporfin was approved for a diagnosis of neovascular AMD with predominately classic subfoveal choroidal neovascularization (CNV) lesions (where the area of classic CNV occupies ≥50% of the area of the entire lesion) at the initial visit as determined by a fluorescein angiogram.

On October 17, 2001, CMS announced its "intent to cover" OPT with verteporfin for AMD patients with occult and no classic subfoveal CNV as determined by a fluorescein angiogram. The October 17, 2001, decision was never implemented.

On March 28, 2002, after thorough review and reconsideration of the October 17, 2001, intent to cover policy, CMS determined that the current noncoverage policy for OPT for verteporfin for AMD patients with occult and no classic subfoveal CNV as determined by a fluorescein angiogram should remain in effect.

Effective August 20, 2002, CMS issued a noncovered instruction for OPT with verteporfin for AMD patients with occult and no classic subfoveal CNV as determined by a fluorescein angiogram.

Indications and Limitations of Coverage

B. Covered Indications

Effective April 1, 2004, OPT with verteporfin continues to be approved for a diagnosis of neovascular AMD with predominately classic subfoveal CNV lesions (where the area of classic CNV occupies ≥50% of the area of the entire lesion) at the initial visit as determined by a fluorescein angiogram. (CNV lesions are comprised of classic and/or occult components.) Subsequent follow-up visits require a fluorescein angiogram prior to treatment. There are no requirements regarding visual acuity, lesion size, and number of re-treatments when treating predominantly classic lesions.

In addition, after thorough review and reconsideration of the August 20, 2002, noncoverage policy, CMS determines that the evidence is adequate to conclude that OPT with verteporfin is reasonable and necessary for treating:

- Subfoveal occult with no classic CNV associated with AMD; and,
- Subfoveal minimally classic CNV (where the area of classic CNV occupies <50% of the area of the entire lesion) associated with AMD.

The above 2 indications are considered reasonable and necessary only when:

- The lesions are small (4 disk areas or less in size) at the time of initial treatment or within the 3 months prior to initial treatment; and,
- The lesions have shown evidence of progression within the 3 months prior to initial treatment. Evidence of progression must be documented by deterioration of visual acuity (at least 5 letters on a standard eye examination chart), lesion growth (an increase in at least 1 disk area), or the appearance of blood associated with the lesion.

C. Noncovered Indications

Other uses of OPT with verteporfin to treat AMD not already addressed by CMS will continue to be noncovered. These include, but are not limited to, the following AMD indications:

- Juxtafoveal or extrafoveal CNV lesions (lesions outside the fovea),
- Inability to obtain a fluorescein angiogram,
- Atrophic or "dry" AMD.

D. Other

OPT with verteporfin for other ocular indications, such as pathologic myopia or presumed ocular histoplasmosis syndrome, continue to be eligible for local coverage determinations through individual contractor discretion.

Pub 100-3, 80.2.1 – Ocular Photodynamic Therapy (OPT)

(Rev 9, 04-01-04)

General

The OPT is used in the treatment of ophthalmologic diseases; specifically, for age-related macular degeneration (AMD), a common eye disease among the elderly. OPT involves the infusion of an intravenous photosensitizing drug called verteporfin followed by exposure to a laser. OPT is only covered when used in conjunction with verteporfin.

Effective July 1, 2001, OPT with verteporfin was approved for a diagnosis of neovascular AMD with predominately classic subfoveal choroidal neovascularization (CNV) lesions (where the area of classic CNV occupies ≥ 50% of the area of the entire lesion) at the initial visit as determined by a fluorescein angiogram. On October 17, 2001, CMS announced its "intent to cover" OPT with verteporfin for AMD patients with occult and no classic subfoveal CNV as determined by a fluorescein angiogram. The October 17, 2001, decision was never implemented.

On March 28, 2002, after thorough review and reconsideration of the October 17, 2001, intent to cover policy, CMS determined that the current noncoverage policy for OPT for verteporfin for AMD patients with occult and no classic subfoveal CNV as determined by a fluorescein angiogram should remain in effect.

Effective August 20, 2002, CMS issued a noncovered instruction for OPT with verteporfin for AMD patients with occult and no classic subfoveal CNV as determined by a fluorescein angiogram.

Covered Indications

Effective April 1, 2004, OPT with verteporfin continues to be approved for a diagnosis of neovascular AMD with predominately classic subfoveal CNV lesions (where the area of classic CNV occupies ≥ 50% of the area of the entire lesion) at the initial visit as determined by a fluorescein angiogram. (CNV lesions are comprised of classic and/or occult components.) Subsequent follow-up visits require a fluorescein angiogram prior to treatment. There are no requirements regarding visual acuity, lesion size, and number of re-treatments when treating predominantly classic lesions.

In addition, after thorough review and reconsideration of the August 20, 2002, noncoverage policy, CMS determines that the evidence is adequate to conclude that OPT with verteporfin is reasonable and necessary for treating:

- Subfoveal occult with no classic CNV associated with AMD; and,

- Subfoveal minimally classic CNV (where the area of classic CNV occupies <50% of the area of the entire lesion) associated with AMD.

The above 2 indications are considered reasonable and necessary only when:

- The lesions are small (4 disk areas or less in size) at the time of initial treatment or within the 3 months prior to initial treatment; and,
- The lesions have shown evidence of progression within the 3 months prior to initial treatment. Evidence of progression must be documented by deterioration of visual acuity (at least 5 letters on a standard eye examination chart), lesion growth (an increase in at least 1 disk area), or the appearance of blood associated with the lesion.

Noncovered Indications

Other uses of OPT with verteporfin to treat AMD not already addressed by CMS will continue to be noncovered. These include, but are not limited to, the following AMD indications:

- Juxtafoveal or extrafoveal CNV lesions (lesions outside the fovea),
- Inability to obtain a fluorescein angiogram,
- Atrophic or "dry" AMD.

Other

OPT with verteporfin for other ocular indications, such as pathologic myopia or presumed ocular histoplasmosis syndrome, continue to be eligible for local coverage determinations through individual contractor discretion.

(This NCD last reviewed March 2004.)

Pub 100-3, 80.3 – Photosensitive Drugs

(Rev. 2, 04-01-04)

Photosensitive drugs are the light-sensitive agents used in photodynamic therapy. Once introduced into the body, these drugs selectively identify and adhere to diseased tissue. The drugs remain inactive until they are exposed to a specific wavelength of light, by means of a laser, that corresponds to their absorption peak. The activation of a photosensitive drug results in a photochemical reaction which treats the diseased tissue without affecting surrounding normal tissue.

A. General

Verteporfin, a benzoporphyrin derivative, is an intravenous lipophilic photosensitive drug with an absorption peak of 690 nm. Verteporfin was first approved by the Food and Drug Administration on April 12, 2000, and subsequently approved for inclusion in the United States Pharmacopoeia on July 18, 2000, meeting Medicare's definition of a drug as defined under §1861(t)(1) of the Social Security Act. Verteporfin is only covered when used in conjunction with ocular photodynamic therapy OPT) when furnished intravenously incident to a physician's service.

Indications and Limitations of Coverage

B. Covered Indications

Effective April 1, 2004, OPT with verteporfin is covered for patients with a diagnosis of neovascular age-related macular degeneration (AMD) with:

- Predominately classic subfoveal choroidal neovascularization (CNV) lesions (where the area of classic CNV occupies ≥ 50% of the area of the entire lesion) at the initial visit as determined by a fluorescein angiogram. (CNV lesions are comprised of classic and/or occult components.) Subsequent follow-up visits require a fluorescein angiogram prior to treatment. There are no requirements regarding visual acuity, lesion size, and number of retreatments when treating predominantly classic lesions.
- Subfoveal occult with no classic associated with AMD.
- Subfoveal minimally classic CNV CNV (where the area of classic CNV occupies <50% of the area of the entire lesion) associated with AMD.

The above 2 indications are considered reasonable and necessary only when:

- The lesions are small (4 disk areas or less in size) at the time of initial treatment or within the 3 months prior to initial treatment;
- The lesions have shown evidence of progression within the 3 months prior to initial treatment. Evidence of progression must be documented by deterioration of visual acuity (at least 5 letters on a standard eye examination chart), lesion growth (an increase in at least 1 disk area), or the appearance of blood associated with the lesion.

C. Noncovered Indications

Other uses of OPT with verteporfin to treat AMD not already addressed by CMS will continue to be noncovered. These include, but are not limited to, the following AMD indications: juxtafoveal or extrafoveal CNV lesions (lesions outside the fovea), inability to obtain a fluorescein angiogram, or atrophic or "dry" AMD.

D. Other

OPT with verteporfin for other ocular indications, such as pathologic myopia or presumed ocular histoplasmosis syndrome, continue to be eligible for local coverage determinations through individual contractor discretion.

Pub 100-3, 80.3.1 – Verteporfin

(Rev 9, 04-01-04)

General

Verteporfin, a benzoporphyrin derivative, is an intravenous lipophilic photosensitive drug with an absorption peak of 690 nm. Verteporfin was first approved by the Food and Drug Administration on April 12, 2000, and subsequently approved for inclusion in the United States Pharmacopoeia on July 18, 2000, meeting Medicare's definition of a drug as defined under §1861(t)(1) of the Social Security Act. Verteporfin is only covered when used in conjunction with ocular photodynamic therapy OPT) when furnished intravenously incident to a physician's service.

Covered Indications

Effective April 1, 2004, OPT with verteporfin is covered for patients with a diagnosis of neovascular age-related macular degeneration (AMD) with:

- Predominately classic subfoveal choroidal neovascularization (CNV) lesions (where the area of classic CNV occupies ≥ 50% of the area of the entire lesion) at the initial visit as determined by a fluorescein angiogram. (CNV lesions are comprised of classic and/or occult components.) Subsequent follow-up visits require a fluorescein angiogram prior to treatment. There are no requirements regarding visual acuity, lesion size, and number of retreatments when treating predominantly classic lesions.
- Subfoveal occult with no classic associated with AMD.
- Subfoveal minimally classic CNV CNV (where the area of classic CNV occupies <50% of the area of the entire lesion) associated with AMD.
- The above 2 indications are considered reasonable and necessary only when:
  - The lesions are small (4 disk areas or less in size) at the time of initial treatment or within the 3 months prior to initial treatment; and,
  - The lesions have shown evidence of progression within the 3 months prior to initial treatment. Evidence of progression must be documented by deterioration of visual acuity (at least 5 letters on a standard eye examination chart), lesion growth (an increase in at least 1 disk area), or the appearance of blood associated with the lesion.

Noncovered Indications

Other uses of OPT with verteporfin to treat AMD not already addressed by CMS will continue to be noncovered. These include, but are not limited to, the following AMD indications: juxtafoveal or extrafoveal CNV lesions (lesions outside the fovea), inability to obtain a fluorescein angiogram, or atrophic or "dry" AMD.

Other

OPT with verteporfin for other ocular indications, such as pathologic myopia or presumed ocular histoplasmosis syndrome, continue to be eligible for local coverage determinations through individual contractor discretion.

(This NCD last reviewed March 2004.)

Pub 100-3, 80.4 – Hydrophilic Contact Lenses

(Rev. 1, 10-03-03)

Hydrophilic contact lenses are eyeglasses within the meaning of the exclusion in §1862(a)(7) of the Act and are not covered when used in the treatment of nondiseased eyes with spherical ametrophia, refractive astigmatism, and/or corneal astigmatism. Payment may be made under the prosthetic device benefit, however, for hydrophilic contact lenses when prescribed for an aphakic patient.

Contractors are authorized to accept an FDA letter of approval or other FDA published material as evidence of FDA approval. (See §80.1 for coverage of a hydrophilic lens as a corneal bandage.)

Cross-references:

The **Medicare Benefit Policy Manual**, Chapter 15, "Covered Medical and Other Health Services," §100 and §120.

The **Medicare Benefit Policy Manual**, Chapter 16, "General Exclusions from Coverage," §20 and §90.

Pub 100-3, 80.5 – Scleral Shell

(Rev. 1, 10-03-03)

Scleral shell (or shield) is a catchall term for different types of hard scleral contact lenses.

A scleral shell fits over the entire exposed surface of the eye as opposed to a corneal contact lens which covers only the central non-white area encompassing the pupil and iris. Where an eye has been rendered sightless and shrunken by inflammatory disease, a scleral shell may, among other things, obviate the need for surgical enucleation and prosthetic implant and act to support the surrounding orbital tissue.

In such a case, the device serves essentially as an artificial eye. In this situation, payment may be made for a scleral shell under §1861(s)(8) of the Act.

Scleral shells are occasionally used in combination with artificial tears in the treatment of "dry eye" of diverse etiology. Tears ordinarily dry at a rapid rate, and are continually replaced by the lacrimal gland. When the lacrimal gland fails, the half-life of artificial tears may be greatly prolonged by the use of the scleral contact lens as a protective barrier against the drying action of the atmosphere. Thus, the difficult and sometimes hazardous process of frequent installation of artificial tears may be avoided. The lens acts in this instance to substitute, in part, for the functioning of the diseased lacrimal gland and would be covered as a prosthetic device in the rare case when it is used in the treatment of "dry eye."

Cross-references:

The **Medicare Benefit Policy Manual**, Chapter 15, "Covered Medical and Other Health Services," §120 and §130

The **Medicare Benefit Policy Manual**, Chapter 1, "Inpatient Hospital Services," §40 and §120.1.

Pub 100-3, 80.12 – Intraocular Lenses (IOLs)

(Rev. 1, 10-03-03)

An intraocular lens, or pseudophakos, is an artificial lens which may be implanted to replace the natural lens after cataract surgery. Intraocular lens implantation services, as well as the lens itself, may be covered if reasonable and necessary for the individual. Implantation services may include hospital, surgical, and other medical services, including preimplantation ultrasound (A-scan) eye measurement of one or both eyes.

Cross-reference:

The **Medicare Benefit Policy Manual**, Chapter 6,"Hospital Services Covered Under Part B," §10.

The **Medicare Benefit Policy Manual**, Chapter 15, "Covered Medical and Other Health Services," §120.

The **Medicare Benefit Policy Manual**, Chapter 16, "General Exclusions from Coverage," §20 and §90.

100.6 – Gastric Freezing

(Rev. 1, 10-03-03)

Gastric freezing for chronic peptic ulcer disease is a non-surgical treatment which was popular about 20 years ago but now is seldom done. It has been abandoned due to a high complication rate, only temporary improvement experienced by patients, and lack of effectiveness when tested by double-blind, controlled clinical trials. Since the procedure is now considered obsolete, it is not covered.

Pub 100-3, 110.2 – Certain Drugs Distributed by the National Cancer Institute

(Rev. 1, 10-03-03)

Under its Cancer Therapy Evaluation, the Division of Cancer Treatment of the National Cancer Institute (NCI), in cooperation with the Food and Drug Administration, approves and distributes certain drugs for use in treating terminally ill cancer patients. One group of these drugs, designated as Group C drugs, unlike other drugs distributed by the NCI, are not limited to use in clinical trials for the purpose of testing their efficacy. Drugs are classified as Group C drugs only if there is sufficient evidence demonstrating their efficacy within a tumor type and that they can be safely administered.

A physician is eligible to receive Group C drugs from the Division of Cancer Treatment only if the following requirements are met:

- A physician must be registered with the NCI as an investigator by having completed an FD-Form 1573;
- A written request for the drug, indicating the disease to be treated, must be submitted to the NCI;
- The use of the drug must be limited to indications outlined in the NCIs guidelines; and
- All adverse reactions must be reported to the Investigational Drug Branch of the Division of Cancer Treatment.

In view of these NCI controls on distribution and use of Group C drugs, intermediaries may assume, in the absence of evidence to the contrary, that a Group C drug and the related hospital stay are covered if all other applicable coverage requirements are satisfied.

If there is reason to question coverage in a particular case, the matter should be resolved with the assistance of the Quality Improvement Organization (QIO), or if there is none, the assistance of the contractor's medical consultants.

Information regarding those drugs which are classified as Group C drugs may be obtained from:

Office of the Chief, Investigational Drug Branch
Division of Cancer Treatment, CTEP, Landow Building
Room 4C09, National Cancer Institute
Bethesda, Maryland 20205

Pub 100-3, 110.3 – Anti-Inhibitor Coagulant Complex (AICC)

(Rev. 1, 10-03-03)

Anti-inhibitor coagulant complex, AICC, is a drug used to treat hemophilia in patients with factor VIII inhibitor antibodies. AICC has been shown to be safe and effective and has Medicare coverage when furnished to patients with hemophilia A and inhibitor antibodies to factor VIII who have major bleeding episodes and who fail to respond to other, less expensive therapies.

Pub 100-3, 110.8 – Blood Platelet Transfusions

(Rev. 1, 10-03-03)

Blood platelet transplants are safe and effective for the correction of thrombocytopenia and other blood defects. It is covered under Medicare when treatment is reasonable and necessary for the individual patient.

Pub 100-3, 110.8.1 – Stem Cell Transplantation

(Rev. 45, Effective: 11-28-05, Implementation: 01-03-06)

A. General

Stem cell transplantation is a process in which stem cells are harvested from either a patient's or donor's bone marrow or peripheral blood for intravenous infusion. Autologous stem cell transplants (AuSCT) must be used to effect hematopoietic reconstitution following severely myelotoxic doses of chemotherapy (HDCT) and/or radiotherapy used to treat various malignancies. Allogeneic stem cell transplant may also be used to restore function in recipients having an inherited or acquired deficiency or defect.

The CMS is clarifying that bone marrow and peripheral blood stem cell transplantation is a process which includes mobilization, harvesting, and transplant of bone marrow or peripheral blood stem cells and the administration of high dose chemotherapy or radiotherapy prior to the actual transplant. When bone marrow or peripheral blood stem cell transplantation is covered, all necessary steps are included in coverage. When bone marrow or peripheral blood stem cell transplantation is non-covered, none of the steps are covered.

Indications and Limitations of Coverage

1 Allogeneic Stem Cell Transplantation

Allogeneic stem cell transplantation is a procedure in which a portion of a healthy donor's stem cell or bone marrow is obtained and prepared for intravenous infusion.

a. Covered Indications

The following uses of allogeneic bone marrow transplantation are covered under Medicare:

- Effective for services performed on or after August 1, 1978, for the treatment of leukemia, leukemia in remission, or aplastic anemia when it is reasonable and necessary; and
- Effective for services performed on or after June 3, 1985, for the treatment of severe combined immunodeficiency disease (SCID), and for the treatment of Wiskott-Aldrich syndrome.

b. Noncovered Indications

Effective for services performed on or after May 24, 1996, allogeneic stem cell transplantation is not covered as treatment for multiple myeloma.

2. Autologous Stem Cell Transplantation (AuSCT)

Autologous stem cell transplantation (AuSCT) is a technique for restoring stem cells using the patient's own previously stored cells.

a. Covered Indications

Effective for services performed on or after April 28, 1989, AuSCT is considered reasonable and necessary under §1862(a)(1)(A) of the Social Security Act (the Act) for the following conditions and is covered under Medicare for patients with:

- Acute leukemia in remission who have a high probability of relapse and who have no human leucocyte antigens (HLA)-matched;
- Resistant non-Hodgkin's lymphomas or those presenting with poor prognostic features following an initial response;
- Recurrent or refractory neuroblastoma; or
- Advanced Hodgkin's disease who have failed conventional therapy and have no HLA-matched donor.

Effective October 1, 2000, single AuSCT is only covered for Durie-Salmon Stage II or III patients that fit the following requirements:

- Newly diagnosed or responsive multiple myeloma. This includes those patients with previously untreated disease, those with at least a partial response to prior chemotherapy (defined as a 50% decrease either in measurable paraprotein [serum and/or urine] or in bone marrow infiltration, sustained for at least 1 month), and those in responsive relapse; and
- Adequate cardiac, renal, pulmonary, and hepatic function.

Effective for services performed on or after March 15, 2005, when recognized clinical risk factors are employed to select patients for transplantation, high dose melphalan (HDM) together with AuSCT is reasonable and necessary for Medicare beneficiaries of any age group with primary amyloid light chain (AL) amyloidosis who meet the following criteria:

- Amyloid deposition in 2 or fewer organs; and,
- Cardiac left ventricular ejection fraction (EF) greater than 45%.

b. Noncovered Indications

Insufficient data exist to establish definite conclusions regarding the efficacy of AuSCT for the following conditions:

- Acute leukemia not in remission;
- Chronic granulocytic leukemia;
- Solid tumors (other than neuroblastoma);
- Up to October 1, 2000, multiple myeloma;
- Tandem transplantation (multiple rounds of AuSCT) for patients with multiple myeloma;
- Effective October 1, 2000, non primary AL amyloidosis; and,
- Effective October 1, 2000, thru March 14, 2005, primary AL amyloidosis for Medicare beneficiaries age 64 or older.

In these cases, AuSCT is not considered reasonable and necessary within the meaning of §1862(a)(1)(A) of the Act and is not covered under Medicare.

B. Other

All other indications for stem cell transplantation not otherwise noted above as covered or noncovered nationally remain at local contractor discretion.

(This NCD last reviewed November 2005.)

Pub 100-3, 140.2 – Breast Reconstruction Following Mastectomy

(Rev. 1, 10-03-03)

During recent years, there has been a considerable change in the treatment of diseases of the breast such as fibrocystic disease and cancer. While extirpation of the disease remains of primary importance, the quality of life following initial treatment is increasingly recognized as of great concern. The increased use of breast reconstruction procedures is due to several factors:

- A change in epidemiology of breast cancer, including an apparent increase in incidence;
- Improved surgical skills and techniques;
- The continuing development of better prostheses; and
- Increasing awareness by physicians of the importance of postsurgical psychological adjustment.

Reconstruction of the affected and the contralateral unaffected breast following a medically necessary mastectomy is considered a relatively safe and effective noncosmetic procedure. Accordingly, program payment may be made for breast reconstruction surgery following removal of a breast for any medical reason.

Program payment may not be made for breast reconstruction for cosmetic reasons. (Cosmetic surgery is excluded from coverage under §1862(a)(10) of the Act.)

Pub 100-3, 150.2 – Osteogenic Stimulator

(Rev.41, Issued: 06-24-05, Effective: 04-27-05, Implementation: 08-01-05)

Electrical Osteogenic Stimulators

A. General

Electrical stimulation to augment bone repair can be attained either invasively or non-invasively. Invasive devices provide electrical stimulation directly at the fracture site either through percutaneously placed cathodes or by implantation of a coiled cathode wire into the fracture site. The power pack for the latter device is implanted into soft tissue near the fracture site and subcutaneously connected to the cathode, creating a self-contained system with no external components. The power supply for the former device is externally placed and the leads connected to the inserted cathodes. With the non-invasive device, opposing pads, wired to an external power supply, are placed over the cast. An electromagnetic field is created between the pads at the fracture site.

B. Nationally Covered Indications

1. Noninvasive Stimulator

The noninvasive stimulator device is covered only for the following indications:

- Nonunion of long bone fractures;
- Failed fusion, where a minimum of 9 months has elapsed since the last surgery;
- Congenital pseudarthroses;

Medicare References

- Effective July 1, 1996, as an adjunct to spinal fusion surgery for patients at high risk of pseudarthrosis due to previously failed spinal fusion at the same site or for those undergoing multiple level fusion. A multiple level fusion involves 3 or more vertebrae (e.g., L3-L5, L4-S1, etc).
- Effective September 15, 1980, nonunion of long bone fractures is considered to exist only after 6 or more months have elapsed without healing of the fracture.
- Effective April 1, 2000, nonunion of long bone fractures is considered to exist only when serial radiographs have confirmed that fracture healing has ceased for 3 or more months prior to starting treatment with the electrical osteogenic stimulator. Serial radiographs must include a minimum of 2 sets of radiographs, each including multiple views of the fracture site, separated by a minimum of 90 days.

2. Invasive (Implantable) Stimulator

The invasive stimulator device is covered only for the following indications:

- Nonunion of long bone fractures;
- Effective July 1, 1996, as an adjunct to spinal fusion surgery for patients at high risk of pseudarthrosis due to previously failed spinal fusion at the same site or for those undergoing multiple level fusion. A multiple level fusion involves 3 or more vertebrae (e.g., L3-L5, L4-S1, etc).
- Effective September 15, 1980, nonunion of long bone fractures is considered to exist only after 6 or more months have elapsed without healing of the fracture.
- Effective April 1, 2000, nonunion of long bone fractures is considered to exist only when serial radiographs have confirmed that fracture healing has ceased for 3 or more months prior to starting treatment with the electrical osteogenic stimulator. Serial radiographs must include a minimum of 2 sets of radiographs, each including multiple views of the fracture site, separated by a minimum of 90 days.

Ultrasonic Osteogenic Stimulators

A. General

An ultrasonic osteogenic stimulator is a noninvasive device that emits low intensity, pulsed ultrasound. The device is applied to the surface of the skin at the fracture site and ultrasound waves are emitted via a conductive coupling gel to stimulate fracture healing. The ultrasonic osteogenic stimulators are not be used concurrently with other non-invasive osteogenic devices.

B. Nationally Covered Indications

Effective January 1, 2001, ultrasonic osteogenic stimulators are covered as medically reasonable and necessary for the treatment of nonunion fractures. In demonstrating non-union fractures, CMS expects:

- A minimum of 2 sets of radiographs, obtained prior to starting treatment with the osteogenic stimulator, separated by a minimum of 90 days. Each radiograph set must include multiple views of the fracture site accompanied with a written interpretation by a physician stating that there has been no clinically significant evidence of fracture healing between the 2 sets of radiographs; and,
- Indications that the patient failed at least one surgical intervention for the treatment of the fracture.
- Effective April 27, 2005, upon reconsideration of ultrasound stimulation for nonunion fracture healing, CMS determines that the evidence is adequate to conclude that noninvasive ultrasound stimulation for the treatment of nonunion bone fractures prior to surgical intervention is reasonable and necessary. In demonstrating non-union fractures, CMS expects:
- A minimum of 2 sets of radiographs, obtained prior to starting treatment with the osteogenic stimulator, separated by a minimum of 90 days. Each radiograph set must include multiple views of the fracture site accompanied with a written interpretation by a physician stating that there has been no clinically significant evidence of fracture healing between the 2 sets of radiographs.

C. Nationally Non-Covered Indications

- Nonunion fractures of the skull, vertebrae and those that are tumor-related are excluded from coverage.
- Ultrasonic osteogenic stimulators may not be used concurrently with other non-invasive osteogenic devices.
- Ultrasonic osteogenic stimulators for fresh fractures and delayed unions remains non-covered.

(This NCD last reviewed June 2005.)

Pub 100-3, 150.3 – Bone (Mineral) Density Studies

(Rev. 69, Issued: 05-11-07, Effective: 01-01-07, Implementation: 07-02-07))

Conditions for coverage of bone mass measurements are now contained in Chapter 15, Section 80.5 of Pub. 100-02, **Medicare Benefit Policy Manual**. Claims processing instructions can be found in Chapter 13, Section 140 of Pub. 100-04, **Medicare Claims Processing Manual**.

Pub 100-3, 150.6 – Vitamin B12 Injections to Strengthen Tendons, Ligaments, etc., of the Foot

(Rev. 1, 10-03-03)

Not Covered

Vitamin B12 injections to strengthen tendons, ligaments, etc., of the foot are not covered under Medicare because (1) there is no evidence that vitamin B12 injections are effective for the purpose of strengthening weakened tendons and ligaments, and (2) this is nonsurgical treatment under the subluxation exclusion. Accordingly, vitamin B12 injections are not considered reasonable and necessary within the meaning of §1862(a)(1) of the Act.

Cross reference:

The **Medicare Benefit Policy Manual**, Chapter 1, "Inpatient Hospital Services," §30.

The **Medicare Benefit Policy Manual**, Chapter 16, "General Exclusions from Coverage," §100.

Pub 100-3, 150.7 – Prolotherapy, Joint Sclerotherapy, and Ligamentous Injections with Sclerosing Agents

(Rev. 1, 10-03-03)

Not Covered

The medical effectiveness of the above therapies has not been verified by scientifically controlled studies. Accordingly, reimbursement for these modalities should be denied on the ground that they are not reasonable and necessary as required by §1862(a)(1) of the Act.

Pub 100-3, 160.2 – Treatment of Motor Function Disorders with Electric Nerve Stimulation

(Rev. 2, 04-01-06)

Not Covered

While electric nerve stimulation has been employed to control chronic intractable pain for some time, its use in the treatment of motor function disorders, such as multiple sclerosis, is a recent innovation, and the medical effectiveness of such therapy has not been verified by scientifically controlled studies.

Where electric nerve stimulation is employed to treat motor function disorders, no reimbursement may be made for the stimulator or for the services related to its implantation since this treatment cannot be considered reasonable and necessary.

Note: For Medicare coverage of deep brain stimulation for essential tremor and Parkinson's disease, see §160.24 of the NCD Manual.

Pub 100-3, Pub 100-3, 160.7 – Electrical Nerve Stimulators

(Rev. 1, 10-03-03)

Two general classifications of electrical nerve stimulators are employed to treat chronic intractable pain: peripheral nerve stimulators and central nervous system stimulators.

A. Implanted Peripheral Nerve Stimulators

Payment may be made under the prosthetic device benefit for implanted peripheral nerve stimulators. Use of this stimulator involves implantation of electrodes around a selected peripheral nerve. The stimulating electrode is connected by an insulated lead to a receiver unit which is implanted under the skin at a depth not greater than 1/2 inch. Stimulation is induced by a generator connected to an antenna unit which is attached to the skin surface over the receiver unit. Implantation of electrodes requires surgery and usually necessitates an operating room.

Note: Peripheral nerve stimulators may also be employed to assess a patient's suitability for continued treatment with an electric nerve stimulator. As explained in §160.7.1, such use of the stimulator is covered as part of the total diagnostic service furnished to the beneficiary rather than as a prosthesis.

B. Central Nervous System Stimulators (Dorsal Column and Depth Brain Stimulators)

The implantation of central nervous system stimulators may be covered as therapies for the relief of chronic intractable pain, subject to the following conditions:

1. Types of Implantations
   There are two types of implantations covered by this instruction:
   - Dorsal Column (Spinal Cord) Neurostimulation – The surgical implantation of neurostimulator electrodes within the dura mater (endodural) or the percutaneous insertion of electrodes in the epidural space is covered.
   - Depth Brain Neurostimulation – The stereotactic implantation of electrodes in the deep brain (e.g., thalamus and periaqueductal gray matter) is covered.
2. Conditions for Coverage
   No payment may be made for the implantation of dorsal column or depth brain stimulators or services and supplies related to such implantation, unless all of the conditions listed below have been met:
   - The implantation of the stimulator is used only as a late resort (if not a last resort) for patients with chronic intractable pain;
   - With respect to item a, other treatment modalities (pharmacological, surgical, physical, or psychological therapies) have been tried and did not prove satisfactory, or are judged to be unsuitable or contraindicated for the given patient;
   - Patients have undergone careful screening, evaluation and diagnosis by a multidisciplinary team prior to implantation. (Such screening must include psychological, as well as physical evaluation);
   - All the facilities, equipment, and professional and support personnel required for the proper diagnosis, treatment training, and follow up of the patient (including that required to satisfy item c) must be available; and
   - Demonstration of pain relief with a temporarily implanted electrode precedes permanent implantation.

Contractors may find it helpful to work with Quality Improvement Organizatins (QIOs) to obtain the information needed to apply these conditions to claims.

See the **Medicare Benefit Policy Manual**, Chapter 15, "Covered Medical and Other Health Services," §120, and the following sections in this manual, §§160.2 and 30.1.

Pub 100-3, 160.7.1 – Assessing Patients Suitability for Electrical Nerve Stimulation Therapy

(Rev. 48, Issued: 03-17-06; Effective/Implementation Dates: 06-19-06)

Electrical nerve stimulation is an accepted modality for assessing a patient's suitability for ongoing treatment with a transcutaneous or an implanted nerve stimulator.

Accordingly, program payment may be made for the following techniques when used to determine the potential therapeutic usefulness of an electrical nerve stimulator:

A. Transcutaneous Electrical Nerve Stimulation (TENS)

This technique involves attachment of a transcutaneous nerve stimulator to the surface of the skin over the peripheral nerve to be stimulated. It is used by the patient on a trial basis and its effectiveness in modulating pain is monitored by the physician, or physical therapist. Generally, the physician or physical therapist is able to determine whether the patient is likely to derive a significant therapeutic benefit from continuous use of a transcutaneous stimulator within a trial period of one month; in a few cases this determination may take longer to make. Document the medical necessity for such services which are furnished beyond the first month. (See ¤160.13 for an explanation of coverage of medically necessary supplies for the effective use of TENS.)

If TENS significantly alleviates pain, it may be considered as primary treatment; if it produces no relief or greater discomfort than the original pain electrical nerve stimulation therapy is ruled out. However, where TENS produces incomplete relief, further evaluation with percutaneous electrical nerve stimulation may be considered to determine whether an implanted peripheral nerve stimulator would provide significant relief from pain.

Usually, the physician or physical therapist providing the services will furnish the equipment necessary for assessment. Where the physician or physical therapist advises the patient to rent the TENS from a supplier during the trial period rather than supplying it himself/herself, program payment may be made for rental of the TENS as well as for the services of the physician or physical therapist who is evaluating its use. However, the combined program payment which is made for the physician's or physical therapist's services and the rental of the stimulator from a supplier should not exceed the amount which would be payable for the total service, including the stimulator, furnished by the physician or physical therapist alone.

B. Percutaneous Electrical Nerve Stimulation (PENS)

This diagnostic procedure which involves stimulation of peripheral nerves by a needle electrode inserted through the skin is performed only in a physician's office, clinic, or hospital outpatient department. Therefore, it is covered only when performed by a physician or incident to physician's service. If pain is effectively controlled by percutaneous stimulation, implantation of electrodes is warranted.

As in the case of TENS (described in subsection A), generally the physician should be able to determine whether the patient is likely to derive a significant therapeutic benefit from continuing use of an implanted nerve stimulator within a trial period of 1 month. In a few cases, this determination may take longer to make. The medical necessity for such diagnostic services which are furnished beyond the first month must be documented.

NOTE: Electrical nerve stimulators do not prevent pain but only alleviate pain as it occurs. A patient can be taught how to employ the stimulator, and once this is done, can use it safely and effectively without direct physician supervision. Consequently, it is inappropriate for a patient to visit his/her physician, physical therapist, or an outpatient clinic on a continuing basis for treatment of pain with electrical nerve stimulation. Once it is determined that electrical nerve stimulation should be continued as therapy and the patient has been trained to use the stimulator, it is expected that a stimulator will be implanted or the patient will employ the TENS on a continual basis in his/her home. Electrical nerve stimulation treatments furnished by a physician in his/her office, by a physical therapist or outpatient clinic are excluded from coverage by section1862(a)(1) of the Act. (See section 160.7 for an explanation of coverage of the therapeutic use of implanted peripheral nerve stimulators under the prosthetic devices benefit. See section 280.13 for an explanation of coverage of the therapeutic use of TENS under the durable medical equipment benefit.)

Pub 100-3, 160.12 – Neuromuscular Electrical Stimulator (NMES)

(Rev. 55, 10-01-06)

NMES involves the use of a device which transmits an electrical impulse to the skin over selected muscle groups by way of electrodes. There are two broad categories of NMES. One type of device stimulates the muscle when the patient is in a resting state to treat muscle atrophy. The second type is used to enhance functional activity of neurologically impaired patients.

Medicare References

Treatment of Muscle Atrophy

Coverage of NMES to treat muscle atrophy is limited to the treatment of disuse atrophy where nerve supply to the muscle is intact, including brain, spinal cord and peripheral nerves, and other non-neurological reasons for disuse atrophy. Some examples would be casting or splinting of a limb, contracture due to scarring of soft tissue as in burn lesions, and hip replacement surgery (until orthotic training begins). (See §160.13 of the NCD Manual for an explanation of coverage of medically necessary supplies for the effective use of NMES.)

Use for Walking in Patients with Spinal Cord Injury (SCI)

The type of NMES that is use to enhance the ability to walk of SCI patients is commonly referred to as functional electrical stimulation (FES). These devices are surface units that use electrical impulses to activate paralyzed or weak muscles in precise sequence. Coverage for the use of NMES/FES is limited to SCI patients for walking, who have completed a training program which consists of at least 32 physical therapy sessions with the device over a period of three months. The trial period of physical therapy will enable the physician treating the patient for his or her spinal cord injury to properly evaluate the person's ability to use these devices frequently and for the long term. Physical therapy necessary to perform this training must be directly performed by the physical therapist as part of a one-on-one training program.

The goal of physical therapy must be to train SCI patients on the use of NMES/FES devices to achieve walking, not to reverse or retard muscle atrophy.

Coverage for NMES/FES for walking will be covered in SCI patients with all of the following characteristics:

- Persons with intact lower motor unite (L1 and below) (both muscle and peripheral nerve);
- Persons with muscle and joint stability for weight bearing at upper and lower extremities that can demonstrate balance and control to maintain an upright support posture independently;
- Persons that demonstrate brisk muscle contraction to NMES and have sensory perception electrical stimulation sufficient for muscle contraction;
- Persons that possess high motivation, commitment and cognitive ability to use such devices for walking;
- Persons that can transfer independently and can demonstrate independent standing tolerance for at least 3 minutes;
- Persons that can demonstrate hand and finger function to manipulate controls;
- Persons with at least 6-month post recovery spinal cord injury and restorative surgery;
- Persons with hip and knee degenerative disease and no history of long bone fracture secondary to osteoporosis; and
- Persons who have demonstrated a willingness to use the device long-term.

NMES/FES for walking will not be covered in SCI patient with any of the following:

- Persons with cardiac pacemakers;
- Severe scoliosis or severe osteoporosis;
- Skin disease or cancer at area of stimulation;
- Irreversible contracture; or
- Autonomic dysflexia.

The only settings where therapists with the sufficient skills to provide these services are employed, are inpatient hospitals; outpatient hospitals; comprehensive outpatient rehabilitation facilities; and outpatient rehabilitation facilities. The physical therapy necessary to perform this training must be part of a one-on-one training program.

Additional therapy after the purchase of the DME would be limited by our general policies in converge of skilled physical therapy.

Pub 100-3, 160.13 – Supplies Used in the Delivery of Transcutaneous Electrical Nerve Stimulation (TENS) and Neuromuscular Electrical Stimulation (NMES)

(Rev. 1, 10-03-03)

Transcutaneous Electrical Nerve Stimulation (TENS) and/or Neuromuscular Electrical Stimulation (NMES) can ordinarily be delivered to patients through the use of conventional electrodes, adhesive tapes and lead wires. There may be times, however, where it might be medically necessary for certain patients receiving TENS or NMES treatment to use, as an alternative to conventional electrodes, adhesive tapes and lead wires, a form-fitting conductive garment (i.e., a garment with conductive fibers which are separated from the patients' skin by layers of fabric).

A form-fitting conductive garment (and medically necessary related supplies) may be covered under the program only when:

1. It has received permission or approval for marketing by the Food and Drug Administration;
2. It has been prescribed by a physician for use in delivering covered TENS or NMES treatment; and
3. One of the medical indications outlined below is met:
    - The patient cannot manage without the conductive garment because there is such a large area or so many sites to be stimulated and the stimulation would have to be delivered so frequently that it is not feasible to use conventional electrodes, adhesive tapes and lead wires;
    - The patient cannot manage without the conductive garment for the treatment of chronic intractable pain because the areas or sites to be stimulated are inaccessible with the use of conventional electrodes, adhesive tapes and lead wires;
    - The patient has a documented medical condition such as skin problems that preclude the application of conventional electrodes, adhesive tapes and lead wires;
    - The patient requires electrical stimulation beneath a cast either to treat disuse atrophy, where the nerve supply to the muscle is intact, or to treat chronic intractable pain; or
    - The patient has a medical need for rehabilitation strengthening (pursuant to a written plan of rehabilitation) following an injury where the nerve supply to the muscle is intact.

A conductive garment is not covered for use with a TENS device during the trial period specified in §160.7.1 unless:

1. The patient has a documented skin problem prior to the start of the trial period; and
2. The carrier's medical consultants are satisfied that use of such an item is medically necessary for the patient.

(See conditions for coverage of the use of TENS in the diagnosis and treatment of chronic intractable pain in §§160.7.1 and 160.13 and the use of NMES in the treatment of disuse atrophy in §160.12.)

Pub 100-3, 160.23 – Sensory Nerve Conduction Threshold Test (sNCT)

(Rev 15, 06-18-04)

A. General

The sNCT is a psychophysical assessment of both central and peripheral nerve functions. It measures the detection threshold of accurately calibrated sensory stimuli. This procedure is entended to evaluate and quantify function in both large and small caliber fibers for the purpose of detecting neurologic disease. Sensory perception and threshold detection are dependent on the integrity of both the peripheral sensory apparatus and peripheral-central sensory pathways. In theory, an abnormality detected by this procedure may signal dysfunction anywhere in the sensory pathway from the receptors, the sensory tracts, the primary sensory cortex, to the association cortex.

This procedure is different and distinct from assessment of nerve conduction velocity, amplitude and latency. It is also different from short-latency somatosensory evoked potentials.

Effective October 1, 2002, CMS initially concluded that there was insufficient scientific or clinical evidence to consider the sNCT test and the device used in performing this test reasonable and necessary within the meaning of section 1862(a)(1)(A) of the law. Therefore, sNCT was noncovered.

Effective April 1, 2004, based on a reconsideration of current Medicare policy for sNCT, CMS concludes that the use of any type of sNCT device (e.g., "current output" type device used to perform current perception threshold (CPT®), pain perception threshold (PPT), or pain tolerance threshold (PPT) testing or "voltage input" type device used for voltage-nerve conduction threshold (v-NCT) testing) to diagnose sensory neuropathies or radiculopathies in Medicare beneficiaries is not reasonable and necessary.

B. Nationally Covered Indications

Not applicable.

C. Nationally Noncovered Indications

All uses of sNCT to diagnose sensory neuropathies or radiculopathies are noncovered.

(This NCD last reviewed June 2004.)

Pub 100-3, 180.2 – Enteral and Parenteral Nutritional Therapy

(Rev. 1, 10-03-03)

Covered As Prosthetic Device

There are patients who, because of chronic illness or trauma, cannot be sustained through oral feeding. These people must rely on either enteral or parenteral nutritional therapy, depending upon the particular nature of their medical condition.

Coverage of nutritional therapy as a Part B benefit is provided under the prosthetic device benefit provision which requires that the patient must have a permanently inoperative internal body organ or function thereof. Therefore, enteral and parenteral nutritional therapy are not covered under Part B in situations involving temporary impairments. Coverage of such therapy, however, does not require a medical judgment that the impairment giving rise to the therapy will persist throughout the patient's remaining years. If the medical record, including the judgment of the attending physician, indicates that the impairment will be of long and indefinite duration, the test of permanence is considered met.

If the coverage requirements for enteral or parenteral nutritional therapy are met under the prosthetic device benefit provision, related supplies, equipment and nutrients are also covered under the conditions in the following paragraphs and the **Medicare Benefit Policy Manual**, Chapter 15, "Covered Medical and Other Health Services," §120.

Parenteral Nutrition Therapy

Daily parenteral nutrition is considered reasonable and necessary for a patient with severe pathology of the alimentary tract which does not allow absorption of sufficient nutrients to maintain weight and strength commensurate with the patient's general condition.

Since the alimentary tract of such a patient does not function adequately, an indwelling catheter is placed percutaneously in the subclavian vein and then advanced into the superior vena cava where intravenous infusion of nutrients is given for part of the day. The catheter is then plugged by the patient until the next infusion. Following a period of hospitalization which is required to initiate parenteral nutrition and to train the patient in catheter care, solution preparation, and infusion technique, the parenteral nutrition can be provided safely and effectively in the patient's home by nonprofessional persons who have undergone special training. However, such persons cannot be paid for their services, nor is payment available for any services furnished by nonphysician professionals except as services furnished incident to a physician's service.

For parenteral nutrition therapy to be covered under Part B, the claim must contain a physician's written order or prescription and sufficient medical documentation to permit an independent conclusion that the requirements of the prosthetic device benefit are met and that parenteral nutrition therapy is medically necessary. An example of a condition that typically qualifies for coverage is a massive small bowel resection resulting in severe nutritional deficiency in spite of adequate oral intake. However, coverage of parenteral nutrition therapy for this and any other condition must be approved on an individual, case-by-case basis initially and at periodic intervals of no more than three months by the carrier's medical consultant or specially trained staff, relying on such medical and other documentation as the carrier may require. If the claim involves an infusion pump, sufficient evidence must be provided to support a determination of medical necessity for the pump. Program payment for the pump is based on the reasonable charge for the simplest model that meets the medical needs of the patient as established by medical documentation.

Nutrient solutions for parenteral therapy are routinely covered. However, Medicare pays for no more than one month's supply of nutrients at any one time. Payment for the nutrients is based on the reasonable charge for the solution components unless the medical record, including a signed statement from the attending physician, establishes that the beneficiary, due to his/her physical or mental state, is unable to safely or effectively mix the solution and there is no family member or other person who can do so. Payment will be on the basis of the reasonable charge for more expensive premixed solutions only under the latter circumstances.

Enteral Nutrition Therapy

Enteral nutrition is considered reasonable and necessary for a patient with a functioning gastrointestinal tract who, due to pathology to, or nonfunction of, the structures that normally permit food to reach the digestive tract, cannot maintain weight and strength commensurate with his or her general condition. Enteral therapy may be given by nasogastric, jejunostomy, or gastrostomy tubes and can be provided safely and effectively in the home by nonprofessional persons who have undergone special training. However, such persons cannot be paid for their services, nor is payment available for any services furnished by nonphysician professionals except as services furnished incident to a physician's service.

Typical examples of conditions that qualify for coverage are head and neck cancer with reconstructive surgery and central nervous system disease leading to interference with the neuromuscular mechanisms of ingestion of such severity that the beneficiary cannot be maintained with oral feeding. However, claims for Part B coverage of enteral nutrition therapy for these and any other conditions must be approved on an individual, case-by-case basis. Each claim must contain a physician's written order or prescription and sufficient medical documentation (e.g., hospital records, clinical findings from the attending physician) to permit an independent conclusion that the patient's condition meets the requirements of the prosthetic device benefit and that enteral nutrition therapy is medically necessary. Allowed claims are to be reviewed at periodic intervals of no more than 3 months by the contractor's medical consultant or specially trained staff, and additional medical documentation considered necessary is to be obtained as part of this review.

Medicare pays for no more than one month's supply of enteral nutrients at any one time.

If the claim involves a pump, it must be supported by sufficient medical documentation to establish that the pump is medically necessary, i.e., gravity feeding is not satisfactory due to aspiration, diarrhea, dumping syndrome. Program payment for the pump is based on the reasonable charge for the simplest model that meets the medical needs of the patient as established by medical documentation.

Nutritional Supplementation

Some patients require supplementation of their daily protein and caloric intake. Nutritional supplements are often given as a medicine between meals to boost protein-caloric intake or the mainstay of a daily nutritional plan. Nutritional supplementation is not covered under Medicare Part B.

Pub 100-3, 190.2 – Diagnostic Pap Smears

(Rev. 48, 06-19-06)

A diagnostic pap smear and related medically necessary services are covered under Medicare Part B when ordered by a physician under one of the following conditions:

- Previous cancer of the cervix, uterus, or vagina that has been or is presently being treated;
- Previous abnormal pap smear;
- Any abnormal findings of the vagina, cervix, uterus, ovaries, or adnexa;
- Any significant complaint by the patient referable to the female reproductive system; or
- Any signs or symptoms that might in the physician's judgment reasonably be related to a gynecologic disorder.

Screening Pap Smears and Pelvic Examinations for Early Detection of Cervical or Vaginal Cancer. (See section 210.2.)

Pub 100-3, 190.6 – Hair Analysis

(Rev. 1, 10-03-03)

Not Covered

Hair analysis to detect mineral traces as an aid in diagnosing human disease is not a covered service under Medicare.

The correlation of hair analysis to the chemical state of the whole body is not possible at this time, and therefore this diagnostic procedure cannot be considered to be reasonable and necessary under §1862(a)(1) of the Act.

190.23 – Lipid Testing

(Rev.28, Issued: 02-11-05, Effective: 01-01-05, Implementation: 03-11-05)

Lipoproteins are a class of heterogeneous particles of varying sizes and densities containing lipid and protein. These lipoproteins include cholesterol esters and free cholesterol, triglycerides, phospholipids and A, C, and E apoproteins. Total cholesterol comprises all the cholesterol found in various lipoproteins.

Factors that affect blood cholesterol levels include age, sex, body weight, diet, alcohol and tobacco use, exercise, genetic factors, family history, medications, menopausal status, the use of hormone replacement therapy, and chronic disorders such as hypothyroidism, obstructive liver disease, pancreatic disease (including diabetes), and kidney disease.

In many individuals, an elevated blood cholesterol level constitutes an increased risk of developing coronary artery disease. Blood levels of total cholesterol and various fractions of cholesterol, especially low density lipoprotein cholesterol (LDL-C) and high density lipoprotein cholesterol (HDL-C), are useful in assessing and monitoring treatment for that risk in patients with cardiovascular and related diseases. Blood levels of the above cholesterol components including triglyceride have been separated into desirable, borderline and high-risk categories by the National Heart, Lung, and Blood Institute in their report in 1993. These categories form a useful basis for evaluation and treatment of patients with hyperlipidemia. Therapy to reduce these risk parameters includes diet, exercise and medications, and fat weight loss, which is particularly powerful when combined with diet and exercise.

Indications

The medical community recognizes lipid testing as appropriate for evaluating atherosclerotic cardiovascular disease. Conditions in which lipid testing may be indicated include:

- Assessment of patients with atherosclerotic cardio-vascular disease.
- Evaluation of primary dyslipidemia.
- Any form of atherosclerotic disease, or any disease leading to the formation of atherosclerotic disease.
- Diagnostic evaluation of diseases associated with altered lipid metabolism, such as: nephrotic syndrome, pancreatitis, hepatic disease, and hypo and hyperthyroidism.
- Secondary dyslipidemia, including diabetes mellitus, disorders of gastrointestinal absorption, chronic renal failure.
- Signs or symptoms of dyslipidemias, such as skin lesions.
- As follow-up to the initial screen for coronary heart disease (total cholesterol + HDL cholesterol) when total cholesterol is determined to be high (>240 mg/dL), or borderline-high (200-140 mg/dL) plus two or more coronary heart disease risk factors, or an HDL cholesterol, <35 mg/dL.

To monitor the progress of patients on anti-lipid dietary management and pharmacologic therapy for the treatment of elevated blood lipid disorders, total cholesterol, HDL cholesterol and LDL cholesterol may be used. Triglycerides may be obtained if the lipid fraction is also elevated or if the patient is put on drugs (for example, thiazide diuretics, beta blockers, estrogens, glucocorticoids, and tamoxifen) which may raise the triglyceride level.

When monitoring long-term anti-lipid dietary or pharmacologic therapy and when following patients with borderline high total or LDL cholesterol levels, it may be reasonable to perform the lipid panel annually. A lipid panel at a yearly interval will usually be adequate while measurement of the serum total cholesterol or a measured LDL should suffice for interim visits if the patient does not have hypertriglyceridemia.

Any one component of the panel or a measured LDL may be reasonable and necessary up to six times the first year for monitoring dietary or pharmacologic therapy. More frequent total cholesterol, HDL cholesterol, LDL cholesterol and triglyceride testing may be indicated for marked elevations or for changes to anti-lipid therapy due to inadequate initial patient response to dietary or pharmacologic therapy. The LDL cholesterol or total cholesterol may be measured three times yearly after treatment goals have been achieved.

Electrophoretic or other quantitation of lipoproteins may be indicated if the patient has a primary disorder of lipoid metabolism.

Effective January 1, 2005, the Medicare law expanded coverage to cardiovascular screening services. Several of the procedures included in this NCD may be covered for screening purposes subject to specified frequencies. See 42 CFR 410.17 and Section 100, Chapter 18, of the *Medicare Claims Processing Manual*, for a full description of this benefit.

Limitations

Lipid panel and hepatic panel testing may be used for patients with severe psoriasis which has not responded to conventional therapy and for which the retinoid etretinate has been prescribed and who have developed hyperlipidemia or hepatic toxicity. Specific examples include erythrodermia and generalized pustular type and psoriasis associated with arthritis.

Routine screening and prophylactic testing for lipid disorder are not covered by Medicare. While lipid screening may be medically appropriate, Medicare by statute does not pay for it. Lipid testing in asymptomatic individuals is considered to be screening regardless of the presence of other risk factors such as family history, tobacco use, etc.

Once a diagnosis is established, one or several specific tests are usually adequate for monitoring the course of the disease. Less specific diagnoses (for example, other chest pain) alone do not support medical necessity of these tests.

When monitoring long-term anti-lipid dietary of pharmacologic therapy and when following patients with borderline high total or LDL cholesterol levels, it is reasonable to perform the lipid panel annually. A lipid panel at a yearly interval will usually be adequate while measurement of the serum total cholesterol or a measured LDL should suffice for interim visits if the patient does not have hypertriglyceridemia.

Any one component of the panel or a measured LDL may be medically necessary up to six times the first year for monitoring dietary or pharmacologic therapy. More frequent total cholesterol, HDL cholesterol, LDL cholesterol and triglyceride testing may be indicated for marked elevations or for changes to anti-lipid therapy due to inadequate initial patient response to dietary or pharmacologic therapy. The LDL cholesterol or total cholesterol may be measured three times yearly after treatment goals have been achieved.

If no dietary or pharmacologic therapy is advised, monitoring is not necessary.

When evaluating non-specific chronic abnormalities of the liver (for example, elevations of transaminase, alkaline phosphatase, abnormal imaging studies, etc.), a lipid panel would generally not be indicated more than twice per year

Pub 100-3, 210.1 – Prostate Cancer Screening Tests

(Rev. 48, Issued: 03-17-06; Effective/Implementation Dates: 06-19-06)

Covered

A. General

Section 4103 of the Balanced Budget Act of 1997 provides for coverage of certain prostate cancer screening tests subject to certain coverage, frequency, and payment limitations. Medicare will cover prostate cancer screening tests/procedures for the early detection of prostate cancer. Coverage of prostate cancer screening tests includes the following procedures furnished to an individual for the early detection of prostate cancer:

- Screening digital rectal examination; and
- Screening prostate specific antigen blood test

B. Screening Digital Rectal Examinations

Screening digital rectal examinations are covered at a frequency of once every 12 months for men who have attained age 50 (at least 11 months have passed following the month in which the last Medicare-covered screening digital rectal examination was performed). Screening digital rectal examination means a clinical examination of an individual's prostate for nodules or other abnormalities of the prostate. This screening must be performed by a doctor of medicine or osteopathy (as defined in §1861(r)(1) of the Act), or by a physician assistant, nurse practitioner, clinical nurse specialist, or certified nurse midwife (as defined in §1861(aa) and §1861(gg) of the Act) who is authorized under State law to perform the examination, fully knowledgeable about the beneficiary's medical condition, and would be responsible for using the results of any examination performed in the overall management of the beneficiary's specific medical problem.

C. Screening Prostate Specific Antigen Tests

Screening prostate specific antigen tests are covered at a frequency of once every 12 months for men who have attained age 50 (at least 11 months have passed following the month in which the last Medicare-covered screening prostate specific antigen test was performed). Screening prostate specific antigen tests (PSA) means a test to detect the marker for adenocarcinoma of prostate. PSA is a reliable immunocytochemical marker for primary and metastatic adenocarcinoma of prostate. This screening must be ordered by the beneficiary's physician or by the beneficiary's physician assistant, nurse practitioner, clinical nurse specialist, or certified nurse midwife (the term "attending physician" is defined in §1861(r)(1) of the Act to mean a doctor of medicine or osteopathy and the terms "physician assistant, nurse practitioner, clinical nurse specialist, or certified nurse midwife" are defined in §1861(aa) and §1861(gg) of the Act) who is fully knowledgeable about the beneficiary's medical condition, and who would be responsible for using the results of any examination (test) performed in the overall management of the beneficiary's specific medical problem.

Pub 100-3, 210.2 – Screening Pap Smears and Pelvic Examinations for Early Detection of Cervical or Vaginal Cancer

(Rev. 48, Issued: 03-17-06; Effective/Implementation Dates: 06-19-06)

Screening Pap Smear

A screening pap smear and related medically necessary services provided to a woman for the early detection of cervical cancer (including collection of the sample of cells and a physician's interpretation of the test results) and pelvic examination (including clinical breast examination) are covered under Medicare Part B when ordered by a physician (or authorized practitioner) under one of the following conditions:

- She has not had such a test during the preceding two years or is a woman of childbearing age (§1861(nn) of the Act).
- There is evidence (on the basis of her medical history or other findings) that she is at high risk of developing cervical cancer and her physician (or authorized practitioner) recommends that she have the test performed more frequently than every two years.

High risk factors for cervical and vaginal cancer are:

- Early onset of sexual activity (under 16 years of age).
- Multiple sexual partners (five or more in a lifetime).
- History of sexually transmitted disease (including HIV infection).
- Fewer than three negative or any pap smears within the previous 7 years.; and
- DES (diethylstilbestrol) – exposed daughters of women who took DES during pregnancy.

NOTE: Claims for pap smears must indicate the beneficiary's low or high risk status by including the appropriate ICD-9-CM on the line item (Item 24E of the Form CMS-1500).

Definitions

- A woman as described in §1861(nn) of the Act is a woman who is of childbearing age and has had a pap smear test during any of the preceding three years that indicated the presence of cervical or vaginal cancer or other abnormality, or is at high risk of developing cervical or vaginal cancer.
- A woman of childbearing age is one who is premenopausal and has been determined by a physician or other qualified practitioner to be of childbearing age, based upon the medical history or other findings.
- Other qualified practitioner, as defined in 42 CFR 410.56(a) includes a certified nurse midwife (as defined in §1861(gg) of the Act), or a physician assistant, nurse practitioner, or clinical nurse specialist (as defined in §1861(aa) of the Act) who is authorized under State law to perform the examination.

Screening Pelvic Examination

Section 4102 of the Balanced Budget Act of 1997 provides for coverage of screening pelvic examinations (including a clinical breast examination) for all female beneficiaries, subject to certain frequency and other limitations. A screening pelvic examination (including a clinical breast examination) should include at least seven of the following eleven elements:

- Inspection and palpation of breasts for masses or lumps, tenderness, symmetry, or nipple discharge.
- Digital rectal examination including sphincter tone, presence of hemorrhoids, and rectal masses. Pelvic examination (with or without specimen collection for smears and cultures) including:
- External genitalia (for example, general appearance, hair distribution, or lesions).
- Urethral maetus (for example, size, location, lesions, or prolapse).
- Urethra (for example, masses, tenderness, or scarring).
- Bladder (for example, fullness, masses, or tenderness).
- Vagina (for example, general appearance, estrogen effect, discharge lesions, pelvic support, cystocele, or rectocele).
- Cervix (for example, general appearance, lesions, or discharge).
- Uterus (for example, size, contour, position, mobility, tenderness, consistency, descent, or support).
- Adnexa/parametria (for example, masses, tenderness, organomegaly, or nodularity).
- Anus and perineum.

This description is from Documentation Guidelines for Evaluation and Management Services, published in May 1997 and was developed by the Centers for Medicare and Medicaid Services and the American Medical Association.

Pub 100-3, 210.3 – Colorectal Cancer Screening Tests

(Rev. 105, Issued: 08-07-09, Effective: 05-12-09, Implementation: 09-08-09)

A. General

Section 4104 of the Balanced Budget Act of 1997 provides for coverage of screening colorectal cancer procedures under Medicare Part B. Medicare currently covers: (1) annual fecal occult blood tests (FOBTs); (2) flexible sigmoidoscopy over 4 years; (3) screening colonoscopy for persons at average risk for colorectal cancer every 10 years, or for persons at high risk for colorectal cancer every 2 years; (4) barium enema every 4 years as an alternative to flexible sigmoidoscopy, or every 2 years as an alternative to colonoscopy for persons at high risk for colorectal cancer; and, (5) other procedures the Secretary finds appropriate based on consultation with appropriate experts and organizations.

Coverage of the above screening examinations was implemented in regulations through a final rule that was published on October 31, 1997 (62 FR 59079), and was effective January 1, 1998. At that time, based on consultation with appropriate experts and organizations, the definition of the term "FOBT" was defined in 42 CFR §410.37(a)(2) of the regulation to mean a "guaiac-based test for peroxidase activity, testing two samples from each of three consecutive stools."

In the 2003 Physician Fee Schedule Final Rule (67 FR 79966) effective March 1, 2003, the Centers for Medicare & Medicaid Services (CMS) amended the FOBT screening test regulation definition to provide that it could include either: (1) a guaiac-based FOBT, or, (2) other tests determined by the Secretary through a national coverage determination.

B. Nationally Covered Indications

Fecal Occult Blood Tests (FOBT) (effective for services performed on or after January 1, 2004).

1. History

The FOBTs are generally divided into two types: immunoassay and guaiac types. Immunoassay (or immunochemical) fecal occult blood tests (iFOBT) use "antibodies directed against human globin epitopes. While most iFOBTs use spatulas to collect stool samples, some use a brush to

Medicare References

collect toilet water surrounding the stool. Most iFOBTs require laboratory processing.

Guaiac fecal occult blood tests (gFOBT) use a peroxidase reaction to indicate presence of the heme portion of hemoglobin. Guaiac turns blue after oxidation by oxidants or peroxidases in the presence of an oxygen donor such as hydrogen peroxide. Most FOBTs use sticks to collect stool samples and may be developed in a physician's office or a laboratory. In 1998, Medicare began reimbursement for guaiac FOBTs, but not immunoassay type tests for colorectal cancer screening. Since the fundamental process is similar for other iFOBTs, CMS evaluated colorectal cancer screening using immunoassay FOBTs in general.

2. Expanded Coverage

Medicare covers one screening FOBT per annum for the early detection of colorectal cancer. This means that Medicare will cover one guaiac-based (gFOBT) or one immunoassay-based (iFOBT) at a frequency of every 12 months; i.e., at least 11 months have passed following the month in which the last covered screening FOBT was performed, for beneficiaries aged 50 years and older. The beneficiary completes the existing gFOBT by taking samples from two different sites of three consecutive stools; the beneficiary completes the iFOBT by taking the appropriate number of stool samples according to the specific manufacturer's instructions. This screening requires a written order from the beneficiary's attending physician. ("Attending physician means a doctor of medicine or osteopathy (as defined in §1861(r)(1) of the Social Security Act) who is fully knowledgeable about the beneficiary's medical condition, and who would be responsible for using the results of any examination performed in the overall management of the beneficiary's specific medical problem.)

C. Nationally Non-Covered Indications

All other indications for colorectal cancer screening not otherwise specified above remain non-covered. Non-coverage specifically includes:

(1) Screening DNA (Deoxyribonucleic acid) stool tests, effective April 28, 2008, and,

(2) Screening computed tomographic colonography (CTC), effective May 12, 2009.

D. Other

N/A (This NCD last reviewed May 2009)

Noncovered Indications

All other indications for colorectal cancer screening not otherwise specified above remain noncovered.

Pub 100-3, 210.4 – Smoking and Tobacco-Use Cessation Counseling

(Rev. 36, Issued: 05-20-05; Effective: 03-22-05; Implementation: 07-05-05)

A. General

Tobacco use continues to be the leading cause of preventable death in the United States. In 1964, the Surgeon General of the U.S. Public Health Service (PHS) issued the report of his Advisory Committee on Smoking and Health, officially recognizing that cigarette smoking is a cause of cancer and other serious diseases. Though smoking rates have significantly declined, 9.3% of the population age 65 and older smokes cigarettes. Approximately 440,000 people die annually from smoking related disease, with 68% (300,000) age 65 or older. Many more people of all ages suffer from serious illness caused from smoking, leading to disability and decreased quality of life. Reduction in smoking prevalence is a national objective in Healthy People 2010.

B. Nationally Covered Indications

Effective March 22, 2005, the Centers for Medicare and Medicaid Services (CMS) has determined that the evidence is adequate to conclude that smoking and tobacco use cessation counseling, based on the current PHS Guideline, is reasonable and necessary for a patient with a disease or an adverse health effect that has been found by the U.S. Surgeon General to be linked to tobacco use, or who is taking a therapeutic agent whose metabolism or dosing is affected by tobacco use as based on FDA-approved information.

Patients must be competent and alert at the time that services are provided. Minimal counseling is already covered at each evaluation and management (E&M) visit. Beyond that, Medicare will cover 2 cessation attempts per year. Each attempt may include a maximum of 4 intermediate or intensive sessions, with the total annual benefit covering up to 8 sessions in a 12-month period. The practitioner and patient have flexibility to choose between intermediate or intensive cessation strategies for each attempt.

Intermediate and intensive smoking cessation counseling services will be covered for outpatient and hospitalized beneficiaries who are smokers and who qualify as above, as long as those services are furnished by qualified physicians and other Medicare-recognized practitioners.

C. Nationally Non-Covered Indications

Inpatient hospital stays with the principal diagnosis of Tobacco Use Disorder are not reasonable and necessary for the effective delivery of tobacco cessation counseling services. Therefore, we will not cover tobacco cessation services if tobacco cessation is the primary reason for the patient's hospital stay.

(This NCD last reviewed May 2005.)

Pub 100-3, 220.2 – Magnetic Resonance Imaging

(Various Effective Dates Below)

A. General

1. Method of Operation

Magnetic Resonance Imaging (MRI), formerly called nuclear magnetic resonance (NMR), is a non-invasive method of graphically representing the distribution of water and other hydrogen-rich molecules in the human body. In contrast to conventional radiographs or computed tomography (CT) scans, in which the image is produced by x-ray beam attenuation by an object, MRI is capable of producing images by several techniques. In fact, various combinations of MRI image production methods may be employed to emphasize particular characteristics of the tissue or body part being examined. The basic elements by which MRI produces an image are the density of hydrogen nuclei in the object being examined, their motion, and the relaxation times, and the period of time required for the nuclei to return to their original states in the main, static magnetic field after being subjected to a brief additional magnetic field. These relaxation times reflect the physical-chemical properties of tissue and the molecular environment of its hydrogen nuclei. Only hydrogen atoms are present in human tissues in sufficient concentration for current use in clinical MRI.

Magnetic Resonance Angiography (MRA) is a non-invasive diagnostic test that is an application of MRI. By analyzing the amount of energy released from tissues exposed to a strong magnetic field, MRA provides images of normal and diseased blood vessels, as well as visualization and quantification of blood flow through these vessels.

2. General Clinical Utility

Overall, MRI is a useful diagnostic imaging modality that is capable of demonstrating a wide variety of soft-tissue lesions with contrast resolution equal or superior to CT scanning in various parts of the body.

Among the advantages of MRI are the absence of ionizing radiation and the ability to achieve high levels of tissue contrast resolution without injected iodinated radiological contrast agents. Recent advances in technology have resulted in development and Food and Drug Administration (FDA) approval of new paramagnetic contrast agents for MRI which allow even better visualization in some instances. Multislice imaging and the ability to image in multiple planes, especially sagittal and coronal, have provided flexibility not easily available with other modalities. Because cortical (outer layer) bone and metallic prostheses do not cause distortion of MR images, it has been possible to visualize certain lesions and body regions with greater certainty than has been possible with CT. The use of MRI on certain soft tissue structures for the purpose of detecting disruptive, neoplastic, degenerative, or inflammatory lesions has now become established in medical practice.

Phase contrast (PC) and time-of-flight (TOF) are some of the available MRA techniques at the time these instructions are being issued. PC measures the difference between the phases of proton spins in tissue and blood and measures both the venous and arterial blood flow at any point in the cardiac cycle. TOF measures the difference between the amount of magnetization of tissue and blood and provides information on the structure of blood vessels, thus indirectly indicating blood flow. Two-dimensional (2D) and three-dimensional (3D) images can be obtained using each method.

Contrast-enhanced MRA (CE-MRA) involves blood flow imaging after the patient receives an intravenous injection of a contrast agent. Gadolinium, a non-ionic element, is the foundation of all contrast agents currently in use. Gadolinium affects the way in which tissues respond to magnetization, resulting in better visualization of structures when compared to un-enhanced studies. Unlike ionic (i.e., iodine-based) contrast agents used in conventional contrast angiography (CA), allergic reactions to gadolinium are extremely rare. Additionally, gadolinium does not cause the kidney failure occasionally seen with ionic contrast agents. Digital subtraction angiography (DSA) is a computer-augmented form of CA that obtains digital blood flow images as contrast agent courses through a blood vessel. The computer "subtracts" bone and other tissue from the image, thereby improving visualization of blood vessels. Physicians elect to use a specific MRA or CA technique based upon clinical information from each patient.

B. Nationally Covered MRI and MRA Indications

1. MRI

Although several uses of MRI are still considered investigational and some uses are clearly contraindicated (see subsection C), MRI is considered medically efficacious for a number of uses. Use the following descriptions as general guidelines or examples of what may be considered covered rather than as a restrictive list of specific covered indications. Coverage is limited to MRI units that have received FDA premarket approval, and such units must be operated within the parameters specified by the approval. In addition, the services must be reasonable and necessary for the diagnosis or treatment of the specific patient involved.

a. Effective November 22, 1985, MRI is useful in examining the head, central nervous system, and spine. Multiple sclerosis can be diagnosed with MRI and the contents of the posterior fossa are visible. The inherent tissue contrast resolution of MRI makes it an appropriate standard diagnostic modality for general neuroradiology.

b. Effective November 22, 1985, MRI can assist in the differential diagnosis of mediastinal and retroperitoneal masses, including abnormalities of the large vessels such as aneurysms and dissection. When a clinical need exists to visualize the parenchyma of solid organs to detect anatomic disruption or neoplasia, this can be accomplished in the liver, urogenital system, adrenals, and pelvic organs without the use of radiological contrast materials. When MRI is considered reasonable and necessary, the use of paramagnetic contrast materials may be covered as part of the study. MRI may also be used to detect and stage pelvic and retroperitoneal neoplasms and to evaluate disorders of cancellous bone and soft tissues. It may also be used in the detection of pericardial thickening. Primary and secondary bone neoplasm and aseptic necrosis can be detected at an early stage and monitored with MRI. Patients with metallic prostheses, especially of the hip, can be imaged in order to detect the early stages of infection of the bone to which the prosthesis is attached.

c. Effective March 22, 1994, MRI may also be covered to diagnose disc disease without regard to whether radiological imaging has been tried first to diagnose the problem.

d. Effective March 4, 1991, MRI with gating devices and surface coils, and gating devices that eliminate distorted images caused by cardiac and respiratory movement cycles are now considered state of the art techniques and may be covered. Surface and other specialty coils may also be covered, as they are used routinely for high resolution imaging where small limited regions of the body are studied. They produce high signal-to-noise ratios resulting in images of enhanced anatomic detail.

2. MRA (MRI for Blood Flow)

Currently covered indications include using MRA for specific conditions to evaluate flow in internal carotid vessels of the head and neck, peripheral arteries of lower extremities, abdomen and pelvis, and the chest. Coverage is limited to MRA units that have received FDA premarket approval, and such units must be operated within the parameters specified by the approval. In addition, the services must be reasonable and necessary for the diagnosis or treatment of the specific patient involved.

a. Head and Neck

Effective April 15, 2003, studies have proven that MRA is effective for evaluating flow in internal carotid vessels of the head and neck. However, not all potential applications of MRA have been shown to be reasonable and necessary. All of the following criteria must apply in order for Medicare to provide coverage for MRA of the head and neck:

- MRA is used to evaluate the carotid arteries, the circle of Willis, the anterior, middle or posterior cerebral arteries, the vertebral or basilar arteries or the venous sinuses;
- MRA is performed on patients with conditions of the head and neck for which surgery is anticipated and may be found to be appropriate based on the MRA. These conditions include, but are not limited to, tumor, aneurysms, vascular malformations, vascular occlusion or thrombosis. Within this broad category of disorders, medical necessity is the underlying determinant of the need for an MRA in specific diseases. The medical records should clearly justify and demonstrate the existence of medical necessity; and
- MRA and CA are not expected to be performed on the same patient for diagnostic purposes prior to the application of anticipated therapy. Only one of these tests will be covered routinely unless the physician can demonstrate the medical need to perform both tests.

b. Peripheral Arteries of Lower Extremities

Effective April 15, 2003, studies have proven that MRA of peripheral arteries is useful in determining the presence and extent of peripheral vascular disease in lower extremities. This procedure is non-invasive and has been shown to find occult vessels in some patients for which those vessels were not apparent when CA was performed. Medicare will cover either MRA or CA to evaluate peripheral arteries of the lower extremities. However, both MRA and CA may be useful in some cases, such as:

- A patient has had CA and this test was unable to identify a viable run-off vessel for bypass. When exploratory surgery is not believed to be a reasonable medical course of action for this patient, MRA may be performed to identify the viable runoff vessel; or
- A patient has had MRA, but the results are inconclusive.

c. Abdomen and Pelvis

i. Pre-operative Evaluation of Patients Undergoing Elective Abdominal Aortic Aneurysm (AAA) Repair

Effective July 1, 1999, MRA is covered for pre-operative evaluation of patients undergoing elective AAA repair if the scientific evidence reveals MRA is considered comparable to CA in determining the extent of AAA, as well as in evaluating aortoiliac occlusion disease and renal artery pathology that may be necessary in the surgical planning of AAA repair. These studies also reveal that MRA could provide a net benefit to the patient. If preoperative CA is avoided, then patients are not exposed to the risks associated with invasive procedures, contrast media, end-organ damage, or arterial injury.

ii. Imaging the Renal Arteries and the Aortoiliac Arteries in the Absence of AAA or Aortic Dissection

Effective July 1, 2003, MRA coverage is expanded to include imaging the renal arteries and the aortoiliac arteries in the absence of AAA or aortic dissection. MRA should be obtained in those circumstances in which using MRA is expected to avoid obtaining CA, when physician history, physical examination, and standard assessment tools provide insufficient information for patient management, and obtaining an MRA has a high probability of positively affecting patient management. However, CA may be ordered after obtaining the results of an MRA in those rare instances where medical necessity is demonstrated.

d. Chest

i. Diagnosis of Pulmonary Embolism

Current scientific data has shown that diagnostic pulmonary MRAs are improving due to recent developments such as faster imaging capabilities and gadolinium-enhancement. However, these advances in MRA are not significant enough to warrant replacement of pulmonary angiography in the diagnosis of pulmonary embolism for patients who have no contraindication to receiving intravenous iodinated contrast

Medicare References

material. Patients who are allergic to iodinated contrast material face a high risk of developing complications if they undergo pulmonary angiography or computed tomography angiography. Therefore, Medicare will cover MRA of the chest for diagnosing a suspected pulmonary embolism when it is contraindicated for the patient to receive intravascular iodinated contrast material.

ii. Evaluation of Thoracic Aortic Dissection and Aneurysm
Studies have shown that MRA of the chest has a high level of diagnostic accuracy for pre-operative and post-operative evaluation of aortic dissection of aneurysm. Depending on the clinical presentation, MRA may be used as an alternative to other non-invasive imaging technologies, such as transesophageal echocardiography and CT. Generally, Medicare will provide coverage only for MRA or for CA when used as a diagnostic test. However, if both MRA and CA of the chest are used, the physician must demonstrate the medical need for performing these tests.

While the intent of this policy is to provide reimbursement for either MRA or CA, CMS is also allowing flexibility for physicians to make appropriate decisions concerning the use of these tests based on the needs of individual patients. CMS anticipates, however, low utilization of the combined use of MRA and CA. As a result, CMS encourages contractors to monitor the use of these tests and, where indicated, require evidence of the need to perform both MRA and CA.

C. Contraindications and Nationally Noncovered Indications

1. Contraindications

The MRI is not covered when the following patient-specific contraindications are present:

- It is not covered for patients with cardiac pacemakers or with metallic clips on vascular aneurysms.
- MRI during a viable pregnancy is also contraindicated at this time.
- The danger inherent in bringing ferromagnetic materials within range of MRI units generally constrains the use of MRI on acutely ill patients requiring life support systems and monitoring devices that employ ferromagnetic materials.
- In addition, the long imaging time and the enclosed position of the patient may result in claustrophobia, making patients who have a history of claustrophobia unsuitable candidates for MRI procedures.

2. Nationally Noncovered Indications

The Centers for Medicare & Medicaid Services (CMS) has determined that MRI of cortical bone and calcifications, and procedures involving spatial resolution of bone and calcifications, are not considered reasonable and necessary indications within the meaning of section 1862(a)(1)(A) of the Social Security Act, and are therefore non-covered.

D. Other

Effective June 3, 2010, all other uses of MRI or MRA for which CMS has not specifically indicated coverage or non-coverage continue to be eligible for coverage through individual local contractor discretion.

(This NCD last reviewed June 2010.)

Pub 100-3, 220.2.1 – Magnetic Resonance Spectroscopy

(Rev. 21, Issued: 09-10-04, Effective: 09-10-04, Implementation: 09-10-04)

A. General

Magnetic Resonance Spectroscopy (MRS) is an application of magnetic resonance imaging (MRI). It is a non-invasive diagnostic test that uses strong magnetic fields to measure and analyze the chemical composition of human tissues. On March 22, 1994, CMS considered MRS an investigational procedure and issued a national noncoverage determination for all indications of MRS.

B. Nationally Covered Indications

Not applicable.

C. Nationally Noncovered Indications

After thorough review and reconsideration of the existing national noncoverage determination for MRS, as well as the available evidence for the use of MRS as a diagnostic tool for distinguishing indeterminate brain lesions, and/or as an aid in conducting brain biopsies, CMS has determined that the evidence is not adequate to conclude that MRS is reasonable and necessary within the meaning of Section 1862(a)(1)(A) of the Social Security Act, for use in the diagnosis of brain tumors. Therefore, CMS reaffirms its current national noncoverage determination for all indications of MRS.

D. Other

Not applicable. (This NCD last reviewed September 2004.)

Pub 100-3, 220.3 – Magnetic Resonance Angiography

(replaced with section 220.2)

(Rev. 123, Issued: 07-09-10, Effective: 06-03-10, Implementation: 08-09, 2010)

Pub 100-3, 220.4 – Mammograms

(Rev. 1, 10-03-03)

A diagnostic mammography is a radiologic procedure furnished to a man or woman with signs and symptoms of breast disease, or a personal history of breast cancer, or a personal history of biopsy – proven benign breast disease, and includes a physician's interpretation of the results of the procedure. A diagnostic mammography is a covered service if it is ordered by a doctor of medicine or osteopathy as defined in §1861 (r) (1) of the Act. A screening mammography is a radiologic procedure furnished to a woman without signs or symptoms of breast disease, for the purpose of early detection of breast cancer, and includes a physician's interpretation of the results of the procedure. A screening mammography has limitations as it must be, at a minimum a two-view exposure (cranio-caudal and a medial lateral oblique view) of each breast. Payment may not be made for a screening mammography performed on a woman under age 35. Payment may be made for only one screening mammography performed on a woman over age 34, but under age 40. For an asymptomatic woman over age 39, payment may be made for a screening mammography performed after at least 11 months have passed following the month in which the last screening mammography was performed.

A radiological mammogram is a covered diagnostic test under the following conditions:

- A patient has distinct signs and symptoms for which a mammogram is indicated.
- A patient has a history of breast cancer.
- A patient is asymptomatic but, on the basis of the patient's history and other factors the physician considers significant, the physician's judgment is that a mammogram is appropriate.

Use of mammograms in routine screening of:

1. Asymptomatic women aged 50 and over.
2. Asymptomatic women aged 40 or over whose mothers or sisters have had the disease, is considered medically appropriate, but would not be covered for Medicare purposes.

Cross-reference:

The **Medicare Benefit Policy Manual**, Chapter 15, "Covered Medical and Other Health Services," §80.

The **Medicare Benefit Policy Manual**, Chapter 1, "Inpatient Hospital Services," §50

Pub 100-3, 220.5 – Ultrasound Diagnostic Procedures

(Rev. 76, Issued: 09-12-07, Effective: 05-22-07, Implementation: 09-28-07)

A. General

Ultrasound diagnostic procedures utilizing low energy sound waves are being widely employed to determine the composition and contours of nearly all body tissues except bone and air-filled spaces. This technique permits noninvasive visualization of even the deepest structures in the body. The use of the ultrasound technique is sufficiently developed that it can be considered essential to good patient care in diagnosing a wide variety of conditions.

Ultrasound diagnostic procedures are listed below and are divided into two categories. Medicare coverage is extended to the procedures listed in Category I. Periodic claims review by the intermediary's medical consultants should be conducted to ensure that the techniques are medically appropriate and the general indications specified in these categories are met. Techniques in Category II are considered experimental and should not be covered at this time.

B. Nationally Covered Indications

Category I—(Clinically effective, usually part of initial patient evaluation, may be an adjunct to radiologic and nuclear medicine diagnostic technique)

- Echoencephalography, (Diencephalic Midline) (A-Mode)
- Echoencephalography, Complete (Diencephalic Midline and Ventricular Size)
- Ocular and Orbital Echography (A-Mode)
- Covered procedures include efforts to determine the suitability of aphakic patients for implantation of an artificial lens (pseudophakoi) following cataract surgery.
- Ocular and Orbital Sonography (B-Mode)
- Echocardiography, Pericardial Effusion (M-Mode)
- Pericardiocentesis, by Ultrasonic Guidance
- Echocardiography, Cardiac Valve(s) (M-Mode)
- Echocardiography, Complete (M-Mode)
- Echocardiography, limited (e.g., follow-up or limited study) (M-Mode)
- Pleural Effusion Echography
- Thoracentesis, by Ultrasonic Guidance
- Abdominal Sonography, complete survey study (B-Scan)
- Abdominal Sonography, limited (e.g., follow-up or limited study) (B-Scan)
- Abdominal Sonography is not synonymous with ultrasound examination of individual organs.
- Renal Cyst Aspiration, by Ultrasonic Guidance
- Renal Biopsy, by Ultrasonic Guidance
- Pancreas Sonography (B-Scan)
- Pancreatic Sonography has proven effective in diagnosing pseudocysts.
- Spleen Sonography (B-Scan)
- Abdominal Aorta Echography (A-Mode)
- Abdominal Aorta Sonography (B-Scan)
- Retroperitoneal Sonography (B-Scan)
- Retroperitoneal Sonography does not include planning of fields for radiation therapy.
- Urinary Bladder Sonography (B-Scan)
- Urinary bladder Sonography does not include staging of bladder tumors.
- Pregnancy Diagnosis Sonography (B-Scan)
- Fetal Age Determination (Biparietal Diameter) Sonography (B-Scan)
- Fetal Growth Rate Sonography (B-Scan)
- Placenta Localization Sonography (B-Scan)
- Pregnancy Sonography, Complete (B-Scan)
- Molar Pregnancy Diagnosis Sonography (B-Scan)
- Ectopic Pregnancy Diagnosis Sonography (B-Scan)
- Passive Testing (Antepartum Monitoring of Fetal Heart Rate In the Resting Fetus)
- Intrauterine Contraceptive Device Sonography (B-Scan)
- Pelvic Mass Diagnosis Sonography (B-Scan)
- Amniocentesis, by Ultrasonic Guidance
- Arterial Flow Study, Peripheral (Doppler)
- Venous Flow Study, Peripheral (Doppler)
- Arterial Aneurysm, Peripheral (B-Scan)
- Radiation Therapy Planning Sonography (B-Scan)
- Thyroid Echography (A-Mode)
- Thyroid Sonography (B-Scan)
- Breast Echography (A-Mode)
- Breast Sonography (B-Scan)
- Hepatic Sonography (B-Scan)
- Gallbladder Sonography
- Renal Sonography
- Two-Dimensional Echocardiography (B-Mode)
- Monitoring of cardiac output (Esophageal Doppler) for ventilated patients in the ICU and operative patients with a need for intra-operative fluid optimization

C. Nationally Non-Covered Indications

Category II—(Clinical reliability and efficacy not proven)

- B-Scan for atherosclerotic narrowing of peripheral arteries

D. Other

Uses for ultrasound diagnostic procedures not listed in Category I or II above are left to local contractor discretion. In view of the rapid changes in the field of ultrasound diagnosis, uses for ultrasound diagnostic procedures other than those listed under Categories I and II should be carefully reviewed before payment. Medical justification may be required.

(This NCD last reviewed June 2007)

Cross reference: §20.17.

Pub 100-3, 220.6 – Positron Emission Tomography (PET) Scans

(Effective April 6, 2009)

(Rev. 120; Issued: 05-06-10; Effective Date: 04-03-09; Implementation Date: 10-30-09)

Positron Emission Tomography (PET) is a minimally invasive diagnostic imaging procedure used to evaluate metabolism in normal tissue as well as in diseased tissues in conditions such as cancer, ischemic heart disease, and some neurologic disorders. A radiopharmaceutical is injected into the patient that gives off sub-atomic particles, known as positrons, as it decays. PET uses a positron camera (tomograph) to measure the decay of the radiopharmaceutical. The rate of decay provides biochemical information on the metabolism of the tissue being studied.

NOTE: This manual section 220.6 lists all Medicare-covered uses of PET scans. Except as set forth below in cancer indications listed as "Coverage with Evidence Development," a particular use of PET scans is not covered unless this manual specifically provides that such use is covered. Although this section 220.6 lists some non-covered uses of PET scans, it does not constitute an exhaustive list of all non-covered uses.

(This NCD last reviewed March 2009.)

Pub 100-3, 220.6.1 – PET for Perfusion of the Heart

(Various Effective Dates)

(Rev. 120; Issued: 05-06-10; Effective Date: 04-03-09; Implementation Date: 10-30-09)

1. Rubidium 82 (Effective March 14, 1995)

Effective for services performed on or after March 14, 1995, PET scans performed at rest or with pharmacological stress used for noninvasive imaging of the perfusion of the heart for the diagnosis and management of patients with known or suspected coronary artery disease using the FDA-approved radiopharmaceutical Rubidium 82 (Rb 82) are covered, provided the requirements below are met:

- The PET scan, whether at rest alone, or rest with stress, is performed in place of, but not in addition to, a single photon emission computed tomography (SPECT); or
- The PET scan, whether at rest alone or rest with stress, is used following a SPECT that was found to be inconclusive. In these cases, the PET scan must have been considered necessary in order to determine what medical or surgical intervention is required to treat the patient. (For purposes of this requirement, an inconclusive test is a test(s) whose results are equivocal, technically uninterpretable, or discordant with a patient's other clinical data and must be documented in the beneficiary's file.)

- For any PET scan for which Medicare payment is claimed for dates of services prior to July 1, 2001, the claimant must submit additional specified information on the claim form (including proper codes and/or modifiers), to indicate the results of the PET scan. The claimant must also include information on whether the PET scan was performed after an inconclusive non-invasive cardiac test. The information submitted with respect to the previous noninvasive cardiac test must specify the type of test performed prior to the PET scan and whether it was inconclusive or unsatisfactory. These explanations are in the form of special G codes used for billing PET scans using Rb 82. Beginning July 1, 2001, claims should be submitted with the appropriate codes.

2. Ammonia N-13 (Effective October 1, 2003)

Effective for services performed on or after October 1, 2003, PET scans performed at rest or with pharmacological stress used for noninvasive imaging of the perfusion of the heart for the diagnosis and management of patients with known or suspected coronary artery disease using the FDA-approved radiopharmaceutical ammonia N-13 are covered, provided the requirements below are met:

- The PET scan, whether at rest alone, or rest with stress, is performed in place of, but not in addition to, a SPECT; or
- The PET scan, whether at rest alone or rest with stress, is used following a SPECT that was found to be inconclusive. In these cases, the PET scan must have been considered necessary in order to determine what medical or surgical intervention is required to treat the patient. (For purposes of this requirement, an inconclusive test is a test whose results are equivocal, technically uninterpretable, or discordant with a patient's other clinical data and must be documented in the beneficiary's file.)

(This NCD last reviewed March 2005)

Pub 100-3, 220.6.2 – FDG PET for Lung Cancer

(Replaced with Section 220.6.17)

(Rev. 120; Issued: 05-06-10; Effective Date: 04-03-09; Implementation Date: 10-30-09)

Pub 100-3, 220.6.3 – FDG PET for Esophageal Cancer

(Replaced with Section 220.6.17)

(Rev. 120; Issued: 05-06-10; Effective Date: 04-03-09; Implementation Date: 10-30-09)

Pub 100-3, 220.6.4 – FDG PET for Colorectal Cancer

(Replaced with Section 220.6.17)

(Rev. 120; Issued: 05-06-10; Effective Date: 04-03-09; Implementation Date: 10-30-09)

Pub 100-3, 220.6.5 – FDG PET for Lymphoma

(Replaced with Section 220.6.17)

(Rev. 120; Issued: 05-06-10; Effective Date: 04-03-09; Implementation Date: 10-30-09)

Pub 100-3, 220.6.6 – FDG PET for Melanoma

(Replaced with Section 220.6.17)

(Rev. 120; Issued: 05-06-10; Effective Date: 04-03-09; Implementation Date: 10-30-09)

Pub 100-3, 220.6.7 – FDG PET for Head and Neck Cancers

(Replaced with Section 220.6.17)

(Rev. 120; Issued: 05-06-10; Effective Date: 04-03-09; Implementation Date: 10-30-09)

Pub 100-3, 220.6.8 – FDG PET for Myocardial Viability

(Various Effective Dates Below)

(Rev. 31, Issued: 04-04-05; Effective: 01-28-05; Implementation: 04-18-05)

The identification of patients with partial loss of heart muscle movement or hibernating myocardium is important in selecting candidates with compromised ventricular function to determine appropriateness for revascularization. Diagnostic tests such as FDG PET distinguish between dysfunctional but viable myocardial tissue and scar tissue in order to affect management decisions in patients with ischemic cardiomyopathy and left ventricular dysfunction.

1. FDG PET is covered for the determination of myocardial viability following an inconclusive single photon emission computed tomography (SPECT) test from July 1, 2001, through September 30, 2002. Only full ring PET scanners are covered from July 1, 2001, through December 31, 2001. However, as of January 1, 2002, full and partial ring scanners are covered.
2. Beginning October 1, 2002, Medicare covers FDG PET for the determination of myocardial viability as a primary or initial diagnostic study prior to revascularization, or following an inconclusive SPECT. Studies performed by full and partial ring scanners are covered.

Limitations: In the event a patient receives a SPECT test with inconclusive results, a PET scan may be covered. However, if a patient receives a FDG PET study with inconclusive results, a follow up SPECT test is not covered.

Documentation that these conditions are met should be maintained by the referring physician in the beneficiary's medical record, as is normal business practice.

(See §220.12 for SPECT coverage.)

(This NCD last reviewed September 2002.)

Pub 100-3, 220.6.9 – FDG PET for Refractory Seizures

(Effective July 1, 2001)

(Rev. 120; Issued: 05-06-10; Effective Date: 04-03-09; Implementation Date: 10-30-09)

Beginning July 1, 2001, Medicare covers FDG PET for pre-surgical evaluation for the purpose of localization of a focus of refractory seizure activity.

Limitations: Covered only for pre-surgical evaluation.

Documentation that these conditions are met should be maintained by the referring physician in the beneficiary's medical record, as is normal business practice.

(This NCD last reviewed June 2001.)

Pub 100-3, 220.6.10 – FDG PET for Breast Cancer

(Effective October 1, 2002)

(Replaced with Section 220.6.17)

(Rev. 120; Issued: 05-06-10; Effective Date: 04-03-09; Implementation Date: 10-30-09)

Pub 100-3, 220.6.11 – FDG PET for Thyroid Cancer

(Various Effective Dates Below) (Replaced with Section 220.6.17)

(Rev. 120; Issued: 05-06-10; Effective Date: 04-03-09; Implementation Date: 10-30-09)

Pub 100-3, 220.6.12 – FDG PET for Soft Tissue Sarcoma

(Various Effective Dates Below) (Replaced with Section 220.6.17)

(Rev. 120; Issued: 05-06-10; Effective Date: 04-03-09; Implementation Date: 10-30-09)

Pub 100-3, 220.6.13 – FDG PET for Dementia and Neurodegenerative Diseases

(Effective September 15, 2004)

(Rev. 120; Issued: 05-06-10; Effective Date: 04-03-09; Implementation Date: 10-30-09)

A. General

Medicare covers FDG PET scans for either the differential diagnosis of fronto-temporal dementia (FTD) and Alzheimer's disease (AD) under specific requirements; OR, its use in a Centers for Medicare & Medicaid Services (CMS)-approved practical clinical trial focused on the utility of FDG PET in the diagnosis or treatment of dementing neurodegenerative diseases. Specific requirements for each indication are clarified below:

B. Nationally Covered Indications

1. FDG-PET Requirements for Coverage in the Differential Diagnosis of AD and FTD

An FDG PET scan is considered reasonable and necessary in patients with a recent diagnosis of dementia and documented cognitive decline of at least 6 months, who meet diagnostic criteria for both AD and FTD. These patients have been evaluated for specific alternate neurodegenerative diseases or other causative factors, but the cause of the clinical symptoms remains uncertain.

The following additional conditions must be met before an FDG PET scan will be covered:

a. The patient's onset, clinical presentation, or course of cognitive impairment is such that FTD is suspected as an alternative neurodegenerative cause of the cognitive decline. Specifically, symptoms such as social disinhibition, awkwardness, difficulties with language, or loss of executive function are more prominent early in the course of FTD than the memory loss typical of AD;

b. The patient has had a comprehensive clinical evaluation (as defined by the American Academy of Neurology (AAN)) encompassing a medical history from the patient and a well-acquainted informant (including assessment of activities of daily living), physical and mental status examination (including formal documentation of cognitive decline occurring over at least 6 months) aided by cognitive scales or neuropsychological testing, laboratory tests, and structural imaging such as magnetic resonance imaging (MRI) or computed tomography (CT);

c. The evaluation of the patient has been conducted by a physician experienced in the diagnosis and assessment of dementia;

d. The evaluation of the patient did not clearly determine a specific neurodegenerative disease or other cause for the clinical symptoms, and information available through FDG PET is reasonably expected to help clarify the diagnosis between FTD and AD and help guide future treatment;

e. The FDG PET scan is performed in a facility that has all the accreditation necessary to operate nuclear medicine equipment. The reading of the scan should be done by an expert in nuclear medicine, radiology, neurology, or psychiatry, with experience interpreting such scans in the presence of dementia;

f. A brain single photon emission computed tomography (SPECT) or FDG PET scan has not been obtained for the same indication. (The indication can be considered to be different in patients who exhibit important changes in scope or severity of cognitive decline, and meet all other qualifying criteria listed above and below (including the judgment that the likely diagnosis remains uncertain). The results of a prior SPECT or FDG PET scan must have been inconclusive or, in the case of SPECT, difficult to interpret due to immature or inadequate technology. In these instances, an FDG PET scan may be covered after 1 year has passed from the time the first SPECT or FDG PET scan was performed.)

g. The referring and billing provider(s) have documented the appropriate evaluation of the Medicare beneficiary. Providers should establish the medical necessity of an FDG PET scan by ensuring that the following:
   - Date of onset of symptoms.
   - Diagnosis of clinical syndrome (normal aging; mild cognitive impairment or MCI; mild, moderate or severe dementia.)
   - Mini mental status exam (MMSE) or similar test score.
   - Presumptive cause (possible, probable, uncertain AD.)
   - Any neuropsychological testing performed.
   - Results of any structural imaging (MRI or CT) performed.
   - Relevant laboratory tests (B12, thyroid hormone.)
   - Number and name of prescribed medications.

The billing provider must furnish a copy of the FDG PET scan result for use by CMS and its contractors upon request. These verification requirements are consistent with federal requirements set forth in 42 Code of Federal Regulations section 410.32 generally for diagnostic x-ray tests, diagnostic laboratory tests, and other tests. In summary, section 410.32 requires the billing physician and the referring physician to maintain information in the medical record of each patient to demonstrate medical necessity [410.32(d) (2)] and submit the information demonstrating medical necessity to CMS and/or its agents upon request [410.32(d)(3)(I)] (OMB number 0938-0685).

2. FDG PET Requirements for Coverage in the Context of a CMS-approved Practical Clinical Trial Utilizing a Specific Protocol to Demonstrate the Utility of FDG PET in the Diagnosis, and Treatment of Neurodegenerative Dementing Diseases

An FDG PET scan is considered reasonable and necessary in patients with MCI or early dementia (in clinical circumstances other than those specified in subparagraph 1) only in the context of an approved clinical trial that contains patient safeguards and protections to ensure proper administration, use and evaluation of the FDG PET scan.

The clinical trial must compare patients who do and do not receive an FDG PET scan and have as its goal to monitor, evaluate, and improve clinical outcomes. In addition, it must meet the following basic criteria:

a. Written protocol on file.
b. Institutional Review Board review and approval.
c. Scientific review and approval by two or more qualified individuals who are not part of the research team.
d. Certification that investigators have not been disqualified.

C. Nationally Non-covered Indications

All other uses of FDG PET for patients with a presumptive diagnosis of dementia-causing neurodegenerative disease (e.g., possible or probable AD, clinically typical FTD, dementia of Lewy bodies, or Creutzfeld-Jacob disease) for which CMS has not specifically indicated coverage continue to be non-covered.

D. Other

Not applicable.

(This NCD last reviewed September 2004.)

Pub 100-3, 220.6.14 – FDG PET for Brain, Cervical, Ovarian, Pancreatic, Small Cell Lung, and Testicular Cancers

(Effective January 28, 2005)

(Replaced with Section 220.6.17)

(Rev. 120; Issued: 05-06-10; Effective Date: 04-03-09; Implementation Date: 10-30-09)

Pub 100-3, 220.6.15 – FDG PET for All Other Cancer Indications Not Previously Specified

(Effective January 28, 2005)

(Replaced with Section 220.6.17)

(Rev. 120; Issued: 05-06-10; Effective Date: 04-03-09; Implementation Date: 10-30-09)

Pub 100-3, 220.6.16 – FDG PET for Infection and Inflammation

(Effective March 19, 2008)

(Rev. 84; Issued: 06-27-08; Effective Date: 03-19-08; Implementation Date: 07-28-08)

A. General

The Centers for Medicare & Medicaid Services (CMS) received a formal, complete request to reconsider the current, de facto non-coverage for FDG PET imaging for the following off-label uses, each in lieu of bone, leukocyte, and/or gallium scintigraphy:

1. Suspected chronic osteomyelitis in patients with: (a) previously documented osteomyelitis with suspected recurrence, or, (b) symptoms of osteomyelitis for more than 6 weeks (including diabetic foot ulcers)
2. Investigation of patients with suspected infection of hip prosthesis
3. Fever of unknown origin in patients with a febrile illness of >3 weeks duration, a temperature of >38.3 degrees Centigrade on at least two occasions, and uncertain diagnosis after a thorough history, physical examination, and one week of proper investigation.

B. Nationally Covered Indications

N/A

C. Nationally Non-Covered Indications

The CMS is continuing its national non-coverage of FDG PET for the requested indications. Based upon our review, CMS has determined that the evidence is inadequate to conclude that FDG PET for chronic osteomyelitis, infection of hip arthroplasty, and fever of unknown origin improves health outcomes in the Medicare populations, and therefore has determined that FDG PET for chronic osteomyelitis, infection of hip arthroplasty, and fever of unknown origin is not reasonable and necessary under section 1862(a)(1)(A) of the Social Security Act.

D. Other

The CMS has also determined that the request for coverage is not appropriate for the Coverage with Evidence Development (CED) paradigm.

(This NCD last reviewed March 2008.)

Pub 100-3, 220.6.17 – Positron Emission Tomography (PET) (FDG) for Oncologic Conditions

(Various Effective Dates)

(Rev. 124; Issued: 09-24-10; Effective Date: 08-04-10; Implementation Date: 10-25-10)

A. General

The Centers for Medicare and Medicaid Services (CMS) was asked to reconsider section 220.6, of the National Coverage Determinations (NCD) Manual, to end the prospective data collection requirements across all oncologic indications of FDG PET except for monitoring response to treatment. Section 220.6 of the NCD Manual, establishes the requirement for prospective data collection for FDG PET used in the diagnosis, staging, restaging, and monitoring response to treatment for brain, cervical, ovarian, pancreatic, small cell lung and testicular cancers, as well as for cancer indications not previously specified in section 220.6 in its entirety.

The CMS received public input indicating that the current coverage framework, which required cancer-by-cancer consideration of diagnosis, staging, restaging, and monitoring response to treatment should be replaced by a more omnibus consideration. Thus, CMS broadened the scope of this review through an announcement on the Web site and solicited additional public comment on the use of FDG PET imaging for solid tumors so that it could transparently consider this possibility.

1. Framework

Effective for claims with dates of service on and after April 3, 2009, CMS is adopting a coverage framework that replaces the four-part diagnosis, staging, restaging and monitoring response to treatment categories with a two-part framework that differentiates FDG PET imaging used to inform the initial antitumor treatment strategy from other uses related to guiding subsequent antitumor treatment strategies after the completion of initial treatment. CMS is making this change for all NCDs that address coverage of FDG PET for the specific oncologic conditions addressed in this decision.

2. Initial Anti-tumor Treatment Strategy

Effective for claims with dates of service on and after April 3, 2009, CMS has determined that the evidence is adequate to determine that the results of FDG PET imaging are useful in determining the appropriate initial treatment strategy for beneficiaries with suspected solid tumors and myeloma and improve health outcomes and thus are reasonable and necessary under §1862(a)(1)(A) of the Social Security Act (the Act).

Therefore, effective for claims with dates of service on and after August 4, 2010, CMS will continue to nationally cover one FDG PET study for beneficiaries who have solid tumors that are biopsy proven or strongly suspected based on other diagnostic testing when the beneficiary's treating physician determines that the FDG PET study is needed to determine the location and/or extent of the tumor for the following therapeutic purposes related to the initial treatment strategy:

- To determine whether or not the beneficiary is an appropriate candidate for an invasive diagnostic or therapeutic procedure; or
- To determine the optimal anatomic location for an invasive procedure; or
- To determine the anatomic extent of tumor when the recommended anti-tumor treatment reasonably depends on the extent of the tumor.

In addition, effective for claims with dates of service on and after August 4, 2010, CMS believes that an NCD is not appropriate for addressing coverage for additional FDG PET scans for the therapeutic purposes related to the initial treatment strategy. Therefore, local Medicare contractors will have discretion to cover (or not cover) within their jurisdictions any additional PET scan for the therapeutic purposes related to the initial treatment strategy as described above.

As exceptions to the April 3, 2009, initial treatment strategy section above:

a. The CMS has reviewed evidence on the use of FDG PET imaging to determine initial anti-tumor treatment in patients with adenocarcinoma of the prostate. CMS has determined that the available evidence does not demonstrate that FDG PET imaging improves physician decision making in the determination of initial anti-tumor treatment strategy in Medicare beneficiaries who have adenocarcinoma of the prostate, does not improve health outcomes and is thus not reasonable and necessary under §1862(a)(1)(A) of the Act. Therefore, FDG PET is nationally non-covered for this indication of this tumor type.

b. The CMS received no new evidence demonstrating a change was warranted with respect to the use of FDG PET imaging to determine initial anti-tumor treatment in breast cancer; thus CMS is not making any change to the current coverage policy for FDG PET in breast cancer. CMS is continuing to nationally cover FDG PET imaging for the initial treatment strategy for male and female breast cancer only when used in staging distant metastasis. FDG PET imaging for diagnosis and initial staging of axillary nodes will remain nationally non-covered.

c. The CMS received no new evidence demonstrating a change was warranted with respect to use of FDG PET imaging of regional lymph nodes in melanoma; thus CMS is not changing the current NCD for FDG PET in melanoma. CMS will continue national non-coverage of FDG PET for the evaluation of regional lymph nodes in melanoma. Other uses of FDG PET to determine initial treatment for melanoma strategy remain nationally covered.

d. The CMS received no new evidence demonstrating a change was warranted with respect to use of FDG PET imaging in the initial treatment strategy for cervical cancer. CMS is continuing to nationally cover FDG PET imaging as an adjunct test for the detection of pre-treatment metastasis (i.e., staging) in newly diagnosed cervical cancers following conventional imaging that is negative for extra-pelvic metastasis. All other uses of FDG PET for the initial treatment strategy for beneficiaries diagnosed with cervical cancer will continue to only be covered nationally as research under §1862(a)(1)(E) of the Act through Coverage with Evidence Development (CED). Therefore, CMS will cover nationally one initial FDG PET study for newly diagnosed cervical cancer when not used as an adjunct test for the detection of

Medicare References

pre-treatment metastases following conventional imaging that is negative for extra-pelvic metastasis only when the beneficiary's treating physician determines that the FDG PET study is needed to inform the initial anti-tumor treatment strategy and the beneficiary is enrolled in, and the FDG PET provider is participating in, the specific type of prospective clinical study outlined under subsequent treatment strategy below.

e. Effective November 10, 2009, as a result of a reconsideration request, CMS ended the prospective data collection requirements, or CED, for the use of FDG PET imaging in the initial staging of cervical cancer related to initial treatment strategy. CMS is continuing to nationally cover FDG PET imaging as an adjunct test for the detection of pre-treatment metastasis (i.e., staging) in newly diagnosed cervical cancers following conventional imaging that is negative for extra-pelvic metastasis.

Therefore, CMS will nationally cover one initial FDG PET study for staging in beneficiaries who have biopsy-proven cervical cancer when the beneficiary's treating physician determines that the FDG PET study is needed to determine the location and/or extent of the tumor for the following therapeutic purposes related to initial treatment strategy:

- To determine whether or not the beneficiary is an appropriate candidate for an invasive diagnostic or therapeutic procedure; or
- To determine the optimal anatomic location for an invasive procedure; or
- To determine the anatomic extent of the tumor when the recommended anti-tumor treatment reasonably depends on the extent of the tumor.

In addition, effective for claims with dates of service on and after August 4, 2010, CMS believes that an NCD is not appropriate for addressing coverage for additional FDG PET scans for the therapeutic purposes related to the initial treatment strategy. Therefore, local Medicare contractors will have discretion to cover (or not cover) within their jurisdictions any additional PET scan for the therapeutic purposes related to the initial treatment strategy as described above.

Additionally, effective November 10, 2009, following a reconsideration request, CMS determines that there is no credible evidence that the results of FDG PET imaging are useful to make the initial diagnoses of cervical cancer, does not improve health outcomes, and is not reasonable and necessary under section 1862(a)(1)(A) of the Social Security Act. Therefore, CMS will non-cover FDG PET imaging for initial diagnosis of cervical cancer related to initial treatment strategy.

3. Subsequent Anti-tumor Treatment Strategy

As part of its April 3, 2009, NCD, the CMS reviewed evidence on the use of FDG PET in the subsequent treatment strategy for patients with tumor types other than those seven indications currently covered without exception (breast, colorectal, esophagus, head and neck (non-CNS/thyroid), lymphoma, melanoma, and non-small cell lung).

As a result, CMS determined that the available evidence is adequate to determine that FDG PET imaging also improves physician decision making in the determination of subsequent treatment strategy in Medicare beneficiaries who have ovarian cancer, cervical cancer, and myeloma, improves health outcomes, and is thus reasonable and necessary under §1862(a)(1)(A) of the Act.

Therefore, effective for claims with dates of service on and after April 3, 2009, for tumor types other than breast, colorectal, esophagus, head and neck (non-CNS/thyroid), lymphoma, melanoma, non-small cell lung, ovarian, cervical, and myeloma, CMS has determined that the available evidence is not adequate to determine that FDG PET imaging improves physician decision making in the determination of subsequent anti-tumor treatment strategy or improves health outcomes in Medicare beneficiaries and thus is not reasonable and necessary under §1862(a)(1)(A) of the Act.

However, CMS has determined that the available evidence is sufficient to determine that FDG PET imaging for subsequent anti-tumor treatment strategy for all other tumor types other than the 10 indications noted above may be nationally covered as research under §1862(a)(1)(E) of the Act through CED. Therefore, CMS will nationally cover a subsequent FDG PET study for all other tumor types other than the 10 indications noted above, when the beneficiary's treating physician determines that the FDG PET study is needed to inform the subsequent anti-tumor treatment strategy and the beneficiary is enrolled in, and the FDG PET provider is participating in, the following type of prospective clinical study:

An FDG PET clinical study that is designed to collect additional information at the time of the scan to assist in patient management. Qualifying clinical studies must ensure that specific hypotheses are addressed; appropriate data elements are collected; hospitals and providers are qualified to provide the FDG PET scan and interpret the results; participating hospitals and providers accurately report data on all enrolled patients not included in other qualifying trials through adequate auditing mechanisms; and all patient confidentiality, privacy, and other Federal laws must be followed.

The clinical studies for which CMS will provide coverage must answer one or more of the following three questions:

Prospectively, in Medicare beneficiaries whose treating physician determines that the FDG PET study is needed to inform the subsequent anti-tumor treatment strategy, does the addition of FDG PET imaging lead to:

- A change in the likelihood of appropriate referrals for palliative care?
- Improved quality of life?
- Improved survival?

The study must adhere to the following standards of scientific integrity and relevance to the Medicare population:

a. The principal purpose of the research study is to test whether a particular intervention potentially improves the participants' health outcomes.

b. The research study is well-supported by available scientific and medical information or it is intended to clarify or establish the health outcomes of interventions already in common clinical use.

c. The research study does not unjustifiably duplicate existing studies.

d. The research study design is appropriate to answer the research question being asked in the study.

e. The research study is sponsored by an organization or individual capable of executing the proposed study successfully.

f. The research study is in compliance with all applicable Federal regulations concerning the protection of human subjects found in the Code of Federal Regulations (CFR) at 45 CFR Part 46. If a study is regulated by the Food and Drug Administration (FDA), it also must be in compliance with 21 CFR Parts 50 and 56.

g. All aspects of the research study are conducted according to the appropriate standards of scientific integrity.

h. The research study has a written protocol that clearly addresses, or incorporates by reference, the Medicare standards.

i. The clinical research study is not designed to exclusively test toxicity or disease pathophysiology in healthy individuals. Trials of all medical technologies measuring therapeutic outcomes as one of the objectives meet this standard only if the disease or condition being studied is life-threatening as defined in 21 CFR 312.81(a) and the patient has no other viable treatment options.

j. The clinical research study is registered on the www.ClinicalTrials.gov Web site by the principal sponsor/investigator prior to the enrollment of the first study subject.

k. The research study protocol specifies the method and timing of public release of all pre-specified outcomes to be measured including release of outcomes if outcomes are negative or study is terminated early. The results must be made public within 24 months of the end of data collection. If a report is planned to be published in a peer-reviewed journal, then that initial release may be an abstract that meets the requirements of the International Committee of Medical Journal Editors. However, a full report of the outcomes must be made public no later than 3 years after the end of data collection.

l. The research study protocol must explicitly discuss subpopulations affected by the treatment under investigation, particularly traditionally underrepresented groups in clinical studies, how the inclusion and exclusion criteria affect enrollment of these populations, and a plan for the retention and reporting of said populations on the trial. If the inclusion and exclusion criteria are expected to have a negative effect on the recruitment or retention of underrepresented populations, the protocol must discuss why these criteria are necessary.

m. The research study protocol explicitly discusses how the results are or are not expected to be generalizable to the Medicare population to infer whether Medicare patients may benefit from the intervention. Separate discussions in the protocol may be necessary for populations eligible for Medicare due to age, disability or Medicaid eligibility.

Consistent with section 1142 of the Act, the Agency for Healthcare Research and Quality (AHRQ) supports clinical research studies that CMS determines meet the above-listed standards and address the above-listed research questions.

4. Synopsis of New Framework

Effective for claims with dates of service on and after April 3, 2009, the CMS transitioned the prior framework—diagnosis, staging, restaging, and monitoring response to treatment—into the initial treatment strategy and subsequent treatment strategy framework. The chart below summarizes national FDG PET coverage as of November 10, 2009:

FDG PET Coverage for Solid Tumors and Myeloma

Tumor Type	Initial Treatment Strategy (formerly "diagnosis" & "staging")	Subsequent Treatment Strategy (formerly "restaging" & "monitoring response to treatment")
Colorectal	Cover	Cover
Tumor Type	Initial Treatment Strategy (formerly "diagnosis" & "staging")	Subsequent Treatment Strategy (formerly "restaging" & "monitoring response to treatment")
Esophagus	Cover	Cover
Head & Neck (not Thyroid, CNS)	Cover	Cover
Lymphoma	Cover	Cover
Non-Small Cell Lung	Cover	Cover
Ovary	Cover	Cover
Brain	Cover	CED
Cervix	Cover w/exception*	Cover
Small Cell Lung	Cover	CED
Soft Tissue Sarcoma	Cover	CED
Pancreas	Cover	CED
Testes	Cover	CED
Breast (female and male)	Cover w/exception*	Cover
Melanoma	Cover w/exception*	Cover
Prostate	Non-Cover	CED
Thyroid	Cover	Cover w/exception or CED*
All Other Solid Tumors	Cover	CED
Myeloma	Cover	Cover
All other cancers not listed	CED	CED

**Cervix: Nationally non-covered for the initial diagnosis of cervical cancer related to initial treatment strategy. All other indications for initial treatment strategy for cervical cancer are nationally covered.*

**Breast: Nationally non-covered for initial diagnosis and/or staging of axillary lymph nodes. Covered for initial staging of metastatic disease. All other indications for breast cancer initial treatment strategy are nationally covered.*

**Melanoma: Nationally non-covered for initial staging of regional lymph nodes. All other indications for initial treatment strategy for melanoma are nationally covered.*

**Thyroid: Nationally covered for subsequent treatment strategy of recurrent or residual thyroid cancer of follicular cell origin previously treated by thyroidectomy and radioiodine ablation and have a serum thyroglobulin >10ng/ml and have a negative I-131 whole body scan. All other indications for subsequent treatment strategy for thyroid cancer are nationally covered under CED.*

(This NCD last reviewed November 2009.)

Pub 100-3, 220.6.19 – Positron Emission Tomography NaF-18 (NaF-18 PET) to Identify Bone Metastasis of Cancer

(Effective February 26, 2010)

(Rev. 119, Issued: 03-26-10, Effective: 02-26-10, Implementation: 07-06-10)

A. General

Positron Emission Tomography (PET) is a non-invasive, diagnostic imaging procedure that assesses the level of metabolic activity and perfusion in various organ systems of the body. A positron camera (tomograph) is used to produce cross-sectional tomographic images, which are obtained from positron-emitting radioactive tracer substances (radiopharmaceuticals) such as F-18 sodium fluoride. NaF-18 PET has been recognized as an excellent technique for imaging areas of altered osteogenic activity in bone. The clinical value of detecting and assessing the initial extent of metastatic cancer in bone is attested by a number of professional guidelines for oncology. Imaging to detect bone metastases is also recommended when a patient, following completion of initial treatment, is symptomatic with bone pain suspicious for metastases from a known primary tumor.

B. Nationally Covered Indications

Effective February 26, 2010, the Centers for Medicare & Medicaid Services (CMS) will cover NaF-18 PET imaging when the beneficiary's treating physician determines that the NaF-18 PET study is needed to inform to inform the initial antitumor treatment strategy or to guide subsequent antitumor treatment strategy after the completion of initial treatment, and when the beneficiary is enrolled in, and the NaF-18 PET provider is participating in, the following type of prospective clinical study:

A NaF-18 PET clinical study that is designed to collect additional information at the time of the scan to assist in initial antitumor treatment planning or to guide subsequent treatment strategy by the identification, location and quantification of bone metastases in beneficiaries in whom bone metastases are strongly suspected based on clinical symptoms or the results of other diagnostic studies. Qualifying clinical studies must ensure that specific hypotheses are addressed; appropriate data elements are collected; hospitals and providers are qualified to provide the PET scan and interpret the results; participating hospitals and providers accurately report data on all enrolled patients not included in other qualifying trials through adequate auditing mechanisms; and all patient confidentiality, privacy, and other Federal laws must be followed.

The clinical studies for which Medicare will provide coverage must answer one or more of the following questions:

Prospectively, in Medicare beneficiaries whose treating physician determines that the NaF-18 PET study results are needed to inform the initial antitumor treatment strategy or to guide subsequent antitumor treatment strategy after the completion of initial treatment, does the addition of NaF-18 PET imaging lead to:

- A change in patient management to more appropriate palliative care; or
- A change in patient management to more appropriate curative care; or
- Improved quality of life; or
- Improved survival?

The study must adhere to the following standards of scientific integrity and relevance to the Medicare population:

a. The principal purpose of the research study is to test whether a particular intervention potentially improves the participants' health outcomes.

b. The research study is well-supported by available scientific and medical information or it is intended to clarify or establish the health outcomes of interventions already in common clinical use.

c. The research study does not unjustifiably duplicate existing studies.

d. The research study design is appropriate to answer the research question being asked in the study.

e. The research study is sponsored by an organization or individual capable of executing the proposed study successfully.

f. The research study is in compliance with all applicable Federal regulations concerning the protection of human subjects found in the Code of Federal Regulations (CFR) at 45 CFR Part 46. If a study is regulated by the Food and Drug Administration (FDA), it also must be in compliance with 21 CFR Parts 50 and 56.

g. All aspects of the research study are conducted according to the appropriate standards of scientific integrity.

h. The research study has a written protocol that clearly addresses, or incorporates by reference, the Medicare standards.

i. The clinical research study is not designed to exclusively test toxicity or disease pathophysiology in healthy individuals. Trials of all medical technologies measuring therapeutic outcomes as one of the objectives meet this standard only if the disease or condition being studied is life-threatening as defined in 21 CFR §312.81(a) and the patient has no other viable treatment options.

j. The clinical research study is registered on the www.ClinicalTrials.gov Web site by the principal sponsor/investigator prior to the enrollment of the first study subject.

k. The research study protocol specifies the method and timing of public release of all pre-specified outcomes to be measured including release of outcomes if outcomes are negative or study is terminated early. The results must be made public within 24 months of the end of data collection. If a report is planned to be published in a peer-reviewed journal, then that initial release may be an abstract that meets the requirements of the International Committee of Medical Journal Editors. However, a full report of the outcomes must be made public no later than three (3) years after the end of data collection.

l. The research study protocol must explicitly discuss subpopulations affected by the treatment under investigation, particularly traditionally underrepresented groups in clinical studies, how the inclusion and exclusion criteria affect enrollment of these populations, and a plan for the retention and reporting of said populations on the trial. If the inclusion and exclusion criteria are expected to have a negative effect on the recruitment or retention of underrepresented populations, the protocol must discuss why these criteria are necessary.

m. The research study protocol explicitly discusses how the results are or are not expected to be generalizable to the Medicare population to infer whether Medicare patients may benefit from the intervention. Separate discussions in the protocol may be necessary for populations eligible for Medicare due to age, disability or Medicaid eligibility.

Consistent with section 1142 of the Social Security Act (the Act), the Agency for Healthcare Research and Quality (AHRQ) supports clinical research studies that the Centers for Medicare and Medicaid Services (CMS) determines meet the above-listed standards and address the above-listed research questions.

C. Nationally Non-Covered Indications

Effective February 26, 2010, CMS determines that the evidence is not sufficient to determine that the results of NaF-18 PET imaging to identify bone metastases improve health outcomes of beneficiaries with cancer and is not reasonable and necessary under §1862(a)(1)(A) of the Act unless it is to inform initial antitumor treatment strategy or to guide subsequent antitumor treatment strategy after completion of initial treatment, and then only under CED. All other uses and clinical indications of NaF-18 PET are nationally non-covered.

D. Other

The only radiopharmaceutical diagnostic imaging agents covered by Medicare for PET cancer imaging are 2-[F-18] Fluoro-D-Glucose (FDG) and NaF-18 (sodium fluoride-18). All other PET radiopharmaceutical diagnostic imaging agents are non-covered for this indication.

(This NCD was last reviewed in February 2010.)

Pub 100-3, 220.12 – Single Photon Emission Computed Tomograph (SPECT)

(Rev. 1, 10-03-03)

SPECT acquires information on the concentration of radionuclides introduced into the patient's body. It is useful in the diagnosis of several clinical conditions including:

- Stress fracture
- Spondylosis
- Infection (e.g., discitis)
- Tumor (e.g., osteoid osteoma)
- Analyze blood flow to an organ, as in the case of myocardial viability
- Differentiate ischemic heart disease from dilated cardiomyopathy.

Frequency limitations: Contractor discretion.

In the case of myocardial viability, FDG PET may be used following a SPECT that was found to be inconclusive. However, SPECT may not be used following an inconclusive FDG PET performed to evaluate myocardial viability.

Pub 100-3, 230.5 – Gravlee Jet Washer

(Rev. 1, 10-03-03)

The Gravlee Jet Washer is a sterile, disposable, diagnostic device for detecting endometrial cancer. The use of this device is indicated where the patient exhibits clinical symptoms or signs suggestive of endometrial disease, such as irregular or heavy vaginal bleeding.

Program payment cannot be made for the washer or the related diagnostic services when furnished in connection with the examination of an asymptomatic patient. Payment for routine physical checkups is precluded under the statute. (See §1862(a)(7) of the Act.) (See the **Medicare Benefit Policy Manual**, Chapter 16, "General Exclusions From Coverage," §90).

Pub 100-3, 230.6 – Vabra Aspirator

(Rev. 1, 10-03-03)

The VABRA aspirator is a sterile, disposable, vacuum aspirator which is used to collect uterine tissue for study to detect endometrial carcinoma. The use of this device is indicated where the patient exhibits clinical symptoms or signs suggestive of endometrial disease, such as irregular or heavy vaginal bleeding.

Program payment cannot be made for the aspirator or the related diagnostic services when furnished in connection with the examination of an asymptomatic patient. Payment for routine physical checkups is precluded under the statute (§1862(a)(7) of the Act).

Cross-reference:

See the **Medicare Benefit Policy Manual**, Chapter 16, "General Exclusions From Coverage," §90, and §230.5 of this manual.

Pub 100-3, 230.7 – Water Purification and Softening Systems Used in Conjunction With Home Dialysis

(Rev. 1, 10-03-03)

A Water Purification Systems

Water used for home dialysis should be chemically free of heavy trace metals and/or organic contaminants that could be hazardous to the patient. It should also be as free of bacteria as possible but need not be biologically sterile. Since the characteristics of natural water supplies in most areas of the country are such that some type of water purification system is needed, such a system used in conjunction with a home dialysis (either peritoneal or hemodialysis) unit is covered under Medicare.

There are two types of water purification systems that will satisfy these requirements:

- Deionization – The removal of organic substances, mineral salts of magnesium and calcium (causing hardness), compounds of fluoride and chloride from tap water using the process of filtration and ion exchange; or
- Reverse Osmosis – The process used to remove impurities from tap water utilizing pressure to force water through a porous membrane.

Use of both a deionization unit and reverse osmosis unit in series, theoretically to provide the advantages of both systems, has been determined medically unnecessary since either system can provide water which is both chemically and bacteriologically pure enough for acceptable use in home dialysis. In addition, spare deionization tanks are not covered since they are essentially a precautionary supply rather than a current requirement for treatment of the patient.

Activated carbon filters used as a component of water purification systems to remove unsafe concentrations of chlorine and chloramines are covered when prescribed by a physician.

B Water Softening System

Medicare References

Except as indicated below, a water softening system used in conjunction with home dialysis is excluded from coverage under Medicare as not being reasonable and necessary within the meaning of §1862(a)(1) of the Act. Such a system, in conjunction with a home dialysis unit, does not adequately remove the hazardous heavy metal contaminants (such as arsenic) which may be present in trace amounts.

A water softening system may be covered when used to pretreat water to be purified by a reverse osmosis (RO) unit for home dialysis where:

The manufacturer of the RO unit has set standards for the quality of water entering the RO (e.g., the water to be purified by the RO must be of a certain quality if the unit is to perform as intended);

The patients water is demonstrated to be of a lesser quality than required; and

The softener is used only to soften water entering the RO unit, and thus, used only for dialysis. (The softener need not actually be built into the RO unit, but must be an integral part of the dialysis system.)

C Developing Need When a Water Softening System is Replaced with a Water Purification Unit in an Existing Home Dialysis System

The medical necessity of water purification units must be care fully developed when they replace water softening systems in existing home dialysis systems. A purification system may be ordered under these circumstances for a number of reasons. For example, changes in the medical community's opinions regarding the quality of water necessary for safe dialysis may lead the physician to decide the quality of water previously used should be improved, or the water quality itself may have deteriorated. Patients may have dialyzed using only an existing water softener previous to Medicare ESRD coverage because of inability to pay for a purification system. On the other hand, in some cases, the installation of a purification system is not medically necessary. Thus, when such a case comes to the contractor's attention, the contractor asks the physician to furnish the reason for the changes. Supporting documentation, such as the suppliers recommendations or water analysis, may be required. All such cases should be reviewed by the contractor's medical consultants.

Cross reference:

The **Medicare Benefit Policy Manual**, Chapter 15, "Covered Medical and Other Health Services," §110.

Pub 100-3, Pub 100-3, 230.8 – Non-Implantable Pelvic Flood Electrical Stimulator

(Rev. 48, 06-19-06)

Non-implantable pelvic floor electrical stimulators provide neuromuscular electrical stimulation through the pelvic floor with the intent of strengthening and exercising pelvic floor musculature. Stimulation is generally delivered by vaginal or anal probes connected to an external pulse generator.

The methods of pelvic floor electrical stimulation vary in location, stimulus frequency (Hz), stimulus intensity or amplitude (mA), pulse duration (duty cycle), treatments per day, number of treatment days per week, length of time for each treatment session, overall time period for device use and between clinic and home settings. In general, the stimulus frequency and other parameters are chosen based on the patient's clinical diagnosis.

Indications and Limitations of Coverage

Pelvic floor electrical stimulation with a non-implantable stimulator is covered for the treatment of stress and/or urge urinary incontinence in cognitively intact patients who have failed a documented trial of pelvic muscle exercise (PME) training.

A failed trial of PME training is defined as no clinically significant improvement in urinary continence after completing 4 weeks of an ordered plan of pelvic muscle exercises designed to increase periurethral muscle strength.

Pub 100-3, 230.10 – Incontinence Control Devices

(Rev. 1, 10-03-03)

A Mechanical/Hydraulic Incontinence Control Devices

Mechanical/hydraulic incontinence control devices are accepted as safe and effective in the management of urinary incontinence in patients with permanent anatomic and neurologic dysfunctions of the bladder. This class of devices achieves control of urination by compression of the urethra. The materials used and the success rate may vary somewhat from device to device. Such a device is covered when its use is reasonable and necessary for the individual patient.

B Collagen Implant

A collagen implant which is injected into the submucosal tissues of the urethra and/or the bladder neck and into tissues adjacent to the urethra, is a prosthetic device used in the treatment of stress urinary incontinence resulting from intrinsic sphincter deficiency (ISD). ISD is a cause of stress urinary incontinence in which the urethral sphincter is unable to contract and generate sufficient resistance in the bladder, especially during stress maneuvers.

Prior to collagen implant therapy, a skin test for collagen sensitivity must be administered and evaluated over a 4-week period.

In male patients, the evaluation must include a complete history and physical examination and a simple cystometrogram to determine that the bladder fills and stores properly. The patient then is asked to stand upright with a full bladder and to cough or otherwise exert abdominal pressure on his bladder. If the patient leaks, the diagnosis of ISD is established.

In female patients, the evaluation must include a complete history and physical examination (including a pelvic exam) and a simple cystometrogram to rule out abnormalities of bladder compliance and abnormalities of urethral support. Following that determination, an abdominal leak point pressure (ALLP) test is performed. Leak point pressure, stated in cm H2O, is defined as the intra-abdominal pressure at which leakage occurs from the bladder (around a catheter) when the bladder has been filled with a minimum of 150 cc fluid. If the patient has an ALLP of less than 100 cm H2O, the diagnosis of ISD is established.

To use a collagen implant, physicians must have urology training in the use of a cystoscope and must complete a collagen implant training program.

Coverage of a collagen implant, and the procedure to inject it, is limited to the following types of patients with stress urinary incontinence due to ISD:

- Male or female patients with congenital sphincter weakness secondary to conditions such as myelomeningocele or epispadias;
- Male or female patients with acquired sphincter weakness secondary to spinal cord lesions;
- Male patients following trauma, including prostatectomy and/or radiation; and
- Female patients without urethral hypermobility and with abdominal leak point pressures of 100 cm H2O or less.

Patients whose incontinence does not improve with five injection procedures (five separate treatment sessions) are considered treatment failures, and no further treatment of urinary incontinence by collagen implant is covered. Patients who have a reoccurrence of incontinence following successful treatment with collagen implants in the past (e.g., 6-12 months previously) may benefit from additional treatment sessions. Coverage of additional sessions may be allowed but must be supported by medical justification. See the **Medicare Benefit Policy Manual**, Chapter 15, "Covered Medical and Other Health Services," §120. (See §230.8.)

Pub 100-3, 230.11 – Diagnostic Pap Smears

(Rev. 1, 10-03-03)

The guide in §190.2 applies.

Pub 100-3, 230.12 – Dimethyl Sulfoxide (DMSO)

(Rev. 1, 10-03-03)

DMSO is an industrial solvent produced as a chemical byproduct of paper production from wood pulp. The Food and Drug Administration has determined that the only purpose for which DMSO is safe and effective for humans is in the treatment of the bladder condition, interstitial cystitis. Therefore, the use of DMSO for all other indications is not considered to be reasonable and necessary. Payment may be made for its use only when reasonable and necessary for a patient in the treatment of interstitial cystitis.

Pub 100-3, 240.1 – Lung Volume Reduction Surgery (Reduction Pneumoplasty)

(Rev. 44, Effective 11-17-05, Implementation 03-02-06)

A. General

Lung volume reduction surgery (LVRS) or reduction pneumoplasty, also referred to as lung shaving or lung contouring, is performed on patients with severe emphysema in order to allow the remaining compressed lung to expand, and thus, improve respiratory function. Medicare-covered LVRS approaches are limited to bilateral excision of a damaged lung with stapling performed via median sternotomy or video-assisted thoracoscopic surgery.

Indications and Limitations of Coverage

B. Nationally Covered Indications

Effective for services performed on or after January 1, 2004 Medicare will only consider LVRS reasonable and necessary when all of the following requirements are met (note varying dates for facility criteria in section 3. below):

1. The patient satisfies all the criteria outlined in the following table:

Assessment	Criteria
History and physical examination	Consistent with emphysema
	BMI, ≤ 31.1 kg/m2 (men) or ≤ 32.3 kg/m2 (women)
	Stable with ≤20 mg prednisone (or equivalent) qd
Radiographic	High Resolution Computer Tomography (HRCT) scan evidence of bilateral emphysema
Pulmonary function (pre-rehabilitation)	Forced expiratory volume in one second (FEV1) ≤ 45% predicted (≥ 15% predicted if age ≥70 years)
	Total lung capacity (TLC) ≥100% predicted post-bronchodilator
	Residual volume (RV) ≥150% predicted post-bronchodilator
Arterial blood gas level (pre-rehabilitation)	PCO2, ≤ 60 mm Hg (PCO2, ≤ 55 mm Hg if 1-mile above sea level)
	PO2, ≥ 45 mm Hg on room air (PO2, ≥ 30 mm Hg if 1-mile above sea level)
Cardiac assessment	Approval for surgery by cardiologist if any of the following are present: Unstable angina; left-ventricular ejection fraction (LVEF) cannot be estimated from the echocardiogram; LVEF < 45%; dobutamine-radionuclide cardiac scan indicates coronary artery disease or ventricular dysfunction; arrhythmia (> 5 premature ventricular contractions per minute; cardiac rhythm other than sinus; premature ventricular contractions on EKG at rest)
Surgical assessment	Approval for surgery by pulmonary physician, thoracic surgeon, and anesthesiologist post-rehabilitation
Exercise	Post-rehabilitation 6-min walk of ≥140 m; able to complete 3 min unloaded pedaling in exercise tolerance test (pre- and post-rehabilitation)
Consent	Signed consents for screening and rehabilitation
Smoking	Plasma cotinine level ≤ 13.7 ng/mL (or arterial carboxyhemoglobin ≤ 2.5% if using nicotine products)
	Nonsmoking for 4 months prior to initial interview and throughout evaluation for surgery
Preoperative diagnostic and therapeutic program adherence	Must complete assessment for and program of preoperative services in preparation for surgery

2. In addition, the patient must have:
   - Severe upper lobe predominant emphysema (as defined by radiologist assessment of upper lobe predominance on CT scan), or
   - Severe non-upper lobe emphysema with low exercise capacity.

   Patients with low exercise capacity are those whose maximal exercise capacity is at or below 25 watts for women and 40 watts (w) for men after completion of the preoperative therapeutic program in preparation for LVRS. Exercise capacity is measured by incremental, maximal, symptom-limited exercise with a cycle ergometer utilizing 5 or 10 watt/minute ramp on 30% oxygen after 3 minutes of unloaded pedaling.
3. Effective for services performed on or after November 17, 2005, CMS determines that LVRS is reasonable and necessary when performed at facilities that are:

(1) certified by the Joint Commission on Accreditation of Healthcare Organizations (Joint Commission) under the LVRS Disease Specific Care Certification Program (program standards and requirements as printed in the Joint Commission's October 25, 2004, Disease Specific Care Certification Program packet); or (2) approved as Medicare lung or heart-lung transplantation hospitals.

In addition, LVRS performed between January 1, 2004, and May 17, 2007, is reasonable and necessary when performed at facilities that: (1) were approved by the National Heart Lung and Blood Institute to participate in the National Emphysema Treatment Trial (NETT); or (2) are approved as Medicare lung or heart-lung transplantation hospitals.

A list of approved facilities and their approval dates will be listed and maintained on the CMS Web site at http://www.cms.hhs.gov/MedicareApprovedFacilitie/04_lvrs.asp#TopOfPage.

The surgery must be preceded and followed by a program of diagnostic and therapeutic services consistent with those provided in the NETT and designed to maximize the patient's potential to successfully undergo and recover from surgery. The program must include a 6- to 10-week series of at least 16, and no more than 20, preoperative sessions, each lasting a minimum of 2 hours. It must also include at least 6, and no more than 10, postoperative sessions, each lasting a minimum of 2 hours, within 8 to 9 weeks of the LVRS. This program must be consistent with the care plan developed by the treating physician following performance of a comprehensive evaluation of the patient's medical, psychosocial and nutritional needs, be consistent with the preoperative and postoperative services provided in the NETT, and arranged, monitored, and performed under the coordination of the facility where the surgery takes place.

C. Nationally Non-covered Indications

1. LVRS is not covered in any of the following clinical circumstances:

   Patient characteristics carry a high risk for perioperative morbidity and/or mortality;

   The disease is unsuitable for LVRS;

   Medical conditions or other circumstances make it likely that the patient will be unable to complete the preoperative and postoperative pulmonary diagnostic and therapeutic program required for surgery;

   The patient presents with FEVõ <20% of predicted value, and either homogeneous distribution of emphysema on CT scan, or carbon monoxide diffusing capacity of <20% of predicted value (high-risk group identified October 2001 by the NETT); or

The patient satisfies the criteria outlined above in section B(1), and has severe, non-upper lobe emphysema with high exercise capacity. High exercise capacity is defined as a maximal workload at the completion of the preoperative diagnostic and therapeutic program that is above 25 w for women and 40 w for men (under the measurement conditions for cycle ergometry specified above).

2. All other indications for LVRS not otherwise specified remain noncovered.

(This NCD last reviewed November 2005.)

Pub 100-3, 240.2 – Home Use of Oxygen

(Rev. 1, 10-03-03)

A. General

Medicare coverage of home oxygen and oxygen equipment under the durable medical equipment (DME) benefit (see §1861(s)(6) of the Act) is considered reasonable and necessary only for patients with significant hypoxemia who meet the medical documentation, laboratory evidence, and health conditions specified in subsections B, C, and D. This section also includes special coverage criteria for portable oxygen systems. Finally, a statement on the absence of coverage of the professional services of a respiratory therapist under the DME benefit is included in subsection F.

B. Medical Documentation

Initial claims for oxygen services must include a completed Form CMS-484 (Certificate of Medical Necessity: Oxygen) to establish whether coverage criteria are met and to ensure that the oxygen services provided are consistent with the physician's prescription or other medical documentation. The treating physician's prescription or other medical documentation must indicate that other forms of treatment (e.g., medical and physical therapy directed at secretions, bronchospasm and infection) have been tried, have not been sufficiently successful, and oxygen therapy is still required. While there is no substitute for oxygen therapy, each patient must receive optimum therapy before long-term home oxygen therapy is ordered. Use Form CMS-484 for recertifications. (See the **Medicare Program Integrity Manual**, Chapter 5, for completion of Form CMS-484.)

The medical and prescription information in section B of Form CMS-484 can be completed only by the treating physician, the physician's employee, or another clinician (e.g., nurse, respiratory therapist, etc.) as long as that person is not the DME supplier. Although hospital discharge coordinators and medical social workers may assist in arranging for physician-prescribed home oxygen, they do not have the authority to prescribe the services. Suppliers may not enter this information. While this section may be completed by non-physician clinician or a physician employee, it must be reviewed and the Form CMS-484 signed by the attending physician.

A physician's certification of medical necessity for oxygen equipment must include the results of specific testing before coverage can be determined.

Claims for oxygen must also be supported by medical documentation in the patient's record. Separate documentation is used with electronic billing. This documentation may be in the form of a prescription written by the patient's attending physician who has recently examined the patient (normally within a month of the start of therapy) and must specify:

- A diagnosis of the disease requiring home use of oxygen;
- The oxygen flow rate; and
- An estimate of the frequency, duration of use (e.g., 2 liters per minute, 10 minutes per hour, 12 hours per day), and duration of need (e.g., 6 months or lifetime).

Note: A prescription for "Oxygen PRN" or "Oxygen as needed" does not meet this last requirement. Neither provides any basis for determining if the amount of oxygen is reasonable and necessary for the patient.

A member of the carrier's medical staff should review all claims with oxygen flow rates of more than four liters per minute before payment can be made.

The attending physician specifies the type of oxygen delivery system to be used (i.e., gas, liquid, or concentrator) by signing the completed Form CMS-484. In addition, the supplier or physician may use the space in section C for written confirmation of additional details of the physician's order. The additional order information contained in section C may include the means of oxygen delivery (mask, nasal, cannula, etc.), the specifics of varying flow rates, and/or the noncontinuous use of oxygen as appropriate. The physician confirms this order information with their signature in section D.

New medical documentation written by the patient's attending physician must be submitted to the carrier in support of revised oxygen requirements when there has been a change in the patient's condition and need for oxygen therapy.

Carriers are required to conduct periodic, continuing medical necessity reviews on patients whose conditions warrant these reviews and on patients with indefinite or extended periods of necessity as described in the **Medicare Program Integrity Manual**, Chapter 5, "Items and Services Having Special DMERC Review Considerations." When indicated, carriers may also request documentation of the results of a repeat arterial blood gas or oximetry study.

Note: Section 4152 of OBRA 1990 requires earlier recertification and retesting of oxygen patients who begin coverage with an arterial blood gas result at or above a partial pressure of 55 or an arterial oxygen saturation percentage at or above 89. (See the Medicare Claims Processing Manual, Chapter 20, "Durable Medical Equipment, Prosthetics and Orthotics, and Supplies (DMEPOS)," §100.2.3, for certification and retesting schedules.)

C. Laboratory Evidence

Initial claims for oxygen therapy must also include the results of a blood gas study that has been ordered and evaluated by the attending physician. This is usually in the form of a measurement of the partial pressure of oxygen (PO2) in arterial blood. A measurement of arterial oxygen saturation obtained by ear or pulse oximetry, however, is also acceptable when ordered and evaluated by the attending and performed under his or her supervision or when performed by a qualified provider or supplier of laboratory services. When the arterial blood gas and the oximetry studies are both used to document the need for home oxygen therapy and the results are conflicting, the arterial blood gas study is the preferred source of documenting medical need. A DME supplier is not considered a qualified provider or supplier of laboratory services for purposes of these guidelines. This prohibition does not extend to the results of blood gas test conducted by a hospital certified to do such tests. The conditions under which the laboratory tests are performed must be specified in writing and submitted with the initial claim, i.e., at rest, during exercise, or during sleep.

The preferred sources of laboratory evidence are, existing physician and/or hospital records that reflect the patient's medical condition. Since it is expected that virtually all patients who qualify for home oxygen coverage for the first time under these guidelines have recently been discharged from a hospital where they submitted to arterial blood gas tests, the carrier needs to request that such test results be submitted in support of their initial claims for home oxygen. If more than one arterial blood gas test is performed during the patient's hospital stay, the test result obtained closest to, but no earlier than two days prior to the hospital discharge date is required as evidence of the need for home oxygen therapy.

For those patients whose initial oxygen prescription did not originate during a hospital stay, blood gas studies should be done while the patient is in the chronic stable state, i.e., not during a period of an acute illness or an exacerbation of their underlying disease.

Carriers may accept an attending physician's statement of recent hospital test results for a particular patient, when appropriate, in lieu of copies of actual hospital records.

A repeat arterial blood gas study is appropriate when evidence indicates that an oxygen recipient has undergone a major change in their condition relevant to home use of oxygen. If the carrier has reason to believe that there has been a major change in the patient's physical condition, it may ask for documentation of the results of another blood gas or oximetry study.

D. Health Conditions

Coverage is available for patients with significant hypoxemia in the chronic stable state, i.e, not during a period of acute illness or an exacerbation of their underlying disease, if:

1. The attending physician has determined that the patient has a health condition outlined in subsection D.1,

2. The patient meets the blood gas evidence requirements specified in subsection D.3, and
3. The patient has appropriately tried other treatment without complete success. (See subsection B.)

1 Conditions for Which Oxygen Therapy May Be Covered

- A severe lung disease, such as chronic obstructive pulmonary disease, diffuse interstitial lung disease, cystic fibrosis, bronchiectasis, widespread pulmonary neoplasm, or
- Hypoxia-related symptoms or findings that might be expected to improve with oxygen therapy. Examples of these symptoms and findings are pulmonary hypertension, recurring congestive heart failure due to chronic cor pulmonale, erythrocytosis, impairment of the cognitive process, nocturnal restlessness, and morning headache.

2 Conditions for Which Oxygen Therapy Is Not Covered

- Angina pectoris in the absence of hypoxemia. This condition is generally not the result of a low oxygen level in the blood, and there are other preferred treatments;
- Breathlessness without cor pulmonale or evidence of hypoxemia. Although intermittent oxygen use is sometimes prescribed to relieve this condition, it is potentially harmful and psychologically addicting;
- Severe peripheral vascular disease resulting in clinically evident desaturation in one or more extremities. There is no evidence that increased PO2 improves the oxygenation of tissues with impaired circulation; or
- Terminal illnesses that do not affect the lungs.

3 Covered Blood Gas Values

If the patient has a condition specified in subsection D.1, the carrier must review the medical documentation and laboratory evidence that has been submitted for a particular patient (see subsections B and C) and determine if coverage is available under one of the three group categories outlined below.

(a) Group I – Except as modified in subsection d, coverage is provided for patients with significant hypoxemia evidenced by any of the following:

- An arterial PO2 at or below 55 mm Hg, or an arterial oxygen saturation at or below 88 percent, taken at rest, breathing room air.
- An arterial PO2 at or below 55 mm Hg, or an arterial oxygen saturation at or below 88 percent, taken during sleep for a patient who demonstrates an arterial PO2 at or above 56 mm Hg, or an arterial oxygen saturation at or above 89 percent, while awake; or a greater than normal fall in oxygen level during sleep (a decrease in arterial PO2 more than 10 mm Hg, or decrease in arterial oxygen saturation more than 5 percent) associated with symptoms or signs reasonably attributable to hypoxemia (e.g., impairment of cognitive processes and nocturnal restlessness or insomnia). In either of these cases, coverage is provided only for use of oxygen during sleep, and then only one type of unit will be covered. Portable oxygen ,therefore, would not be covered in this situation.
- An arterial PO2 at or below 55 mm Hg or an arterial oxygen saturation at or below 88 percent, taken during exercise for a patient who demonstrates an arterial PO2 at or above 56 mm Hg, or an arterial oxygen saturation at or above 89 percent, during the day while at rest. In this case, supplemental oxygen is provided for during exercise if there is evidence the use of oxygen improves the hypoxemia that was demonstrated during exercise when the patient was breathing room air.

(b) Group II – Except as modified in subsection d, coverage is available for patients whose arterial PO2 is 56-59 mm Hg or whose arterial blood oxygen saturation is 89 percent, if there is evidence of:

- Dependent edema suggesting congestive heart failure;
- Pulmonary hypertension or cor pulmonale, determined by measurement of pulmonary artery pressure, gated blood pool scan, echocardiogram, or "P" pulmonale on EKG (P wave greater than 3 mm in standard leads II, III, or AVF); or
- Erythrocythemia with a hematocrit greater than 56 percent.

(c) Group III – Except as modified in subsection d, carriers must apply a rebuttable presumption that a home program of oxygen use is not medically necessary for patients with arterial PO2 levels at or above 60 mm Hg, or arterial blood oxygen saturation at or above 90 percent. In order for claims in this category to be reimbursed, the carrier's reviewing physician needs to review any documentation submitted in rebuttal of this presumption and grant specific approval of the claims. The CMS expects few claims to be approved for coverage in this category.

(d) Variable Factors That May Affect Blood Gas Values – In reviewing the arterial PO2 levels and the arterial oxygen saturation percentages specified in subsections D. 3.a, b and c, the carrier's medical staff must take into account variations in oxygen measurements that may result from such factors as the patient's age, the altitude level, or the patient's decreased oxygen carrying capacity.

E. Portable Oxygen Systems

A patient meeting the requirements specified below may qualify for coverage of a portable oxygen system either (1) by itself or (2) to use in addition to a stationary oxygen system. Portable oxygen is not covered when it is provided only as a backup to a stationary oxygen system. A portable oxygen system is covered for a particular patient if:

- The claim meets the requirements specified in subsections A-D, as appropriate; and
- The medical documentation indicates that the patient is mobile in the home and would benefit from the use of a portable oxygen system in the home. Portable oxygen systems are not covered for patients who qualify for oxygen solely based on blood gas studies obtained during sleep

F. Respiratory Therapists

Respiratory therapists' services are not covered under the provisions for coverage of oxygen services under the Part B durable medical equipment benefit as outlined above. This benefit provides for coverage of home use of oxygen and oxygen equipment, but does not include a professional component in the delivery of such services.

(See §280.1, and the **Medicare Benefit Policy Manual**, Chapter 15, "Covered Medical and Other Health Services," §110)

Pub 100-3, 240.3 – Heat Treatment, Including the Use of Diathermy and Ultra-Sound for Pulmonary Conditions

(Rev. 1, 10-03-03)

Not Covered

There is no physiological rationale or valid scientific documentation of effectiveness of diathermy or ultrasound heat treatments for asthma, bronchitis, or any other pulmonary condition and for such purpose this treatment cannot be considered reasonable and necessary within the meaning of §1862(a)(1) of the Act.

Cross-reference: §150.5.

Pub 100-3, 240.4 – Continuous Positive Airway Pressure (CPAP) Therapy For Obstructive Sleep Apnea (OSA)

(Rev. 96, Issued: 10-15-08, Effective: 03-13-08, Implementation: 08-04-08)

A. General

Continuous Positive Airway Pressure (CPAP) is a non-invasive technique for providing single levels of air pressure from a flow generator, via a nose mask, through the nares. The purpose is to prevent the collapse of the oropharyngeal walls and the obstruction of airflow during sleep, which occurs in obstructive sleep apnea (OSA).

The apnea hypopnea index (AHI) is equal to the average number of episodes of apnea and hypopnea per hour. The respiratory disturbance index (RDI) is equal to the average number of respiratory disturbances per hour.

Apnea is defined as a cessation of airflow for at least 10 seconds. Hypopnea is defined as an abnormal respiratory event lasting at least 10 seconds with at least a 30% reduction in thoracoabdominal movement or airflow as compared to baseline, and with at least a 4% oxygen desaturation.

The AHI and/or RDI may be measured by polysomnography (PSG) in a facility based sleep study laboratory or by a Type II home sleep test (HST) monitor, a Type III HST monitor, or a Type IV HST monitor measuring at least 3 channels.

B. Nationally Covered Indications

Effective for claims with dates of service on and after March 13, 2008, the Centers for Medicare & Medicaid Services (CMS) determines that CPAP therapy when used in adult patients with OSA is considered reasonable and necessary under the following situations:

1. The use of CPAP is covered under Medicare when used in adult patients with OSA. Coverage of CPAP is initially limited to a 12-week period to identify beneficiaries diagnosed with OSA as subsequently described who benefit from CPAP. CPAP is subsequently covered only for those beneficiaries diagnosed with OSA who benefit from CPAP during this 12-week period.
2. The provider of CPAP must conduct education of the beneficiary prior to the use of the CPAP device to ensure that the beneficiary has been educated in the proper use of the device. A caregiver, for example a family member, may be compensatory, if consistently available in the beneficiary's home and willing and able to safely operate the CPAP device.
3. A positive diagnosis of OSA for the coverage of CPAP must include a clinical evaluation and a positive:
   - attended PSG performed in a sleep laboratory; or
   - unattended HST with a Type II home sleep monitoring device; or
   - unattended HST with a Type III home sleep monitoring device; or
   - unattended HST with a Type IV home sleep monitoring device that measures at least 3 channels.
4. The sleep test must have been previously ordered by the beneficiary's treating physician and furnished under appropriate physician supervision.
5. An initial 12-week period of CPAP is covered in adult patients with OSA if either of the following criterion using the AHI or RDI are met:
   - AHI or RDI greater than or equal to 15 events per hour, or,
   - AHI or RDI greater than or equal to 5 events and less than or equal to 14 events per hour, with documented symptoms of excessive daytime sleepiness, impaired cognition, mood disorders or insomnia, or documented hypertension, ischemic heart disease, or history of stroke.
6. The AHI or RDI is calculated on the average number of events per hour. If the AHI or RDI is calculated based on less than 2 hours of continuous recorded sleep, the total number of recorded events to calculate the AHI or RDI during sleep testing must be at a minimum the number of events that would have been required in a 2-hour period.
7. Apnea is defined as a cessation of airflow for at least 10 seconds. Hypopnea is defined as an abnormal respiratory event lasting at least 10 seconds with at least a 30% reduction in thoracoabdominal movement or airflow as compared to baseline, and with at least a 4% oxygen desaturation.
8. Coverage with Evidence Development (CED): Medicare provides the following limited coverage for CPAP in adult beneficiaries who do not qualify for CPAP coverage based on criteria 1-7 above. A clinical study seeking Medicare payment for CPAP provided to a beneficiary who is an enrolled subject in that study must address one or more of the following questions

   In Medicare-aged subjects with clinically identified risk factors for OSA, how does the diagnostic accuracy of a clinical trial of CPAP compare with PSG and Type II, III & IV HST in identifying subjects with OSA who will respond to CPAP?

   In Medicare-aged subjects with clinically identified risk factors for OSA who have not undergone confirmatory testing with PSG or Type II, III & IV HST, does CPAP cause clinically meaningful harm?

   The study must meet the following additional standards: The principal purpose of the research study is to test whether a particular intervention potentially improves the participants' health outcomes.

   The research study is well-supported by available scientific and medical information or it is intended to clarify or establish the health outcomes of interventions already in common clinical use.

   The research study does not unjustifiably duplicate existing studies.

   The research study design is appropriate to answer the research question being asked in the study.

   The research study is sponsored by an organization or individual capable of executing the proposed study successfully.

   The research study is in compliance with all applicable Federal regulations concerning the protection of human subjects found at 45 CFR Part 46. If a study is Food and Drug Administration-regulated, it also must be in compliance with 21 CFR Parts 50 and 56.

   All aspects of the research study are conducted according to the appropriate standards of scientific integrity.

   The research study has a written protocol that clearly addresses, or incorporates by reference, the Medicare standards.

   The clinical research study is not designed to exclusively test toxicity or disease pathophysiology in healthy individuals. Trials of all medical technologies measuring therapeutic outcomes as one of the objectives meet this standard only if the disease or condition being studied is life-threatening as defined in 21 CFR § 312.81(a) and the patient has no other viable treatment options.

   The clinical research study is registered on the ClinicalTrials.gov website by the principal sponsor/investigator prior to the enrollment of the first study subject.

   The research study protocol specifies the method and timing of public release of all pre-specified outcomes to be measured, including release of outcomes if outcomes are negative or study is terminated early. The results must be made public within 24 months of the end of data collection. If a report is planned for publication in a peer-reviewed journal, then that initial release may be an abstract that meets the requirements of the International Committee of Medical Journal Editors. However, a full report of the outcomes must be made public no later than three (3) years after the end of data collection.

   The research study protocol must explicitly discuss subpopulations affected by the treatment under investigation, particularly traditionally underrepresented groups in

   clinical studies, how the inclusion and exclusion criteria affect enrollment of these populations, and a plan for the retention and reporting of said populations in the trial. If the inclusion and exclusion criteria are expected to have a negative effect on the recruitment or retention of underrepresented populations, the protocol must discuss why these criteria are necessary.

   The research study protocol explicitly discusses how the results are or are not expected to be generalizable to the Medicare population to infer whether Medicare patients may benefit from the intervention. Separate discussions in the protocol may be necessary for populations eligible for Medicare due to age, disability, or Medicaid eligibility.

C. Nationally Non-covered Indications

Effective for claims with dates of services on and after March 13, 2008, other diagnostic tests for the diagnosis of OSA other than those noted above for prescribing CPAP are not sufficient for the coverage of CPAP

D. Other

N/A

(This NCD last reviewed March 2008.)

Pub 100-3, 240.4.1 – Sleep Testing for Obstructive Sleep Apnea (OSA)

(Effective March 3, 2009)

(Rev. 103, Issued: 07-10-09, Effective: 03-03-09, Implementation: 08-10-09)

A. General

Obstructive sleep apnea (OSA) is the collapse of the oropharyngeal walls and the obstruction of airflow occurring during sleep. Diagnostic tests for OSA have historically been classified into four types. The most comprehensive is designated Type I attended facility based polysomnography (PSG), which is considered the reference standard for diagnosing OSA. Attended facility based polysomnogram is a comprehensive diagnostic sleep test including at least electroencephalography (EEG), electro-oculography (EOG), electromyography (EMG), heart rate or electrocardiography (ECG), airflow, breathing/respiratory effort, and arterial oxygen saturation (SaO2) furnished in a sleep laboratory facility in which a technologist supervises the recording during sleep time and has the ability to intervene if needed. Overnight PSG is the conventional diagnostic test for OSA. The American Thoracic Society and the American Academy of Sleep Medicine have recommended supervised PSG in the sleep laboratory over 2 nights for the diagnosis of OSA and the initiation of continuous positive airway pressure (CPAP).

Three categories of portable monitors (used both in attended and unattended settings) have been developed for the diagnosis of OSA. Type II monitors have a minimum of 7 channels (e.g., EEG, EOG, EMG, ECG-heart rate, airflow, breathing/respiratory effort, SaO2)-this type of device monitors sleep staging, so AHI can be calculated). Type III monitors have a minimum of 4 monitored channels including ventilation or airflow (at least two channels of respiratory movement or respiratory movement and airflow), heart rate or ECG, and oxygen saturation. Type IV devices may measure one, two, three or more parameters but do not meet all the criteria of a higher category device. Some monitors use an actigraphy algorithm to identify periods of sleep and wakefulness.

B. Nationally Covered Indications

Effective for claims with dates of service on and after March 3, 2009, the Centers for Medicare & Medicaid Services finds that the evidence is sufficient to determine that the results of the sleep tests identified below can be used by a beneficiary's treating physician to diagnose OSA, that the use of such sleep testing technologies demonstrates improved health outcomes in Medicare beneficiaries who have OSA and receive the appropriate treatment, and that these tests are thus reasonable and necessary under section 1862(a)(1)(A) of the Social Security Act.

1. Type I PSG is covered when used to aid the diagnosis of OSA in beneficiaries who have clinical signs and symptoms indicative of OSA if performed attended in a sleep lab facility.
2. Type II or Type III sleep testing devices are covered when used to aid the diagnosis of OSA in beneficiaries who have clinical signs and symptoms indicative of OSA if performed unattended in or out of a sleep lab facility or attended in a sleep lab facility.
3. Type IV sleep testing devices measuring three or more channels, one of which is airflow, are covered when used to aid the diagnosis of OSA in beneficiaries who have signs and symptoms indicative of OSA if performed unattended in or out of a sleep lab facility or attended in a sleep lab facility.
4. Sleep testing devices measuring three or more channels that include actigraphy, oximetry, and peripheral arterial tone, are covered when used to aid the diagnosis of OSA in beneficiaries who have signs and symptoms indicative of OSA if performed unattended in or out of a sleep lab facility or attended in a sleep lab facility.

C. Nationally Non-Covered Indications

Effective for claims with dates of services on and after March 3, 2009, other diagnostic sleep tests for the diagnosis of OSA, other than those noted above for prescribing CPAP, are not sufficient for the coverage of CPAP and are not covered.

D. Other

N/A

(This NCD last reviewed March 2009.)

Pub 100-3, 240.5 – Intrapulmonary Percussive Ventilator (IPV)

(Rev. 1, 10-03-03)

Not Covered

IPV is a mechanized form of chest physical therapy. Instead of a therapist clapping or slapping the patient's chest wall, the IPV delivers mini-bursts (more than 200 per minute) of respiratory gasses to the lungs via a mouthpiece. Its intended purpose is to mobilize endobronchial secretions and diffuse patchy atelectasis. The patient controls variables such as inspiratory time, peak pressure and delivery rates.

Studies do not demonstrate any advantage of IPV over that achieved with good pulmonary care in the hospital environment and there are no studies in the home setting. There are no data to support the effectiveness of the device. Therefore, IPV in the home setting is not covered.

Pub 100-3, 260.3 – Pancreas Transplants

(Rev. 56, Issued 05-19-06, Effective: 04-26-06, Implementation: 07-03-06)

CIM 35-82

Pancreas transplantation is performed to induce an insulin-independent, euglycemic state in diabetic patients. The procedure is generally limited to those patients with severe secondary complications of diabetes, including kidney failure. However, pancreas transplantation is sometimes performed on patients with labile diabetes and hypoglycemic unawareness.

B. Nationally Covered Indications

Effective for services performed on or after July 1, 1999, whole organ pancreas transplantation is nationally covered by Medicare when performed simultaneous with or after a kidney transplant. If the pancreas transplant occurs after the kidney transplant, immunosuppressive therapy begins with the date of discharge from the inpatient stay for the pancreas transplant.

Effective for services performed on or after April 26, 2006, pancreas transplants alone (PA) are reasonable and necessary for Medicare beneficiaries in the following limited circumstances:

1. PA will be limited to those facilities that are Medicare-approved for kidney transplantation. (Approved centers can be found at http://www.cms.hhs.gov/ESRDGeneralInformation/02_Data.asp#TopOfPage
2. Patients must have a diagnosis of type I diabetes:
   - Patient with diabetes must be beta cell autoantibody positive; or
   - Patient must demonstrate insulinopenia defined as a fasting C-peptide level that is less than or equal to 110% of the lower limit of normal of the laboratory's measurement method. Fasting C-peptide levels will only be considered valid with a concurrently obtained fasting glucose <225 mg/dL;
3. Patients must have a history of medically-uncontrollable labile (brittle) insulin-dependent diabetes mellitus with documented recurrent, severe, acutely life-threatening metabolic complications that require hospitalization. Aforementioned complications include frequent hypoglycemia unawareness or recurring severe ketoacidosis, or recurring severe hypoglycemic attacks;
4. Patients must have been optimally and intensively managed by an endocrinologist for at least 12 months with the most medically-recognized advanced insulin formulations and delivery systems;
5. Patients must have the emotional and mental capacity to understand the significant risks associated with surgery and to effectively manage the lifelong need for immunosuppression; and,
6. Patients must otherwise be a suitable candidate for transplantation.

C. Nationally Non-Covered Indications

The following procedure is not considered reasonable and necessary within the meaning of section 1862(a)(1)(A) of the Social Security Act:

Transplantation of partial pancreatic tissue or islet cells (except in the context of a clinical trial (see section 260.3.1 of the National Coverage Determinations Manual).

D. Other

Not applicable.

(This NCD last reviewed April 2006.)

Medicare References

Pub 100-3, 260.6 – Dental Examination Prior to Kidney Transplantation

(Rev. 1, 10-03-03)

Despite the "dental services exclusion" in §1862(a)(12) of the Act (see the **Medicare Benefit Policy Manual**, Chapter 16, "General Exclusions From Coverage," §140;), an oral or dental examination performed on an inpatient basis as part of a comprehensive workup prior to renal transplant surgery is a covered service. This is because the purpose of the examination is not for the care of the teeth or structures directly supporting the teeth. Rather, the examination is for the identification, prior to a complex surgical procedure, of existing medical problems where the increased possibility of infection would not only reduce the chances for successful surgery but would also expose the patient to additional risks in undergoing such surgery.

Such a dental or oral examination would be covered under Part A of the program if performed by a dentist on the hospital's staff, or under Part B if performed by a physician. (When performing a dental or oral examination, a dentist is not recognized as a physician under §1861(r) of the Act.) (See the Medicare General Information, Eligibility, and Entitlement Manual, Chapter 5, "Definitions," §70.2, and the **Medicare Benefit Policy Manual**, Chapter 15, "Covered Medical and Other Health Services," §150.)

Pub 100-3, 260.7 – Lymphocyte Immune Globulin, Anti-Thymocyte Globulin (Equine)

(Rev. 1, 10-03-03)

The lymphocyte immune globulin preparations are biologic drugs not previously approved or licensed for use in the management of renal allograft rejection. A number of other lymphocyte immune globulin products of equine, lapine, and murine origin are currently under investigation for their potential usefulness in controlling allograft rejections in human transplantation. These biologic drugs are viewed as adjunctive to traditional immunosuppressive products such as steroids and anti-metabolic drugs. At present, lymphocyte immune globulin preparations are not recommended to replace conventional immunosuppressive drugs, but to supplement them and to be used as alternatives to elevated or accelerated dosing with conventional immunosuppressive agents.

The FDA has approved one lymphocyte immune globulin preparation for marketing, lymphocyte immune globulin, anti-thymocyte globulin (equine). This drug is indicated for the management of allograft rejection episodes in renal transplantation. It is covered under Medicare when used for this purpose. Other forms of lymphocyte globulin preparation which the FDA approves for this indication in the future may be covered under Medicare.

Pub 100-3, 270.1 – Electrical Stimulation (ES) and Electromagnetic Therapy for the Treatment of Wounds

(Rev 7, 07-01-06)

Electrical stimulation (ES) and electromagnetic therapy have been used or studied for many different applications, one of which is accelerating wound healing. ES for the treatment of wounds is the application of electrical current through electrodes placed directly on the skin in close proximity to the wound. Electromagnetic therapy uses a pulsed magnetic field to induce current. CMS was asked to reconsider its national noncoverage determination for electromagnetic therapy. After thorough review, CMS determined that the results from the use of electromagnetic therapy for the treatment of wounds were similar to the results from the use of ES. Therefore, effective July 1, 2004, Medicare will cover electromagnetic therapy for the same settings and conditions for which ES is covered. This means Medicare will allow either one covered ES therapy or one covered electromagnetic therapy for the treatment of wounds.

Indications and Limitations of Coverage

A. Nationally Covered Indications

The use of ES and electromagnetic therapy for the treatment of wounds are considered adjunctive therapies, and will only be covered for chronic Stage III or Stage IV pressure ulcers, arterial ulcers, diabetic ulcers, and venous stasis ulcers. Chronic ulcers are defined as ulcers that have not healed within 30 days of occurrence. ES or electromagnetic therapy will be covered only after appropriate standard wound therapy has been tried for at least 30 days and there are no measurable signs of improved healing. This 30-day period may begin while the wound is acute.

Standard wound care includes: optimization of nutritional status, debridement by any means to remove devitalized tissue, maintenance of a clean, moist bed of granulation tissue with appropriate moist dressings, and necessary treatment to resolve any infection that may be present. Standard wound care based on the specific type of wound includes: frequent repositioning of a patient with pressure ulcers (usually every 2 hours), offloading of pressure and good glucose control for diabetic ulcers, establishment of adequate circulation for arterial ulcers, and the use of a compression system for patients with venous ulcers.

Measurable signs of improved healing include: a decrease in wound size (either surface area or volume), decrease in amount of exudates, and decrease in amount of necrotic tissue. ES or electromagnetic therapy must be discontinued when the wound demonstrates 100% epitheliliazed wound bed.

ES and electromagnetic therapy services can only be covered when performed by a physician, physical therapist, or incident to a physician service. Evaluation of the wound is an integral part of wound therapy. When a physician, physical therapist, or a clinician incident to a physician, performs ES or electromagnetic therapy, the practitioner must evaluate the wound and contact the treating physician if the wound worsens. If ES or electromagnetic therapy is being used, wounds must be evaluated at least monthly by the treating physician.

B. Nationally Noncovered Indications

1. ES and electromagnetic therapy will not be covered as an initial treatment modality.
2. Continued treatment with ES or electromagnetic therapy is not covered if measurable signs of healing have not been demonstrated within any 30-day period of treatment.
3. Unsupervised use of ES or electromagnetic therapy for wound therapy will not be covered, as this use has not been found to be medically reasonable and necessary.

C. Other

All other uses of ES and electromagnetic therapy not otherwise specified for the treatment of wounds remain at local contractor discretion. (This NCD last reviewed March 2004.)

Pub 100-3, 270.3 – Blood-Derived Products for Chronic Non-Healing Wounds

(Rev. 83, Issued: 05-02-08, Effective: 03-19-08, Implementation: 06-02-08)

A. General

Wound healing is a dynamic, interactive process that involves multiple cells and proteins. There are three progressive stages of normal wound healing, and the typical wound healing duration is about 4 weeks. While cutaneous wounds are a disruption of the normal, anatomic structure and function of the skin, subcutaneous wounds involve tissue below the skin's surface. Wounds are categorized as either acute, in where the normal wound healing stages are not yet completed but it is presumed they will be, resulting in orderly and timely wound repair, or chronic, in where a wound has failed to progress through the normal wound healing stages and repair itself within a sufficient time period.

Platelet-rich plasma (PRP) is produced in an autologous or homologous manner. Autologous PRP is comprised of blood from the patient who will ultimately receive the PRP. Alternatively, homologous PRP is derived from blood from multiple donors.

Blood is donated by the patient and centrifuged to produce an autologous gel for treatment of chronic, non-healing cutaneous wounds that persists for 30 days or longer and fail to properly complete the healing process. Autologous blood derived products for chronic, non-healing wounds includes both: (1) platelet derived growth factor (PDGF) products (such as Procuren), and (2) PRP.

The PRP is different from previous products in that it contains whole cells including white cells, red cells, plasma, platelets, fibrinogen, stem cells, macrophages, and fibroblasts.

The PRP is used by physicians in clinical settings in treating chronic, non-healing wounds, open, cutaneous wounds, soft tissue, and bone. Alternatively, PDGF does not contain cells and was previously marketed as a product to be used by patients at home.

B. Nationally Covered Indications

Not applicable.

C. Nationally Non-Covered Indications

1. Effective December 28, 1992, the Centers for Medicare & Medicaid Services (CMS) issued a national non-coverage determination for platelet-derived wound-healing formulas intended to treat patients with chronic, non-healing wounds. This decision was based on a lack of sufficient published data to determine safety and efficacy, and a public health service technology assessment.
2. Effective July 23, 2004, upon reconsideration, the clinical effectiveness of autologous PDGF products continues to not be adequately proven in scientific literature. As the evidence is insufficient to conclude that autologous PDGF in a platelet-poor plasma is reasonable and necessary, it remains non-covered for treatment of chronic, non-healing cutaneous wounds. Also, the clinical evidence does not support a benefit in the application of autologous PRP for the treatment of chronic, non-healing, cutaneous wounds. Therefore, CMS determines it is not reasonable and necessary and is nationally non-covered.
3. Effective April 27, 2006, coverage for treatments utilizing becaplermin, a non-autologous growth factor for chronic, non-healing subcutaneous wounds, remains nationally non-covered under Part B based on section 1861(s)(2)(A) and (B) of the Social Security Act because this product is usually administered by the patient.
4. Effective March 19, 2008, upon reconsideration, the evidence is not adequate to conclude that autologous PRP is reasonable and necessary and remains non-covered for the treatment of chronic non-healing, cutaneous wounds. Additionally, upon reconsideration, the evidence is not adequate to conclude that autologous PRP is reasonable and necessary for the treatment of acute surgical wounds when the autologous PRP is applied directly to the closed incision, or for dehiscent wounds.

D. Other

In accordance with Section 310.1, of the **National Coverage Determination Manual**, the routine costs in Federally sponsored or approved clinical trials assessing the efficacy of autologous PRP in treating chronic, non-healing cutaneous wounds are covered by Medicare. (This NCD last reviewed March 2008.)

Pub 100-3, 280.1 – Durable Medical Equipment Reference List

(Rev. 37, Issued: 06-03-05; Effective: 05-05-05; Implementation: 07-05-05)

The durable medical equipment (DME) list that follows is designed to facilitate the contractor's processing of DME claims. This section is designed as a quick reference tool for determining the coverage status of certain pieces of DME and especially for those items commonly referred to by both brand and generic names. The information contained herein is applicable (where appropriate) to all DME national coverage determinations (NCDs) discussed in the DME portion of this manual. The list is organized into two columns. The first column lists alphabetically various generic categories of equipment on which NCDs have been made by the Centers for Medicare & Medicaid Services (CMS); the second column notes the coverage status.

In the case of equipment categories that have been determined by CMS to be covered under the DME benefit, the list outlines the conditions of coverage that must be met if payment is to be allowed for the rental or purchase of the DME by a particular patient, or cross-refers to another section of the manual where the applicable coverage criteria are described in more detail. With respect to equipment categories that cannot be covered as DME, the list includes a brief explanation of why the equipment is not covered. This DME list will be updated periodically to reflect any additional NCDs that CMS may make with regard to other categories of equipment.

When the contractor receives a claim for an item of equipment which does not appear to fall logically into any of the generic categories listed, the contractor has the authority and responsibility for deciding whether those items are covered under the DME benefit.

These decisions must be made by each contractor based on the advice of its medical consultants, taking into account:

- The **Medicare Claims Processing Manual**, Chapter 20, "Durable Medical Equipment, Prosthetics and Orthotics, and Supplies (DMEPOS)."
- Whether the item has been approved for marketing by the Food and Drug Administration (FDA) and is otherwise generally considered to be safe and effective for the purpose intended; and
- Whether the item is reasonable and necessary for the individual patient.

The term DME is defined as equipment which:

- Can withstand repeated use; i.e., could normally be rented and used by successive patients;
- Is primarily and customarily used to serve a medical purpose;
- Generally is not useful to a person in the absence of illness or injury; and,
- Is appropriate for use in a patient's home.

Durable Medical Equipment Reference List

Item	Coverage
Air Cleaners	Deny—environmental control equipment; not primarily medical in nature (§1861(n) of the Act).
Air Conditioners	Deny—environmental control equipment; not primarily medical in nature (§1861(n) of the Act).
Air-Fluidized Beds	(See Air-Fluidized Beds §280.8 of this manual.)
Alternating Pressure Pads, Mattresses and Lambs Wool Pads	Covered if patient has, or is highly susceptible to, decubitus ulcers and patient's physician specifies that he/she will be supervising the course of treatment.
Audible/Visible Signal/ Pacemaker Monitors	(See Self-Contained Pacemaker Monitors.)
Augmentative Communication Devices	(See Speech-Generating Devices §50.1 of this manual.)
Bathtub Lifts	Deny—convenience item; not primarily medical in nature (§1861(n) of the Act).
Bathtub Seats	Deny—comfort or convenience item; hygienic equipment; not primarily medical in nature (§1861(n) of the Act).
Bead Beds	(See §280.8.)
Bed Baths (home type)	Deny—hygienic equipment; not primarily medical in nature (§1861(n) of the Act).
Bed Lifters (bed elevators)	Deny—not primarily medical in nature (§1861(n) of the Act).
Bedboards	Deny—not primarily medical in nature (§1861(n) of the Act).
Bed Pans (autoclavable hospital type)	Covered if patient is bed-confined.
Bed Side Rails	(See Hospital Beds §280.7 of this manual.)
Beds-Lounges (power or manual)	Deny—not a hospital bed; comfort or convenience item; not primarily medical in nature (§1861(n) of the Act).
Beds (Oscillating)	Deny—institutional equipment; inappropriate for home use.
Bidet Toilet Seats	(See Toilet Seats.)
Blood Glucose Analyzers (Reflectance Colorimeter)	Deny—unsuitable for home use (see §40.2 of this manual).
Blood Glucose Monitors	Covered if patient meets certain conditions (see §40.2 of this manual).
Braille Teaching Texts	Deny—educational equipment; not primarily medical in nature (§1861(n) of the Act).
Canes	Covered if patient meets Mobility Assistive Equipment clinical criteria (see §280.3 of this manual).
Carafes	Deny—convenience item; not primarily medical in nature (§1861(n) of the Act).
Catheters	Deny—non-reusable disposable supply (§1861(n) of the Act). (See Medicare Claims Processing Manual, Chapter 20, DMEPOS).

Item	Coverage
Commodes	Covered if patient is confined to bed or room. NOTE: The term "room-confined" means that patient's condition is such that leaving the room is medically contraindicated. The accessibility of bathroom facilities generally would not be a factor in this determination. However, confinement of a patient to a home in a case where there are no toilet facilities in the home may be equated to room confinement. Moreover, payment may also be made if a patient's medical condition confines him to a floor of the home and there is no bathroom located on that floor.
Communicators	(See §50.1 of this manual, Speech Generating Devices.)
Continuous Passive Motion Devices	Continuous passive motion devices are devices covered for patients who have received a total knee replacement. To qualify for coverage, use of the device must commence within 2 days following surgery. In addition, coverage is limited to that portion of the 3-week period following surgery during which the device is used in the patient's home. There is insufficient evidence to justify coverage for longer periods of time or for other applications.
Continuous Positive Airway Pressure (CPAP) Devices	(See §240.4 of this manual.)
Crutches	Covered if patient meets Mobility Assistive Equipment clinical criteria (see section 280.3 of this manual).
Cushion Lift Power Seats	(See Seat Lifts.)
Dehumidifiers (room or central heating system type)	Deny—environmental control equipment; not primarily medical in nature (§1861(n) of the Act.
Diathermy Machines (standard pulses wave types)	Deny—inappropriate for home use (see §150.5 of this manual).
Digital Electronic Pacemaker Monitors	(See Self-Contained Pacemaker Monitors).
Disposable Sheets and Bags	Deny—nonreusable disposable supplies (§1861(n) of the Act).
Elastic Stockings	Deny—nonreusable supply; not rental-type items (§1861(n) of the Act.) (See §270.5 of this manual.)
Electric Air Cleaners	Deny—(see Air Cleaners.) (§1861(n) of the Act).
Electric Hospital Beds	(See Hospital Beds §280.7 of this manual.)
Electrical Stimulation for Wounds	Deny—inappropriate for home use. (See §270.1 of this manual.)
Electrostatic Machines	Deny—(see Air Cleaners and Air Conditioners.) (§1861(n) of the Act).
Elevators	Deny—convenience item; not primarily medical in nature (§1861(n) of the Act).
Emesis Basins	Deny—convenience item; not primarily medical in nature (§1861(n) of the Act).
Esophageal Dilators	Deny—physician instrument; inappropriate for patient use.
Exercise Equipment	Deny—not primarily medical in nature (§1861(n) of the Act).
Fabric Supports	Deny—non-reusable supplies; not rental-type items (§1861(n) of the Act).
Face Masks (oxygen)	Covered if oxygen is covered. (See §240.2 of this manual.)
Face Masks (surgical)	Deny—non-reusable disposable items (§1861(n) of the Act).
Flowmeters	(See Medical Oxygen Regulators.) (See §240.2 of this manual.)
Fluidic Breathing Assisters	(See Intermittent Positive Pressure Breathing Machines.)
Fomentation Devices	(See Heating Pads.)
Gel Flotation Pads and Mattresses	(See Alternating Pressure Pads and Mattresses.)
Grab Bars	Deny—self-help device; not primarily medical in nature (§1861(n) of the Act).
Heat and Massage Foam Cushion Pads	Deny—not primarily medical in nature; personal comfort item (§1861(n) and 1862(a)(6) of the Act).
Heating and Cooling Plants	Deny—environmental control equipment not primarily medical in nature (§1861(n) of the Act).
Heating Pads	Covered if contractor's medical staff determines patient's medical condition is one for which the application of heat in the form of a heating pad is therapeutically effective.
Heat Lamps	Covered if contractor's medical staff determines patient's medical condition is one for which the application of heat in the form of a heat lamp is therapeutically effective.
Hospital Beds	(See §280.7 of this manual.)
Hot Packs	(See Heating Pads.)
Humidifiers (oxygen)	(See Oxygen Humidifiers.)
Humidifiers (room or central heating system types)	Deny—environmental control equipment; not medical in nature (§1861(n) of the Act).
Hydraulic Lifts	(See Patient Lifts.)
Incontinent Pads	Deny—non-reusable supply; hygienic item (§1861(n) of the Act).
Infusion Pumps	For external and implantable pumps, see §40.2 of this manual. If pump is used with an enteral or parenteral nutritional therapy system, see §180.2 of this manual for special coverage rules.
Injectors (hypodermic jet)	Deny—not covered self-administered drug supply; pressure-powered devices (§1861(s)(2)(A) of the Act) for injection of insulin.
Intermittent Positive Pressure Breathing Machines	Covered if patient's ability to breathe is severely impaired.
Iron Lungs	(See Ventilators.)
Irrigating Kits	Deny—non-reusable supply; hygienic equipment (§1861(n) of the Act).
Lambs Wool Pads	(See Alternating Pressure Pads, Mattresses, and Lambs Wool Pads.)
Leotards	Deny—(See Pressure Leotards.) (§1861(n) of the Act).
Lymphedema Pumps	Covered (See Pneumatic Compression Devices §280.6 of this manual.)
Massage Devices	Deny—personal comfort items; not primarily medical in nature (§1861(n) and 1862(a)(6) of the Act).
Mattresses	Covered only where hospital bed is medically necessary. (Separate Charge for replacement mattress should not be allowed where hospital bed with mattress is rented.) (See §280.7 of this manual.)
Medical Oxygen Regulators	Covered if patient's ability to breathe is severely impaired. (See §240.2 of this manual.)
Mobile Geriatric Chairs	Covered if patient meets Mobility Assistive Equipment clinical criteria (see §280.3 of this manual). (See Rolling Chairs).
Motorized Wheelchairs	Covered if patient meets Mobility Assistive Equipment clinical criteria (see §280.3 of this manual).
Muscle Stimulators	Covered for certain conditions. (See §250.4 of this manual.)
Nebulizers	Covered if patient's ability to breathe is severely impaired.
Oscillating Beds	Deny—institutional equipment; inappropriate for home use.
Over-bed Tables	Deny—convenience item; not primarily medical in nature (§1861(n) of the Act).
Oxygen	Covered if oxygen has been prescribed for use in connection with medically necessary DME. (See §240.2 of this manual.)
Oxygen Humidifiers	Covered if oxygen has been prescribed for use in connection with medically necessary DME for purposes of moisturizing oxygen. (See §240.2 of this manual.)
Oxygen Regulators (Medical)	(See Medical Oxygen Regulators.)
Oxygen Tents	(See §240.2 of this manual.)
Paraffin Bath Units (Portable)	(See Portable Paraffin Bath Units.)
Paraffin Bath Units (Standard)	Deny—institutional equipment; inappropriate for home use.
Parallel Bars	Deny—support exercise equipment; primarily for institutional use; in the home setting other devices (e.g., walkers) satisfy patient's need.

Medicare References

Item	Coverage
Patient Lifts	Covered if contractor's medical staff determines patient's condition is such that periodic movement is necessary to effect improvement or to arrest/retard deterioration in condition.
Percussors	Covered for mobilizing respiratory tract secretions in patients with chronic obstructive lung disease, chronic bronchitis, or emphysema, when patient/operator of powered percussor receives appropriate training by a physician/therapist, and no one competent to administer manual therapy is available.
Portable Oxygen Systems	1. Regulated Covered (adjustable covered under conditions specified in a flow rate). Refer all claims to medical staff for this determination. 2. Preset Deny (flow rate deny emergency, first-aid, or not adjustable) precautionary equipment; essentially not therapeutic in nature.
Portable Paraffin Bath Units	Covered when patient has undergone a successful trial period of paraffin therapy ordered by a physician and patient's condition is expected to be relieved by long-term use of this modality.
Portable Room Heaters	Deny—environmental control equipment; not primarily medical in nature (§1861(n) of the Act).
Portable Whirlpool Pumps	Deny—not primarily medical in nature; personal comfort items (§§1861(n) and 1862(a)(6) of the Act).
Postural Drainage Boards	Covered if patient has a chronic pulmonary condition.
Preset Portable Oxygen Units	Deny—emergency, first-aid, or precautionary equipment; essentially not therapeutic in nature.
Pressure Leotards	Deny—non-reusable supply, not rental-type item (§1861(n) of the Act).
Pulse Tachometers	Deny—not reasonable or necessary for monitoring pulse of homebound patient with/without a cardiac pacemaker.
Quad-Canes	Covered if patient meets Mobility Assistive Equipment clinical criteria (see §280.3 of this manual).
Raised Toilet Seats	Deny—convenience item; hygienic equipment; not primarily medical in nature (§1861(n) of the Act).
Reflectance Colorimeters	(See Blood Glucose Analyzers.)
Respirators	(See Ventilators.)
Rolling Chairs	Covered if patient meets Mobility Assistive Equipment clinical criteria (see §280.3 of this manual). Coverage is limited to those roll-about chairs having casters of at least 5 inches in diameter and specifically designed to meet the needs of ill, injured, or otherwise impaired individuals. Coverage is denied for the wide range of chairs with smaller casters as are found in general use in homes, offices, and institutions for many purposes not related to the care/treatment of ill/injured persons. This type is not primarily medical in nature. (§1861(n) of the Act.)
Safety Rollers	Covered if patient meets Mobility Assistive Equipment clinical criteria (see §280.3 of this manual).
Sauna Baths	Deny—not primarily medical in nature; personal comfort items (§§1861(n) and (1862(a)(6) of the Act).
Seat Lifts	Covered under conditions specified in §280.4 of this manual. Refer all to medical staff for this determination.
Self-Contained Pacemaker Monitors	Covered when prescribed by a physician for a patient with a cardiac pacemaker. (See §§20.8.1 and 280.2 of this manual.)
Sitz Baths	Covered if contractor's medical staff determines patient has an infection/injury of the perineal area and the item has been prescribed by the patient's physician as part of planned regimen of treatment in patient's home.
Spare Tanks of Oxygen	Deny—convenience or precautionary supply.
Speech Teaching Machines	Deny—education equipment; not primarily medical in nature (§1861(n) of the Act).
Stairway Elevators	Deny—(See Elevators.) (§1861(n) of the Act).
Standing Tables	Deny—convenience item; not primarily medical in nature (§1861(n) of the Act).
Steam Packs	These packs are covered under same conditions as heating pads. (See Heating Pads.)
Suction Machines	Covered if contractor's medical staff determines that the machine specified in the claim is medically required and appropriate for home use without technical/professional supervision.
Support Hose	Deny (See Fabric Supports.) (§1861(n) of the Act).
Surgical Leggings	Deny—non-reusable supply; not rental-type item (§1861(n) of the Act).
Telephone Alert Systems	Deny—these are emergency communications systems and do not serve a diagnostic/therapeutic purpose.
Toilet Seats	Deny—not medical equipment (§1861(n) of the Act).
Traction Equipment	Covered if patient has orthopedic impairment requiring traction equipment that prevents ambulation during period of use. (Consider covering devices usable during ambulation; e.g., cervical traction collar, under brace provision.)
Trapeze Bars	Covered if patient is bed-confined and needs a trapeze bar to sit up because of respiratory condition, to change body position for other medical reasons, or to get in/out of bed.
Treadmill Exercisers	Deny—exercise equipment; not primarily medical in nature (§1861(n) of the Act).
Ultraviolet Cabinets	Covered for selected patients with generalized intractable psoriasis. Using appropriate consultation, contractor should determine whether medical/other factors justify treatment at home rather than at alternative sites, e.g., outpatient department of a hospital.
Urinals autoclavable	Covered if patient is bed-confined (hospital type).
Vaporizers	Covered if patient has a respiratory illness.
Ventilators	Covered for treatment of neuromuscular diseases, thoracic restrictive diseases, and chronic respiratory failure consequent to chronic obstructive pulmonary disease. Includes both positive/negative pressure types. (See §240.5 of this manual.)
Walkers	Covered if patient meets Mobility Assistive Equipment clinical criteria (see §280.3 of this manual).
Water and Pressure Pads and Mattresses	(See Alternating Pressure Pads, Mattresses, and Lambs Wool Pads.)
Wheelchairs (manual)	Covered if patient meets Mobility Assistive Equipment clinical criteria (see §280.3 of this manual).
Wheelchairs (power-operated)	Covered if patient meets Mobility Assistive Equipment clinical criteria (see §280.3 of this manual).
Wheelchairs (scooter/POV)	Covered if patient meets Mobility Assistive Equipment clinical criteria (see §280.3 of this manual).
Wheelchairs (specially-sized)	Covered if patient meets Mobility Assistive Equipment clinical criteria (see §280.3 of this manual).
Whirlpool Bath Equipment	Covered if patient is homebound and has a (standard) condition for which the whirlpool bath can be expected to provide substantial therapeutic benefit justifying its cost. Where patient is not homebound but has such a condition, payment is restricted to the cost of providing the services elsewhere; e.g., an outpatient department of a participating hospital, if that alternative is less costly. In all cases, refer claim to medical staff for determination.
Whirlpool Pumps	Deny—(See Portable Whirlpool Pumps.) (§1861(n) of the Act).
White Canes	Deny— (See §280.2 of this manual.) (Not considered Mobility Assistive Equipment)

Cross-references:: **Medicare Benefit Policy Manual**, Chapters 13, "Rural Health Clinic (RHC) and Federally Qualified Health Center (FQHC) Services," 15, "Covered Medical and Other Health Services."

Medicare **Claims Processing Manual**, Chapters 12, "Physician/Practitioner Billing," 20, "Durable Medical Equipment, Prosthetics and Orthotics, and Supplies (DMEPOS)," 23, "Fee Schedule Administration and Coding Requirements."

Pub 100-3, 280.2 – White Cane for Use by a Blind Person

(Rev. 1, 10-03-03)

Not Covered

A white cane for use by a blind person is more an identifying and self-help device than an item which makes a meaningful contribution in the treatment of an illness or injury.

Pub 100-3, 280.3 – Mobility Assistive Equipment (MAE)

(Rev. 37, Issued: 06-03-05; Effective: 05-05-05; Implementation: 07-05-05)

A. General

The Centers for Medicare & Medicaid Services (CMS) addresses numerous items that it terms "mobility assistive equipment" (MAE) and includes within that category canes, crutches, walkers, manual wheelchairs, power wheelchairs, and scooters. This list, however, is not exhaustive.

Medicare beneficiaries may require mobility assistance for a variety of reasons and for varying durations because the etiology of the disability may be due to a congenital cause, injury, or disease. Thus, some beneficiaries experiencing temporary disability may need mobility assistance on a short-term basis, while in contrast, those living with chronic conditions or enduring disabilities will require mobility assistance on a permanent basis.

Medicare beneficiaries who depend upon mobility assistance are found in varied living situations. Some may live alone and independently while others may live with a caregiver or in a custodial care facility. The beneficiary's environment is relevant to the determination of the appropriate form of mobility assistance that should be employed. For many patients, a device of some sort is compensation for the mobility deficit. Many beneficiaries experience co-morbid conditions that can impact their ability to safely utilize MAE independently or to successfully regain independent function even with mobility assistance.

The functional limitation as experienced by a beneficiary depends on the beneficiary's physical and psychological function, the availability of other support, and the beneficiary's living environment. A few examples include muscular spasticity, cognitive deficits, the availability of a caregiver, and the physical layout, surfaces, and obstacles that exist in the beneficiary's living environment.

B. Nationally Covered Indications

Effective May 5, 2005, CMS finds that the evidence is adequate to determine that MAE is reasonable and necessary for beneficiaries who have a personal mobility deficit sufficient to impair their participation in mobility-related activities of daily living (MRADLs) such as toileting, feeding, dressing, grooming, and bathing in customary locations within the home. Determination of the presence of a mobility deficit will be made by an algorithmic process, Clinical Criteria for MAE Coverage, to provide the appropriate MAE to correct the mobility deficit.

Clinical Criteria for MAE Coverage

The beneficiary, the beneficiary's family or other caregiver, or a clinician, will usually initiate the discussion and consideration of MAE use. Sequential consideration of the questions below provides clinical guidance for the coverage of equipment of appropriate type and complexity to restore the beneficiary's ability to participate in MRADLs such as toileting, feeding, dressing, grooming, and bathing in customary locations in the home. These questions correspond to the numbered decision points on the accompanying flow chart. In individual cases where the beneficiary's condition clearly and unambiguously precludes the reasonable use of a device, it is not necessary to undertake a trial of that device for that beneficiary.

1. Does the beneficiary have a mobility limitation that significantly impairs his/her ability to participate in one or more MRADLs in the home? A mobility limitation is one that:
   a. Prevents the beneficiary from accomplishing the MRADLs entirely, or,
   b. Places the beneficiary at reasonably determined heightened risk of morbidity or mortality secondary to the attempts to participate in MRADLs, or,
   c. Prevents the beneficiary from completing the MRADLs within a reasonable time frame.
2. Are there other conditions that limit the beneficiary's ability to participate in MRADLs at home?
   a. Some examples are significant impairment of cognition or judgment and/or vision.
   b. For these beneficiaries, the provision of MAE might not enable them to participate in MRADLs if the comorbidity prevents effective use of the wheelchair or reasonable completion of the tasks even with MAE.
3. If these other limitations exist, can they be ameliorated or compensated sufficiently such that the additional provision of MAE will be reasonably expected to significantly improve the beneficiary's ability to perform or obtain assistance to participate in MRADLs in the home?
   a. A caregiver, for example a family member, may be compensatory, if consistently available in the beneficiary's home and willing and able to safely operate and transfer the beneficiary to and from the wheelchair and to transport the beneficiary using the wheelchair. The caregiver's need to use a wheelchair to assist the beneficiary in the MRADLs is to be considered in this determination.
   b. If the amelioration or compensation requires the beneficiary's compliance with treatment, for example medications or therapy, substantive non-compliance, whether willing or involuntary, can be grounds for denial of MAE coverage if it results in the beneficiary continuing to have a significant limitation. It may be determined that partial compliance results in adequate amelioration or compensation for the appropriate use of MAE.
4. Does the beneficiary or caregiver demonstrate the capability and the willingness to consistently operate the MAE safely?
   a. Safety considerations include personal risk to the beneficiary as well as risk to others. The determination of safety may need to occur several times during the process as the consideration focuses on a specific device.
   b. A history of unsafe behavior in other venues may be considered.
5. Can the functional mobility deficit be sufficiently resolved by the prescription of a cane or walker?
   a. The cane or walker should be appropriately fitted to the beneficiary for this evaluation.
   b. Assess the beneficiary's ability to safely use a cane or walker.
6. Does the beneficiary's typical environment support the use of wheelchairs including scooters/power-operated vehicles (POVs)?
   a. Determine whether the beneficiary's environment will support the use of these types of MAE.
   b. Keep in mind such factors as physical layout, surfaces, and obstacles, which may render MAE unusable in the beneficiary's home.
7. Does the beneficiary have sufficient upper extremity function to propel a manual wheelchair in the home to participate in MRADLs during a typical day? The manual wheelchair should be optimally configured (seating options, wheelbase, device weight, and other appropriate accessories) for this determination.
   a. Limitations of strength, endurance, range of motion, coordination, and absence or deformity in one or both upper extremities are relevant.
   b. A beneficiary with sufficient upper extremity function may qualify for a manual wheelchair. The appropriate type of manual wheelchair, i.e. light weight, etc., should be determined based on the beneficiary's physical characteristics and anticipated intensity of use.
   c. The beneficiary's home should provide adequate access, maneuvering space and surfaces for the operation of a manual wheelchair.
   d. Assess the beneficiary's ability to safely use a manual wheelchair.

NOTE: If the beneficiary is unable to self-propel a manual wheelchair, and if there is a caregiver who is available, willing, and able to provide assistance, a manual wheelchair may be appropriate.

8. Does the beneficiary have sufficient strength and postural stability to operate a POV/scooter?
   a. A POV is a 3- or 4-wheeled device with tiller steering and limited seat modification capabilities. The beneficiary must be able to maintain stability and position for adequate operation.
   b. The beneficiary's home should provide adequate access, maneuvering space and surfaces for the operation of a POV.
   c. Assess the beneficiary's ability to safely use a POV/scooter.
9. Are the additional features provided by a power wheelchair needed to allow the beneficiary to participate in one or more MRADLs?
   a. The pertinent features of a power wheelchair compared to a POV are typically control by a joystick or alternative input device, lower seat height for slide transfers, and the ability to accommodate a variety of seating needs.
   b. The type of wheelchair and options provided should be appropriate for the degree of the beneficiary's functional impairments.
   c. The beneficiary's home should provide adequate access, maneuvering space and surfaces for the operation of a power wheelchair.
   d. Assess the beneficiary's ability to safely use a power wheelchair.

   NOTE: If the beneficiary is unable to use a power wheelchair, and if there is a caregiver who is available, willing, and able to provide assistance, a manual wheelchair is appropriate. A caregiver's inability to operate a manual wheelchair can be considered in covering a power wheelchair so that the caregiver can assist the beneficiary.

C. Nationally Non-Covered Indications

Medicare beneficiaries not meeting the clinical criteria for prescribing MAE as outlined above, and as documented by the beneficiary's physician, would not be eligible for Medicare coverage of the MAE.

D. Other

All other durable medical equipment (DME) not meeting the definition of MAE as described in this instruction will continue to be covered, or noncovered, as is currently described in the NCD Manual, in Section 280, Medical and Surgical Supplies. Also, all other sections not altered here and the corresponding policies regarding MAEs which have not been discussed here remain unchanged.

(This NCD last reviewed May 2005).

Cross-references: section 280.1 of the NCD Manual.

Clinical Criteria for MAE Coverage

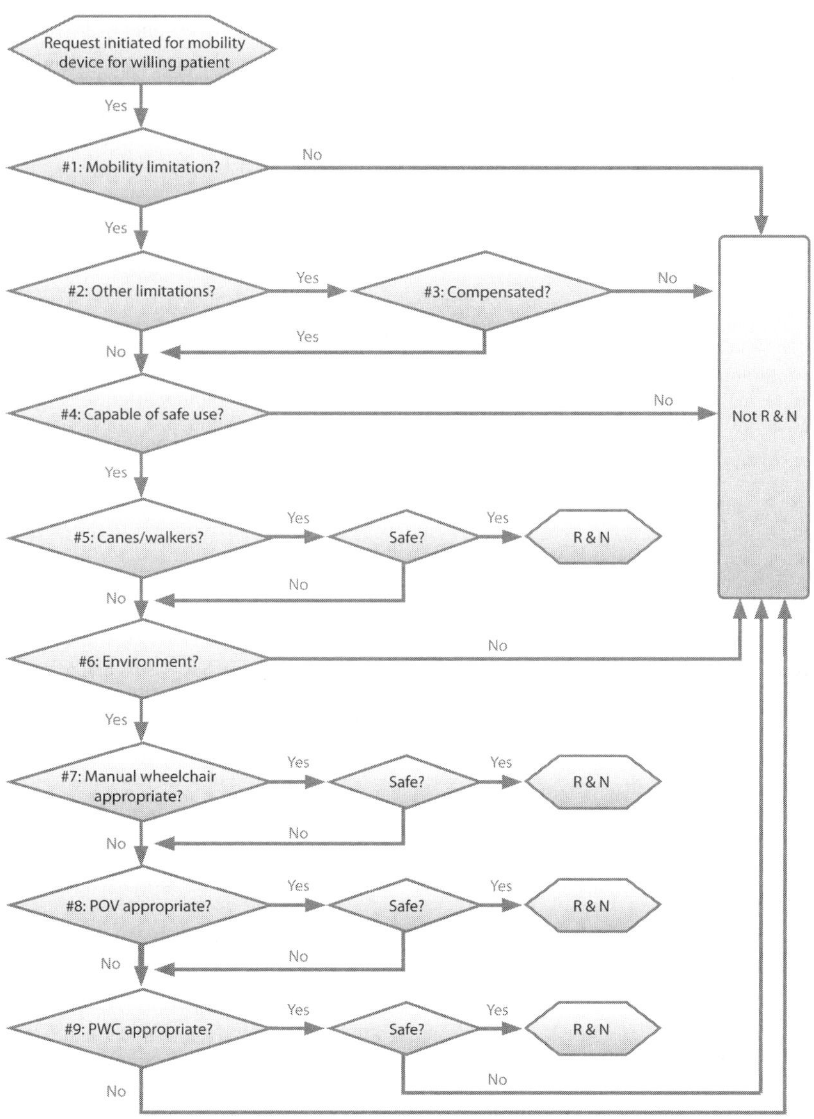

Pub 100-3, 280.4 – Seat Lift

(Rev. 1, 10-03-03)

Reimbursement may be made for the rental or purchase of a medically necessary seat lift when prescribed by a physician for a patient with severe arthritis of the hip or knee and patients with muscular dystrophy or other neuromuscular disease when it has been determined the patient can benefit therapeutically from use of the device. In establishing medical necessity for the seat lift, the evidence must show that the item is included in the physician's course of treatment, that it is likely to effect improvement, or arrest or retard deterioration in the patient's condition, and that the severity of the condition is such that the alternative would be chair or bed confinement.

Coverage of seat lifts is limited to those types which operate smoothly, can be controlled by the patient, and effectively assist a patient in standing up and sitting down without other assistance. Excluded from coverage is the type of lift which operates by a spring release mechanism with a sudden, catapult-like motion and jolts the patient from a seated to a standing position. Limit the payment for units which incorporate a recliner feature along with the seat lift to the amount payable for a seat lift without this feature.

Cross Reference:

The Medicare **Claims Processing Manual**, Chapter 20, "Durable Medical Equipment, Prosthetics and Orthotics, and Supplies (DMEPOS)," §90.

Pub 100-3, 280.6 – Pneumatic Compression Devices

(Rev. 1, 10-03-03)

Pneumatic compression devices consist of an inflatable garment for the arm or leg and an electrical pneumatic pump that fills the garment with compressed air. The garment is intermittently inflated and deflated with cycle times and pressures that vary between devices. Pneumatic devices are covered for the treatment of lymphedema or for the treatment of chronic venous insufficiency with venous stasis ulcers.

Lymphedema

Lymphedema is the swelling of subcutaneous tissues due to the accumulation of excessive lymph fluid. The accumulation of lymph fluid results from impairment to the normal clearing function of the lymphatic system and/or from an excessive production of lymph. Lymphedema is divided into two broad classes according to etiology. Primary lymphedema is a relatively uncommon, chronic condition which may be due to such causes as Milroy's Disease or congenital anomalies. Secondary lymphedema which is much more common, results from the destruction of or damage to formerly functioning lymphatic channels, such as surgical removal of lymph nodes or post radiation fibrosis, among other causes.

Pneumatic compression devices are covered in the home setting for the treatment of lymphedema if the patient has undergone a four-week trial of conservative therapy and the treating physician determines that there has been no significant improvement or if significant symptoms remain after the trial. The trial of conservative therapy must include use of an appropriate compression bandage system or compression garment, exercise, and elevation of the limb. The garment may be prefabricated or custom-fabricated but must provide adequate graduated compression.

Chronic Venous Insufficiency With Venous Stasis Ulcers

Chronic venous insufficiency (CVI) of the lower extremities is a condition caused by abnormalities of the venous wall and valves, leading to obstruction or reflux of blood flow in the veins. Signs of CVI include hyperpigmentation, stasis dermatitis, chronic edema, and venous ulcers.

Pneumatic compression devices are covered in the home setting for the treatment of CVI of the lower extremities only if the patient has one or more venous stasis ulcer(s) which have failed to heal after a six month trial of conservative therapy directed by the treating physician. The trial of conservative therapy must include a compression bandage system or compression garment, appropriate dressings for the wound, exercise, and elevation of the limb.

General Coverage Criteria

Pneumatic compression devices are covered only when prescribed by a physician and when they are used with appropriate physician oversight, i.e., physician evaluation of the patient's condition to determine medical necessity of the device, assuring suitable instruction in the operation of the machine, a treatment plan defining the pressure to be used and the frequency and duration of use, and ongoing monitoring of use and response to treatment.

The determination by the physician of the medical necessity of a pneumatic compression device must include:

1. The patient's diagnosis and prognosis;
2. Symptoms and objective findings, including measurements which establish the severity of the condition;
3. The reason the device is required, including the treatments which have been tried and failed; and
4. The clinical response to an initial treatment with the device.

The clinical response includes the change in pretreatment measurements, ability to tolerate the treatment session and parameters, and ability of the patient (or caregiver) to apply the device for continued use in the home.

The only time that a segmented, calibrated gradient pneumatic compression device (HCPCS code E0652) would be covered is when the individual has unique characteristics that prevent them from receiving satisfactory pneumatic compression treatment using a nonsegmented device in conjunction with a segmented appliance or a segmented compression device without manual control of pressure in each chamber.

Cross Reference: §280.1.

Pub 100-3, 280.7 – Hospital Beds

(Rev. 1, 10-03-03)

A General Requirements for Coverage of Hospital Beds

A physician's prescription, and such additional documentation as the contractors' medical staffs may consider necessary, including medical records and physicians' reports, must establish the medical necessity for a hospital bed due to one of the following reasons:

- The patient's condition requires positioning of the body; e.g., to alleviate pain, promote good body alignment, prevent contractures, avoid respiratory infections, in ways not feasible in an ordinary bed; or
- The patient's condition requires special attachments that cannot be fixed and used on an ordinary bed.

B Physician's Prescription

The physician's prescription which must accompany the initial claim, and supplementing documentation when required, must establish that a hospital bed is medically necessary. If the stated reason for the need for a hospital bed is the patient's condition requires positioning, the prescription or other documentation must describe the medical condition, e.g., cardiac disease, chronic obstructive pulmonary disease, quadriplegia or paraplegia, and also the severity and frequency of the symptoms of the condition, that necessitates a hospital bed for positioning.

If the stated reason for requiring a hospital bed is the patient's condition requires special attachments, the prescription must describe the patient's condition and specify the attachments that require a hospital bed.

C Variable Height Feature

In well documented cases, the contractors' medical staffs may determine that a variable height feature of a hospital bed, approved for coverage under subsection A above, is medically necessary and, therefore, covered, for one of the following conditions:

- Severe arthritis and other injuries to lower extremities; e.g., fractured hip – The condition requires the variable height feature to assist the patient to ambulate by enabling the patient to place his or her feet on the floor while sitting on the edge of the bed;
- Severe cardiac conditions – For those cardiac patients who are able to leave bed, but who must avoid the strain of "jumping" up or down;
- Spinal cord injuries, including quadriplegic and paraplegic patients, multiple limb amputee and stroke patients. For those patients who are able to transfer from bed to a wheelchair, with or without help; or
- Other severely debilitating diseases and conditions, if the variable height feature is required to assist the patient to ambulate.

D Electric Powered Hospital Bed Adjustments

Medicare References

Electric powered adjustments to lower and raise head and foot may be covered when the contractor's medical staff determines that the patient's condition requires frequent change in body position and/or there may be an immediate need for a change in body position (i.e., no delay can be tolerated) and the patient can operate the controls and cause the adjustments. Exceptions may be made to this last requirement in cases of spinal cord injury and brain damaged patients.

E Side Rails

If the patient's condition requires bed side rails, they can be covered when an integral part of, or an accessory to, a hospital bed.

Pub 100-3, 280.8 – Air-Fluidized Bed

(Rev. 1, 10-03-03)

Air fluidized beds are covered for services rendered on or after: July 30, 1990.

An air-fluidized bed uses warm air under pressure to set small ceramic beads in motion which simulate the movement of fluid. When the patient is placed in the bed, his body weight is evenly distributed over a large surface area which creates a sensation of "floating." Medicare payment for home use of the air-fluidized bed for treatment of pressure sores can be made if such use is reasonable and necessary for the individual patient.

A decision that use of an air-fluidized bed is reasonable and necessary requires that:

- The patient has a stage 3 (full thickness tissue loss) or stage 4 (deep tissue destruction) pressure sore;
- The patient is bedridden or chair bound as a result of severely limited mobility;
- In the absence of an air-fluidized bed, the patient would require institutionalization;
- The air-fluidized bed is ordered in writing by the patient's attending physician based upon a comprehensive assessment and evaluation of the patient after completion of a course of conservative treatment designed to optimize conditions that promote wound healing. This course of treatment must have been at least one month in duration without progression toward wound healing. This month of prerequisite conservative treatment may include some period in an institution as long as there is documentation available to verify that the necessary conservative treatment has been rendered.
- Use of wet-to-dry dressings for wound debridement, begun during the period of conservative treatment and which continue beyond 30 days, will not preclude coverage of air-fluidized bed. Should additional debridement again become necessary, while a patient is using an air-fluidized bed (after the first 30-day course of conservative treatment) that will not cause the air-fluidized bed to become noncovered. In all instances documentation verifying the continued need for the bed must be available.
- A trained adult caregiver is available to assist the patient with activities of daily living, fluid balance, dry skin care, repositioning, recognition and management of altered mental status, dietary needs, prescribed treatments, and management and support of the air-fluidized bed system and its problems such as leakage;
- A physician directs the home treatment regimen, and reevaluates and recertifies the need for the air-fluidized bed on a monthly basis; and
- All other alternative equipment has been considered and ruled out.

Conservative treatment must include:

- Frequent repositioning of the patient with particular attention to relief of pressure over bony prominences (usually every 2 hours);
- Use of a specialized support surface (Group II) designed to reduce pressure and shear forces on healing ulcers and to prevent new ulcer formation;
- Necessary treatment to resolve any wound infection;
- Optimization of nutrition status to promote wound healing;
- Debridement by any means (including wet to dry dressings-which does not require an occlusive covering) to remove devitalized tissue from the wound bed;
- Maintenance of a clean, moist bed of granulation tissue with appropriate moist dressings protected by an occlusive covering, while the wound heals.

Home use of the air-fluidized bed is not covered under any of the following circumstances:

- The patient has coexisting pulmonary disease (the lack of firm back support makes coughing ineffective and dry air inhalation thickens pulmonary secretions);
- The patient requires treatment with wet soaks or moist wound dressings that are not protected with an impervious covering such as plastic wrap or other occlusive material;
- The caregiver is unwilling or unable to provide the type of care required by the patient on an air-fluidized bed;
- Structural support is inadequate to support the weight of the air-fluidized bed system (it generally weighs 1600 pounds or more);
- Electrical system is insufficient for the anticipated increase in energy consumption; or
- Other known contraindications exist.

Coverage of an air-fluidized bed is limited to the equipment itself. Payment for this covered item may only be made if the written order from the attending physician is furnished to the supplier prior to the delivery of the equipment. Payment is not included for the caregiver or for architectural adjustments such as electrical or structural improvement.

Cross reference:

The Medicare **Claims Processing Manual**, Chapter 23, "Fee Schedule Administration and Coding Requirements," §§60.

Pub 100-3, 280.9 – Power Operated Vehicles That May Be Used as Wheelchairs

(Rev. 1, 10-03-03)

Power-operated vehicles that may be appropriately used as wheelchairs are covered under the durable medical equipment provision.

These vehicles have been appropriately used in the home setting for vocational rehabilitation and to improve the ability of chronically disabled persons to cope with normal domestic, vocational and social activities. They may be covered if a wheelchair is medically necessary and the patient is unable to operate a wheelchair manually.

A specialist in physical medicine, orthopedic surgery, neurology, or rheumatology must provide an evaluation of the patient's medical and physical condition and a prescription for the vehicle to assure that the patient requires the vehicle and is capable of using it safely. When a Durable Medical Equipment Regional Carrier (DMERC) determines that such a specialist is not reasonably accessible, e.g., more than one day's round trip from the beneficiary's home, or the patient's condition precludes such travel, a prescription from the beneficiary's physician is acceptable.

The DMERC's medical staff reviews all claims for a power-operated vehicle, including the specialists' or other physicians' prescriptions and evaluations of the patient's medical and physical conditions, to insure that all coverage requirements are met. (See §280.1 and the Medicare **Claims Processing Manual**, Chapter 20,"Durable Medical Equipment, Prosthetics and Orthotics, and Supplies (DMEPOS)," §§110, 120, 130, 140, 150, 160, and 170.)

Pub 100-3, 280.10 – Prosthetic Shoe

(Rev. 1, 10-03-03)

A prosthetic shoe (a device used when all or a substantial portion of the front part of the foot is missing) can be covered as a terminal device; i.e., a structural supplement replacing a totally or substantially absent hand or foot. The coverage of artificial arms and legs includes payment for terminal devices such as hands or hooks even though the patient may not require an artificial limb. The function of the prosthetic shoe is quite distinct from that of excluded orthopedic shoe and supportive foot devices which are used by individuals whose feet, although impaired, are essentially intact. (Section 1862(a)(8) of the Act excludes payment for orthopedic shoes or other supportive devices for the feet.) See the **Medicare Benefit Policy Manual**, Chapter 15, "Covered Medical and Other Services," §130.

Pub 100-3, 280.11 – Corset Used as Hernia Support

(Rev. 1, 10-03-03)

A hernia support (whether in the form of a corset or truss) which meets the definition of a brace is covered under Part B under §1861(s)(9) of the Act. See the **Medicare Benefit Policy Manual**, Chapter 15, "Covered Medical and Other Services," §130.

Pub 100-3, 280.12 – Sykes Hernia Control

(Rev. 1, 10-03-03)

Based on professional advice, it has been determined that the sykes hernia control (a spring-type, U-shaped, strapless truss) is not functionally more beneficial than a conventional truss. Make program reimbursement for this device only when an ordinary truss would be covered. (Like all trusses, it is only of benefit when dealing with a reducible hernia). Thus, when a charge for this item is substantially in excess of that which would be reasonable for a conventional truss used for the same condition, base reimbursement on the reasonable charges for the conventional truss. See the **Medicare Benefit Policy Manual**, Chapter 15, "Covered Medical and Other Services," §130.

Pub 100-3, 280.14 – Infusion Pumps

(Rev. 27, Issued: 02-04-05, Effective: 12-17-04, Implementation: 02-18-05)

A. General

Infusion pumps are medical devices used to deliver solutions containing parenteral drugs under pressure at a regulated flow rate.

B. Nationally Covered Indications

The following indications for treatment using infusion pumps are covered under Medicare:

1. External Infusion Pumps

a. Iron Poisoning (Effective for Services Performed On or After September 26, 1984)

When used in the administration of deferoxamine for the treatment of acute iron poisoning and iron overload, only external infusion pumps are covered.

b. Thromboembolic Disease (Effective for Services Performed On or After September 26, 1984)

When used in the administration of heparin for the treatment of thromboembolic disease and/or pulmonary embolism, only external infusion pumps used in an institutional setting are covered.

c. Chemotherapy for Liver Cancer (Effective for Services Performed On or After January 29, 1985)

The external chemotherapy infusion pump is covered when used in the treatment of primary hepatocellular carcinoma or colorectal cancer where this disease is unresectable; OR, where the patient refuses surgical excision of the tumor.

d. Morphine for Intractable Cancer Pain (Effective for Services Performed On or After April 22, 1985)

Morphine infusion via an external infusion pump is covered when used in the treatment of intractable pain caused by cancer (in either an inpatient or outpatient setting, including a hospice).

e. Continuous Subcutaneous Insulin Infusion (CSII) Pumps (Effective for Services Performed On or after December 17, 2004)

Continuous subcutaneous insulin infusion (CSII) and related drugs/supplies are covered as medically reasonable and necessary in the home setting for the treatment of diabetic patients who: (1) either meet the updated fasting C-Peptide testing requirement, or, are beta cell autoantibody positive; and, (2) satisfy the remaining criteria for insulin pump therapy as described below. Patients must meet either Criterion A or B as follows:

Criterion A: The patient has completed a comprehensive diabetes education program, and has been on a program of multiple daily injections of insulin (i.e., at least 3 injections per day), with frequent self-adjustments of insulin doses for at least 6 months prior to initiation of the insulin pump, and has documented frequency of glucose self-testing an average of at least 4 times per day during the 2 months prior to initiation of the insulin pump, and meets one or more of the following criteria while on the multiple daily injection regimen:

- Glycosylated hemoglobin level (HbAlc) > 7.0 percent;
- History of recurring hypoglycemia;
- Wide fluctuations in blood glucose before mealtime;
- Dawn phenomenon with fasting blood sugars frequently exceeding 200 mg/dl; or,
- History of severe glycemic excursions.

Criterion B: The patient with diabetes has been on a pump prior to enrollment in Medicare and has documented frequency of glucose self-testing an average of at least 4 times per day during the month prior to Medicare enrollment.

General CSII Criteria

In addition to meeting Criterion A or B above, the following general requirements must be met:

The patient with diabetes must be insulinopenic per the updated fasting C-peptide testing requirement, or, as an alternative, must be beta cell autoantibody positive.

Updated fasting C-peptide testing requirement:

- Insulinopenia is defined as a fasting C-peptide level that is less than or equal to 110% of the lower limit of normal of the laboratory's measurement method.
- For patients with renal insufficiency and creatinine clearance (actual or calculated from age, gender, weight, and serum creatinine) ≤50 ml/minute, insulinopenia is defined as a fasting C-peptide level that is less than or equal to 200% of the lower limit of normal of the laboratory's measurement method.
- Fasting C-peptide levels will only be considered valid with a concurrently obtained fasting glucose ≤225 mg/dL.
- Levels only need to be documented once in the medical records.

Continued coverage of the insulin pump would require that the patient be seen and evaluated by the treating physician at least every 3 months.

The pump must be ordered by and follow-up care of the patient must be managed by a physician who manages multiple patients with CSII and who works closely with a team including nurses, diabetes educators, and dietitians who are knowledgeable in the use of CSII.

Other Uses of CSII

The CMS will continue to allow coverage of all other uses of CSII in accordance with the Category B investigational device exemption (IDE) clinical trials regulation (42 CFR 405.201) or as a routine cost under the clinical trials policy (Medicare National Coverage Determinations (NCD) Manual 310.1).

f. Other Uses

Other uses of external infusion pumps are covered if the contractor's medical staff verifies the appropriateness of the therapy and the prescribed pump for the individual patient.

NOTE: Payment may also be made for drugs necessary for the effective use of a covered external infusion pump as long as the drug being used with the pump is itself reasonable and necessary for the patient's treatment.

2. Implantable Infusion Pumps

a. Chemotherapy for Liver Cancer (Effective for Services Performed On or After September 26, 1984)

The implantable infusion pump is covered for intra-arterial infusion of 5-FUdR for the treatment of liver cancer for patients with primary hepatocellular carcinoma or Duke's Class D colorectal cancer, in whom the metastases are limited to the liver, and where: (1) the disease is unresectable, or (2) the patient refuses surgical excision of the tumor.

b. Anti-Spasmodic Drugs for Severe Spasticity

An implantable infusion pump is covered when used to administer anti-spasmodic drugs intrathecally (e.g., baclofen) to treat chronic intractable spasticity in patients who have proven unresponsive to less invasive medical therapy as determined by the following criteria:

As indicated by at least a 6-week trial, the patient cannot be maintained on noninvasive methods of spasm control, such as oral anti-spasmodic drugs, either because these methods fail to control adequately the spasticity or produce intolerable side effects, and prior to pump implantation, the patient must have responded favorably to a trial intrathecal dose of the anti-spasmodic drug.

c. Opioid Drugs for Treatment of Chronic Intractable Pain

An implantable infusion pump is covered when used to administer opioid drugs (e.g., morphine) intrathecally or epidurally for treatment of severe chronic intractable pain of malignant or nonmalignant origin in patients who have a life expectancy of at least 3 months, and who have proven unresponsive to less invasive medical therapy as determined by the following criteria:

The patient's history must indicate that he/she would not respond adequately to noninvasive methods of pain control, such as systemic opioids (including attempts to eliminate physical and behavioral abnormalities which may cause an exaggerated reaction to pain); and a preliminary trial of intraspinal opioid drug administration must be undertaken with a temporary intrathecal/epidural catheter to substantiate adequately acceptable pain relief and degree of side effects (including effects on the activities of daily living) and patient acceptance.

d. Coverage of Other Uses of Implanted Infusion Pumps

Determinations may be made on coverage of other uses of implanted infusion pumps if the contractor's medical staff verifies that:

- The drug is reasonable and necessary for the treatment of the individual patient;
- It is medically necessary that the drug be administered by an implanted infusion pump; and,
- The Food and Drug Administration (FDA)-approved labeling for the pump must specify that the drug being administered and the purpose for which it is administered is an indicated use for the pump.

e. Implantation of Infusion Pump Is Contraindicated

The implantation of an infusion pump is contraindicated in the following patients:

- With a known allergy or hypersensitivity to the drug being used (e.g., oral baclofen, morphine, etc.);
- Who have an infection;
- Whose body size is insufficient to support the weight and bulk of the device; and,
- With other implanted programmable devices since crosstalk between devices may inadvertently change the prescription.

NOTE: Payment may also be made for drugs necessary for the effective use of an implantable infusion pump as long as the drug being used with the pump is itself reasonable and necessary for the patient's treatment.

C. Nationally Noncovered Indications

The following indications for treatment using infusion pumps are not covered under Medicare:

1. External Infusion Pumps

a. Vancomycin (Effective for Services Beginning On or After September 1, 1996)

Medicare coverage of vancomycin as a durable medical equipment infusion pump benefit is not covered. There is insufficient evidence to support the necessity of using an external infusion pump, instead of a disposable elastomeric pump or the gravity drip method, to administer vancomycin in a safe and appropriate manner.

2. Implantable Infusion Pump

a. Thromboembolic Disease (Effective for Services Performed On or After September 26, 1984)

According to the Public Health Service, there is insufficient published clinical data to support the safety and effectiveness of the heparin implantable pump. Therefore, the use of an implantable infusion pump for infusion of heparin in the treatment of recurrent thromboembolic disease is not covered.

b. Diabetes

An implanted infusion pump for the infusion of insulin to treat diabetes is not covered. The data does not demonstrate that the pump provides effective administration of insulin.

D. Other

Not applicable.

(This NCD last reviewed January 2005.)

Pub 100-3, 300.1 – Obsolete or Unreliable Diagnostic Tests

(Rev. 48, 06-19-06)

A. Diagnostic Tests

Do not routinely pay for the following diagnostic tests because they are obsolete and have been replaced by more advanced procedures. The listed tests may be paid for only if the medical need for the procedure is satisfactorily justified by the physician who performs it.

When the services are subject to the Quality Improvement Organization (QIO) Review, the QIO is responsible for determining that satisfactory medical justification exists. When the services are not subject to QIO review, the intermediary or carrier is responsible for determining that satisfactory medical justification exists. This includes:

- Amylase, blood isoenzymes, electrophoretic,
- Chromium, blood,
- Guanase, blood,
- Zinc sulphate turbidity, blood,
- Skin test, cat scratch fever,
- Skin test, lymphopathia venereum,
- Circulation time, one test,
- Cephalin flocculation,
- Congo red, blood,
- Hormones, adrenocorticotropin quantitative animal tests,
- Hormones, adrenocorticotropin quantitative bioassay,
- Thymol turbidity, blood,
- Skin test, actinomycosis,
- Skin test, brucellosis,
- Skin test, psittacosis,
- Skin test, trichinosis,
- Calcium, feces, 24-hour quantitative,
- Starch, feces, screening,
- Chymotrypsin, duodenal contents,
- Gastric analysis, pepsin,
- Gastric analysis, tubeless,
- Calcium saturation clotting time,
- Capillary fragility test (Rumpel-Leede),
- Colloidal gold,
- Bendien's test for cancer and tuberculosis,
- Bolen's test for cancer,
- Rehfuss test for gastric acidity, and
- Serum seromucoid assay for cancer and other diseases.

B. Cardiovascular Tests

Do not pay for the following phonocardiography and vectorcardiography diagnostic tests because they have been determined to be outmoded and of little clinical value. They include:

Medicare References

- Phonocardiogram with or without ECG lead; with supervision during recording with interpretation and report (when equipment is supplied by the physician),
- Phonocardiogram; tracing only, without interpretation and report (e.g., when equipment is supplied by the hospital, clinic),
- Phonocardiogram; interpretation and report,
- Phonocardiogram with ECG lead, with indirect carotid artery and/or jugular vein tracing, and/or apex cardiogram; with interpretation and report,
- Phonocardiogram; without interpretation and report,
- Phonocardiogram; interpretation and report only,
- Intracardiac,
- Vectorcardiogram (VCG), with or without ECG; with interpretation and report,
- Vectorcardiogram; tracing only, without interpretation and report, and
- Vectorcardiogram; interpretation and report only.

Pub 100-4 – Medicare Claims Processing Manual

Pub 100-4, 8, 60.1 – Lab Services

(Rev. 1655, Issued: 12-31-08, Effective: 01-01-09, Implementation: 02-02-09)

See the Medicare Benefit Policy Manual, Chapter 11, for a description of lab services included in the composite rate.

Independent laboratories and independent dialysis facilities with the appropriate clinical laboratory certification in accordance with CLIA may be paid for ESRD clinical laboratory tests that are separately billable. The laboratories and independent dialysis facilities are paid for separately billable clinical laboratory tests according to the Medicare laboratory fee schedule for independent laboratories. (See Chapter 16, section 40.3 for details on Part B hospital billing rules for laboratory services and Chapter 16, section 40.6 for details on ESRD billing.)

Hospital-based laboratories providing separately billable laboratory services to dialysis patients of the hospital's dialysis facility or another dialysis facility bill and are paid in accordance with the hospital outpatient laboratory provisions in Chapter 16, section 40.3. If the ESRD patient also receives other hospital outpatient services on the same day as aspecimen collection and/or laboratory test, then the patient is considered to be a registered hospital outpatient and cannot be considered to be a non-patient on that day for purposes of the specimen collection and laboratory test. When the patient does not also receive hospital outpatient services on the same day as the specimen collection and/or laboratory test, then the hospital may choose to register the beneficiary as an outpatient for the specimen collection or bill for these services as non-patient on the 14x bill type.

Clinical laboratory tests are performed individually. Automated profiles and application of the "50 percent rule" can be found in Chapter 16 of this manual.

A specimen collection fee determined by CMS (as of this writing, up to $3.00) will be allowed for ESRD Method II billing only in the following circumstances:

- Drawing a blood sample through venipuncture (i.e., inserting into a vein a needle with a syringe or vacutainer to draw the specimen).
- Collecting a urine sample by catheterization.

Laboratory tests for Hemodialysis, Intermittent Peritoneal Dialysis (IPD), Continuous Cycling Peritoneal Dialysis (CCPD), and Hemofiltration (as specified in the ***Medicare Benefit Policy Manual*** Pub. 100-02, Chapter 11, Section 30.2) are usually performed for dialysis patients and are routinely covered at the frequency specified in the absence of indications to the contrary, i.e., no documentation of medical necessity is required other than knowledge of the patient's status as an ESRD beneficiary. When any of these tests is performed at a frequency greater than that specified, the additional tests are separately billable and are covered only if they are medically justified by accompanying documentation. A diagnosis of ESRD alone is not sufficient medical evidence to warrant coverage of the additional tests. The nature of the illness or injury (diagnosis, complaint, or symptom) requiring the performance of the test(s) must be present on the claim. Such information must be furnished using the ICD-9-CM coding system.

Pub 100-4, 8, 60.2.4 – Intravenous Iron Therapy

(Rev. 1, 10-01-03)

RDF-319.4, A3-3644.E

Iron deficiency is a common condition in ESRD patients undergoing dialysis. Iron is a critical structural component of hemoglobin, a key protein found in normal red blood cells (RBCs) which transports oxygen. Without this important building block, anemic patients experience difficulty in restoring adequate, healthy RBC (hematocrit) levels. Clinical management of iron deficiency involves treating patients with iron replacement products while they undergo hemodialysis.

Pub 100-4, 8, 60.2.4.1 – Facility Billing Requirements to the Intermediary

(Rev. 1, 10-01-03)

A3-3644

See **Medicare Benefit Policy Manual**, Chapter 11 for coverage and effective dates applicable to intravenous iron therapy services.

For claims with dates of service on or after December 1, 2000, sodium ferric gluconate complex in sucrose injection is covered by Medicare for first line treatment of iron deficiency anemia in patients undergoing chronic hemodialysis who are receiving supplemental erythropoeitin therapy. Payment is made on a reasonable cost basis for claims with dates of service on or after December 1, 2000 in renal dialysis centers (freestanding facilities). Payment is made pursuant to 42 CFR 405.517 for claims with dates of service on or after January 1, 2001.

For claims with dates of service on or after October 1, 2001, Medicare also covers iron sucrose injection as a first line treatment of iron deficiency anemia when furnished intravenously to patients undergoing chronic hemodialysis who are receiving supplemental erythropoeitin therapy. Payment is made under the outpatient prospective payment system for hospital outpatient departments. Payment is made on a reasonable cost basis in CAHs and in renal dialysis centers (freestanding facilities). See Chapter 17. Deductible and coinsurance apply.

Facilities bill the FI using type of bill 72X and revenue code 0636. For claims with dates of service on or after December 1, 2000, report HCPCS code J3490 (Unclassified drugs) for sodium ferric gluconate complex in sucrose injection. For claims with dates of service on or after January 1, 2001, facilities report HCPCS code J2915 for sodium ferric gluconate complex in sucrose injection. Until a specific code is developed for iron sucrose injection, report HCPCS code J3490 (Unclassified drugs).

Pub 100-4, 8, 60.2.4.2 – Physician Billing Requirements to the Carrier

(Rev. 1, 10-01-03)

B3-4461.1, B3-4461.2, B3-4461.3

A. Sodium Ferric Gluconate Complex in Sucrose Injection

Sodium Ferric Gluconate Complex in sucrose injection may be payable for claims with dates of service on or after December 1, 2000 when furnished intravenously, for first line treatment of iron deficiency anemia in patients undergoing chronic hemodialysis who are receiving supplemental erythropoeitin therapy. Physicians bill and carriers pay for HCPCS codes J1755 or J1756 when submitted with a primary diagnosis for chronic renal failure and a secondary diagnosis for iron deficiency anemia in Item 21. The ICD-9-CM diagnosis codes are:

- 585 – Primary diagnosis for chronic renal failure, and
- 280.0, 280.1, 280.8, or 280.9 – Only one is necessary as a secondary diagnosis for iron deficiency anemia.

This benefit is subject to the Part B deductible and coinsurance and should be paid per current Medicare drug payment reimbursement rules. Carriers may cover other uses of this drug at their discretion.

B. Iron Sucrose Injection

Iron Sucrose injections are payable for claims with dates of service on or after October 1, 2001, when furnished intravenously, for first line treatment of iron deficiency anemia in patients undergoing chronic hemodialysis who are receiving supplemental erythropoeitin therapy. Until a specific code for iron sucrose injection is developed, providers must submit HCPCS code J3490, with the appropriate explanation of drug name and dosage entered in Item 19 of the form CMS-1500 or the corresponding electronic format. The primary diagnosis code ICD-9-CM 585 for chronic renal failure and one of the following secondary diagnosis codes for iron deficiency anemia ICD-9-CM codes 280.0, 280.1, 280.8, or 280.9 must be entered in Item 21. Iron sucrose injection is subject to the Part B deductible and coinsurance and should be paid per current Medicare drug payment reimbursement rules. Carriers may cover other uses of this drug at their discretion.

C. Messages for Use with Denials

The following denial messages should be used to deny claims for sodium ferric gluconate complex in sucrose injection or iron sucrose injection due to a missing diagnosis code.

Remittance Advice: Claim adjustment reason code 16, Claim/service lacks information which is needed for adjudication, along with remark code M76, Incomplete/invalid patient's diagnosis(es) and condition (s).

Explanation of Medicare Benefits: 9.8, Medicare cannot pay for this service because the claim is missing information/documentation.

Medicare Summary Notice: 9.2, This item or service was denied because information required to make payment was missing.

Pub 100-4, 8, 60.4.2 – Epoetin Alfa (EPO) Supplier Billing Requirements (Method II) on the Form CMS-1500

(Rev 118, 03-05-04)

A. Claims With Dates of Service Prior to January 1, 2004

For claims with dates of service prior to January 1, 2004, the correct EPO code to use is the one that indicates the patient's most recent hematocrit (HCT) (rounded to the nearest whole percent) or hemoglobin (Hgb) (rounded to the nearest g/dl) prior to the date of service of the EPO. For example, if the patient's most recent hematocrit was 20.5 percent, bill Q9921; if it was 28.4 percent, bill Q9928.

To convert actual hemoglobin to corresponding hematocrit for Q code reporting, multiply the Hgb value by 3 and round to the nearest whole number. For example, if Hgb = 8.4, report as Q9925 (8.4 X 3 = 25.2, rounded down to 25).

One unit of service of EPO is reported for each 1000 units dispensed. For example if 20,000 units are dispensed, bill 20 units. If the dose dispensed is not an even multiple of 1,000, rounded down for 1 – 499 units (e.g. 20,400 units dispensed = 20 units billed), round up for 500 – 999 units (e.g. 20,500 units dispensed = 21 units billed).

Q9920 Injection of EPO, per 1,000 units, at patient HCT of 20 or less

Q9921 Injection of EPO, per 1,000 units, at patient HCT of 21

Q9922 Injection of EPO, per 1,000 units, at patient HCT of 22

Q9923 Injection of EPO, per 1,000 units, at patient HCT of 23

Q9924 Injection of EPO, per 1,000 units, at patient HCT of 24

Q9925 Injection of EPO, per 1,000 units, at patient HCT of 25

Q9926 Injection of EPO, per 1,000 units, at patient HCT of 26

Q9927 Injection of EPO, per 1,000 units, at patient HCT of 27

Q9928 Injection of EPO, per 1,000 units, at patient HCT of 28

Q9929 Injection of EPO, per 1,000 units, at patient HCT of 29

Q9930 Injection of EPO, per 1,000 units, at patient HCT of 30

Q9931 Injection of EPO, per 1,000 units, at patient HCT of 31

Q9932 Injection of EPO, per 1,000 units, at patient HCT of 32

Q9933 Injection of EPO, per 1,000 units, at patient HCT of 33

Q9934 Injection of EPO, per 1,000 units, at patient HCT of 34

Q9935 Injection of EPO, per 1,000 units, at patient HCT of 35

Q9936 Injection of EPO, per 1,000 units, at patient HCT of 36

Q9937 Injection of EPO, per 1,000 units, at patient HCT of 37

Q9938 Injection of EPO, per 1,000 units, at patient HCT of 38

Q9939 Injection of EPO, per 1,000 units, at patient HCT of 39

Q9940 Injection of EPO, per 1,000 units, at patient HCT of 40 or above.

B. Claims with Dates of Service January 1, 2004 and after

The above codes were replaced effective January 1, 2004 by Q4055. This Q code is for the injection of EPO furnished to ESRD Beneficiaries on Dialysis. The new code does not include the hematocrit. See §60.7.

Q4055 Injection, Epoetin alfa, 1,000 units (for ESRD on Dialysis).

The DMERC shall return to provider (RTP) assigned claims for EPO, Q4055, that do not contain a HCT value. For unassigned claims, the DMERC shall deny claims for EPO, Q4055 that do not contain a HCT value.

DMERCs must use the following messages when payment for the injection (Q4055) does not meet the coverage criteria and is denied:

Medicare References

MSN Message 6.5—English: Medicare cannot pay for this injection because one or more requirements for coverage were not met

MSN Message 6.5—Spanish: Medicare no puede pagar por esta inyeccion porque uno o mas requisitos para la cubierta no fueron cumplidos. (MSN Message 6.5 in Spanish).

Adjustment Reason Code B:5 Payment adjusted because coverage/ program guidelines were not met or were exceeded.

The DMERCs shall use the following messages when returning as unprocessable assigned claims without a HCT value:

The ANSI Reason Code 16 – Claim/service lacks information, which is needed for adjudication.

Additional information is supplied using remittance advice remarks codes whenever appropriate.

Remark Code M58 – Missing/incomplete/invalid claim information. Resubmit claim after corrections.

Deductibles and coinsurance apply.

Pub 100-4, 8, 60.4.2.1 – Other Information Required on the Form CMS-1500 for Epoetin Alfa (EPO)

(Rev 118, 03-05-04)

The following information is required for EPO. Incomplete assigned claims are returned to providers for completion. Incomplete unassigned claims are rejected. The rejection will be due to a lack of a HCT value. Note that when a claim is submitted on paper Form CMS-1500, these items are submitted on a separate document. It is not necessary to enter them into the claims processing system. This information is used in utilization review.

A. Diagnoses

The diagnoses must be submitted according to ICD-9-CM and correlated to the procedure. This information is in Item 21, of the Form CMS-1500.

B. Hematocrit (HCT)/Hemoglobin (Hgb)

There are special HCPCS codes for reporting the injection of EPO for claims with dates of service prior to January 1, 2004. These allow the simultaneous reporting of the patient's latest HCT or Hgb reading before administration of EPO.

The physician and/or staff are instructed to enter a separate line item for injections of EPO at different HCT/Hgb levels. The Q code for each line items is entered in Item 24D.

1. Code Q9920 – Injection of EPO, per 1,000 units, at patient HCT of 20 or less/Hgb of 6.8 or less.
2. Codes Q9921 through Q9939 – Injection of EPO, per 1,000 units, at patient HCT of 21 to 39/Hgb of 6.9 to 13.1. For HCT levels of 21 or more, up to a HCT of 39/Hgb of 6.9 to 13.1, a Q code that includes the actual HCT levels is used. To convert actual Hgb to corresponding HCT values for Q code reporting, multiply the Hgb value by 3 and round to the nearest whole number. Use the whole number to determine the appropriate Q code.

   EXAMPLES: If the patient's HCT is 25/Hgb is 8.2-8.4, Q9925 must be entered on the claim. If the patient's HCT is 39/Hgb is 12.9-13.1, Q9939 is entered.
3. Code Q9940 – Injection of EPO, per 1,000 units at patient HCT of 40 or above.

   A single line item may include multiple doses of EPO administered while the patient's HCT level remained the same.

   Codes Q9920-Q9940 will no longer be recognized by the system if submitted after March 31, 2004. If claims for dates of service prior to January 1, 2004 are submitted after March 31, 2004, then code Q4055 must be used.

C. Units Administered

The standard unit of EPO is 1,000. The number of 1,000 units administered per line item is included on the claim. The physician's office enters 1 in the units field for each multiple of 1,000 units. For example, if 12,000 units are administered, 12 is entered. This information is shown in Item 24G (Days/Units) on Form CMS-1500.

In some cases, the dosage for a single line item does not total an even multiple of 1,000. If this occurs, the physician's office rounds down supplemental dosages of 0 to 499 units to the prior 1,000 units. Supplemental dosages of 500 to 999 are rounded up to the next 1,000 units.

EXAMPLES:

A patient's HCT reading on August 6 was 22/Hgb was 7.3. The patient received 5,000 units of EPO on August 7, August 9, and August 11, for a total of 15,000 units. The first line of Item 24 of Form CMS-1500 shows:

Dates of Service	Procedure Code	Days or Units
8/7 – 8/11	Q9922	15

On September 13, the patient's HCT reading increased to 27/Hgb increased to 9. The patient received 5,100 units of EPO on September 13, September 15, and September 17, for a total of 15,300 units. Since less than 15,500 units were given, the figure is rounded down to 15,000. This line on the claim form shows:

Dates of Service	Procedure Code	Days or Units
9/13 – 9/17	Q9927	15

On October 16, the HCT level increased to 33/Hgb increased to 11. The patient received doses of 4,850 units on October 16, October 18, and October 20 for a total of 14,550 units. Since more than 14,500 units were administered, the figure is rounded up to 15,000. Form CMS-1500 shows:

Dates of Service	Procedure Code	Days or Units
10/16 – 10/20	Q9933	15

NOTE: Creatinine and weight identified below are required on EPO claims as applicable.

D. Date of the Patient's most recent HCT or Hgb

E. Most recent HCT or Hgb level – (prior to initiation of EPO therapy)

F. Date of most recent HCT or Hgb level – (prior to initiation of EPO therapy)

G. Patient's most recent serum creatinine – (within the last month, prior to initiation of EPO therapy)

H. Date of most recent serum creatinine – (prior to initiation of EPO therapy)

I. Patient's weight in kilograms

J. Patient's starting dose per kilogram – (The usual starting dose is 50-100 units per kilogram)

Pub 100-4, 8, 60.4.2.2 – Completion of Subsequent Form CMS-1500 Claims for Epoetin Alfa (EPO)

(Rev 118, 03-05-04)

Subsequent claims are completed as initial claims in §60.4.2, except the following fields:

A. Diagnoses.

B. Hematocrit or Hemoglobin

For dates of service prior to January 1, 2004, this is indicated by the appropriate Q code. For dates of service January 1, 2004, and after, suppliers must indicate the beneficiary's hematocrit on the claim. (See 60.4.2.) Claims include an EJ modifier to the Q code. This allows the contractor to identify subsequent claims, which do not require as much information as initial claims and prevent unnecessary development.

Number of Units Administered – Subsequent claims may be submitted electronically.

Pub 100-4, 8, 60.4.3 – Payment Amount for Epoetin Alfa (EPO)

(Rev. 1084, Issued: 07-13-07; Effective: 01-01-08; Implementation: 01-07-08)

Dates of service prior to January 1, 2005, the FI pays the facility $10 per 1,000 units of EPO administered, rounded to the nearest 100 units (i.e., $1.00 per 100 units). Effective January 1, 2005, EPO will be paid based on the ASP Pricing File. Also effective January 1, 2005, the cost of supplies to administer EPO may be billed to the FI. HCPCS A4657 and Revenue

Code 270 should be used to capture the charges for syringes used in the administration of EPO. Where EPO is furnished by a supplier that is not a facility, the DMERC pays at the same rate.

Physician payment is calculated through the drug payment methodology described in Chapter 17 of the **Claims Processing Manual**.

EXAMPLE: The billing period is 2/1/94 – 2/28/94.

The facility provides the following:

Date	Units	Date	Units
2/1	3000	2/15	2500
2/4	3000	2/18	2500
2/6	3000	2/20	2560
2/8	3000	2/22	2500
2/11	2500	2/25	2000
2/13	2500	2/27	2000

Total 31,060 units

For value code 68, the facility enters 31,060. The 31,100 are used to determine the rate payable. This is 31,060 rounded to the nearest 100 units. The amount payable is 31.1 x $10 =$311.00. In their systems, FIs have the option of setting up payment of $1.00 per 100 units. Effective January 1, 2005, EPO will be paid based on the ASP Pricing File.

EXAMPLE: 311 x $1.00 = $311.00

If an ESRD beneficiary requires 10,000 units or more of EPO per administration, special documentation must be made in the medical records. It must consist of a narrative report that addresses the following:

- Iron deficiency. Most patients need supplemental iron therapy while being treated, even if they do not start out iron deficient;
- Concomitant conditions such as infection, inflammation, or malignancy. These conditions must be addressed to assure that EPO has maximum effect;
- Unrecognized blood loss. Patients with kidney disease and anemia may easily have chronic blood loss (usually gastrointestinal) as a major cause of anemia. In those circumstances, EPO is limited in effectiveness;
- Concomitant hemolysis, bone morrow dysplasia, or refractory anemia for a reason other than renal disease, e.g., aluminum toxicity;
- Folic acid or vitamin B12 deficiencies;
- Circumstances in which the bone morrow is replaced with other tissue, e.g., malignancy or osteitis fibrosa cystica; and

Patient's weight, the current dose required, a historical record of the amount that has been given, and the hematocrit response to date.

Pub 100-4, 8, 60.4.3.1 – Payment for Epoetin Alfa (EPO) in Other Settings

(Rev. 1041, Issued: 08-25-06; Effective: 01-01-07; Implementation: 01-02-07)

In the hospital inpatient setting, payment under Part A is included in the DRG.

In the hospital inpatient setting, payment under Part B is made on bill type 12x. Hospitals report the drug units based on the units defined in the HCPCS description. Hospitals do not report value code 68 for units of EPO. For dates of service prior to April 1, 2006, report EPO under revenue code 0636. For dates of service from April 1, 2006 report EPO under the respective revenue code 0634 for EPO less than 10,000 units and revenue code 0635 for EPO over 10,000 units. Payment will be based on the ASP Pricing File.

In a skilled nursing facility (SNF), payment for EPO covered under the Part B EPO benefit is not included in the prospective payment rate for the resident's Medicare-covered SNF stay.

In a hospice, payment is included in the hospice per diem rate.

For a service furnished by a physician or incident to a physician's service, payment is made to the physician by the carrier in accordance with the rules for 'incident to" services. When EPO is administered in the renal facility, the service is not an "incident to" service and not under the "incident to" provision.

Pub 100-4, 8, 60.4.3.2 – Epoetin Alfa (EPO) Provided in the Hospital Outpatient Departments

(Rev. 1503; Issued: 05-16-08; Effective Date: 10-01-08; Implementation Date: 10- 06-08)

When ESRD patients come to the hospital for an unscheduled or emergency dialysis treatment they may also require the administration of EPO. Effective January 1, 2005, EPO will be paid based on the ASP Pricing File.

Hospitals use type of bill 13X (or 85X for Critical Access Hospitals) and report charges under the respective revenue code 0634 for EPO less than 10,000 units and revenue code 0635 for EPO over 10,000 units. Hospitals report the drug units based on the units defined in the HCPCS description. Hospitals do not report value code 68 for units of EPO. Value code 49 must be reported with the hematocrit value for the hospital outpatient visits prior to January 1, 2006, and for all claims with dates of service on or after January 1, 2008.

Pub 100-4, 8, 60.4.4 – Epoetin Alfa (EPO) Furnished to Home Patients

(Rev. 447, Issued: 01-21-05, Effective: 07-01-05, Implementation: 07-05-05)

Medicare covers EPO for dialysis patients who use EPO in the home, when requirements for a patient care plan and patient selection as described in the **Medicare Benefit Policy Manual**, Chapter 11, are met.

When EPO is prescribed for a home patient, it may be either administered in a facility, e.g., the one shown on the Form CMS-382 (ESRD Beneficiary Method Selection Form) or furnished by a facility or Method II supplier for self-administration to a home patient determined to be competent to administer this drug. For EPO furnished for self-administration to Method I and Method II home patients determined to be competent, the renal facility bills its FI and the Method II supplier bills its DMERC. No additional payment is made for training a prospective self-administering patient or retraining an existing home patient to self-administer EPO.

Method II patients who self-administer may obtain EPO only from either their Method II supplier, or a Medicare certified ESRD facility.

In this case, the DMERC makes payment at the same rate that applies to facilities. Program payment may not be made for EPO furnished by a physician to a patient for self-administration.

The DMERCs pay for EPO for Method II ESRD beneficiaries only. DMERCs shall deny claims for EPO where the beneficiary is not a Method II home dialysis patient.

When denying line items for patients that are not Method II, use the following message on the remittance advice:

> The ANSI message 7011: Claim not covered by this payer contractor. You must send the claim to the correct payer contractor.

When denying line items for patients that are not Method II, use the following message on the Medicare Summary Notice (MSN):

> English: 8.59 – Durable Medical Equipment Regional Carriers pay for Epoetin Alfa and Darbepoetin Alfa only for Method II End Stage Renal Disease home dialysis patients.
>
> Spanish: 8.59 – Las Empresas Regionales de Equipo Médico Duradero pagan por los medicamentos Epoetina Alfa y Darbepoetina Alfa sólo a pacientes del Método II de diálisis con enfermedad renal en etapa final que están confinados al hogar.

Pub 100-4, 8, 60.4.4.1 – Self Administered EPO Supply

(Rev. 1581; Issued: 08-29-08; Effective/Implementation Date: 12-01-08)

Initially, facilities may bill for up to a 2-month supply of EPO for Method I beneficiaries who meet the criteria for selection for self-administration. After the initial two months' supply, the facility will bill for one month's supply at a time. Condition code 70 is used to indicate payment requested for a supply of EPO furnished a beneficiary. Usually, revenue code 0635 would apply since the supply would be over 10,000 units. Facilities leave FL 46, Units of Service, blank since they are not administering the drug. For value code 68, they enter the total amount of the supply.

For claims with dates of service on or after January 1, 2008, supplies of EPO for self administration should be billed according to the predetermined plan of care schedule provided to the beneficiary. Submit a separate line item for each date an administration is expected to be performed with the expected dosage. In the event that the schedule was changed, the provider should note the changes in the medical record and bill according to the revised schedule. For patients beginning to self administer EPO at home receiving an extra month supply of the drug, bill the one month reserve supply on one claim line and include modifier EM defined as "Emergency Reserve Supply (for ESRD benefit only)".

When billing for drug wastage in accordance with the policy in chapter 17 of this manual, section 40.1 the provider must show the wastage on a separate line item with the modifier JW. The line item date of service should be the date of the last covered administration according to the plan of care or if the patient dies use the date of death.

Condition code 70 should be reported on claims billing for home dialysis patients that self administer anemia management drugs including epoetin alfa and darbepoetin alfa.

Pub 100-4, 8, 80 – Home Dialysis Method I Billing to the Intermediary

(Rev. 1, 10-01-03)

A3-3644.A, PRM-1-2710, PRM-1-2710.4, A3-3169, RDF-318, RO2-3440, B3-4270, B3-4271

If the Medicare home dialysis patient chooses Method I, the dialysis facility with which the Medicare home patient is associated assumes responsibility for providing all home dialysis equipment and supplies, and home support services. For these services, the facility receives the same Medicare dialysis payment rate as it would receive for an in-facility patient under the composite rate system. The beneficiary is responsible for paying any unmet Part B deductible and the 20-percent coinsurance. After the beneficiary's Part B deductible is met, the FI pays 80 percent of the specific facility's composite rate for each in-facility outpatient maintenance dialysis treatment.

Under Method I items and services included in the composite rate must be furnished by the facility, either directly or under arrangement. The cost of an item or service is included under the composite rate unless specifically excluded. Therefore, the determination as to whether an item or service is covered under the composite rate payment does not depend on the frequency that dialysis patients require the item or service, or the number of patients who require it. If the facility fails to provide (either directly or under arrangement) any part of the items and services covered under the rate, the facility cannot be paid any amount for the items and services that it does furnish. New items or services developed after the rate applicable for that particular year was computed are included in the composite rate payments. As such, ESRD facilities assume the responsibility for providing a dialysis service and must decide whether a particular item or service is medically appropriate and cost effective. Since the composite rate is adjusted, as necessary, based on the most recent cost data available to CMS, the costs of new items and services are taken into account in setting future rates. Similarly, any savings attributable to advancements in the treatment of ESRD accrue to the facility because no adjustment to any individual facility's rate is made.

Pub 100-4, 8, 90 – Method II Billing

(Rev. 1, 10-01-03)

A3-3644.A, RO-2-3440.C, B

1-2740, A3-3644.3

Physicians and independent laboratories, must submit claims (Form CMS-1500 or electronic equivalent) to their local carrier for services furnished to end stage renal disease (ESRD) beneficiaries. Suppliers of Method II dialysis equipment and supplies will submit their claims (Form CMS-1500 or electronic equivalent) to the appropriate Durable Medical Equipment Regional Carriers (DMERCs). All ESRD facilities must submit their claims to their appropriate FI. The amount of Medicare payment under Method II for home dialysis equipment and supplies may NOT exceed $1974.45 for continuous cycling peritoneal dialysis (CCPD) and $1490.85 for all other methods of dialysis.

All laboratory tests furnished to home dialysis patients who have selected payment Method II (see §70.1 above), are billed to and paid by the carrier at the fee schedule, if the tests are performed by an independent laboratory for an independent dialysis facility patient.

If the beneficiary elects to deal directly with a supplier and make arrangements for securing the necessary supplies and equipment to dialyze at home, and chooses Method II, he/she deals directly with a supplier of home dialysis equipment and supplies (this supplier is not a dialysis facility). A supplier other than a facility bills the DMERC. There can be only one supplier per beneficiary, and the supplier must accept assignment. The beneficiary is responsible for any unmet Part B deductible and the 20 percent coinsurance. Only a supplier that is not a dialysis facility may submit a claim to a DMERC for home dialysis supplies and equipment. Suppliers will submit these claims on Form CMS 1500, or electronic equivalent. Under Method II, beneficiaries may not submit any claims and cannot receive payment for any benefits for home dialysis equipment and supplies.

The supplier must have a written agreement with a Medicare approved dialysis facility that will provide all necessary support, backup, and emergency dialysis services. The dialysis facility will not receive a regular per treatment payment for a patient who chooses Method II.

However, if the facility provides any support services, backup, and emergency dialysis services to a beneficiary who selects this option, the facility is reimbursed for the items or services it furnishes. Hospital-based facilities are paid the reasonable cost of support services, subject to the lesser of cost or charges provisions of §1833(a)(2)(A) of the Act. Independent facilities are paid on a reasonable charge basis for any home dialysis support services they furnish.

A. Description of Support Services Support services specifically applicable to home patients include but are not limited to:
   - Surveillance of the patient's home adaptation, including provisions for visits to the home in accordance with a written plan prepared and periodically reviewed by a team that includes the patient's physician and other professionals familiar with the patient's condition;
   - Furnishing dialysis-related emergency services; Consultation for the patient with a qualified social worker and a qualified dietician;
   - Maintaining a record-keeping system which assures quality of care;
   - Maintaining and submitting all required documentation to the ESRD network;
   - Assuring that the water supply is of the appropriate quality;
   - Assuring that the appropriate supplies are ordered on an ongoing basis;
   - Arranging for the provision of all ESRD laboratory tests;
   - Testing and appropriate treatment of water used in dialysis;
   - Monitoring the functioning of dialysis equipment;
   - All other necessary dialysis services as required under the ESRD conditions for coverage;
   - Watching the patient perform CAPD and assuring that it is done correctly, and reviewing with the patient any aspects of the technique he/she may have forgotten, or informing the patient of modification in apparatus or technique;
   - Documenting whether the patient has or has not had peritonitis that requires physician intervention or hospitalization, (unless there is evidence of peritonitis, a culture for peritonitis is not necessary); Inspection of the catheter site; and
   - Since home dialysis support services include maintaining a medical record for each home dialysis patient, the Method II supplier must report to the support service dialysis facility within 30 days all items and services that it furnished to the patient so that the facility can record this information in the patient's medical record.

   The services must be furnished in accordance with the written plan required for home dialysis patients. See the **Medicare Benefit Policy Manual**, Chapter 15, for coverage of telehealth services, and this manual, Chapter 12 for billing telehealth.

   Each of the support services may be paid routinely at a frequency of once per month. Any furnished in excess of this frequency must be documented for being reasonable and necessary. For example, the patient may contract peritonitis and require an unscheduled connecting tube change.

B. Reasonableness Determinations Support services (which include the laboratory services included under the composite rate for in-facility patients) are paid on a reasonable charge basis to independent facilities and a reasonable cost basis to hospital-based facilities, subject to the Method II payment cap (refer to §140). A reasonable cost/charge determination must be made for each individual support service furnished to home patients. With respect to the connecting tube change, facilities may bill Medicare for the personnel services required to change the connecting tube, but must look to the Method II supplier for payment for the connecting tube itself. The payment cap is not a payment rate that is paid automatically each month. Accordingly, in no case may the FI routinely pay any monthly amount for support services without a claim that shows the services actually furnished.

Pub 100-4, 8, 130 – Physicians and Supplier (Nonfacility) Billing for ESRD Services – General

(Rev. 1, 10-01-03)

B3-4270 updated with Transmittal 1729

Payment for renal-related physicians' services to ESRD patients is made in either of the following ways:

- Under the Monthly Capitation Payment (MCP) (see §140 below for an explanation of the MCP); or
- Using the daily codes for ESRD services (CPT codes 90922-90925) with units that represent the number of days services were furnished.
- Under the Initial method (IM)

The carrier receives bills (Form CMS--1500 or electronic equivalent) from physicians for services furnished ESRD beneficiaries. DMERCs receive bills for equipment and supplies for Method II beneficiaries. Intermediaries receive bills from ESRD facilities.

Lab bills from CLIA certified independent dialysis facilities were billed to the carrier before September 1, 1997, and to the FI beginning on that date. Other certified labs continue to bill the carrier.

Pub 100-4, 8, 130.1 – Initial Method for Physician's Services to Maintenance Dialysis Patients

(Rev. 1, 10-01-03)

B3-4275, B3-4275.1, B3-4275.2, PRM-1-2715, PRM-1-2715.1, PRM-1-2715.2

Under the Initial Method (IM), do not pay for physician's routine professional dialysis services. Instead, the dialysis facility's FI pays the dialysis facility for them as part of the facility's composite rate. Physician's professional services that are not routine professional dialysis services are billed to the contractor and paid in the same way as any other Medicare covered physician professional service.

1. For the physician to be paid under the IM, the following requirements must be met:

   All physicians of the facility must choose the IM with respect to all of the patients treated at the facility and all of the facility's Method I home dialysis patients. (See §70.1 for a description of Method I). All of the facility's physicians must file a written statement with their carrier and the facility's FI to this effect. For example:

   The physicians practicing at ________________ dialysis facility are listed below. The signature of each physician indicates the physician's election to be paid for their routine professional dialysis services under the Initial Method. This election is effective for services furnished beginning with the second month after the month in which this statement is filed with the carrier(s) and the facility's intermediary.

   This written statement must be signed and dated by each physician.

2. The physician may bill the carrier only those physician's professional services that are not routine professional dialysis services. (See paragraph 3 below).

   The election of the IM is effective for services furnished beginning with the second calendar month after the month in which all the physicians of a facility elect it. A physician may terminate the election by written notice to the carrier and to the facility's FI that the physician thereby terminates the IM. If the carrier and the FI receive the termination notice on or before November 1, it is effective the following January 1. If the carrier or the FI receives it after November 1, it is effective January 1 of the second year after the calendar year in which the notice of termination is received. Note that if the IM is terminated by one physician, it is thereby terminated for all physicians at the same facility with respect to the patients treated through that facility.

3. Definitions

   A. Administrative Services

   Physician services that are differentiated from routine professional services and other physician services. They include supervision, as described in the definition of "supervision of staff," are not related directly to the care of an individual patient and are supportive of the facility as a whole and of benefit to patients in general. Examples of administrative services include supervision of staff, staff training, participation in staff conferences and in the management of the facility, and advising staff on the procurement of supplies.

   B. Dialysis Session

   The period of time that begins when the patient arrives at the facility and ends when the patient departs from the facility. In the case of home dialysis, the period begins when the patient prepares for dialysis and generally ends when the patient is disconnected from the machine. In this context, a dialysis facility includes only those parts of the building used as a facility. It does not include any areas used as a physician's private office.

   C. Medical Direction

   Routine professional service that entails substantial direct involvement and the physical presence of the physician in the delivery of services directly to the patient.

   D. Routine Professional Services

   Physicians' services furnished during a dialysis session and all services listed under "Types of routine professional services" that:

   - Are personally furnished by a physician to an individual patient.
   - Contribute directly to the diagnosis or treatment of an individual patient.
   - Ordinarily must be performed by a physician.

   E. Supervision of Staff

   Administrative services that do not necessarily require the physician to be present at the dialysis session. It is a general activity primarily concerned with monitoring performance of and giving guidance to other health care personnel (such as nurses and dialysis technicians) who deliver services to patients.

   F. Types of Routine Professional Services

   Routine professional services include at least the following services when medically appropriate:

   - Visits to the patient during dialysis, and in conjunction with review of laboratory test results,
   - Nurses' notes and any other medical documentation, as a basis for:
     - Adjustment of the patient's medication, diet or the dialysis procedure;
     - Prescription of medical supplies; and
     - Evaluation of the patient's psychosocial status and the appropriateness of the modality,
     - Medical direction of staff in delivering services to a patient during a dialysis session, and
     - Pre-dialysis and post-dialysis examinations or examinations that could have been furnished on a pre-dialysis or post-dialysis basis.

Pub 100-4, 12, 20.4.4 – Supplies

(Rev. 1, 10-01-03)

B3-15900.2

Carriers make a separate payment for supplies furnished in connection with a procedure only when one of the two following conditions exists:

A. HCPCS code A4300 is billed in conjunction with the appropriate procedure in the Medicare Physician Fee Schedule Data Base (place of service is physician's office). However, A4550, A4300, and A4263 are no longer separately payable as of 2002. Supplies have been incorporated into the practice expense RVU for 2002. Thus, no payment may be made for these supplies for serviced provided on or after January 1, 2002.

Medicare References

B. The supply is a pharmaceutical or radiopharmaceutical diagnostic imaging agent (including codes A4641 through A4647); pharmacologic stressing agent (code J1245); or therapeutic radionuclide (CPT code 79900). Other agents may be used which do not have an assigned HCPCS code. The procedures performed are:
- Diagnostic radiologic procedures (including diagnostic nuclear medicine) requiring pharmaceutical or radiopharmaceutical contrast media and/or pharmacologic stressing agent;
- Other diagnostic tests requiring a pharmacologic stressing agent;
- Clinical brachytherapy procedures (other than remote after-loading high intensity brachytherapy procedures (CPT codes 77781 through 77784) for which the expendable source is included in the TC RVUs); or
- Therapeutic nuclear medicine procedures.

Drugs are not supplies, and may be paid incidental to physicians' services as described in Chapter 17.

Pub 100-4, 12, 30 – Correct Coding Policy

(Rev. 1, 10-01-03)

The Correct Coding Initiative was developed to promote national correct coding methodologies and to control improper coding leading to inappropriate payment in Part B claims. Refer to Chapter 23 for additional information on the initiative.

The principles for the correct coding policy are:

- The service represents the standard of care in accomplishing the overall procedure.
- The service is necessary to successfully accomplish the comprehensive procedure. Failure to perform the service may compromise the success of the procedure.
- The service does not represent a separately identifiable procedure unrelated to the comprehensive procedure planned.

For a detailed description of the correct coding policy, refer to http://www.cms.hhs.gov/medlearn/ncci.asp.

The CMS as well as many third party payers have adopted the HCPCS/CPT coding system for use by physicians and others to describe services rendered. The system contains three levels of codes. Level I contain the American Medical Association's Current Procedural Terminology (CPT) numeric codes. Level II contains alpha-numeric codes primarily for items and services not included in CPT. Level III contains carrier specific codes that are not included in either Level I or Level II. For a list of CPT and HCPCS codes refer to the CMS Web site.

The following general coding policies encompass coding principles that are to be applied in the review of Medicare claims. They are the basis for the correct coding edits that are installed in the claims processing systems effective January 1, 1996.

A. Coding Based on Standards of Medical/Surgical Practice

All services integral to accomplishing a procedure are considered bundled into that procedure and, therefore, are considered a component part of the comprehensive code. Many of these generic activities are common to virtually all procedures and, on other occasions, some are integral to only a certain group of procedures, but are still essential to accomplish these particular procedures. Accordingly, it is inappropriate to separately report these services based on standard medical and surgical principles.

Because many services are unique to individual CPT coding sections, the rationale for rebundling is described in that particular section of the detailed coding narratives that are transmitted to carriers periodically.

B. CPT Procedure Code Definition

The format of the CPT manual includes descriptions of procedures, which are, in order to conserve space, not listed in their entirety for all procedures. The partial description is indented under the main entry. The main entry then encompasses the portion of the description preceding the semicolon. The main entry applies to and is a part of all indented entries, which follow with their codes.

In the course of other procedure descriptions, the code definition specifies other procedures that are included in this comprehensive code. In addition, a code description may define a rebundling relationship where one code is a part of another based on the language used in the descriptor.

C. CPT Coding Manual Instruction/Guideline

Each of the six major subsections includes guidelines that are unique to that section. These directions are not all inclusive of nor limited to, definitions of terms, modifiers, unlisted procedures or services, special or written reports, details about reporting separate, and multiple or starred procedures and qualifying circumstances.

D. Coding Services Supplemental to Principal Procedure (Add-On Codes) Code

Generally, these are identified with the statement "list separately in addition to code for primary procedure" in parentheses, and other times the supplemental code is used only with certain primary codes, which are parenthetically identified. The reason for these CPT codes is to enable physicians and others to separately identify a service that is performed in certain situations as an additional service. Incidental services that are necessary to accomplish the primary procedure (e.g., lysis of adhesions in the course of an open cholecystectomy) are not separately billed.

E. Separate Procedures

The narrative for many CPT codes includes a parenthetical statement that the procedure represents a "separate procedure."

The inclusion of this statement indicates that the procedure, while possible to perform separately, is generally included in a more comprehensive procedure, and the service is not to be billed when a related, more comprehensive, service is performed. The "separate procedure" designation is used with codes in the surgery (CPT codes 10000-69999), radiology (CPT codes 70000-79999), and medicine (CPT codes 90000-99199) sections. When a related procedure from the same section, subsection, category, or subcategory is performed, a code with the designation of "separate procedure" is not to be billed with the primary procedure.

F. Designation of Sex

Many procedure codes have a sex designation within their narrative. These codes are not billed with codes having an opposite sex designation because this would reflect a conflict in sex classification either by the definition of the code descriptions themselves, or by the fact that the performance of these procedures on the same beneficiary would be anatomically impossible.

G. Family of Codes

In a family of codes, there are two or more component codes that are not billed separately because they are included in a more comprehensive code as members of the code family. Comprehensive codes include certain services that are separately identifiable by other component codes. The component codes as members of the comprehensive code family represent parts of the procedure that should not be listed separately when the complete procedure is done. However, the component codes are considered individually if performed independently of the complete procedure and if not all the services listed in the comprehensive codes were rendered to make up the total service.

H. Most Extensive Procedures

When procedures are performed together that are basically the same or performed on the same site but are qualified by an increased level of complexity, the less extensive procedure is bundled into the more extensive procedure.

I. Sequential Procedures

An initial approach to a procedure may be followed at the same encounter by a second, usually more invasive approach. There may be separate CPT codes describing each service. The second procedure is usually performed because the initial approach was unsuccessful in accomplishing the medically necessary service. These procedures are considered "sequential procedures." Only the CPT code for one of the services, generally the more invasive service, should be billed.

J. With/Without Procedures

In the CPT manual, there are various procedures that have been separated into two codes with the definitional difference being "with" versus "without" (e.g., with and without contrast). Both procedure codes cannot be billed. When done together, the "without" procedure is bundled into the "with" procedure.

K. Laboratory Panels

When components of a specific organ or disease oriented laboratory panel (e.g., codes 80061 and 80059) or automated multi-channel tests (e.g., codes 80002 - 80019) are billed separately, they must be bundled into the comprehensive panel or automated multi-channel test code as appropriate that includes the multiple component tests. The individual tests that make up a panel or can be performed on an automated multi-channel test analyzer are not to be separately billed.

L. Mutually Exclusive Procedures

There are numerous procedure codes that are not billed together because they are mutually exclusive of each other. Mutually exclusive codes are those codes that cannot reasonably be done in the same session.

An example of a mutually exclusive situation is when the repair of the organ can be performed by two different methods. One repair method must be chosen to repair the organ and must be billed. Another example is the billing of an "initial" service and a "subsequent" service. It is contradictory for a service to be classified as an initial and a subsequent service at the same time.

CPT codes which are mutually exclusive of one another based either on the CPT definition or the medical impossibility/improbability that the procedures could be performed at the same session can be identified as code pairs. These codes are not necessarily linked to one another with one code narrative describing a more comprehensive procedure compared to the component code, but can be identified as code pairs which should not be billed together.

M. Use of Modifiers

When certain component codes or mutually exclusive codes are appropriately furnished, such as later on the same day or on a different digit or limb, it is appropriate that these services be reported using a HCPCS code modifier. Such modifiers are modifiers E1 - E4, FA, F1 - F9, TA, T1 - T9, LT, RT, LC, LD, RC, 58, 78, and 79.

Modifier 59 is not appropriate to use with weekly radiation therapy management codes (77427) or with evaluation and management services codes (99201 - 99499).

Application of these modifiers prevent erroneous denials of claims for several procedures performed on different anatomical sites, on different sides of the body, or at different sessions on the same date of service. The medical record must reflect that the modifier is being used appropriately to describe separate services.

Pub 100-4, 12, 30.1 – Digestive System (Codes 40000 – 49999)

(Rev. 1, 10-01-03)

A. Upper Gastrointestinal Endoscopy Including Endoscopic Ultrasound (EUS) (Code 43259)

If the person performing the original diagnostic endoscopy has access to the EUS and the clinical situation requires an EUS, the EUS may be done at the same time. The procedure, diagnostic and EUS, is reported under the same code, CPT 43259. This code conforms to CPT guidelines for the indented codes. The service represented by the indented code, in this case code 43259 for EUS, includes the service represented by the unintended code preceding the list of indented codes. Therefore, when a diagnostic examination of the upper gastrointestinal tract "including esophagus, stomach, and either the duodenum or jejunum as appropriate," includes the use of endoscopic ultrasonography, the service is reported by a single code, namely 43259.

Interpretation, whether by a radiologist or endoscopist, is reported under CPT code 76975-26. These codes may both be reported on the same day.

B. Incomplete Colonoscopies (Codes 45330 and 45378)

An incomplete colonoscopy, e.g., the inability to extend beyond the splenic flexure, is billed and paid using colonoscopy code 45378 with modifier 53. The Medicare physician fee schedule database has specific values for code 45378-53. These values are the same as for code 45330, sigmoidoscopy, as failure to extend beyond the splenic flexure means that a sigmoidoscopy rather than a colonoscopy has been performed. However, code 45378-53 should be used when an incomplete colonoscopy has been done because other MPFSDB indicators are different for codes 45378 and 45330.

Pub 100-4, 12, 30.2 – Urinary and Male Genital Systems (Codes 50010 – 55899)

(Rev. 1, 10-01-03)

A. Cystourethroscopy With Ureteral Catheterization (Code 52005)

Code 52005 has a zero in the bilateral field (payment adjustment for bilateral procedure does not apply) because the basic procedure is an examination of the bladder and urethra (cystourethroscopy), which are not paired organs. The work RVUs assigned take into account that it may be necessary to examine and catheterize one or both ureters. No additional payment is made when the procedure is billed with bilateral modifier 50. Neither is any additional payment made when both ureters are examined and code 52005 is billed with multiple surgery modifier 51. It is inappropriate to bill code 52005 twice, once by itself and once with modifier 51, when both ureters are examined.

B. Cystourethroscopy With Fulgration and/or Resection of Tumors (Codes 52234, 52235, and 52240)

The descriptors for codes 52234 through 52240 include the language "tumor(s)."

This means that regardless of the number of tumors removed; only one unit of a single code can be billed on a given date of service. It is inconsistent to allow payment for removal of a small (code 52234) and a large (code 52240) tumor using two codes when only one code is allowed for the removal of more than one large tumor. For these three codes only one unit may be billed for any of these codes, only one of the codes may be billed, and the billed code reflects the size of the largest tumor removed.

Pub 100-4, 12, 30.3 – Audiological Services

(Rev. 2044, Issued: 09-03-10, Effective: 09-30-10, Implementation: 09-30-10)

Section 1861(ll)(3)of the Social Security Act (the Act) defines "audiology services" as such hearing and balance assessment services furnished by a qualified audiologist as the audiologist is legally authorized to perform under State law (or the State regulatory mechanism provided by State law), as would otherwise by covered if furnished by a physician. In this section, these hearing and balance assessment services are termed "audiology services," regardless of whether they are furnished by an audiologist, physician, nonphysician practitioner (NPP), or hospital.

Because audiology services are diagnostic tests, when furnished in an office or hospital outpatient department, they must be furnished by or under the appropriate level of supervision of a physician as established in 42 CFR 410.32(b)(1) and 410.28(e). If not personally furnished by a physician, audiologist, or NPP, audiology services must be performed under direct physician supervision. As specified in 42 CFR 410.32(b)(2)(ii) or (v), respectively, these services are excepted from physician supervision when they are personally furnished by a qualified audiologist or performed by a nurse practitioner or clinical nurse specialist authorized to perform the tests under applicable State laws.

References to technicians apply also to other qualified clinical staff. See Pub. 100-02, chapter 15, section 80.3.D.

A. Correct Reporting

1. **General**. Contact the contractor for guidance if the CPT codebook changes the description of codes mentioned in this section.

   Other policies concerning audiological services are found in Pub. 100-02, chapter 15, section 80.3.

   See chapter 26 of this manual for place of service and type of service coding.

   Section 4541(a)(2) of the Balanced Budget Act (BBA) (P.L. 105-33), which added section 1834(k)(5) to (the Act), required that all claims for certain audiology services be reported using a uniform coding system. CMS chose HCPCS (Healthcare Common Procedure Coding System) as the coding system for the reporting of these services. This coding requirement is effective for all claims for audiology services submitted on or after April 1, 1998.

   The BBA also required payment under a prospective payment system for audiology services. Effective for claims with dates of service on or after January 1, 1999, the Medicare Physician Fee Schedule (MPFS) became the method of payment for audiology services furnished in the office setting and for the associated professional services furnished in physician's office and hospital outpatient settings.

2. **Use of the NPI.** For audiologists who are enrolled and bill independently for services they render, the audiologist's NPI is required on all claims they submit. For example, in offices and private practice settings, an enrolled audiologist shall use his or her own NPI in the rendering loop to bill under the MPFS for the services the audiologist furnished. If an enrolled audiologist furnishing services to hospital outpatients reassigns his/her benefits to the hospital, the hospital may bill the carrier or Medicare administrative contractor for the professional services of the audiologist under the MPFS using the NPI of the audiologist. If an audiologist is employed by a hospital but is not enrolled in Medicare, the only payment for a hospital outpatient audiology service that can be made is the payment to the hospital for its facility services under the hospital Outpatient Prospective Payment System (OPPS) or other applicable hospital payment system. No payment can be made under the MPFS for professional services of an audiologist who is not enrolled.

   Audiologists must be enrolled and use their NPI on claims for services they render in office settings on or after October 1, 2008 (for additional information about enrollment, refer to Pub. 100-08, Medicare Program Integrity Manual, chapter 15). Before October 1, 2008, the services of audiologists who were not yet enrolled in Medicare were billed by a physician or group who employed the audiologist. Audiologists shall use the billing instructions in the Medicare manuals; for example, see this manual, chapter 1, section 30.

   See the most recent MPFS for pricing and physician supervision levels for audiology services: http://www.cms.hhs.gov/PFSlookup/01_Overview.asp#TopOfPage. The NPI of the supervising physician shall be used to bill audiology services when supervision is appropriate.

   The most recent OPPS pricing for audiology services is available in Addendum B at:

   http://www.cms.gov/HospitalOutpatientPPS/AU/list.asp#TopOfPage.

B. Billing for Audiology Services

See the CMS Web site at: http://www.cms.gov/PhysicianFeeSched/50_Audiology.asp for a listing of all CPT codes for audiology services. For information concerning codes that are not on the list, and which codes may be billed when furnished by technicians, contractors shall provide guidance. The Physician Fee Schedule at http://www.cms.gov/PFSlookup/01_Overview.asp#TopOfPage allows you to search pricing amounts, various payment policy indicators, RVUs, and GPCIs.

Audiology services may not be billed when the place of service is a comprehensive outpatient rehabilitation facility (CORF) or a rehabilitation agency.

Audiology services may be furnished and billed by audiologists and, when these services are furnished by an audiologist, no physician supervision is required.

The interpretation and report shall be written in the medical record by the audiologist, physician, or NPP who personally furnished any audiology service, or by the physician who supervised the service. Technicians shall not interpret audiology services, but may record objective test results of those services they may furnish under direct physician supervision. Payment for the interpretation and report of the services is included in payment for all audiology services, and specifically in the professional component if the audiology service has a professional component/technical component split.

1. *Billing under the MPFS for Audiology Services Outside the Facility Setting*

The individuals who furnish audiology services in all settings must be qualified to furnish those services. The qualifications of the individual performing the services must be consistent with the number, type and complexity of the tests, the abilities of the individual, and the patient's ability to interact to produce valid and reliable results. The physician who supervises and bills for the service is responsible for assuring the qualifications of the technician, if applicable are appropriate to the test.

a. Professional Skills.

   When a professional personally furnishes an audiology service, that individual must interact with the patient to provide professional skills and be directly involved in decision-making and clinical judgment during the test.

   The skills required when professionals furnish audiology services for payment under the MPFS are masters or doctoral level skills that involve clinical judgment or assessment and specialized knowledge and ability including, but not limited to, knowledge of anatomy and physiology, neurology, psychology, physics, psychometrics, and interpersonal communication. The interactions of these knowledge bases are required to attain the clinical expertise for audiology tests. Also required are skills to administer valid and reliable tests safely, especially when they involve stimulating the auditory nerve and testing complex brain functions.

   Diagnostic audiology services also require skills and judgment to administer and modify tests, to make informed interpretations about the causes and implications of the test results in the context of the history and presenting complaints, and to provide both objective results and professional knowledge to the patient and to the ordering physician.

   Examples include, but are not limited to:

   - Comparison or consideration of the anatomical or physiological implications of test results or patient responsiveness to stimuli during the test;
   - Development and modification of the test battery and test protocols;
   - Clinical judgment, assessment, evaluation, and decision-making;
   - Interpretation and reporting observations, in addition to the objective data, that may influence interpretation of the test outcomes;
   - Tests related to implantation of auditory prosthetic devices, central auditory processing, contralateral masking; and/or
   - Tests to identify central auditory processing disorders, tinnitus, or nonorganic hearing loss.

   Audiology codes may be billed under the MPFS by audiologists, physicians, and NPPs using their own NPI in the rendering loop when those professionals personally furnish the test. Physicians and NPPs may not bill for these codes when an audiologist has furnished the service.

b. Technician Skills.

   There may be subtests, or parts of a battery of tests, that may be appropriately furnished by an educated and experienced technician using a specific protocol under the direction of a supervising physician. These services are identified by local contractor determination as services that do not require professional skills. They may be furnished by a qualified technician under the direct supervision of a physician, but not under the supervision of an audiologist or an NPP. The supervising physician is responsible for rendering and documenting all clinical judgment and for the appropriate provision of the service by the technician.

   A technician may not perform any part of a service that requires professional skills. A technician also may not perform a global service. For example, a technician may not interpret test results or engage in clinical decision-making.

c. Professional Component (PC)/Technical Component (TC) Split Codes.

   The PC of a PC/TC split code may be billed by the audiologist, physician, or NPP who personally furnishes the service. (Note this is also true in the facility setting.) A physician or NPP may bill for the PC when the physician or NPP furnish the PC and an (unsupervised) audiologist furnishes and bills for the TC. The PC may not be billed if a technician furnishes the service. A physician or NPP may not bill for a PC service furnished by an audiologist.

   The TC of a PC/TC split code may be billed by the audiologist, physician, or NPP who personally furnishes the service. Physicians may bill the TC for services furnished by technicians when the technician furnishes the service under the direct supervision of that physician. Audiologists and NPPs may not bill for the TC of the service when a technician furnishes the service, even if the technician is supervised by the NPP or audiologist.

   The "global" service is billed when both the PC and TC of a service are personally furnished by the same audiologist, physician, or

NPP. The global service may also be billed by a physician, but not an audiologist or NPP, when a technician furnishes the TC of the service under direct physician supervision and that physician furnishes the PC, including the interpretation and report.

d. Tests that are Not Described by Specific CPT Codes. Tests that have no appropriate CPT code may be reported under CPT code 92700 (Unlisted otorhinolaryngological service or procedure).

e. Tests that are Contractor-Priced. For codes valued by contractors, the contractor determines whether and how much, if applicable, to pay for the service. The contractor sets the requirements for personnel furnishing the tests.

2. ***Billing for Audiology Services Furnished to Hospital Outpatients.*** All codes may be reported for audiology services furnished in the hospital outpatient setting and, in such cases, the code represents the facility service for the diagnostic test. All audiology services furnished to hospital outpatients must be billed and paid to the hospital under the OPPS or other applicable hospital payment system. The hospital bills its fiscal intermediary or Medicare administrative contractor (A/B MAC) and is paid for the facility resources required to furnish the services, regardless of whether the service is furnished by a physician, NPP, audiologist, or technician.

   Physicians, NPPs, and audiologists cannot bill and be paid for the TC of PC/TC split codes when these services are furnished to hospital outpatients. The associated professional services (represented by the PC or the CPT code for the audiology test which has no PC/TC split) of an enrolled audiologist, physician, or NPP who has reassigned benefits may be billed by the hospital to the carrier or A/B MAC, as appropriate. Alternatively, if the physician, NPP, or audiologist has not assigned benefits, the professional would bill his/her carrier or A/B MAC for the professional services furnished.

   The appropriate revenue code for reporting audiology services is 0470 (Audiology; General Classification). Providers are required to report a line-item date of service per revenue code line for audiology services.

3. ***Billing for Audiology Services Furnished to Skilled Nursing Facility (SNF) Patients.*** Payment for the facility resources (including the TC of PC/TC split codes) of audiology services provided to Part A inpatients of SNFs is included in the PPS rate. For SNFs, if the beneficiary has Part B but not Part A coverage (e.g., Part A benefits are exhausted), the SNF may elect to bill for audiology services but is not required to do so. As explained in Pub. 100-04, chapter 7, section 40.1, since audiology services furnished during a noncovered SNF stay are not bundled with speech-language pathology services, payment can be made either to the SNF or to the audiology service provider/supplier.

   Audiologists, physicians, and NPPs enrolled in Medicare may bill directly for services rendered to Medicare beneficiaries who are in a SNF stay that is not covered by Part A but who have Part B eligibility. Payment is made based on the MPFS, whether on an institutional or professional claim. For beneficiaries in a noncovered SNF stay, audiology services are payable under Part B when billed by the SNF on an institutional

   claim as type of bill 22X, or when billed directly by the provider or supplier of the service (the audiologist, physician, or NPP who personally furnishes the test) on a professional claim. For PC/TC split codes, the SNF may elect to bill for the TC of the test on an institutional claim but is not required to bill for the service.

C. Implant Processing

Payment for diagnostic testing of implants, such as cochlear, osseointegrated or brainstem implants, including programming or reprogramming following implantation surgery is not included in the global fee for the surgery.

The diagnostic analysis of a cochlear implant shall be billed using CPT codes 92601 through 92604.

Osseointegrated prosthetic devices should be billed and paid for under provisions of the applicable payment system. For example, payment may differ depending upon whether the device is furnished on an inpatient or outpatient basis, and by a hospital subject to the OPPS, or by a Critical Access Hospital, physician's clinic, or a Federally Qualified Health Center

D Aural Rehabilitation Services

General policy for evaluation and treatment of conditions related to the auditory system.

For evaluation of auditory processing disorders and speech-reading or lip-reading by a speech-language pathologist, use the untimed code 92506 with "1" as the unit of service, regardless of the duration of the service on a given day. This "always therapy" evaluation code must be provided by speech-language pathologists according to the policies in Pub. 100-02, chapter 15, sections 220 and 230. The codes 92620 and 92621 are diagnostic audiological tests and may not be used for SLP services.

For treatment of auditory processing disorders or auditory rehabilitation/ auditory training (including speech-reading or lip-reading), 92507, and 92508 are used to report a single encounter with "1" as the unit of service, regardless of the duration of the service on a given day. These codes always represent SLP services. See Pub. 100-02, chapter 15, sections 220 and 230 for SLP policies. These SLP evaluation and treatment services are not covered when performed or billed by audiologists, even if they are supervised by physicians or qualified NPPs.

For evaluation of auditory rehabilitation to instruct the use of residual hearing provided by an implant or hearing aid related to hearing loss, the timed codes 92626 and 92627 are used. These are not "always therapy" codes. Evaluation of auditory rehabilitation shall be appropriately provided and billed by an audiologist or speech-language pathologist. Also, these services may be provided incident to a physician's or qualified NPP's service by a speech-language pathologist, or personally by a physician or qualified NPP within their scope of practice. Evaluation of auditory rehabilitation is a covered diagnostic test when performed and billed by an audiologist and is an SLP evaluation service covered under the SLP benefit when performed by a speech-language pathologist.

General policies for post implant services.

The services of a speech-language pathologist may be covered for SLP services provided after implantation of auditory devices. For example, a speech-language pathologist may provide evaluation and treatment of speech, language, cognition, voice, and auditory processing using code 92506 and 92507. Use 92626 and 92627 for auditory (aural) rehabilitation evaluation following cochlear implantation or for other hearing impairments.

For diagnostic testing of cochlear implants, audiologists use codes 92601, 92602, 92603 and 92604. These services may not be provided by speech-language pathologists or others, with the exception of physicians and NPPs who may personally provide the services that are within their scope of practice.

Pub 100-4, 12, 30.4 – Cardiovascular System (Codes 92950-93799)

(Rev. 979, Issued: 06-09-06, Effective: 07-10-06, Implementation: 07-10-06)

A. Echocardiography Contrast Agents

Effective October 1, 2000, physicians may separately bill for contrast agents used in echocardiography. Physicians should use HCPCS Code A9700 (Supply of Injectable Contrast Material for Use in Echocardiography, per study). The type of service code is 9. This code will be carrier-priced.

B. Electronic Analyses of Implantable Cardioverter-defibrillators and Pacemakers

The CPT codes 93731, 93734, 93741 and 93743 are used to report electronic analyses of single or dual chamber pacemakers and single or dual chamber implantable cardioverter-defibrillators.

In the office, a physician uses a device called a programmer to obtain information about the status and performance of the device and to evaluate the patient's cardiac rhythm and response to the implanted device.

Advances in information technology now enable physicians to evaluate patients with implanted cardiac devices without requiring the patient to be present in the physician's office. Using a manufacturer's specific monitor/transmitter, a patient can send complete device data and specific cardiac data to a distant receiving station or secure Internet server. The electronic analysis of cardiac device data that is remotely obtained provides immediate and long-term data on the device and clinical data on the patient's cardiac functioning equivalent to that obtained during an in-office evaluation. Physicians should report the electronic analysis of an implanted cardiac device using remotely obtained data as described above with CPT code 93731, 93734, 93741 or 93743, depending on the type of cardiac device implanted in the patient.

Pub 100-4, 12, 30.6 – Evaluation and Management Service Codes – General (Codes 99201–99499)

Pub 100-4, 12, 30.6.1 – Selection of Level of Evaluation and Management Service

(Rev. 1875, Issued: 12-14-09, Effective: 01-01-10, Implementation: 01-04-10)

A. Use of CPT Codes

Advise physicians to use CPT codes (level 1 of HCPCS) to code physician services, including evaluation and management services. Medicare will pay for E/M services for specific non-physician practitioners (i.e., nurse practitioner (NP), clinical nurse specialist (CNS) and certified nurse midwife (CNM)) whose Medicare benefit permits them to bill these services. A physician assistant (PA) may also provide a physician service, however, the physician collaboration and general supervision rules as well as all billing rules apply to all the above non-physician practitioners. The service provided must be medically necessary and the service must be within the scope of practice for a non-physician practitioner in the State in which he/she practices. Do not pay for CPT evaluation and management codes billed by physical therapists in independent practice or by occupational therapists in independent practice.

Medical necessity of a service is the overarching criterion for payment in addition to the individual requirements of a CPT code. It would not be medically necessary or appropriate to bill a higher level of evaluation and management service when a lower level of service is warranted. The volume of documentation should not be the primary influence upon which a specific level of service is billed. Documentation should support the level of service reported. The service should be documented during, or as soon as practicable after it is provided in order to maintain an accurate medical record.

B. Selection of Level of Evaluation and Management Service

Instruct physicians to select the code for the service based upon the content of the service. The duration of the visit is an ancillary factor and does not control the level of the service to be billed unless more than 50 percent of the face-to-face time (for non-inpatient services) or more than 50 percent of the floor time (for inpatient services) is spent providing counseling or coordination of care as described in subsection C.

Any physician or non-physician practitioner (NPP) authorized to bill Medicare services will be paid by the carrier at the appropriate physician fee schedule amount based on the rendering UPIN/PIN.

"Incident to" Medicare Part B payment policy is applicable for office visits when the requirements for "incident to" are met (refer to sections 60.1, 60.2, and 60.3, chapter 15 in IOM 100-02).

SPLIT/SHARED E/M SERVICE

Office/Clinic Setting

In the office/clinic setting when the physician performs the E/M service the service must be reported using the physician's UPIN/PIN. When an E/M service is a shared/split encounter between a physician and a non-physician practitioner (NP, PA, CNS or CNM), the service is considered to have been performed "incident to" if the requirements for "incident to" are met and the patient is an established patient. If "incident to" requirements are not met for the shared/split E/M service, the service must be billed under the NPP's UPIN/PIN, and payment will be made at the appropriate physician fee schedule payment.

Hospital Inpatient/Outpatient/Emergency Department Setting

When a hospital inpatient/hospital outpatient or emergency department E/M is shared between a physician and an NPP from the same group practice and the physician provides any face-to-face portion of the E/M encounter with the patient, the service may be billed under either the physician's or the NPP's UPIN/PIN number. However, if there was no face-to-face encounter between the patient and the physician (e.g., even if the physician participated in the service by only reviewing the patien'ts medical record) then the service may only be billed under the NPP's UPIN/PIN. Payment will be made at the appropriate physician fee schedule rate based on the UPIN/PIN entered on the claim.

Examples Of Shared Visits

1. If the NPP sees a hospital inpatient in the morning and the physician follows with a later face-to-face visit with the patient on the same day, the physician or the NPP may report the service.
2. In an office setting the NPP performs a portion of an E/M encounter and the physician completes the E/M service. If the "incident to" requirements are met, the physician reports the service. If the "incident to" requirements are not met, the service must be reported using the NPP's UPIN/PIN.

In the rare circumstance when a physician (or NPP) provides a service that does not reflect a CPT code description, the service must be reported as an unlisted service with CPT code 99499. A description of the service provided must accompany the claim. The carrier has the discretion to value the service when the service does not meet the full terms of a CPT code description (e.g., only a history is performed). The carrier also determines the payment based on the applicable percentage of the physician fee schedule depending on whether the claim is paid at the physician rate or the non-physician practitioner rate. CPT modifier 52 (reduced services) must not be used with an evaluation and management service. Medicare does not recognize modifier 52 for this purpose.

C. Selection Of Level Of Evaluation and Management Service Based On Duration Of Coordination Of Care and/or Counseling

Advise physicians that when counseling and/or coordination of care dominates (more than 50 percent) the face-to-face physician/patient encounter or the floor time (in the case of inpatient services), time is the key or controlling factor in selecting the level of service. In general, to bill an E/M code, the physician must complete at least 2 out of 3 criteria applicable to the type/level of service provided. However, the physician may document time spent with the patient in conjunction with the medical decision-making involved and a description of the coordination of care or counseling provided. Documentation must be in sufficient detail to support the claim.

EXAMPLE: A cancer patient has had all preliminary studies completed and a medical decision to implement chemotherapy. At an office visit the physician discusses the treatment options and subsequent lifestyle effects of treatment the patient may encounter or is experiencing. The physician need not complete a history and physical examination in order to select the level of service. The time spent in counseling/coordination of care and medical decision-making will determine the level of service billed.

The code selection is based on the total time of the face-to-face encounter or floor time, not just the counseling time. The medical record must be documented in sufficient detail to justify the selection of the specific code if time is the basis for selection of the code.

In the office and other outpatient setting, counseling and/or coordination of care must be provided in the presence of the patient if the time spent providing those services is used to determine the level of service reported. Face-to-face time refers to the time with the physician only. Counseling by other staff is not considered to be part of the face-to-face physician/patient encounter time. Therefore, the time spent by the other staff is not considered in selecting the appropriate level of service. The code used depends upon the physician service provided.

In an inpatient setting, the counseling and/or coordination of care must be provided at the bedside or on the patient's hospital floor or unit that is associated with an individual patient. Time spent counseling the patient or coordinating the patient's care after the patient has left the office or the physician has left the patient's floor or begun to care for another patient on the floor is not considered when selecting the level of service to be reported.

The duration of counseling or coordination of care that is provided face-to-face or on the floor may be estimated but that estimate, along with the total duration of the visit, must be recorded when time is used for the selection of the level of a service that involves predominantly coordination of care or counseling.

D. Use of Highest Levels of Evaluation and Management Codes

Contractors must advise physicians that to bill the highest levels of visit codes, the services furnished must meet the definition of the code (e.g., to bill a Level 5 new patient visit, the history must meet CPT's definition of a comprehensive history).

The comprehensive history must include a review of all the systems and a complete past (medical and surgical) family and social history obtained at that visit. In the case of an established patient, it is acceptable for a physician to review the existing record and update it to reflect only changes in the patient's medical, family, and social history from the last encounter, but the physician must review the entire history for it to be considered a comprehensive history.

The comprehensive examination may be a complete single system exam such as cardiac, respiratory, psychiatric, or a complete multi-system examination.

Pub 100-4, 12, 30.6.1.1 – Initial Preventive Physical Examination

(Rev. 1615, Issued: 10-17-08, Effective: 01-01-09, Implementation: 01-05-09)

A. Definition

The initial preventive physical examination (IPPE), or "Welcome to Medicare Visit" (WMV) is a preventive evaluation and management service (E/M), allowed by Section 611 of the Medicare Prescription Drug Improvement and Modernization Act (MMA) of 2003, that includes: (1) review of the individual's medical and social history with attention to modifiable risk factors for disease detection, (2) review of the individual's potential (risk factors) for depression or other mood disorders, (3) review of the individual's functional ability and level of safety, (4) a physical examination to include measurement of the individual's height, weight, blood pressure, a visual acuity screen, and other factors as deemed appropriate by the examining physician or qualified nonphysician practitioner (NPP), (5) performance and interpretation of an electrocardiogram (EKG), (6) education, counseling, and referral, as deemed appropriate, based on the results of the review and evaluation services described in the previous 5 elements, and, (7) education, counseling, and referral including a brief written plan (e.g., a checklist or alternative) provided to the individual for obtaining the appropriate screening and other preventive services.

Effective January 1, 2007, Section 5112 of the Deficit Reduction Act of 2005 allows for one ultrasound screening for Abdominal Aortic Aneurysm (AAA), HCPCS code G0389, as a result of a referral from an IPPE. This service is not subject to the Part B annual deductible. For AAA physician/practitioner billing, correct coding, and payment policy, refer to Chapter 18, §110, of this manual.

Effective January 1, 2009, Section 101 (b) of the Medicare Improvement for Patients and Providers Act (MIPPA) of 2008 requires the addition of the measurement of an individual's body mass index and, upon an individual's consent, end-of-life planning, to the IPPE. Also, effective January 1, 2009, MIPPA removes the screening electrocardiogram (EKG) as a mandatory service of the IPPE. MIPPA requires that there be education, counseling, and referral for an EKG, as appropriate. This is a once-in-a-lifetime screening EKG as a result of a referral from an IPPE.

The MIPPA of 2008 allows for possible future payment for additional preventive services not otherwise described in Title XVIII of the Social Security Act (the Act) that identify medical conditions or risk factors for eligible individuals if the Secretary determines through the national coverage determination (NCD) process (as defined in Section 1869(f) (1)(B) of the Act) that they are: (1) reasonable and necessary for the prevention or early detection of illness or disability, (2) recommended with a grade of A or B by the United States Preventive Services Task Force, and, (3) appropriate for individuals entitled to benefits under Part A or enrolled under Part B, or both. MIPPA requires that there be education, counseling, referral for additional preventive services, as appropriate, under the IPPE, if the Secretary determines in the future that such services are covered.

Preventive services are separately covered under Medicare Part B benefits.

(For billing requirements, refer to Chapter 18, §80, of this manual.)

B. Who May Perform

The IPPE may be performed by a doctor of medicine or osteopathy as defined in Section 1861(r)(1) of the Act or by a qualified NPP (nurse practitioner, physician assistant and clinical nurse specialist). The contractor will pay the appropriate physician fee schedule amount based on the rendering National Provider Identification (NPI) number.

C. Eligibility

As a result of the MMA 2003, Medicare will pay for one IPPE per beneficiary per lifetime. A beneficiary is eligible when he first enrolls in Medicare Part B on or after January 1, 2005, and receives the IPPE benefit within the first 6 months of the effective date of the initial Part B coverage period.

The Medicare deductible for the IPPE performed before January 1, 2009, (HCPCS code G0344) applies.

The MIPPA of 2008 extends the eligibility period for an IPPE from 6 months to 12 months after an individual's Medicare Part B enrollment. A beneficiary is eligible for IPPE benefits identified in MIPPA if the IPPE is performed on or after January 1, 2009 and within the 12-month period of his/her effective date of the initial enrollment in Medicare Part B.

For a Medicare beneficiary who has the IPPE performed on or after January 1, 2009, and it occurs within the 12-month period of his/her effective date of the initial enrollment in Medicare Part B, the Medicare deductible for the IPPE (HCPCS code G0402) is waived and no longer applies.

Medicare continues to pay for only one IPPE per beneficiary per lifetime. Co-insurance for these services applies both prior to and after January 1, 2009.

D. The EKG Component

Under the MMA of 2003, if the physician or qualified NPP is not able to perform both the examination and the screening EKG, an arrangement may be made to ensure that another physician or entity performs the screening EKG and reports the EKG separately using the appropriate HCPCS G code(s) identified in E. When the screening EKG is performed, the primary physician or qualified NPP shall document the results of the screening EKG into the beneficiary's medical record to complete and bill for the IPPE benefit. NOTE: Both components of the IPPE (the examination and the screening EKG) must be performed before the claims can be submitted by the physician, qualified NPP, and/or entity.

MIPPA 2008 changes the once-in-a-lifetime screening EKG from a mandated service to a service that may be performed, as appropriate, with a referral from an IPPE. The waived deductible for the IPPE, effective January 1, 2009, does not apply to the screening EKG service irrespective of the codes used or date of service.

E. Codes Used to Bill the IPPE

For IPPE and EKG services provided prior to January 1, 2009, the physician or qualified NPP shall bill HCPCS code G0344 for the physical examination performed face-to-face, and HCPCS code G0366 for performing a screening EKG that includes both the interpretation and report. If the primary physician or qualified NPP performs only the examination, he/she shall bill HCPCS code G0344 only. The physician or entity that performs the screening EKG that includes both the interpretation and report shall bill HCPCS code G0366. The physician or entity that performs the screening EKG tracing only (without interpretation and report) shall bill HCPCS code G0367. The physician or entity that performs the interpretation and report only (without the EKG tracing) shall bill HCPCS code G0368. Medicare will pay for a screening EKG only as part of the IPPE. HCPCS codes G0344, G0366, G0367 and G0368 will not be billable codes effective on or after January 1, 2009.

Effective for a beneficiary who has the IPPE on or after January 1, 2009 and within his/her 12-month enrollment period of Medicare Part B, the IPPE and screening EKG services are billable with the appropriate HCPCS G code(s).

The physician or qualified NPP shall bill HCPCS code G0402 for the physical examination performed face-to-face with the patient.

The physician or entity shall bill HCPCS code G0403 for performing the complete screening EKG that includes the tracing, interpretation and report.

The physician or entity that performs the screening EKG tracing only (without interpretation and report) shall bill HCPCS code G0404.

The physician or entity that performs the screening EKG interpretation and report only, (without the EKG tracing) shall bill HCPCS code G0405.

For an IPPE performed during the global period of surgery refer to Chapter 12, §30.6.6, of this manual for reporting instructions.

F. Documentation

The physician and qualified NPP shall use the appropriate screening tools typically used in routine physician practice. Physicians and qualified NPPs are required to use the 1995 and 1997 E/M documentation guidelines to document the medical record with the appropriate clinical information. (http://www.cms.hhs.gov/MLNEdWebGuide/25_EMDOC.asp)

All referrals and a written medical plan must be included in this documentation.

G. Reporting A Medically Necessary E/M at Same IPPE Visit

When the physician or qualified NPP provides a medically necessary E/M service in addition to the IPPE, CPT codes 99201 – 99215 may be used depending on the clinical appropriateness of the circumstances. CPT Modifier –25 shall be appended to the medically necessary E/M service identifying this service as a significant, separately identifiable service from the IPPE code reported (G0344 or G0402, whichever applies based on the date the IPPE is performed). NOTE: Some of the components of a medically necessary E/M service (e.g., a portion of history or physical exam portion) may have been part of the IPPE and should not be included when determining the most appropriate level of E/M service to be billed for the medically necessary E/M service.

Pub 100-4, 12, 190 – Medicare Payment for Telehealth Services

Pub 100-4, 12, 190.1 – Background

(Rev. 1635, Issued: 11-14-08, Effective: 01-01-09, Implementation: 01-05-09)

Section 223 of the Medicare, Medicaid and SCHIP Benefits Improvement and Protection Act of 2000 (BIPA) - Revision of Medicare Reimbursement for Telehealth Services amended §1834 of the Act to provide for an expansion of Medicare payment for telehealth services.

Effective October 1, 2001, coverage and payment for Medicare telehealth includes consultation, office visits, individual psychotherapy, and pharmacologic management delivered via a telecommunications system. Eligible geographic areas include rural health professional shortage areas (HPSA) and counties not classified as a metropolitan statistical area (MSA). Additionally, Federal telemedicine demonstration projects as of December 31, 2000, may serve as the originating site regardless of geographic location.

An interactive telecommunications system is required as a condition of payment; however, BIPA does allow the use of asynchronous "store and forward" technology in delivering these services when the originating site is a Federal telemedicine demonstration program in Alaska or Hawaii. BIPA does not require that a practitioner present the patient for interactive telehealth services.

With regard to payment amount, BIPA specified that payment for the professional service performed by the distant site practitioner (i.e., where the expert physician or practitioner is physically located at time of telemedicine encounter) is equal to what would have been paid without the use of telemedicine. Distant site practitioners include only a physician as described in §1861(r) of the Act and a medical practitioner as described in §1842(b)(18)(C) of the Act. BIPA also expanded payment under Medicare to include a $20 originating site facility fee (location of beneficiary).

Previously, the Balanced Budget Act of 1997 (BBA) limited the scope of Medicare telehealth coverage to consultation services and the implementing regulation prohibited the use of an asynchronous, 'store and forward' telecommunications system. BBA 1997 also required the professional fee to be shared between the referring and consulting practitioners, and prohibited Medicare payment for facility fees and line charges associated with the telemedicine encounter.

BIPA required that Medicare Part B (Supplementary Medical Insurance) pay for this expansion of telehealth services beginning with services furnished on October 1, 2001.

Section 149 of the Medicare Improvements for Patients and Providers Act of 2008 (MIPPA) amended §1834 of the Act to add certain entities as originating sites for payment of telehealth services. Effective for services furnished on or after January 1, 2009, eligible originating sites include a hospital-based or critical access hospital-based renal dialysis center (including satellites); a skilled nursing facility (as defined in §1819(a) of the Act); and a community mental health center (as defined in §1861(ff)(3)(B) of the Act). MIPPA also amended§1888(e)(2)(A)(ii) of the Act to exclude telehealth services furnished under §1834(m)(4)(C)(ii)(VII) from the consolidated billing provisions of the skilled nursing facility prospective payment system (SNF PPS).

NOTE: MIPPA did not add independent renal dialysis facilities as originating sites for payment of telehealth services.

The telehealth provisions authorized by §1834(m) of the Act are implemented in 42 CFR 410.78 and 414.65.

Pub 100-4, 12, 190.2 – Eligibility Criteria

(Rev. 1635, Issued: 11-14-08, Effective: 01-01-09, Implementation: 01-05-09)

1. Beneficiaries eligible for telehealth services.

Medicare beneficiaries are eligible for telehealth services only if they are presented from an originating site located in either a rural health professional shortage area (HPSA) as defined by §332(a)(1) (A) of the Public Health Services Act or in a county outside of an MSA as defined by §1886(d)(2)(D) of the Act.

2. Exception to rural HPSA and non MSA geographic requirements.

Entities participating in a Federal telemedicine demonstration project that were approved by or were receiving funding from the Secretary of Health and Human Services as of December 31, 2000, qualify as originating sites regardless of geographic location. Such entities are not required to be in a rural HPSA or non-MSA.

3. Originating site defined.

The term originating site means the location of an eligible Medicare beneficiary at the time the service being furnished via a telecommunications system occurs. Originating sites authorized by law are listed below:

- The office of a physician or practitioner
- A hospital (inpatient or outpatient)
- A critical access hospital (CAH)
- A rural health clinic (RHC)
- A federally qualified health center (FQHC)
- A hospital-based or critical access hospital-based renal dialysis center (including satellites) (effective January 1, 2009)
- A skilled nursing facility (SNF) (effective January 1, 2009)
- A community mental health center (CMHC) (effective January 1, 2009)

NOTE: Independent renal dialysis facilities are not eligible originating sites.

For asynchronous, store and forward telecommunications technologies, an originating site is only a Federal telemedicine demonstration program conducted in Alaska or Hawaii.

Pub 100-4, 12, 190.3 – List of Medicare Telehealth Services

(Rev. 1881; Issued: 12-18-09; Effective Date: 01-01-10; Implementation Date: 01-04-10)

The use of a telecommunications system may substitute for a face-to-face, "hands on" encounter for professional consultations, office visits, office psychiatry services, and a limited number of other physician fee schedule (PFS) services. The various services and corresponding current procedure terminology (CPT) or Healthcare Common Procedure Coding System (HCPCS) codes are listed below.

- Consultations (CPT codes 99241 - 99275) - Effective October 1, 2001 – December 31, 2005;
- Consultations (CPT codes 99241 - 99255) - Effective January 1, 2006 – December 31, 2009;
- Initial inpatient telehealth consultations (HCPCS codes G0425 – G0427) - Effective January 1, 2010;
- Follow-up inpatient telehealth consultations (HCPCS codes G0406, G0407, and G0408) - Effective January 1, 2009;
- Office or other outpatient visits (CPT codes 99201 - 99215);
- Individual psychotherapy (CPT codes 90804 - 90809);
- Pharmacologic management (CPT code 90862);

- Psychiatric diagnostic interview examination (CPT code 90801) – Effective March 1, 2003;
- End Stage Renal Disease (ESRD) related services (HCPCS codes G0308, G0309, G0311, G0312, G0314, G0315, G0317, and G0318) – Effective January 1, 2005 – December 31, 2008;
- End Stage Renal Disease (ESRD) related services (CPT codes 90951, 90952, 90954, 90955, 90957, 90958, 90960, and 90961) – Effective January 1, 2009;
- Individual Medical Nutrition Therapy (HCPCS codes G0270, 97802, and 97803) - Effective January 1, 2006;
- Neurobehavioral status exam (CPT code 96116) - Effective January 1, 2008; and
- Individual health and behavior assessment and intervention (CPT codes 96150 – 96152) - Effective January 1, 2010.

NOTE: Beginning January 1, 2010, CMS eliminated the use of all consultation codes, except for inpatient telehealth consultation G-codes. CMS will no longer recognize office/outpatient consultation CPT codes for payment of office/outpatient visits. Instead, physicians and practitioners are instructed to bill a new or established patient visit CPT code (in the range of CPT codes 99201-99215), as appropriate to the particular patient, for all office/outpatient visits.

190.3.1 – Follow-Up Inpatient Telehealth Consultations Defined

(Rev. 1881; Issued: 12-18-09; Effective Date: 01-01-10; Implementation Date: 01-04-10)

A consultation service is an evaluation and management (E/M) service furnished to evaluate and possibly treat a patient's problem(s). It can involve an opinion, advice, recommendation, suggestion, direction, or counsel from a physician or qualified nonphysician practitioner (NPP) at the request of another physician or appropriate source.

Section 1834(m) of the Social Security Act includes "professional consultations" in the definition of telehealth services. Inpatient consultations furnished via telehealth can facilitate the provision of certain services and/or medical expertise that might not otherwise be available to a patient located at an originating site.

The use of a telecommunications system may substitute for a face-to-face, "hands on" encounter for initial and follow-up inpatient consultations. E/M inpatient visits may not be furnished via telehealth.

Medicare contractors pay for reasonable and medically necessary inpatient telehealth consultation services furnished to beneficiaries in hospitals or SNFs when all of the following criteria for the use of a consultation code are met:

- An inpatient consultation service is distinguished from other inpatient evaluation and management (E/M) visits because it is provided by a physician or qualified NPP whose opinion or advice regarding evaluation and/or management of a specific problem is requested by another physician or other appropriate source. The qualified NPP may perform consultation services within the scope of practice and licensure requirements for NPPs in the State in which he/she practices;
- A request for an inpatient telehealth consultation from an appropriate source and the need for an inpatient telehealth consultation (i.e., the reason for a consultation service) shall be documented by the consultant in the patient's medical record and included in the requesting physician or qualified NPP's plan of care in the patient's medical record; and
- After the inpatient telehealth consultation is provided, the consultant shall prepare a written report of his/her findings and recommendations, which shall be provided to the referring physician.

The intent of an inpatient telehealth consultation service is that a physician or qualified NPP or other appropriate source is asking another physician or qualified NPP for advice, opinion, a recommendation, suggestion, direction, or counsel, etc. in evaluating or treating a patient because that individual has expertise in a specific medical area beyond the requesting professional's knowledge.

190.3.2 – Initial Inpatient Telehealth Consultations Defined

(Rev. 1881; Issued: 12-18-09; Effective Date: 01-01-10; Implementation Date: 01-04-10)

Initial inpatient telehealth consultations are furnished to beneficiaries in hospitals or SNFs via telehealth at the request of the physician of record, the attending physician, or another appropriate source. The physician or practitioner who furnishes the initial inpatient consultation via telehealth cannot be the physician of record or the attending physician, and the initial inpatient telehealth consultation would be distinct from the care provided by the physician of record or the attending physician. Counseling and coordination of care with other providers or agencies is included as well, consistent with the nature of the problem(s) and the patient's needs. Initial inpatient telehealth consultations are subject to the criteria for inpatient telehealth consultation services, as described in §190.3.1.

Payment for initial inpatient telehealth consultations includes all consultation related services furnished before, during, and after communicating with the patient via telehealth. Pre-service activities would include, but would not be limited to, reviewing patient data (for example, diagnostic and imaging studies, interim labwork) and communicating with other professionals or family members. Intra-service activities must include the three key elements described below for each procedure code. Post-service activities would include, but would not be limited to, completing medical records or other documentation and communicating results of the consultation and further care plans to other health care professionals. No additional E/M service could be billed for work related to an initial inpatient telehealth consultation.

Initial inpatient telehealth consultations could be provided at various levels of complexity:

- Practitioners taking a problem focused history, conducting a problem focused examination, and engaging in medical decision making that is straightforward, would bill HCPCS G0425. At this level of service, practitioners would typically spend 30 minutes communicating with the patient via telehealth.
- Practitioners taking a detailed history, conducting a detailed examination, and engaging in medical decision making that is of moderate complexity, would bill HCPCS G0426. At this level of service, practitioners would typically spend 50 minutes communicating with the patient via telehealth.
- Practitioners taking a comprehensive history, conducting a comprehensive examination, and engaging in medical decision making that is of high complexity, would bill HCPCS G0427. At this level of service, practitioners would typically spend 70 minutes or more communicating with the patient via telehealth.

Although initial inpatient telehealth consultations are specific to telehealth, these services must be billed with either the "GT" or "GQ" modifier to identify the telehealth technology used to provide the service. (See §190.6 et. al. for instructions on how to use these modifiers.)

190.3.3 – Follow-Up Inpatient Telehealth Consultations Defined

(Rev. 1881; Issued: 12-18-09; Effective Date: 01-01-10; Implementation Date: 01-04-10)

Follow-up inpatient telehealth consultations are furnished to beneficiaries in hospitals or SNFs via telehealth to follow up on an initial consultation, or subsequent consultative visits requested by the attending physician. The initial inpatient consultation may have been provided in person or via telehealth.

Follow-up inpatient telehealth consultations include monitoring progress, recommending management modifications, or advising on a new plan of care in response to changes in the patient's status or no changes on the consulted health issue. Counseling and coordination of care with other providers or agencies is included as well, consistent with the nature of the problem(s) and the patient's needs.

The physician or practitioner who furnishes the inpatient follow-up consultation via telehealth cannot be the physician of record or the attending physician, and the follow-up inpatient consultation would be distinct from the follow-up care provided by the physician of record or the attending physician. If a physician consultant has initiated treatment at an initial consultation and participates thereafter in the patient's ongoing care management, such care would not be included in the definition of a follow-up inpatient consultation and is not appropriate for delivery via telehealth. Follow-up inpatient telehealth consultations are subject to the criteria for inpatient telehealth consultation services, as described in §190.3.1

Payment for follow-up inpatient telehealth consultations includes all consultation related services furnished before, during, and after communicating with the patient via telehealth. Pre-service activities would include, but would not be limited to, reviewing patient data (for example, diagnostic and imaging studies, interim labwork) and communicating with other professionals or family members. Intra-service activities must include at least two of the three key elements described below for each procedure code. Post-service activities would include, but would not be limited to, completing medical records or other documentation and communicating results of the consultation and further care plans to other health care professionals. No additional evaluation and management service could be billed for work related to a follow-up inpatient telehealth consultation.

Follow-up inpatient telehealth consultations could be provided at various levels of complexity:

- Practitioners taking a problem focused interval history, conducting a problem focused examination, and engaging in medical decision making that is straightforward or of low complexity, would bill a limited service, using HCPCS G0406, Follow-up inpatient telehealth consultation, limited. At this level of service, practitioners would typically spend 15 minutes communicating with the patient via telehealth.
- Practitioners taking an expanded focused interval history, conducting an expanded problem focused examination, and engaging in medical decision making that is of moderate complexity, would bill an intermediate service using HCPCS G0407, Follow-up inpatient telehealth consultation, intermediate. At this level of service, practitioners would typically spend 25 minutes communicating with the patient via telehealth.
- Practitioners taking a detailed interval history, conducting a detailed examination, and engaging in medical decision making that is of high complexity, would bill a complex service, using HCPCS G0408, Follow-up inpatient telehealth consultation, complex. At this level of service, practitioners would typically spend 35 minutes or more communicating with the patient via telehealth.

Although follow-up inpatient telehealth consultations are specific to telehealth, these services must be billed with either the "GT" or "GQ" modifier to identify the telehealth technology used to provide the service. *(See §190.6 et. al. for instructions on how to use these modifiers.)*

Pub 100-4, 12, 190.4 – Conditions of Payment

(Rev. 1, 10-01-03)

1. Technology

For Medicare payment to occur, interactive audio and video telecommunications must be used, permitting real-time communication between the distant site physician or practitioner and the Medicare beneficiary. As a condition of payment, the patient must be present and participating in the telehealth visit.

2. Exception to the interactive telecommunications requirement

In the case of Federal telemedicine demonstration programs conducted in Alaska or Hawaii, Medicare payment is permitted for telemedicine when asynchronous "store and forward technology" in single or multimedia formats is used as a substitute for an interactive telecommunications system. The originating site and distant site practitioner must be included within the definition of the demonstration program.

3. "Store and forward" defined

For purposes of this instruction, "store and forward" means the asynchronous transmission of medical information to be reviewed at a later time by physician or practitioner at the distant site. A patient's medical information may include, but not limited to, video clips, still images, x-rays, MRIs, EKGs and EEGs, laboratory results, audio clips, and text. The physician or practitioner at the distant site reviews the case without the patient being present. Store and forward substitutes for an interactive encounter with the patient present; the patient is not present in real-time.

NOTE: Asynchronous telecommunications system in single media format does not include telephone calls, images transmitted via facsimile machines and text messages without visualization of the patient (electronic mail). Photographs must be specific to the patients' condition and adequate for rendering or confirming a diagnosis and or treatment plan. Dermatological photographs, e.g., a photograph of a skin lesion, may be considered to meet the requirement of a single media format under this instruction.

4. Telepresenters

A medical professional is not required to present the beneficiary to physician or practitioner at the distant site unless medically necessary. The decision of medical necessity will be made by the physician or practitioner located at the distant site.

Pub 100-4, 12, 190.5 – Payment Methodology for Physician/Practitioner at the Distant Site

(Rev. 790, Issued: 12-23-05; Effective: 01-01-06; Implementation: 04-03-06)

1. Distant Site Defined

The term "distant site" means the site where the physician or practitioner, providing the professional service, is located at the time the service is provided via a telecommunications system.

2. Payment Amount (professional fee)

The payment amount for the professional service provided via a telecommunications system by the physician or practitioner at the distant site is equal to the current fee schedule amount for the service provided. Payment for an office visit, consultation, individual psychotherapy or pharmacologic management via a telecommunications system should be made at the same amount as when these services are furnished without the use of a telecommunications system. For Medicare payment to occur, the service must be within a practitioner's scope of practice under State law. The beneficiary is responsible for any unmet deductible amount and applicable coinsurance.

3. Medicare Practitioners Who May Receive Payment at the Distant Site (i.e., at a site other than where beneficiary is)

As a condition of Medicare Part B payment for telehealth services, the physician or practitioner at the distant site must be licensed to provide the service under State law. When the physician or practitioner at the distant site is licensed under State law to provide a covered telehealth service (i.e., professional consultation, office and other outpatient visits, individual psychotherapy, and pharmacologic management) then he or she may bill for and receive payment for this service when delivered via a telecommunications system.

If the physician or practitioner at the distant site is located in a critical access hospital (CAH) that has elected Method II, and the physician or practitioner has reassigned his/her benefits to the CAH, the CAH bills its regular FI for the professional services provided at the distant site via a telecommunications system, in any of the revenue codes 096x, 097x or 098x. All requirements for billing distant site telehealth services apply.

4. Medicare Practitioners Who May Bill for Covered Telehealth Services are Listed Below (subject to State law)

- Physician
- Nurse practitioner
- Physician assistant
- Nurse-midwife
- Clinical nurse specialist
- Clinical psychologist*
- Clinical social worker*
- Registered dietitian or nutrition professional

*Clinical psychologists and clinical social workers cannot bill for psychotherapy services that include medical evaluation and management services under Medicare. These practitioners may not bill or receive payment for the following CPT codes: 90805, 90807, and 90809.

Pub 100-4, 12, 190.6 – Originating Site Facility Fee Payment Methodology

(Rev. 1635, Issued: 11-14-08, Effective: 01-01-09, Implementation: 01-05-09)

1. Originating site defined

The term originating site means the location of an eligible Medicare beneficiary at the time the service being furnished via a telecommunications system occurs. For asynchronous, store and forward telecommunications technologies, an originating site is only a Federal telemedicine demonstration program conducted in Alaska or Hawaii.

2. Facility fee for originating site

The originating site facility fee is a separately billable Part B payment. The contractor pays it outside of other payment methodologies. This fee is subject to post payment verification.

For telehealth services furnished from October 1, 2001, through December 31, 2002, the originating site facility fee is the lesser of $20 or the actual charge. For services furnished on or after January 1 of each subsequent year, the originating site facility fee is updated by the Medicare Economic Index. The updated fee is included in the Medicare Physician Fee Schedule (MPFS) Final Rule, which is published by November 1 prior to the start of the calendar year for which it is effective.

3. Payment amount:

The originating site facility fee is a separately billable Part B payment. The payment amount to the originating site is the lesser of 80 percent of the actual charge or 80 percent of the originating site facility fee, except CAHs. The beneficiary is responsible for any unmet deductible amount and Medicare coinsurance.

The originating site facility fee payment methodology for each type of facility is clarified below.

Hospital outpatient department. When the originating site is a hospital outpatient department, payment for the originating site facility fee must be made as described above and not under the outpatient prospective payment system (OPPS). Payment is not based on the OPPS payment methodology.

Hospital inpatient. For hospital inpatients, payment for the originating site facility fee must be made outside the diagnostic related group (DRG) payment, since this is a Part B benefit, similar to other services paid separately from the DRG payment, (e.g., hemophilia blood clotting factor).

Critical access hospitals. When the originating site is a critical access hospital, make payment separately from the cost-based reimbursement methodology. For CAH's, the payment amount is 80 percent of the originating site facility fee.

Federally qualified health centers (FQHCs) and rural health clinics (RHCs). The originating site facility fee for telehealth services is not an FQHC or RHC service. When an FQHC or RHC serves as the originating site, the originating site facility fee must be paid separately from the center or clinic all-inclusive rate.

Physicians' and practitioners' offices. When the originating site is a physician's or practitioner's office, the payment amount, in accordance with the law, is the lesser of 80 percent of the actual charge or 80 percent of the originating site facility fee, regardless of geographic location. The carrier shall not apply the geographic practice cost index (GPCI) to the originating site facility fee. This fee is statutorily set and is not subject to the geographic payment adjustments authorized under the MPFS.

Hospital-based or critical access-hospital based renal dialysis center (or their satellites). When a hospital-based or critical access hospital-based renal dialysis center (or their satellites) serves as the originating site, the originating site facility fee is covered in addition to any composite rate or MCP amount.

Skilled nursing facility (SNF). The originating site facility fee is outside the SNF prospective payment system bundle and, as such, is not subject to SNF consolidated billing. The originating site facility fee is a separately billable Part B payment.

Community Mental Health Center (CMHC). The originating site facility fee is not a partial hospitalization service. The originating site facility fee does not count towards the number of services used to determine payment for partial hospitalization services. The originating site facility fee is not bundled in the per diem payment for partial hospitalization. The originating site facility fee is a separately billable Part B payment.

To receive the originating facility site fee, the provider submits claims with HCPCS code "Q3014, telehealth originating site facility fee"; short description "telehealth facility fee." The type of service for the telehealth originating site facility fee is "9, other items and services." For carrier-processed claims, the "office" place of service (code 11) is the only payable setting for code Q3014. There is no participation payment differential for code Q3014. Deductible and coinsurance rules apply to Q3014. By submitting Q3014 HCPCS code, the originating site authenticates they are located in either a rural HPSA or non-MSA county.

This benefit may be billed on bill types 12X, 13X, 22X, 23X, 71X, 72X, 73X, 76X, and 85X. Unless otherwise applicable, report the originating site facility fee under revenue code 078X and include HCPCS code "Q3014, telehealth originating site facility fee."

Hospitals and critical access hospitals bill their intermediary for the originating site facility fee. Telehealth bills originating in inpatient hospitals must be submitted on a 12X TOB using the date of discharge as the line item date of service.

Independent and provider-based RHCs and FQHCs bill the appropriate intermediary using the RHC or FQHC bill type and billing number. HCPCS code Q3014 is the only non-RHC/FQHC service that is billed using the clinic/center bill type and provider number. All RHCs and FQHCs must use revenue code 078X when billing for the originating site facility fee. For all other non-RHC/FQHC services, provider based RHCs and FQHCs must bill using the base provider's bill type and billing number. Independent RHCs and FQHCs must bill the carrier for all other non-RHC/FQHC services. If an RHC/FQHC visit occurs on the same day as a telehealth service, the RHC/FQHC serving as an originating site must bill for HCPCS code Q3014 telehealth originating site facility fee on a separate revenue line from the RHC/FQHC visit using revenue code 078X.

Hospital-based or CAH-based renal dialysis centers (including satellites) bill their local FIs and/or Part A MACs for the originating site facility fee. Telehealth bills originating in renal dialysis centers must be submitted on a 72X TOB. All hospital-based or CAH-based renal dialysis centers (including satellites) must use revenue code 078X when billing for the originating site facility fee. The renal dialysis center serving as an originating site must bill for HCPCS code Q3014, telehealth originating site facility fee, on a separate revenue line from any other services provided to the beneficiary.

Skilled nursing facilities (SNFs) bill their local FIs and/or Part A MACs for the originating site facility fee. Telehealth bills originating in SNFs must be submitted on TOB 22X or 23X. For SNF inpatients in a covered Part A stay, the originating site facility fee must be submitted on a 22X TOB. All SNFs must use revenue code 078X when billing for the originating site facility fee. The SNF serving as an originating site must bill for HCPCS code Q3014, telehealth originating site facility fee, on a separate revenue line from any other services provided to the beneficiary.

Community mental health centers (CMHCs) bill their local FIs and/or Part A MACs for the originating site facility fee. Telehealth bills originating in CMHCs must be submitted on a 76X TOB. All CMHCs must use revenue code 078X when billing for the originating site facility fee. The CMHC serving as an originating site must bill for HCPCS code Q3014, telehealth originating site facility fee, on a separate revenue line from any other services provided to the beneficiary. Note that Q3014 does not count towards the number of services used to determine per diem payments for partial hospitalization services.

The beneficiary is responsible for any unmet deductible amount and Medicare coinsurance.

Pub 100-4, 12, 190.6.1 –Submission of Telehealth Claims for Distant Site Practitioners

(Rev. 1716, Issued: 04-24-09; Effective: 01-01-09; Implementation: 05-26-09)

Claims for telehealth services are submitted to the contractors that process claims for the performing physician/practitioner's service area. Physicians/practitioners submit the appropriate HCPCS procedure code for covered professional telehealth services along with the "GT" modifier ("via interactive audio and video telecommunications system"). By coding and billing the "GT" modifier with a covered telehealth procedure code, the distant site physician/practitioner certifies that the beneficiary was present at an eligible originating site when the telehealth service was furnished. By coding and billing the "GT" modifier with a covered ESRD-related service telehealth code, the distant site physician/practitioner certifies that 1 visit per month was furnished face-to-face "hands on" to examine the vascular access site. Refer to Pub. 100-02, chapter 15, section 270.4.1 for the conditions of telehealth payment for ESRD-related services.

In situations where a CAH has elected payment Method II for CAH outpatients, and the practitioner has reassigned his/her benefits to the CAH, FIs should make payment for telehealth services provided by the physician or practitioner at 80 percent of the MPFS amount for the distant site service. In all other cases, except for MNT services as discussed in Section 190.7-Contractor Editing of Telehealth Claims, telehealth services provided by the physician or practitioner at the distant site are billed to the carrier.

Physicians and practitioners at the distant site bill their local Medicare carrier for covered telehealth services, for example, "99245 GT." Physicians' and practitioners' offices serving as a telehealth originating site bill their local Medicare carrier for the originating site facility fee.

Pub 100-4, 12, 190.6.2 – Exception for Store and Forward (Noninteractive) Telehealth

(Rev. 1, 10-01-03)

In the case of Federal telemedicine demonstration programs conducted in Alaska or Hawaii, store and forward technologies may be used as a substitute for an interactive telecommunications system. Covered store and forward telehealth services are billed with the "GQ" modifier, "via asynchronous telecommunications system." By using the "GQ" modifier, the distant site physician/practitioner certifies that the asynchronous medical file was collected and transmitted to them at their distant site from a Federal telemedicine demonstration project conducted in Alaska or Hawaii.

Pub 100-4, 12, 190.7 – Contractor Editing of Telehealth Claims

(Rev. 997, Issued: 07-07-06; Effective: 01-01-06; Implementation: 08-07-06)

Medicare telehealth services (as listed in Section 190.3) are billed with either the GT or GQ modifier. The contractor shall approve covered telehealth services if the physician or practitioner is licensed under State law to provide the service. Contractors must familiarize themselves with licensure provisions of States for which they process claims and disallow telehealth services furnished by physicians or practitioners who are not authorized to furnish the applicable telehealth service under State law. For example, if a nurse practitioner is not licensed to provide individual psychotherapy under State law, he or she would not be permitted to receive payment for individual psychotherapy under Medicare. The contractor shall install edits to ensure that only properly licensed physicians and practitioners are paid for covered telehealth services.

If a contractor receives claims for professional telehealth services coded with the GQ modifier (representing "via asynchronous telecommunications system"), it shall approve/pay for these services only if the physician or practitioner is affiliated with a Federal telemedicine demonstration conducted in Alaska or Hawaii. The contractor may require the physician or practitioner at the distant site to document his or her participation in a Federal telemedicine demonstration program conducted in Alaska or Hawaii prior to paying for telehealth services provided via asynchronous, store and forward technologies.

If a contractor denies telehealth services because the physician or practitioner may not bill for them, the contractor uses MSN message 21.18: "This item or service is not covered when performed or ordered by this practitioner." The contractor uses remittance advice message 52 when denying the claim based upon MSN message 21.18.

If a service is billed with one of the telehealth modifiers and the procedure code is not designated as a covered telehealth service, the contractor denies the service using MSN message 9.4: "This item or service was denied because information required to make payment was incorrect." The remittance advice message depends on what is incorrect, e.g., B18 if procedure code or modifier is incorrect, 125 for submission billing errors, 4-12 for difference inconsistencies. The contractor uses B18 as the explanation for the denial of the claim.

The only claims from institutional facilities that FIs shall pay for telehealth services at the distant site, except for MNT services, are for physician or practitioner services when the distant site is located in a CAH that has elected Method II, and the physician or practitioner has reassigned his/her benefits to the CAH. The CAH bills its regular FI for the professional services provided at the distant site via a telecommunications system, in any of the revenue codes 096x, 097x or 098x. All requirements for billing distant site telehealth services apply.

Claims from hospitals or CAHs for MNT services are submitted to the hospital's or CAH's regular FI. Payment is based on the non-facility amount on the Medicare Physician Fee Schedule for the particular HCPCS codes.

Pub 100-4, 13, 20 – Payment Conditions for Radiology Services

(Rev. 1, 10-01-03)

B3-15022

Pub 100-4, 13, 20.1 – Professional Component (PC)

(Rev. 1, 10-01-03)

Carriers must pay for the PC of radiology services furnished by a physician to an individual patient in all settings under the fee schedule for physician services regardless of the specialty of the physician who performs the service. For services furnished to hospital patients, carriers pay only if the services meet the conditions for fee schedule payment and are identifiable, direct, and discrete diagnostic or therapeutic services to an individual patient, such as an interpretation of diagnostic procedures and the PC of therapeutic procedures. The interpretation of a diagnostic procedure includes a written report.

Pub 100-4, 13, 20.2 – Technical Component (TC)

(Rev. 1, 10-01-03)

Pub 100-4, 13, 20.2.1 – Hospital and Skilled Nursing Facility (SNF) Patients

(Rev. 1221, Issued: 04-18-07, Effective: 04-01-07, Implementation: 04-02-07)

Carriers may not pay for the technical component (TC) of radiology services furnished to hospital patients. Payment for physicians' radiological services to the hospital, e.g., administrative or supervisory services, and for provider services needed to produce the radiology service, is made by the fiscal intermediary (FI) as a provider service.

FIs include the TC of radiology services for hospital inpatients except Critical Access Hospitals (CAH) in the prospective payment system (PPS) payment to hospitals.

Hospital bundling rules exclude payment to suppliers of the Technical Component (TC) of a radiology service for beneficiaries in a hospital inpatient stay. CWF performs reject edits to incoming claims from suppliers of radiology services.

Upon receipt of a hospital inpatient claim at the CWF, CWF searches paid claim history and compares the period between the hospital inpatient admission and discharge dates to the line item service date on a line item TC of a radiology service billed by a supplier. The CWF will generate an unsolicited response when the line item service date falls within the admission and discharge dates of the hospital inpatient claim.

Upon receipt of an unsolicited response, the carrier will adjust the TC of the radiology service and recoup the payment.

For CAHs, payment is made by the FI based on reasonable cost.

Radiology and other diagnostic services furnished to hospital outpatients are paid under the Outpatient Prospective Payment System (OPPS) to the hospital. This applies to bill types 12X and13Xthat are submitted to the FI. Effective 4/1/06, type of bill 14X is for non-patient laboratory specimens and is no longer applicable for radiology services.

As a result of SNF Consolidated Billing (Section 4432(b) of the Balanced Budget Act (BBA) of 1997), carriers may not pay for the TC of radiology services furnished to Skilled Nursing Facility (SNF) inpatients during a Part A covered stay. The SNF must bill radiology services furnished its inpatients in a Part A covered stay and payment is included in the SNF Prospective Payment System (PPS).

Radiology services furnished to outpatients of SNFs may be billed by the supplier performing the service or by the SNF under arrangements with the supplier. If billed by the SNF, FIs pay according to the Medicare Physician Fee Schedule. SNFs submit claims to the FI with type of bill 22X or 23X.

Pub 100-4, 13, 20.2.2 – Services Not Furnished in Hospitals

(Rev. 1, 10-01-03)

Carriers must pay under the fee schedule for the TC of radiology services furnished to beneficiaries who are not patients of any hospital, and who receive services in a physician's office, a freestanding imaging or radiation oncology center, or other setting that is not part of a hospital.

Pub 100-4, 13, 20.2.3 – Services Furnished in Leased Departments

(Rev. 1, 10-01-03)

In the case of procedures furnished in a leased hospital radiology department to a beneficiary who is neither an inpatient nor an outpatient of any hospital, e.g., the patient is referred by an outside physician and is not registered as a hospital outpatient, both the PC and the TC of the services are payable under the fee schedule by the carrier.

Pub 100-4, 13, 20.2.4 – Purchased Diagnostic Tests – Carriers

(Rev. 1, 10-01-03)

B3-15048

Section 1842(n) of the Social Security Act (the Act) establishes payment rules for diagnostic tests billed by a physician but performed by an outside supplier. For this purpose, diagnostic tests are tests covered under §1861(s)(3) of the Act other than clinical diagnostic laboratory tests. These include, but are not limited to, such tests as x-rays, EKGs, EEGs, cardiac monitoring, ultrasound, and the technical component of physician pathology services furnished on or after January 1, 1994. (Note that screening mammography services are covered under another provision of the Act and are not subject to the purchased services limitation.) These rules apply to the purchased test itself (the TC) and not to physicians' services associated with the test.

Pub 100-4, 13, 20.2.4.1 – Carrier Payment Rules

(Rev. 135, 04-02-04)

If a test is personally performed by a physician or is supervised by a physician, such physician may bill under the normal physician fee schedule rules. This includes situations in which the test is performed or supervised by another physician with whom the billing physician shares a practice. Section 80, chapter 15, of Pub. 100-02, Medicare Benefit Polity, sets forth the various levels of physician supervision required for diagnostic tests. The supervision requirement for physician billing is not met when the test is administered by supplier personnel regardless of whether the test is performed at the physician's office or at another location.

If a physician bills for a diagnostic test performed by an outside supplier, the fee schedule amount for the purchased service equals the lower of the billing physician's fee schedule or the price he or she paid for the service. The lower figure is the fee schedule amount for purposes of the limiting charge. (See §30.3.12.1, chapter 1 of this publication.) The billing physician must identify the supplier (including the supplier's provider number) and the amount the supplier charged the billing physician (net of any discounts). A physician who accepts assignment is permitted to bill and collect from the beneficiary only the applicable deductible and coinsurance for the purchased test. A physician who does not accept assignment is permitted to bill and collect from the beneficiary only the fee schedule amount (as defined above) for the purchased test. The limiting charge provision is not applicable.

If the physician does not identify the supplier and provide the other required information, no payment is allowed, and the physician may not bill the beneficiary any amount for the test.

Pub 100-4, 13, 20.2.4.2 – Payment to Physician for Purchased Diagnostic Tests

(Rev. 135, 04-02-04)

A physician or a medical group may submit the claim and (if assignment is accepted) receive the Part B payment, for the technical component of diagnostic tests which the physician or group purchases from an independent physician, medical group, or other supplier. (This claim and payment procedure does not extend to clinical diagnostic laboratory tests.) The purchasing physician or group may be the same physician or group as ordered the tests or may be a different physician or group. An example of the latter situation is when the attending physician orders radiology tests from a radiologist and the radiologist purchases the tests from an imaging center. The purchasing physician or group may not mark up the charge for a test from the purchase price and must accept the lowest of the fee schedule amount if the supplier had billed directly; the physician's actual charge; or the supplier's net charge to the purchasing physician or group, as full payment for the test even if assignment is not accepted.

In order to purchase a diagnostic test, the purchaser must perform the interpretation. The physician or other supplier that furnished the technical component must be enrolled in the Medicare program. No formal reassignment is necessary.

A. Purchased TC Services

Carriers must apply the purchased services limitation to the TC of radiologic services other than screening mammography procedures.

B. Payment to Supplier of Diagnostic Tests for Purchased Interpretations

A person or entity that provides diagnostic tests may submit the claim, and (if assignment is accepted) receive the Part B payment, for diagnostic test interpretations which that person or entity purchases from an independent physician or medical group if:

- The tests are initiated by a physician or medical group which is independent of the person or entity providing the tests and of the physician or medical group providing the interpretations;
- The physician or medical group providing the interpretations does not see the patient; and
- The purchaser (or employee, partner, or owner of the purchaser) performs the technical component of the test. The interpreting physician must be enrolled in the Medicare program. No formal reassignment is necessary.

The purchaser must keep on file the name, the provider identification number and address of the interpreting physician. The rules permitting claims by a facility or clinic for services of an independent contractor physician on the physical premises of the facility or clinic are set forth in Chapter 1.

C. Sanctions

Physicians who knowingly and willfully, in repeated cases, bill Medicare beneficiaries amounts beyond those outlined in this chapter are subject to the penalties contained under §1842(j)(2) of the Act. Penalties are assigned after post-pay review depending on the severity.

D. Questionable Business Arrangements

No special charge or payment constraints are imposed on tests performed by a physician or a technician under the physician's supervision. There are two requirements for all diagnostic tests under §1861(s)(3) of the Act, as implemented by 42 CFR §410.32 and section 10 of chapter13 of this publication and section 80, chapter 15 of Pub. 100-02BP. Namely, the test must be ordered by the treating practitioner, and the test must be supervised by a physician. However, attempts may be made by the medical diagnostic community to adjust or establish arrangements which continue to allow physicians to profit from other's work or by creating the appearance that the physician has performed or supervised his/her technicians who are employed, contracted, or leased. Some of these arrangements may involve cardiac scanning services and mobile ultrasound companies leasing their equipment to physicians for the day the equipment is used, and hiring out their staff to the physicians to meet the supervision requirement.

The bonafides of such arrangements may be suspect and could be an attempt to circumvent the prohibition against the mark-up on purchased diagnostic tests. If you have any doubt that a particular arrangement is a valid relationship where the physician is performing or supervising the services, this should be investigated. The Office of the Inspector General (OIG) has responsibility for investigating violations of §1842(n) of the Act.

Another arrangement to circumvent the purchased diagnostic service provision is for the ordering physician to reassign his/her payment for the interpretation of the test to the supplier. The supplier, in turn, bills for both the test and the interpretation and pays the ordering physician a fee for the interpretation. This arrangement violates §1842(b)(6) of the Act, which prohibits Medicare from paying benefits due the person that furnished the service to any other person, subject to limited exceptions discussed in §3060.D. Also, this arrangement could constitute a violation of §1128 B (b) of the Act, which prohibits remuneration for referrals (i.e., kickbacks).

Violations of §1128B (b) of the Act may subject the physician or supplier to criminal penalties or exclusion from the Medicare and Medicaid programs. Illegal remuneration for referrals can be found even when the ordering physician performs some service for the remuneration.

Pub 100-4, 13, 50.2 – Stressing Agent

(Rev. 1, 10-01-03)

Carriers must make separate payment under code J1245 for pharmacologic stressing agents used in connection with nuclear medicine and cardiovascular stress testing procedures furnished to beneficiaries in settings in which TCs are payable. Such an agent is classified as a supply and covered as an integral part of the diagnostic test. However, carriers pay for code J1245 under the policy for determining payments for "incident to" drugs. See Chapter 17 for payment for drugs.

Pub 100-4, 13, 60 – Positron Emission Tomography (PET) Scans – General Information

(Rev. 1833; Issued: 10-16-09; Effective Date: 04-03-09; Implementation Date: 10-30-09)

Positron emission tomography (PET) is a noninvasive imaging procedure that assesses perfusion and the level of metabolic activity in various organ systems of the human body. A positron camera (tomograph) is used to produce cross-sectional tomographic images which are obtained by detecting radioactivity from a radioactive tracer substance (radiopharmaceutical) that emits a radioactive tracer substance (radiopharmaceutical FDG) such as 2 –[F-18] flouro-D-glucose FDG, that is administered intravenously to the patient.

The ***Medicare National Coverage Determinations (NCD) Manual***, chapter 1, §220.6, contains additional coverage instructions to indicate the conditions under which a PET scan is performed.

A. Definitions

For all uses of PET, excluding Rubidium 82 for perfusion of the heart, myocardial viability and refractory seizures, the following definitions apply:

- **Diagnosis:** PET is covered only in clinical situations in which the PET results may assist in avoiding an invasive diagnostic procedure, or in which the PET results may assist in determining the optimal anatomical location to perform an invasive diagnostic procedure. In general, for most solid tumors, a tissue diagnosis is made prior to the performance of PET scanning. PET scans following a tissue diagnosis are generally performed for the purpose of staging, rather than diagnosis. Therefore, the use of PET in the diagnosis of lymphoma, esophageal and colorectal cancers, as well as in melanoma, should be rare. PET is not covered for other diagnostic uses, and is not covered for screening (testing of patients without specific signs and symptoms of disease).
- **Staging:** PET is covered in clinical situations in which (1) (a) the stage of the cancer remains in doubt after completion of a standard diagnostic workup, including conventional imaging (computed tomography, magnetic resonance imaging, or ultrasound) or, (b) the use of PET would also be considered reasonable and necessary if it could potentially replace one or more conventional imaging studies when it is expected that conventional study information is insufficient for the clinical management of the patient and, (2) clinical management of the patient would differ depending on the stage of the cancer identified.

  NOTE: Effective for services on or after April 3, 2009, the terms "diagnosis" and "staging" will be replaced with "Initial Treatment Strategy." For further information on this new term, refer to Pub. 100-03, NCD Manual, section 220.6.17.
- **Restaging:** PET will be covered for restaging: (1) after the completion of treatment for the purpose of detecting residual disease, (2) for detecting suspected recurrence, or metastasis, (3) to determine the extent of a known recurrence, or (4) if it could potentially replace one or more conventional imaging studies when it is expected that conventional study information is to determine the extent of a known recurrence, or if study information is insufficient for the clinical management of the patient. Restaging applies to testing after a course of treatment is completed and is covered subject to the conditions above.
- **Monitoring:** Use of PET to monitor tumor response to treatment during the planned course of therapy (i.e., when a change in therapy is anticipated).

  NOTE: Effective for services on or after April 3, 2009, the terms "restaging" and "monitoring" will be replaced with "Subsequent Treatment Strategy." For further information on this new term, refer to Pub. 100-03, NCD Manual, section 220.6.17.

B. Limitations

For staging and restaging: PET is covered in either/or both of the following circumstances:

- The stage of the cancer remains in doubt after completion of a standard diagnostic workup, including conventional imaging (computed tomography, magnetic resonance imaging, or ultrasound)
- The clinical management of the patient would differ depending on the stage of the cancer identified. PET will be covered for restaging after the completion of treatment for the purpose of detecting residual disease, for detecting suspected recurrence, or to determine the extent of a known recurrence. Use of PET would also be considered reasonable and necessary if it could potentially replace one or more conventional imaging studies when it is expected that conventional study information is insufficient for the clinical management of the patient.

The PET is not covered for other diagnostic uses, and is not covered for screening (testing of patients without specific symptoms). Use of PET to monitor tumor response during the planned course of therapy (i.e., when no change in therapy is being contemplated) is not covered.

Pub 100-4, 13, 60.1 – Billing Instructions

(Rev. 527, Issued: 04-15-05, Effective: 01-28-05, Implementation: 04-18-05)

A. Billing and Payment Instructions or Responsibilities for Carriers

Claims for PET scan services must be billed on Form-CMS 1500 or the electronic equivalent with the appropriate HCPCS or CPT code and diagnosis codes to the local carrier. Effective for claims received on or after July 1, 2001, PET modifiers were discontinued and are no longer a claims processing requirement for PET scan claims. Therefore, July 1, 2001, and after the MSN messages regarding the use of PET modifiers can be discontinued. The type of service (TOS) for the new PET scan procedure codes is TOS 4, Diagnostic Radiology. Payment is based on the Medicare Physician Fee Schedule.

B. Billing and Payment Instructions or Responsibilities for FIs

Claims for PET scan procedures must be billed to the FI on Form CMS-1450 (UB-92) or the electronic equivalent with the appropriate diagnosis and HCPCS "G" code or CPT code to indicate the conditions under which a PET scan was done. These codes represent the technical component costs associated with these procedures when furnished to hospital and SNF outpatients. They are paid as follows:

- under OPPS for hospitals subject to OPPS
- under current payment methodologies for hospitals not subject to OPPS
- on a reasonable cost basis for critical access hospitals.
- on a reasonable cost basis for skilled nursing facilities.

Institutional providers bill these codes under Revenue Code 0404 (PET Scan).

Medicare contractors shall pay claims submitted for services provided by a critical access hospital (CAH) as follows: Method I technical services are paid at 101% of reasonable cost; Method II technical services are paid at 101% of reasonable cost, and professional services are paid at 115% of the Medicare Physician Fee Schedule Data Base.

C. Frequency

In the absence of national frequency limitations, for all indications covered on and after July 1, 2001, contractors can, if necessary, develop frequency limitations on any or all covered PET scan services.

D. Post-Payment Review for PET Scans

As with any claim, but particularly in view of the limitations on this coverage, Medicare may decide to conduct post-payment reviews to determine that the use of PET scans is consistent with coverage instructions. Pet scanning facilities must keep patient record information on file for each Medicare patient for whom a PET scan claim is made. These medical records can be used in any post-payment reviews and must include the information necessary to substantiate the need for the PET scan. These records must

include standard information (e.g., age, sex, and height) along with sufficient patient histories to allow determination that the steps required in the coverage instructions were followed. Such information must include, but is not limited to, the date, place and results of previous diagnostic tests (e.g., cytopathology and surgical pathology reports, CT), as well as the results and reports of the PET scan(s) performed at the center. If available, such records should include the prognosis derived from the PET scan, together with information regarding the physician or institution to which the patient proceeded following the scan for treatment or evaluation. The ordering physician is responsible for forwarding appropriate clinical data to the PET scan facility.

Effective for claims received on or after July 1, 2001, CMS no longer requires paper documentation to be submitted up front with PET scan claims. Contractors shall be aware and advise providers of the specific documentation requirements for PET scans for dementia and neurodegenerative diseases. This information is outlined in section 60.12. Documentation requirements such as physician referral and medical necessity determination are to be maintained by the provider as part of the beneficiary's medical record. This information must be made available to the carrier or FI upon request of additional documentation to determine appropriate payment of an individual claim.

Pub 100-4, 13, 60.2 – Use of Gamma Cameras and Full Ring and Partial Ring PET Scanners for PET Scans

(Rev. 527, Issued: 04-15-05, Effective: 01-28-05, Implementation: 04-18-05)

See the Medicare NCD Manual, Section 220.6, concerning 2-[F-18] Fluoro-D-Glucose (FDG) PET scanners and details about coverage.

On July 1, 2001, HCPCS codes G0210 – G0230 were added to allow billing for all currently covered indications for FDG PET. Although the codes do not indicate the type of PET scanner, these codes were used until January 1, 2002, by providers to bill for services in a manner consistent with the coverage policy.

Effective January 1, 2002, HCPCS codes G0210 – G0230 were updated with new descriptors to properly reflect the type of PET scanner used. In addition, four new HCPCS codes became effective for dates of service on and after January 1, 2002, (G0231, G0232, G0233, G0234) for covered conditions that may be billed if a gamma camera is used for the PET scan. For services performed from January 1, 2002, through January 27, 2005, providers should bill using the revised HCPCS codes G0210 – G0234. Beginning January 28, 2005 providers should bill using the appropriate CPT code.

Pub 100-4, 13, 60.2.1 – Coverage for Myocardial Viability

(Rev. 1, 10-01-03)

AB-02-065

The FDG PET is covered for the determination of myocardial viability following an inconclusive single photon computed tomography test (SPECT) from July 1, 2001, through September 30, 2002. Only full ring scanners are covered as the scanning medium for this service from July 1, 2001, through December 31, 2001. However, as of January 1, 2002, full and partial ring scanners are covered for myocardial viability following an inconclusive SPECT.

Beginning October 1, 2002, Medicare will cover FDG PET for the determination of myocardial viability as a primary or initial diagnostic study prior to revascularization, and will continue to cover FDG PET when used as a follow-up to an inconclusive SPECT. However, if a patient received a FDG PET study with inconclusive results, a follow-up SPECT is not covered. FDA full and partial ring PET scanners are covered.

In the event that a patient receives a SPECT with inconclusive results, a PET scan may be performed and covered by Medicare. However, a SPECT is not covered following a FDG PET with inconclusive results. See the **Medicare National Coverage Determinations Manual** for specific frequency limitations for Myocardial Viability following an inconclusive SPECT.

In the absence of national frequency limitations, contractors can, if necessary develop reasonable frequency limitations for myocardial viability.

Documentation that these conditions are met should be maintained by the referring physician as part of the beneficiary's medical record.

Pub 100-4, 13, 60.3 – PET Scan Qualifying Conditions and HCPCS Code Chart

(Rev. 527, Issued: 04-15-05, Effective: 01-28-05, Implementation: 04-18-05)

Below is a summary of all covered PET scan conditions, with effective dates.

NOTE: The G codes below except those a # can be used to bill for PET Scan services through January 27, 2005. Effective for dates of service on or after January 28, 2005, providers must bill for PET Scan services using the appropriate CPT codes. See section 60.3.1. The G codes with a # can continue to be used for billing after January 28, 2005 and these remain non-covered by Medicare. (NOTE: PET Scanners must be FDA-approved.)

Conditions	Coverage Effective Date	****HCPCS/CPT
*Myocardial perfusion imaging (following previous PET G0030-G0047) single study, rest or stress (exercise and/or pharmacologic)	3/14/95	G0030
*Myocardial perfusion imaging (following previous PET G0030-G0047) multiple studies, rest or stress (exercise and/or pharmacologic)	3/14/95	G0031
*Myocardial perfusion imaging (following rest SPECT, 78464); single study, rest or stress (exercise and/or pharmacologic)	3/14/95	G0032
*Myocardial perfusion imaging (following rest SPECT 78464); multiple studies, rest or stress (exercise and/or pharmacologic)	3/14/95	G0033
*Myocardial perfusion (following stress SPECT 78465); single study, rest or stress (exercise and/or pharmacologic)	3/14/95	G0034
*Myocardial Perfusion Imaging (following stress SPECT 78465); multiple studies, rest or stress (exercise and/or pharmacologic)	3/14/95	G0035
*Myocardial Perfusion Imaging (following coronary angiography 93510-93529); single study, rest or stress (exercise and/or pharmacologic)	3/14/95	G0036
*Myocardial Perfusion Imaging, (following coronary angiography), 93510-93529); multiple studies, rest or stress (exercise and/or pharmacologic)	3/14/95	G0037

Medicare References

Conditions	Coverage Effective Date	****HCPCS/CPT
*Myocardial Perfusion Imaging (following stress planar myocardial perfusion, 78460); single study, rest or stress (exercise and/or pharmacologic)	3/14/95	G0038
*Myocardial Perfusion Imaging (following stress planar myocardial perfusion, 78460); multiple studies, rest or stress (exercise and/or pharmacologic)	3/14/95	G0039
*Myocardial Perfusion Imaging (following stress echocardiogram 93350); single study, rest or stress (exercise and/or pharmacologic)	3/14/95	G0040
*Myocardial Perfusion Imaging (following stress echocardiogram, 93350); multiple studies, rest or stress (exercise and/or pharmacologic)	3/14/95	G0041
*Myocardial Perfusion Imaging (following stress nuclear ventriculogram 78481 or 78483); single study, rest or stress (exercise and/or pharmacologic)	3/14/95	G0042
*Myocardial Perfusion Imaging (following stress nuclear ventriculogram 78481 or 78483); multiple studies, rest or stress (exercise and/or pharmacologic)	3/14/95	G0043
*Myocardial Perfusion Imaging (following stress ECG, 93000); single study, rest or stress (exercise and/or pharmacologic)	3/14/95	G0044
*Myocardial perfusion (following stress ECG, 93000), multiple studies; rest or stress (exercise and/or pharmacologic)	3/14/95	G0045
*Myocardial perfusion (following stress ECG, 93015), single study; rest or stress (exercise and/or pharmacologic)	3/14/95	G0046
*Myocardial perfusion (following stress ECG, 93015); multiple studies, rest or stress (exercise and/or pharmacologic)	3/14/95	G0047
PET imaging regional or whole body; single pulmonary nodule	1/1/98	G0125
Lung cancer, non-small cell (PET imaging whole body) Diagnosis, Initial Staging, Restaging	7/1/01	G0210 G0211 G0212
Colorectal cancer (PET imaging whole body) >p>Diagnosis, Initial Staging, Restaging	7/1/01	G0213 G0214 G0215
Melanoma (PET imaging whole body) Diagnosis, Initial Staging, Restaging	7/1/01	G0216 G0217 G0218
Melanoma for non-covered indications	7/1/01	#G0219
Lymphoma (PET imaging whole body) Diagnosis, Initial Staging, Restaging	7/1/01	G0220 G0221 G0222
Head and neck cancer; excluding thyroid and CNS cancers (PET imaging whole body or regional) Diagnosis, Initial Staging, Restaging	7/1/01	G0223 G0224 G0225
Esophageal cancer (PET imaging whole body) Diagnosis, Initial Staging, Restaging	7/1/01	G0226 G0227 G0228
Metabolic brain imaging for pre-surgical evaluation of refractory seizures	7/1/01	G0229
Metabolic assessment for myocardial viability following inconclusive SPECT study	7/1/01	G0230
Recurrence of colorectal or colorectal metastatic cancer (PET whole body, gamma cameras only)	1/1/02	G0231
Staging and characterization of lymphoma (PET whole body, gamma cameras only)	1/1/02	G0232

Conditions	Coverage Effective Date	****HCPCS/CPT
Recurrence of melanoma or melanoma metastatic cancer (PET whole body, gamma cameras only)	1/1/02	G0233
Regional or whole body, for solitary pulmonary nodule following CT, or for initial staging of non-small cell lung cancer (gamma cameras only)	1/1/02	G0234
Non-Covered Service PET imaging, any site not otherwise specified	1/28/05	#G0235
Non-Covered Service Initial diagnosis of breast cancer and/or surgical planning for breast cancer (e.g., initial staging of axillary lymph nodes), not covered (full- and partial-ring PET scanners only)	10/1/02	#G0252
Breast cancer, staging/restaging of local regional recurrence or distant metastases, i.e., staging/restaging after or prior to course of treatment (full- and partial-ring PET scanners only)	10/1/02	G0253
Breast cancer, evaluation of responses to treatment, performed during course of treatment (full- and partial-ring PET scanners only)	10/1/02	G0254
Myocardial imaging, positron emission tomography (PET), metabolic evaluation)	10/1/02	78459
Restaging or previously treated thyroid cancer of follicular cell origin following negative I-131 whole body scan (full- and partial-ring PET scanner only)	10/1/03	G0296
Tracer Rubidium**82 (Supply of Radiopharmaceutical Diagnostic Imaging Agent) (This is only billed through Outpatient Perspective Payment System, OPPS.) (Carriers must use HCPCS Code A4641).	10/1/03	Q3000
Supply of Radiopharmaceutical Diagnostic Imaging Agent, Ammonia N-13	1/1/04	A9526
PET imaging, brain imaging for the differential diagnosis of Alzheimer's disease with aberrant features vs. fronto-temporal dementia	9/15/04	Appropriate CPT Code from section 60.3.1
PET Cervical Cancer Staging as adjunct to conventional imaging, other staging, diagnosis, restaging, monitoring	1/28/05	Appropriate CPT Code from section 60.3.1

*__NOTE:__ Carriers must report A4641 for the tracer Rubidium 82 when used with PET scan codes G0030 through G0047 for services performed on or before January 27, 2005

**__NOTE:__ Not FDG PET

***__NOTE:__ For dates of service October 1, 2003, through December 31, 2003, use temporary code Q4078 for billing this radiopharmaceutical.

Pub 100-4, 13, 60.3.1 – Appropriate CPT Codes Effective for PET Scans for Services Performed on or After January 28, 2005

(Rev. 1301, Issued: 07-20-07, Effective: 01-28-05 CPT Code 78609/01-01-08 HCPCS Code A4641, Implementation: 01-07-08)

NOTE: All PET scan services require the use of a radiopharmaceutical diagnostic imaging agent (tracer). The applicable tracer code should be billed when billing for a PET scan service. See Section 60.3.2 below for applicable tracer codes.

CPT Code	Description
78459	Myocardial imaging, positron emission tomography (PET), metabolic evaluation
78491	Myocardial imaging, positron emission tomography (PET), perfusion, single study at rest or stress
78492	Myocardial imaging, positron emission tomography (PET), perfusion, multiple studies at rest and/or stress
78608	Brain imaging, positron emission tomography (PET); metabolic evaluation
78609	Brain imaging, positron emission tomography (PET); perfusion evaluation
78811	Tumor imaging, positron emission tomography (PET); limited area (eg, chest, head/neck)
78812	Tumor imaging, positron emission tomography (PET); skull base to mid-thigh
78813	Tumor imaging, positron emission tomography (PET); whole body
78814	Tumor imaging, positron emission tomography (PET) with concurrently acquired computed tomography (CT) for attenuation correction and anatomical localization; limited area (eg, chest, head/neck)
78815	Tumor imaging, positron emission tomography (PET) with concurrently acquired computed tomography (CT) for attenuation correction and anatomical localization; skull base to mid-thigh
78816	Tumor imaging, positron emission tomography (PET) with concurrently acquired computed tomography (CT) for attenuation correction and anatomical localization; whole body

Pub 100-4, 13, 60.3.2 – Tracer Codes Required for PET Scans

(Rev. 1937, Issued: 03-26-10, Effective: 02-26-10, Implementation: 07-06-10)

The following tracer codes are applicable only to CPT 78491 and 78492. They can not be reported with any other code.

Institutional providers billing the fiscal intermediary

HCPCS	Description
*A9555	Rubidium Rb-82, Diagnostic, Per study dose, Up to 60 Millicuries
*Q3000 (Deleted effective 12/31/05)	Supply of Radiopharmaceutical Diagnostic Imaging Agent, Rubidium Rb-82, per dose
A9526	Nitrogen N-13 Ammonia, Diagnostic, Per study dose, Up To 40 Millicuries

NOTE: For claims with dates of service prior to 1/01/06, providers report Q3000 for supply of radiopharmaceutical diagnostic imaging agent, Rubidium Rb-82. For claims with dates of service 1/01/06 and later, providers report A9555 for radiopharmaceutical diagnostic imaging agent, Rubidium Rb-82 in place of Q3000.

Physicians/practitioners billing the carrier:

HPCPS	Description
*A4641	Supply of Radiopharmaceutical Diagnostic Imaging Agent, Not Otherwise Classified
A9526	Nitrogen N-13 Ammonia, Diagnostic, Per study dose, Up To 40 Millicuries
A9555	Rubidium Rb-82, Diagnostic, Per study dose, Up To 60 Millicuries

***NOTE**: Effective January 1, 2008, tracer code A4641 is not applicable for PET Scans.

The following tracer codes are applicable only to CPT 78459, 78608, 78811-78816. They cannot be reported with any other code:

Institutional providers billing the fiscal intermediary:

HCPCS	Description
*A9552	Fluorodeoxyglucose F18, FDG, Diagnostic, Per study dose, Up to 45 Millicuries
*C1775 (Deleted effective 12/31/05)	Supply of Radiopharmaceutical Diagnostic Imaging Agent, Fluorodeoxyglucose F18 (2-Deoxy-2-18F Fluoro-D-Glucose), Per dose (4-40 Mci/Ml)
**A4641	Supply of Radiopharmaceutical Diagnostic Imaging Agent, Not Otherwise Classified
A9580	Sodium Fluoride F-18, Diagnostic, per study dose, up to 30 Millicuries

***NOTE:** For claims with dates of service prior to 1/01/06, OPPS hospitals report C1775 for supply of radiopharmaceutical diagnostic imaging agent, Fluorodeoxyglucose F18. For claims with dates of service January 1, 2006 and later, providers report A9552 for radiopharmaceutical diagnostic imaging agent, Fluorodeoxyglucose F18 in place of C1775.

** **NOTE:** Effective January 1, 2008, tracer code A4641 is not applicable for PET Scans.

*****NOTE:** Effective for claims with dates of service February 26, 2010 and later, tracer code A9580 is applicable for PET Scans.

Physicians/practitioners billing the carrier:

HCPCS	Description
*A4641	Supply of Radiopharmaceutical Diagnostic Imaging Agent, Not Otherwise Classified
A9552	Fluorodeoxyglucose F18, FDG, Diagnostic, Per study dose, Up to 45 Millicuries
A9580	Sodium Fluoride F-18, Diagnostic, per study dose, up to 30 Millicuries

***NOTE:** Effective January 1, 2008, tracer code A4641 is not applicable for PET Scans.

*****NOTE:** Effective for claims with dates of service February 26, 2010 and later, tracer code A9580 is applicable for PET Scans.

Pub 100-4, 13, 60.4 – PET Scans for Imaging of the Perfusion of the Heart Using Rubidium 82 (Rb 82)

(Rev. 223, Issued: 07-02-04) (Effective/Implementation: Not Applicable)

For dates of service on or after March 14, 1995, Medicare covers one PET scan for imaging of the perfusion of the heart using Rubidium 82 (Rb 82), provided that the following conditions are met:

- The PET is done at a PET imaging center with a PET scanner that has been approved by the FDA;
- The PET scan is a rest alone or rest with pharmacologic stress PET scan, used for noninvasive imaging of the perfusion of the heart for the diagnosis and management of patients with known or suspected coronary artery disease, using Rb 82; and
- Either the PET scan is used in place of, but not in addition to, a single photon emission computed tomography (SPECT) or the PET scan is used following a SPECT that was found inconclusive.

Pub 100-4, 13, 60.11 – Coverage of PET Scans for Perfusion of the Heart Using Ammonia N-13

(Rev. 223, Issued: 07-02-04) (Effective/Implementation: Not Applicable)

Effective for service performed on or after October 1, 2003, PET scans performed at rest or with pharmacological stress used for noninvasive imaging of the perfusion of the heart for the diagnosis and management of patients with known or suspected coronary artery disease using the FDA-approved radiopharmaceutical ammonia N-13 are covered, provided the following requirements are met.

Medicare References

Pub 100-4, 13, 90 – Services of Portable X-Ray Suppliers

(Rev. 1, 10-01-03)

B3-2070.4, B3-15022.G, B3-4131, B3-4831

Services furnished by portable x-ray suppliers may have as many as four components. Carriers must follow the following rules.

Pub 100-4, 13, 90.1 – Professional Component

(Rev. 1, 10-01-03)

Pay the PC of radiologic services furnished by portable x-ray suppliers on the same basis as other physician fee schedule services.

Pub 100-4, 13, 90.2 – Technical Component

(Rev. 1, 10-01-03)

Pay the TC of radiology services furnished by portable x-ray suppliers under the fee schedule on the same basis as TC services generally.

Pub 100-4, 13, 90.3 – Transportation Component (HCPCS Codes R0070 – R0076)

(Rev. 343, Issued: 10-29-04, Effective: 04-01-05, Implementation: 04-04-05)

This component represents the transportation of the equipment to the patient. Establish local RVUs for the transportation R codes based on carrier knowledge of the nature of the service furnished. Carriers shall allow only a single transportation payment for each trip the portable x-ray supplier makes to a particular location. When more than one Medicare patient is x-rayed at the same location, e.g., a nursing home, prorate the single fee schedule transportation payment among all patients receiving the services. For example, if two patients at the same location receive x-rays, make one-half of the transportation payment for each.

R0075 must be billed in conjunction with the CPT radiology codes (7000 series) and only when the x-ray equipment used was actually transported to the location where the x-ray was taken. R0075 would not apply to the x-ray equipment stored in the location where the x-ray was done (e.g., a nursing home) for use as needed.

Below are the definitions for each modifier that must be reported with R0075. Only one of these five modifiers shall be reported with R0075. NOTE: If only one patient is served, R0070 should be reported with no modifier since the descriptor for this code reflects only one patient seen.

UN – Two patients served

UP – Three patients served

UQ – Four patients served

UR – Five Patients served

US – Six or more patients served

Payment for the above modifiers must be consistent with the definition of the modifiers. Therefore, for R0075 reported with modifiers, -UN, -UP, -UQ, and –UR, the total payment for the service shall be divided by 2, 3, 4, and 5 respectively. For modifier –US, the total payment for the service shall be divided by 6 regardless of the number of patients served. For example, if 8 patients were served, R0075 would be reported with modifier –US and the total payment for this service would be divided by 6.

The units field for R0075 shall always be reported as "1" except in extremely unusual cases. The number in the units field should be completed in accordance with the provisions of 100-04, chapter 23, section 10.2 item 24 G which defines the units field as the number of times the patient has received the itemized service during the dates listed in the from/to field. The units field must never be used to report the number of patients served during a single trip. Specifically, the units field must reflect the number of services that the specific beneficiary received, not the number of services received by other beneficiaries.

As a carrier priced service, carriers must initially determine a payment rate for portable x-ray transportation services that is associated with the cost of providing the service. In order to determine an appropriate cost, the carrier should, at a minimum, cost out the vehicle, vehicle modifications, gasoline and the staff time involved in only the transportation for a portable x-ray service. A review of the pricing of this service should be done every five years.

Direct costs related to the vehicle carrying the x-ray machine are fully allocable to determining the payment rate. This includes the cost of the vehicle using a recognized depreciation method, the salary and fringe benefits associated with the staff who drive the vehicle, the communication equipment used between the vehicle and the home office, the salary and fringe benefits of the staff who determine the vehicles route (this could be proportional of office staff), repairs and maintenance of the vehicle(s), insurance for the vehicle(s), operating expenses for the vehicles and any other reasonable costs associated with this service as determined by the carrier. The carrier will have discretion for allocating indirect costs (those costs that cannot be directly attributed to portable x-ray transportation) between the transportation service and the technical component of the x-ray tests.

Suppliers may send carriers unsolicited cost information. The carrier may use this cost data as a comparison to its carrier priced determination. The data supplied should reflect a year's worth (either calendar or corporate fiscal) of information. Each provider who submits such data is to be informed that the data is subject to verification and will be used to supplement other information that is used to determine Medicare's payment rate.

Carriers are required to update the rate on an annual basis using independently determined measures of the cost of providing the service. A number of readily available measures (e.g., ambulance inflation factor, the Medicare economic index) that are used by the Medicare program to adjust payment rates for other types of services may be appropriate to use to update the rate for years that the carrier does not recalibrate the payment. Each carrier has the flexibility to identify the index it will use to update the rate. In addition, the carrier can consider locally identified factors that are measured independently of CMS as an adjunct to the annual adjustment.

NOTE: No transportation charge is payable unless the portable x-ray equipment used was actually transported to the location where the x-ray was taken. For example, carriers do not allow a transportation charge when the x-ray equipment is stored in a nursing home for use as needed. However, a set-up payment (see §90.4, below) is payable in such situations. Further, for services furnished on or after January 1, 1997, carriers may not make separate payment under HCPCS code R0076 for the transportation of EKG equipment by portable x-ray suppliers or any other entity.

Pub 100-4, 13, 90.4 – Set-Up Component (HCPCS Code Q0092)

(Rev. 1, 10-01-03)

Carriers must pay a set-up component for each radiologic procedure (other than retakes of the same procedure) during both single patient and multiple patient trips under Level II HCPCS code Q0092. Carriers do not make the set-up payment for EKG services furnished by the portable x-ray supplier.

Pub 100-4, 13, 90.5 – Transportation of Equipment Billed by a SNF to an FI

(Rev. 716, Issued: 10-21-05; Effective Date: 04-01-06; Implementation Date: 04-03-06)

SNF 533.1.J

When a SNF bills for portable x-ray equipment transported to a site by van or other vehicle, the SNF should bill for the transportation costs using one of the following HCPCS codes along with the appropriate revenue code:

HCPCS	Description
R0070	Transportation of Portable x-ray Equipment and Personnel to Home or Nursing Home, Per Trip to Facility or Location, One Patient Seen.
R0075	Transportation of Portable x-ray Equipment and Personnel to Home or Nursing Home, Per Trip to Facility or Location, More than One Patient Seen, Per Patient.

These HCPCS codes are subject to the fee schedule.

Effective April 1, 2006, SNFs are required to report the appropriate modifiers to identify the number of patients served when billing for

Medicare References

R0075. See section 90.3, of this chapter for the list of modifiers used to identify on the claim the number of patients served.

Fiscal intermediaries shall ensure that payment for R0075 is consistent with the definition of the modifiers.

Pub 100-4, 13, 140 – Bone Mass Measurements BMMs)

(Rev. 1416; Issued: 01-18-08; Effective: 01-01-07; Implementation: 02-20-08)

Sections 1861(s)(15) and (rr)(1) of the Social Security Act (the Act) (as added by §4106 of the Balanced Budget Act (BBA) of 1997) standardize Medicare coverage of medically necessary bone mass measurements by providing for uniform coverage under Medicare Part B. This coverage is effective for claims with dates of service furnished on or after July 1, 1998.

Effective for dates of service on and after January 1, 2007, the CY 2007 Physician Fee Schedule final rule expanded the number of beneficiaries qualifying for BMM by reducing the dosage requirement for glucocorticoid (steroid) therapy from 7.5 mg of prednisone per day to 5.0 mg. It also changed the definition of BMM by removing coverage for a single-photon absorptiometry as it is not considered reasonable and necessary under section 1862 (a)(1)(A) of the Act.

Conditions of Coverage for BMMs are located in Pub.100-02, Medicare Benefit Policy Manual, chapter 15.

Pub 100-4, 13, 140.1 – Payment Methodology and HCPCS Coding

(Rev. 1472, Issued: 03-06-08, Effective: 05-23-07, Implementation: 04-07-08)

Carriers pay for BMM procedures based on the Medicare physician fee schedule. Claims from physicians, other practitioners, or suppliers where assignment was not taken are subject to the Medicare limiting charge.

The FIs pay for BMM procedures under the current payment methodologies for radiology services according to the type of provider.

Do not pay BMM procedure claims for dual photon absorptiometry, CPT procedure code 78351.

Deductible and coinsurance apply.

Any of the following CPT procedure codes may be used when billing for BMMs through December 31, 2006. All of these codes are bone densitometry measurements except code 76977, which is bone sonometry measurements. CPT procedure codes are applicable to billing FIs and carriers.

76070	76071	76075	76076
76078	76977	78350	G0130

Effective for dates of services on and after January 1, 2007, the following changes apply to BMM:

- New 2007 CPT bone mass procedure codes have been assigned for BMM. The following codes will replace current codes, however the CPT descriptors for the services remain the same:
  77078 replaces 76070
  77079 replaces 76071
  77080 replaces 76075
  77081 replaces 76076
  77083 replaces 76078
- Certain BMM tests are covered when used to screen patients for osteoporosis subject to the frequency standards described in chapter 15, section 80.5.5 of the Medicare Benefit Policy Manual.
- Contractors will pay claims for screening tests when coded as follows:
  - Contains CPT procedure code 77078, 77079, 77080, 77081, 77083, 76977 or G0130
  - Contains a valid ICD-9-CM diagnosis code indicating the reason for the test is postmenopausal female, vertebral fracture, hyperparathyroidism, or steroid therapy. Contractors are to maintain local lists of valid codes for the benefit's screening categories.
- Contractors will deny claims for screening tests when coded as follows:
  - Contains CPT procedure code 77078, 77079, 77081, 77083, 76977 or G0130, but
  - Does not contain a valid ICD-9-CM diagnosis code from the local lists of valid ICD-9-CM diagnosis codes maintained by the contractor for the benefit's screening categories indicating the reason for the test is postmenopausal female, vertebral fracture, hyperparathyroidism, or steroid therapy.
  - Dual-energy x-ray absorptiometry (axial) tests are covered when used to monitor FDA-approved osteoporosis drug therapy subject to the 2-year frequency standards described in chapter 15, section 80.5.5 of the ***Medicare Benefit Policy Manual***.
- Contractors will pay claims for monitoring tests when coded as follows:
  - Contains CPT procedure code 77080, and
  - Contains 733.00, 733.01, 733.02, 733.03, 733.09, 733.90, or 255.0 as the ICD-9-CM diagnosis code.
- Contractors will deny claims for monitoring tests when coded as follows:
  - Contains CPT procedure code 77078, 77079, 77081, 77083, 76977 or G0130, and
  - Contains 733.00, 733.01, 733.02, 733.03, 733.09, 733.90, or 255.0 as the ICD-9-CM diagnosis code, but
  - Does not contain a valid ICD-9-CM diagnosis code from the local lists of valid ICD-9-CM diagnosis codes maintained by the contractor for the benefit's screening categories indicating the reason for the test is postmenopausal female, vertebral fracture, hyperparathyroidism, or steroid therapy.
  - Single photon absorptiometry tests are not covered. Contractors will deny CPT procedure code 78350

The FIs are billed using the ANSI X12N 837 I or hardcopy Form CMS-1450. The appropriate bill types are: 12X, 13X, 22X, 23X, 34X, 71X (Provider-based and independent), 72X, 73X (Provider-based and freestanding), 83X, and 85X. Effective April 1, 2006, type of bill 14X is for non-patient laboratory specimens and is no longer applicable for bone mass measurements. Information regarding the claim form locators that correspond to the HCPCS/CPT code or Type of Bill and a table to crosswalk its CMS-1450 form locators to the 837 transaction are found in Chapter 25.

Providers must report HCPCS codes for bone mass measurements under revenue code 320 with number of units and line item dates of service per revenue code line for each bone mass measurement reported.

Carriers are billed for bone mass measurement procedures using the ANSI X12N 837 P or hardcopy Form CMS-1500.

Pub 100-4, 13, 140.2 – Medicare Summary Notice (MSN) Messages

(Rev. 1236, Issued: 05-11-07, Effective: 01-01-07, Implementation: 07-02-07)

Use appropriate MSN messages when processing claims.

For denials effective January 1, 2007, use the following MSN messages:

Include the following messages if an ABN was issued:

- MSN# 16.10: "Medicare does not pay for this item or service." (English version) or "Medicare no paga por este articulo o servicio." (Spanish version)
- MSN# 36.1: "Our records show that you were informed in writing, before receiving the service, that Medicare would not pay. You are liable for this charge. If you do not agree with this statement, you may ask for a review." (English version) or "Nuestros archivos indican que usted fue informado por escrito, antes de recibir el servicio, que Medicare no pagaría. Usted es responsable por esta cantidad. Si usted no está de acuerdo, usted puede pedir una revisión." (Spanish version)

NOTE: FIs are not to include MSN 16.10.

Include the following messages if an ABN was not issued:

- MSN# 16.10: "Medicare does not pay for this item or service." (English version) or "Medicare no paga por este articulo o servicio." (Spanish Version)
- MSN number 36.2: "It appears that you did not know that we would not pay for this service, so you are not liable. Do not pay your provider for this service. If you have paid your provider for this service, you should submit to this office three things: (1) a copy of this notice, (2) your provider's bill, and (3) a receipt or proof that you have paid the bill. You must file your written request for payment within 6 months of the date of this notice. Future services of this

type provided to you will be your responsibility." (English version) or "Aparentemente, usted no sabia que nosotros no pagamos por este servicio, por lo tanto usted no es responsable. Si usted le pagó al proveedor por este servicio debe enviarnos lo siguiente: (1) Copia de esta notificación; (2) Factura del proveedor; (3) El recibo o prueba de que usted le pagó. Debe enviar su petición por escrito dentro de 6 meses de la fecha de esta notificación. Servicios de este tipo prestados en el futuro serán su responsabilidad." (Spanish Version)

NOTE: FIs are not to include MSN 16.10.

Pub 100-4, 13, 140.3 – Remittance Advice (RA) Messages

(Rev. 1236, Issued: 05-11-07, Effective: 01-01-07, Implementation: 07-02-07))

Use appropriate RA messages when processing claims.

For denials effective January 1, 2007, use the following RA messages:

Claim adjustment reason code 50:

"These are non-covered services because this is not deemed a "medical necessity" by the payer".

Include the following RA messages if an ABN was issued:

- RA remark code M38:

  "The patient is liable for the charges for this service as you informed the patient in writing before the service was furnished that we would not pay for it, and the patient agreed to pay."

- Group code PR:

  "Patient Responsibility."

If an ABN was not issued include the following messages:

- RA remark code M27:

  "The patient has been relieved of liability of payment of these items and services under the limitation of liability provision of the law. You, the provider, are ultimately liable for the patient's waived charges, including any charges for coinsurance, since the items or services were not reasonable and necessary or constituted custodial care, and you knew or could reasonably have been expected to know, that they were not covered.

  You may appeal this determination. You may ask for an appeal regarding both the coverage determination and the issue of whether you exercised due care. The appeal request must be filed within 120 days of the date you receive this notice. You must make the request through this office."

- Group code CO:

  "Contractual Obligations."

Pub 100-4, 13, 140.4 – Advance Beneficiary Notices (ABNs)

(Rev. 1236, Issued: 05-11-07, Effective: 01-01-07, Implementation: 07-02-07

For the denial situations listed in Section 140.1, physicians, practitioners and hospitals are liable for payment unless they issue an appropriate ABN. Contractors will utilize the appropriate messages, see sections 140.2 and 140.3

Pub 100-4, 16, 10 – Background

(Rev. 1, 10-01-03)

B3-2070, B3-2070.1, B3-4110.3, B3-5114

Diagnostic X-ray, laboratory, and other diagnostic tests, including materials and the services of technicians, are covered under the Medicare program. Some clinical laboratory procedures or tests require Food and Drug Administration (FDA) approval before coverage is provided.

A diagnostic laboratory test is considered a laboratory service for billing purposes, regardless of whether it is performed in:

- A physician's office, by an independent laboratory;
- By a hospital laboratory for its outpatients or nonpatients;
- In a rural health clinic; or
- In an HMO or Health Care Prepayment Plan (HCPP) for a patient who is not a member.

When a hospital laboratory performs laboratory tests for nonhospital patients, the laboratory is functioning as an independent laboratory, and still bills the fiscal intermediary (FI). Also, when physicians and laboratories perform the same test, whether manually or with automated equipment, the services are deemed similar.

Laboratory services furnished by an independent laboratory are covered under SMI if the laboratory is an approved Independent Clinical Laboratory. However, as is the case of all diagnostic services, in order to be covered these services must be related to a patient's illness or injury (or symptom or complaint) and ordered by a physician. A small number of laboratory tests can be covered as a preventive screening service.

See the ***Medicare Benefit Policy Manual***, Chapter 15, for detailed coverage requirements.

See the ***Medicare Program Integrity Manual,*** Chapter 10, for laboratory/supplier enrollment guidelines.

See the Medicare State Operations Manual for laboratory/supplier certification requirements.

Pub 100-4, 16, 10.1 – Definitions

(Rev. 85, 02-06-04)

B3-2070.1, B3-2070.1.B, RHC-406.4

"Independent Laboratory" – An independent laboratory is one that is independent both of an attending or consulting physician's office and of a hospital that meets at least the requirements to qualify as an emergency hospital as defined in §1861(e) of the Social Security Act (the Act.) (See the ***Medicare Benefit Policy Manual,*** Chapter 15, for detailed discussion.)

"Physician Office Laboratory" – A physician office laboratory is a laboratory maintained by a physician or group of physicians for performing diagnostic tests in connection with the physician practice.

"Clinical Laboratory" – See the ***Medicare Benefit Policy Manual,*** Chapter 15.

"Qualified Hospital Laboratory" – A qualified hospital laboratory is one that provides some clinical laboratory tests 24 hours a day, 7 days a week, to serve a hospital's emergency room that is also available to provide services 24 hours a day, 7 days a week. For the qualified hospital laboratory to meet this requirement, the hospital must have physicians physically present or available within 30 minutes through a medical staff call roster to handle emergencies 24 hours a day, 7 days a week; and hospital laboratory technologists must be on duty or on call at all times to provide testing for the emergency room.

"Hospital Outpatient" – See the ***Medicare Benefit Policy Manual***, Chapter 2.

"Referring laboratory" – A Medicare-approved laboratory that receives a specimen to be tested and that refers the specimen to another laboratory for performance of the laboratory test.

"Reference laboratory" – A Medicare-enrolled laboratory that receives a specimen from another, referring laboratory for testing and that actually performs the test.

"Billing laboratory" – The laboratory that submits a bill or claim to Medicare.

"Service" – A clinical diagnostic laboratory test. Service and test are synonymous.

"Test" – A clinical diagnostic laboratory service. Service and test are synonymous.

"CLIA" – The Clinical Laboratory Improvement Act and CMS implementing regulations and processes.

"Certification" – A laboratory that has met the standards specified in the CLIA.

"Draw Station' – A place where a specimen is collected but no Medicare-covered clinical laboratory testing is performed on the drawn specimen.

"Medicare-approved laboratory – A laboratory that meets all of the enrollment standards as a Medicare provider including the certification by a CLIA certifying authority.

Pub 100-4, 16, 70.6 – Certificate for Provider-Performed Microscopy Procedures

(Rev. 865, Issued: 02-17-06; Effective: 01-01-06; Implementation: 07-03-06)

Effective January 19, 1993, a laboratory that holds a certificate for provider-performed microscopy procedures may perform only those tests specified as provider-performed microscopy procedures and waived tests, as described below, and no others.

HCPCS Code	Test
Q0111	Wet mounts, including preparations of vaginal, cervical or skin specimens
Q0112	All potassium hydroxide (KOH) preparations
Q0113	Pinworm examinations
Q0114	Fern test
Q0115	Post-coital direct, qualitative examinations of vaginal or cervical mucous
81015	Urinalysis; microscopic only
81000	Urinalysis, by dipstick or tablet reagent for bilirubin, glucose, hemoglobin, ketones, leukocytes, nitrite, pH, protein, specific gravity, urobilinogen, any number of these constituents; non-automated, with microscopy
81001	Urinalysis, by dipstick or tablet reagent for bilirubin, glucose, hemoglobin, ketones, leukocytes, nitrite, pH, protein, specific gravity, urobilinogen, any number of these constituents; automated, with microscopy (NOTE: May only be used when the lab is using an automated dipstick urinalysis instrument approved as waived.)
81020	Urinalysis; two or three glass test
89055	Fecal leukocyte examination
89190	Nasal smears for eosinophils
G0027	Semen analysis; presence and/or motility of sperm excluding Huhner

Pub 100-4, 17, 10 – Payment Rules for Drugs and Biologicals

(Rev. 1445, Issued: 02-08-08; Effective: 01-01-08; Implementation: 03-10-08)

Drugs for inpatient hospital and inpatient skilled nursing facility (SNF) beneficiaries are included in the respective prospective payment system (PPS) rates, except for hemophilia clotting factors for hospital inpatients under Part A.

All hospital outpatient drugs are excluded from SDP because the payment allowance for such drugs is determined by a different methodology. Non pass-through drugs with estimated per day costs less than or equal to the applicable drug packaging threshold that are furnished to hospital outpatients are packaged under the outpatient prospective payment system (OPPS). Their costs are recognized and included but paid as part of the ambulatory payment classification (APC) group payment for the service with which they are billed. Non pass-through drugs with estimated per day costs greater than the applicable drug packaging threshold are paid separately.

Drugs that are granted "pass through" payment status are required by law to be paid at either the amount paid under the physician fee schedule, or, if the drug is included in the Part B drug competitive acquisition program (CAP), at the Part B drug CAP rate. Drugs that have pass-through status may have coinsurance amounts that are less than 20 percent of the OPPS payment amount. This is because pass-through payment amounts, by law, are not subject to coinsurance. CMS considers the amount of the pass-through drug payment rate that exceeds the otherwise applicable OPPS payment rate to be the pass-through payment amount. Thus, in situations where the pass-through payment rate exceeds the otherwise applicable OPPS payment rate, the coinsurance is based on a portion of the total drug payment rate, not the full payment rate.

Hospitals must report all appropriate HCPCS codes and charges for separately payable drugs, in addition to reporting the applicable drug administration codes. Hospitals should also report the HCPCS codes and charges for drugs that are packaged into payments for the corresponding drug administration or other separately payable services. Historical hospital cost data may assist with future payment packaging decisions for such drugs. Drugs are billed in multiples of the dosage specified in the HCPCS code long descriptor. If the drug dose used in the care of a patient is not a multiple of the HCPCS code dosage descriptor, the provider rounds to the next highest unit based on the HCPCS long descriptor for the code in order to report the dose provided.

If the full dosage provided is less than the dosage for the HCPCS code descriptor specifying the minimum dosage for the drug, the provider reports one unit of the HCPCS code for the minimum dosage amount.

OPPS Pricer includes a table of drugs and prices and provides the contractor with the appropriate prices.

Section H90H relates specifically to billing for hospital outpatients. The remainder of this chapter relates to procedures for pricing and paying DME recipients, and to beneficiaries who receive drugs under special benefits such as pneumococcal, flu and hepatitis vaccines; clotting factors, immunosuppressive therapy, self administered cancer and antiemetic drugs, and drugs incident to physicians' services.

The Medicare Prescription Drug, Improvement, and Modernization Act (MMA) of 2003 defines a Specified Covered Outpatient Drug (SCOD) as a covered outpatient drug for which a separate APC has been established and that is either a radiopharmaceutical agent, or a drug or biological for which payment was made on a pass-through basis on or before December 31, 2002.

Payment for SCODs is set, by law, at the average acquisition cost. Under the OPPS, a single payment is made for SCODs that represents payment for both the acquisition cost of the drug and any associated pharmacy overhead or nuclear medicine handling costs.

Drugs or biologicals must meet the coverage requirements in Chapter 15 of the Medicare Benefit Policy Manual. Additionally, for end stage renal disease (ESRD) patients, see the Medicare Benefit Policy Manual, Chapter 11. For ESRD patient billing for drugs and claims processing, see Chapter 8 of this manual. The following chart describes the payment provisions for drugs.

Table – Drug Payment Methodology

(Rev. 1445, Issued: 02-08-08; Effective: 01-01-08; Implementation: 03-10-08)

In the table below, if the item does not have an asterisk ("*") the bill is submitted to the contractor. An asterisk ("*") indicates the bill is submitted to the local carrier or DMERC, as applicable.

Key to the Following Table:

* Bills carrier; no asterisk means bills the hospital's contractor or RHHI NOTE: DMERCs do not process claims for blood clotting factors.

† Drugs and biologicals outside the composite rate are paid as described in 2 below. Those inside the composite rate are paid as described in 1.

1 Included in PPS rate, or other provider-type all inclusive encounter rate

2 Price taken from CMS drug/biological pricing file effective on the specific date of service.

3 Reasonable cost.

4 Lower of cost or 95% AWP paid for drug in addition to PPS rate, or in addition to reasonable cost if excluded from PPS.

5 OPPS-APC, whether pass-thru drug or not.

6 Can not furnish as that "provider" type;

7 $10.00 per 1000 units (Payment rate for EPO set in statute).

8 May get carrier billing number if qualified and bill carrier.

++ Except in the State of Washington, where CMS permits the RDF to bill immunosuppressives due to the unique State assistance to the beneficiary provided only via the RDF.

Medicare References

Provider/Drug	Hepatitis B Vaccine	Pneumococcal & Flu Vaccines	Hemophilia Clotting Factors	Immuno Suppressive	Erythro- (EPO)	Self Admin Anti-Cancer Anti-Emetic	Other
Hospital Inpatient (IP) A ¬Prospective Payment System (IPPS)	1	1	4	1	1	1	1
Hospital IP A - not IPPS	3	3	3	3	3	3	3
Hospital IP B Outpatient Prospective Payment System (OPPS)	5	3	5	5	5	5	5
Hospital IP B - not OPPS I	3	3	3	3	3	3	3
Hospital Outpatient (OP) - OPPS I	5	3	5	5 (30 day supply)	5	5	5
Hospital OP - not OPPS hospital	3	3	3	3	3	3	5
Skilled Nursing Facility (SNF)	1	1	1	1	1	1	1
SNF IP B	3	3	3	3	6	6	6
SNF OP	3	3	3	3	6	6	6
Independent Renal Dialysis Facility (RDF)	3	3	6	6++	7	6	1/2†
Hospital based RDF	5	5	5	6	7	6	3
Comprehensive Outpatient Rehabilitation Facility (CORF)/ Outpatient Rehabilitation Facility (ORF)	5	2	6	2*	2	6	2
Community Mental Health Clinic (CMHC)	6	6	6	6	6	6	6
Rural Health Clinical (RHC)/Federally Qualified Health Clinic (FQHC) -hospital based	1	1	5	5	5	5	5
RHC/FQHC-independent	1	1	8,2*	8,2*	8,2*	8,2*	8,2*
Home Health Agencies (HHA)	5	3	5	5	5	5	5
Hospice	6 1	6 1	6 1	6 1	6 1	6 1	6 1
Physicians	2*	2*	2*	2*	2*	2*	2*
Pharmacy	2*	2*	2*	2*	7*	2*	2*
Durable Medical Equipment, Prosthetics, Orthotics, and Supplies (DMEPOS) Supplier	2*	2*	2*	2*	7*	2	2*
Critical Access Hospital (CAH) Outpt-Method I	3	3	3	3	3	3	3
CAH Outpt-Method II	3	3	3	3	3	3	3
CAH Inpt	3	3	3	3	3	3	3

NOTE: RHCs do not bill for vaccines. These are paid on the cost report. Vaccine payment to FQHCs is bundled into the encounter rate. Hepatitis B vaccine is paid on a reasonable cost basis in a hospital outpatient department. Deductible and coinsurance apply. Influenza and pneumococcal vaccines are also paid on a reasonable cost basis in a hospital outpatient department. Neither deductible nor coinsurance apply. HHAs cannot bill for vaccines, except on TOB 34X, since vaccines are not part of the HH benefit and cannot be paid under HH PPS. Pneumococcal and influenza are paid once for the vaccine and once for the administration of the vaccine. The provider or supplier (including physician) must enter each of the HCPCS on separate lines of the claim.

A Part B blood clotting factor claim from a Part B supplier is processed by the Local Part B Carrier.

A Part A blood clotting factor claim from a Part A provider, including a hospital-based hemophilia center, is processed by the hospital's Medicare contractor.

Pub 100-4, 17, 80 – Claims Processing for Special Drug Categories

(Rev. 1, 10-01-03)

NOTE: Preventive vaccines, influenza, pneumococcal and hepatitis B, are covered in Chapter 18 of this manual.

NOTE: The definition of Off-Label and its uses are described in the **Medicare Benefit Policy Manual**, Chapter 15.

Pub 100-4, 17, 80.1 – Oral Cancer Drugs

(Rev. 1, 10-01-03)

A3 3660.13, SNF 536.1

Effective January 1, 1994, oral self administered versions of covered injectable cancer drugs furnished may be paid if other coverage requirements are met. To be covered the drug must have had the same active ingredient as the injectable drug. Effective January 1, 1999, this coverage was expanded to include FDA approved Prodrugs used as anticancer drugs. A Prodrug may have a different chemical composition than the injectable drug but body metabolizing of the Prodrug results in the same chemical composition in the body.

Pub 100-4, 17, 80.1.1 – HCPCS Service Coding for Oral Cancer Drugs

(Rev. 1, 10-01-03)

The following codes may be used for drugs other than Prodrugs, when covered:

Generic/Chemical Name	How Supplied	HCPCS
Busulfan 2 mg	ORAL	J8510
Capecitabine 150mg	ORAL	J8520
Capecitabine 500mg	ORAL	J8521
Methotrexate 2.5 mg	ORAL	J8610
Cyclophosphamide * 25 mg	ORAL	J8530
Cyclophosphamide * (Treat 50 mg. as 2 units) 50 mg	ORAL	J8530
Etoposide 50 mg	ORAL	J8560
Melphalan 2 mg	ORAL	J8600
Prescription Drug chemotherapeutic NOC	ORAL	J8999

Each tablet or capsule is equal to one unit, except for 50 mg./ORAL of cyclophosphamide (J8530), which is shown as 2 units. The 25m and 50 mg share the same code. NOTE: HIPAA requires that drug claims submitted to DMERCs be identified by NDC.

Pub 100-4, 17, 80.1.2 – HCPCS and NDC Reporting for Prodrugs

(Rev. 136, 04-09-04)

FI claims

For oral anti-cancer Prodrugs HCPCS code J8999 is reported with revenue code 0636.

DMERC claims

The supplier reports the NDC code on the claim. The DMERC converts the NDC code to a "WW" HCPCS code for CWF. As new "WW" codes are established for oral anticancer drugs they will be communicated in a Recurring Update Notification.

Pub 100-4, 17, 80.1.3 – Other Claims Processing Issues for Oral Cancer Drugs

(Rev. 1, 10-01-03)

Deductible and coinsurance apply. A cancer diagnosis code must be reported when billing for these HCPCS codes. If there is no cancer diagnosis the claims is denied. The number of tablets or capsules is reported as units.

Pub 100-4, 17, 80.1.4 – MSN/ANSI X12N Message Codes for Oral Cancer Drug Denials

(Rev. 1, 10-01-03)

If the claim for an oral cancer drug is denied because it was not approved by FDA, is not considered to be a medically accepted treatment for cancer, or is not the chemical equivalent of a covered injectable cancer drug (or a covered Prodrug), use the appropriate message on the MSN:

6.2 Drugs not specifically classified as effective by the Food and Drug Administration are not covered. (ANSI X12 Adjustment Code 114)

6.3 Payment cannot be made for oral drugs that do not have the same active ingredients as they would have if given by injection. (ANSI X12 Group Code-PR 46)

Pub 100-4, 17, 80.2 – Oral Anti-Emetic Drugs Used as Full Replacement for Intravenous Anti-Emetic Drugs as Part of a Cancer Chemotherapeutic Regimen

(Rev. 1599, Issued: 09-19-08, Effective: 10-01-08, Implementation: 10-06-08)

See the ***Medicare Benefits Policy Manual***, Chapter 15, for detailed coverage requirements.

Effective for dates of service on or after January 1, 1998, FIs and carriers pay for oral anti-emetic drugs when used as full therapeutic replacement for intravenous dosage forms as part of a cancer chemotherapeutic regimen when the drug(s) is administered or prescribed by a physician for use immediately before, at, or within 48 hours after the time of administration of the chemotherapeutic agent.

The allowable period of covered therapy includes day one, the date of service of the chemotherapy drug (beginning of the time of treatment), plus a period not to exceed two additional calendar days, or a maximum period up to 48 hours. Some drugs are limited to 24 hours; some to 48 hours. The hour limit is included in the narrative description of the HCPCS code.

The oral three drug combination is aprepitant, a 5-HT3 antagonist, e.g. granisetron, ondansetron, or dolasetron, and dexamethasone, a corticosteroid.

The oral anti-emetic drug(s) should be prescribed only on a per chemotherapy treatment basis. For example, only enough of the oral anti-emetic(s) for one 24- or 48-hour dosage regimen (depending upon the drug) should be prescribed/supplied for each incidence of chemotherapy treatment. The three drug combination protocol requires the first dose to be administered before, during, or immediately after the anti-cancer chemotherapy administration. The second day is defined as "within 24 hours" and the third day is defined as "within 48 hours" of the chemotherapy administration. These drugs may be supplied by the physician in the office, by an inpatient or outpatient provider (e.g., hospital, CAH, SNF), or through a supplier (e.g., a pharmacy).

The physician must indicate on the prescription that the beneficiary is receiving the oral anti-emetic drug(s) as full therapeutic replacement for an intravenous anti-emetic drug as part of a cancer chemotherapeutic regimen. Where the drug is provided by a facility, the beneficiary's medical record maintained by the facility must be documented to reflect that the beneficiary is receiving the oral anti-emetic drug(s) as full therapeutic replacement for an intravenous anti-emetic drug as part of a cancer chemotherapeutic regimen.

Payment for these drugs is made under Part B. Beginning 1/1/05, the payment allowance limit for these Part B drugs (the term "drugs" includes biologicals) will be based on the Average Sales Price (ASP) plus 6%. Hospital outpatient department providers may either:

(1) Bill the entire Tri-Pak to the FI (three days of aprepitant, 57 units of J8501), or (2) Bill the first day's drug to their local FI or A/B MAC, and give a prescription for the second and third days' supply of aprepitant.

If billed to the FI, all three drugs in the combination oral anti-emetic must be on the same claim. Providers subject to the hospital outpatient PPS will be paid on the basis of an APC. If the hospital outpatient department dispenses the aprepitant for days two and three to the beneficiary and bills the DME MAC for the take home drugs, the hospital's billing department should review all instructions for billing oral anti-emetics. Follow this link to reach the LCD for oral anti-emetics:

http://www.cms.hhs.gov/mcd/viewlcd.asp?lcd_id=5058&lcd_version=27&show=all

In the case of IV Emend provided on day 1, payment for days 2 and 3 would not be made under Part B.

Payment allowances for these drugs dispensed in physician offices will be based on the lower of the submitted charge or the ASP file price. These drugs continue to be priced based on the date of service. The drug payment allowance limit pricing file is distributed to contractors by CMS on a quarterly basis.

The HCPCS codes shown in section 80.2.1 are used.

The CWF edits claims with these codes to assure that the beneficiary is receiving the oral anti-emetic(s) as part of a cancer chemotherapeutic regimen by requiring a diagnosis of cancer.

Most drugs furnished as an outpatient hospital service are packaged under OPPS. However, chemotherapeutic agents and the supportive and adjunctive drugs used with them are paid separately.

Effective for dates of service on or after April 4, 2005, coverage for the use of the oral anti-emetic 3-drug combination of aprepitant (Emend®), a 5-HT3 antagonist, and dexamethasone is considered reasonable and necessary for only those patients who are receiving one or more of the following anti-cancer chemotherapeutic agents:

- Carmustine
- Cisplatin
- Cyclophosphamide
- Dacarbazine
- Mechlorethamine
- Streptozocin
- Doxorubicin
- Epirubicin

Pub 100-4, 17, 80.2.1 – HCPCS Codes for Oral Anti-Emetic Drugs

(Rev. 590, Issued: 06-24-05, Effective: 04-04-05, Implementation: 07-05-05)

The physician/supplier bills for these drugs on Form CMS-1500 or its electronic equivalent. The facility bills for these drugs on Form CMS-1450 or its electronic equivalent. The following HCPCS codes are assigned:

Medicare References

HCPCS Code	Drug Name	Notes
J8501	APREPITANT, 5mg, Oral	(Code is Effective 1/1/05 but coverage is effective 4/4/05, Note: Aprepitant is only covered in combination with a 5-HT3 antagonist, and dexamethasone for beneficiaries who have received one or more of the specified anti-cancer chemotherapeutic agents.
Q0163	DIPHENHYDRAMINE HYDROCHLORIDE 50mg, oral	FDA-approved prescription anti-emetic, for use as a complete therapeutic substitute for an IV anti-emetic at time of chemotherapy treatment not to exceed a 48-hour dosage regimen.
Q0164	PROCHLORPERAZINE MALEATE 5mg, oral	FDA-approved prescription anti-emetic, for use as a complete therapeutic substitute for an IV anti-emetic at the time of chemotherapy treatment, not to exceed a 48-hour dosage regimen.
Q0165	PROCHLORPERAZINE MALEATE 10mg, oral	FDA-approved prescription anti-emetic, for use as a complete therapeutic substitute for an IV anti-emetic at the time of chemotherapy treatment, not to exceed a 48-hour dosage regimen.
Q0166	GRANISETRON HYDROCHLORIDE 1mg, oral	FDA-approved prescription anti-emetic, for use as a complete therapeutic substitute for an IV anti-emetic at the time of chemotherapy treatment, not to exceed a 24-hour dosage regimen.
Q0167	DRONABINOL 2.5mg, oral	FDA-approved prescription anti-emetic, for use as a complete therapeutic substitute for an IV anti-emetic at the time of chemotherapy treatment, not to exceed a 48-hour dosage regimen.
Q0168	DRONABINOL 5mg, oral	FDA-approved prescription anti-emetic, for use as a complete therapeutic substitute for an IV anti-emetic at the time of chemotherapy treatment, not to exceed a 48-hour dosage regimen.
Q0169	PROMETHAZINE HYDROCHLORIDE 12.5mg, oral	FDA-approved prescription anti-emetic, for use as a complete therapeutic substitute for an IV anti-emetic at the time of chemotherapy treatment, not to exceed a 48-hour dosage regimen.
Q0170	PROMETHAZINE HYDROCHLORIDE 25mg, oral	FDA-approved prescription anti-emetic, for use as a complete therapeutic substitute for an IV anti-emetic at the time of chemotherapy treatment, not to exceed a 48-hour dosage regimen.
Q0171	CHLORPROMAZINE HYDROCHLORIDE 10mg, oral	FDA-approved prescription anti-emetic, for use as a complete therapeutic substitute for an IV anti-emetic at the time of chemotherapy treatment, not to exceed a 48-hour dosage regimen.
Q0172	CHLORPROMAZINE HYDROCHLORIDE 25mg, oral	FDA-approved prescription anti-emetic, for use as a complete therapeutic substitute for an IV anti-emetic at the time of chemotherapy treatment, not to exceed a 48-hour dosage regimen.
Q0173	TRIMETHOBENZAMIDE HYDROCHLORIDE 250mg, oral	FDA-approved prescription anti-emetic, for use as a complete therapeutic substitute for an IV anti-emetic at the time of chemotherapy treatment, not to exceed a 48-hour dosage regimen.
Q0174	THIETHYLPERAZINE MALEATE 10mg, oral	FDA-approved prescription anti-emetic, for use as a complete therapeutic substitute for an IV anti-emetic at the time of chemotherapy treatment, not to exceed a 48-hour dosage regimen.
Q0175	PERPHENAZINE 4mg, oral	FDA-approved prescription anti-emetic, for use as a complete therapeutic substitute for an IV anti-emetic at the time of chemotherapy treatment, not to exceed a 48-hour dosage regimen.
Q0176	PERPHENAZINE 8mg, oral	FDA-approved prescription anti-emetic, for use as a complete therapeutic substitute for an IV anti-emetic at the time of chemotherapy treatment, not to exceed a 48-hours dosage regimen.
Q0177	HYDROXYZINE PAMOATE 25mg, oral	FDA-approved prescription antiemetic, for use as a complete therapeutic substitute for an IV anti-emetic at the time of chemotherapy treatment, not to exceed a 48-hour dosage regimen.
Q0178	HYDROXYZINE PAMOATE 50mg, oral	FDA-approved prescription antiemetic, for use as a complete therapeutic substitute for an IV anti-emetic at the time of chemotherapy treatment, not to exceed a 48-hour dosage regimen.
Q0179	ONDANSETRON HYDROCHLORIDE 8mg, oral	FDA-approved prescription anti-emetic, for use as a complete therapeutic substitute for an IV anti-emetic at the time of chemotherapy treatment, not to exceed a 48-hour dosage regimen.
Q0180	DOLASETRON MESYLATE 100mg, oral	FDA-approved prescription antiemetic, for use as a complete therapeutic substitute for an IV anti-emetic at the time of chemotherapy treatment, not to exceed a 24-hour dosage regimen.
Q0181	UNSPECIFIED ORAL DOSAGE FORM	FDA-approved prescription antiemetic, for use as a complete therapeutic substitute for an IV anti-emetic at the time of chemotherapy treatment, not to exceed a 48-hour dosage regimen

NOTE: The 24-hour maximum drug supply limitation on dispensing, for HCPCS Codes Q0166 and Q0180, has been established to bring the Medicare benefit as it applies to these two therapeutic entities in conformity with the "Indications and Usage" section of currently FDA-approved product labeling for each affected drug product.

Pub 100-4, 17, 80.2.2 – Claims Processing Jurisdiction for Oral Anti-Emetic Drugs

(Rev. 882, Issued: 03-03-06; Effective: 07-01-06; Implementation: 07-03-06)

The following chart shows which drugs are billed to the local carrier or FI and which to the DMERC.

Per the BBA '97, effective for claims with dates of service on or after January 1, 1998, the claims processing jurisdiction rules in Chart 1 apply. Effective July 1, 2006, claims from institutional (hospital) pharmacies are also billed as shown in this chart.

CHART 1

COMBINATION	JURISDICTION
Oral anti-cancer chemotherapy drug with oral anti-emetic drug	DMERC maintains processing responsibility for the NDC oral anti-cancer chemotherapy drug and the K0415 oral anti-emetic drug code combinations. DMERC processes the NDC oral anti-cancer chemotherapy drug and Q code oral anti-emetic drug(s) when provided in the physician's office. DMERC processes the NDC oral anti-cancer chemotherapy drug and/or Q code oral anti-emetic drug(s) when supplied by a pharmacy, including a hospital pharmacy.
Oral anti-cancer chemotherapy drug with rectal anti-emetic drug	DMERC maintains responsibility for processing both the NDC oral anti-cancer chemotherapy drug and the K0416 rectal anti-emetic drug.
Oral anti-cancer chemotherapy drug with intravenous anti-emetic drug	DMERC maintains responsibility for processing the NDC oral anti-cancer chemotherapy drug and the local carrier or FI for processing the intravenous anti-emetic J code drug(s).
Intravenous anti-cancer chemotherapy drug with oral anti-emetic drug	Local carrier or FI processes the intravenous J code anticancer chemotherapy drug. The oral anti-emetic Q code drug(s) is processed by the DMERC when provided in the physician's office, hospital, or when provided by a supplier.
Intravenous anti-cancer chemotherapy drug with intravenous anti-emetic drug	Local carrier or FI processes both intravenous anticancer chemotherapy J code drug and intravenous antiemetic J code drug(s).

For claims with dates of service prior to January 1, 1998, per OBRA '93, the claims processing jurisdiction rules in Chart 2 apply.

Medicare References

CHART 2

COMBINATION	UNDER OBRA '93
Oral anti-cancer chemotherapy drug with oral anti-emetic drug	DMERC processes both oral anti-cancer chemotherapy drug (NDC) [1] and the oral anti-emetic drug (HCPCS code J8498) [2].
Oral anti-cancer chemotherapy drug with rectal anti-emetic drug	DMERC processes both the oral anti-cancer chemotherapy drug (NDC) [1] and the anti-emetic drug (HCPCS code J8498) [2].
Oral anti-cancer chemotherapy drug with intravenous anti-emetic drug	DMERC processes the oral anti-cancer chemotherapy drug (NDC) [1] and the local carrier or FI processes the intravenous anti-emetic drug (NDC) [3].
Intravenous anti-cancer chemotherapy drug with oral anti-emetic drug	Local carrier or FI processes intravenous anti-cancer chemotherapy drug (NDC) [3] and self-administered oral anti-emetic drug is noncovered.
Intravenous anti-cancer chemotherapy drug with intravenous anti-emetic drug	Local carrier or FI processes both intravenous anticancer chemotherapy drug (NDC) [3] and intravenous anti-emetic drug (NDC) [3].

Key:
1 = OBRA '93 Legislation (Coverage for Oral Anti-Cancer Drugs)
2 = Carrier Manual Transmittal No. 1528 (November 1995) (Adds oral/rectal anti-emetic)
3 = "Incident to" a physician service

Providers (HIPAA definition) that bill the DMERC require a supplier number issued by the NSC in order to submit claims. Medicare Carriers and Fiscal Intermediaries (FIs) should instruct providers without a supplier number to contact the National Supplier Clearinghouse (NSC) service center at 1-866-238-9652 to request an enrollment package for a supplier number. Alternatively, providers may go to the CMS Web site, cms.hhs.gov/providers/enrollment/default.asp, and download the Form CMS-855-S in Adobe Acrobat format. The application can be completed hard copy and submitted to the NSC.

Pub 100-4, 17, 80.2.3 – MSN /ANSI X12N Denial Messages for Anti-Emetic Drugs

(Rev. 684, Issued: 09-23-05; Effective and Implementation Dates: 12-23-05)

If the claim for an anti-emetic drug is denied because FDA did not approve it or because the drug is not being used as part of an anticancer chemotherapeutic regimen, the contractor uses one of the following appropriate messages on the MSN:

6.2 Drugs not specifically classified as effective by the Food and Drug Administration are not covered. (ANSI X12 Adjustment Code 114)

6.4 Medicare does not pay for an oral anti-emetic drug that is not administered for use immediately before, at, or within 48 hours after administration of a Medicare covered chemotherapy drug. (ANSI X12 Group Code PR 96 with Remark Code M100)

Pub 100-4, 17, 80.2.4 – Billing and Payment Instructions for FIs

(Rev.1472, Issued: 03-06-08, Effective: 05-23-07, Implementation: 04-07-08)

Claims for the initial dose of the oral anti-emetic drug aprepitant must be billed to the FI on the ASC 837I or on hard copy Form CMS-1450 (UB-92) with the appropriate cancer diagnosis and HCPCS code or CPT code. The following payment methodologies apply when furnished to hospital and SNF outpatients:

- Based on APC for hospitals subject to OPPS.
- Under current payment methodologies for hospitals not subject to OPPS.
- On a reasonable cost basis for SNFs.

Institutional providers bill for aprepitant under Revenue Code 0636 (Drugs requiring detailed coding).

Medicare contractors shall pay claims submitted for services provided by a CAH as follows: Method I technical services are paid at 101% of reasonable cost; Method II technical services are paid at 101% of reasonable cost, and, Professional services are paid at 115% of the Medicare Physician Fee Schedule Data Base.

NOTE: Inpatient claims submitted for oral anti-emetic drugs are processed under the current payment methodologies.

Pub 100-4, 17, 80.3 – Billing for Immunosuppressive Drugs

(Rev. 1448; Issued: 02-15-08; Effective: 07-01-08; Implementation: 07-07-08)

B3-4471, A3-3660.8, PM AB-01-10

Beginning January 1, 1987, Medicare pays for FDA approved immunosuppressive drugs and for drugs used in immunosuppressive therapy. (See the ***Medicare Benefit Policy Manual***, Chapter 15 for detailed coverage requirements.) Generally, contractors pay for self-administered immunosuppressive drugs that are specifically labeled and approved for marketing as such by the FDA, or identified in FDA-approved labeling for use in conjunction with immunosuppressive drug therapy. This benefit is subject to the Part B deductible and coinsurance provision.

Contractors are expected to keep informed of FDA additions to the list of the immunosuppressive drugs and notify providers. Prescriptions for immunosuppressive drugs generally should be nonrefillable and limited to a 30-day supply. The 30-day guideline is necessary because dosage frequently diminishes over a period of time, and further, it is not uncommon for the physician to change the prescription from one drug to another. Also, these drugs are expensive and the coinsurance liability on unused drugs could be a financial burden to the beneficiary. Unless there are special circumstances, contractors will not consider a supply of drugs in excess of 30 days to be reasonable and necessary and should deny payment accordingly.

Entities that normally bill the carrier bill the DMERC. Entities that normally bill the FI continue to bill the FI, except for hospitals subject to OPPS, which must bill the DMERC.

Prior to December 21, 2000 coverage was limited to immunosuppressive drugs received within 36 months of a transplant. ESRD beneficiaries continue to be limited to 36 months of coverage after a Medicare covered kidney transplant. For all other beneficiaries, BBA '97 increased the length of time a beneficiary could receive immunosuppressives by a sliding method. So for the period 8/97 thru 12/00 a longer period of time MAY apply for a transplant. Effective with immunosuppressive drugs furnished on or after December 21, 2000, there is no time limit, but an organ transplant must have occurred for which immunosuppressive therapy is appropriate. That is, the time limit for immunosuppressive drugs was eliminated for transplant beneficiaries that will continue Medicare coverage after 36 months based on disability or age. The date of transplant is reported to the FI with occurrence code 36.

CWF will edit claim records to determine if a history of a transplant is on record. If not an error will be returned. See Chapter 27 for edit codes and resolution.

Pub 100-4, 17, 80.3.1 – Requirements for Billing FI for Immunosuppressive Drugs

(Rev. 1472, Issued: 03-06-08, Effective: 05-23-07, Implementation: 04-07-08)

Beginning January 1, 1987, Medicare pays for FDA approved immunosuppressive drugs and for drugs used in immunosuppressive therapy. (See the ***Medicare Benefit Policy Manual***, Chapter 15 for detailed coverage requirements.) Generally, contractors pay for self-administered immunosuppressive drugs that are specifically labeled and approved for marketing as such by the FDA, or identified in FDA-approved labeling for use in conjunction with immunosuppressive drug therapy. This benefit is subject to the Part B deductible and coinsurance provision.

Contractors are expected to keep informed of FDA additions to the list of the immunosuppressive drugs and notify providers. Prescriptions for immunosuppressive drugs generally should be nonrefillable and limited to a 30-day supply. The 30-day guideline is necessary because dosage frequently diminishes over a period of time, and further, it is not uncommon for the physician to change the prescription from one drug to another. Also, these drugs are expensive and the coinsurance liability on unused drugs could be a financial burden to the beneficiary. Unless there are special circumstances, contractors will not consider a supply of drugs in excess of 30 days to be reasonable and necessary and should deny payment accordingly.

Entities that normally bill the carrier bill the DME MAC. Entities that normally bill the FI continue to bill the FI, except for hospitals subject to OPPS, which must bill the DME MAC.

Prior to December 21, 2000 coverage was limited to immunosuppressive drugs received within 36 months of a transplant. ESRD beneficiaries continue to be limited to 36 months of coverage after a Medicare covered kidney transplant. For all other beneficiaries, BBA '97 increased the length of time a beneficiary could receive immunosuppressives by a sliding method. So for the period 8/97 thru 12/00 a longer period of time MAY apply for a transplant. Effective with immunosuppressive drugs furnished on or after December 21, 2000, there is no time limit, but an organ transplant must have occurred for which immunosuppressive therapy is appropriate. That is, the time limit for immunosuppressive drugs was eliminated for transplant beneficiaries that will continue Medicare coverage after 36 months based on disability or age. The date of transplant is reported to the FI with occurrence code 36.

CWF will edit claim records to determine if a history of a transplant is on record. If not, an error will be returned.

For claims filed on and after July 1, 2008, suppliers that furnish an immunosuppressive drug to a Medicare beneficiary, when such drug has been prescribed due to the beneficiary having undergone an organ transplant, shall: 1) secure from the prescriber the date of such organ transplant, 2) retain documentation of such transplant date in its files, and 3) annotate the Medicare claim for such drug with the "KX" modifier to signify both that the supplier retains such documentation of the beneficiary's transplant date and that such transplant date precedes the Date of Service (DOS) for furnishing the drug.

For claims received on and after July 1, 2008, contractors shall accept claims for immunosuppressive drugs without a KX modifier but shall deny such claims unless a query of the Master Beneficiary Record (MBR) shows that Medicare has made payment for an organ transplant on a date that precedes the DOS of the immunosuppressive drug claim.

In the context of a claim for an immunosuppressive drug that is submitted to Medicare in order to receive payment, the use of the KX modifier signifies that the supplier has documentation on file to the effect that the beneficiary has undergone an organ transplant on a date certain and that the immunosuppressive drug has been prescribed incident to such transplant.

If a supplier has not determined (or does not have documentation on file to support a determination) that either the beneficiary did not receive an organ transplant or that the beneficiary was not enrolled in Medicare Part A as of the date of the transplant, then the supplier may not, with respect to furnishing an immunosuppressive drug: 1) bill Medicare, 2) bill or collect any amount from the beneficiary, or 3) issue an Advance Beneficiary Notice (ABN) to the beneficiary.

Pub 100-4, 17, 80.3.1 – Requirements for Billing FI for Immunosuppressive Drugs

(Rev. 1472, Issued: 03-06-08, Effective: 05-23-07, Implementation: 04-07-08)

Hospitals not subject to OPPS bill on a Form CMS-1450 with bill type 12x (hospital inpatient Part B) or l3x (hospital outpatient) as appropriate. For claims with dates of service prior to April 1, 2000, providers report the following entries:

- Occurrence code 36 and date
- Revenue code 0250
- Narrative description

NOTE: Information regarding the claim form locators that correspond with these fields and a table to crosswalk the CMS-1450 form locators to the 837 transaction is found in Chapter 25.

For claims with dates of service on or after April 1, 2000, hospitals report

- Occurrence code 36 and date
- Revenue code 0636
- HCPCS code of the immunosuppressive drug
- Number of units (the number of units billed must accurately reflect the definition of one unit of service in each code narrative. E.g.,: If fifty 10-mg. Prednisone tablets are dispensed, the hospital bills J7506, 100 units (1 unit of J7506 = 5 mg.)

NOTE: Information regarding the claim form locators that correspond with these fields and a table to crosswalk the CMS-1450 form locators to the 837 transaction is found in Chapter 25. The hospital completes the remaining items in accordance with regular billing instructions.

Pub 100-4, 17, 80.3.2 – MSN/Remittance Messages for Immunosuppressive Drugs

(Rev. 1, 10-01-03)

A. MSN

MSN messages for denied Immunosuppressive Drugs are as follows: If no transplant use:

6.2 Drugs not specifically classified as effective by the Food and Drug Administration are not covered.

If the claim for an immunosuppressive drug is partially denied because of the 30-day supply limitation, use the following message:

4.3 Prescriptions for immunosuppressive drugs are limited to a 30-day supply.

B. Remittance

Remittance codes/messages for denied Immunosuppressive Drugs are as follows:

- If the claim is denied because the immunosuppressive drug is not approved by the FDA, the FI uses existing American National Standard Institute (ANSI) X-12-835 claim adjustment reason code/message 114, Procedure/product not approved by the Food and Drug Administration.
- If the claim is denied because the benefit period has expired or because of the 30 day limitation, the FI uses existing ANSI X12N 835 claim adjustment reason code/message 35, Benefit maximum has been reached.
- If the claim is denied for the immunosuppressive drug because a transplant was not covered, the FI uses existing ANSI X12N 835 claim adjustment reason code/message 107, Claim/service denied because the related or qualifying claim/service was not paid or identified on the claim.

Pub 100-4, 17, 80.4 – Billing for Hemophilia Clotting Factors

(Rev. 1564, Issued: 07-25-08, Effective: 04-01-08, Implementation: 01-05-09)

Blood clotting factors not paid on a cost or prospective payment system basis are priced as a drug/biological under the drug pricing fee schedule effective for the specific date of service. As of January 1, 2005, the average sales price (ASP) plus 6 percent shall be used.

If a beneficiary is in a covered part A stay in a PPS hospital, the clotting factors are paid in addition to the DRG/HIPPS payment. For FY 2005, this payment is based on 95 percent of AWP. For FY 2006, the add-on payment for blood clotting factor administered to hemophilia inpatients is based on average sales price (ASP) + 6 percent and a furnishing fee. The furnishing fee is updated each calendar year. For a SNF subject to SNF/PPS, the payment is bundled into the SNF/PPS rate.

For hospitals subject to OPPS, the clotting factors, when paid under Part B, are paid the APC. For SNFs the clotting factors, when paid under Part B, are paid based on cost.

Local carriers and Part B MACs shall process non-institutional blood clotting factor claims. The FIs and Part A MACs shall process institutional blood clotting factor claims (Part A and Part B institutional).The FIs shall process institutional blood clotting factor claims (Part A and Part B institutional).

Pub 100-4, 17, 80.4.1 – Clotting Factor Furnishing Fee

(Rev. 1908; Issued: 02-05-10; Effective Date: 01-01-05; Implementation Date: 03-05-10)

The Medicare Modernization Act section 303(e)(1) added section 1842(o)(5)(C) of the Social Security Act which requires that, beginning January 1, 2005, a furnishing fee will be paid for items and services associated with clotting factor.

Medicare References

Beginning January 1, 2005, a clotting factor furnishing fee is separately payable to entities that furnish clotting factor unless the costs associated with furnishing the clotting factor is paid through another payment system.

The clotting factor furnishing fee is updated each calendar year based on the percentage increase in the consumer price index (CPI) for medical care for the 12-month period ending with June of the previous year. The clotting factor furnishing fees applicable for dates of service in each calendar year (CY) are listed below:

CY 2005 - $0.140 per unit

CY 2006 - $0.146 per unit

CY 2007 - $0.152 per unit

CY 2008 - $0.158 per unit

CY 2009 - $0.164 per unit

CY 2010 - $0.170 per unit

Annual updates to the clotting factor furnishing fee are subsequently communicated by a Recurring Update Notification.

CMS includes this clotting factor furnishing fee in the nationally published payment limit for clotting factor billing codes. When the clotting factor is not included on the Average Sales Price (ASP) Medicare Part B Drug Pricing File or Not Otherwise Classified (NOC) Pricing File, the contractor must make payment for the clotting factor as well as make payment for the furnishing fee.

Pub 100-4, 17, 80.5 – Self-Administered Drugs

(Rev. 1539: Issued: 06-20-08; Effective/Implementation Date: 07-21-08)

See Pub. 100-02, ***Medicare Benefit Policy Manual***, chapter 15, section 50.2.

A. Reporting Requirement

Each carrier and FI must report to CMS every September 1 and April 1 (i.e., every 6 months) its complete list of injectable drugs that are excluded when furnished incident to a physician's service on the basis that the drug is usually self-administered by the patient. Contractors must E-mail this list along with the contractor's name, Medicare identification number and the State(s) affected by the list to: drugdata@cms.hhs.gov.

Pub 100-4, 17, 80.6 – Intravenous Immune Globulin

(Rev. 74, 01-23-04)

Beginning for dates of service on or after January 1, 2004, Medicare pays for intravenous immune globulin administered in the home. (See the **Medicare Benefit Policy Manual**, Chapter 15 for coverage requirements.) Contractors pay for the drug, but not the items or services related to the administration of the drug when administered in the home, if deemed medically appropriate.

Contractors may pay any entity licensed in the State to furnish intravenous immune globulin. Payment will be furnished to the entity with the authority to furnish the drug. Beneficiaries are ineligible to receive payment for the drug. Pharmacies and hospitals dispensing intravenous immune globulin would bill the DMERC. Home Health Agencies dispensing intravenous immune globulin would bill the RHHI. Physicians furnishing intravenous immune globulin for the refilling of an external pump for home infusion would bill the DMERC.

The appropriate ICD-9 codes are as follows: 279.04, 279.05, 279.06, 279.12, and 279.2. The appropriate HCPCs codes are J1563 and J1564.

Pub 100-4, 17, 80.7 – Pharmacy Supplying Fee and Inhalation Drug Dispensing Fee

(Rev. 754, Issued: 11-10-05, Effective: 01-01-06, Implementation: 01-03-06)

Section 303(e) (2) of the MMA implements a supplying fee for immunosuppressive drugs, oral anti-cancer chemotherapeutic drugs, and oral anti-emetic drugs used as part of an anti-cancer chemotherapeutic regimen. Effective January 1, 2005, Medicare paid a separately billable supplying fee of $24.00 to a pharmacy, dialysis facility in the State of Washington or any hospital outpatient department not subject to the OPPS for each supplied prescription of the above-mentioned drugs. In addition, Medicare also paid a separately billable supplying fee of $50.00 for the initial supplied prescription of the immunosuppressive drugs during the first month following the patient's transplant. Effective January 1, 2006, we are changing the supplying fee when multiple prescriptions are supplied in a 30-day period. Medicare will pay $24 for the first prescription of the above-mentioned drugs supplied by a pharmacy in a 30-day period, and will pay $16 for each subsequent prescription, after the first one, supplied in that 30-day period. A pharmacy will be limited to one $24 fee per 30-day period even if the pharmacy supplies more than one category of the abovementioned drugs (for example, an oral-anticancer drug and an oral anti-emetic drug) to a beneficiary. If two different pharmacies supply the above-mentioned drugs to a beneficiary during a 30-day period, each pharmacy will be eligible for one $24 supplying fee for the first prescription supplied during that 30-day period, and a supplying fee of $16 for each subsequent prescription supplied in that 30- day period. For a refill prescription, Medicare will allow payment of a $24 supplying fee to a particular supplier up to seven days before the end of the 30-day period for which the last $24 supplying fee was paid to that supplier; however, each supplier will be limited to twelve $24 supplying fees per beneficiary per year. Medicare will pay a supplying fee for each prescription, including prescriptions for different strengths of the same drug supplied on the same day (for example, a prescription for 100 mg tablets and 5 mg Tablets). These changes do not alter the one-time $50 supplying fee for the first immunosuppressive prescription after a transplant.

We are also changing the dispensing fee for inhalation drugs furnished through durable medical equipment. Effective January 1, 2006, Medicare will pay an initial dispensing fee of $57 to a pharmacy for the initial 30-day period of inhalation drugs furnished through DME regardless of the number of shipments or drugs dispensed during that time and regardless of the number of pharmacies used by a beneficiary during that time. This initial 30-day dispensing fee is a one-time fee applicable only to beneficiaries who are using inhalation drugs for the first time as a Medicare beneficiary. Except in those circumstances where an initial 30-day dispensing fee is applicable, Medicare will pay a dispensing fee of $33 to a pharmacy/supplier for each 30-day supply of inhalation drugs furnished through DME regardless of the number of shipments or drugs dispensed during the 30 day period. Medicare will pay a dispensing fee of $66 to a pharmacy/supplier for each 90-day period of inhalation drugs furnished through DME regardless of the number of shipments or drugs dispensed during the 90 days. Only one 30-day dispensing fee will be payable per 30-day period, and only one 90-day dispensing fee will be payable per 90- day period, regardless of the numbers of suppliers used during the respective periods. A 30-day and 90-day supplying fee cannot be paid for drug supplied for the same month. For a refill prescription, Medicare will allow payment of the dispensing fee no sooner than 7 days before the end of usage for the current 30-day or 90-day period for which a dispensing fee was previously paid. Each inhalation drug supplier will be allowed no more than 12 months of dispensing fees per beneficiary per year. Medicare will not pay separately for compounding drugs. This cost is in the dispensing fees. Supply fees and dispensing fees must be billed on the same claim as the drug.

HCPCS Codes and Fees:

GO369, G0370, G0371, G0374 – not recognized by Medicare as of 1/1/06.

Q0510 First immunosuppressive prescription after a transplant, $50.00 fee

Q0511 Pharmacy supplying fee for immunosuppressive, oral-anti-cancer, and oral antiemetic drugs, first prescription in a one month period. Each pharmacy may receive this fee once in a 30-day period. Fee is $24.00.

Q0512 Pharmacy supplying fee for immunosuppressive, oral anti-cancer, and oral antiemetic drugs – each subsequent prescription in a 30-day period. Fee is $16.00.

Q0513 Pharmacy dispensing fee for inhalation drug(s); per 30-days.

Effective 1/1/06, Medicare will pay a dispensing fee of $33.00 to a pharmacy for a 30- day period of inhalation drugs furnished through DME regardless of the number of shipments or drugs dispensed during that time and regardless of the number of pharmacies used by a beneficiary during that period. Payment will be made on the first claim received.

Q0514 Pharmacy dispensing fee for inhalation drugs(s); per 90-days.

Effective 1/1/06, Medicare will pay a dispensing fee of $66.00 to a pharmacy for a 90- day period of inhalation drugs furnished through DME regardless of the number of shipments or drugs dispensed during that time and regardless of the number of pharmacies used by a beneficiary during that period. Payment will be made on the first claim received.

G0333 Pharmacy dispensing fee for initial inhalation drug(s); initial 30 day supply to a beneficiary.

Effective January 1, 2006, Medicare will pay an initial dispensing fee of $57.00 to a pharmacy for the initial 30-day period of inhalation drugs furnished through DME regardless of the number of shipments or drugs dispensed during that time and regardless of the number of pharmacies used by a beneficiary during that time. This initial 30-day dispensing fee is a one-time fee applicable only to beneficiaries who are using inhalation drugs for the first time as a Medicare beneficiary.

Based on the code descriptions above, a supplying fee and a dispensing fee is not appropriate for one drug. The supplying fee is for immunosuppressives, oral anti-cancer drugs and oral anti-emetic drugs. The dispensing fee is for inhalation drugs only. A supplier cannot be paid for more than one of the following -- an initial dispensing fee (G0333), a 30-day dispensing fee (Q0513), or a 90-day dispensing fee (Q0514) – for a beneficiary for the same period.

Pub 100-4, 17, 80.9 – Hospitals Billing for Epoetin Alfa (EPO) for Non-ESRD Patients

(Rev. 1412, Issued: 01-11-08, Effective: 01-01-08, Implementation: 04-07-08)

Effective January 1, 2008, all non-ESRD claims billing HCPCS J0881 and J0885 must begin reporting one of the following modifiers:

EA: ESA, anemia, chemo-induced

EB: ESA, anemia, radio-induced

EC: ESA, anemia, non-chemo/radio

Institutional claims that do not report one of the above modifiers will be returned to the provider.

Professional claims that are billed without the required modifiers will be returned as unprocessable.

Use Reason code 4 and Remark code MA 130 to return ESA services billed without one of the required modifiers.

ESAs administered for more than one of the indicated therapies are billed as separate line items (i.e., ESAs for chemo-induced anemia (EA modifier) are reported as separate line items (e.g., J0881EA); ESAs for radio-induced anemia (EB modifier) are reported as separate line items (e.g., J0885EB); ESAs for non-chemo/radio induced anemia (EC modifier) are reported as separate line items (e.g., J0881EC). Only one of the three ESA modifiers may be reported at the line item level.

Use Reason code 125 and Remark code N63 to return HCPCS J0881 or J0885 billed with more than one ESA modifier at the line item level.

Pub 100-4, 17, 80.10 – Hospitals Billing for Darbepoetin Alfa (Aranesp) for Non-ESRD Patients

(Rev. 1412, Issued: 01-11-08, Effective: 01-01-08, Implementation: 04-07-08)

NOTE: For EPO and Aranesp billing instructions for beneficiaries with ESRD, see the ***Claims Processing Manual,*** Chapter 8, sections 60.4 and 60.7.

For patients with chronic renal failure who are not yet on a regular course of dialysis, EPO and Aranesp administered in a hospital and billed as an outpatient service on type of bill 13x or inpatient Part B bill type 12x are paid under the Outpatient Prospective Payment System (OPPS). Non-OPPS hospitals are paid on reasonable charges.

Hospitals report charges under revenue code 0636. For EPO, hospitals report charges under revenue code 0636 with HCPCS code J0885 effective January 1, 2006. Aranesp is reported with HCPCS code J0881 effective January 1, 2006.

Pub 100-4, 17, 80.11 – Requirement for Providing Route of Administration Codes for Erythropoiesis Stimulating Agents (ESAs)

(Rev. 1212; Issued: 03-30-07; Effective: 01-01-07; Implementation: 06-29-07)

Patients with end stage renal disease (ESRD) receiving administrations of erythropoiesis stimulating agents (ESA), such as epoetin alfa (EPO) and Darbepoetin alfa (Aranesp) for the treatment of anemia may receive intravenous administration or subcutaneous administrations of the ESA.

Effective for claims submitted on or after February 1, 2007 with dates of services on or after January 1, 2007, all providers billing for injections of ESA for ESRD beneficiaries are encouraged to include the modifier JA on the claim to indicate an intravenous administration or modifier JB to indicate a subcutaneous administration. All providers billing for injections of ESAs for ESRD beneficiaries will be required to include route of administration when claims processing system changes are completed. Renal dialysis facilities claim including charges for administrations of the ESA by both methods must report separate lines to identify the number of administration provided using each method.

Pub 100-4, 18, 10 – Pneumococcal Pneumonia, Influenza Virus, and Hepatitis B Vaccines

(Rev. 1586, Issued: 09-05-08, Effective: 10-06-08, Implementation: 10-06-08)

For Carriers/AB MACs, Part B of Medicare pays 100 percent of the Medicare allowed amount for pneumococcal vaccines and influenza virus vaccines and their administration.

Part B deductible and coinsurance do not apply for pneumococcal and influenza virus vaccine.

Part B of Medicare also covers the hepatitis B vaccine and its administration. Part B deductible and coinsurance do apply for hepatitis B vaccine.

State laws governing who may administer pneumococcal and influenza virus vaccinations and how the vaccines may be transported vary widely. Medicare contractors should instruct physicians, suppliers, and providers to become familiar with State regulations for all vaccines in the areas where they will be immunizing.

Pub 100-4, 18, 10.1 – Coverage Requirements

(Rev. 1586, Issued: 09-05-08, Effective: 10-06-08, Implementation: 10-06-08)

Pneumococcal vaccine, influenza virus vaccine, and hepatitis B vaccine and their administration are covered only under Medicare Part B, regardless of the setting in which they are furnished, even when provided to an inpatient during a hospital stay covered under Part A.

See Pub. 100-02, ***Medicare Benefit Policy Manual***, chapter 15, for additional coverage requirements for pneumococcal vaccine, hepatitis B vaccine, and influenza virus vaccine.

Pub 100-4, 18, 10.1.1 – Pneumococcal Pneumonia Vaccine (PPV)

(Rev. 1586, Issued: 09-05-08, Effective: 10-06-08, Implementation: 10-06-08)

Effective for services furnished on or after July 1, 2000, Medicare does not require for coverage purposes, that a doctor of medicine or osteopathy order the pneumococcal vaccine and its administration. Therefore, the beneficiary may receive the vaccine upon request without a physician's order and without physician supervision.

See Pub. 100-02, ***Medicare Benefit Policy Manual***, chapter 15, section 50.4.4.2 for additional coverage requirements for pneumococcal vaccine.

A. Frequency of PPV Vaccinations

Typically, the pneumococcal vaccine is administered once in a lifetime. Claims are paid for beneficiaries who are at high risk of pneumococcal disease and have not received the pneumococcal vaccine within the last 5 years or are revaccinated because they are unsure of their vaccination status.

An initial pneumococcal vaccination may be administered only to persons at high risk (see below) of pneumococcal disease. Revaccination may be administered only to persons at highest risk of serious pneumococcal infection and those likely to have a rapid decline in pneumococcal antibody levels, provided that at least 5 years have passed since receipt of a previous dose of pneumococcal vaccine.

B. High Risk of Pneumococcal Disease

Persons at high risk for whom an initial vaccine may be administered include:

- All people age 65 and older;
- Immunocompetent adults who are at increased risk of pneumococcal disease or its complications because of chronic illness (e.g., cardiovascular disease, pulmonary disease, diabetes mellitus, alcoholism, cirrhosis, or cerebrospinal fluid leaks); and
- Individuals with compromised immune systems (e.g., splenic dysfunction or anatomic asplenia, Hodgkin's disease, lymphoma, multiple myeloma, chronic renal failure, Human Immunodeficiency Virus (HIV) infection, nephrotic syndrome, sickle cell disease, or organ transplantation).

Persons at highest risk and those most likely to have rapid declines in antibody levels are those for whom revaccination may be appropriate. This group includes persons with functional or anatomic asplenia (e.g., sickle cell disease, splenectomy), HIV infection, leukemia, lymphoma, Hodgkin's disease, multiple myeloma, generalized malignancy chronic renal failure, nephrotic syndrome, or other conditions associated with immunosuppression such as organ or bone marrow transplantation, and those receiving immunosuppressive chemotherapy. Routine revaccinations of people age 65 or older that are not at highest risk are not appropriate.

Those administering the vaccine should not require the patient to present an immunization record prior to administering the pneumococcal vaccine, nor should they feel compelled to review the patient's complete medical record if it is not available. Instead, if the patient is competent, it is acceptable for them to rely on the patient's verbal history to determine prior vaccination status. If the patient is uncertain about their vaccination history in the past 5 years, the vaccine should be given. However, if the patient is certain he/she was vaccinated in the last 5 years, the vaccine should not be given. If the patient is certain that the vaccine was given and that more than 5 years have passed since receipt of the previous dose, revaccination is not appropriate unless the patient is at highest risk.

Pub 100-4, 18, 10.1.2 – Influenza Virus Vaccine

(Rev. 1586, Issued: 09-05-08, Effective: 10-06-08, Implementation: 10-06-08)

Effective for services furnished on or after May 1, 1993, the influenza virus vaccine and its administration is covered when furnished in compliance with any applicable State law. Typically, this vaccine is administered once a year in the fall or winter. Medicare does not require for coverage purposes that a doctor of medicine or osteopathy order the vaccine. Therefore, the beneficiary may receive the vaccine upon request without a physician's order and without physician supervision.

Typically, one influenza vaccination is allowable per influenza virus season. Contractors edit to identify more than one influenza virus vaccine in a 12-month period, and determine medical necessity of services failing the edit. Since there is no yearly limit, contractors determine whether such services are reasonable and necessary (e.g., a patient receives an influenza injection in January for the current influenza season and is vaccinated again in November of the same year for the next influenza season) and allow payment if appropriate.

See Pub. 100-02, ***Medicare Benefit Policy Manual***, chapter 15, section 50.4.4.2 for additional coverage requirements for influenza virus vaccines.

Pub 100-4, 18, 10.2 – Billing Requirements

(Rev. 1586, Issued: 09-05-08, Effective: 10-06-08, Implementation: 10-06-08)

A Edits Not Applicable to PPV or Influenza Virus Vaccine Bills and Their Administration

The Common Working File (CWF) and shared systems bypass all Medicare Secondary Payer (MSP) utilization edits in CWF on all claims when the only service provided is pneumococcal or influenza virus vaccine and/or their administration. This waiver does not apply when other services (e.g., office visits) are billed on the same claim as pneumococcal or influenza virus vaccinations. If the provider knows or has reason to believe that a particular group health plan covers pneumococcal or influenza virus vaccine and their administration, and all other MSP requirements for the Medicare beneficiary are met, the primary payer must be billed.

First claim development alerts from CWF are not generated for pneumococcal or influenza virus vaccines. However, first claim development is performed if other services are submitted along with pneumococcal or development is performed if other services are submitted along with pneumococcal or influenza virus vaccines.

See Pub. 100-05, ***Medicare Secondary Payer Manual***, chapters 4 and 5, for responsibilities for MSP development where applicable.

B Intermediary (FI) Bills

Chapter 25 of this manual provides general billing instructions that must be followed for bills submitted to FIs/AB MACs.

The following "providers of services" may administer and bill the FI/AB MACs for these vaccines:

- Hospitals;
- Critical Access Hospitals (CAHs);
- Skilled Nursing Facilities (SNFs);
- Home Health Agencies (HHAs);
- Comprehensive Outpatient Rehabilitation Facilities (CORFs); and
- Indian Health Service (IHS)/Tribally owned and/or operated hospitals and hospital-based facilities.

Other billing entities that may bill the FIs/AB MACs are:

- Independent Renal Dialysis Facilities (RDFs).

All providers bill the FIs/AB MACs for hepatitis B on Form CMS-1450. Providers other than independent RHCs and freestanding FQHCs bill the FIs/AB MACs for influenza virus and pneumococcal vaccinations on Form CMS-1450. (See §10.2.2.2 of this chapter for special instructions for independent RHCs and freestanding FQHCs and §10.2.4 of this chapter for hospice instruction.)

FIs/AB MACs instruct providers, other than independent RHCs and freestanding FQHCs, to bill for the vaccines and their administration on the same bill. Separate bills for vaccines and their administration are not required. The only exceptions to this rule occur when the vaccine is administered during the course of an otherwise covered home health visit since the vaccine or its administration is not included in the visit charge. (See §10.2.3 of this chapter).

C Carrier Claims

1 Billing for Additional Services

If a physician sees a beneficiary for the sole purpose of administering the influenza virus vaccine, the pneumococcal vaccine, and/or the hepatitis B vaccine, they may not routinely bill for an office visit. However, if the beneficiary actually receives other services constituting an "office visit" level of service, the physician may bill for a visit in addition to the vaccines and their administration, and Medicare will pay for the visit in addition to the vaccines and their administration if it is reasonable and medically necessary.

2. Nonparticipating Physicians and Suppliers

Nonparticipating physicians and suppliers (including local health facilities) that do not accept assignment may collect payment from the beneficiary for the administration of the vaccines, but must submit an unassigned claim on the beneficiary's behalf. Effective for claims with dates of service on or after February 1, 2001, per §114 of the Benefits Improvement and Protection Act of 2000, all drugs and biologicals must be paid based on mandatory assignment. Therefore, regardless of whether the physician and supplier usually accept assignment, they must accept assignment for the vaccines, may not collect any fee up front, and must submit the claim for the beneficiary.

Entities, such as local health facilities, that have never submitted Medicare claims must obtain a National Provider Identifier (NPI) for Part B billing purposes.

3. Separate Claims for Vaccine and Their Administration

In situations in which the vaccine and the administration are furnished by two different entities, the entities should submit separate claims. For example, a supplier (e.g., a pharmacist) may bill separately for the vaccine, using the Healthcare Common Procedural Coding System (HCPCS) code for the vaccine, and the physician or supplier (e.g., a drugstore) who actually administers the vaccine may bill separately for the administration, using the HCPCS code for the administration. This procedure results in contractors receiving two claims, one for the vaccine and one for its administration.

For example, when billing for influenza virus vaccine administration only, billers should list only HCPCS code G0008 in block 24D of the Form CMS-1500. When billing for the influenza virus vaccine only, billers should list only HCPCS code 90658 in block 24D of the Form CMS-1500. The same applies for pneumococcal and hepatitis B billing using pneumococcal and hepatitis B HCPCS codes.

Pub 100-4, 18, 10.2.1 – Healthcare Common Procedure Coding System (HCPCS) and Diagnosis Codes

(Rev. 1586, Issued: 09-05-08, Effective: 10-06-08, Implementation: 10-06-08)

Vaccines and their administration are reported using separate codes. The following codes are for reporting the vaccines only.

HCPCS	Definition
90655	Influenza virus vaccine, split virus, preservative free, for children 6-35 months of age, for intramuscular use;
90656	Influenza virus vaccine, split virus, preservative free, for use in individuals 3 years and above, for intramuscular use;
90657	Influenza virus vaccine, split virus, for children 6-35 months of age, for intramuscular use;
90658	Influenza virus vaccine, split virus, for use in individuals 3 years of age and above, for intramuscular use;
90659	Influenza virus vaccine, whole virus, for intramuscular or jet injection use (Discontinued December 31, 2003);
90660	Influenza virus vaccine, live, for intranasal use;
90669	Pneumococcal conjugate vaccine, polyvalent, for children under 5 years, for intramuscular use
90732	Pneumococcal polysaccharide vaccine, 23-valent, adult or immunosuppressed patient dosage, for use in individuals 2 years or older, for subcutaneous or intramuscular use;
90740	Hepatitis B vaccine, dialysis or immunosuppressed patient dosage (3 dose schedule), for intramuscular use;
90743	Hepatitis B vaccine, adolescent (2 dose schedule), for intramuscular use;
90744	Hepatitis B vaccine, pediatric/adolescent dosage (3 dose schedule), for intramuscular use;
90746	Hepatitis B vaccine, adult dosage, for intramuscular use; and
90747	Hepatitis B vaccine, dialysis or immunosuppressed patient dosage (4 dose schedule), for intramuscular use.

The following codes are for reporting administration of the vaccines only. The administration of the vaccines is billed using:

HCPCS	Definition
G0008	Administration of influenza virus vaccine;
G0009	Administration of pneumococcal vaccine; and
*G0010	Administration of Hepatitis B vaccine.
*90471	Immunization administration. (For OPPS hospitals billing for the Hepatitis B vaccine administration)
*90472	Each additional vaccine. (For OPPS hospitals billing for the Hepatitis B vaccine administration)

** Note: For claims with dates of service prior to January 1, 2006, OPPS and non-OPPS hospitals report G0010 for Hepatitis B vaccine administration. For claims with dates of service January 1, 2006 and later, OPPS hospitals report 90471 or 90472 for hepatitis B vaccine administration as appropriate in place of G0010.*

One of the following diagnosis codes must be reported as appropriate. If the sole purpose for the visit is to receive a vaccine or if a vaccine is the only service billed on a claim the applicable following diagnosis code may be used.

Diagnosis Code	Description
V03.82	PPV
V04.81**	Influenza
V06.6***	PPV and Influenza
V05.3	Hepatitis B

***Effective for influenza virus claims with dates of service October 1, 2003 and later.*

****Effective October 1, 2006, providers may report diagnosis code V06.6 on claims for pneumococcus and/or influenza virus vaccines when the purpose of the visit was to receive both vaccines.*

If a diagnosis code for pneumococcus, hepatitis B, or influenza virus vaccination is not reported on a claim, contractors may not enter the diagnosis on the claim. Contractors must follow current resolution processes for claims with missing diagnosis codes.

If the diagnosis code and the narrative description are correct, but the HCPCS code is incorrect, the carrier or intermediary may correct the HCPCS code and pay the claim. For example, if the reported diagnosis code is V04.81 and the narrative description (if annotated on the claim) says "flu shot" but the HCPCS code is incorrect, contractors may change the HCPCS code and pay for the flu vaccine. Effective October 1, 2006, carriers/AB MACs should follow the instructions in Pub. 100-04, Chapter 1, Section 80.3.2.1.1 (Carrier Data Element Requirements) for claims submitted without a HCPCS code.

Claims for Hepatitis B vaccinations must report the I.D. Number of referring physician. In addition, if a doctor of medicine or osteopathy does not order the influenza virus vaccine, the intermediary claims require:

- UPIN code SLF000 to be reported on claims submitted prior to the date when Medicare will no longer accept identifiers other than NPIs, or
- The provider's own NPI to be reported in the NPI field for the attending physician on claims submitted when NPI requirements are implemented.

Pub 100-4, 18, 10.2.2 – Bills Submitted to FIs

(Rev. 1586, Issued: 09-05-08, Effective: 10-06-08, Implementation: 10-06-08)

The applicable types of bills acceptable when billing for influenza virus and pneumococcal vaccines are 12X, 13X, 22X, 23X, 34X, 72X, 75X, 83X and 85X.

The following revenue codes are used for reporting vaccines and administration of the vaccines for all providers except RHCs and FQHCs. Independent and provider based RHCs and FQHCs follow §10.2.2.2 below when billing for influenza virus, pneumococcal and hepatitis B vaccines.

Units and HCPCS codes are required with revenue code 0636:

Revenue Code	Description
0636	Pharmacy, Drugs requiring detailed coding (a)
0771	Preventive Care Services, Vaccine Administration

In addition, for the influenza virus vaccine, providers report condition code M1 in Form Locator (FLs) 24-30 when roster billing. See roster billing instructions in §10.3 of this chapter.

When vaccines are provided to inpatients of a hospital or SNF, they are covered under the vaccine benefit. However, the hospital bills the FI on bill type 12X using the discharge date of the hospital stay or the date benefits are exhausted. A SNF submits type of bill 22X for its Part A inpatients.

Pub 100-4, 18, 10.2.2.1 – FI Payment for Pneumococcal Pneumonia Virus, Influenza Virus, and Hepatitis B Virus Vaccines and Their Administration

(Rev. 1586, Issued: 09-05-08, Effective: 10-06-08, Implementation: 10-06-08)

Payment for Vaccines

Payment for all of these vaccines is on a reasonable cost basis for hospitals, home health agencies (HHAs), skilled nursing facilities (SNFs), critical access hospitals (CAHs), and hospital-based renal dialysis facilities (RDFs). Payment for comprehensive outpatient rehabilitation facilities (CORFs), Indian Health Service hospitals (IHS), IHS CAHs and independent RDFs is based on 95 percent of the average wholesale price (AWP). Section 10.2.4

Medicare References

of this chapter contains information on payment of these vaccines when provided by RDFs or hospices. See §10.2.2.2 for payment to independent and provider- based Rural Health Centers and Federally Qualified Health Clinics.

Payment for these vaccines is as follows:

Facility	Type of Bill	Payment
Hospitals, other than Indian Health Service (IHS) Hospitals and Critical Access Hospitals (CAHs)	12x, 13x	Reasonable cost
IHS Hospitals	12x, 13x, 83x	95% of AWP
IHS CAHs	85x	95% of AWP
CAHs Method I and Method II	85x	Reasonable cost
Skilled Nursing Facilities	22x, 23x	Reasonable cost
Home Health Agencies	34x	Reasonable cost
Comprehensive Outpatient Rehabilitation Facilities	75x	95% of the AWP
Independent Renal Dialysis Facilities	72x	95% of the AWP
Hospital-based Renal Dialysis Facilities	72x	Reasonable cost

Payment for Vaccine Administration

Payment for the administration of Influenza Virus and pneumococcal vaccines is as follows:

Facility	Type of Bill	Payment
Hospitals, other than IHS Hospitals and CAHs.	12x, 13x	Outpatient Prospective Payment System (OPPS) for hospitals subject to OPPS Reasonable cost for hospitals not subject to OPPS
IHS Hospitals	12x, 13x, 83x	MPFS as indicated in guidelines below.
IHS CAHs	85x	MPFS as indicated in guidelines below.
CAHs Method I and II	85x	Reasonable cost
Skilled Nursing Facilities	22x, 23x	MPFS as indicated in the guidelines below
Home Health Agencies	34x	OPPS
Comprehensive Outpatient Rehabilitation Facilities	75x	MPFS as indicated in the guidelines below
Independent RDFs	72x	MPFS as indicated in the guidelines below
Hospital-based RDFs	72x	Reasonable cost

Guidelines for pricing pneumococcal and influenza virus vaccine administration under the MPFS.

Make reimbursement based on the rate in the MPFS associated with the CPT code 90782 or 90471 as follows:

HCPCS	Effective prior to March 1, 2003	Effective on and after March 1, 2003
G0008	90782	90471
G0009	90782	90471

See §10.2.2.2 for payment to independent and provider based Rural Health Centers and Federally Qualified Health Clinics.

Payment for the administration of hepatitis B vaccine is as follows:

Facility	Type of Bill	Payment
Hospitals other than IHS hospitals and CAHs.	12x, 13x	Outpatient Prospective Payment System (OPPS) for hospitals subject to OPPS Reasonable cost for hospitals not subject to OPPS
IHS Hospitals	12x, 13x, 83x	MPFS as indicated in the guidelines below
CAHs Method I and II	85x	Reasonable cost
IHS CAHs	85x	MPFS as indicated in guidelines below.
Skilled Nursing Facilities	22x, 23x	MPFS as indicated in the chart below
Home Health Agencies	34x	OPPS
Comprehensive Outpatient Rehabilitation Facilities	75x	MPFS as indicated in the guidelines below
Independent RDFs	72x	MPFS as indicated in the chart below
Hospital-based RDFs	72x	Reasonable cost

Guidelines for pricing Hepatitis B vaccine administration under the MPFS

Make reimbursement based on the rate in the MPFS associated with the CPT code 90782 or 90471 as follows:

HCPCS	Effective prior to March 1, 2003	Effective on and after March 1, 2003
G0010	90782	90471

See §10.2.2.2 for payment to independent and provider based Rural Health Centers and Federally Qualified Health Clinics.

Pub 100-4, 18, 10.2.2.2 – Special Instructions for Independent and Provider-Based Rural Health Clinics/Federally Qualified Health Center (RHCs/FQHCs)

(Rev. 1586, Issued: 09-05-08, Effective: 10-06-08, Implementation: 10-06-08)

Independent and provider-based RHCs and FQHCs do not include charges for influenza virus and pneumococcal vaccines on Form CMS-1450. Administration of these vaccines does not count as a visit when the only service involved is the administration of influenza virus and/ or pneumococcal vaccine(s). If there was another reason for the visit, the RHC/FQHC should bill for the visit without adding the cost of the influenza virus and pneumococcal vaccines to the charge for the visit on the bill. FIs/AB MACs pay at the time of cost settlement and adjust interim rates to account for this additional cost if they determine that the payment is more than a negligible amount.

Payment for the hepatitis B vaccine is included in the all-inclusive rate. However, RHCs/FQHCs do not bill for a visit when the only service involved is the administration of the hepatitis B vaccine. As with other vaccines administered during an otherwise payable encounter, no line items specifically for this service are billed on the RHC/FQHC claims in addition to the encounter.

Pub 100-4, 18, 10.2.3 – Bills Submitted to Regional Home Health Intermediaries (RHHIs)

(Rev. 1586, Issued: 09-05-08, Effective: 10-06-08, Implementation: 10-06-08)

The following provides billing instructions for Home Health Agency (HHAs) in various situations:

- Where the sole purpose for an HHA visit is to administer a vaccine (influenza virus, pneumococcal, or hepatitis B), Medicare will not pay for a skilled nursing visit by an HHA nurse under the HHA benefit. However, the vaccine and its administration are covered under the vaccine benefit. The administration should include charges only for the supplies being used and the cost of the injection. RHHIs do not allow HHAs to charge for travel time or other expenses (e.g., gasoline). In this situation, the HHA bills under bill type 34X and reports revenue code 0636 along with the appropriate HCPCS code for the vaccine and revenue code 0771 along with the appropriate HCPCS code for the administration.

NOTE: A separate bill is not allowed for the visit

- If a vaccine (influenza virus, pneumococcal, or hepatitis B) is administered during the course of an otherwise covered home health visit (e.g., to perform wound care), the visit would be covered as normal but the HHA must not include the vaccine or its administration in their visit charge. In this case, the HHA is entitled to payment for the vaccine and its administration under the vaccine benefit. In this situation, the HHA bills under bill type 34X and reports revenue code 0636 along with the appropriate HCPCS code for the vaccine and revenue code 0771 along with the appropriate HCPCS code for the administration.

NOTE: A separate bill is required for the visit

- Where a beneficiary does not meet the eligibility criteria for home health coverage, a home health nurse may be paid for the vaccine (influenza virus, pneumococcal, or hepatitis B) and its administration. No skilled nursing visit charge is billable. Administration of the services should include charges only for the supplies being used and the cost of the injection. RHHIs do not pay for travel time or other expenses (e.g., gasoline). In this situation, the HHA bills under bill type 34X and reports revenue code 0636 along with the appropriate HCPCS code for the vaccine and revenue code 0771 along with the appropriate HCPCS code for the administration.

If a beneficiary meets the eligibility criteria for coverage, but his or her spouse does not, and the spouse wants an injection the same time as a nursing visit, HHAs bill in accordance with the bullet point above.

Pub 100-4, 18, 10.2.4 – Bills Submitted by Hospices and Payment Procedures for Renal Dialysis Facilities (RDF)

(Rev. 1586, Issued: 09-05-08, Effective: 10-06-08, Implementation: 10-06-08)

Hospices can provide the influenza virus, pneumococcal, and hepatitis B vaccines to those beneficiaries who request them including those who have elected the hospice benefit. These services may be covered when furnished by the hospice. Services for the vaccines should be billed to the local carrier/AB MAC on the Form CMS-1500. Payment is made using the same methodology as if they were a supplier. Hospices that do not have a supplier number should contact their local carrier/AB MAC to obtain one in order to bill for these benefits.

FIs/AB MACs pay for pneumococcal, influenza virus, and hepatitis B virus vaccines for freestanding Renal Dialysis facilities (RDFs) based on the lower of the actual charge or 95 percent of the average wholesale price and based on reasonable cost for provider-based RDFs. Deductible and coinsurance do not apply for influenza virus and pneumococcal vaccines. FIs/AB MACs must contact their carrier/AB MAC to obtain information in order to make payment for the administration of these vaccines.

Deductible and coinsurance apply for hepatitis B vaccine.

Pub 100-4, 18, 10.2.4.1 – Hepatitis B Vaccine Furnished to ESRD Patients

(Rev. 1586, Issued: 09-05-08, Effective: 10-06-08, Implementation: 10-06-08)

Hepatitis B vaccine and its administration (including staff time and supplies such as syringes) are paid to ESRD facilities in addition to, and separately from, the dialysis composite rate payment.

Payment for the hepatitis B vaccine for ESRD patients follows the same general principles that are applicable to any injectable drug or biological. Hospital-based facilities are paid for their direct and indirect costs on a reasonable cost basis, and independent facilities are paid the lower of the actual charge or 95 percent of the AWP. The allowance for injectables is based on the cost of the injectable and any supplies used for administration, plus a maximum $2 for the labor involved, if the facility's staff administers the vaccine. In addition, the FI/AB MAC makes an appropriate allowance for facility overhead.

Where the vaccine is administered in a hospital outpatient department for home dialysis patients or for patients with chronic renal failure (but not yet on dialysis), payment is on a reasonable cost basis. Outpatient hospital vaccines for nondialysis purposes are paid under hospital outpatient PPS rules.

Pub 100-4, 18, 10.2.5 – Claims Submitted to Carriers/ AB MACs

(Rev. 1586, Issued: 09-05-08, Effective: 10-06-08, Implementation: 10-06-08)

Medicare does not require that the influenza virus vaccine be administered under a physician's order or supervision. Effective for claims with dates of service on or after July 1, 2000, Medicare does not require that pneumococcal vaccinations be administered under a physician's order or supervision. Medicare still requires that the hepatitis B vaccine be administered under a physician's order with supervision. As a physician order is still required for claims for hepatitis B vaccinations, information on the ordering and/or referring physician must be entered on the claim.

A. Reporting Specialty Code/Place of Service (POS) to CWF Specialty

Contractors use specialty code 60 (Public Health or Welfare Agencies (Federal, State, and Local)) for Public Health Service Clinics (PHCs).

Contractors use specialty code 73 (Mass Immunization Roster Billers) for centralized billers and specialty code 87 for pharmacists (all other suppliers (drug stores, department stores)).

Entities and individuals other than PHCs and pharmacists use the CMS specialty code that best defines their provider type. A list of specialty codes can be found in chapter 26. The CMS specialty code 99 (Unknown Physician Specialty) is acceptable where no other code fits.

Place of Service (POS)

State or local PHCs use POS code 71 (State or Local Public Health Clinic). POS 71 is not used for individual offices/entities other than PHCs (e.g., a mobile unit that is non-PHC affiliated should use POS 99). Preprinted Form CMS-1500s (08-05) used for simplified roster billing should show POS 60 (Mass Immunization Center) regardless of the site where vaccines are given (e.g., a PHC or physician's office that roster claims should use POS 60). Individuals/entities administering influenza virus and pneumococcal vaccinations in a mass immunization setting (including centralized flu billers), regardless of the site where vaccines are given, should use POS 60 for roster claims, paper claims, and electronically filed claims.

Normal POS codes should be used in other situations.

Providers use POS 99 (Other Unlisted Facility) if no other POS code applies.

Pub 100-4, 18, 10.2.5.1 – Carrier/AB MAC Indicators for the Common Working File (CWF)

(Rev. 1586, Issued: 09-05-08, Effective: 10-06-08, Implementation: 10-06-08)

The carrier/AB MAC record submitted to CWF must contain the following indicators:

Description	Payment Indicator	Payment	Deductible Indicator	Deductible	Type of Service
Pneumococcal	"1"	100 percent	"1"	Zero deductible	"V"
Influenza	"1"	100 percent	"1"	Zero deductible	"V"
Hepatitis B	"0"	80 percent	"0"	Deductible	"1"

A payment indicator of "1" represents 100 percent payment. A deductible indicator of "1" represents a zero deductible. A payment indicator of "0" represents 80 percent payment. A deductible indicator of "0" indicates that a deductible applies to the claim.

The record must also contain a "V" in the type of service field, which indicates that this is a pneumococcal or influenza virus vaccine. Carriers/ AB MACs use a "1" in the type of service field which indicates medical care for a hepatitis B vaccine.

Pub 100-4, 18, 10.2.5.2 – Carrier/AB MAC Payment Requirements

(Rev. 1586, Issued: 09-05-08, Effective: 10-06-08, Implementation: 10-06-08)

Payment for pneumococcal, influenza virus, and hepatitis B vaccines follows the same standard rules that are applicable to any injectable drug or biological. (See chapter 17 for procedures for determining the payment rates for pneumococcal and influenza virus vaccines.)

Effective for claims with dates of service on or after February 1, 2001, §114, of the Benefits Improvement and Protection Act of 2000 mandated that all drugs and biologicals be paid based on mandatory assignment. Therefore, all providers of influenza virus and pneumococcal vaccines must accept assignment for the vaccine.

Prior to March 1, 2003, the administration of pneumococcal, influenza virus, and hepatitis B vaccines, (HCPCS codes G0008, G0009, and G0010), though not reimbursed directly through the MPFS, were reimbursed at the same rate as HCPCS code 90782 on the MPFS for the year that corresponded to the date of service of the claim.

Prior to March 1, 2003, HCPCS codes G0008, G0009, and G0010 are reimbursed at the same rate as HCPCS code 90471. Assignment for the administration is not mandatory, but is applicable should the provider be enrolled as a provider type "Mass Immunization Roster Biller," submits roster bills, or participates in the centralized billing program.

Carriers/AB MACs may not apply the limiting charge provision for pneumococcal, influenza virus vaccine, or hepatitis B vaccine and their administration in accordance with §§1833(a)(1) and 1833(a)(10)(A) of the Social Security Act (the Act.) The administration of the influenza virus vaccine is covered in the influenza virus vaccine benefit under §1861(s)(10)(A) of the Act, rather than under the physicians' services benefit. Therefore, it is not eligible for the 10 percent Health Professional Shortage Area (HPSA) incentive payment or the 5 percent Physician Scarcity Area (PSA) incentive payment.

A. No Legal Obligation to Pay

Nongovernmental entities that provide immunizations free of charge to all patients, regardless of their ability to pay, must provide the immunizations free of charge to Medicare beneficiaries and may not bill Medicare. (See Pub. 100-02, ***Medicare Benefit Policy Manual***, chapter 16.) Thus, for example, Medicare may not pay for influenza virus vaccinations administered to Medicare beneficiaries if a physician provides free vaccinations to all non-Medicare patients or where an employer offers free vaccinations to its employees. Physicians also may not charge Medicare beneficiaries more for a vaccine than they would charge non-Medicare patients. (See §1128(b)(6)(A) of the Act.) When an employer offers free vaccinations to its employees, it must also offer the free vaccination to an employee who is also a Medicare beneficiary. It does not have to offer free vaccinations to its non-Medicare employees.

Nongovernmental entities that do not charge patients who are unable to pay or reduce their charges for patients of limited means, yet expect to be paid if the patient has health insurance coverage for the services provided, may bill Medicare and expect payment.

Governmental entities (such as PHCs) may bill Medicare for pneumococcal, hepatitis B, and influenza virus vaccines administered to Medicare beneficiaries when services are rendered free of charge to non-Medicare beneficiaries.

Pub 100-4, 18, 10.3 – Simplified Roster Claims for Mass Immunizers

(Rev. 1586, Issued: 09-05-08, Effective: 10-06-08, Implementation: 10-06-08)

The simplified roster billing process was developed to enable Medicare beneficiaries to participate in mass pneumococcal and influenza virus vaccination programs offered by

PHCs and other individuals and entities that give the vaccine to a group of beneficiaries, e.g. at PHCs, shopping malls, grocery stores, senior citizen homes, and health fairs. Roster billing is not available for hepatitis B vaccinations.

Properly licensed individuals and entities conducting mass immunization programs may submit claims using a simplified claims filing procedure known as roster billing to bill for the influenza virus vaccine benefit for multiple beneficiaries if they agree to accept assignment for these claims. They may not collect any payment from the beneficiary. Effective November 1, 1996, roster billing is also available to individuals and entities billing for pneumococcal vaccinations.

Effective July 1, 1998, immunization of at least five beneficiaries on the same date is no longer required for any individual or entity to qualify for roster billing to carriers. However, the rosters should not be used for single patient claims and the date of service for each vaccination administered must be entered.

Entities that submit claims on roster claims must accept assignment and may not collect any "donation" or other cost sharing of any kind from Medicare beneficiaries for pneumococcal or influenza virus vaccinations. However, the entity may bill Medicare for the amount, which is not subsidized from its own budget. For example, an entity that incurs a cost of $7.50 per vaccination and pays $2.50 of the cost from its budget may bill Medicare the $5.00 cost which is not paid out of its budget.

A. Provider Enrollment Criteria for Mass Immunizers

B3-4480.8.A

Those entities and individuals that desire to provide mass immunization services, but may not otherwise be able to qualify as a Medicare provider, may be eligible to enroll as a provider type "Mass Immunization Roster Biller."

These individuals and entities must enroll by completing the Provider/Supplier Enrollment Application, Form CMS-855. Individuals and entities that enroll as this provider type may not bill Medicare for any services other than pneumococcal and/or influenza virus vaccines and their administration. In addition, claims submitted by the provider type "Mass Immunization Roster Biller" are always reimbursed at the assigned payment rate.

B. Payment Floor for Roster Claims

Roster claims are considered paper claims and are not paid as quickly as electronic media claims (EMC). If available, offer electronic billing software free or at-cost to PHCs and other properly licensed individuals and entities. Contractors must ensure that the software is as user friendly as possible for the pneumococcal and influenza virus vaccine benefits.

C. Medicare Advantage Plans Processing Requirements

Medicare Advantage Plans may use roster billing only if vaccinations are the only Medicare-covered services furnished by the Medicare Advantage Plans to Medicare patients who are not members of the Medicare Advantage Plans. Medicare Advantage Plans must use Place of Service (POS) code 60 for processing roster claims.

Pub 100-4, 18, 10.3.1 – Roster Claims Submitted to Carriers/AB MACs for Mass Immunization

(Rev. 1586, Issued: 09-05-08, Effective: 10-06-08, Implementation: 10-06-08)

If the PHC or other individual or entity qualifies to submit roster claims, it may use a preprinted Form CMS-1500 (08-05) that contains standardized information about the entity and the benefit. Key information from the beneficiary roster list and the abbreviated Form CMS-1500 (08-05) is used to process pneumococcal and influenza virus vaccination claims.

Separate Form CMS-1500 (08-05) claim forms, along with separate roster bills, must be submitted for pneumococcal and influenza roster billing.

If other services are furnished to a beneficiary along with pneumococcal or influenza virus vaccine, individuals and entities must submit claims using normal billing procedures, e.g., submission of a Form CMS-1500 (08-05) or electronic billing for each beneficiary.

Contractors must create and count one claim per beneficiary from roster bills. They must split claims for each beneficiary if there are multiple beneficiaries included in a roster bill. Providers must show the unit cost for one service on the claim. The contractor must replicate the claim for each beneficiary listed on the roster.

Contractors must provide Palmetto-Railroad Retirement Board (RRB) with local pricing files for pneumococcal and influenza virus vaccine and their administration. If PHCs or other individuals or entities inappropriately bill pneumococcal or influenza virus vaccinations using the roster billing method, contractors return the claim to the provider with a cover letter explaining why it is being returned and the criteria for the roster billing process. Contractors may not deny these claims.

Providers must retain roster bills with beneficiaries' signatures at their permanent location for a time period consistent with Medicare regulations.

A. Modified Form CMS-1500 (08-05) for Cover Document

Entities submitting roster claims to carriers/AB MACs must complete the following blocks on a single modified Form CMS-1500 (08-05), which serves as the cover document for the roster for each facility where services are furnished. In order for carriers/AB MACs to reimburse by correct payment locality, a separate Form CMS-1500 (08-05) must be used for each different facility or physical location where services are furnished.

Item 1: An X in the Medicare block
Item 2: (Patient's Name): "SEE ATTACHED ROSTER"
Item 11: (Insured's Policy Group or FECA Number): "NONE"
Item 20: (Outside Lab?): An "X" in the NO block

Medicare References

Item 21: (Diagnosis or Nature of Illness): Line 1: Choose appropriate diagnosis code from §10.2.1

Item 24B: (Place of Service (POS)): Line 1: "60"; Line 2: "60"; NOTE: POS Code '60" must be used for roster billing.

Item 24D: (Procedures, Services or Supplies): Line 1: PPV vaccine: "90732" or Influenza Virus vaccine: "Select appropriate influenza vaccine code"; Line 2: PPV Administration: "G0009" or Influenza Virus Administration: "G0008"

Item 24E: (Diagnosis Code): Lines 1 and 2: "1"

Item 24F: ($ Charges): The entity must enter the charge for each listed service. If the entity is not charging for the vaccine or its administration, it should enter 0.00 or "NC" (no charge) on the appropriate line for that item. If your system is unable to accept a line item charge of 0.00 for an immunization service, do not key the line item. Likewise, electronic media claim (EMC) billers should submit line items for free immunization services on EMC PPV or influenza virus vaccine claims only if your system is able to accept them.

Item 27: (Accept Assignment): An "X" in the YES block.

Item 29: (Amount Paid): "$0.00"

Item 31: (Signature of Physician or Supplier): The entity's representative must sign the modified Form CMS-1500 (08-05).

Item 32: Enter the name, address, and Zip Code of the location where the service was provided. (including centralized billers).

Item32a: Enter the NPI of the service facility as soon as it is available. The NPI may be reported on the Form CMS-1500 (08-05) as early as October 1, 2006.

Item 33: (Physician's, Supplier's Billing Name): The entity must complete this item to include the Provider Identification Number (not the Unique Physician Identification Number) or NPI when required.

Item 33a: Effective May 23, 2007, and later, enter the NPI of the billing provider or group. (The NPI may be reported on the Form CMS-1500 (08-05) as early as October 1, 2006.)

B. Format of Roster Claims

Qualifying individuals and entities must attach to the Form CMS-1500 (08-05) claim form, a roster which contains the variable claims information regarding the supplier of the service and individual beneficiaries. While qualifying entities must use the modified Form CMS-1500 (08-05) without deviation, contractors must work with these entities to develop a mutually suitable roster that contains the minimum data necessary to satisfy claims processing requirements for these claims. Contractors must key information from the beneficiary roster list and abbreviated Form CMS-1500 (08-05) to process pneumococcal and influenza virus vaccination claims.

The roster must contain at a minimum the following information:

- Provider name and number;
- Date of service;

NOTE: Although physicians who provide pneumococcal or influenza virus vaccinations may roster bill if they vaccinate fewer than five beneficiaries per day, they must include the individual date of service for each beneficiary's vaccination on the roster form.

- Control number for contractor;
- Patient's health insurance claim number;
- Patient's name;
- Patient's address;
- Date of birth;
- Patient's sex; and
- Beneficiary's signature or stamped "signature on file".

NOTE: A stamped "signature on file" qualifies as an actual signature on a roster claim form if the provider has a signed authorization on file to bill Medicare for services rendered. In this situation, the provider is not required to obtain the patient signature on the roster, but instead has the option of reporting signature on file in lieu of obtaining the patient's actual signature.

The pneumococcal roster must contain the following language to be used by providers as a precaution to alert beneficiaries prior to administering the pneumococcal vaccination.

WARNING: Beneficiaries must be asked if they have received a pneumococcal vaccination.

- Rely on patients' memory to determine prior vaccination status.
- If patients are uncertain whether they have been vaccinated within the past 5 years, administer the vaccine.

If patients are certain that they have been vaccinated within the past 5 years, do not revaccinate.

Pub 100-4, 18, 10.3.1.1 – Centralized Billing for Flu and Pneumococcal (PPV) Vaccines to Medicare Carriers/AB MACs

(Rev. 1586, Issued: 09-05-08, Effective: 10-06-08, Implementation: 10-06-08)

The CMS currently authorizes a limited number of providers to centrally bill for influenza virus and pneumococcal immunization claims. Centralized billing is an optional program available to providers who qualify to enroll with Medicare as the provider type "Mass Immunization Roster Biller," as well as to other individuals and entities that qualify to enroll as regular Medicare providers. Centralized billers must roster bill, must accept assignment, and must bill electronically.

To qualify for centralized billing, a mass immunizer must be operating in at least three payment localities for which there are three different contractors processing claims. Individuals and entities providing the vaccine and administration must be properly licensed in the State in which the immunizations are given and the contractor must verify this through the enrollment process.

Centralized billers must send all claims for influenza virus and pneumococcal immunizations to a single contractor for payment, regardless of the jurisdiction in which the vaccination was administered. (This does not include claims for the Railroad Retirement Board, United Mine Workers or Indian Health Services. These claims must continue to go to the appropriate processing entity.) Payment is made based on the payment locality where the service was provided. This process is only available for claims for the influenza virus and pneumococcal vaccines and their administration. The general coverage and coding rules still apply to these claims.

This section applies only to those individuals and entities that provide mass immunization services for influenza virus and pneumococcal vaccinations and that have been authorized by CMS to centrally bill. All other providers, including those individuals and entities that provide mass immunization services that are not authorized to centrally bill, must continue to bill for these claims to their regular carrier/AB MAC per the instructions in §10.3.1 of this chapter.

The claims processing instructions in this section apply only to the designated processing contractor. However, all carriers/AB MACs must follow the instructions in §10.3.1.1.J, below, "Provider Education Instructions for All Carriers/AB MACs."

A. Processing Carrier

Trailblazers Health Enterprises is designated as the sole contractor for the payment of influenza virus and pneumococcal claims for centralized billers from October 1, 2000, through the length of the contract. The CMS central office will notify centralized billers of the appropriate contractor to bill when they receive their notification of acceptance into the centralized billing program.

B. Request for Approval

Approval to participate in the CMS centralized billing program is a two part approval process. Individuals and corporations who wish to enroll as a CMS mass immunizer centralized biller must send their request in writing. CMS will complete Part 1 of the approval process by reviewing preliminary demographic information included in the request for participation letter. Completion of Part 1 is not approval to set up vaccination clinics, vaccinate beneficiaries, and bill Medicare for reimbursement. All new participants must complete Part 2 of the approval process (Form CMS-855 Application) before they may set up vaccination clinics, vaccinate Medicare beneficiaries, and bill Medicare for reimbursement. If an individual or entity's request is approved for centralized billing, the approval is limited to 12 months from September to August 31 of the next year. It is the responsibility of the centralized biller to reapply for approval each year. The designated contractor shall provide in writing to CMS and approved centralized billers notification of completion and approval of Part 2 of the approval process. The designated contractor may not process claims for any centralized biller who has not completed Parts 1 and 2 of the approval process. If claims are submitted by a provider who has not received approval of Parts 1 and 2 of the approval process to participate as a centralized biller, the contractor must return the claims to the provider to submit to the local carrier/AB MAC for payment.

C. Notification of Provider Participation to the Processing Contractor

Before September 1 of every year, CMS will provide the designated contractor with the names of the entities that are authorized to participate in centralized billing for the 12 month period beginning September 1 and ending August 31 of the next year.

D. Enrollment

Though centralized billers may already have a Medicare provider number, for purposes of centralized billing, they must also obtain a provider number from the processing contractor for centralized billing through completion of the Form CMS-855 (Provider Enrollment Application). Providers/suppliers are encouraged to apply to enroll as a centralized biller early as possible. Applicants who have not completed the entire enrollment process and received approval from CMS and the designated contractor to participate as a Medicare mass immunizer centralized biller will not be allowed to submit claims to Medicare for reimbursement.

Whether an entity enrolls as a provider type "Mass Immunization Roster Biller" or some other type of provider, all normal enrollment processes and procedures must be followed. Authorization from CMS to participate in centralized billing is dependent upon the entity's ability to qualify as some type of Medicare provider. In addition, as under normal enrollment procedures, the contractor must verify that the entity is fully qualified and certified per State requirements in each State in which they plan to operate.

The contractor will activate the provider number for the 12-month period from September 1 through August 31 of the following year. If the provider is authorized to participate in the centralized billing program the next year, the contractor will extend the activation of the provider number for another year. The entity need not re-enroll with the contractor every year. However, should there be changes in the States in which the entity plans to operate, the contractor will need to verify that the entity meets all State certification and licensure requirements in those new States.

E. Electronic Submission of Claims on Roster Bills

Centralized billers must agree to submit their claims on roster bills in an Electronic Media Claims standard format using the appropriate version of American National Standards Institute (ANSI) format. Contractors should refer to the appropriate ANSI Implementation Guide to determine the correct location for this information on electronic claims. The processing contractor must provide instructions on acceptable roster billing formats to the approved centralized billers. Paper claims will not be accepted.

F. Required Information on Roster Bills for Centralized Billing

In addition to the roster billing instructions found in §10.3.1 of this chapter, centralized billers must complete on the electronic format the area that corresponds to Item 32 and 33 on Form CMS 1500 (08-05). The contractor must use the ZIP Code in Item 32 to determine the payment locality for the claim. Item 33 must be completed to report the provider of service/supplier's billing name, address, ZIP Code, and telephone number. In addition, the NPI of the billing provider or group must be appropriately reported.

For electronic claims, the name, address, and ZIP Code of the facility are reported in:

- The HIPAA compliant ANSI X12N 837: Claim level loop 2310D NM101=FA. When implemented, the facility (e.g., hospitals) NPI will be captured in the loop 2310D NM109 (NM108=XX) if one is available. Prior to NPI, enter the tax information in loop 2310D NM109 (NM108=24 or 34) and enter the Medicare legacy facility identifier in loop 2310D REF02 (REF01=1C). Report the address, city, state, and ZIP Code in loop 2310D N301 and N401, N402, and N403. Facility data is not required to be reported at the line level for centralized billing.

G. Payment Rates and Mandatory Assignment

The payment rates for the administration of the vaccinations are based on the Medicare Physician Fee Schedule (MPFS) for the appropriate year. Payment made through the MPFS is based on geographic locality. Therefore, payments vary based on the geographic locality where the service was performed.

The HCPCS codes G0008 and G0009 for the administration of the vaccines are not paid on the MPFS. However, prior to March 1, 2003, they must be paid at the same rate as HCPCS code 90782, which is on the MPFS. The designated contractor must pay per the correct MPFS file for each calendar year based on the date of service of the claim. Beginning March 1, 2003, HCPCS codes G0008, G0009, and G0010 are to be reimbursed at the same rate as HCPCS code 90471.

In order to pay claims correctly for centralized billers, the designated contractor must have the correct name and address, including ZIP Code, of the entity where the service was provided.

The following remittance advice and Medicare Summary Notice (MSN) messages apply:

> Claim adjustment reason code 16, "Claim/service lacks information which is needed for adjudication. At least one Remark Code must be provided (may be comprised of either the Remittance Advice Remark Code or NCPDP Reject Reason Code.)" and
>
> Remittance advice remark code MA114, "Missing/incomplete/invalid information on where the services were furnished." and
>
> MSN 9.4 - "This item or service was denied because information required to make payment was incorrect."

The payment rates for the vaccines must be determined by the standard method used by Medicare for reimbursement of drugs and biologicals. (See chapter 17 for procedures for determining the payment rates for vaccines.)

Effective for claims with dates of service on or after February 1, 2001, §114, of the Benefits Improvement and Protection Act of 2000 mandated that all drugs and biologicals be paid based on mandatory assignment. Therefore, all providers of influenza virus and pneumococcal vaccines must accept assignment for the vaccine. In addition, as a requirement for both centralized billing and roster billing, providers must agree to accept assignment for the administration of the vaccines as well. This means that they must agree to accept the amount that Medicare pays for the vaccine and the administration. Also, since there is no coinsurance or deductible for the influenza virus and pneumococcal benefit, accepting assignment means that Medicare beneficiaries cannot be charged for the vaccination.

H. Common Working File Information

To identify these claims and to enable central office data collection on the project, special processing number 39 has been assigned. The number should be entered on the HUBC claim record to CWF in the field titled Demonstration Number.

I. Provider Education Instructions for the Processing Contractor

The processing contractor must fully educate the centralized billers on the processes for centralized billing as well as for roster billing. General information on influenza virus and pneumococcal coverage and billing instructions is available on the CMS Web site for providers.

J. Provider Education Instructions for All Carriers/AB MACs

By April 1 of every year, all carriers/AB MACs must publish in their bulletins and put on their Web sites the following notification to providers. Questions from interested providers should be forwarded to the central office address below. Carriers/AB MACs must enter the name of the assigned processing contractor where noted before sending.

> NOTIFICATION TO PROVIDERS
>
> Centralized billing is a process in which a provider, who provides mass immunization services for influenza virus and pneumococcal pneumonia virus (PPV) immunizations, can send all claims to a single contractor for payment regardless of the geographic locality in which the vaccination was administered. (This does not include claims for the Railroad Retirement Board, United Mine Workers or Indian Health Services. These claims must continue to go to the appropriate processing entity.) This process is only available for claims for the influenza virus and pneumococcal vaccines and their administration. The administration of the vaccinations is reimbursed at the assigned rate based on the Medicare physician fee schedule for the appropriate locality. The vaccines are reimbursed at the assigned rate using the Medicare standard method for reimbursement of drugs and biologicals.

Medicare References

Individuals and entities interested in centralized billing must contact CMS central office, in writing, at the following address by June 1 of the year they wish to begin centrally billing.

Center for Medicare & Medicaid Services
Division of Practitioner Claims Processing
Provider Billing and Education Group
7500 Security Boulevard
Mail Stop C4-10-07
Baltimore, Maryland 21244

By agreeing to participate in the centralized billing program, providers agree to abide by the following criteria.

CRITERIA FOR CENTRALIZED BILLING

- To qualify for centralized billing, an individual or entity providing mass immunization services for influenza virus and pneumococcal vaccinations must provide these services in at least three payment localities for which there are at least three different carriers processing claims.
- Individuals and entities providing the vaccine and administration must be properly licensed in the State in which the immunizations are given.
- Centralized billers must agree to accept assignment (i.e., they must agree to accept the amount that Medicare pays for the influenza virus and pneumococcal benefit, accepting assignment means that Medicare beneficiaries cannot be charged for the vaccination, i.e., beneficiaries may not incur any out-of-pocket expense. For example, a drugstore may not charge a Medicare beneficiary $10 for an influenza vaccination and give the beneficiary a coupon for $10 to be used in the drugstore.

  NOTE: The practice of requiring a beneficiary to pay for the vaccination upfront and to file their own claim for reimbursement is inappropriate. All Medicare providers are required to file claims on behalf of the beneficiary per §1848(g)(4)(A) of the Social Security Act and centralized billers may not collect any payment.
- The contractor assigned to process the claims for centralized billing is chosen at the discretion of CMS based on such considerations as workload, user-friendly software developed by the contractor for billing claims, and overall performance. The assigned contractor for this year is [Fill in name of contractor.]
- The payment rates for the administration of the vaccinations are based on the Medicare physician fee schedule (MPFS) for the appropriate year. Payment made through the MPFS is based on geographic locality. Therefore, payments received may vary based on the geographic locality where the service was performed. Payment is made at the assigned rate.
- The payment rates for the vaccines are determined by the standard method used by Medicare for reimbursement of drugs and biologicals. Payment is made at the assigned rate.
- Centralized billers must submit their claims on roster bills in an approved Electronic Media Claims standard format. Paper claims will not be accepted.
- Centralized billers must obtain certain information for each beneficiary including name, health insurance number, date of birth, sex, and signature. [Fill in name of contractor] must be contacted prior to the season for exact requirements. The responsibility lies with the centralized biller to submit correct beneficiary Medicare information (including the beneficiary's Medicare Health Insurance Claim Number) as the contractor will not be able to process incomplete or incorrect claims.
- Centralized billers must obtain an address for each beneficiary so that a Medicare Summary Notice (MSN) can be sent to the beneficiary by the contractor. Beneficiaries are sometimes confused when they receive an MSN from a contractor other than the contractor that normally processes their claims which results in unnecessary beneficiary inquiries to the Medicare contractor. Therefore, centralized billers must provide every beneficiary receiving an influenza virus or pneumococcal vaccination with the name of the processing contractor. This notification must be in writing, in the form of a brochure or handout, and must be provided to each beneficiary at the time he or she receives the vaccination.
- Centralized billers must retain roster bills with beneficiary signatures at their permanent location for a time period consistent with Medicare regulations. [Fill in name of contractor] can provide this information.
- Though centralized billers may already have a Medicare provider number, for purposes of centralized billing, they must also obtain a provider number from [Fill in name of contractor]. This can be done by completing the Form CMS-855 (Provider Enrollment Application), which can be obtained from [Fill in name of contractor].
- If an individual or entity's request for centralized billing is approved, the approval is limited to the 12 month period from September 1 through August 31 of the following year. It is the responsibility of the centralized biller to reapply to CMS CO for approval each year by June 1. Claims will not be processed for any centralized biller without permission from CMS.
- Each year the centralized biller must contact [Fill in name of contractor] to verify understanding of the coverage policy for the administration of the pneumococcal vaccine, and for a copy of the warning language that is required on the roster bill.
- The centralized biller is responsible for providing the beneficiary with a record of the pneumococcal vaccination.

The information in items 1 through 8 below must be included with the individual or entity's annual request to participate in centralized billing:

1. Estimates for the number of beneficiaries who will receive influenza virus vaccinations;
2. Estimates for the number of beneficiaries who will receive pneumococcal vaccinations;
3. The approximate dates for when the vaccinations will be given;
4. A list of the States in which influenza virus and pneumococcal clinics will be held;
5. The type of services generally provided by the corporation (e.g., ambulance, home health, or visiting nurse);
6. Whether the nurses who will administer the influenza virus and pneumococcal vaccinations are employees of the corporation or will be hired by the corporation specifically for the purpose of administering influenza virus and pneumococcal vaccinations;
7. Names and addresses of all entities operating under the corporation's application;
8. Contact information for designated contact person for centralized billing program.

Pub 100-4, 18, 10.3.2 – Claims Submitted to FIs/AB MACs for Mass Immunizations of Influenza Virus and Pneumococcal Vaccinations

(Rev. 1586, Issued: 09-05-08, Effective: 10-06-08, Implementation: 10-06-08)

Some potential "mass immunizers," such as hospital outpatient departments and HHAs, have expressed concern about the complexity of billing for the influenza virus vaccine and its administration. Consequently, to increase the number of beneficiaries who obtain needed preventive immunizations, simplified (roster) billing procedures are available to mass immunizers. The simplified (roster) claims filing procedure has been expanded for the pneumococcal vaccine. A mass immunizer is defined as any entity that gives the influenza virus vaccine or pneumococcal vaccine to a group of beneficiaries, e.g., at public health clinics, shopping malls, grocery stores, senior citizen homes, and health fairs. To qualify for roster billing, immunizations of at least five beneficiaries on the same date are required. (See §10.3.2.2 for an exception to this requirement for inpatient hospitals.)

The simplified (roster) claims filing procedure applies to providers other than RHCs and FQHCs that conduct mass immunizations. Since independent and provider based RHCs and FQHCs do not submit individual Form CMS-1450s for the influenza virus vaccine, they do not utilize the simplified billing process. Instead, payment is made for the vaccine at the time of cost settlement.

The simplified process involves use of the provider billing form (Form CMS-1450) with preprinted standardized information relative to the provider and the benefit. Mass immunizers attach a standard roster to a single pre-printed Form CMS-1450 that contains the variable claims information regarding the service provider and individual beneficiaries.

Qualifying individuals and entities must attach a roster, which contains the variable claims information regarding the supplier of the service and individual beneficiaries.

The roster must contain at a minimum the following information:

- Provider name and number;
- Date of service;
- Patient name and address;
- Patient date of birth;
- Patient sex;
- Patient health insurance claim number; and
- Beneficiary signature or stamped "signature on file."

In addition, for inpatient Part B services (12x and 22X) the following data elements are also needed:

- Admission date;
- Admission type;
- Admission diagnosis;
- Admission source code; and
- Patient status code.

NOTE: A stamped "signature on file" can be used in place of the beneficiary's actual signature for all institutional providers that roster bill from an inpatient or outpatient department provided the provider has a signed authorization on file to bill Medicare for services rendered. In this situation, they are not required to obtain the patient signature on the roster. However, the provider has the option of reporting "signature on file" in lieu of obtaining the patient's actual signature on the roster.

The pneumococcal vaccine roster must contain the following language to be used by providers as a precaution to alert beneficiaries prior to administering the pneumococcal vaccine.

The PPV roster must contain the following language to be used by providers as a precaution to alert beneficiaries prior to administering PPV.

Warning: Beneficiaries must be asked if they have been vaccinated with the pneumococcal vaccine.

- Rely on the patients' memory to determine prior vaccination status.
- If patients are uncertain whether they have been vaccinated within the past 5 years, administer the vaccine,
- If patients are certain that they have been vaccinated within the past 5 years, do not revaccinate.

For providers using the simplified billing procedure, the modified Form CMS-1450 shows the following preprinted information in the specific form locators (FLs). Information regarding the form locator numbers that correspond to the data element names below and a table to crosswalk the CMS-1450 form locators to the 837 transaction is found in chapter 25:

- The words "See Attached Roster" (Patient Name);
- Patient Status code 01 (Patient Status);
- Condition code M1 (Condition Code) (See NOTE below);
- Condition code A6 (Condition Code);
- Revenue code 636 in (Revenue Code), along with the appropriate HCPCS code in (HCPCS Code);
- Revenue code 771 (Revenue Code), along with the appropriate "G" HCPCS code (HCPCS Code);
- "Medicare" (Payer, line A);
- The words "See Attached Roster" on line A of FL 51 (Provider Number); and
- Diagnosis code V03.82 for the pneumococcal vaccine or V04.8 for Influenza Virus vaccine in FL 67 (Principal Diagnosis Code). For influenza virus vaccine claims with dates of service October 1, 2003 and later, use diagnosis code V04.81.
- Influenza virus vaccines require:
- the UPIN SLF000 in FL 82 on claims submitted before May 23, 2007, or
- the provider's own NPI to be reported in the NPI field for the attending physician on claims submitted on or after May 23, 2007.

Providers conducting mass immunizations are required to complete the following FLs on the preprinted Form CMS-1450:

- Type of Bill
- Total Charges
- Provider Representative
- Date

NOTE: Medicare Secondary Payer (MSP) utilization editing is bypassed in CWF for all mass immunization roster bills. However, if the provider knows that a particular group health plan covers the pneumococcal vaccine and all other MSP requirements for the Medicare beneficiary are met, the primary payer must be billed. First claim development alerts from CWF are not generated for the pneumococcal and influenza virus vaccines.

Contractors use the beneficiary roster list to generate Form CMS-1450s to process the pneumococcal vaccine claims by mass immunizers indicating condition code M1 to avoid MSP editing. Standard System Maintainers must develop the necessary software to generate Form CMS-1450 records that will process through their system.

Providers that do not mass immunize must continue to bill for the pneumococcal and influenza virus vaccines using the normal billing method, e.g., submission of a Form CMS-1450 or electronic billing for each beneficiary.

Pub 100-4, 18, 10.3.2.1 – Simplified Billing for Influenza Virus and Pneumococcal Vaccine Services by HHAs

(Rev. 1586, Issued: 09-05-08, Effective: 10-06-08, Implementation: 10-06-08)

The following billing instructions apply to HHAs that roster bill for influenza virus and pneumococcal vaccines.

- When an HHA provides the influenza virus vaccine or the pneumococcal vaccine in a mass immunization setting, it does not have the option to pick and choose whom to bill for this service. If it is using employees from the certified portion, and as a result will be reflecting these costs on the cost report, it must bill the FI/AB MAC on the Form CMS-1450.
- If the HHA is using employees from the noncertified portion of the agency (employees of another entity that are not certified as part of the HHA), and as a result, will not be reflecting these costs on the cost report, it must obtain a provider number and bill their carrier/AB MAC on the Form CMS-1500.
- If employees from both certified and noncertified portions of the HHA furnish the vaccines at a single mass immunization site, they must prepare two separate rosters, e.g., one for employees of the certified portion to be submitted to the FI/AB MAC and one roster for employees of the noncertified portion to be submitted to the carrier/AB MAC.

Pub 100-4, 18, 10.3.2.2 – Hospital Inpatient Roster Billing

(Rev. 1586, Issued: 09-05-08, Effective: 10-06-08, Implementation: 10-06-08)

The following billing instructions apply to hospitals that roster bill for the influenza virus vaccine and the pneumococcal vaccine provided to inpatients:

- Hospitals do not have to wait until patients are discharged to provide the vaccine. They may provide it anytime during the patient's stay;
- The roster should reflect the actual date of service;
- The requirement to provide the vaccine to five or more patients at the same time to meet the requirements for mass immunizers is waived when vaccines are provided to hospital inpatients. Therefore, the roster may contain fewer than five patients or fewer than five patients on the same day; and
- The roster should contain information indicating that the vaccines were provided to inpatients to avoid questions regarding the number of patients or various dates.

Pub 100-4, 18, 10.3.2.3 – Electronic Roster Claims

(Rev. 1586, Issued: 09-05-08, Effective: 10-06-08, Implementation: 10-06-08)

As for all other Medicare-covered services, FIs/AB MACs pay electronic claims more quickly than paper claims. For payment floor purposes, roster bills are paper bills and may not be paid as quickly as EMC. (See chapter 1.) If available, FIs/AB MACs must offer free, or at-cost, electronic billing software and ensure that the software is as user friendly as possible for the influenza virus vaccine benefit.

Pub 100-4, 18, 10.4 – CWF Edits

(Rev. 1617, Issued: 10-24-08, Effective: 04-06-09, Implementation: 04-06-09)

In order to prevent duplicate payments for influenza virus and pneumococcal vaccination claims by the local contractor/AB MAC and the centralized billing contractor, effective for claims received on or after July 1, 2002, CWF has implemented a number of edits.

NOTE: 90659 was discontinued December 31, 2003.

CWF returns information in Trailer 13 information from the history claim. The following fields are returned to the contractor:

- Trailer Code
- Contractor Number
- Document Control Number
- First Service Date
- Last Service Date
- Provider, Physician, Supplier Number
- Claim Type
- Procedure code
- Alert Code (where applicable)
- More history (where applicable))

Pub 100-4, 18, 10.4.1 – CWF Edits on FI/AB MAC Claims

(Rev.1617, Issued: 10-24-08, Effective: 04-06-09, Implementation: 04-06-09)

In order to prevent duplicate payment by the same FI/AB MAC, CWF edits by line item on the FI/AB MAC number, the beneficiary Health Insurance Claim (HIC) number, and the date of service, the influenza virus procedure codes 90655, 90656, 90657, 90658, 90659, or 90660 the pneumococcal procedure codes 90669 or 90732, and the administration codes G0008 or G0009.

If CWF receives a claim with either HCPCS codes 90655, 90656, 90657, 90658, 90659, or 90660 and it already has on record a claim with the same HIC number, same FI/AB MAC number, same date of service, and any one of those HCPCS codes, the second claim submitted to CWF rejects.

If CWF receives a claim with HCPCS codes 90669 or 90732 and it already has on record a claim with the same HIC number, same FI/AB MAC number, same date of service, and the same HCPCS code, the second claim submitted to CWF rejects when all four items match.

If CWF receives a claim with HCPCS administration codes G0008 or G0009 and it already has on record a claim with the same HIC number, same FI/AB MAC number, same date of service, and same procedure code, CWF rejects the second claim submitted when all four items match.

CWF returns to the FI/AB MAC a reject code "7262" for this edit. FIs/AB MACs must deny the second claim and use the same messages they currently use for the denial of duplicate claims.

Pub 100-4, 18, 10.4.2 – CWF Edits on Carrier/AB MAC Claims

(Rev. 1617, Issued: 10-24-08, Effective: 04-06-09, Implementation: 04-06-09)

In order to prevent duplicate payment by the same carrier/AB MAC, CWF will edit by line item on the carrier/AB MAC number, the HIC number, the date of service, the influenza virus procedure codes 90655, 90656, 90657, 90658, 90659, or 90660; the pneumococcal procedure codes 90669 or 90732; and the administration code G0008 or G0009.

If CWF receives a claim with either HCPCS codes 90655, 90656, 90657, 90658, 90659, or 90660 and it already has on record a claim with the same HIC number, same carrier/AB MAC number, same date of service, and any one of those HCPCS codes, the second claim submitted to CWF will reject.

If CWF receives a claim with HCPCS codes 90669 or 90732 and it already has on record a claim with the same HIC number, same carrier/AB MAC number, same date of service, and the same HCPCS code, the second claim submitted to CWF will reject when all four items match.

If CWF receives a claim with HCPCS administration codes G0008 or G0009 and it already has on record a claim with the same HIC number, same carrier/AB MAC number, same date of service, and same procedure code, CWF will reject the second claim submitted.

CWF will return to the carrier/AB MAC a specific reject code for this edit. Carriers/AB MACs must deny the second claim and use the same messages they currently use for the denial of duplicate claims.

In order to prevent duplicate payment by the centralized billing contractor and local carrier/AB MAC, CWF will edit by line item for carrier number, same HIC number, same date of service, the influenza virus procedure codes 90655, 90656, 90657, 90658, 90659, or 90660; the pneumococcal procedure codes 90669 or 90732; and the administration code G0008 or G0009.

If CWF receives a claim with either HCPCS codes 90655, 90656, 90657, 90658, 90659, or 90660 and it already has on record a claim with a different carrier/AB MAC number, but same HIC number, same date of service, and any one of those same HCPCS codes, the second claim submitted to CWF will reject.

If CWF receives a claim with HCPCS codes 90669 or 90732 and it already has on record a claim with the same HIC number, different carrier/AB MAC number, same date of service, and the same HCPCS code, the second claim submitted to CWF will reject.

If CWF receives a claim with HCPCS administration codes G0008 or G0009 and it already has on record a claim with a different carrier/AB MAC number, but the same HIC number, same date of service, and same procedure code, CWF will reject the second claim submitted.

CWF will return a specific reject code for this edit. Carriers/AB MACs must deny the second claim. For the second edit, the reject code should automatically trigger the following Medicare Summary Notice (MSN) and Remittance Advice (RA) messages.

MSN: 7.2 – "This is a duplicate of a claim processed by another contractor. You should receive a Medicare Summary Notice from them."

Claim adjustment reason code 18 – duplicate claim or service.

Pub 100-4, 18, 10.4.3 – CWF A/B Crossover Edits for FI/AB MAC and Carrier/AB MAC Claims

(Rev. 1617, Issued: 10-24-08, Effective: 04-06-09, Implementation: 04-06-09)

When CWF receives a claim from the carrier/AB MAC, it will review Part B outpatient claims history to verify that a duplicate claim has not already been posted.

CWF will edit on the beneficiary HIC number; the date of service; the influenza virus procedure codes 90655, 90656, 90657, 90658, 90659, or 90660; the pneumococcal procedure codes 90669 or 90732; and the administration code G0008 or G0009.

CWF will return a specific reject code for this edit. Contractors must deny the second claim and use the same messages they currently use for the denial of duplicate claims.

Pub 100-4, 18, 10.5 – Medicare Summary Notice (MSN)

(Rev. 1586, Issued: 09-05-08, Effective: 10-06-08, Implementation: 10-06-08)

Contractors must generate a Medicare Summary Notice (MSN) for the pneumococcal, influenza virus, hepatitis B vaccines, and their administration.

For vaccines rendered to beneficiaries other than pneumococcal, influenza virus or hepatitis B, which are not covered by Medicare, they must send the following MSN message.

MSN: 18.2:

This immunization and/or preventive care is not covered.

The Spanish version of this MSN message should read:

Esta inmunización y/o servicios preventivos no están cubiertos.

Pub 100-4, 18, 20.2 – HCPCS and Diagnosis Codes for Mammography Services

(Rev. 1472, Issued: 03-06-08, Effective: 05-23-07, Implementation: 04-07-08)

The following HCPCS and TOS codes are used to bill for mammography services.

HCPCS Code	TOS	Definition
77051* (76082*)	4	Computer aided detection (computer algorithm analysis of digital image data for lesion detection) with further physician review for interpretation, with or without digitization of film radiographic images, diagnostic mammography (list separately in addition to code for primary procedure). Code 76082 is effective January 1, 2004 thru December 31, 2006. Code 77051 is effective January 1, 2007.
77052* (76083*)	1	Computer aided detection (computer algorithm analysis of digital image data for lesion detection) with further physician review for interpretation, with or without digitization of film radiographic images, screening mammography (list separately in addition to code for primary procedure). Code 76083 is effective January 1, 2004 thru December 31, 2006. Code 77052 is effective January 1, 2007.
76085	1	Digitization of film radiographic images with computer analysis for lesion detection and further physician review for interpretation screening mammography (list separately in addition to code for primary procedure). Use with CPT code 76092. Code 76085 was effective January 1, 2002 for all claims submitted to a carrier or an FI, except hospital outpatient prospective payment (OPPS) claims, which are billed to the FI. For OPPS claims billed to the FI, this code is effective April 1, 2002. Deleted as of December 31, 2003.
77055* (76090*)	4	Diagnostic mammography, unilateral.
77056* (76091*)	4	Diagnostic mammography, bilateral.
77057* (76092*)	1	Screening mammography, bilateral (two view film study of each breast).
G0202	1	Screening mammography, producing direct digital image, bilateral, all views. Code Effective April 1, 2001.
G0203		Screening mammography film processed to produce digital images analyzed for potential abnormalities, bilateral all views; Code Effective April 1, 2001 and terminated December 31, 2001, with the exception of hospitals subject to OPPS, who may bill this code through March 31, 2002.
G0204	4	Diagnostic mammography, direct digital image, bilateral, all views; Code Effective April 1, 2001.
G0205		Diagnostic mammography, film processed to produce digital image analyzed for potential abnormalities, bilateral, all views; Code Effective April 1, 2001 and terminated December 31, 2001, with the exception of hospitals subject to OPPS, who may bill this code through March 31, 2002.
G0206	1	Diagnostic mammography, producing direct digital image, unilateral, all views; Code Effective April 1, 2001.
G0207		Diagnostic mammography, film processed to produce digital image analyzed for potential abnormalities, unilateral, all views; Code Effective April 1, 2001 and terminated December 31, 2001, with the exception of hospitals subject to OPPS, who may bill this code through March 31, 2002.
G0236		Digitization of film radiographic images with computer analysis for lesion detection and further physician review for interpretation, diagnostic mammography (List separately in addition to code for primary procedure). Use with CPT Codes 76090 or 76091. Code G0236 was effective January 1, 2002 for all claims submitted to a carrier or an FI except hospital OPPS claims, which are billed to the FI. For OPPS claims billed to the FI, the code is effective April 1, 2002. Deleted as of December 31, 2003.

**For claims with dates of service prior to January 1, 2007, providers report CPT codes 76082, 76083, 76090, 76091, and 76092. For claims with dates of service January 1, 2007 and later, providers report CPT codes 77051, 77052, 77055, 77056, and 77057 respectively.*

New Modifier "GG": Performance and payment of a screening mammography and diagnostic mammography on same patient same day – This is billed with the Diagnostic Mammography code to show the test changed from a screening test to a diagnostic test. Contractors will pay both the screening and diagnostic mammography tests. This modifier is for tracking purposes only. This applies to claims with dates of service on or after January 1, 2002.

A. Diagnosis for Services On or After January 1, 1998

The BBA of 1997 eliminated payment based on high-risk indicators. However, to assure proper coding, one of the following diagnosis codes should be reported on screening mammography claims as appropriate:

V76.11 Special screening for malignant neoplasm, screening mammogram for high-risk patients

V76.12 Special screening for malignant neoplasm, other screening mammography

Beginning October 1, 2003, carriers are no longer permitted to plug the ICD-9-CM code for a screening mammography when the screening mammography claim has no diagnosis code. Screening mammography claims with no diagnosis code must be returned as unprocessable for assigned claims. For unassigned claims, deny the claim.

Providers report on Form CMS-1450 diagnosis code V76.11 or V76.12 in FL 67, "Principal Diagnosis Code" or in Loop 2300 of ANSI-X12 837 if the screening mammography is the only services reported on the claim. If the claim contains other services in addition to the screening mammography, diagnostic codes V76.11 or V76.12 are reported, as appropriate, in FL's 68-75, "Other Diagnostic Codes" or in Loop 2300 of ANSI-X12 837. Carriers receive this diagnosis in field 21 and field 24E with the appropriate pointer code of Form CMS-1500 or in Loop 2300 of ANSI- X12 837.

Diagnosis codes for a diagnostic mammography will vary according to diagnosis.

B. Diagnoses for Services October 1, 1997 Through December 31, 1997

On every screening mammography claim where the patient is not a high-risk individual, diagnosis code V76.12 is reported on the claim.

If the screening is for a high risk individual, the provider reports the principal diagnosis code as V76.11 – "Screening mammogram for high risk patient."

In addition, for high-risk individuals, one of the following applicable diagnoses codes is reported as "Other Diagnoses codes" (Form CMS-1450, FL 68)

- V10.3 "Personal history – Malignant neoplasm female breast";
- V16.3 "Family history – Malignant neoplasm breast"; or
- V15.89 "Other specified personal history representing hazards to health."

The following chart indicates the ICD-9 diagnosis codes reported for each high-risk category:

High Risk Category	Appropriate Diagnosis Code
A personal history of breast cancer	V10.3
A mother, sister, or daughter who has breast cancer	V16.3
Not given birth prior to age 30	V15.89
A personal history of biopsy-proven benign breast disease	V15.89

Pub 100-4, 18, 20.2.1 – Computer-Aided Detection (CAD) Add-On Codes

(Rev. 1070, Issued: 09-29-06, Effective: 01-01-07, Implementation: 01-02-07)

Screening Add-on Codes 76085 and 77052* (76083*)

Effective for services on or after January 1, 2002 through December 31, 2003, (or April 1, 2002 for hospitals subject to OPPS) a new CPT code 76085, CAD conversion of standard film images to digital images has been established as an add-on code that can be billed only in conjunction with the primary service screening mammography code 76092. The definition of 76085 is: "Digitization of film radiographic images with computer analysis for lesion detection and further physician review for interpretation, mammography (list separately in addition to code for primary procedure)."

NOTE: For claims with dates of service April 1, 2003 – December 31, 2003, code G0202 may be billed in conjunction with 76085.

Carriers and FIs make payment under the Medicare physician fee schedule. There is no Part B deductible. However, coinsurance is applicable.

For claims with dates of service April 1, 2005, and later, hospitals bill for code 76082* (77051*) under the 13X bill type. The 14X bill type is no longer applicable. Appropriate TOBs for providers other than hospitals are 22X, 23X, and 85X.

Contractors must assure that claims containing code 76085 also contain HCPCS code 76092 or G0202. If not, FIs return claims to the provider with an explanation that payment for code 76085 cannot be made when billed alone. Carriers deny payment for 76085 when billed without 76092 or G0202.

NOTE: When screening CAD 76085 is billed in conjunction with a screening mammography (76092 or G0202) and the screening mammography (76092 or G0202) fails the age and frequency edits in CWF, both services will be rejected by CWF.

Effective with claims with dates of service January 1, 2004 thru December 31, 2006, HCPCS code 76083, "Computer aided detection (computer algorithm analysis of digital image data for lesion detection) with further physician review for interpretation with or without digitization of film radiographic images; screening mammography (list separately in addition to code for primary procedure)," can be billed in conjunction with the primary service mammography code 76092 or G0202.

Effective with claims with dates of service January 1, 2007 and later, HCPCS code 77052, which replaces code 76083 "Computer aided detection (computer algorithm analysis of digital image data for lesion detection) with further physician review for interpretation with or without digitization of film radiographic images; screening mammography (list separately in addition to code for primary procedure)," can be billed in conjunction with the primary service mammography code 77057 or G0202.

Contractors must assure that claims containing code 77052* (76083*) also contain HCPCS code 77057* (76092*) or G0202. FIs return claims containing code 77052* (76083*) that do not also contain HCPCS code 77057* (76092*) or G0202 with an explanation that payment for code 77052* (76083*) cannot be made when billed alone. Carriers deny payment for 77052* (76083*) when billed without 77057* (76092*) or G0202.

NOTE: When screening CAD 77052* (76083*) is billed in conjunction with a screening mammography (77057* (76092*) or G0202) and the screening mammography (77057* (76092*) or G0202) fails the age and frequency edits in CWF, both services will be rejected by CWF.

**For claims with dates of service prior to January 1, 2007, providers report CPT codes 76083 and 76092 or G0202. For claims with dates of service January 1, 2007 and later, providers report CPT codes 77052 and 77057 or G0202, respectively.*

Diagnostic Add-on Codes G0236 and 77051* (76082*)

Effective for services on or after January 1, 2002 thru December 31, 2003, (or April 1, 2002 for hospital claims subject to OPPS), HCPCS code G0236 was established for diagnostic mammography CAD that can be billed only on the same claim with the primary service of either 76090 or 76091. The definition of G0236 is: "Digitization of film radiographic images with computer analysis for lesion detection and further physician review for interpretation." The code must be listed separately in addition to code for the primary procedure.

NOTE: For claims with dates of service April 1, 2003 – December 31, 2003, code G0204 and G0206 may be billed in conjunction with G0236.

For claims with dates of service April 1, 2005, and later, hospitals bill for code 76082* (77051*) under the 13X bill type. The 14X bill type is no longer applicable. Appropriate TOBs for providers other than hospitals are 22X, 23X, and 85X.

There are no frequency limitations on film or digital diagnostic tests or CAD-diagnostic tests.

Contractors must assure that claims containing code G0236 also contain HCPCS code 76090, 76091, G0204, or G0206. If not, FIs return claims to the provider with an explanation that payment for code G0236 cannot be made when billed alone. Carriers deny payment for G0236 when billed without 76090, 76091, G0204, or G0206.

Effective with claims with dates of service January 1, 2004 thru December 31, 2006, HCPCS code 76082, "Computer aided detection (computer algorithm analysis of digital image data for lesion detection) with further physician review for interpretation with or without digitization of film radiographic images; diagnostic mammography (list separately in addition to code for primary procedure)," can be billed in conjunction with the primary service mammography code 76090, 76091, G0204, or G0206.

Effective for claims with dates of service January 1, 2007 and later, HCPCS code 77051, which replaces code 76082,"Computer aided detection (computer algorithm analysis of digital image data for lesion detection) with further physician review for interpretation with or without digitization of film radiographic images; diagnostic mammography (list separately in addition to code for primary procedure)," can be billed in conjunction with the primary service mammography code 77055, 77056, G0204, or G0206.

Contractors must assure that claims containing code 77051* (76082*) also contain HCPCS codes 77055*(76090*), 77056* (76091*), G0204 or G0206. FIs return claims containing code 77051* (76082*) that do not also contain HCPCS code 77055* (76090*), 77056* (76091*), G0204, or G0206 with an explanation that payment for code 77051* (76082*), cannot be made when billed alone. Carriers deny payment for 77051* (76082*) when billed without 77055* (76090*), 77056* (76091*), G0204, or G0206.

**For claims with dates of service prior to January 1, 2007, providers report CPT codes 76090, 76091, G0204 or G0206 with 76082. For claims with dates of service January 1, 2007 and later, providers report CPT codes 77055, 77056, G0204, or G0206 with 77051, respectively.*

Pub 100-4, 18, 20.2.1.1 – CAD Billing Charts

(Rev. 1070, Issued: 09-29-06, Effective: 01-01-07, Implementation: 01-02-07)

The following chart provides guidance for billing of CAD add-on codes. It reflects appropriate coding combinations that may be billed and the time frames associated with each.

Chart I – Screening CAD Codes

CAD Codes	Effective 01-01-02 thru 03-31-03	Effective 04-01-03 thru 12-31-03	Effective 01-01-04 thru 12-31-06	Effective 01-01-07 and later
76085	76092	76092, G0202	N/A	N/A
76083	N/A	N/A	76092, G0202	N/A
77052	N/A	N/A	N/A	77057, G0202

Chart II – Diagnostic CAD Codes

CAD Codes	Effective 01-01-02 thru 03-31-03	Effective 04-01-03 thru 12-31-03	Effective 01-01-04 thru 12-31-06	Effective 01-01-07 and later
G0236	76090	76090	N/A	N/A
	76091	76091		
		G0204		
		G0206		
76082	N/A	N/A	76090	N/A
			76091	N/A
			G0204	N/A
			G0206	N/A
77051	N/A	N/A	N/A	G0204
				G0206
				77055
				77056

**For claims with dates of service prior to January 1, 2007, providers report CPT codes 76090, 76091, G0204 or G0206 with 76082. For claims with dates of service January 1, 2007 and later, providers report CPT codes 77055, 77056, G0204, or G0206 with 77051, respectively.*

The CWF Application of Age and Frequency Edits,--The following chart reflects proper application of CWF age and frequency edits applied to CAD HCPCS codes billed in conjunction with screening mammographies HCPCS codes.

CAD Codes	Effective 01-01-02 thru 03-31-03	Effective 04-01-03 thru 12-31-03	Effective 01-01-04 thru 12-31-06	Effective 01-01-07 and later
76085	76092	76092, G0202	N/A	N/A
76083	N/A	N/A	76092, G0202	N/A
77052	N/A	N/A	N/A	77057, G0202

See section 20.5.1, for carrier CWF edits

**For claims with dates of service prior to January 1, 2007, providers report CPT codes 76083 and 76092. For claims with dates of service January 1, 2007 and later, providers report CPT codes 77052 and 77057 respectively.*

Pub 100-4, 18, 20.3 – Payment

(Rev. 1931, Issued: 03-12-10, Effective: 06-14-10, Implementation: 06-14-10)

There is no Part B deductible for screening mammographies, however, coinsurance is applicable. The anti-markup payment limitation on physician billing for diagnostic tests does not apply to these services. Following are three categories of billing for mammography services:

- Professional component of mammography services (that is the physician's interpretation of the results of the examination)
- Technical component (all other services)
- Both professional and technical components (global). However, global billing is not permitted for services furnished in provider outpatient departments, except for CAHs electing the optional method of payment for mammography services furnished on or after January 1, 2002.

Pub 100-4, 18, 20.3.1 – Payment for Screening Mammography Services Provided Prior to January 1, 2002

(Rev. 1070, Issued: 09-29-06, Effective: 01-01-07, Implementation: 01-02-07)

Claims with dates of service prior to January 1, 2002, are subject to a payment limitation. The professional component is 32 percent of the total limit for the complete service. The technical component is 68 percent.

When the technical and professional components of the screening mammography are billed separately, the payment limit is adjusted to reflect either the professional or technical component only. That is, the limitation applicable to global billing for screening is allocated between the professional and technical components as set forth by regulations. Below are the limitation amounts applicable each calendar year:

Calendar Year	Global Payment Limit	Technical Component Amount	Professional Component Amount
1996	$62.10	$42.23	$19.87
1997	$63.34	$43.07	$20.27
1998	$64.73	$44.02	$20.71
1999	$66.22	$45.03	$21.19
2000	$67.81	$46.11	$21.69
2001	$69.23	$47.08	$22.15

NOTE: The CMS annually updates the overall limit annually by the percentage increase in the Medicare Economic Index.

EXAMPLE: In calendar year 2001, 32 percent of the $69.23 limit, or $22.15, is used in determining payment for the professional component; and 68 percent of the $69.23 limit, or $47.08, is used in determining payment for the technical component.

FI Payment

Payment for the technical component equals 80 percent of the least of:

- The actual charge for the technical component (HCPCS code 77057* (76092*)) of the service;
- The physicians' fee schedule amount for the technical component of HCPCS code 77056* (76091*) (a bilateral diagnostic mammogram); or
- The technical portion of the screening mammography limit as identified in the chart above.

**For claims with dates of service prior to January 1, 2007, providers report CPT codes 76091 and 76092. For claims with dates of service January 1, 2007 and later, providers report CPT codes 77056 and 77057 respectively.*

Carrier Payment – Technical Component

Payment for the technical component equals 80 percent of the least of:

- The actual charge for the technical component of the service;
- The amount determined with respect to the technical component for the service under Medicare Physicians' Fee Schedule; or
- The technical portion of the screening mammography limit as identified in the chart above.

Carrier Payment – Professional Component

The amount of payment for the professional charge equals 80 percent of the least of:

- The actual charge for the professional component;
- The amount determined with respect to the professional component for the service under the Medicare Physician Fee Schedule; or
- The professional portion of the screening mammography limit based on the year of service according to the chart above.

FI or Carrier Payment – Global

The amount of payment for the global charge equals 80 percent of the least of:

- The actual charge for the procedure;
- The amount determined with respect to the global procedure under the Medicare Fee Schedule; or
- The limit for the procedure based on the year of service according to the chart above.

Carriers may receive bills for global, professional, or technical components. If mammography services are furnished by nonparticipating physicians and suppliers, there is a special limiting charge. Carriers must apply the appropriate payment reductions to screening mammography procedures furnished by new physicians.

Providers bill the technical component of mammography services to FIs. Only a CAH may bill globally if the CAH elected the optional method of payment for mammography services furnished on or after January 1, 2002.

FI Payment Example

$90.00 Provider charges for HCPCS;

$75.00 Physician' fee schedule amount; and

$47.08 Technical portion of the screening mammography limit (68% of $69.23 (year 2001))

Payment is 80 percent of the lower of the following amounts. To calculate the payment, select the lower of:

$90.00 Provider charges;

$75.00 Physician' fee schedule amount for the technical component; or

$47.08 Technical portion of the screening mammography limit (year 2001).

Payment is 80 percent of the remainder. FIs do not apply the provider's interim rate. This is a final payment to the provider. In this example, payment is calculated as follows:

$47.08 x 80% = $ 37.66 payment to the provider

To determine the patient's liability, multiply the actual charge by 20 percent. The result is the patient's liability. In this example, the calculation is:

$90.00 x 20% = $18.00 (coinsurance).

Pub 100-4, 18, 20.3.2 – Payment for Screening Mammography Services Provided On and After January 1, 2002

(Rev. 1070, Issued: 09-29-06, Effective: 01-01-07, Implementation: 01-02-07)

The payment limitation methodology does not apply to claims with dates of service on or after January 1, 2002.

FI Claims

For claims with dates of service on or after January 1, 2002, §104 of the Benefits Improvement and Protection Act (BIPA) 2000, provides for payment of screening mammography under the Medicare physician fee schedule (MPFS) when furnished in hospitals, skilled nursing facilities (SNFs), and CAHs not electing the optional method of payment for outpatient services. However, payment under the physician fee schedule is not applicable to hospitals subject to the Outpatient Prospective Payment System (OPPS) until April 1, 2002.

The payment for code 77057* (76092*) is equal to the lower of:

- The actual charge or
- Locality specific technical component payment amount under the MPFS.

Program payment for the service is 80 percent of the lower amount and coinsurance is 20 percent. Part B deductible does not apply. This is a final payment.

FIs use the benefit-pricing file provided by CMS to pay mammography codes.

Payment for the add-on code 76085 is made under the Medicare Physician Fee Schedule. Deductible does not apply, however, coinsurance is applicable.

**For claims with dates of service prior to January 1, 2007, providers report CPT code 76092. For claims with dates of service January 1, 2007 and later, providers report CPT code 77057.*

Carrier Claims

Physicians and suppliers are paid by the carrier for all mammography tests (including screening mammography) under the MPFS. Separate prices for the technical component, the professional component and the global service are included on the MPFS.

The Medicare allowed charge is the lower of:

- The actual charge, or
- The MPFS amount for the service billed.

The Medicare payment for the service is 80 percent of the allowed charge. Coinsurance is 20 percent of the lower of the actual charge or the MPFS amount. Part B deductible is waived and does not apply to screening mammography.

As with other MPFS services, the nonparticipating provider reduction and the limiting charge provisions apply to all mammography tests (including screening mammography).

Pub 100-4, 18, 20.3.2.1 – Outpatient Hospital Mammography Payment Table

(Rev. 1070, Issued: 09-29-06, Effective: 01-01-07, Implementation: 01-02-07)

Payment for Mammography in the Hospital Outpatient PPS Setting. For all other hospitals, the effective date for column 1 is April 1, 2001, through December 31, 2001, and for column 2, the effective date is January 2002.

PAYMENT FOR SCREENING MAMMOGRAPHY

Screening Mammography (Revenue Code 403)	Year 2000	2001 (April 1, 01 thru March 31, 2002)	April 1, 2002 – forward
77057* (76092*) Screening Mammography, bilateral No deductible, Coinsurance applies	Lesser of: 1. Charges, 2. TC of PFS for 76091, or 3. Annual payment limit	Lesser of: 1. Charge, 2. TC of MPFS for code 76091, or 3. Annual payment limit $47.08	Lesser of: 1. Charge, or 2. TC of MPFS for code 77057* (76092*)
G0202 Screening Mammography, producing direct digital image, bilateral, all views. No deductible Coinsurance applies	N/A	Lesser of: 1. Charge, or 2. 150% TC of MPFS for code 76091	Lesser of: 1. Actual charge, or 2. TC of MPFS for code G0202
G0203 Screening mammography, film processed to produce digital image analyzed for potential abnormalities, bilateral, all views. No Deductible Coinsurance Applies	N/A	Lesser of: 1. Charge, 2. TC of MPFS for code 76091, or 3. $57.28 (annual $ limit of $47.08 plus $10.20TC add on)	N/A

**For claims with dates of service prior to January 1, 2007, providers report CPT codes 76091 and 76092. For claims with dates of service January 1, 2007 and later, providers report CPT codes 77056 and 77057 respectively.*

PAYMENT FOR DIAGNOSTIC MAMMOGRAPHY

Diagnostic Mammography (Revenue Code 401)	Year 2000	April 1, 2001 thru March 31, 2002	April 1, 2002 thru December 31, 2004	January 1, 2005 – forward
77056* (76091*) Mammography, bilateral Deductible and coinsurance apply	OPPS (beginning Aug.1, 2000)	OPPS	OPPS	Lesser of charge or TC or the MPFS for 77056* (76091*)
77055* (76090*) Mammography, bilateral Deductible and coinsurance apply	OPPS (beginning Aug.1, 2000)	OPPS	OPPS	Lesser of charge or TC or the MPFS for 77055* (76090*)
G0204 Diagnostic Mammography, direct digital image, bilateral, all views Deductible and coinsurance apply	N/A	Lesser of: 1. Charge, or 2. 150% TC of MPFS for code 76091	OPPS	Lesser of charge or TC or the MPFS for G0204
G0206 Diagnostic Mammography, direct digital image, unilateral, all views Deductible and coinsurance apply	N/A	OPPS (same APC as 76090)	OPPS	Lesser of charge or TC or the MPFS for G0206
G0205 Diagnostic Mammography, film processed to produce digital image analyzed for potential abnormalities, unilateral, all views Deductible and coinsurance apply	N/A	Lesser of: 1. Charge, 2. TC of MPFS for code 76091, or 3. $57.28 (annual $ limit of $47.08 plus $10.20TC add on)	N/A	N/A

Medicare References

Diagnostic Mammography (Revenue Code 401)	Year 2000	April 1, 2001 thru March 31, 2002	April 1, 2002 thru December 31, 2004	January 1, 2005 – forward
G0207 Diagnostic Mammography, film processed to produce digital image analyzed for potential abnormalities, unilateral, all views Deductible and coinsurance apply	N/A	OPPS (same APC as 76090)	N/A	N/A

For claims with dates of service prior to January 1, 2007, providers report CPT codes 76090 and 76091. For claims with dates of service January 1, 2007 and later, providers report CPT codes 77055 and 77056 respectively.

Beginning January 1, 2005, Medicare Prescription Drug, Improvement, and Modernization Act (MMA) of 2003, §644, Public Law 108-173 has changed the way Medicare pays for diagnostic mammography. Medicare payment will be based on the MPFS. Payment will no longer be made under the OPPS.

COMPUTER-AIDED DETECTION (CAD) DEVICES

Computer-aided Detection (CAD)	Year 2000	2001 (April 1 – Dec 31)	Year 2002 – 2003	January 1, 2004	January 1, 2005 – forward
76085* CAD with screening mammography (may bill with 76092) No deductible coinsurance applies	N/A	N/A	Lesser of: 1. Charge, or 2. TC of MPFS for code 76085	N/A	N/A
G0236* CAD with diagnostic mammography (may bill with 76090 or 76091) Deductible and coinsurance apply	N/A	N/A	OPPS	N/A	N/A
77052* (76083*) CAD with screening mammography (may bill with 77057* (76092*) or G0202) No deductible applies	N/A	N/A	N/A	Lesser of: 1. Charge, or 2. TC of MPFS for code 76083	Lesser of: 1. Charge, or 2. TC of MPFS for code 77052* (76083*)
77051* (76082*) CAD with diagnostic mammography (may bill with 77055* (76090*), 77056* (76091*), G0204, or G0206) Deductible and coinsurance apply	N/A	N/A	N/A	OPPS	Lesser of: 1. Charge, or 2. TC of MPFS for code 77051* (76082*)

TC = technical component
MPFS= Medicare Physician Fee Schedule
OPPS= Outpatient Prospective Payment System
APC= Ambulatory Payment Classification

** Code 76085 is a deleted code as of December 31, 2003. The code to be used for dates of service beginning January 1, 2004 thru December 31, 2006, is 76083. For claims with dates of service January 1, 2007 and later, the new code is 77052. Code G0236 is a deleted code as of December 31, 2003. The code to be used for dates of service beginning January 1, 2004 thru December 31, 2006, is 76082. For claims with dates of service January 1, 2007 and later, the new code is 77051.*

Beginning January 1, 2005, Medicare Prescription Drug, Improvement, and Modernization Act (MMA) of 2003, §644, Public Law 108-173 has changed the way Medicare pays for diagnostic CAD services. Medicare payment will be based on the MPFS. Payment will no longer be made under the OPPS.

Pub 100-4, 18, 20.3.2.2 – Payment for Computer Add-On Diagnostic and Screening Mammograms for FIs and Carriers

(Rev. 1070, Issued: 09-29-06, Effective: 01-01-07, Implementation: 01-02-07)

Payment for computer add-on diagnostic mammogram HCPCS code G0236 or 77051* (76082*) when billed with CPT code 77055* (76090*), 77056* (76091*), G0204, or G0206 is as follows:

Place/Provider of Service	Payment
Physician	Medicare physicians' fee schedule
Outpatient Hospital	Outpatient Prospective Payment System (OPPS)
Critical Access Hospital (CAH)	Reasonable Cost
SNF	Medicare physicians' fee schedule – technical component
Independent RHC	All-inclusive rate for professional component (codes 76090 and 76091)**
Freestanding FQHC	All-inclusive rate for professional component (codes 76090 and 76091)**

*** Only for dates of service prior to April 1, 2005.*

NOTE: Effective for claims with dates of service on or after January 1, 2005, computer add-on diagnostic mammography services provided in a hospital are paid under the MPFS. Payment is no longer made under the OPPS.

Code G0236, "Digitization of film radiographic images with computer analysis for lesion detection and further physician review for interpretation, diagnostic mammography," for CAD has been established as an add on code that can be billed in conjunction with primary service code G0204 or G0206, as well as existing codes 76090 or 76091. The Part B deductible and coinsurance apply. HCPCS code G0236 is deleted as of December 31, 2003.

Effective for claims with dates of service January 1, 2004 thru December 31, 2006, add-on HCPCS code 76082, "Computer aided detection (computer algorithm analysis of digital image data for lesion detection) with further physician review for interpretation, with or without digitization of film radiographic images; diagnostic mammography (list separately in addition to code for primary procedure)," can be billed in conjunction with primary service codes G0204 or G0206 as well as codes 76090 or 76091. The Part B deductible and coinsurance apply.

Effective for claims with dates of service January 1, 2007 and later, add-on HCPCS code 77051, "Computer aided detection (computer algorithm analysis of digital image data for lesion detection) with further physician review for interpretation, with or without digitization of film radiographic images; diagnostic mammography (list separately in addition to code for primary procedure)," can be billed in conjunction with primary service codes G0204 or G0206 as well as codes 77055 or 77056. The Part B deductible and coinsurance apply.

The add-on code cannot be billed alone. FIs return to provider claims containing only codes G0236 or 77051* (76082*) with an explanation that payment for code G0236 or 77051* (76082*) cannot be made when billed alone.

Carriers deny the claim using remark code N122, "Mammography add-on code can not be billed by itself" (effective September 12, 2002).

Payment for computer add-on screening mammogram HCPCS code 76085 or 77052* (76083*) when billed with CPT code 77057* (76092*) or G0202 is as follows:

Place/Provider of Service	Payment
Physician	Medicare physicians' fee schedule
Outpatient Hospital	Medicare physicians' fee schedule
Critical Access Hospital (CAH)	Reasonable Cost
SNF	Medicare physicians' fee schedule – technical component
Independent RHC	All-inclusive rate for professional component (code 76092**)
Freestanding FQHC	All-inclusive rate for professional component (code 76092**)

*** Only for dates of service prior to April 1, 2005.*

Code 76085, "Digitization of film radiographic images with computer analysis for lesion detection and further physician review for interpretation, screening mammography," for CAD has been established as an add on code that can be billed in conjunction with primary service code G0202 as well as 76092. HCPCS code 76085 is deleted as of December 31, 2003. The Part B Deductible does not apply. However, coinsurance is applicable. FIs use the benefit pricing file provided by CMS to pay the above codes where payment is based on the technical component of the Medicare physician fee schedule.

Effective for claims with dates of service January 1, 2004 thru December 31, 2006, HCPCS code 76083, "Computer aided detection (computer algorithm analysis of digital image data for lesion detection) with further physician review for interpretation, with or without digitization of film radiographic images; screening mammography (list separately in addition to code for primary procedure)," can be billed in conjunction with the primary service code G0202 as well as code 76092. There is no Part B deductible but coinsurance applies.

Effective for claims with dates of service January 1, 2007 and later, HCPCS code 77052, "Computer aided detection (computer algorithm analysis of digital image data for lesion detection) with further physician review for interpretation, with or without digitization of

film radiographic images; screening mammography (list separately in addition to code for primary procedure)," can be billed in conjunction with the primary service code G0202 as well as code 77057. There is no Part B deductible but coinsurance applies.

The add-on code cannot be billed alone. FIs return to provider claims containing only codes 76085 or 77052* (76083*) with an explanation that payment for code 76085 or 77052* (76083*) cannot be made when billed alone.

Carriers deny the claim using remark code N122 "Mammography add-on code cannot be billed by itself" (effective September 12, 2002).

**For claims with dates of service prior to January 1, 2007, providers report CPT codes 76082, 76083, 76090, 76091, and 76092. For claims with dates of service January 1, 2007 and later, providers report CPT codes 77051, 77052, 77055, 77056, and 77057 respectively.*

Pub 100-4, 18, 20.3.2.3 – Critical Access Hospital Payment

(Rev. 1070, Issued: 09-29-06, Effective: 01-01-07, Implementation: 01-02-07)

Payment to a CAH for screening mammography is not subject to applicable Part B deductible, but coinsurance does apply. Any deductible or coinsurance collected is deducted from the payment.

A. Under the Optional (All Inclusive) Method

Section 403(d) of the BBRA amended §1834(g) of the Act to permit a CAH to elect an optional method of payment for outpatient services. This option is effective for cost reporting periods beginning on or after October 1, 2001. A CAH may elect to be paid for outpatient services by reasonable costs for facility services and §202 of BIPA allows an amount equal to 115 percent of the allowed amount for professional component. (Costs related to professional services are excluded from the cost payment.)

CAHs electing the optional method of reimbursement bill the FI with type of bill 85X, revenue code 0403 and HCPCS code 77057* (76092*). They also include the professional component on a separate line, with revenue code 96X, 97X, or 98X and HCPCS code 77057* (76092*).

**For claims with dates of service prior to January 1, 2007, providers report CPT codes 76083 and 76092. For claims with dates of service January 1, 2007 and later, providers report CPT codes 77052 and 77057 respectively.*

B. Under the Standard Method

CAHs reimbursed on the standard method of payment bill the technical component of a screening mammography to the FI on type of bill 85X, revenue code 0403 and HCPCS code 77057* (76092*).

Professional services are billed to the carrier and paid based on the fee schedule by the carrier.

For claims with dates of service on or after January 1, 2002, §104 of the Benefits Improvement and Protection Act (BIPA) 2000, provides for payment of screening mammographies under the Medicare physician fee schedule (MPFS) in CAHs not electing the optional method of payment for outpatient services.

**For claims with dates of service prior to January 1, 2007, providers report CPT code 76092. For claims with dates of service January 1, 2007 and later, providers report CPT code 77057.*

Pub 100-4, 18, 20.3.2.3.1 – CAH Screening Mammography Payment Table

(Rev. 1070, Issued: 09-29-06, Effective: 01-01-07, Implementation: 01-02-07)

Payment for Screening Mammography in the Critical Access Hospital Outpatient Setting

Method 1 (Standard)

	TOB	Rev Code	HCPCS	Payment
Services prior to cost reporting periods ending October 1, 2001 and services prior to July 1, 2001 (BIPA)				
Technical Component Deductible does not apply. Coinsurance based on charge.	85X	403	76092	FI payment is 80% of the reasonable cost.
Professional Component Deductible does not apply. Coinsurance based on lower of MPFS or charge.			76092	Carrier payment is 80% of the lower of the charge or MPFS amount for the technical component.
Services on or after July 1, 2001 to January 1, 2002				
Technical Component Deductible does not apply. Coinsurance based on charge.	85X	403	76092	FI payment is 80% of the reasonable cost.
Professional Component Deductible does not apply. Coinsurance based on lower of MPFS or charge.			76092	Carrier payment is 80% of the lower of the charge or MPFS amount.
Services on or after January 1 2002				
Technical Component Deductible does not apply. Coinsurance based on charge.	85X	403	*76092 *76085 G0202	FI payment is 80% of the lower of the charge or the fee schedule amount.
Professional Component Deductible does not apply. Coinsurance based on lower of MPFS or charge.			*76092 *76085 G0202	Carrier payment is 80% of the lower of the charge or MPFS amount for the technical component. The new A3 states payment for 76092 is lower of charge or locality specific TECHNICAL component amount under MPFS.

*Codes must be billed together on the same claim. Also note that 76085 is deleted after December 31, 2003. Use code 76083 for claims with dates of service January 1, 2004 and later.

Method 2 (Optional Method)

Option available with cost reporting periods starting on or after October 1, 2001 and dates of service on or after July 1, 2001.

	TOB	Rev Code	HCPCS	Payment
Services for cost reporting periods on or after October 1, 2001 and service dates on or after July 1 and prior to January 1, 2002				
Technical Component Deductible does not apply. Coinsurance based on charge.	85X	403	76092	FI payment is 80% of the reasonable cost. (Interim rate times charge)
Professional Component Deductible does not apply. Coinsurance based on charge.	85X	96X, or 97X or 98X	76092	FI payment is 115% of the lower of the charge or MPFS amount after coinsurance is deducted.
Professional Component service in a rural or urban HPSA area. Deductible does not apply. Coinsurance based on charge	85X	96X, or 97X or 98X	Modifier "QB" or "QU" for dates of service prior to January 1, 2006. For more information on HPSA modifiers see chapter 4, section 250.2.2 in Pub. 100-04.	If HPSA area, FI payment is 115% of 110% of the lower of the charge or MPFS amount after coinsurance is deducted times 110%.
Services on or after January 1 2002				
Technical Component Deductible does not apply. Coinsurance based on charge.	85X	403	*76085 77057* (76092*) G0202	FI payment is 80% of the lower of the charge or the fee schedule amount.
Professional Component Deductible does not apply. Coinsurance based on lower of MPFS or charge.	85X	96X, 97X, or 98X	*76085 77057* (76092*) G0202	FI pays 115% of 80% (that is 92%) of the lower of the charge or the MPFS amount.

* Codes must be billed together on the same claim. Also note that 76085 is deleted after December 31, 2003. Use code 76083 for claims with dates of service January 1, 2004 thru December 31, 2006, and 77052 for claims with dates of service January 1, 2007 and later. Also, for claims with dates of service prior to January 1, 2007, CAHs report CPT code 76092. For claims of service with dates of service January 1, 2007 and later, CAHs report CPT code 77057.

Pub 100-4, 18, 20.3.2.4 – SNF Mammography Payment Table

(Rev. 1070, Issued: 09-29-06, Effective: 01-01-07, Implementation: 01-02-07)

Payment for Screening Mammography

Screening Mammography (Revenue Code 0403)	Year 2000	2001 (April 1 – March 31, 2002)	April 1, 2002 and later
77057* (76092*) Screening Mammography, bilateral No deductible, Coinsurance applies	Lesser of: 1. Charges or, 2. TC of MPFS 76091, or 3. Annual payment limit	Lesser of: 1. Charge or, 2. TC of MPFS for code 76091, or 3.Annual payment limit $47.08	Lower of: 1. Charge, or 2. TC of MPFS for code 77057* (76092*)
G0202 Screening Mammography, producing direct digital image, bilateral, all views. No deductible Coinsurance applies	N/A	Lower of: 1. Charge, or 2. 150% TC of MPFS for code 76091	Lower of: 1. Charge, or 2. TC of MPFS for code G0202
G0203 Screening mammography, film processed to produce digital image analyzed for potential abnormalities, bilateral, all views. No Deductible Coinsurance Applies	N/A	Lesser of: 1. Charge, 2. TC of MPFS for code 76091,or 3. $57.28 (annual $ limit of $47.08 plus $10.20TC add on)	N/A

* *For claims with dates of service prior to January 1, 2007, SNFs report CPT codes 76091 and 76092. For claims with dates of service January 1, 2007 and later, SNFs report CPT codes 77056 and 77057 respectively.*

Payment for Diagnostic Mammography

Diagnostic Mammography (Revenue Code 401)	Year 2000	2001 (April 1-March 31, 2002)	April 1, 2002 and later
77056* (76091*) Mammography, bilateral Deductible and coinsurance apply	Lower of charge or TC of MPFS	Lower of charge or TC of MPFS	Lower of charge or TC of MPFS
77055* (76090*) Mammography, bilateral Deductible and coinsurance apply	Lower of charge or TC of MPFS	Lower of charge or TC of MPFS	Lower of charge or TC of MPFS
G0204 Diagnostic Mammography, direct digital image, bilateral, all views Deductible and coinsurance apply	N/A	Lower of: 1. Charge, or 2. 150% TC of MPFS for code 76091	Lower of charge or MPFS
G0206 Diagnostic Mammography, direct digital image, unilateral, all views Deductible and coinsurance apply	N/A	Lower of charge or MPFS	Lower of charge or MPFS
G0205 Diagnostic Mammography, film processed to produce digital image analyzed for potential abnormalities, unilateral, all views Deductible and coinsurance apply	N/A	Lesser of: 1. Charge, 2. TC of MPFS for code 76091 or 3. $57.28 (annual $ limit of $47.08 plus $10.20TC add on)	N/A
G0207 Diagnostic Mammography, film processed to produce digital image analyzed for potential abnormalities, unilateral, all views Deductible and coinsurance apply	N/A	Lower of charge or MPFS	N/A

* *For claims with dates of service prior to January 1, 2007, SNFs report CPT codes 76090 and 76091. For claims with dates of service January 1, 2007 and later, SNFs report CPT codes 77055 and 77056 respectively.*

Payment for Screening and Diagnostic Computer-Aided Detection (CAD)

Computer-aided Detection (CAD)	Year 2000	2001 (April 1- Dec 31)	Year 2002 and later
76085** CAD with screening mammography (may bill with 77057* (76092*)) No Deductible Coinsurance Applies	N/A	N/A	Lower of: 1. Charge or, 2. TC of MPFS for code 76085
G0236 CAD with diagnostic mammography Deductible and coinsurance apply	N/A	N/A	SNFs cannot be paid for this service

TC = technical component
MPFS= Medicare Physician Fee Schedule

* *76085 is a deleted code after December 31, 2003. Use code 76083* instead of 76085 for claims with dates of service through December 31, 2006, and code 77052 for claims with dates of service January 1, 2007 and later.*

* *For claims with dates of service prior to January 1, 2007, SNFs report CPT codes 76082, 76083, 76090, 76091, and 76092. For claims with dates of service January 1, 2007 and later, SNFs report CPT codes 77051, 77052, 77055, 77056, and 77057 respectively.*

Pub 100-4, 18, 20.4 – Billing Requirements – FI/A MAC Claims

(Rev. 1519, Issued: 05-30-08, Effective: 05-23-08, Implementation: 06-30-08)

Contractors use the weekly-updated MQSA file to verify that the billing facility is certified by the FDA to perform mammography services, and has the appropriate certification to perform the type of mammogram billed (film and/or digital). (See §20.1.) FIs/A/B MACs use the provider number submitted on the claim to identify the facility and use the MQSA data file to verify the facility's certification(s). FIs/A/B MACs complete the following activities in processing mammography claims:

- If the provider number on the claim does not correspond with a certified mammography facility on the MQSA file, then intermediaries/ A/B MACs deny the claim.
- When a film mammography HCPCS code is on a claim, the claim is checked for a "1" film indicator.
- If a film mammography HCPCS code comes in on a claim and the facility is certified for film mammography, the claim is paid if all other relevant Medicare criteria are met.
- If a film mammography HCPCS code is on a claim and the facility is certified for digital mammography only, the claim is denied.
- When a digital mammography HCPCS code is on a claim, the claim is checked for "2" digital indicator.
- If a digital mammography HCPCS code is on a claim and the facility is certified for digital mammography, the claim is paid if all other relevant Medicare criteria are met.
- If a digital mammography HCPCS code is on a claim and the facility is certified for film mammography only, the claim is denied.

NOTE: The Common Working File (CWF) no longer receives the mammography file for editing purposes.

Except as provided in the following sections for RHCs and FQHCs, the following procedures apply to billing for screening mammographies:

The technical component portion of the screening mammography is billed on Form CMS-1450 under bill type 12X, 13X, 14X**, 22X, 23X or 85X using revenue code 0403 and HCPCS code 77057* (76092*).

The technical component portion of the diagnostic mammography is billed on Form CMS-1450 under bill type 12X, 13X, 14X**, 22X, 23X or 85X using revenue code 0401 and HCPCS code 77055* (76090*), 77056* (76091*), G0204 and G0206.

Separate bills are required for claims for screening mammographies with dates of service prior to January 1, 2002. Providers include on the bill only charges for the screening mammography. Separate bills are not required for claims for screening mammographies with dates of service on or after January 1, 2002.

See separate instructions below for rural health clinics (RHCs) and federally qualified health centers (FQHCs).

** For claims with dates of service prior to January 1, 2007, providers report CPT codes 76090, 76091, and 76092. For claims with dates of service January 1, 2007 and later, providers report CPT codes 77055, 77056, and 77057 respectively.*

*** For claims with dates of service April 1, 2005 and later, hospitals bill for all mammography services under the 13X type of bill or for dates of service April 1, 2007 and later, 12X or 13X as appropriate. The 14X type of bill is no longer applicable. Appropriate bill types for providers other than hospitals are 22X, 23X, and 85X.*

In cases where screening mammography services are self-referred and as a result an attending physician NPI is not available, the provider shall duplicate their facility NPI in the attending physician identifier field on the claim.

Pub 100-4, 18, 20.4.1 – Rural Health Clinics and Federally Qualified Health Centers

(Rev. 1, 10-01-03)

Pub 100-4, 18, 20.4.1.1 – RHC/FQHC Claims With Dates of Service Prior to January 1, 2002

(Rev. 371, Issued 11-19-04, Effective: 04-01-05, Implementation: 04-04-05)

A. Provider-Based RHC and FQHC

For claims with dates of service prior to January 1, 2002, provider-based RHCs and FQHCs bill the FI for the technical component and their carrier for the professional component of the screening and diagnostic mammography. Provider-based RHCs and FQHCs use the base provider number and bill type (13X, 22X, 23X or 85X as appropriate) when billing the FI for this service. Payment is based on the payment method for the base provider – the limitation.

B. Independent RHCs and Freestanding FQHCs

Independent RHCs and freestanding FQHCs bill their carrier for both the technical and professional components. Payment is made based on the limitation.

Pub 100-4, 18, 20.4.1.2 – RHC/FQHC Claims With Dates of Service on or After January 1, 2002

(Rev. 1070, Issued: 09-29-06, Effective: 01-01-07, Implementation: 01-02-07)

A. Provider-Based RHC & FQHC – Technical Component

The technical component of a screening or diagnostic mammography for provider-based RHCs/FQHCs is typically furnished by the base provider. The provider of that service bills the FI under bill type 12X, 13X, 22X, 23X or 85X as appropriate using their outpatient provider number (not the RHC/FQHC provider number since these services are not covered as RHC/FQHC services). The appropriate revenue code for a screening mammography is 0403, and the appropriate HCPCS codes are 77057*, (76092)*, G0202, 76085, 77052*, and (76083)*. Payment is based on the payment method for the base provider.

The appropriate revenue code for a diagnostic mammography is 0401, and the appropriate HCPCS codes are 77055* (76090*), 77056* (76091*), G0204, G0206, 77051*, (76082)*, and G0236**.

***G0236 is a deleted code after December 31, 2003. Use 76082* for claims with dates of service January 1, 2004 through December 31, 2006, and code 77051 for claims with dates of service January 1, 2007 and later.*

** For claims with dates of service prior to January 1, 2007, report CPT codes 76082, 76090, 76091, and 76092. For claims with dates of service January 1, 2007 and later, report CPT codes 77051, 77055, 77056, and 77057 respectively.*

B. Independent RHCs and Freestanding FQHCs – Technical Component

The technical component of a screening or diagnostic mammography is outside the scope of the RHC/FQHC benefit. The practitioner that renders the technical service bills their carrier on Form CMS-1500. Payment is based on the MPFS.

C. Provider-Based RHC & FQHC, Independent RHCs and Freestanding FQHCs – Professional Component

For claims with dates of service on or after January 1, 2002 but before April 1, 2005, the professional component of a screening mammography furnished within an RHC/FQHC by a physician or nonphysician is considered an RHC/FQHC service. RHCs and FQHCs bill the FI under bill type 71X or 73X for the professional component along with revenue code 0403 and HCPCS code 76085* or 76092. Payment is made under the all-inclusive rate. Specific revenue coding and HCPCS coding is required for this service in order for CWF to perform age and frequency editing.

**76085 is a deleted code after December 31, 2003. Use 76083 for claims with dates of service on or after January 1, 2004 but before April 1, 2005.*

For claims with dates of service on or after January 1, 2002 but before April 1, 2005, RHCs and FQHCs bill the FI under bill type 71X or 73X for the professional component of a diagnostic mammography along with revenue code 0401 and HCPCS codes 76090 or 76091.

Payment should not be made for a screening or diagnostic mammography unless the claim contains a related visit code. FIs should assure payment is not made for revenue code 0403 (screening mammography) or 0401(diagnostic mammography). The claim must also contain a visit revenue code 0520 or 0521. Payment is made for the professional component under the all-inclusive rate for the line item reporting revenue code 0520 or 0521. No payment is made on the line item reporting revenue code 0403. For claims with dates of service on or after April 1, 2005, the professional component of a screening mammography furnished within an RHC/FQHC by a physician or nonphysician is considered an RHC/FQHC service. RHCs and FQHCs bill the FI under bill type 71X or 73X for the professional component. Payment is made for the professional component under the all-inclusive rate. Additional revenue and HCPCS coding is no longer required for this service when RHCs/FQHCs are billing for the professional component. Use revenue code 0520 or 0521 as appropriate.

For claims with dates of service on or after April 1, 2005, RHCs and FQHCs bill the FI under bill type 71X or 73X for the professional component of a diagnostic mammography. Use revenue code 0520 or 0521 as appropriate. No HCPCS coding is required for the diagnostic mammography.

Pub 100-4, 18, 20.4.2 – FI Requirements for Nondigital Screening Mammographies

(Rev. 1070, Issued: 09-29-06, Effective: 01-01-07, Implementation: 01-02-07)

The FI will consider the following when determining whether payment may be made:

- Presence of revenue code 0403;
- Presence of HCPCS code 77057* (76092*);
- Presence of high risk diagnosis code indicator where appropriate;
- Date of last screening mammography; and
- Age of beneficiary.

The FIs must accept revenue code 0403 for bill types 13X, 22X, 23X, 71X, 73X, or 85X.

** For claims with dates of service prior to January 1, 2007, providers report CPT code 76092. For claims with dates of service January 1, 2007 and later, providers report CPT code 77057.*

Pub 100-4, 18, 20.4.2.1 – FI Data for CWF and the Provider Statistical and Reimbursement Report (PS&R)

(Rev. 1070, Issued: 09-29-06, Effective: 01-01-07, Implementation: 01-02-07)

The CWF records are annotated with the date of the first (technical) screening mammography claim received. The record is updated based on the next covered (technical) claim received. Contractors assume the claim is the first received for the beneficiary where records do not contain a date of last screening and process accordingly.

The FIs include revenue code, HCPCS code, units, and covered charges in the CWF record fields with the same name. They report the payment amount for revenue code 0403 in the CWF field named "Rate" and the billed charges in the field named "Charges" of the CWF record. In addition, FIs report special override code 1 in the field named "Special Action" of the CWF record to avoid application of the Part B deductible.

When a screening CAD (76085**) is billed in conjunction with a screening mammography (77057* (76092*)) and the screening mammography (77057* (76092*) or G0202) fails the age and frequency edits in CWF, both services will be rejected by CWF.

***76085 is a deleted code after December 31, 2003. Use 76083* for claims with dates of service January 1, 2004 through December 31, 2006, and code 77052 for claims with dates of service January 1, 2007 and later.*

The FIs include in the financial data portion of the PS&R record, revenue code, HCPCS code, units, charges, and rate (fee schedule amount).

The PS&R system will include screening mammographies on a separate report from cost-based payments. See the PS&R guidelines for specific information.

** For claims with dates of service prior to January 1, 2007, providers report CPT codes 76083 and 76092. For claims with dates of service January 1, 2007 and later, providers report CPT codes 77052 and 77057 respectively.*

Pub 100-4, 18, 20.5 – Billing Requirements – Carrier/B MAC Claims

(Rev. 1931, Issued: 03-12-10, Effective: 06-14-10, Implementation: 06-14-10)

Contractors use the weekly-updated file to verify that the billing facility is certified by the FDA to perform mammography services, and has the appropriate certification to perform the type of mammogram billed (film and/or digital). Carriers/B MACs match the FDA assigned, 6-digit mammography certification number on the claim to the FDA mammography certification number appearing on the file for the billing facility. Carriers/B MACs complete the following activities in processing mammography claims:

- If the claim does not contain the facility's 6-digit certification number, or if a 6-digit certification number is not reported in item 32 of the Form CMS-1500 for paper claims, or in the 2400 loop (REF 02 segment, where 01=EW segment) of the ASC X12N 837 professional claim format, version 4010A1, for electronic claims, then carriers/B MACs return the claim as unprocessable.
- If the claim contains a 6-digit certification number that is reported in the proper field or segment (as specified in the previous bullet) but such number does not correspond to the number specified in the MQSA file for the facility, then carriers/B MACs deny the claim.
- When a film mammography HCPCS code is on a claim, the claim is checked for a "1" film indicator.
- If a film mammography HCPCS code comes in on a claim and the facility is certified for film mammography, the claim is paid if all other relevant Medicare criteria are met.
- If a film mammography HCPCS code is on a claim and the facility is certified for digital mammography only, the claim is denied.
- When a digital mammography HCPCS code is on a claim, the claim is checked for "2" digital indicator.
- If a digital mammography HCPCS code is on a claim and the facility is certified for digital mammography, the claim is paid if all other relevant Medicare criteria are met.
- If a digital mammography HCPCS code is on a claim and the facility is certified for film mammography only, the claim is denied.
- Process the claim to the point of payment based on the information provided on the claim and in carrier claims history.
- Identify the claim as a screening mammography claim by the CPT-4 code listed in field 24D and the diagnosis code(s) listed in field 21 of Form CMS-1500.
- Assign physician specialty code 45 to facilities that are certified to perform only screening mammography.
- Ensure that entities that bill globally for screening mammography contain a blank in modifier modifier position #1.
- Ensure that entities that bill for the technical component use only HCPCS modifier "-TC."
- Ensure that physicians who bill the professional component separately use HCPCS modifier "-26."
- Send the mammography modifier to CWF in the first modifier position on the claim. If more than one modifier is necessary, e.g., if the service was performed in a rural Health Manpower Shortage Area (HMSA) facility, instruct providers to bill the mammography modifier in modifier position 1 and the rural (or other) modifier in modifier position 2.
- Ensure all those who are qualified include the 6-digit FDA-assigned certification number of the screening center in field 32 of Form CMS-1500 and in the REF02 segment (where 01 = EW segment) of the 2400 loop for the ASC X12N 837 professional claim format, version 4010A1. Carriers/B MACs retain this number in their provider files.
- Waive Part B deductible and apply coinsurance for a screening mammography.
- Add diagnosis code V76.12 if a claim comes in for screening mammography without a diagnosis and the carrier file data shows this is appropriate. If there are other diagnoses on the claim, but not code V76.12, add it. (Do not change or overlay code V76.12 but ADD it.) At a minimum, edit for age, frequency, and place of service (POS).
- After May 23, 2008, accept the screening mammography facility's NPI number in place of the attending/referring physician NPI number for self-referred mammography claims.
- When a mammography claim contains services subject to the anti-markup payment limitation and the service was acquired from another billing jurisdiction, the provider must submit their own NPI with the name, address, and zip code of the performing physician/supplier.
- Refer to Pub. 100-04, chapter 1, section 10.1.1.1., for claims processing instructions for payment jurisdiction on Form CMS-1500 and electronic form ANSI X12 837P.

NOTE: Beginning October 1, 2003, carriers/B MACs are no longer permitted to add the ICD-9 code for a screening mammography when the screening mammography claim has no diagnosis code. Screening mammography claims with no diagnosis code must be returned as unprocessable for assigned claims. For unassigned claims, deny the claim.

Carrier Provider Education

- Educate providers that when a screening mammography turns to a diagnostic mammography on the same day for the same beneficiary, add the "-GG" modifier to the diagnostic code and bill both codes on the same claim. Both services are reimbursable by Medicare.
- Educate providers that they cannot bill an add-on code without also billing for the appropriate mammography code. If just the add-on code is billed, the service will be denied. Both the add-on code and the appropriate mammography code should be on the same claim.
- Educate providers to submit their own NPI in place of an attending/referring physician NPI in cases where screening mammography services are self-referred.

Pub 100-4, 18, 20.5.1 – Part B Carrier Claim Record for CWF

(Rev. 60, 01-09-04)

B3-4601.3.B

Carriers complete the type of service field in the CWF Part B claim record with a "B" if the patient is a high risk screening mammography patient or a "C" if she is a low risk screening mammography patient for services prior to January 1, 1998.

For services on or after January 1, 1998, the type of service field on CWF must have a value of "1" for medical care (screening) or a "4" for diagnostic radiology (diagnostic). Fill in POS. Fill in deductible indicator field with a "1"; not subject to deductible if screening mammography. Submit the claim to the CWF host. Trailer 17 of the Part B Basic Reply record will give the date of the last screening mammography.

The CWF edits for age and frequency for screening mammography. There are no frequency limitations on diagnostic tests or CAD-diagnostic tests. When a screening CAD is billed in conjunction with a screening mammogram and the screening mammogram fails the age or frequency edits then both services will be rejected.

Pub 100-4, 18, 20.5.1.1 – Carrier and CWF Edits

(Rev. 1070, Issued: 09-29-06, Effective: 01-01-07, Implementation: 01-02-07)

The CWF will not edit for POS for screening mammography. Disable 76X1 edit.

Add-on CAD Code 76083 must be billed in conjunction with screening mammography code 76092 or G0202 for claims with dates of service on or after January 1, 2004 through December 31, 2006. For claims with dates of service January 1, 2007 and later, add on CAD code 77052 must be billed in conjunction with screening mammography code 77057 or G0202. Use Type of Service "1".

Add-on CAD Code 76082 must be billed in conjunction with diagnostic mammography code 76090, 76091, G0204, or G0206 for claims with dates of service on or after January 1, 2004 through December 31, 2006. For claims with dates of service January 1, 2007 and later, add- on CAD code 77051 must be billed in conjunction with diagnostic mammography codes 77055, 77056, G0204 and G0206. Use Type of Service "4".

Frequency edits apply to screening mammography with or without the CAD code.

Screening and diagnostic mammographies (film and digital) are subject to the FDA certification. However, CAD equipment does not require FDA Certification.

Pub 100-4, 18, 20.5.2 – Transportation Costs for Mobile Units

(Rev. 1, 10-01-03)

B3-4601.2.J

Transportation costs are associated with mobile units for diagnostic mammography tests only. CMS formally added diagnostic mammography to the regulation language of the portable x-ray benefit in 42 CFR 410.32(c)(3). These units are usually reserved for screening tests only. For the screening tests performed in a mobile unit, there is no separate transportation cost allowed. Carriers should investigate transportation costs associated with the mobile mammography diagnostic tests that exceed data analysis guidelines.

To receive transportation payments, the approved portable x-ray supplier must also meet the certification requirements of §354 of the Public Health Service Act.

Pub 100-4, 18, 20.6 – Instructions When an Interpretation Results in Additional Films

(Rev. 1070, Issued: 09-29-06, Effective: 01-01-07, Implementation: 01-02-07)

A. Claims With Dates of Service October 1, 1998 Through December 31, 2001

A radiologist who interprets a screening mammography is allowed to order and interpret additional films based on the results of the screening mammogram while the beneficiary is still at the facility for the screening exam. Where a radiologist interpretation results in additional films, the mammography is no longer considered a screening exam for application of age and frequency standards or for payment purposes. This can be done without an additional order from the treating physician. When this occurs, the claim will be billed and paid as a diagnostic mammography instead of a screening mammography. However, since the original intent for the exam was for screening, for statistical purposes, the claim is considered a screening.

The claim should be prepared for FI processing reflecting the diagnostic revenue code (0401) along with HCPCS code 76090, 76091, G0204, G0206 or G0236 as appropriate and modifier GH "Diagnostic mammogram converted from screening mammogram on same day." Statistics will be collected based on the presence of modifier GH. A separate claim is not required. Regular billing instructions remain in place for mammograms that do not fit this situation.

Carriers should receive a claim for a screening mammogram with CPT code 76092 (screening mammography, bilateral) (Type of Service = 1) but, if the screening mammogram turns into a diagnostic mammogram, the claim is billed with CPT code 76090 (unilateral) or 76091 (bilateral), (TOS= 4), with modifier GH. Carriers pay the claim as a diagnostic mammography instead of a screening mammography.

NOTE: However, the ordering of a diagnostic test by a radiologist following a screening test that shows a potential problem need not be on the same date of service.

In this case, where additional diagnostic tests are performed for the same beneficiary, same visit on the same day, the UPIN of the treating physician is needed on the carrier claim. The radiologist must refer back to the treating physician for his/her UPIN and also report to the treating physician the condition of the patient. Carriers need to educate radiologists and treating physicians that the treating physician's UPIN is required whenever a physician refers or orders a diagnostic lab or radiology service. If no UPIN is present for the diagnostic mammography code, the carrier will reject the claim.

B. Claims With Dates of Service On or After January 1, 2002, (or On or After April 1, 2002 for Hospitals Subject to OPPS)

A radiologist who interprets a screening mammography is allowed to order and interpret additional films based on the results of the screening mammogram while a beneficiary is still at the facility for the screening exam. When a radiologist's interpretation results in additional films, Medicare will pay for both the screening and diagnostic mammogram.

Carrier Claims – For carrier claims, providers submitting a claim for a screening mammography and a diagnostic mammography for the same patient on the same day, attach modifier GG to the diagnostic mammography. A modifier GG is appended to the claim for the diagnostic mammogram for tracking and data collection purposes. Medicare will reimburse both the screening mammography and the diagnostic mammography.

FI Claims – FIs require the diagnostic claim be prepared reflecting the diagnostic revenue code (0401) along with HCPCS code 77055* (76090*), 77056* (76091*), G0204, G0206 or G0236 and modifier GG "Performance and payment of a screening mammogram and diagnostic mammogram on the same patient, same day." Reporting of this modifier is needed for data collection purposes. Regular billing instructions remain in place for a screening mammography that does not fit this situation.

Both carrier and FI systems must accept the GH and GG modifiers where appropriate.

** For claims with dates of service prior to January 1, 2007, providers report CPT codes 76090 and 76091. For claims with dates of service January 1, 2007 and later, providers report CPT codes 77055 and 77056 respectively.*

Pub 100-4, 18, 20.7 – Mammograms Performed With New Technologies

(Rev. 1070, Issued: 09-29-06, Effective: 01-01-07, Implementation: 01-02-07)

Section 104 of the Benefits Improvement and Protection Act 2000, (BIPA) entitled Modernization of Screening Mammography Benefit, provides for new payment methodologies for both diagnostic and screening mammograms that utilize advanced new technologies for the period April 1, 2001, to December 31, 2001 (to March 31, 2002 for hospitals subject to OPPS). Under this provision, payment for technologies that directly take digital images would equal 150 percent of the amount that would otherwise be paid for a bilateral diagnostic mammography. For technologies that convert standard film images to digital form, payment will be derived from the statutory screening mammography limit plus an additional payment of $15.00 for carrier claims and $10.20 for FI (technical component only) claims.

Payment restrictions for digital screening and diagnostic mammography apply to those facilities that meet all FDA certifications as provided under the Mammography Quality Standards Act. However, CAD codes billed in conjunction with digital mammographies or film mammographies are not subject to FDA certification requirements.

Mammography related CAD equipment does not require FDA certification. Mammography utilizes a direct x-ray of the breast. By contrast, the CAD process uses laser beam to scan the mammography film from a film (analog) mammography, converts it into digital data for the computer, and analyzes the video display for areas suspicious for cancer. The CAD process used with digital mammography analyzes the data from the mammography on a video display for suspicious areas. The patient is not required to be present for the CAD process.

Only one screening mammogram, either 77057* (76092*) or G0202, may be billed in a calendar year. Therefore, providers/suppliers must not submit claims reflecting both a film screening mammography (77057* (76092*)) and a digital screening mammography G0202. Also, they must not submit claims reflecting HCPCS codes 77055* (76090*) or 77056* (76091*) (diagnostic mammography-film) and G0204 or G0206 (diagnostic mammography-digital). Contractors deny the claim when both a film and digital screening or diagnostic mammography is reported. However, a screening and diagnostic mammography can be billed together.

** For claims with dates of service prior to January 1, 2007, providers report CPT codes 76090, 76091, and 76092. For claims with dates of service January 1, 2007 and later, providers report CPT codes 77055, 77056, and 77057 respectively.*

A. Payment Requirements for FI Claims With Dates of Service On or After April 1, 2001 Through December 31, 2001 (Through March 31, 2002 for Hospitals Subject to OPPS).

Providers bill the FI for the technical component of screening and diagnostic mammographies that utilize advanced technologies with one of six new HCPCS codes, G0202 – G0207. See payment methodology below for each of the codes during the period April 1, 2001 through December 31, 2001 (or March 31, 2002 for hospitals subject to OPPS). Payments for codes G0202 through G0205 are based, in part, on the MPFS payment amounts. The amounts that are based on the MPFS that both carriers and FIs use in calculating the payments for these codes were furnished in a BIPA mammography benefit pricing file for implementation on April 1, 2001.

HCPCS	Definition
G0202	Screening mammography producing direct digital image, bilateral, all views

Payment Method:

Payment will be the lesser of the provider's charge or the amount that will be provided for this code in the pricing file. (That amount is 150 percent of the locality specific technical component payment amount under the physician fee schedule for CPT code 76091, the code for bilateral diagnostic mammogram, during 2001.) Part B deductible does not apply. Coinsurance will equal 20 percent of the lesser of the actual charge or 150 percent of the locality specific payment of CPT code 76091.

HCPCS	Definition
G0203	Screening mammography, film processed to produce digital image analyzed for potential abnormalities, bilateral, all views

Payment Method:

Payment will be equal to the lesser of the actual charge for the procedure, the amount that is provided in the pricing file (which represents 68 percent of the locality specific global payment amount for a bilateral diagnostic mammography (CPT 76091) under the physician fee schedule), or $57.28 (which represents the amount of the 2001 statutory limit for a screening mammography attributable to the technical component of the service, plus the technical portion of the $15.00 add-on for 2001 which is provided under the new legislation). Part B deductible does not apply. Coinsurance is 20 percent of the charge.

HCPCS	Definition
G0204	Diagnostic mammography, direct digital image, bilateral, all views

Payment Method:

Payment will be the lesser of the provider's charge or the amount that will be provided for this code in the pricing file. (That amount is 150 percent of the locality specific amount paid under the physician fee schedule for the technical component (TC) of CPT code 76091, the code for a bilateral diagnostic mammogram.) Deductible is applicable. Coinsurance will equal 20 percent of the lesser of the actual charge or 150 percent of the locality specific payment of CPT code 76091.

NOTE: Effective January 1, 2005, payment will be made under MPFS for claims from hospitals subject to OPPS.

HCPCS	Definition
G0205	Diagnostic mammography, film processed to produce digital image analyzed for potential abnormalities, bilateral, all views.

Payment Method:

Payment will be equal to the lesser of the actual charge for the procedure, the amount that will be provided in the pricing file (which represents 68 percent of the locality specific global payment amount for a bilateral diagnostic mammography (CPT 76091) under the physician fee schedule), or $57.28 (which represents the amount of the 2001 statutory limit for a screening mammography attributable to the technical component of the service, plus the technical portion of the $15.00 add-on for 2001 which is provided under the new legislation). Deductible applies. Coinsurance is 20 percent of the charge.

HCPCS	Definition
G0206	Diagnostic mammography, direct digital image, unilateral, all views.

Payment Method:

Payment will be made based on the same amount that is paid to the provider, under the payment method applicable to the specific provider type (e.g., hospital, rural health clinic, etc.) for CPT code 76090, the code for a mammogram, and one breast. For example, this service, when furnished as a hospital outpatient service, will be paid the amount under the outpatient prospective payment system (OPPS) for CPT code 76090. Deductible applies. Coinsurance is the national unadjusted coinsurance for the APC wage adjusted for the specific hospital.

NOTE: Effective January 1, 2005, payment will be made under MPFS for claims from hospitals subject to OPPS.

HCPCS	Definition
G0207	Diagnostic mammography, film processed to produce digital image analyzed for potential abnormalities, unilateral, all views.

Payment Method:

Payment will be based on the same amount that is paid to the provider, under the payment method applicable to the specific provider type (e.g., hospital, rural health clinic, etc.) for CPT code 76090, the code for mammogram, and one breast. For example, this service, when furnished as a hospital outpatient service, will be paid the amount payable under the OPPS for CPT code 76090. Deductible applies. Coinsurance is the

Medicare References

national unadjusted coinsurance for the APC wage adjusted for the specific hospital.

B. Payment Requirements for Claims with Dates of Service on or After January 1, 2002 (April 1, 2002 for hospitals subject to OPPS).

Codes G0203, G0205 and G0207 are not billable codes for claims with dates of service on or after January 1, 2002 (April 1, 2002 for hospitals subject to OPPS).

FI Payment

Code	Payment
G0202	Payment will be equal to the lower of the actual charge or the locality specific technical component payment amount under the MPFS when performed in a hospital outpatient department, CAH, or SNF. Coinsurance is 20 percent of the lower amount; the Program pays 80 percent. Deductible does not apply.
G0204	Payment will be made under OPPS for hospital outpatient departments. Coinsurance is the national unadjusted coinsurance for the APC wage adjusted for the specific hospital. Payment will be made on a reasonable cost basis for CAHs and coinsurance is based on charges. Payment is made under the MPFS when performed in a SNF and coinsurance is 20 percent of the lower of the actual charge or the MPFS amount. Deductible applies. NOTE: Effective January 1, 2005, payment will be made under MPFS for claims from hospitals subject to OPPS.
G0206	Payment will be made under OPPS for hospital outpatient departments. Coinsurance is the national unadjusted coinsurance for the APC wage adjusted for the specific hospital. Payment will be made on a reasonable cost basis for CAHs and coinsurance is based on charges. Payment is made under the MPFS when performed in a SNF. Coinsurance is 20 percent of the lower of the actual charge or the MPFS amount. Deductible applies. NOTE: Effective January 1, 2005, payment will be made under MPFS for claims from hospitals subject to OPPS.

Providers bill for the technical portion of screening and diagnostic mammograms on Form CMS-1450 under bill type 13X, 22X, 23X, or 85X. The professional component is billed to the carrier on Form CMS-1500 (or electronic equivalent).

Providers bill for digital screening mammographies on Form CMS-1450, utilizing revenue code 0403 and HCPCS G0202 or G0203.

Providers bill for digital diagnostic mammographies on Form CMS-1450, utilizing revenue code 0401 and HCPCS G0204, G0205, G0206 or G0207.

NOTE: Codes G0203, G0205 and G0207 are not billable codes for claims with dates of service on or after January 1, 2002.

CAHs electing the optional method of payment for outpatient services are paid according to §20.3.2.3 of this chapter.

Carrier Payment

All codes paid by the carrier are based on the Medicare Physician Fee Schedule (MPFS).

Code	Payment
G0202	Payment is the lesser of the provider's charge or the MPFS amount provided for this code in the pricing file. Part B deductible does not apply, however, coinsurance applies.
G0204	Payment is the lesser of the provider's charge or the MPFS amount provided for this code in the pricing file. Deductible and coinsurance apply.
G0206	Payment is the lesser of the provider's charge or the MPFS amount provided for this code in the pricing file. Deductible and coinsurance apply.

Contractors were furnished a mammography benefit pricing file to pay claims containing the above codes.

Pub 100-4, 18, 20.8 – Beneficiary and Provider Notices

(Rev. 1, 10-01-03)

B3-4601.4, A3-3660.10.I, SNF-537.2.G

20.8.1 – MSN Messages

(Rev. 298, Issued: 09-10-04, Effective/Implementation: 09-25-04)

B3-4601.4, A3-3660.10.I

The following messages are used on the MSN.

If the claim is denied because the beneficiary is under 35 years of age, use the following MSN:

MSN 18.3:

> Screening mammography is not covered for women under 35 years of age.

The Spanish version of this MSN message should read:

> Las pruebas de mamografía para mujeres menores de 35 años no están cubiertas.

If the claim is denied for a woman 35-39 because she has previously received this examination, use the following MSN:

MSN 18.6:

> A screening mammography is covered only once for women age 35-39.

The Spanish version of this MSN message should read:

> Una mamografía de cernimiento es cubierta una vez solamente para mujeres entre las edades de 35-39.

If the claim is denied because the period of time between screenings for the woman based on age has not passed, use the following MSN:

MSN 18.4:

> This service is being denied because it has not been 12 months since your last examination of this kind. (NOTE: Insert appropriate number of months.)

The Spanish version of this MSN message should read:

> Este servicio se denegó debido a que no han transcurrido 12 meses desde su último examen de este tipo.

If the claim is denied because the provider is not certified to perform this service (film mammography) or if the claim is denied because the provider is not certified to perform this service (digital mammography), use the following MSN:

MSN 16.2:

> This service cannot be paid when provided in this location/facility.

The Spanish version of this MSN message should read:

> Este servicio no se puede pagar cuando es suministrado en este sitio/facilidad.

In addition to the above denial messages, the FI/carrier may add the following:

MSN 18.12:

> Screening mammograms are covered annually for women 40 years of age and older.

The Spanish version of this MSN message should read:

> El examen de mamografía de cernimiento se cubre una vez al año para mujeres de 40 años de edad o más.

For Carriers only:

> For claims submitted with invalid or missing certification number, use the following MSN:

MSN 9.2:

> This item or service was denied because information required to make payment was missing.

The Spanish version of this MSN message should read:

> Este artículo o servicio fue denegado porque la información requerida para hacer el pago fue omitida.

Pub 100-4, 18, 20.8.2 – Remittance Advice Messages

(Rev. 1387, Issued: 12-07-07, Effective: 04-01-08, Implementation: 04-07-08)

If the claim is denied because the beneficiary is under 35 years of age, contractors must use existing ASC X12N 835 claim adjustment reason code/message 6, "The procedure/revenue code is inconsistent with the patient's age" along with the remark code M37 (at the line item level), "Service is not covered when the patient is under age 35."

If the claim is denied for a woman 35-39 because she has previously received this examination, contractors must use existing ASC X12N 835 claim adjustment reason code/message 119, "Benefit maximum for this time period or occurrence has been reached" along with the remark code M89 (at the line item level), "Not covered more than once under age 40."

If the claim is denied for a woman age 40 and above because she has previously received this examination within the past 12 months, contractors must use existing ASC X12N 835 claim adjustment reason code/message 119, "Benefit maximum for this time period or occurrence has been reached" along with remark code M90 (at the line item level), "Not covered more than once in a 12-month period."

For Intermediaries/A MACs only:

If the claim is denied because the provider that performed the screening is not certified to perform the type of mammography billed (film and/or digital) use existing ASC X12N 835 claim adjustment reason code/message B7, "This provider was not certified/eligible to be paid for this procedure/service on this date of service."

For Carriers/B MACs only:

For claims submitted by a facility not certified to perform film mammography, use existing reason code 171, "Payment is denied when performed/billed by this type of provider in this type of facility." along with remark code N110, "This facility is not certified for film mammography."

For claims submitted by a facility not certified to perform digital mammograms, use existing reason code 171, "This payment is adjusted when performed/billed by this type of provider, by this type of provider in this type of facility, or by a provider of this specialty" along with remark code N92,"This facility is not certified for digital mammography."

For claims that were submitted without the facility's FDA-assigned certification number, use existing reason code 16, "Claim/service lacks information which is needed for adjudication" along with remark code MA128 "Missing/incomplete/invalid FDA approval number."

For claims that were submitted with an invalid facility certification number, use existing reason code 125, "Payment adjusted due to a submission/billing error(s) along with remark code MA128 "Missing/incomplete/invalid FDA approval number."

Pub 100-4, 18, 30 – Screening Pap Smears

(Rev. 1, 10-01-03)

A3-3628.1, B3-4603.1, B3-4603.1A, SNF-541.2

Effective January 1, 1998, §1861(nn) of the Act (42 USC 1395x(nn)) provides Medicare Part B coverage for a screening Pap smear for women under certain conditions. See the **Medicare Benefit Policy Manual**, Chapter 15, for coverage of screening PAP smears.

To be covered screening Pap smears must be ordered and collected by a doctor of medicine or osteopathy (as defined in §1861(r)(l) of the Act), or other authorized practitioner (e.g., a certified nurse midwife, physician assistant, nurse practitioner, or clinical nurse specialist, who is authorized under State law to perform the examination) under one of the conditions identified in §30.1, below.

Pub 100-4, 18, 30.1 – Pap Smears From January 1, 1998, Through June 30 2001

(Rev. 1, 10-01-03)

B3-4603.1A.1, B3-4603.1A.2, B3-4603.1A.3, A3-3628.1A

The following requirements must be met.

1. The beneficiary has not had a screening Pap smear test during the preceding three years (i.e., 35 months have passed following the month that the woman had the last covered Pap smear. Use one of the following ICD-9-CM codes V76.2, V76.47, or V76.49; or
2. There is evidence (on the basis of her medical history or other findings) that she is of childbearing age and has had an examination that indicated the presence of cervical or vaginal cancer or other abnormalities during any of the preceding 3 years; and at least 11 months have passed following the month that the last covered Pap smear was performed; or
3. She is at high risk of developing cervical or vaginal cancer (use ICD-9-CM code V15.89, other specified personal history presenting hazards to health) and at least 11 months have passed following the month that the last covered screening Pap smear was performed. The high risk factors for cervical and vaginal cancer are:
   a. Cervical Cancer High Risk Factors:
      - Early onset of sexual activity (under 16 years of age)
      - Multiple sexual partners (5 or more in a lifetime)
      - History of a sexually transmitted disease (including HIV infection)
      - Fewer than three negative or any Pap smears within the previous 7 years

   b. Vaginal Cancer High Risk Factors:
      - DES (diethylstilbestrol)-exposed daughters of women who took DES during pregnancy.

   NOTE: The term "woman of childbearing age" means a woman who is premenopausal, and has been determined by a physician, or qualified practitioner, to be of childbearing age, based on her medical history or other findings.

COUNTING: To determine the 11-, 23-, and 35-month periods, start counts beginning with the month after the month in which a previous test/procedure was performed.

COUNTING EXAMPLE: A beneficiary identified as being at high risk for developing cervical cancer received a screening Pap smear in January 2000. Start counts beginning with February 2000. The beneficiary is eligible to receive another screening Pap smear in January 2001 (the month after 11 full months have passed).

Pub 100-4, 18, 30.2 – Pap Smears On and After July 1, 2001

(Rev. 1, 10-01-03)

B3-4603.1.B, A3-3628.1.A.1

If the beneficiary does not qualify for more frequent screening based on paragraphs (2) and (3) above, for services performed on or after July 1, 2001, payment may be made for a screening PAP smear after 23 months have passed after the end of the month of the last covered smear. All other coverage and payment requirements remain the same.

Pub 100-4, 18, 30.3 – Deductible and Coinsurance

(Rev. 1, 10-01-03)

B3-4603.4, A3-3628.1.A.3

Neither the Part B deductible nor coinsurance apply for services paid under the laboratory fee schedule. The Part B deductible for screening Pap smear and services paid for under the physician fee schedule is waived effective January 1, 1998. Coinsurance applies.

A. Carrier Action for Submitting Claim to CWF and CWF Edit

B3-4603.4, B3-4603.6, B3-4603.1.B

When a carrier receives a claim for a screening Pap smear, performed on or after January 1, 1998, it must enter a deductible indicator of 1 (not subject to deductible) in field 67 of the HUBC record.

CWF will edit for screening pelvic examinations performed more frequently than allowed according to the presence of high risk factors.

Pub 100-4, 18, 30.4 – Payment Method

(Rev. 1, 10-01-03)

B3-4603.1.C.1 and 2

Payment may be under the clinical diagnostic lab fee schedule or the MPFS, depending upon the code billed. See the categories in §30.5 of this chapter for a description.

Pub 100-4, 18, 30.4.1 – Payment Method for RHCs and FQHCs

(Rev. 795, Issued: 12-30-05; Effective: 10-01-04; Implementation: 04-03-06)

The professional component of a screening Pap smear furnished within an RHC/FQHC by a physician or non physician is considered an RHC/FQHC service. RHCs and FQHCs bill the FI under bill type 71X or 73X for the professional component along with revenue code 052X. See Chapter 9, for RHC and FQHC bill processing instructions.

The technical component of a screening Pap smear is outside the scope of the RHC/FQHC benefit. If the technical component of this service is furnished within an independent RHC or freestanding FQHC, the provider of that technical service bills the carrier on Form CMS-1500.

If the technical component of a screening Pap smear is furnished within a provider-based RHC/FQHC, the provider of that service bills the FI under bill type 13X, 14X, 22X, 23X, or 85X as appropriate using their outpatient provider number (not the RHC/FQHC provider number since these services are not covered as RHC/FQHC services). The appropriate revenue code is 311. Effective 4/1/06, type of bill 14X is for non-patient laboratory specimens.

Pub 100-4, 18, 30.5 – HCPCS Codes for Billing

(Rev. 795, Issued: 12-30-05; Effective: 10-01-04; Implementation: 04-03-06)

The following HCPCS codes can be used for screening Pap smear:

A. Codes Billed to the Carrier and Paid Under the Physician Fee Schedule

The following HCPCS codes are submitted by those providers/entities that submit claims to carriers. The deductible is waived for these services effective January 1, 1998, however, coinsurance applies.

NOTE: These codes are not billed on FI claims except for HCPCS code Q0091 which may be submitted to FIs. Payment for code Q0091 performed in a hospital outpatient department is under OPPS, (see 30.5C).

- Q0091 – Screening Papanicolaou (Pap) smear, obtaining, preparing and conveyance of cervical or vaginal smear to laboratory;
- P3001 – Screening Papanicolaou smear, cervical or vaginal, up to three smears requiring interpretation by a physician;
- G0124 – Screening cytopathology, cervical or vaginal (any reporting system), collected in preservative fluid, automated thin layer preparation, requiring interpretation by physician; and
- G0141 – Screening cytopathology smears, cervical or vaginal, performed by automated system, with manual re-screening, requiring interpretation by physician.

B. Codes Paid Under the Clinical Lab Fee Schedule by FI and Carriers

The following codes are billed to FIs by providers they serve, or billed to carriers by the physicians/suppliers they service. Deductible and coinsurance do not apply.

- P3000 – Screening Papanicolaou smear, cervical or vaginal, up to three smears, by a technician under the physician supervision;
- G0123 – Screening cytopathology, cervical or vaginal (any reporting system) collected in preservative fluid; automated thin layer preparation, screening by cytotechnologist under physician supervision;
- G0143 – Screening cytopathology, cervical or vaginal, (any reporting system), collected in preservative fluid, automated thin layer preparation, with manual screening and re-screening, by cytotechnologist under physician supervision;
- G0144 – Screening cytopathology, cervical or vaginal, (any reporting system), collected in preservative fluid, automated thin layer preparation, with screening by automated system under physician supervision;
- G0145 – Screening cytopathology, cervical or vaginal, (any reporting system), collected in preservative fluid, automated thin layer preparation, with screening by automated system and manual re-screening under physician supervision;
- G0147 – Screening cytopathology smears, cervical or vaginal, performed by automated system under physician supervision; and
- G0148 – Screening cytopathology smears, cervical or vaginal, performed by automated system with manual reevaluation.

C. Payment of Q0091 When Billed to FIs

Payment for code Q0091 in a hospital outpatient department is under OPPS. A SNF is paid using the technical component of the MPFS. For a CAH, payment is on a reasonable cost basis. For RHC/FQHCs payment is made under the all inclusive rate for the professional component. Deductible is not applicable, however, coinsurance applies.

The technical component of a screening Pap smear is outside the RHC/FQHC benefit. If the technical component of a screening Pap smear is furnished within a provider-based RHC/FQHC, the provider of that service bills the FI under the bill type 13X, 14X, 22X, 23X, or 85X as appropriate using their base provider number (not the RHC/FQHC provider number since these services are not covered as RHC/FQHC services). For independent RHCs/FQHCs, the practitioner bills the technical component to the carrier on Form CMS-1500 or the ANSI X12N 837 P. Effective 4/1/06, type of bill 14X is for non-patient laboratory specimens.

D. Payment of Q0091 When Billed to Carriers

Payment for Q0091 is paid under the Medicare physician fee schedule. Deductible is not applicable, however the coinsurance applies.

Effective for services on and after July 1, 2005, on those occasions when physicians must perform a screening Pap smear (Q0091) that they know will not be covered by Medicare because the low risk patient has already received a covered Pap smear (Q0091) in the past 2 years, the physician can bill Q0091 and the claim will be denied appropriately. The physician shall obtain an advance beneficiary notice (ABN) in these situations as the denial will be considered a not reasonable and necessary denial. The physician indicates on the claim that an ABN has been obtained by using the GA modifier.

Effective for services on or after April 1, 1999, a covered evaluation and management (E/M) visit and code Q0091 may be reported by the same physician for the same date of service if the E/M visit is for a separately identifiable service. In this case, the modifier "-25" must be reported with the E/M service and the medical records must clearly document the E/M reported. Both procedure codes should be shown as separate line items on the claim. These services can also be performed separately on separate office visits.

E. Common Working File (CWF) Editing for Q0091

The CWF will edit for claims containing the HCPCS code Q0091 effective for dates of service on and after July 1, 2005. Previously, the editing for Q0091 had been removed from the CWF. Medicare pays for a screening Pap smear every 2 years for low risk patients based on the low risk diagnoses, see sections 30.2 and 30.6. Medicare pays for a screening Pap smear every year for a high risk patient based on the high risk diagnosis, see sections 30.1 and 30.6. This criteria will be the CWF parameters for editing Q0091.

In those situations where unsatisfactory screening Pap smear specimens have been collected and conveyed to clinical labs that are unable to interpret the test results, another specimen will have to be collected. When the physician bills for this reconveyance, the physician should annotate the claim with Q0091 along with modifier -76, (repeat procedure by same physician).

Pub 100-4, 18, 30.6 – Diagnoses Codes

(Rev. 1472, Issued: 03-06-08, Effective: 05-23-07, Implementation: 04-07-08)

Below is the current diagnoses that should be used when billing for screening Pap smear services. Effective, July 1, 2005, V72.31 is being added to the CWF edit as an additional low risk diagnosis. The following chart lists the diagnosis codes that CWF must recognize for low risk or high risk patients for screening Pap smear services.

Low Risk Diagnosis Codes	Definitions
V76.2	Special screening for malignant neoplasms, cervix
V76.47	Special screening for malignant neoplasm, vagina
V76.49	Special screening for malignant neoplasm, other sites NOTE: providers use this diagnosis for women without a cervix.
V72.31	Routine gynecological examination NOTE: This diagnosis should only be used when the provider performs a full gynecological examination.
High Risk Diagnosis Code	**Definition**
V15.89	Other

A. Applicable Diagnoses for Billing a Carrier

There are a number of appropriate diagnosis codes that can be used in billing for screening Pap smear services that the provider can list on the claim to give a true picture of the patient's condition. Those diagnoses can be listed in Item 21 of Form CMS-1500 or the electronic equivalent (see Chapter 26 for electronic equivalent formats). In addition, one of the following diagnoses shall appear on the claim: the low risk diagnosis of V76.2, V76.47, V76.49 and (effective July 1, 2005, V72.31) or the high risk diagnosis of V15.89 (for high risk patients). One of the above diagnoses must be listed in item 21of the Form CMS-1500 or the electronic equivalent to indicate either low risk or high risk depending on the patient's condition. Then either the low risk or high risk diagnosis must also be pointed to in Item 24E of Form CMS-1500 or the electronic equivalent. Providers must make sure that for screening Pap smears for a high risk beneficiary, that the high risk diagnosis code of V15.89 appears in Item 21 and V15.89 is the appropriate diagnosis code that must be pointed to in Item 24E or the electronic equivalent. If Pap smear claims do not point to one of these specific diagnoses in Item 24E or the electronic equivalent, the claim will reject in the CWF. Periodically, carriers should do provider education on diagnosis coding of Pap smear claims.

If these pointers are not present on claims submitted to carriers, CWF will reject the record.

B. Applicable Diagnoses for Billing an FI

Providers report one of the following diagnosis codes in Form CMS-1450 or the electronic equivalent (NOTE: Information regarding the form locator numbers that correspond to the diagnosis codes and a table to crosswalk its CMS-1450 form locator to the 837 transaction is found in Chapter 25.):

Low risk diagnosis codes:

V76.2

V76.47

V76.49

V72.31

High risk diagnosis codes:

V15.89

Periodically provider education should be done on diagnosis coding of Pap Smear claims.

Pub 100-4, 18, 30.7 – Type of Bill and Revenue Codes for Form CMS-1450

(Rev. 827, Issued: 02-01-06; Effective Date: 07-01-06; Implementation Date: 07-03-06)

The applicable bill types for screening Pap smears are 12X, 13X, 14X, 22X, 23X, and 85X. Use revenue code 0311 (laboratory, pathology, cytology). Report the screening pap smear as a diagnostic clinical laboratory service using one of the HCPCS codes shown in §30.5.B.

In addition, CAHs electing method II report professional services under revenue codes 096X, 097X, or 098X.

Effective April 1, 2006, type of bill 14X is for non-patient laboratory specimens.

Pub 100-4, 18, 30.8 – MSN Messages

(Rev. 1, 10-01-03)

If there are no high risk factors, and the screening Pap smear and/or screening pelvic examination is being denied because the procedure/examination is performed more frequently than allowed, use MSN 18.17:

> Medicare pays for a screening Pap smear and/or screening pelvic examination only once every (2, 3) years unless high risk factors are present.

Pub 100-4, 18, 30.9 – Remittance Advice Codes

If high risk factors are not present, and the screening Pap smear and/or screening pelvic examination is being denied because the procedure/examination is performed more frequently than allowed, use existing ANSI X12N 835:

- Claim adjustment reason code 119 – "Benefit maximum for this time period has been reached" at the line level, and
- Remark code M83 – "Service is not covered unless the patient is classified as at high risk: at the line item level.

Pub 100-4, 18, 40 – Screening Pelvic Examinations

(Rev. 1541, Issued: 06-20-08, Effective: 09-23-08, Implementation: 09-23-08)

Section 4102 of the BBA of 1997 (P.L. 105-33) amended §1861(nn) of the Act (42 USC 1395X(nn)) to include Medicare Part B coverage of screening pelvic examinations (including a clinical breast examination) for all female beneficiaries for services provided January 1, 1998 and later. Effective July 1, 2001, the Consolidated Appropriations Act of 2001 (P.L. 106-554) modifies §1861(nn) to provide Medicare Part B coverage for biennial screening pelvic examinations. A screening pelvic examination with or without specimen collection for smears and cultures, should include at least seven of the following eleven elements:

- Inspection and palpation of breasts for masses or lumps, tenderness, symmetry, or nipple discharge; and
- Digital rectal examination including sphincter tone, presence of hemorrhoids, and rectal masses.
- External genitalia (for example, general appearance, hair distribution, or lesions);
- Urethral meatus (for example, size, location, lesions, or prolapse);
- Urethra (for example, masses, tenderness, or scarring);
- Bladder (for example, fullness, masses, or tenderness);
- Vagina (for example, general appearance, estrogen effect, discharge, lesions, pelvic support, cystocele, or rectocele);
- Cervix (for example, general appearance, lesions or discharge)
- Uterus (for example, size, contour, position, mobility, tenderness, consistency, descent, or support);
- Adnexa/parametria (for example, masses, tenderness, organomegaly, or nodularity); and
- Anus and perineum.

Pub 100-4, 18, 40.1 – Screening Pelvic Examinations From January 1, 1998, Through June 30 2001

(Rev. 1, 10-01-03)

B3-4603.2.A, B3-4603.5, A3-3628.1.B.1, R1888.A.3 Dated 6-3-2003

The following requirements must be met:

The exam must be performed by a doctor of medicine or osteopathy (as defined in §1861(r)(1) of the Act), or by a certified nurse midwife (as defined in §1861(gg) of the Act), or a physician assistant, nurse practitioner, or clinical nurse specialist (as defined in §1861(aa) of the Act) who is authorized under State law to perform the examination.

This examination does not have to be ordered by a physician or other authorized practitioner.

Payment may be made: Once every three years on an asymptomatic woman only if the individual has not had a screening pelvic examination paid for by Medicare during the preceding 35 months following the month in which the last Medicare-covered screening pelvic examination was performed. The provider uses one of the

Medicare References

following ICD-9-CM codes V76.2, V76.47, or V76.49. Exceptions are as follows:

- Payment may be made for a screening pelvic examination performed more frequently than once every 35 months if the test is performed by a physician or other practitioner and there is evidence that the woman is at high risk (on the basis of her medical history or other findings) of developing cervical cancer, or vaginal cancer. (providers use ICD-9-CM code V15.89, other specified personal history presenting hazards to health.) The high risk factors for cervical and vaginal cancer are:
  - Cervical Cancer High Risk Factors
    - Early onset of sexual activity (under 16 years of age)
    - Multiple sexual partners (five or more in a lifetime)
    - History of a sexually transmitted disease (including HIV infection)
    - Fewer than three negative or any Pap smears within the previous seven years
  - Vaginal Cancer High Risk Factors
    - DES (diethylstilbestrol)-exposed daughters of women who took DES during pregnancy.

ICD-9-CM code V15.89, other specified personal history presenting hazards to health is used to indicate that one or more of these factors is present; or

- Payment may also be made for a screening pelvic examination performed more frequently than once every 36 months if the examination is performed by a physician or other practitioner, for a woman of childbearing age, who has had such an examination that indicated the presence of cervical or vaginal cancer or other abnormality during any of the preceding three years. The term "women of childbearing age" means a woman who is premenopausal, and has been determined by a physician, or qualified practitioner, to be of childbearing age, based on her medical history or other findings. Payment is not made for a screening pelvic examination for women at high risk or who qualify for coverage under the childbearing provision more frequently than once every 11 months after the month that the last screening pelvic examination covered by Medicare was performed.
- For claims with dates of service on or after July 1, 2001, if the beneficiary does not qualify for an annual screening pelvic exam as noted above, pay for the screening pelvic exam only after at least 23 months have passed following the month during which the beneficiary received her last covered screening pelvic exam. All other coverage and payment requirements remain the same.

Calculating the Frequency Limitations

To determine the screening periods, start counts beginning with the month after the month in which a previous test/procedure was performed.

Frequency Limitation Example

A beneficiary identified as being at high risk for developing cervical cancer received a pelvic exam in January 2002. Start counts beginning with February 2002. The beneficiary is eligible to receive another screening exam, if high risk, in January 2003 (the month after 11 full months have passed).

Pub 100-4, 18, 40.2 – Screening Pelvic Examinations on and After July 1, 2001

(Rev. 1, 10-01-03)

B3-4603.2.B and C, A3-3628.1.B.1

When the beneficiary does not qualify for a more frequently performed screening pelvic exam noted in §40.1 of this chapter, items 2, or 3, the screening pelvic exam may be paid only after at least 23 months have passed following the month during which the beneficiary received her last covered screening pelvic exam. All other coverage and payment requirements remain the same.

A HCPCS code has been established for the pelvic and clinical breast examinations. Use code G0101 (cervical or vaginal cancer screening, pelvic and clinical breast examination).

Pub 100-4, 18, 40.3 – Deductible and Coinsurance

(Rev. 1, 10-01-03)

B3-4603.2.C, A3-3628.1.B.3

The Part B deductible for screening pelvic examinations is waived effective January 1, 1998. Coinsurance is applicable.

A. Action When Submitting Claims to CWF and CWF Edit

B3-4603.4, B3-4603.6, A3-3628.1.C.1

When a carrier receives a claim for a pelvic examination, performed on or after January 1, 1998, it must enter a deductible indicator of 1 (not subject to deductible) in field 65 of the HUBC record.

When an FI receives a claim for a screening pelvic examination (including a clinical breast examination), performed on or after January 1, 1998, it reports special override Code 1 in the "Special Action Code/Override Code" field of the CWF record for the line item, indicating the Part B deductible does not apply.

CWF edits for screening pelvic examinations performed more frequently than allowed according to the presence of high risk factors.

Pub 100-4, 18, 40.4 – Diagnoses Codes

(Rev. 440, Issued: 01-21-05, Effective: 07-01-05, Implementation: 07-05-05)

Below is the current diagnoses that should be used when billing for screening pelvic examination services. Effective, July 1, 2005, V72.31 is being added to the CWF edit as an additional low risk diagnosis. The following chart lists the diagnosis codes that CWF must recognize for low risk or high risk patients for screening pelvic examination services.

Low Risk Diagnosis Codes	Definitions
V76.2	Special screening for malignant neoplasm, cervix
V76.47	Special screening for malignant neoplasm, vagina
V76.49	Special screening for malignant neoplasm, other sites NOTE: Providers use this diagnosis for women without a cervix.
V72.31	Routine gynecological examination NOTE: This diagnosis should only be used when the provider performs a full gynecological examination.
High Risk Diagnosis Code	**Definitions**
V15.89	Other

A. Applicable Diagnoses for Billing a Carrier

There are a number of appropriate diagnosis codes that can be used in billing for screening pelvic examinations that the provider can list on the claim to give a true picture of the patient's condition. Those diagnoses can be listed in Item 21 of Form CMS-1500 or the electronic equivalent (see Chapter 26 for electronic equivalent formats). In addition, one of the following diagnoses shall appear on the claim: the low risk diagnosis of V76.2, V76.47, V76.49 and (effective July 1, 2005, V72.31) or the high risk diagnosis of V15.89 (for high risk patients). One of the above diagnoses must be listed in item 21 to indicate either low risk or high risk depending on the patient's condition. Then either the low risk or high risk diagnosis must also be pointed to in Item 24E of Form CMS-1500 or the electronic equivalent. Providers must make sure that for screening pelvic exams for a high risk beneficiary, that the high risk diagnosis code of V15.89 appears in Item 21 and V15.89 is the appropriate diagnosis code that must be pointed to in Item 24E or electronic equivalent. If pelvic examination claims do not point to one of these specific diagnoses in Item 24E or the electronic equivalent, the claim will reject in the CWF. Periodically, carriers should do provider education on diagnosis coding of screening pelvic examination claims.

If these pointers are not present on claims submitted to carriers, CWF will reject the record.

B – Applicable Diagnoses for Billing an FI

Providers report one of the following diagnosis codes in FL 67 of Form CMS-1450 or the electronic equivalent (see Chapter 25 for electronic equivalent format):

Low risk diagnosis codes:

V76.2

V76.47

V76.49

V72.31

High risk diagnosis code

V15.89

Periodically provider education should be done on diagnosis coding of pelvic exam claims.

Pub 100-4, 18, 40.5 – Payment Method

(Rev 440, Issued: 01-21-05, Effective: 07-01-05, Implementation: 07-05-05)

Pelvic examinations are paid under the MPFS, whether billed to the FI or carrier except:

- Hospital outpatient services are paid under OPPS;
- See §40.5.B of this chapter for proper billing by RHC/FQHCs for the professional and technical components of a screening pelvic examination. RHCs/FQHCs are paid under the all-inclusive rate for the professional component; or based on the provider's payment method for the technical component;
- CAH payment is under reasonable cost.

NOTE: SNFs are paid under the MPFS and bill the FI. Physicians and other individual practitioners bill the carrier.

Pub 100-4, 18, 40.6 – Revenue Code and HCPCS Codes for Billing

(Rev. 827, Issued: 02-01-06; Effective Date: 07-01-06; Implementation Date: 07-03-06)

A. Billing to the Carrier

Code G0101 (cervical or vaginal cancer screening, pelvic and clinical breast examination) is used.

Effective for services on or after January 1, 1999, a covered evaluation and management (E/M) visit and code G0101 may be reported by the same physician for the same date of service if the E/M visit is for a separately identifiable service. In this case, the modifier "-25" must be reported with the E/M service and the medical records must clearly document the E/M service reported. Both procedure codes should be shown as separate line items on the claim. These services can also be performed separately on separate office visits.

B. Billing to the FI

The applicable bill types for a screening pelvic examination (including breast examination) are 12X, 13X, 22X, 23X, and 85X. The applicable revenue code is 0770. (See §70.1.1.2 for RHCs and FQHCs.) Effective April 1, 2006, type of bill 14X is for non-patient laboratory specimens and is no longer applicable for a screening pelvic examination.

The professional component of a screening pelvic examination furnished within an RHC/FQHC by a physician or nonphysician is considered an RHC/FQHC service. RHCs and FQHCs bill the FI under bill type 71X or 73X for the professional component along with revenue code 052X.

The technical component of a screening pelvic examination is outside the scope of the RHC/FQHC benefit. If the technical component of this service is furnished within an independent RHC or freestanding FQHC, the provider of that technical service bills the carrier on ANSI X12N 837 P or hardcopy Form CMS-1500.

If the technical component of a screening pelvic examination is furnished within a provider-based RHC/FQHC, the provider of that service bills the FI under bill type 12X, 13X, 22X, 23X, or 85X as appropriate using their outpatient provider number (not the RHC/FQHC provider number since these services are not covered as RHC/FQHC services). The appropriate revenue code is 0770. Effective April 1, 2006, type of bill 14X is for non-patient laboratory specimens and is no longer applicable for a screening pelvic examination.

Pub 100-4, 18, 40.7 – MSN Messages

(Rev. 440, Issued: 01-21-05, Effective: 07-01-05, Implementation: 07-05-05)

If there are no high risk factors, and the screening Pap smear and/or screening pelvic examination is being denied because the procedure/ examination is performed more frequently than allowed, contractors use MSN 18-17:

- Medicare pays for a screening Pap smear and/or screening pelvic examination only once every (2, 3) years unless high risk factors are present.

Pub 100-4, 18, 40.8 – Remittance Advice Codes

(Rev. 440, Issued: 01-21-05, Effective: 07-01-05, Implementation: 07-05-05)

If high risk factors are not present, and the screening Pap smear and/ or screening pelvic examination is being denied because the procedure/ examination is performed more frequently than allowed, use existing ANSI X12N 835:

- Claim adjustment reason code 119 – "Benefit maximum for this time period has been reached" at the line level, and

Remark code M83 – "Service is not covered unless the patient is classified as at high risk." At the line item level.

Pub 100-4, 18, 50 – Prostate Cancer Screening Tests and Procedures

(Rev. 1, 10-01-03)

B3-4182, A3-3616

Sections 1861(s)(2)(P) and 1861(oo) of the Act (as added by §4103 of the Balanced Budget Act of 1997), provide for Medicare Part B coverage of certain prostate cancer screening tests subject to certain coverage, frequency, and payment limitations. Effective for services furnished on or after January 1, 2000, Medicare Part B covers prostate cancer screening tests/procedures for the early detection of prostate cancer. Coverage of prostate cancer screening tests includes the following procedures furnished to an individual for the early detection of prostate cancer:

- Screening digital rectal examination, and
- Screening prostate specific antigen (PSA) blood test.

Each test may be paid at a frequency of once every 12 months for men who have attained age 50 (i.e., starting at least one day after they have attained age 50), if at least 11 months have passed following the month in which the last Medicare-covered screening digital rectal examination was performed (for digital rectal exams) or PSA test was performed (for PSA tests).

Pub 100-4, 18, 50.1 – Definitions

(Rev. 1, 10-01-03)

A3-3616.A.1 and 2

A. Screening Digital Rectal Examination

Screening digital rectal examination means a clinical examination of an individual's prostate for nodules or other abnormalities of the prostate. This screening must be performed by a doctor of medicine or osteopathy (as defined in §186l(r)(1) of the Act), or by a physician assistant, nurse practitioner, clinical nurse specialist, or by a certified nurse mid-wife (as defined in §1861(aa) and §1861(gg) of the Act), who is authorized under State law to perform the examination, fully knowledgeable about the beneficiary, and would be responsible for explaining the results of the examination to the beneficiary.

B. Screening Prostate Specific Antigen (PSA) Tests

Screening prostate specific antigen (PSA) is a test that measures the level of prostate specific antigen in an individual's blood. This screening must be ordered by the beneficiary's physician or by the beneficiary's physician assistant, nurse practitioner, clinical nurse specialist, or certified nurse midwife (the term "physician" is defined in §1861(r)(1) of the Act to mean a doctor of medicine or osteopathy and the terms "physician assistant, nurse practitioner, clinical nurse specialist, or certified nurse midwife" are defined in §1861(aa) and §1861(gg) of the Act) who is fully knowledgeable about the beneficiary, and who would be responsible for explaining the results of the test to the beneficiary.

Pub 100-4, 18, 50.2 – Deductible and Coinsurance

(Rev. 1, 10-01-03)

B3-4182.3

The screening PSA test is a lab test to which neither deductible nor coinsurance apply.

Both deductible (if unmet) and coinsurance are applicable to screening rectal examinations.

Pub 100-4, 18, 50.3 – Payment Method – FIs and Carriers

(Rev. 795, Issued: 12-30-05; Effective: 10-01-04; Implementation: 04-03-06)

Screening PSA tests (G0103) are paid under the clinical diagnostic lab fee schedule.

Screening rectal examinations (G0102) are paid under the MPFS except for the following bill types identified (FI only). Bill types not identified are paid under the MPFS.

12X = Outpatient Prospective Payment System

13X = Outpatient Prospective Payment System

14X-=Outpatient Prospective Payment System

71X = Included in All Inclusive Rate

73X = Included in All Inclusive Rate

85X = Cost (Payment should be consistent with amounts paid for code 84153 or code 86316.)

Effective 4/1/06 the type of bill 14X is for non-patient laboratory specimens.

The RHCs and FQHCs should include the charges on the claims for future inclusion in encounter rate calculations.

Pub 100-4, 18, 50.3.1 – Correct Coding Requirements for Carrier Claims

(Rev. 1, 10-01-03)

B3-4182.6

Billing and payment for a Digital Rectal Exam (DRE) (G0102) is bundled into the payment for a covered E/M service (CPT codes 99201 – 99456 and 99499) when the two services are furnished to a patient on the same day. If the DRE is the only service or is provided as part of an otherwise noncovered service, HCPCS code G0102 would be payable separately if all other coverage requirements are met.

Pub 100-4, 18, 50.4 – HCPCS, Revenue, and Type of Service Codes

(Rev. 795, Issued: 12-30-05; Effective: 10-01-04; Implementation: 04-03-06)

The appropriate bill types for billing the FI on Form CMS-1450 or its electronic equivalent are 12X, 13X, 14X, 22X, 23X, 71X, 73X, 75X, and 85X. Effective 4/1/06, type of bill 14X is for non-patient laboratory specimens.

The HCPCS code G0102 – for prostate cancer screening digital rectal examination.

- Carrier TOS is 1
- FI revenue code is 0770

The HCPCS code G0103 – for prostate cancer screening PSA tests

- Carrier TOS is 5
- FI revenue code is 030X

Pub 100-4, 18, 50.5 – Diagnosis Coding

(Rev. 1, 10-01-03)

B3-4182.7

Prostate cancer screening digital rectal examinations and screening Prostate Specific Antigen (PSA) blood tests must be billed using screening ("V") code V76.44 (Special Screening for Malignant Neoplasms, Prostate).

Pub 100-4, 18, 50.6 – Calculating Frequency

(Rev. 1, 10-01-03)

A3-3616.D and E, B3-4182.4, B3-4182.5

Calculating Frequency – To determine the 11-month period, the count starts beginning with the month after the month in which a previous test/procedure was performed.

EXAMPLE: The beneficiary received a screening prostate specific antigen test in January 2002. Start counts beginning February 2002. The beneficiary is eligible to receive another screening prostate specific antigen test in January 2003 (the month after 11 months have passed).

Common Working File (CWF) Edits

Beginning October 1, 2000, the following CWF edits were implemented for dates of service January 1, 2000, and later, for prostate cancer screening tests and procedures for the following:

- Age;
- Frequency;
- Sex; and
- Valid HCPCS code.

Pub 100-4, 18, 50.7 – MSN Messages

(Rev. 1, 10-01-03)

B3-4182.8.B, A3-3616.F

If a claim for screening prostate specific antigen test or a screening digital rectal examination is being denied because of the age of the beneficiary, FIs use MSN message 18.13:

> This service is not covered for patients under 50 years of age.

The Spanish version of this MSN message should read:

> Este servicio no está cubierto hasta después de que el beneficiario cumpla 50 años.

Carriers use MSN Message 18.19:

> This service is not covered until after the patient's 50th birthday.

The Spanish version of this MSN message should read:

> Este servicio no está cubierto hasta después de que el beneficiario cumpla 50 años.

If the claim for screening prostate specific antigen test or screening digital rectal examination is being denied because the time period between the same test or procedure has not passed, FIs and carriers use MSN message 18.14:

> Service is being denied because it has not been 12 months since your last test/procedure) of this kind.

The Spanish version of this MSN message should read:

> Este servicio está siendo denegado ya que no han transcurrido (12, 24, 48) meses desde el último (examen/procedimiento) de esta clase.

Pub 100-4, 18, 50.8 – Remittance Advice Notices

(Rev. 1, 10-01-03)

B3-4182.8, A3-3616.G

If the claim for a screening prostate antigen test or screening digital rectal examination is being denied because the patient is less than 50 years of age, ANSI X12N 835.

- Claim adjustment reason code 6 "the procedure/revenue code is inconsistent with the patient's age," at the line level; and
- Remark code M140 "Service is not covered until after the patient's 50th birthday, i.e., no coverage prior to the day after the 50th birthday."

If the claim for a screening prostate specific antigen test or screening digital rectal examination is being denied because the time period between the test/procedure has not passed, contractors use ANSI X12N 835 claim adjustment reason code 119 "Benefit maximum for this time period has been reached" at the line level.

If the claim for a screening prostate antigen test or screening digital rectal examination is being denied due to the absence of diagnosis code V76.44

on the claim, use ANSI X12N 835 claim adjustment reason code 47, "This (these) diagnosis(es) is (are) not covered, missing, or invalid."

Pub 100-4, 18, 60 – Colorectal Cancer Screening

(Rev. 52, 12-19-03)

B3-4180, B3-4180.6, A3-3660.17

See the **Medicare Benefit Policy Manual**, Chapter 1, for Medicare Part B coverage and effective dates of colorectal rectal screening services.

Effective for services furnished on or after January 1, 1998, payment may be made for colorectal cancer screening for the early detection of cancer. For screening colonoscopy services (one of the types of services included in this benefit) prior to July 2001, coverage was limited to high-risk individuals. For services July 1, 2001, and later screening colonoscopies are covered for individuals not at high risk.

The following services are considered colorectal cancer screening services:

- Fecal-occult blood test, 1-3 simultaneous determinations (guaiac-based);
- Flexible sigmoidoscopy;
- Colonoscopy; and,
- Barium enema

Effective for services on or after January 1, 2004, payment may be made for the following colorectal cancer screening service as an alternative for the guaiac-based fecal-occult blood test, 1-3 simultaneous determinations:

- Fecal-occult blood test, immunoassay, 1-3 simultaneous determinations

Pub 100-4, 18, 60.1 – Payment

(Rev. 1217, Issued: 03-30-07, Effective: 07-01-07, Implementation: 07-02-07)

Payment (contractor) is under the MPFS except as follows:

- Fecal occult blood tests (82270* (G0107*) and G0328) are paid under the clinical diagnostic lab fee schedule except reasonable cost is paid to all non-OPPS hospitals, including CAHs, but not IHS hospitals billing on TOB 83x. IHS hospitals billing on TOB 83x are paid the ASC payment amount. Other IHS hospitals (billing on TOB 13x) are paid the OMB approved AIR, or the facility specific per visit amount as applicable. Deductible and coinsurance do not apply for these tests. See section A below for payment to Maryland waiver on TOB 13X. Payment from all hospitals for non-patient laboratory specimens on TOB 14X will be based on the clinical diagnostic fee schedule, including CAHs and Maryland waiver hospitals.
- Flexible sigmoidoscopy (code G0104) is paid under OPPS for hospital outpatient departments and on a reasonable cost basis for CAHs; or current payment methodologies for hospitals not subject to OPPS.
- Colonoscopies (G0105 and G0121) and barium enemas (G0106 and G0120) are paid under OPPS for hospital outpatient departments and on a reasonable costs basis for CAHs or current payment methodologies for hospitals not subject to OPPS. Also colonoscopies may be done in an Ambulatory Surgical Center (ASC) and when done in an ASC the ASC rate applies. The ASC rate is the same for diagnostic and screening colonoscopies. The ASC rate is paid to IHS hospitals when the service is billed on TOB 83x.

Prior to January 1, 2007, deductible and coinsurance apply to HCPCS codes G0104, G0105, G0106, G0120, and G0121. Beginning with services provided on or after January 1, 2007, Section 5113 of the Deficit Reduction Act of 2005 waives the requirement of the annual Part B deductible for these screening services. Coinsurance still applies. Coinsurance and deductible applies to the diagnostic colorectal service codes listed below.

The following screening codes must be paid at rates consistent with the diagnostic codes indicated.

Screening Code	Diagnostic Code
G0104	45330
G0105 and G0121	45378
G0106 and G0120	74280

A. Special Payment Instructions for TOB 13X Maryland Waiver Hospitals

For hospitals in Maryland under the jurisdiction of the Health Services Cost Review Commission, screening colorectal services

HCPCS codes G0104, G0105, G0106, 82270* (G0107*), G0120, G0121 and G0328 are paid according to the terms of the waiver, that is 94% of submitted charges minus any unmet existing deductible, co-insurance and non-covered charges. Maryland Hospitals bill TOB 13X for outpatient colorectal cancer screenings.

B. Special Payment Instructions for Non-Patient Laboratory Specimen (TOB 14X) for all hospitals

Payment for colorectal cancer screenings (82270* (G0107*) and G0328) to a hospital for a non-patient laboratory specimen (TOB 14X), is the lesser of the actual charge, the fee schedule amount, or the National Limitation Amount (NLA), (including CAHs and Maryland Waiver hospitals). Part B deductible and coinsurance do not apply.

*NOTE: For claims with dates of service prior to January 1, 2007, physicians, suppliers, and providers report HCPCS code G0107. Effective January 1, 2007, code G0107 is discontinued and replaced with CPT code 82270.

Pub 100-4, 18, 60.1.1 – Deductible and Coinsurance

(Rev. 1325; Issued: 08-29-07; Effective: 01-01-08; Implementation: 01-07-08)

There is no deductible and no coinsurance or copayment for the fecal occult blood tests (G0107 and G0328). Prior to January 1, 2007 deductible and coinsurance apply to other colorectal procedures (G0104, G0105, G0106, G0120, and G0121). After January 1, 2007, the deductible is waived for those tests.

NOTE: A 25 percent coinsurance applies for all colorectal cancer screening colonoscopies (G0105 and G0121) performed in ASCs and non-OPPS hospitals effective for services performed on or after January 1, 2007. The 25 percent coinsurance was implemented in the OPPS PRICER for OPPS hospitals effective for services performed on or after January 1, 1999.

A 25 percent coinsurance also applies for colorectal cancer screening sigmoidoscopies (G0104) performed in non-OPPS hospitals effective for services performed on or after January 1, 2007. Beginning January 1, 2008, colorectal cancer screening sigmoidoscopies (G0104) are payable in ASCs, and a 25 percent coinsurance applies. The 25 percent coinsurance for colorectal cancer screening sigmoidoscopies was implemented in OPPS PRICER for OPPS hospitals effective for services performed on or after January 1, 1999.

Pub 100-4, 18, 60.2 – HCPCS Codes, Frequency Requirements, and Age Requirements (If Applicable)

(Rev. 1062, Issued: 09-22-06, Effective: 01-01-07, Implementation: 01-02-07)

Effective for services furnished on or after January 1, 1998, the following codes are used for colorectal cancer screening services:

- 82270* (G0107*) – Colorectal cancer screening; fecal-occult blood tests, 1-3 simultaneous determinations;
- G0104 – Colorectal cancer screening; flexible sigmoidoscopy;
- G0105 – Colorectal cancer screening; colonoscopy on individual at high risk;
- G0106 – Colorectal cancer screening; barium enema; as an alternative to G0104, screening sigmoidoscopy;
- G0120 – Colorectal cancer screening; barium enema; as an alternative to G0105, screening colonoscopy.

Effective for services furnished on or after July 1, 2001, the following codes are used for colorectal cancer screening services:

- G0121 – Colorectal cancer screening; colonoscopy on individual not meeting criteria for high risk. Note that the description for this code has been revised to remove the term "noncovered."
- G0122 – Colorectal cancer screening; barium enema (noncovered).

Effective for services furnished on or after January 1, 2004, the following code is used for colorectal cancer screening services as an alternative to 82270* (G0107*):

Medicare References

- G0328 – Colorectal cancer screening; immunoassay, fecal-occult blood test, 1-3 simultaneous determinations

**NOTE: For claims with dates of service prior to January 1, 2007, physicians, suppliers, and providers report HCPCS code G0107. Effective January 1, 2007, code G0107 is discontinued and replaced with CPT code 82270.*

G0104 Colorectal Cancer Screening; Flexible Sigmoidoscopy

Screening flexible sigmoidoscopies (code G0104) may be paid for beneficiaries who have attained age 50, when performed by a doctor of medicine or osteopathy at the frequencies noted below.

For claims with dates of service on or after January 1, 2002, contractors pay for screening flexible sigmoidoscopies (code G0104) for beneficiaries who have attained age 50 when these services were performed by a doctor of medicine or osteopathy, or by a physician assistant, nurse practitioner, or clinical nurse specialist (as defined in §1861(aa)(5) of the Act and in the Code of Federal Regulations at 42 CFR 410.74, 410.75, and 410.76) at the frequencies noted above. For claims with dates of service prior to January 1, 2002, contractors pay for these services under the conditions noted only when a doctor of medicine or osteopathy performs them.

For services furnished from January 1, 1998, through June 30, 2001, inclusive:

- Once every 48 months (i.e., at least 47 months have passed following the month in which the last covered screening flexible sigmoidoscopy was done).

For services furnished on or after July 1, 2001:

- Once every 48 months as calculated above unless the beneficiary does not meet the criteria for high risk of developing colorectal cancer (refer to §60.3 of this chapter) and he/she has had a screening colonoscopy (code G0121) within the preceding 10 years. If such a beneficiary has had a screening colonoscopy within the preceding 10 years, then he or she can have covered a screening flexible sigmoidoscopy only after at least 119 months have passed following the month that he/she received the screening colonoscopy (code G0121).

NOTE: If during the course of a screening flexible sigmoidoscopy a lesion or growth is detected which results in a biopsy or removal of the growth; the appropriate diagnostic procedure classified as a flexible sigmoidoscopy with biopsy or removal should be billed and paid rather than code G0104.

G0105 Colorectal Cancer Screening; Colonoscopy on Individual at High Risk

Screening colonoscopies (code G0105) may be paid when performed by a doctor of medicine or osteopathy at a frequency of once every 24 months for beneficiaries at high risk for developing colorectal cancer (i.e., at least 23 months have passed following the month in which the last covered G0105 screening colonoscopy was performed). Refer to §60.3 of this chapter for the criteria to use in determining whether or not an individual is at high risk for developing colorectal cancer.

NOTE: If during the course of the screening colonoscopy, a lesion or growth is detected which results in a biopsy or removal of the growth, the appropriate diagnostic procedure classified as a colonoscopy with biopsy or removal should be billed and paid rather than code G0105.

A. Colonoscopy Cannot be Completed Because of Extenuating Circumstances

1. FIs

When a covered colonoscopy is attempted but cannot be completed because of extenuating circumstances, Medicare will pay for the interrupted colonoscopy as long as the coverage conditions are met for the incomplete procedure. However, the frequency standards associated with screening colonoscopies will not be applied by CWF. When a covered colonoscopy is next attempted and completed, Medicare will pay for that colonoscopy according to its payment methodology for this procedure as long as coverage conditions are met, and the frequency standards will be applied by CWF. This policy is applied to both screening and diagnostic colonoscopies. When submitting a facility claim for the interrupted colonoscopy, providers are to suffix the colonoscopy HCPCS codes with a modifier of 73 or 74 as appropriate to indicate that the procedure was interrupted. Payment for covered incomplete screening colonoscopies shall be consistent with payment methodologies currently in place for complete screening colonoscopies, including those contained in 42 CFR 419.44(b). In situations where a critical access hospital (CAH) has elected payment Method II for CAH patients, payment shall be consistent with payment methodologies currently in place as outlined in Chapter 3. As such, instruct CAHs that elect Method II payment to use modifier 53 to identify an incomplete screening colonoscopy (physician professional service(s) billed in revenue

code 096X, 097X, and/or 098X). Such CAHs will also bill the technical or facility component of the interrupted colonoscopy in revenue code 075X (or other appropriate revenue code) using the 73 or 74 modifier as appropriate.

Note that Medicare would expect the provider to maintain adequate information in the patient's medical record in case it is needed by the contractor to document the incomplete procedure.

2. Carriers

When a covered colonoscopy is attempted but cannot be completed because of extenuating circumstances (see Chapter 12), Medicare will pay for the interrupted colonoscopy at a rate consistent with that of a flexible sigmoidoscopy as long as coverage conditions are met for the incomplete procedure. When a covered colonoscopy is next attempted and completed, Medicare will pay for that colonoscopy according to its payment methodology for this procedure as long as coverage conditions are met. This policy is applied to both screening and diagnostic colonoscopies. When submitting a claim for the interrupted colonoscopy, professional providers are to suffix the colonoscopy code with a modifier of "–53" to indicate that the procedure was interrupted. When submitting a claim for the facility fee associated with this procedure, Ambulatory Surgical Centers (ASCs) are to suffix the colonoscopy code with "–73" or "–74" as appropriate. Payment for covered screening colonoscopies, including that for the associated ASC facility fee when applicable, shall be consistent with payment for diagnostic colonoscopies, whether the procedure is complete or incomplete.

Note that Medicare would expect the provider to maintain adequate information in the patient's medical record in case it is needed by the contractor to document the incomplete procedure.

G0106 Colorectal Cancer Screening; Barium Enema; as an Alternative to G0104, Screening Sigmoidoscopy

Screening barium enema examinations may be paid as an alternative to a screening sigmoidoscopy (code G0104). The same frequency parameters for screening sigmoidoscopies (see those codes above) apply.

In the case of an individual aged 50 or over, payment may be made for a screening barium enema examination (code G0106) performed after at least 47 months have passed following the month in which the last screening barium enema or screening flexible sigmoidoscopy was performed. For example, the beneficiary received a screening barium enema examination as an alternative to a screening flexible sigmoidoscopy in January 1999. Start counts beginning February 1999. The beneficiary is eligible for another screening barium enema in January 2003.

The screening barium enema must be ordered in writing after a determination that the test is the appropriate screening test. Generally, it is expected that this will be a screening

double contrast enema unless the individual is unable to withstand such an exam. This means that in the case of a particular individual, the attending physician must determine that the estimated screening potential for the barium enema is equal to or greater than the screening potential that has been estimated for a screening flexible sigmoidoscopy for the same individual. The screening single contrast barium enema also requires a written order from the beneficiary's attending physician in the same manner as described above for the screening double contrast barium enema examination.

82270* (G0107*) – Colorectal Cancer Screening; Fecal-Occult Blood Test, 1-3 Simultaneous Determinations

Effective for services furnished on or after January 1, 1998, screening FOBT (code 82270* (G0107*) may be paid for beneficiaries who have attained age 50, and at a frequency of once every 12 months (i.e., at least 11 months have passed following the month in which the last covered screening FOBT was performed). This screening FOBT means a guaiac-based test for peroxidase activity, in which the beneficiary completes it by taking samples from two different sites of three consecutive stools. This screening requires a written order from the beneficiary's attending physician. (The term "attending physician" is defined to mean a doctor of medicine or osteopathy (as defined in §1861(r)(1) of the Act) who is fully knowledgeable about the beneficiary's medical condition, and who would be responsible for using the results of any examination performed in the overall management of the beneficiary's specific medical problem.)

Effective for services furnished on or after January 1, 2004, payment may be made for a immunoassay-based FOBT (G0328, described below) as an alternative to the guaiac-based FOBT, 82270* (G0107*). Medicare will pay for only one covered FOBT per year, either 82270* (G0107*) or G0328, but not both.

*NOTE: For claims with dates of service prior to January 1, 2007, physicians, suppliers, and providers report HCPCS code G0107. Effective January 1, 2007, code G0107 is discontinued and replaced with CPT code 82270.

G0328 Colorectal Cancer Screening; Immunoassay, Fecal-Occult Blood Test, 1-3 Simultaneous Determinations

Effective for services furnished on or after January 1, 2004, screening FOBT, (code G0328) may be paid as an alternative to 82270* (G0107*) for beneficiaries who have attained age 50. Medicare will pay for a covered FOBT (either 82270* (G0107*) or G0328, but not both) at a frequency of once every 12 months (i.e., at least 11 months have passed following the month in which the last covered screening FOBT was performed). Screening FOBT, immunoassay, includes the use of a spatula to collect the appropriate number of samples or the use of a special brush for the collection of samples, as determined by the individual manufacturer's instructions. This screening requires a written order from the beneficiary's attending physician. (The term "attending physician" is defined to mean a doctor of medicine or osteopathy (as defined in §1861(r)(1) of the Act) who is fully knowledgeable about the beneficiary's medical condition, and who would be responsible for using the results of any examination performed in the overall management of the beneficiary's specific medical problem.)

G0120 Colorectal Cancer Screening; Barium Enema; as an Alternative to or G0105, Screening Colonoscopy

Screening barium enema examinations may be paid as an alternative to a screening colonoscopy (code G0105) examination. The same frequency parameters for screening colonoscopies (see those codes above) apply.

In the case of an individual who is at high risk for colorectal cancer, payment may be made for a screening barium enema examination (code G0120) performed after at least 23 months have passed following the month in which the last screening barium enema or the last screening colonoscopy was performed. For example, a beneficiary at high risk for developing colorectal cancer received a screening barium enema examination (code G0120) as an alternative to a screening colonoscopy (code G0105) in January 2000. Start counts beginning February 2000. The beneficiary is eligible for another screening barium enema examination (code G0120) in January 2002.

The screening barium enema must be ordered in writing after a determination that the test is the appropriate screening test. Generally, it is expected that this will be a screening double contrast enema unless the individual is unable to withstand such an exam. This means that in the case of a particular individual, the attending physician must determine that the estimated screening potential for the barium enema is equal to or greater than the screening potential that has been estimated for a screening colonoscopy, for the same individual. The screening single contrast barium enema also requires a written order from the beneficiary's attending physician in the same manner as described above for the screening double contrast barium enema examination.

G0121 Colorectal Screening; Colonoscopy on Individual Not Meeting Criteria for High Risk – Applicable On and After July 1, 2001

Effective for services furnished on or after July 1, 2001, screening colonoscopies (code G0121) performed on individuals not meeting the criteria for being at high risk for developing colorectal cancer (refer to §60.3 of this chapter) may be paid under the following conditions:

- At a frequency of once every 10 years (i.e., at least 119 months have passed following the month in which the last covered G0121 screening colonoscopy was performed.)
- If the individual would otherwise qualify to have covered a G0121 screening colonoscopy based on the above but has had a covered screening flexible sigmoidoscopy (code G0104), then he or she may have covered a G0121 screening colonoscopy only after at least 47 months have passed following the month in which the last covered G0104 flexible sigmoidoscopy was performed.

NOTE: If during the course of the screening colonoscopy, a lesion or growth is detected which results in a biopsy or removal of the growth, the appropriate diagnostic procedure classified as a colonoscopy with biopsy or removal should be billed and paid rather than code G0121.

G0122 Colorectal Cancer Screening; Barium Enema

The code is not covered by Medicare.

Pub 100-4, 18, 60.2.1 – Common Working Files (CWF) Edits

(Rev. 1062, Issued: 09-22-06, Effective: 01-01-07, Implementation: 01-02-07)

Effective for dates of service January 1, 1998, and later, CWF will edit all colorectal screening claims for age and frequency standards. The CWF will also edit FI claims for valid procedure codes (G0104, G0105, G0106, 82270* (G0107*), G0120, G0121, G0122, and G0328) and for valid bill types. The CWF currently edits for valid HCPCS codes for carriers. (See §60.6 of this chapter for bill types.)

*NOTE: For claims with dates of service prior to January 1, 2007, physicians, suppliers, and providers report HCPCS code G0107. Effective January 1, 2007, code G0107 is discontinued and replaced with CPT code 82270.

Pub 100-4, 18, 60.2.2 – Ambulatory Surgical Center (ASC) Facility Fee

(Rev. 1160, Issued: 01-19-07, Effective: 01-01-07, Implementation: 07-02-07)

CPT code 45378, which is used to code a diagnostic colonoscopy, is on the list of procedures approved by Medicare for payment of an ambulatory surgical center facility under §1833(I) of the Act. CPT code 45378 is currently assigned to ASC payment group 2. Code G0105, colorectal cancer screening; colonoscopy on individuals at high risk, was added to the ASC list effective for services furnished on or after January 1, 1998. Code G0121, colorectal cancer screening; colonoscopy on individual not meeting criteria for high risk, was added to the ASC list effective for services furnished on or after July 1, 2001. Codes G0105 and G0121 are assigned to ASC payment group 2. The ASC facility service is the same whether the procedure is a screening or a diagnostic colonoscopy. If during the course of the screening colonoscopy performed at an ASC, a lesion or growth is detected which results in a biopsy or removal of the growth, the appropriate diagnostic procedure classified as a colonoscopy with biopsy or removal should be billed rather than code G0105. Effective for services performed on or after January 1, 2007, a 25 percent coinsurance payment will apply for the colorectal cancer screening services (G0105 and G0121).

Pub 100-4, 18, 60.3 – Determining High Risk for Developing Colorectal Cancer

(Rev. 1, 10-01-03)

B3-4180.3, A3-3660.17, HO-456.B

A. Characteristics of the High Risk Individual

An individual at high risk for developing colorectal cancer has one or more of the following:

- A close relative (sibling, parent, or child) who has had colorectal cancer or an adenomatous polyp;
- A family history of familial adenomatous polyposis;
- A family history of hereditary nonpolyposis colorectal cancer;
- A personal history of adenomatous polyps;
- A personal history of colorectal cancer; or
- Inflammatory bowel disease, including Crohn's Disease, and ulcerative colitis.

B. Partial List of ICD-9-CM Codes Indicating High Risk

Listed below are some examples of diagnoses that meet the high-risk criteria for colorectal cancer. This is not an all-inclusive list. There may be more instances of conditions, which may be coded and could be considered high risk at the medical directors' discretion.

Personal History

V10.05 Personal history of malignant neoplasm of large intestine

V10.06 Personal history of malignant neoplasm of rectum, rectosigmoid junction, and anus

Chronic Digestive Disease Condition:

555.0 Regional enteritis of small intestine

555.1 Regional enteritis of large intestine

555.2 Regional enteritis of small intestine with large intestine

555.9 Regional enteritis of unspecified site
556.0 Ulcerative (chronic) enterocolitis
556.1 Ulcerative (chronic) ileocolitis
556.2 Ulcerative (chronic) proctitis
556.3 Ulcerative (chronic) proctosigmoiditis
556.8 Other ulcerative colitis
556.9 Ulcerative colitis, unspecified (non-specific PDX on the MCE)

Inflammatory Bowel:

558.2 Toxic gastroenteritis and colitis
558.9 Other and unspecified non-infectious gastroenteritis and colitis

Pub 100-4, 18, 60.4 – Determining Frequency Standards

(Rev. 1, 10-01-03)

B3-4180.4, A3-3660.17.D, HO-456.D

To determine the 11, 23, 47, and 119 month periods, start counts beginning with the month after the month in which a previous test/procedure was performed.

EXAMPLE: The beneficiary received a fecal-occult blood test in January 2000. Start counts beginning with February 2000. The beneficiary is eligible to receive another blood test in January 2001 (the month after 11 full months have passed).

Pub 100-4, 18, 60.5 – Noncovered Services

(Rev. 1, 10-01-03)

B3-4180.5, A3-3660.17, HO-456.C

The following noncovered HCPCS codes are used to allow claims to be billed and denied for beneficiaries who need a Medicare denial for other insurance purposes for the dates of service indicated:

A. From January 1, 1998 Through June 30, 2001, Inclusive

Code G0121 (colorectal cancer screening; colonoscopy on an individual not meeting criteria for high risk) should be used when this procedure is performed on a beneficiary who does not meet the criteria for high risk. This service should be denied as noncovered because it fails to meet the requirements of the benefit for these dates of service. The beneficiary is liable for payment. Note that this code is a covered service for dates of service on or after July 1, 2001.

B. On or After January 1, 1998

Code G0122 (colorectal cancer screening; barium enema) should be used when a screening barium enema is performed not as an alternative to either a screening colonoscopy (code G0105) or a screening flexible sigmoidoscopy (code G0104). This service should be denied as noncovered because it fails to meet the requirements of the benefit. The beneficiary is liable for payment.

Pub 100-4, 18, 60.6 – Billing Requirements for Claims Submitted to FIs

(Rev. 1953, Issued: 04-28-10, Effective: 10-01-10, Implementation: 10-04-10)

Follow the general bill review instructions in Chapter 25. Hospitals use the ANSI X12N 837I to bill the FI or on the hardcopy Form CMS-1450. Hospitals bill revenue codes and HCPCS codes as follows:

Screening Test/ Procedure	Revenue Code	HCPCS Code	TOB
Fecal Occult blood test	030X	82270*** (G0107***), G0328	12X, 13X, 14X**, 22X, 23X, 83X, 85X
Barium enema	032X	G0106, G0120, G0122	12X, 13X, 22X, 23X, 85X****
Flexible Sigmoidoscopy	*	G0104	12X, 13X, 22X, 23X, 83X, 85X****
Colonoscopy-high risk	*	G0105, G0121	12X, 13X, 22X, 23X, 83X, 85X****

** The appropriate revenue code when reporting any other surgical procedure.*
*** 14X is only applicable for non-patient laboratory specimens.*
**** For claims with dates of service prior to January 1, 2007, physicians, suppliers, and providers report HCPCS code G0107. Effective January 1, 2007, code G0107, is discontinued and replaced with CPT code 82270.*
***** CAHs that elect Method II bill revenue code 096X, 097X, and/or 098X for professional services and 075X (or other appropriate revenue code) for the technical or facility component.*

Special Billing Instructions for Hospital Inpatients

When these tests/procedures are provided to inpatients of a hospital or when Part A benefits have been exhausted, they are covered under this benefit. However, the provider bills on bill type 12X using the discharge date of the hospital stay to avoid editing in the Common Working File (CWF) as a result of the hospital bundling rules.

Pub 100-4, 18, 60.7 – MSN Messages

(Rev. 1062, Issued: 09-22-06, Effective: 01-01-07, Implementation: 01-02-07)

The following MSN messages are used (See Chapter 21 for the Spanish versions of these messages):

A. If a claim for a screening fecal-occult blood test, a screening flexible sigmoidoscopy, or a barium enema is being denied because of the age of the beneficiary, MSN message 18.13 is used.

This service is not covered for patients under 50 years of age.

B. If the claim for a screening fecal-occult blood test, a screening colonoscopy, a screening flexible sigmoidoscopy, or a barium enema is being denied because the time period between the same test or procedure has not passed, MSN message 18.14 is used:

Service is being denied because it has not been (12, 24, 48, 120) months since your last (test/procedure) of this kind.

C. If the claim is being denied for a screening colonoscopy or a barium enema because the beneficiary is not at a high risk, MSN message 18.15 is used:

Medicare covers this procedure only for patients considered to be at a high risk for colorectal cancer.

D. If the claim is being denied because payment has already been made for a screening fecal-occult blood test (82270* (G0107*) or G0328), flexible sigmoidoscopy (code G0104), screening colonoscopy (code G0105), or a screening barium enema (codes G0106 or G0120), MSN message 18.16 is used:

This service is denied because payment has already been made for a similar procedure within a set timeframe.

NOTE: MSN message 18-16 should only be used when a certain screening procedure is performed as an alternative to another screening procedure. For example: If the claims history indicates a payment has been made for code G0120 and an incoming claim is submitted for code G0105 within 24 months, the incoming claim should be denied.

E. If the claim is being denied for a noncovered screening procedure code such as G0122, the following MSN message 16.10 is used:

Medicare does not pay for this item or service.

If an invalid procedure code is reported, the contractor will return the claim as unprocessable to the provider under current procedures.

*NOTE: For claims with dates of service prior to January 1, 2007, physicians, suppliers, and providers report HCPCS code G0107. Effective January 1, 2007, code G0107 is discontinued and replaced with CPT code 82270.

Pub 100-4, 18, 60.8 – Remittance Advice Notices

(Rev. 1, 10-01-03)

B3-4180.9, A3-3660.17.J, HO-456.J

All messages refer to ANSI X12N 835 coding.

A. If the claim for a screening fecal-occult blood test, a screening flexible sigmoidoscopy, or a screening barium enema is being denied because the patient is less than 50 years of age, use:

- Claim adjustment reason code 6 "the procedure code is inconsistent with the patient's age," at the line level; and

- Remark code M82 "Service is not covered when patient is under age 50." at the line level.

B. If the claim for a screening fecal-occult blood test, a screening colonoscopy, a screening flexible sigmoidoscopy, or a screening barium enema is being denied because the time period between the test/procedure has not passed, use:
- Reason code 119 "Benefit maximum for this time period has been reached" at the line level.

C. If the claim is being denied for a screening colonoscopy (code G0105) or a screening barium enema (G0120) because the patient is not at a high risk, use:
- Claim adjustment reason code 46 "This (these) service(s) is (are) not covered" at the line level; and
- Remark code M83 "Service is not covered unless the patient is classified as a high risk." at the line level.

D. If the service is being denied because payment has already been made for a similar procedure within the set time frame, use:
- Claim adjustment reason code 18, "Duplicate claim/service" at the line level; and
- Remark code M86 "Service is denied because payment already made for similar procedure within a set timeframe." at the line level.

E. If the claim is being denied for a noncovered screening procedure such as G0122, use:
- Claim adjustment reason code 49, "These are noncovered services because this is a routine exam or screening procedure done in conjunction with a routine exam."

F. If the claim is being denied because the code is invalid, use the following at the line level:

Claim adjustment reason code B18 "Payment denied because this procedure code/modifier was invalid on the date of service or claim submission."

Pub 100-4, 18, 70 – Glaucoma Screening Services

(Rev. 1, 10-01-03)

B3-4184

Conditions of Medicare Part B coverage for glaucoma screening are located in the **Medicare Benefit Policy Manual**, Chapter 15.

Pub 100-4, 18, 70.1 – Claims Submission Requirements and Applicable HCPCS Codes

(Rev. 1, 10-01-03)

B3-4184.2, A-01-105 (CR 1783), B-01-46 (CR 1717), A-01-132(CR 1914)

Claims for screening for glaucoma should be submitted on Form CMS-1500 to carriers and Form CMS-1450 to FIs or their electronic equivalents. Claims must be prepared and submitted by physicians and providers to the carrier in accordance with the general instructions in Chapter 26. Claims submitted to FIs must be prepared in accordance with the general bill instructions in Chapter 25.

Pub 100-4, 18, 70.1.1 – HCPCS and Diagnosis Coding

(Rev. 1, 10-01-03)

B3-4184.2, A-01-105 (CR 1783), B-01-46 (CR 1717), A-01-132(CR 1914)

The following HCPCS codes should be reported when billing for screening glaucoma services:

G0117 Glaucoma screening for high-risk patients furnished by an optometrist (physician for carrier) or ophthalmologist.

G0118 Glaucoma screening for high-risk patients furnished under the direct supervision of an optometrist (physician for carrier) or ophthalmologist.

The carrier claims type of service for the above G codes is: TOS Q.

Glaucoma screening claims should be billed using screening ("V") code V80.1 (Special Screening for Neurological, Eye, and Ear Diseases, Glaucoma). Claims submitted without a screening diagnosis code may be returned to the provider as unprocessable (refer to Chapter 1 for more information about incomplete or invalid claims).

Pub 100-4, 18, 70.1.1.1 – Additional Coding Applicable to Claims Submitted to FIs

(Rev. 371, Issued 11-19-04, Effective: 04-01-05, Implementation: 04-04-05)

A. Type of Bill

The applicable FI claim bill types for screening glaucoma services are 13X, 22X, 23X, 71X, 73X, 75X, and 85X. (See instructions below for rural health clinics (RHCs) and federally qualified health centers (FQHCs).)

B. Revenue Coding

The following revenue codes should be reported when billing for screening glaucoma services: Comprehensive outpatient rehabilitation facilities (CORFs), critical access hospitals (CAHs), and skilled nursing facilities (SNFs) bill for this service under revenue code 0770. CAHs electing the optional method of payment for outpatient services also report this service under revenue codes 096X, 097X, or 098X. Hospital outpatient departments bill for this service under any valid/appropriate revenue code. They are not required to report revenue code 0770. (See instructions below for RHCs and FQHCs.)

Pub 100-4, 18, 70.1.1.2 – Special Billing Instructions for RHCs and FQHCs

(Rev. 371, Issued 11-19-04, Effective: 04-01-05, Implementation: 04-04-05)

Screening glaucoma services are considered RHC/FQHC services. For claims with dates of service before April 1, 2005, RHCs and FQHCs bill the FI under bill type 71X or 73X along with revenue code 0770 and HCPCS codes G0117 or G0118 and RHC/FQHC revenue code 0520 or 0521 to report the related visit. Reporting of revenue code 0770 and HCPCS codes G0117 and G0118 in addition to revenue code 0520 or 0521 is required for this service in order for CWF to perform frequency editing. Payment should not be made for a screening glaucoma service unless the claim also contains a visit code for the service. FIs must edit to assure payment is not made for revenue code 0770. The claim must also contain a visit revenue code (0520 or 0521). Payment is made for the screening glaucoma service under the all-inclusive rate for the line item reporting revenue code 0520 or 0521. No payment is made on the line item reporting revenue code 0770.

Screening glaucoma services furnished within an RHC/FQHC by a physician or nonphysician are considered RHC/FQHC services. For claims with dates of service on or after April 1, 2005, RHCs and FQHCs bill the FI under bill type 71X or 73X for the service. Payment is made under the all-inclusive rate. Additional revenue and HCPCS coding is no longer required for this service when RHCs/FQHCs are billing for the service. Use revenue code 0520 or 0521, as appropriate.

Pub 100-4, 18, 70.1.2 – Edits

(Rev. 1, 10-01-03)

B3-4184.4, A-01-132 (CR 1914), B3-4184.5

A. Common Working File Edits

Effective January 1, 2002, CWF edits glaucoma screening claims for frequency and valid HCPCS codes for dates of service January 1, 2002, and later.

B. Claims Edits

Nationwide claims processing edits for pre or post payment review of claim(s) for glaucoma screening are not required at this time. Carriers and FIs monitor claims to assure that they are paid only for covered individuals and perform medical review as appropriate. Local medical review policies and edits may be developed for such claims.

Pub 100-4, 18, 70.2 – Payment Methodology

(Rev. 1, 10-01-03)

B3-4184.7, A-01-132 (CR 1914), A-01-105(CR 1783), B-01-46 (CR 1717)

Carriers pay for glaucoma screening based on the Medicare Physician Fee Schedule. Deductible and coinsurance apply. Claims from physicians or other providers where assignment was not taken are subject to the Medicare limiting charge, which means they cannot charge the beneficiary more than 115 percent of the allowed amount.

FI pay the facility expense as follows:

- Independent and provider-based RHC/free standing and provider-based FQHC receive payment under the all-inclusive rate for the screening glaucoma service based on the visit furnished to the RHC/FQHC patient;
- CAHs receive payment on a reasonable cost basis unless the CAH has elected the optional method of payment for outpatient services in which case, procedures outlined in Chapter 4 should be followed;
- CORFs receive payment under the Medicare Physician Fee Schedule;
- Hospital outpatient departments receive payment under the outpatient prospective payment system (OPPS);
- Hospital inpatient Part B services are paid under OPPS;
- SNF outpatient services are paid under the Medicare physician fee schedule (MPFS); and
- SNF inpatient Part B services are paid under MPFS.

Deductible and coinsurance apply.

Pub 100-4, 18, 70.3 – Determining the 11-Month Period

(Rev. 1, 10-01-03)

A-01-132 (CR 1914), B3-4184.3

Once a beneficiary has received a covered glaucoma screening procedure, the beneficiary may receive another procedure after 11 full months have passed. To determine the 11-month period, start counts beginning with the month after the month in which the previous covered screening procedure was performed.

Pub 100-4, 18, 70.4 – Remittance Advice Notices

(Rev. 895, Issued: 03-24-06; Effective: 01-01-06; Implementation: 04-03-06)

Appropriate remittance advice(s) must be used by fiscal intermediaries and carriers when denying payment for glaucoma screening. The following messages are used where applicable:

- If the services were furnished before January 1, 2002, use existing ANSI X12N 835 remittance advice claim adjustment reason code 26 "Expenses incurred prior to coverage" at the line level.
- If the claim for glaucoma screening is being denied because the minimum time period has not elapsed since the performance of the same Medicare covered procedure, use existing ANSI X12N 835 claim adjustment reason code 119 "Benefit maximum for this time period has been reached" at the line level.
- If the service is being denied because the individual is not an African-American age 50 or over, use existing remittance advice claim adjustment reason code 6, "The procedure code is inconsistent with the patient's age," and existing remark codes M83, "Service not covered unless the patient is classified as at high risk," and M82, "Service not covered when patient is under age 50." Report these codes at the line level.
- If the service is being denied because the individual is not a Hispanic-American age 65 or over, use existing remittance advice claim adjustment reason code 96, "Non-covered charge," and existing remark codes M83, "Service not covered unless the patient is classified as at high risk," and N129, "This amount represents the dollar amount not eligible due to patient's age."
- If the service is being denied because the patient does not have diabetes mellitus, or there is no family history of glaucoma, carriers use existing remittance advice claim adjustment reason code B5, "Payment adjusted because coverage/program guidelines were not met or were exceeded." The zero payment for the service will indicate the denial. In addition, report remark code M83, "Service is not covered unless the patient is classified as at high risk" at the line level.

Pub 100-4, 18, 70.5 – MSN Messages

(Rev. 895, Issued: 03-24-06; Effective: 01-01-06; Implementation: 04-03-06)

The following MSN messages where appropriate must be used.

If a claim for a screening for glaucoma is being denied because the service was performed prior to January 1, 2002, use the MSN message:

MSN Message 16.54:

This service is not covered prior to January 1, 2002.

The Spanish version of the MSN message should read:

Este servicio no está cubierto antes del 1 de enero de 2002.

If a claim for screening for glaucoma is being denied because the minimum time period has not elapsed since the performance of the same Medicare-covered procedure, use MSN message:

MSN Message 18.14:

Service is being denied because it has not been [12/24/48] months since your last [test/procedure] of this kind.

The Spanish version of this MSN message should read:

Este servicio está siendo denegado ya que no han transcurrido [12, 24, 48] meses desde el último[examen/procedimiento] de esta clase.

If a claim for a screening for glaucoma is being denied because the age-related and/or ethnic-related coverage criteria are not met, use:

MSN Message 21.21:

This service was denied because Medicare only covers this service under certain circumstances.

The Spanish version of this MSN message should read:

Este servicio fue denegado porque Medicare solamente lo cubre bajo ciertas circunstancias.

Pub 100-4, 18, 80 – Initial Preventive Physical Examination (IPPE)

(Rev. 1615, Issued: 10-17-08, Effective: 01-01-09, Implementation: 01-05-09)

Background: Effective for services furnished on or after January 1, 2005, Section 611 of the Medicare Prescription Drug Improvement and Modernization Act of 2003 (MMA) provides for coverage under Part B of one initial preventive physical examination (IPPE) for new beneficiaries only, subject to certain eligibility and other limitations. We amended §§411.15 (a)(1) and 411.15 (k)(11) of the Code of Federal Regulations (CFR) to permit payment for an IPPE as described at 42 CFR §410.16, added by 69 FR 66236, 66420 (November 15, 2004) not later than 6 months after the date the individual's first coverage period begins under Medicare Part B.

Under the MMA of 2003, the IPPE may be performed by a doctor of medicine or osteopathy as defined in section 1861 (r)(1) of the Social Security Act (the Act) or by a qualified mid-level nonphysician practitioner (NPP) (nurse practitioner, physician assistant or clinical nurse specialist), not later than 6 months after the date the individual's first coverage begins under Medicare Part B. (See section 80.3 for a list of bill types of facilities that can bill fiscal intermediaries (FIs) for this service.) This examination will include: (1) review of the individual's medical and social history with attention to modifiable risk factors for disease detection, (2) review of the individual's potential (risk factors) for depression or other mood disorders, (3) review of the individual's functional ability and level of safety; (4) a physical examination to include measurement of the individual's height, weight, blood pressure, a visual acuity screen, and other factors as deemed appropriate by the examining physician or qualified nonphysician practitioner (NPP), (5) performance and interpretation of an electrocardiogram (EKG); (6) education, counseling, and referral, as deemed appropriate, based on the results of the review and evaluation services described in the previous 5 elements, and (7) education, counseling, and referral including a brief written plan (e.g., a checklist or alternative) provided to the individual for obtaining the appropriate screening and other preventive services, which are separately covered under Medicare Part B benefits. The EKG performed as a component of the IPPE will be billed separately. Medicare will pay for only one IPPE per beneficiary per lifetime. The Common Working File (CWF) will edit for this benefit.

As required by statute under the MMA of 2003, the total IPPE service includes an EKG, but the EKG is billed with its own unique HCPCS code(s). The IPPE does not include other preventive services that are currently separately covered and paid under Section 1861 of the Act under Medicare Part B screening benefits. (That is, pneumococcal, influenza and hepatitis B vaccines and their administration, screening mammography, screening pap smear and screening pelvic examinations, prostate cancer screening tests, colorectal cancer screening tests, diabetes outpatient self-management training services, bone mass measurements, glaucoma screening, medical nutrition therapy for individuals with diabetes or renal disease, cardiovascular screening blood tests, and diabetes screening tests.)

Section 5112 of the Deficit Reduction Act of 2005 allows for one ultrasound screening for Abdominal Aortic Aneurysm (AAA) as a result of a referral from an IPPE effective January 1, 2007. For AAA physician/practitioner billing, correct coding, and payment policy information, refer to Section 110 of this chapter.

Effective January 1, 2009, Section 101 (b) of the Medicare Improvement for Patients and Providers Act (MIPPA) of 2008 updates the IPPE benefit described under the MMA of 2003. The MIPPA allows the IPPE to be performed not later than 12 months after the date the individual's first coverage period begins under Medicare Part B, requires the addition of the measurement of an individual's body mass index to the IPPE, adds end-of-life planning (upon an individual's consent) to the IPPE, and removes the screening electrocardiogram (EKG) as a mandatory service of the IPPE. The screening EKG is optional effective January 1, 2009, and is permitted as a once-in-a-lifetime screening service as a result of a referral from an IPPE.

The MIPPA of 2008 allows for possible future payment for additional preventive services not otherwise described in Title XVIII of the Social Security Act (the Act) that identify medical conditions or risk factors for eligible individuals if the Secretary determines through the national coverage determination (NCD) process (as defined in section 1869(f)(1)(B) of the Act) that they are: (1) reasonable and necessary for the prevention or early detection of illness or disability, (2) recommended with a grade of A or B by the United States Preventive Services Task Force, and, (3) appropriate for individuals entitled to benefits under Part A or enrolled under Part B, or both. MIPPA requires that there be education, counseling, referral for additional preventive services, as appropriate, under the IPPE, if the Secretary determines in the future that such services are covered. For the physician/practitioner billing correct coding and payment policy, refer to Chapter 12, Section 30.6.1.1, of this manual.

Pub 100-4, 18, 80.1 – HCPCS Coding for the IPPE

(Rev. 1615, Issued: 10-17-08, Effective: 01-01-09, Implementation: 01-05-09)

The HCPCS codes listed below were developed for the IPPE benefit effective January 1, 2005, for individual's whose initial enrollment is on or after January 1, 2005.

G0344 Initial preventive physical examination; face-to-face visit, services limited to new beneficiary during the first 6 months of Medicare enrollment

Short Descriptor: Initial Preventive Exam

G0366 Electrocardiogram, routine ECG with 12 leads; performed as a component of the initial preventive examination with interpretation and report

Short Descriptor: EKG for initial prevent exam

G0367 tracing only, without interpretation and report, performed as a component of the initial preventive examination

Short Descriptor: EKG tracing for initial prev

G0368 interpretation and report only, performed as a component of the initial preventive examination

Short Descriptor: EKG interpret and report preve

The following new HCPCS codes have been developed for the IPPE benefit effective January 1, 2009, and replace codes G0344, G0366, G0367, and G0368 shown above beginning with dates of service on or after January 1, 2009:

G0402 Initial preventive physical examination; face-to-face visit, services limited to new beneficiary during the first 12 months of Medicare enrollment

Short Descriptor: Initial Preventive exam

G0403 Electrocardiogram, routine ECG with 12 leads; performed as a screening for the initial preventive physical examination with interpretation and report

Short Descriptor: EKG for initial prevent exam

G0404 Electrocardiogram, routine ECG with 12 leads; tracing only, without interpretation and report, performed as a screening for the initial preventive physical examination

Short Descriptor: EKG tracing for initial prev

G0405 Electrocardiogram, routine ECG with 12 leads; interpretation and report only, performed as a screening for the initial preventive physical examination

Short Descriptor: EKG interpret & report preve

Pub 100-4, 18, 80.2 – Carrier Billing Requirements

(Rev. 1615, Issued: 10-17-08, Effective: 01-01-09, Implementation: 01-05-09)

Effective for dates of service on and after January 1, 2005, through December 31, 2008, contractors shall recognize the HCPCS codes G0344, G0366, G0367, and G0368 shown above in §80.1 for an IPPE. The type of service (TOS) for each of the new codes is as follows:

G0344: TOS = 1
G0366: TOS = 5
G0367: TOS = 5
G0368: TOS = 5

Contractors shall pay physicians or qualified nonphysician practitioners for only one IPPE performed not later than 6 months after the date the individual's first coverage begins under Medicare Part B, but only if that coverage period begins on or after January 1, 2005.

Effective for dates of service on and after January 1, 2009, contractors shall recognize the HCPCS codes G0402, G0403, G0404, and G0405 shown above in § 80.1 for an IPPE. The type of service (TOS) for each of the new codes is as follows:

G0402: TOS = 1
G0403: TOS = 5
G0404: TOS = 5
G0405: TOS = 5

Under the MIPPA of 2008, contractors shall pay physicians or qualified nonphysician practitioners for only one IPPE performed not later than 12 months after the date the individual's first coverage begins under Medicare Part B.

Contractors shall allow payment for a medically necessary Evaluation and Management (E/M) service at the same visit as the IPPE when it is clinically appropriate. Physicians and qualified nonphysician practitioners shall use CPT codes 99201 - 99215 to report an E/M with CPT modifier 25 to indicate that the E/M is a significant, separately identifiable service from the IPPE code reported (G0344 or G0402, whichever applies based on the date the IPPE is performed). Refer to Chapter 12, § 30.6.1.1, of this manual for the physician/practitioner billing correct coding and payment policy regarding E/M services. If the EKG performed as a component of the IPPE is not performed by the primary physician or qualified NPP during the IPPE visit, another physician or entity may perform and/or interpret the EKG. The referring physician or qualified NPP needs to make sure that the performing physician or entity bills the appropriate G code for the screening EKG, and not a CPT code in the 93000 series. Both the IPPE and the EKG should be billed in order for the beneficiary to receive the complete IPPE service. Effective for dates of service on and after January 1, 2009, the screening EKG is optional and is no longer a mandated service of an IPPE if performed as a result of a referral from an IPPE.

Should the same physician or NPP need to perform an additional medically necessary EKG in the 93000 series on the same day as the IPPE, report the appropriate EKG CPT code(s) with modifier 59, indicating that the EKG is a distinct procedural service.

Physicians or qualified nonphysician practitioners shall bill the contractor the appropriate HCPCS codes for IPPE on the Form CMS-1500 claim or an approved electronic format. The HCPCS codes for an IPPE and screening EKG are paid under the Medicare Physician Fee Schedule (MPFS). The appropriate deductible and coinsurance applies to codes G0344, G0366, G0367, G0368, G0403, G0404, and G0405. The deductible is waived for code G0402 (insert new IPPE code), but the coinsurance still applies.

Pub 100-4, 18, 80.3 – Fiscal Intermediary Billing Requirements

(Rev. 1615, Issued: 10-17-08, Effective: 01-01-09, Implementation: 01-05-09)

The FI will pay for IPPE or EKG only when the services are submitted on one of the following type bills (TOB): 12X, 13X, 22X, 71X, 73X and 85X.

Type of facility and setting determines the basis of payment:

- For the IPPE or the screening EKG tracing only performed on a 12X and 13X, for hospitals subject to the outpatient prospective payment system (OPPS), under the OPPS. Hospitals not subject to OPPS shall be paid under current methodologies.
- For services performed on an 85X TOB, Critical Access Hospitals, pay on reasonable cost.
- For services performed in a SNF, TOB 22x, make payment for the technical component of the EKG based on the MPFS.
- For inpatient or outpatient services in hospitals in Maryland, make payment according to the State Cost Containment System.
- For services performed on a 12X, Indian Health Services (IHS) hospitals, payment is made based on an all inclusive ancillary per diem rate.
- For services performed on a 13X, IHS hospitals, payment is made based on the all inclusive rate (AIR).
- For services performed on an 85X, IHS CAHs, payment is made based on an all inclusive facility specific per visit rate.

All CAHs are paid for the technical or facility component of the IPPE itself. They are also paid for the technical component of the EKG, the tracing only, if the EKG is performed.

Only Method II CAHs are paid for the professional component of the IPPE itself (in addition to the facility payment) in rev code 0960. If the EKG is performed, Method II CAHs may also be paid for the interpretation of the EKG (in addition to the payment for the tracing) when billed in revenue codes 0985 or 0986.

Pub 100-4, 18, 80.3.1 – RHC/FQHCs Special Billing Instructions

(Rev. 1719, Issued: 04-24-09, Effective: 10-01-09, Implementation: 10-05-09)

There are Initial Preventive Physical Examination (IPPE) instructions that are unique to Rural Health Clinics (RHCs) and Federally Qualified Health Centers (FQHCs). Please refer to Publication 100-04, Chapter 9, section 150 of this manual for a description of these instructions.

Pub 100-4, 18, 80.3.2 – Indian Health Services (IHS) Hospitals Special Billing Instructions

(Rev. 1615, Issued: 10-17-08, Effective: 01-01-09, Implementation: 01-05-09)

For the period January 1, 2005 through December 31, 2008, the designated FI pays IHS hospitals when G0344 is submitted; this includes the IPPE whether or not the screening EKG is performed at the same time. The designated FI will also pay IHS hospitals for the screening EKG if HCPCS code G0367 is present. For the professional component of the EKG, the designated carrier shall pay the billing physician or other practitioner the established amount.

Effective January 1, 2009 the following new HCPCS codes have been developed for the IPPE benefit and replace the codes in the paragraph above: G0402 for the IPPE itself, and G0404 for the technical component (tracing only) of the EKG.

Pub 100-4, 18, 80.3.3 – OPPS Hospital Billing

(Rev. 1615, Issued: 10-17-08, Effective: 01-01-09, Implementation: 01-05-09)

Hospitals subject to OPPS (TOBs 12X and 13X) must use modifier 25 when billing the IPPE G0344 along with technical component of the EKG, G0367, on the same claim. The same is true when billing IPPE code G0402 along with the technical component of the screening EKG, code G0404. This is due to an Outpatient Prospective Payment System (OPPS) Outpatient Code Editor (OCE) which contains an edit that requires a modifier 25 on any evaluation and management (E/M) HCPCS code if there is also a status "S" or "T" HCPCS procedure code on the claim.

Pub 100-4, 18, 80.4 – Coinsurance and Deductible

(Rev. 1615, Issued: 10-17-08, Effective: 01-01-09, Implementation: 01-05-09)

The MMA did not make any provision for the waiver of the Medicare coinsurance and Part B deductible for the IPPE. Payment for this service would be applied to the required deductible if the deductible has not been met, with the exception of FQHCs, and the usual coinsurance provisions would apply to all providers.

The FQHC encounter is exempt from deductible. The contractors shall apply coinsurance and deductible to payments for the IPPE except for payments by the FI to FQHCs where only co-insurance applies.

Effective January 1, 2009, under the MIPPA of 2008, the deductible is waived for IPPE code G0402 only. The coinsurance is still applicable.

Pub 100-4, 18, 80.5 – Medicare Summary Notices (MSNs)

(Rev. 1615, Issued: 10-17-08, Effective: 01-01-09, Implementation: 01-05-09)

When denying additional claims for G0344, G0366, G0367 and G0368, contractors shall use MSN 18.22 - This service was denied because Medicare only covers the one-time initial preventive physical exam with an electrocardiogram within the first 6 months that you have Part B coverage, and only if that coverage begins on or after January 1, 2005.

The Spanish version is: 18.22 - Este servicio fue denegado porque Medicare solamente cubre un examen fisico preventivo con un electrocardiograma dentro de los primeros 6 meses que usted tenga cobertura de la Parte B, y sólo si esta cobertura comienza en o después del 1 de enero de 2005.

When denying additional claims for G0402 (or claims with dates of service beyond the 12 month period) contractors shall use MSN 20.91 - This service was denied. Medicare covers a one-time initial preventive physical exam (Welcome to Medicare physical exam) if you get it within the first 12 months of the effective date of your Medicare Part B coverage.

The Spanish version is: Este servicio fue negado. Medicare cubre un examen físico de "Bienvenido a Medicare" ofrecido una sola vez si se obtiene dentro de los primeros 12 meses de la fecha efectiva de su inscripción a la Parte B de Medicare.

When denying additional claims for screening EKG codes G0403, G0404 and G0405, contractors shall use MSN 20.12 - This service was denied because Medicare only covers this service once a lifetime.

The Spanish version is: Este servicio fue negado porque Medicare sólo cubre este servicio una vez en la vida.

Pub 100-4, 18, 80.6 – Remittance Advice Remark Codes

(Rev. 1615, Issued: 10-17-08, Effective: 01-01-09, Implementation: 01-05-09)

Contractors shall use the appropriate claim Remittance Advice Remark code, such as N117 (This service is paid only once in a patient's lifetime) when denying additional claims for an IPPE and/or a screening EKG.

Pub 100-4, 18, 80.7 – Claims Adjustment Reason Codes

(Rev. 1615, Issued: 10-17-08, Effective: 01-01-09, Implementation: 01-05-09)

Contractors shall use the appropriate Claim Adjustment Reason code, such as 149 (Lifetime benefit maximum has been reached for this service/benefit category) when denying additional claims for an IPPE and/or a screening EKG.

Pub 100-4, 18, 80.8 – Advanced Beneficiary Notice (ABN) as Applied to the IPPE

(Rev. 1615, Issued: 10-17-08, Effective: 01-01-09, Implementation: 01-05-09)

If a second IPPE is billed for the same beneficiary, it would be denied based on Section 1861(s)(2) of the Act, since the IPPE is a one-time benefit, and an ABN would not be required in order to hold the beneficiary liable for the cost of the second IPPE. However, an ABN should be issued for all IPPEs conducted after the beneficiary's statutory 6-month period has lapsed since based on Section 1862(a)(1)(K), Medicare is statutorily prohibited from paying for an IPPE outside the initial 6-month period under the MMA of 2003. Effective for dates of service on or after January 1, 2009, an ABN should be issued for all IPPEs conducted after the beneficiary's statutory 12-month period has lapsed since based on Section 1862(a)(1)(K), Medicare is statutorily prohibited from paying for an IPPE outside the initial 12-month period under the MIPPA of 2008.

Pub 100-4, 18, 100 – Cardiovascular Disease Screening

(Rev. 408, Issued: 12-17-04, Effective: 01-01-05, Implementation: 01-03-05)

Pub 100-4, 18, 100.1 – HCPCS Coding for Cardiovascular Disease Screening

(Rev. 408, Issued: 12-17-04, Effective: 01-01-05, Implementation: 01-03-05)

The following HCPCS codes are to be billed for Cardiovascular Disease Screening:

80061	Lipid Panel
82465	Cholesterol, serum or whole blood, total
83718	Lipoprotein, direct measurement, high density cholesterol
84478	Triglycerides

Pub 100-4, 18, 100.2 – Carrier Billing Requirements

(Rev. 408, Issued: 12-17-04, Effective: 01-01-05, Implementation: 01-03-05)

Effective for dates of service, January 1, 2005, and later, carriers shall recognize the above HCPCS codes for Cardiovascular Disease Screening.

Carriers shall pay for Cardiovascular Disease Screening once every 60 months.

A claim that is submitted for Cardiovascular Disease Screening shall be submitted in the following manner:

The line item shall contain 80061, 82465, 83718 or 84478 with a diagnosis code of V81.0 – Special screening for ischemic heart disease, V81.1 – Special screening for hypertension or V81.2 – Special screening for other and unspecified cardiovascular conditions reported in the header and pointed to the line item.

Pub 100-4, 18, 100.3 – Fiscal Intermediary (FI) Billing Requirements

(Rev. 408, Issued: 12-17-04, Effective: 01-01-05, Implementation: 01-03-05)

Effective for dates of service, January 1, 2005, and later, intermediaries shall recognize the above HCPCS codes for Cardiovascular Disease Screening.

FIs shall pay for Cardiovascular Disease Screening once every 60 months.

A claim that is submitted for Cardiovascular Disease Screening shall be submitted in the following manner:

The line item shall contain 80061, 82465, 83718 or 84478 with a diagnosis code of V81.0 – Special screening for ischemic heart disease, V81.1 – Special screening for hypertension or V81.2 – Special screening for other and unspecified cardiovascular conditions reported in the header and pointed to the line item.

Pub 100-4, 18, 100.4 – Diagnosis Code Reporting

(Rev. 408, Issued: 12-17-04, Effective: 01-01-05, Implementation: 01-03-05)

A claim that is submitted for Cardiovascular Disease Screening shall be submitted with one or more of the following diagnosis codes in the header and pointed to the line item:

V81.0	Special screening for ischemic heart disease,
V81.1	Special screening for hypertension, or
V81.2	Special screening for other and unspecified cardiovascular conditions

Pub 100-4, 18, 100.5 – Medicare Summary Notice

(Rev. 408, Issued: 12-17-04, Effective: 01-01-05, Implementation: 01-03-05)

When denying claims for cardiovascular screening based upon a CWF reject for 80061, 82465, 83718, or 84478 billed with one or more the following diagnosis codes V81.0, V81.1 and V81.2, contractors shall use MSN 16.54 Medicare does not pay for this many services or supplies.

Pub 100-4, 18, 100.6 – Remittance Advice Remark Codes

(Rev. 408, Issued: 12-17-04, Effective: 01-01-05, Implementation: 01-03-05)

Contractors shall use the appropriate remittance advice notice that appropriately explains the denial of payment.

Pub 100-4, 18, 100.7 – Claim Adjustment Reason Code

(Rev. 408, Issued: 12-17-04, Effective: 01-01-05, Implementation: 01-03-05)

Contractors shall use claims adjustment reason code 119 "Benefit maximum for this time period has been reached."

Pub 100-4, 18, 110 – Ultrasound Screening for Abdominal Aortic Aneurysm (AAA)

(Rev. 1113, Issued: 11-17-06, Effective: 01-01-07, Implementation: 01-02-07)

Section 5112 of the Deficit Reduction Act of 2005 amended the Social Security Act to provide coverage under Part B of the Medicare program for a one-time ultrasound screening for abdominal aortic aneurysms (AAA).

Pub 100-4, 18, 110.1 – Definitions

(Rev. 1113, Issued: 11-17-06, Effective: 01-01-07, Implementation: 01-02-07)

The term `ultrasound screening for abdominal aortic aneurysm' means—

(1) a procedure using sound waves (or such other procedures using alternative technologies, of commensurate accuracy and cost, as specified by the Secretary of Health and Human Services, through the national coverage determination process) provided for the early detection of abdominal aortic aneurysms; and

(2) includes a physician's interpretation of the results of the procedure.

Pub 100-4, 18, 110.2 – Coverage

(Rev. 1113, Issued: 11-17-06, Effective: 01-01-07, Implementation: 01-02-07)

Effective for services furnished on or after January 1, 2007, payment may be made for a one-time ultrasound screening for AAA for beneficiaries who meet the following criteria:

(i) receives a referral for such an ultrasound screening as a result of an initial preventive physical examination (as defined in section 1861(ww)(1));

(ii) receives such ultrasound screening from a provider or supplier who is authorized to provide covered diagnostic services;

(iii) has not been previously furnished such an ultrasound screening under the Medicare Program; and

(vi) is included in at least one of the following risk categories:

- (I) has a family history of abdominal aortic aneurysm; or
- (II) is a man age 65 to 75 who has smoked at least 100 cigarettes in his lifetime
- (III)is a beneficiary who manifests other risk factors in a beneficiary category recommended for screening by the United States Preventive Services Task Force regarding AAA, as specified by the Secretary of Health and Human Services, through the national coverage determination process.

Medicare References

Pub 100-4, 18, 110.3 – Payment

(Rev. 1113, Issued: 11-17-06, Effective: 01-01-07, Implementation: 01-02-07)

If the screening is provided in a physician office, the service is billed to the carrier using the HCPCS code identified in section 110.3.2 below. Payment is under the Medicare Physicians Fee Schedule (MPFS).

Fiscal Intermediaries (FIs) shall pay for the AAA screening only when the services are performed in a hospital, including a critical access hospital (CAH), Indian Health Service (IHS) Facility, Skilled Nursing Facility (SNF), Rural Health Clinic (RHC), or Federally Qualified Health Center (FQHC) and submitted on one of the following types of bills (TOBs): 12X, 13X, 22X, 23X, 71X, 73X, 85X.

The following describes the payment methodology for AAA Screening:

Facility	Type of Bill	Payment
Hospitals subject to OPPS	12X, 13X	OPPS
Method I and Method II Critical Access Hospitals (CAHs)	12X and 85X	101% of reasonable cost
IHS providers	13X, revenue code 051X	OMB-approved outpatient per visit all inclusive rate (AIR)
IHS providers	12X, revenue code 024X	All-inclusive inpatient ancillary per diem rate
IHS CAHs	85X, revenue code 051X	101% of the all-inclusive facility specific per visit rate
IHS CAHs	12X, revenue code 024X	101% of the all-inclusive facility specific per diem rate
SNFs **	22X, 23X	Non-facility rate on the MPFS
RHCs*	71X, revenue code 052X	All-inclusive encounter rate
FQHCs*	73X, revenue code 052X	All-inclusive encounter rate
Maryland Hospitals under jurisdiction of the Health Services Cost Review Commission (HSCRC)	12X, 13X	94% of provider submitted charges or according to the terms of the Maryland Waiver

**If the screening is provided in an RHC or FQHC, the professional portion of the service is billed to the FI using TOBs 71X and 73X, respectively, and the appropriate site of service revenue code in the 052X revenue code series.*

If the screening is provided in an independent RHC or freestanding FQHC, the technical component of the service can be billed by the practitioner to the carrier under the practitioner's ID following instructions for submitting practitioner claims to the Medicare carrier.

If the screening is provided in a provider-based RHC/FQHC, the technical component of the service can be billed by the base provider to the FI under the base provider's ID, following instructions for submitting claims to the FI from the base provider.

***The SNF consolidated billing provision allows separate part B payment for screening services for beneficiaries that are in skilled Part A SNF stays, however, the SNF must submit these services on a 22X bill type. Screening services provided by other provider types must be reimbursed by the SNF.*

Pub 100-4, 18, 110.3.1 – Deductible and Coinsurance

(Rev. 1113, Issued: 11-17-06, Effective: 01-01-07, Implementation: 01-02-07)

The Part B deductible for screening AAA is waived effective January 1, 2007. Coinsurance is applicable.

Pub 100-4, 18, 110.3.2 – HCPCS Code

(Rev. 1113, Issued: 11-17-06, Effective: 01-01-07, Implementation: 01-02-07)

Effective for services furnished on or after January 1, 2007, the following code, modifiers, and type of service (TOS) are used for AAA screening services:

G0389 Ultrasound, B-scan and or real time with image documentation; for abdominal aortic aneurysm (AAA) screening

Short Descriptor: Ultrasound exam AAA screen

Modifiers: TC, 26

TOS: 4

Pub 100-4, 18, 110.3.3 – Advance Beneficiary Notice

(Rev. 1113, Issued: 11-17-06, Effective: 01-01-07, Implementation: 01-02-07)

Medicare contractors will deny an AAA screening service billed more than once in a beneficiary's lifetime.

If a second G0389 is billed for AAA for the same beneficiary or if any of the other statutory criteria for coverage listed in section 1861(s)(2)(AA) of the Social Security Act are not met, the service would be denied as a statutory (technical) denial under section 1861(s)(2)(AA), not a medical necessity denial.

If a provider cannot determine whether or not the beneficiary has previously had an AAA screening, but all of the other statutory requirements for coverage have been met, the provider should issue the ABN-G. Likewise, if all of the statutory requirements for coverage have been met, but a question of medical necessity still exists, the provider should issue the ABN-G.

Pub 100-4, 18, 120 – Diabetes Self-Management Training (DSMT) Services

(Rev. 1255, Issued: 05-25-07; Effective: 07-01-07; Implementation: 07-02-07)

See Pub. 100-02, **Medicare Benefit Policy Manual**, Chapter 15, Covered Medical and Other Health Services, section 300 for information on coverage requirements, certified providers and enrollment.

Pub 100-4, 18, 120.1 – Coding and Payment of DSMT Services

(Rev. 1255, Issued: 05-25-07; Effective: 07-01-07; Implementation: 07-02-07)

The following HCPCS codes are used to report DSMT:

G0108 Diabetes outpatient self-management training services, individual, per 30 minutes.

G0109 Diabetes outpatient self-management training services, group session (2 or more), per 30 minutes.

The type of service for these codes is 1.

Payment to physicians and providers for outpatient DSMT is made as follows:

Type of Facility	Payment Method	Type of Bill
Physician (billed to the carrier)	MPFS	NA
Hospitals subject to OPPS	MPFS	12X, 13X
Method I and Method II Critical Access Hospitals (CAHs) (technical services)	101% of reasonable cost	12X and 85X
Indian Health Service (IHS) providers billing hospital outpatient Part B	OMB-approved outpatient per visit all inclusive rate (AIR)	13X
IHS providers billing inpatient Part B	All-inclusive inpatient ancillary per diem rate	12X
IHS CAHs billing outpatient Part B	101% of the all-inclusive facility specific per visit rate	85X
IHS CAHs billing inpatient Part B	101% of the all-inclusive facility specific per diem rate	12X
FQHCs*	All-inclusive encounter rate with other qualified services. Separate visit payment available with HCPCS.	73X
Skilled Nursing Facilities **	MPFS non-facility rate	22X, 23X
Maryland Hospitals under jurisdiction of the Health Services Cost Review Commission (HSCRC)	94% of provider submitted charges in accordance with the terms of the Maryland Waiver	12X, 13X
Home Health Agencies (can be billed only if the service is provided outside of the treatment plan)	MPFS non-facility rate	34X

**Effective January 1, 2006, payment for DSMT provided in an FQHC that meets all of the requirements as above, may be made in addition to one other visit the beneficiary had during the same day, if this qualifying visit is billed on TOB*

Medicare References

73X, with HCPCS G0108 or G0109, and revenue codes 0520, 0521, 0522, 0524, 0525, 0527, 0528, or 0900.

***The SNF consolidated billing provision allows separate part B payment for training services for beneficiaries that are in skilled Part A SNF stays, however, the SNF must submit these services on a 22 bill type. Training services provided by other provider types must be reimbursed by X the SNF.*

NOTE: An ESRD facility is a reasonable site for this service, however, because it is required to provide dietician and nutritional services as part of the care covered in the composite rate, ESRD facilities are not allowed to bill for it separately and do not receive separate reimbursement. Likewise, an RHC is a reasonable site for this service, however it must be provided in an RHC with other qualifying services and paid at the all-inclusive encounter rate. Deductible and co-insurance apply.

Pub 100-4, 18, 120.2 – Bill Processing Requirements

(Rev. 1255, Issued: 05-25-07; Effective: 07-01-07; Implementation: 07-02-07)

See Pub. 100-04, chapter 25 for instructions for intermediaries.

See Pub. 100-04, chapter 26 for instructions for carriers.

Billing is to the "certified provider's" regular intermediary or carrier, i.e., there are no specialty contractors for this service. (See Pub 100-02, chapter 15, section 300.2 for the definition of "certified provider" in this instance.)

Pub 100-4, 18, 120.2.1 – Special Processing Instructions for Billing Frequency Requirements

(Rev. 1255, Issued: 05-25-07; Effective: 07-01-07; Implementation: 07-02-07)

The frequency editing for DSMT is performed in CWF as follows:

A Initial Training

The initial year for DSMT is the '12' month period following the initial date. When a claim contains a DSMT HCPCS code and the associated units cause the total time for the DSMT initial year to exceed '10' hours, a CWF error will set.

See Pub. 100-02, **Medicare Benefit Policy Manual**, Chapter 15, Covered Medical and Other Health Services, section 300 for information on coverage for initial training.

B Follow-Up Training

Follow-up training for subsequent years are based on a 12 month calendar year after the initial year. However, if the beneficiary exhausts 10 hours in the initial year then the beneficiary would be eligible for follow-up training in the next calendar year. When a claim contains a DSMT HCPCS code and the associated units cause the total time for any follow-up year to exceed 2 hours, a CWF error will set.

See Pub. 100-02, **Medicare Benefit Policy Manual**, Chapter 15, Covered Medical and Other Health Services, section 300 for information on coverage for follow-up training.

C Examples

Example 1 — Beneficiary Exhausts 10 hours in the Initial Year (12 continuous months)

Bene receives first service: April, 2006
Bene completes initial 10 hours DSMT training: April, 2007
Bene is eligible for follow-up training: May 2007 (13th month begins the subsequent year)
Bene completes follow-up training: December, 2007
Bene is eligible for next year follow-up training: January, 2008

Example 2 —Beneficiary Exhausts 10 hours Within the Initial Calendar Year

Bene receives first service: April 2006
Bene completes initial 10 hours of DSMT training, December 2006
Bene is eligible for follow-up training: January, 2007
Bene completes follow-up training: July 2007
Bene is eligible for next year follow-up training: January 2008

Pub 100-4, 18, 120.2.2 – Advance Beneficiary Notice (ABN) Requirements

(Rev. 1255, Issued: 05-25-07; Effective: 07-01-07; Implementation: 07-02-07)

The beneficiary is liable for services denied over the limited number of hours with referrals for DSMT. An ABN should be issued in these situations. In absence of evidence of a valid ABN, the provider will be held liable.

An ABN should not be issued for Medicare-covered services such as those provided by hospital dietitians or nutrition professionals who are qualified to render the service in their State but who have not obtained Medicare Provider Numbers.

Pub 100-4, 20, 10 – Where to Bill DMEPOS and PEN Items and Services

(Rev. 1603, Issued: 09-26-08, Effective: 10-27-08, Implementation: 10-27-08)

Skilled Nursing Facilities, CORFs, OPTs, and hospitals bill the FI for prosthetic/orthotic devices, supplies, and covered outpatient DME and oxygen (refer to §40). The HHAs may bill Durable Medical Equipment (DME) to the RHHI, or may meet the requirements of a DME supplier and bill the DME MAC. This is the HHA's decision. Fiscal Intermediaries (FIs) other than RHHIs will receive claims only for the class "Prosthetic and Orthotic Devices."

Unless billing to the FI is required as outlined in the preceding paragraph, claims for implanted DME, implanted prosthetic devices, replacement parts, accessories and supplies for the implanted DME must be billed to the local carriers/MACs and not the DME MAC. The Healthcare Common Procedure Coding System (HCPCS) codes that describe these categories of service are updated annually in late spring. All other DMEPOS items are billed to the DME MAC. See the Medicare Claims Processing Manual, Chapter 23, §20.3 for additional information.

Parenteral and enteral nutrition, and related accessories and supplies, are covered under the Medicare program as a prosthetic device. See the Medicare Benefit Policy Manual, Chapter 15, for a description of the policy. All Parenteral and Enteral (PEN) services furnished under Part B are billed to the DME MAC. If a provider (see §01) provides PEN items under Part B it must qualify for and receive a supplier number and bill as a supplier. Note that some PEN items furnished to hospital and SNF inpatients are included in the Part A PPS rate and are not separately billable. (If a service is paid under Part A it may not also be paid under Part B.)

Pub 100-4, 20, 10.1 – Definitions

(Rev. 1, 10-01-03)

A3-3313.1, B3-2100.1, HHA-220.1, HO-235.1, SNF-264.1

Pub 100-4, 20, 10.1.1 – Durable Medical Equipment (DME)

(Rev. 1, 10-01-03)

DME is covered under Part B as a medical or other health service (§1861(s)(6) of the Social Security Act [the Act]) and is equipment that:

a. Can withstand repeated use;
b. Is primarily and customarily used to serve a medical purpose;
c. Generally is not useful to a person in the absence of an illness or injury; and
d. Is appropriate for use in the home.

All requirements of the definition must be met before an item can be considered to be durable medical equipment.

A SNF normally is not considered a beneficiary's home. However, a SNF can be considered a beneficiary's home for Method II home dialysis purposes. See the Program Integrity Manual, Chapter 5, for guidelines on when a SNF may be considered a home. For detailed coverage requirements (including definitions and discussion) associated with the following DME terms and circumstances see the **Medicare Benefit Policy Manual**, Chapter 15:

- Durability
- Medical Equipment
- Equipment Presumptively Medical
- Equipment Presumptively Nonmedical

- Special Exception Items
- Necessary and Reasonable
- Necessity for the Equipment
- Reasonableness of the Equipment
- Payment Consistent With What is Necessary and Reasonable
- Beneficiary's Home
- Establishing the Period of Medical Necessity
- Repairs, Maintenance, Replacement and Delivery
- Leased Renal Dialysis Equipment
- Coverage of Supplies and Accessories
- Beneficiary Disposal of Equipment
- New Supplier Effective Billing Date
- Incurred Expense Date
- Partial Months-Monthly Payment
- Purchased Equipment Delivered Outside the U.S.

For coverage information on specific situations and items of DME, see the **Medicare National Coverage Determinations Manual**.

Pub 100-4, 20, 10.1.2 – Prosthetic Devices – Coverage Definition

(Rev. 1, 10-01-03)

Prosthetic devices (other than dental) are covered under Part B as a medical or other health service (§1861(s)(8) of the Act) and are devices that replace all or part of an internal body organ or replace all or part of the function of a permanently inoperative or malfunctioning internal body organ. Replacements or repairs of such devices are covered when furnished incident to physicians' services or on a physician's orders. For detailed coverage requirements (including definitions and discussion) associated with the following prosthetic device terms and circumstances see the **Medicare Benefit Policy Manual**, Chapter 15:

- Test of Permanence
- Prosthetic Lenses
- Intraocular Lenses (IOLs)
- Supplies, Adjustments, Repairs and Replacements

For coverage information on specific situations and prosthetic devices, see the **Medicare National Coverage Determinations Manual**.

Pub 100-4, 20, 10.1.3 – Prosthetics and Orthotics (Leg, Arm, Back, and Neck Braces, Trusses, and Artificial Legs, Arms, and Eyes) – Coverage Definition

(Rev. 1, 10-01-03)

These appliances are covered under Part B as a medical or other health service (§1861(s)(9) of the Act) when furnished incident to physicians' services or on a physician's order. A brace includes rigid and semi-rigid devices that are used for the purpose of supporting a weak or deformed body member or restricting or eliminating motion in a diseased or injured part of the body.

For detailed coverage requirements (including definitions and discussion) associated with the following terms and circumstances see the **Medicare Benefit Policy Manual**, Chapter 15:

Leg, Arm, Back, and Neck Braces, Trusses, and Artificial Legs, Arms, and Eyes

Adjustments and Replacement of Artificial Limbs

For coverage information on specific situations, braces, trusses, and artificial limbs and eyes, see the **Medicare National Coverage Determinations Manual**.

Pub 100-4, 20, 10.1.4 – Payment Definition Variances

(Rev. 1, 10-01-03)

Pub 100-4, 20, 10.1.4.1 – Prosthetic Devices

(Rev. 1, 10-01-03)

Section 1834(h)(1)(G) of the Act, "Replacement of Prosthetic Devices and Parts," refers to prosthetic devices that are artificial limbs. Section 1861(s) of the Act, which defines "medical and other health services," does not define artificial limbs as "prosthetic devices" (§1861(s)(8)). Rather, artificial limbs are included in the §1861(s)(9) category, "orthotics and prosthetics." When discussing replacement, these instructions will use the term "prosthetic device" as intended by §1834(h)(1)(G), i.e., artificial limbs.

Pub 100-4, 20, 10.1.4.2 – Prosthetic and Orthotic Devices (P&O)

(Rev. 1, 10-01-03)

Except as specifically noted (e.g., IOLs), when discussing payment and other policies, instructions in this chapter will use the terms "prosthetic and orthotic devices" and the abbreviation "P&O" interchangeably to refer to both §1861(s)(8) and (9) services.

Pub 100-4, 20, 10.2 – Coverage Table for DME Claims

(Rev. 1, 10-01-03)

B3-2105

Reimbursement may be made for expenses incurred by a patient for the rental or purchase of durable medical equipment (DME) for use in his/her home provided that all the conditions in column A below have been met. Column B indicates the action contractors will take to establish that the conditions have been met.

A – Conditions	B – Review Action
I. Payment may be made for the following:	1. Payment may be made for the following:
(a) Items of DME that are medically necessary	(a) The HCPCS file shows coverage status of items. If item is not listed in the HCPCS file, the contractor will develop LMRP to determine whether the item is covered.
(b) Separate charges for repair, maintenance and delivery	(b) Repairs – only if DME is being purchased or is already owned by patient and repair is necessary to make the equipment serviceable. Medicare pays the least expensive alternative. (See special exception in Chapter 15 of the *Medicare Benefit Policy Manual* for repair of dialysis delivery system.) NOTE: See Chapter 15 of the Medicare Benefit Policy Manual for handling claims suggesting deliberate or malicious damage or destruction. Maintenance – only if the equipment is being purchased, or is already owned by the patient, and if the maintenance is extensive amounting to repairs, i.e., requiring the services of skilled technicians. (Contractors deny claims for routine maintenance and periodic servicing, e.g., testing, cleaning, checking, oiling, etc.) (See special exception in Chapter 15 of the Medicare Benefit Policy Manual for maintenance of dialysis delivery system.) Delivery – of rented or purchased equipment is covered, but the related payment is included in the fee schedule for the item. Additional payment may be made at the discretion of the contractor in special circumstances (see Chapter 15 of the *Medicare Benefit Policy Manual*)
(c) Separate charges for disposable supplies, e.g., oxygen, if essential to the effective use of medically necessary durable medical equipment. Separate charges for replacement of essential accessories such as hoses, tubes, mouthpieces, etc., only if the beneficiary owns or is purchasing durable medical equipment (BPM, Chapter 15, §110). (Medications used in connection with durable medical equipment are covered under certain conditions – see Chapter 15 of the Medicare Benefit Policy Manual)	(c) Claim must indicate that: •The patient has the DME for which the supply is intended; •The DME continues to be medically necessary; and •The items are readily identifiable as the type customarily used with such equipment. NOTE: If the quantity of accessories and/or supplies included in a claim seems excessive or if claims for such items are received from the same claimant with undue frequency, see Chapter 5 of the *Medicare Program Integrity Manual*.

Medicare References

A – Conditions	B – Review Action
2. DME must be for use in patient's residence other than a health care institution. (BPM §110.3 & PIM, Chapter 5, §1)	2. Payment cannot be made for equipment for use in an institution classified as: a. A participating hospital b. An emergency hospital c. Meets §1861(e)(1) of the Act d. A participating SNF or e. Meets §1819(a)(1) of the Act. Except for a distinct part of a SNF, if one of these institutions has a distinct part that does not meet 1819(a)(1), the patient may be considered in his/her residence if he/she was physically located in such distinct part during the use period. DMEPOS (DME, P&O, and supplies) items provided to hospice patients are generally included in the payment for hospice services. Items of DMEPOS are covered by Medicare and paid in addition to the hospice payment only when those items or supplies are provided to the patient for treatment of a condition or illness not related to the patient's terminal illness.
3. Physician's prescription required.	A supplier must maintain and, upon request, make available to the contractor, the detailed written order (or, when required, the Certificate of Medical Necessity (CMN)) from the treating physician. See the *Medicare Program Integrity Manual*, Chapter 5.

Pub 100-4, 20, 40 – Payment for Maintenance and Service for Non-ESRD Equipment

(Rev. 1, 10-01-03)

Pub 100-4, 20, 40.1 – General

(Rev. 1, 10-01-03)

B3-5102.2.G, B3-5102.3

Contractors pay for maintenance and servicing of purchased equipment in the following classes:

- inexpensive or frequently purchased,
- customized items, other prosthetic and orthotic devices, and
- capped rental items purchased in accordance with §30.5.2 or §30.5.3.

They do not pay for maintenance and servicing of purchased items that require frequent and substantial servicing, or oxygen equipment. (Maintenance and servicing may be paid for purchased items in these two classes if they were purchased prior to June 1, 1989). Reasonable and necessary charges include only those made for parts and labor that are not otherwise covered under a manufacturer's or supplier's warranty. Contractors pay on a lump-sum, as needed basis based on their individual consideration for each item. Payment may not be made for maintenance and servicing of rented equipment other than maintenance and servicing for PEN pumps (under the conditions of §40.3) or the maintenance and servicing fee established for capped rental items in §40.2.

Servicing of equipment that a beneficiary is purchasing or already owns is covered when necessary to make the equipment serviceable. The service charge may include the use of "loaner" equipment where this is required. If the expense for servicing exceeds the estimated expense of purchasing or renting another item of equipment for the remaining period of medical need, no payment can be made for the amount of the excess.

Contractors investigate and deny cases suggesting malicious damage, culpable neglect or wrongful disposition of equipment as discussed in BPM Chapter 15 where they determine that it is unreasonable to make program payment under the circumstances. Such cases are referred to the program integrity specialist in the RO.

Pub 100-4, 20, 100 – General Documentation Requirements

(Rev. 1, 10-01-03)

B3-4107.1, B3-4107.8, HHA-463, Medicare Handbook for New Suppliers: Getting

Started, B-02-31

Benefit policies are set forth in the **Medicare Benefit Policy Manual**, Chapter 15, §§110- 130.

Program integrity policies for DMEPOS are set forth in the **Medicare Program Integrity Manual**, Chapter 5.

See Chapter 21 for applicable MSN messages.

See Chapter 22 for Remittance Advice coding.

Pub 100-4, 20, 100.1 – Written Order Prior to Delivery

(Rev. 1, 10-01-03)

See the **Medicare Program Integrity Manual**, Chapter 5, for requirements for written orders for suppliers, including providers billing the DMERC or carrier as suppliers. See §01 for definitions of provider and supplier.

Pub 100-4, 20, 100.1.1 – Written Order Prior to Delivery – HHAs

(Rev. 1, 10-01-03)

See the **Medicare Program Integrity Manual**, Chapter 6. These instructions apply to bill types 32x, 33x and 34x.

Pub 100-4, 20, 100.2 – Certificates of Medical Necessity (CMN)

(Rev. 1, 10-01-03)

B3-3312

For certain items or services billed to the DME Regional Carrier (DMERC), the supplier must receive a signed Certificate of Medical Necessity (CMN) from the treating physician. CMNs are not required for the same items when billed by HHAs to RHHIs. Instead, the items must be included in the physician's signed orders on the home health plan of care. See the **Medicare Program Integrity Manual**, Chapter 6.

The FI will inform other providers (see §01 for definition pf provider) of documentation requirements.

Contractors may ask for supporting documentation beyond a CMN.

Refer to the local DMERC Web site described in §10 for downloadable copies of CMN forms.

See the **Medicare Program Integrity Manual**, Chapter 5, for specific Medicare policies and instructions on the following topics:

- Requirements for supplier retention of original CMNs
- CMN formats, paper and electronic
- List of currently approved CMNs and items requiring CMNs
- Supplier requirements for submitting CMNs
- Requirements for CMNs to also serve as a physician's order
- Civil monetary penalties for violation of CMN requirements
- Supplier requirements for completing portions of CMNs
- Physician requirements for completing portions of CMNs

Pub 100-4, 20, 100.2.1 – Completion of Certificate of Medical Necessity Forms

(Rev. 1, 10-01-03)

1. SECTION A: (This may be completed by supplier.)
   a. Certification Type/Date – If this is an initial certification for this patient, the date (MM/DD/YY) is indicated in the space marked "INITIAL". If this is a revised certification (to be completed when the physician changes the order, based on the patient's changing clinical needs), the initial date is indicated in the space marked "INITIAL", and the revision date is indicated in the space marked "REVISED". If this is a recertification, the initial date is indicated in the space marked "INITIAL", and the recertification date is indicated in the space marked "RECERTIFICATION". Whether a REVISED or RECERTIFIED CMN is submitted, the INITIAL date as well as the REVISED or RECERTIFICATION date is always furnished.
   b. Patient Information – This indicates the patient's name, permanent legal address, telephone number, and his/her health insurance claim number (HICN) as it appears on his/her Medicare card and on the claim form.
   c. Supplier Information – This indicates the name of the company (supplier name), address, telephone number, and the Medicare

Medicare References

supplier number assigned by the National Supplier Clearinghouse (NSC).

d. Place of Service – This indicates the place in which the item is being used, i.e., patient's home is 12, skilled nursing facility (SNF) is 31, or end stage renal disease (ESRD) facility is 65. See chapter 23 for place of service codes.

e. Facility Name – This indicates the name and complete address of the facility, if the place of service is a facility.

f. HCPCS Codes – This is a list of all HCPCS procedure codes for items ordered that require a CMN. Procedure codes that do not require certification are not listed on the CMN.

g. Patient Date of Birth (DOB), Height, Weight, and Sex – This indicates patient's DOB (MM/DD/YY), height in inches, weight in pounds, and sex (male or female).

h. Physician Name and Address – This indicates the treating physician's name and complete mailing address.

i. UPIN – This indicates the treating physician's unique physician identification number (UPIN).

j. Physician's Telephone Number – This indicates the telephone number where the treating physician can be contacted (preferably where records would be accessible pertaining to this patient) if additional information is needed.

2. SECTION B: (This may not be completed by the supplier. While this section may be completed by a non-physician clinician, or a physician employee, it must be reviewed by the treating physician. Contractors publish this requirement about section B in their bulletins at least annually.)

   a. Estimated Length of Need – This indicates the estimated length of need (the length of time (in months) the physician expects the patient to require use of the ordered item). If the treating physician expects that the patient will require the item for the duration of his/her life, 99 is entered. For recertification and revision CMNs, the cumulative length of need (the total length of time in months from the initial date of need) is entered.

   b. Diagnosis Codes – Listed in the first space is the ICD-9 code that represents the primary reason for ordering this item. Additional ICD-9 codes that would further describe the medical need for the item (up to 3 codes) are also listed. A given CMN may have more than one item billed, and for each item, the primary reason for ordering may be different. For example, a CMN is submitted for a manual wheelchair (K0001) and elevating leg rests (K0195). The primary reason for K0001 is stroke, and the primary reason for K0195 is edema.

   c. Question Section – This section is used to gather clinical information regarding the patient's condition, the need for the DME, and supplies.

   d. Name of Person Answering Section B Questions – If a clinical professional other than the treating physician (e.g., home health nurse, physical therapist, dietician, or a physician employee) answers the questions in section B, he/she must print his/her name, give his/her professional title, and the name of his/her employer, where indicated. If the treating physician answered the questions, this space may be left blank.

3. SECTION C: (This is completed by the supplier.)

   a. Narrative Description of Equipment and Cost – The supplier indicates (1) a narrative description of the item(s) ordered, as well as all options, accessories, supplies, and drugs; (2) the supplier's charge for each item, option, accessory, supply, and drug; and (3) the Medicare fee schedule allowance for each item, option, accessory, supply, or drug, if applicable.

4. SECTION D: (This is completed by the treating physician.)

   a. Physician Attestation – The treating physician's signature certifies the CMN that he/she is reviewing includes sections A, B, C, and D, the answers in section B are correct, and the self-identifying information in section A is correct.

   b. Physician Signature and Date – After completion and/or review by the treating physician of sections A, B, and C, the treating physician must sign and date the CMN in section D, verifying the attestation appearing in this section. The treating physician's signature also certifies the items ordered are medically necessary for this patient. Signature and date stamps are not acceptable. Certifications and recertifications may not be altered by "whiting out" or "pasting over" and entering new data. Such claims are denied and suppliers that show a pattern of altering CMNs are identified for educational contact and/or audit. Also suppliers who have questionable utilization or billing practices or who are under sanction are considered for audit.

Pub 100-4, 20, 100.2.2 – Evidence of Medical Necessity for Parenteral and Enteral Nutrition (PEN) Therapy

(Rev. 1, 10-01-03)

B3-3324, B3-4450

The PEN coverage is determined by information provided by the treating physician and the PEN supplier. A completed certification of medical necessity (CMN) must accompany and support initial claims for PEN to establish whether coverage criteria are met and to ensure that the PEN therapy provided is consistent with the attending or ordering physician's prescription. Contractors ensure that the CMN contains pertinent information from the treating physician. Uniform specific medical data facilitate the review and promote consistency in coverage determinations and timelier claims processing.

The medical and prescription information on a PEN CMN can be most appropriately completed by the treating physician or from information in the patient's records by an employee of the physician for the physician's review and signature. Although PEN suppliers sometimes may assist in providing the PEN services, they cannot complete the CMN since they do not have the same access to patient information needed to properly enter medical or prescription information. Contractors use appropriate professional relations issuances, training sessions, and meetings to ensure that all persons and PEN suppliers are aware of this limitation of their role.

When properly completed, the PEN CMN includes the elements of a prescription as well as other data needed to determine whether Medicare coverage is possible. This practice will facilitate prompt delivery of PEN services and timely submittal of the related claim.

Pub 100-4, 20, 100.2.2.1 – Scheduling and Documenting Certifications and Recertifications of Medical Necessity for PEN

(Rev. 1, 10-01-03)

A certification for PEN therapy must accompany the initial claim submitted. The initial certification is valid for six months. Contractors establish the schedule on a case-by-case basis for recertifying the need for PEN therapy. A change in prescription for a beneficiary past the initial certification period does not restart the certification process. A period of medical necessity ends when PEN services are not medically required for 2 consecutive months. The entire certification process, if required, begins after 2 consecutive months have elapsed.

A revised certification or a change in prescription may impact on the payment levels of PEN services. A revised certification is appropriate when there is a change:

- In the treating physician's orders in the category of nutrients and/or calories prescribed;
- By more than one liter in the daily volume of parenteral solutions;
- From home-mix to pre-mix or pre-mix to home-mix parenteral solutions;
- From enteral to parenteral or parenteral to enteral therapy; or
- In the method of infusion (e.g., from gravity-fed to pump-fed).

Pub 100-4, 20, 100.2.2.2 – Completion of the Elements of PEN CMN

(Rev. 1, 10-01-03)

The patient's name, address, and HICN and the nature of the certification (i.e., initial, renewed, or revised) must be entered on all certifications by the supplier, physician, or physician's designated employees. The supplier identifying information is required on all PEN certifications.

All medical and prescription information must be completed from the patient's records by the attending/ordering physician, or an employee of the physician authorized to act on the physician's behalf, and reviewed and signed by the physician.

1. Place of Service – The CMN must identify the site where the patient is receiving PEN services. A patient may receive services at home, in a nursing home setting (e.g., skilled nursing facility), or another site that must be indicated by the supplier/physician.
2. Patient's General Condition – The attending physician must complete information about the patient's age, height, and weight. The general condition of the patient also includes an estimated duration of therapy (i.e., in months, years, or for life), the ambulatory status, and whether the patient is conscious. The physician should also indicate food allergies/sensitivities, other medical treatments, therapies, and/or medical conditions that may affect the patient's nutritional needs.
3. Patient's Clinical Assessment – The attending physician must indicate all the diagnoses related to the PEN therapy and describe the patient's functional impairment of the digestive tract that precludes the enteral patient from swallowing and the parenteral patient from absorbing nutrients. The physician must certify that PEN therapy meets the requirement that a patient is not able to maintain weight and strength due to pathology or nonfunction of the ingestion system and that the enteral therapy serves as the source of nutrition for the patient who has a functioning digestive tract, but whose disability prevents ingestion of sufficient nutrients to the alimentary tract for metabolism. Nutritional supplements for patients capable of ingesting normally, even if required to maintain weight and strength, cannot be covered under the prosthetic device benefit. The physician must have a basis for certifying or recertifying the need for PEN services. The physician is expected to see the patient within 30 days prior to certifying or recertifying PEN services. However, if the physician did not see the patient, he/she must explain why and describe what other monitoring methods were used to evaluate the patient's PEN needs.
4. Patient's Nutritional Prescription – Subsequent to an examination of the patient and/or a review of the patient's medical information, the attending physician must complete the patient's nutritional requirements (prescription) to certify the PEN therapy provided.

   For the parenteral patient, the CMN must contain the following information:

   - The infusion frequency per week,
   - The route of administration,
   - A reason for the use of pre-mixed parenteral formulas,
   - An explanation for the use of special formulas such as hepatic, renal, or stress formulas, and
   - The amino acid/dextrose formula components of the parenteral solution mix.

   Amino acids serve as a source of protein. Adult parenteral nutrition patients generally need 1 to 1.5 grams of protein per day for each kilogram (2.2 pounds) of body weight. Dextrose concentrations less than 10 percent must be explained by the physician. The physician must document the reason for using more than 12 units (@ 500ml per unit) of lipids per month.

   Parenteral nutrition may be either "self-mixed" (i.e., the patient is taught to prepare the nutrient solution aseptically) or "pre-mixed" (i.e., the nutrient solution is prepared by trained professionals employed or contracted by the PEN supplier). The attending physician must provide information to justify the reason for "pre-mixed" parenteral nutrient solutions.

   Renal dialysis patients sometimes undergo parenteral therapy to replace fluids and nutrients lost during dialysis. Patients are usually infused less than daily and parenteral feeding is often supplemental and, therefore, not covered as a PEN benefit. The renal dialysis patient must meet all the requirements for PEN coverage. The attending physician must document that the patient, despite the need for renal dialysis, suffers from a permanently impaired functional impairment that precludes swallowing or absorption of nutrients.

   For the enteral patient, the attending physician must include the following information on the CMN:

   - The name of the nutrient product or nutrient category,
   - The number of calories per day (100 calories = 1 unit),
   - The frequency per day,
   - The method of administration (i.e., syringe, gravity, or pump),
   - The route of administration (i.e., nasogastric tube, gastrostomy tube, jejunostomy tube, percutaneous enteral gastrostomy tube, or naso-intestinal tube), and
   - The reason for the use of a pump.

   Categories of enteral nutrition are based on the composition and source of ingredients in each enteral nutrient product. Category IB of enteral nutrients contains products that are natural intact protein/protein isolates commonly known as blenderized nutrients. Additional documentation is required to justify the necessity of Category IB nutrients. The attending physician must provide sufficient information to indicate that the patient:

   - Has an intolerance to nutritionally equivalent (semi-synthetic) products;
   - Had a severe allergic reaction to a nutritionally equivalent (semi-synthetic) product; or
   - Was changed to a blenderized nutrient to alleviate adverse symptoms expected to be of permanent duration with continued use of semi-synthetic products.

   Enteral nutrient categories III through VI require additional medical justification for coverage. These categories represent formulas for special needs or use.

   - Category III (code B4153): hydrolyzed protein/amino acids. These products contain a high nitrogen availability as a result of chemical treatment to reduce high molecular protein compounds into smaller molecules and amino acids that are easier to digest.
   - Category IV (code B4154): defined formulas for special metabolic needs and conditions such as abnormal glucose tolerance, renal disease, liver disease, HIV, respiratory insufficiency, and malnutrition.
   - Category V (code B4155): modular components (proteins, carbohydrates, fats).
   - Category VI (code B4156): standardized nutrients. These products contain low residue ingredients.

   If the patient exhibits a problem with any particular formula in Nutrient Category I (HCPCS B4150) or II (HCPCS B4152), the physician must document the unfavorable events that resulted in prescribing a higher category formula.

   Generally, daily enteral intake of 750 to 2,000 calories is considered sufficient to maintain body weight. Patients with medical complications may require an intake outside the range. The attending physician must document the reason for prescribing less than 750 calories per day or more than 2000 calories per day.

   Enteral nutrition may be administered by syringe, gravity, or pump. The attending physician must specify the reason that necessitates the use of an enteral feeding pump. Some enteral patients may experience complications associated with syringe or gravity method of administration. Contractors provide coverage for enteral pumps if the medical necessity is documented by the attending physician on the CMN. Examples of circumstances that indicate the need for a pump include, but are not limited to:

   - Aspiration or Dumping Syndrome;
   - Severe diarrhea remedied by regulated feeding;
   - Insulin-dependent diabetics who require a flow rate of less than 100cc's per hour for proper regulation of nutrients;
   - Patients with congestive heart failure who require a pump to prevent circulatory overload; or
   - Patients with a jejunostomy tube for feeding.

   The DMERC reviews the claims to ensure that the equipment for which payment is claimed is consistent with that prescribed (e.g., expect a claim for an I.V. pole, if a pump is used).
5. Attending Physician's Signature and Identification – A handwritten, original signature and date must be on each certification. The form must be dated to show reasonable association to the dates of active PEN therapy. The full name, address, telephone number (including area code), and Unique Physician Identification Number (UPIN) allows the contractor to determine if the prescriber is authorized to order Medicare services and facilitate claims development.

1\. PEN Supplier's Identification – The PEN supplier's name, address, telephone number, and PEN identification number must be on each certification. This information allows the contractor to determine if the supplier is authorized to provide PEN supplies and facilitate claims development.

Pub 100-4, 20, 100.2.2.3 – DMERC Review of Initial PEN Certifications

(Rev. 1, 10-01-03)

B3-4450

In reviewing the claim and the supporting data on the CMN, the DMERC compares certain items, especially pertinent dates of treatment. For example, the start date of PEN coverage cannot precede the date of physician certification. The estimated duration of therapy must be contained on the CMN. This information is used to verify that the test of permanence is met. Once coverage is established, the estimated length of need at the start of PEN services will determine the recertification schedule.

The information shown on the certification must support the need for PEN supplies as billed. A diagnosis must show a functional impairment that precludes the enteral patient from swallowing and the parenteral patient from absorbing nutrients.

Initial assigned claims with the following conditions are denied without development:

- Inappropriate or missing diagnosis or functional impairment;
- Estimated duration of therapy is less than 90 consecutive days;
- Duration of therapy is not listed;
- Supplies have not been provided;
- Supplies were provided prior to onset date of therapy; and
- Stamped physician's signature.

Unassigned claims are developed for missing or incomplete information.

A. Revised Certifications/Change in Prescription

A revised certification is required when:

- There is a change in the attending physician's orders in the category of nutrients and/or calories prescribed;
- There is a change by more than one liter in the daily volume of parenteral solutions;
- There is a change from home-mix to pre-mix or pre-mix to home-mix parenteral solutions;
- There is a change from enteral to parenteral or parenteral to enteral therapy; or
- There is a change in the method of infusion (e.g., from gravity-fed to pump-fed).

The PEN payments are not adjusted unless a revised or renewed certification documents the necessity for the change. Payment levels for the most current certification or recertification may not be changed unless a prescription change is documented by a new recertification.

The DMERC may adjust the recertification schedule as needed.

Pub 100-4, 20, 100.2.3 – Evidence of Medical Necessity for Oxygen

(Rev. 1, 10-01-03)

B3-4105

Oxygen coverage is determined by the results of an arterial blood gas or oximetry test. A CMN for oxygen equipment must include results of specific testing before coverage can be determined.

Suppliers that bill electronically may transmit initial, revised, and recertification CMNs by electronic media using CMS-established standard formats. Information transmitted from a revised or recertification Form CMS-484 must accompany the first claim for monthly benefits submitted after the supplier has received the hard copy Form CMS-484 from the certifying physician. If the supplier submits Form CMS-484 information to the contractor electronically, the supplier must keep the paper certification readily available so that it may be promptly furnished to the contractor if requested for purposes of audits of medical necessity documentation.

Blood Oxygen Testing

The medical necessity of home oxygen is documented by the results of a blood oxygen test. The blood oxygen test may be either an arterial blood gas or an oximetry test. The following timeliness requirements must be met.

Initial Certification:

Groups I and II: Must be tested within 30 days prior to the date of initial certification. If the oxygen is begun immediately following discharge from an acute care facility, the test must be within two days prior to discharge.

Recertification:

Group I: Retesting requirements are to be determined by the contractor.

Group II: Must be retested between the 61st – 90th day after the date of the initial certification.

Revised Certifications:

Group I and II: Must be tested within 30 days prior to the date of the revised certification if the initial certification specified a length of need that is less than lifetime.

Physician Evaluation

Initial Certification:

Groups I and II: Must be seen and evaluated by the treating physician within 30 days prior to the date of initial certification

Recertifications:

Group I and II: Must be seen and re-evaluated by the treating physician within 90 days prior to any recertification date.

A. Initial Certifications

In reviewing the claim and the supporting data, contractors compare certain items, especially pertinent dates of treatment. For example, the start date of home oxygen coverage cannot precede the date of prescription or the date of the test(s) whose results establish that the special coverage criteria are met. Once coverage is established, the estimated length of need in Section B on the Form CMS-484, and the circumstances and the results of testing that established the medical necessity at the start of home oxygen therapy, determines the recertification schedule.

Definitions of "Group" based on blood gas values:

Group I – An arterial PO2 at or below 55 mm Hg, or arterial blood oxygen saturation at or below 88 percent.

Group II – An arterial PO2 is 56 to 59 mm Hg or arterial blood oxygen saturation is 89 percent.

Group III – An arterial PO2 at or above 60 mm Hg, or arterial blood oxygen saturation at or above 90 percent.

When oxygen is prescribed in an institution, in order to establish medical necessity it is necessary that the institution would have to recheck the oxygen level no sooner than 2 days before discharge.

Clinical documentation will be reviewed to confirm the fact that the prescribing of continued oxygen was based upon the "chronic stable state" (was done while the patient was in a chronic stable state – i.e., not during a period of acute illness or an exacerbation of the patient's underlying disease) of the patient.

Contractors verify that the information shown on or accompanying the Form CMS-484 or other CMN supports the need for oxygen as billed.

When both arterial blood gas (ABG) and oxygen saturation (oximetry) tests have recently been performed on the same day, suppliers report only the ABG result. That test is generally acknowledged as the more reliable indicator of hypoxemia.

Test results from oximetry tests performed by a DME supplier, or anyone financially associated with or related to the DME supplier, are not acceptable.

Values in Group III establish a rebuttable presumption of non-coverage. The CMN must be supplemented by additional documentation from the treating physician designed to overcome this presumption and justify the oxygen order, including a summary of other, more conservative therapy that has not relieved the patient's condition. Claims with such documentation are referred to the contractor's medical director for the coverage determination.

The following types of claims are denied without further development:

- Claims where the only qualifying test results came from oximetry tests conducted by a DME suppliers other than a hospital;
- Claims lacking information necessary to justify coverage;
- Hard copy claims where the CMN or Form CMS-484 lacks the treating physician's signature; or

- Electronic claims where the CMN or Form CMS-484 fails to indicate that the treating physician's handwritten signature is on file in the supplier's office.

An initial CMN is also required when there has been a break in medical necessity of 60 days plus whatever days remained in the rental month during which the oxygen was discontinued. (This indication does not apply if there was just a break in billing because the patient was in a hospital, nursing facility, hospice, or HMO, but the patient continued to use oxygen during that time.)

B. Revised Certifications

Contractors encourage treating physicians to file timely, revised CMNs or Form CMS- 484s through the supplier if their order for oxygen changes.

A revised CMN is necessary when:

1. The prescribed maximum flow rate changes from one of the following categories to another: (a) less than 1 LPM, (b) 1-4 LPM, (c) greater than 4 LPM. If the change is from category (a) or (b) to category (c), a repeat blood gas study with the beneficiary on 4 LPM must be performed within 30 days prior to the start of the greater than 4LPM flow.
2. Portable oxygen is added subsequent to initial certification of a stationary system.

   In this situation, there is no requirement for a repeat blood gas study unless the initial qualifying study was performed during sleep, in which case a repeat blood gas study must be performed while the patient is at rest (awake) or during exercise.
3. The initial certification specified an estimated length of need that is less than lifetime and the physician wants to extend the certification.
4. There is a new treating physician (no new testing is required).

   Contractors do not adjust payments on oxygen claims unless a revised certification documents the necessity for the change. Contractors timely adjust payments, if necessary, for services since the oxygen prescription was changed.

Pub 100-4, 20, 100.2.3.1 – Scheduling and Documenting Recertifications of Medical Necessity for Oxygen

(Rev. 1, 10-01-03)

Recertification scheduling and documentation requirements depend on the date when home oxygen therapy began. Contractors request the following information on all recertifications:

- Date and results of the most recent arterial blood gas or oximetry tests prior to the recertification date;
- Name of the provider conducting the most recent arterial blood gas or oximetry tests performed prior to the recertification date and the conditions under which this test were conducted; and
- Estimated length of need for oxygen (Section B on the Form CMS-484).

Contractors establish the schedule for recertifying the need for oxygen for patients beginning home oxygen therapy in accordance with the requirements below:

1. Recertifications

Group I: Recertification requirements are to be determined by the contractor.

Group II: If oxygen test results on the initial certification were in Group II, according to §1834(a)(5) of the Act, recertification of all oxygen patients must be performed within 90 days after initial certification for all patients who begin coverage after January 1, 1991, with an arterial blood gas result at or above a partial pressure of 55 mm Hg or an arterial oxygen saturation percentage at or above 89. Repeat blood gas study must be performed between the 61st – 90th day of home oxygen therapy. Retesting is required only if a claim for oxygen therapy will be filed for the fourth or later months.

If recertification is due, contractors do not pay the next month's claim if the test was not performed during the required time frame. If a qualifying test is not obtained between the 61st and 90th day of home oxygen therapy, but the patient continues to use oxygen and a test is obtained at a later date, contractors instruct suppliers to use the date of the repeat test as the date of service on a subsequent claim, and if that test meets Group II criteria, they resume payments from that point of time.

2. New Orders

In the following situations, a new order must be obtained and kept on file by the supplier, but neither a new CMN nor a repeat blood gas study are required:

- If the prescribed maximum flow rate changes but remains within one of the following categories: (a) less than 1 LPM, (b) 1-4 LPM, (c) greater than 4 LPM
- If the physician has initially specified a delivery system, and a change is made from one type of stationary system to another (i.e., concentrator, liquid, gaseous).

Pub 100-4, 20, 100.2.3.2 – HHA Recertification for Home Oxygen Therapy

(Rev. 1472, Issued: 03-06-08, Effective: 05-23-07, Implementation: 04-07-08)

Section 1834(a)(5) of the Act requires patients who receive home oxygen therapy and who at the time such services are initiated have an initial arterial blood gas value of 56 or higher or an initial oxygen saturation at or above 89 percent to be retested between 60 and 90 days after the start of oxygen therapy in order to continue to receive payment. HHAs must initiate the request for the retesting as promptly as possible because the recertification at three months must reflect the results of an arterial blood gas or oxygen saturation test conducted between the 61st and 90th day of home oxygen therapy. Payment for the fourth month of home oxygen therapy is possible only if the patient's attending physician certifies that retesting results establish the continuing medical necessity for the services. The physician must certify based on the test of the patient's arterial blood gas value or oxygen saturation that there is a medical need for the patient to continue to receive oxygen therapy.

Value codes have been assigned for HHA reporting of the arterial blood gas and oxygen saturation. HHAs report value code 58 or 59 on every initial bill for home oxygen therapy and on the fourth month's bill. Information regarding the form locator numbers that correspond to value codes and a table to crosswalk UB-04 form locators to the 837 transaction is found in Chapter 25.

For patients receiving oxygen therapy, who are not under a plan of care (bill type 34X), HHAs obtain a physicians recertification of the retesting and maintain a copy in their files for verification.

For patients receiving oxygen therapy, who are under a plan of care (bill types 32X and 33X), HHAs obtain a physician's recertification of the retesting and reflect this on Form CMS-485 or CMS-486 for verification.

RHHIs do not continue to make payment where the HHA fails to have the patient retested to determine continuing need of oxygen therapy within the specified time frames.

Pub 100-4, 20, 100.2.3.3 – Contractor Review of Oxygen Certifications

(Rev. 1, 10-01-03)

All claims with initial certifications calling for oxygen flow rates of more than 4 liters per minute must be reviewed before payment is authorized.

Items Requiring Special Attention

a. Oxygen Delivery or Supply Prescribed – If the treating physician has specified the oxygen equipment to be supplied, contractors ensure that the equipment furnished is consistent with that prescribed.
b. Treating Physician Identification – Contractors must ensure that the CMN or Form CMS-484 has been signed by the treating physician. A stamped signature is unacceptable. The physician's identification number must be the Unique Physician Identification Number (UPIN).

Pub 100-4, 20, 100.3 – Limitations on DMERC Collection of Information

(Rev. 1, 10-01-03)

B-02-031

The Paperwork Reduction Act (PRA) of 1995 §44 USC 3500, et seq. requires that the Director of the Office of Management and Budget approve any collections of information performed by or for the Federal Government unless the collection fits within exceptions for audits and investigations. Absent such approval, the collection violates the PRA and agencies may not hold the public to the requirement. Therefore, DMERCs must adhere to the following:

1. Power operated vehicles additional documentation requirements

   A Certificate of Medical Necessity (CMN) must accompany initial claims for power operated vehicles (POV). Except during the course of audits and investigations, DMERCs must not require that additional documentation accompany all POV claims. DMERCs may continue requesting information during the course of audits and investigations and when developing individual claims on either a pre- or a post-payment basis. If DMERCs choose to conduct such investigations, they must follow the guidelines in the Program Integrity Manual, Chapter 3.

2. Power wheelchair additional documentation requirements re: make and model name/number

   There must be no requirement that all claims for power wheelchairs include the make and model name/number of the wheelchair separate from the claim or the CMN.

   The CMN, an OMB approved information collection form, can be used to collect this information. Specifically, DMERCs can require that the make and model name/ number of the power wheelchair be included in Section C of the CMN. Section C requires the supplier to include a narrative description of the items, options and accessories ordered.

3. Power wheelchair additional documentation requirements re: functional abilities

   There must be no requirement for suppliers to submit additional documentation to describe a beneficiary's medical condition and functional abilities when the supplier bills for a higher level of equipment than previously supplied.

While it is appropriate to avoid paying for duplicate equipment, it is inappropriate to require this documentation for all claims for "higher level equipment." DMERCs may choose to perform pre- or post- payment probe samples to review these types of claims individually in order to determine medical necessity. If DMERCs choose to conduct such investigations, they must follow the guidelines in the Program Integrity Manual, Chapter 3.

Pub 100-4, 20, 130.2 – Billing for Inexpensive or Other Routinely Purchased DME

(Rev. 1, 10-01-03)

A3-3629, B3-4107.8

This is equipment with a purchase price not exceeding $150, or equipment that the Secretary determines is acquired by purchase at least 75 percent of the time, or equipment that is an accessory used in conjunction with a nebulizer, aspirator, or ventilators that are either continuous airway pressure devices or intermittent assist devices with continuous airway pressure devices. Suppliers and providers other than HHAs bill the DMERC or, in the case of implanted DME only, the local carrier. HHAs bill the RHHI.

Effective for items and services furnished after January 1, 1991, Medicare DME does not include seat lift chairs. Only the seat lift mechanism is defined under Medicare as DME. Therefore, seat lift coverage is limited to the seat lift mechanism. If a seat lift chair is provided to a beneficiary, contractors pay only for the lift mechanism portion of the chair.

Some lift mechanisms are equipped with a seat that is considered an integral part of the lift mechanism. Contractors do not pay for chairs (HCPCS code E0620) furnished on or after January 1, 1991. The appropriate HCPCS codes for seat lift mechanisms are E0627, E0628, and E0629.

For TENS, suppliers and providers other than HHAs bill the DMERC. HHAs bill the RHHI using revenue code 0291 for the 2-month rental period (see §30.1.2), billing each month as a separate line item and revenue code 0292 for the actual purchase along with the appropriate HCPCS code.

Pub 100-4, 20, 130.3 – Billing for Items Requiring Frequent and Substantial Servicing

(Rev. 1, 10-01-03)

A3-3629, B3-4107.8

These are items such as intermittent positive pressure breathing (IPPB) machines and ventilators, excluding ventilators that are either continuous airway pressure devices or intermittent assist devices with continuous airway pressure devices.

Suppliers and providers other than HHAs bill the DMERC. HHAs bill the RHHI.

Pub 100-4, 20, 130.4 – Billing for Certain Customized Items

(Rev. 1, 10-01-03)

A3-3629, B3-4107.8

Due to their unique nature (custom fabrication, etc.), certain customized DME cannot be grouped together for profiling purposes. Claims for customized items that do not have specific HCPCS codes are coded as E1399 (miscellaneous DME). This includes circumstances where an item that has a HCPCS code is modified to the extent that neither the original terminology nor the terminology of another HCPCS code accurately describes the modified item.

Suppliers and providers other than HHAs bill the DMERC or local carrier. HHAs bill their RHHI, using revenue code 0292 along with the HCPCS.

Pub 100-4, 20, 130.5 – Billing for Capped Rental Items (Other Items of DME)

(Rev. 1, 10-01-03)

A3-3629, B3-4107.8

These are DME items, other than oxygen and oxygen equipment, not covered by the above categories. Suppliers and providers other than HHAs bill the DMERC. HHAs bill the RHHIs.

Pub 100-4, 32, 11 – Wound Treatments

(Rev 124a, 03-19-04)

Pub 100-4, 32, 11.1 – Electrical Stimulation

(Rev. 371, Issued 11-19-04, Effective: 04-01-05, Implementation: 04-04-05)

A. Coding Applicable to Carriers & Fiscal Intermediaries (FIs)

Effective April 1, 2003, a National Coverage Decision was made to allow for Medicare coverage of Electrical Stimulation for the treatment of certain types of wounds. The type of wounds covered are chronic Stage III or Stage IV pressure ulcers, arterial ulcers, diabetic ulcers and venous stasis ulcers. All other uses of electrical stimulation for the treatment of wounds are not covered by Medicare. Electrical stimulation will not be covered as an initial treatment modality.

The use of electrical stimulation will only be covered after appropriate standard wound care has been tried for at least 30 days and there are no measurable signs of healing. If electrical stimulation is being used, wounds must be evaluated periodically by the treating physician but no less than every 30 days by a physician. Continued treatment with electrical stimulation is not covered if measurable signs of healing have not been demonstrated within any 30-day period of treatment. Additionally, electrical stimulation must be discontinued when the wound demonstrates a 100% epithelialzed wound bed.

Coverage policy can be found in Pub. 100-03, **Medicare National Coverage Determinations Manual**, Chapter 1, Section 270.1 (http://www.cms.hhs.gov/manuals/103_cov_determ/ncd103index.asp)

The applicable Healthcare Common Procedure Coding System (HCPCS) code for Electrical Stimulation and the covered effective date is as follows:

HCPCS Definition Effective Date

G0281 Electrical Stimulation, (unattended), to one or more areas for chronic Stage III and Stage IV pressure ulcers, arterial ulcers, diabetic ulcers and venous stasis ulcers not demonstrating measurable signs of healing after 30 days of conventional care as part of a therapy plan of care.

04/01/2003

Medicare will not cover the device used for the electrical stimulation for the treatment of wounds. However, Medicare will cover the service. Unsupervised home use of electrical stimulation will not be covered.

B. FI Billing Instructions

The applicable types of bills acceptable when billing for electrical stimulation services are 12X, 13X, 22X, 23X, 71X, 73X, 74X, 75X, and

85X. Chapter 25 of this manual provides general billing instructions that must be followed for bills submitted to FIs. FIs pay for electrical stimulation services under the Medicare Physician Fee Schedule for a hospital, Comprehensive Outpatient Rehabilitation Facility (CORF), Outpatient Rehabilitation Facility (ORF), Outpatient Physical Therapy (OPT) and Skilled Nursing Facility (SNF).

Payment methodology for independent Rural Health Clinic (RHC), provider-based RHCs, free-standing Federally Qualified Health Center (FQHC) and provider based FQHCs is made under the all-inclusive rate for the visit furnished to the RHC/FQHC patient to obtain the therapy service. Only one payment will be made for the visit furnished to the RHC/FQHC patient to obtain the therapy service. As of April 1, 2005, RHCs/FQHCs are no longer required to report HCPCS codes when billing for these therapy services.

Payment Methodology for a Critical Access Hospital (CAH) is on a reasonable cost basis unless the CAH has elected the Optional Method and then the FI pays115% of the MPFS amount for the professional component of the HCPCS code in addition to the technical component.

In addition, the following revenues code must be used in conjunction with the HCPCS code identified:

Revenue Code Description

420 Physical Therapy

430 Occupational Therapy

520 Federal Qualified Health Center *

521 Rural Health Center *

977, 978 Critical Access Hospital- method II

CAH professional services only

** NOTE: As of April 1, 2005, RHCs/FQHCs are no longer required to report HCPCS codes when billing for these therapy services.*

C. Carrier Claims

Carriers pay for Electrical Stimulation services billed with HCPCS codes G0281 based on the MPFS. Claims for Electrical Stimulation services must be billed on Form CMS-1500 or the electronic equivalent following instructions in chapter 12 of this manual (http://www.cms.hhs.gov/manuals/104_claims/clm104c12.pdf).

D. Coinsurance and Deductible

The Medicare contractor shall apply coinsurance and deductible to payments for these therapy services except for services billed to the FI by FQHCs. For FQHCs, only coinsurance applies.

Pub 100-4, 32, 11.2 – Electromagnetic Therapy

(Rev. 371, Issued 11-19-04, Effective: 04-01-05, Implementation: 04-04-05)

A. HCPCS Coding Applicable to Carriers & Fiscal Intermediaries (FIs)

Effective July 1, 2004, a National Coverage Decision was made to allow for Medicare coverage of electromagnetic therapy for the treatment of certain types of wounds. The type of wounds covered are chronic Stage III or Stage IV pressure ulcers, arterial ulcers, diabetic ulcers and venous stasis ulcers. All other uses of electromagnetic therapy for the treatment of wounds are not covered by Medicare. Electromagnetic therapy will not be covered as an initial treatment modality.

The use of electromagnetic therapy will only be covered after appropriate standard wound care has been tried for at least 30 days and there are no measurable signs of healing. If electromagnetic therapy is being used, wounds must be evaluated periodically by the treating physician but no less than every 30 days by a physician. Continued treatment with electromagnetic therapy is not covered if measurable signs of healing have not been demonstrated within any 30-day period of treatment. Additionally, electromagnetic therapy must be discontinued when the wound demonstrates a 100% epithelialzed wound bed.

Coverage policy can be found in Pub. 100-03, **Medicare National Coverage Determinations Manual**, Chapter 1, Section 270.1 (www.cms.hhs.gov/manuals/103_cov_determ/ncd103index.asp)

The applicable Healthcare Common Procedure Coding System (HCPCS) code for Electrical Stimulation and the covered effective date is as follows:

HCPCS Definition Effective Date

G0329 ElectromagneticTherapy, to one or more areas for chronic Stage III and Stage IV pressure ulcers, arterial ulcers, diabetic ulcers and venous stasis ulcers not demonstrating measurable signs of healing after 30 days of conventional care as part of a therapy plan of care.

07/01/2004

Medicare will not cover the device used for the electromagnetic therapy for the treatment of wounds. However, Medicare will cover the service. Unsupervised home use of electromagnetic therapy will not be covered.

B. FI Billing Instructions

The applicable types of bills acceptable when billing for electromagnetic therapy services are 12X, 13X, 22X, 23X, 71X, 73X, 74X, 75X, and 85X. Chapter 25 of this manual provides general billing instructions that must be followed for bills submitted to FIs. FIs pay for electromagnetic therapy services under the Medicare Physician Fee Schedule for a hospital, CORF, ORF, and SNF.

Payment methodology for independent (RHC), provider-based RHCs, free-standing FQHC and provider based FQHCs is made under the all-inclusive rate for the visit furnished to the RHC/FQHC patient to obtain the therapy service. Only one payment will be made for the visit furnished to the RHC/FQHC patient to obtain the therapy service. As of April 1, 2005, RHCs/FQHCs are no longer required to report HCPCS codes when billing for the therapy service.

Payment Methodology for a CAH is payment on a reasonable cost basis unless the CAH has elected the Optional Method and then the FI pays pay 115% of the MPFS amount for the professional component of the HCPCS code in addition to the technical component.

In addition, the following revenues code must be used in conjunction with the HCPCS code identified:

Revenue Code Description

420 Physical Therapy

430 Occupational Therapy

520 Federal Qualified Health Center *

521 Rural Health Center *

977, 978 Critical Access Hospital- method II

CAH professional services only

** NOTE: As of April 1, 2005, RHCs/FQHCs are no longer required to report HCPCS codes when billing for the therapy service.*

C. Carrier Claims

Carriers pay for Electromagnetic Therapy services billed with HCPCS codes G0329 based on the MPFS. Claims for electromagnetic therapy services must be billed on Form CMS- 1500 or the electronic equivalent following instructions in chapter 12 of this manual (www.cms.hhs.gov/manuals/104_claims/clm104index.asp).

Payment information for HCPCS code G0329 will be added to the July 2004 update of the Medicare Physician Fee Schedule Database (MPFSD).

D. Coinsurance and Deductible

The Medicare contractor shall apply coinsurance and deductible to payments for electromagnetic therapy services except for services billed to the FI by FQHCs. For FQHCs only co-insurance applies.

Pub 100-4, 32, 60 – Coverage and Billing for Home Prothrombin Time (PT/INR) Monitoring for Home Anticoagulation Management

(Rev. 1562, Issued: 07-25-08, Effective: 03-19-08, Implementation: 08-25-08)

The prothrombin time (PT) test is an in-vitro test to assess coagulation. PT testing and its normalized correlate, the International Normalized Ratio (INR), are the standard measurements for therapeutic effectiveness of warfarin therapy. Warfarin, Coumadin®, and others, are self-administered, oral anticoagulant, or blood thinner, medications that affect a person's Vitamin K-dependent clotting factors.

Use of the INR allows physicians to determine the level of anticoagulation in a patient independent of the laboratory reagents used. The INR is the ratio of the patient's prothrombin time compared to the mean prothrombin time for a group of normal individuals.

Pub 100-4, 32, 60.1 – Coverage Requirements

(Rev. 1562, Issued: 07-25-08, Effective: 03-19-08, Implementation: 08-25-08)

For services furnished on or after July 1, 2002, Medicare will cover the use of home INR monitoring for anticoagulation management for patients with mechanical heart valves on warfarin. The monitor and the home testing must be prescribed by a physician and the following patient requirements must be met:

- Must have been anticoagulated for at least three months prior to use of the home INR device;
- Must undergo an educational program on anticoagulation management and the use of the device prior to its use in the home; and
- Self testing with the device is limited to a frequency of once per week.

For services furnished on or after March 19, 2008, the Centers for Medicare & Medicaid Services revised its national coverage determination (NCD) on PT/INR Monitoring for Home Anticoagulation Management as follows:

Medicare will cover the use of home PT/INR monitoring for chronic, oral anticoagulation management for patients with mechanical heart valves, chronic atrial fibrillation, or venous thromboembolism (inclusive of deep venous thrombosis and pulmonary embolism) on warfarin. The monitor and the home testing must be prescribed by a treating physician as provided at 42 CFR 410.32(a), and all of the following requirements must be met:

1. The patient must have been anticoagulated for at least 3 months prior to use of the home INR device; and,
2. The patient must undergo a face-to-face educational program on anticoagulation management and must have demonstrated the correct use of the device prior to its use in the home; and,
3. The patient continues to correctly use the device in the context of the management of the anticoagulation therapy following the initiation of home monitoring; and,
4. Self-testing with the device should not occur more frequently than once a week.

NOTE: Porcine valves are not included in this NCD, so Medicare will not make payment on home INR monitoring for patients with porcine valves unless covered by local Medicare contractors.

Pub 100-4, 32, 60.2 – Intermediary Payment Requirements

(Rev. 216, 06-25-04)

Pub 100-4, 32, 60.2.1 – Part A Payment Methods

(Rev. 216, 06-25-04)

Payment is as follows:

- Hospital outpatient departments – Outpatient Prospective Payment System (OPPS)
- Critical Access Hospital (CAH) – Reasonable cost or Medicare Physician Fee Schedule (MPFS)

Deductible and coinsurance apply.

Pub 100-4, 32, 60.3 – Intermediary Billing Procedures

(Rev. 216, 06-25-04)

Pub 100-4, 32, 60.3.1 – Bill Types

(Rev. 216, 06-25-04)

The applicable bill types are 13X and 85X.

Pub 100-4, 32, 60.3.2 – Revenue Codes

(Rev. 216, 06-25-04)

Hospitals may report these services under revenue code 920 or they may report HCPCS codes G0248 and G0249 under the revenue center where they are performed.

Pub 100-4, 32, 60.4 – Intermediary Allowable Codes

(Rev. 216, 06-25-04)

Pub 100-4, 32, 60.4.1 – Allowable Covered Diagnosis Codes

(Rev. 1663; Issued: 01-08-09; Effective Date: 03-19-08; Implementation Date: 02-09-09)

For services furnished on or after July 1, 2002, the applicable ICD-9-CM diagnosis code for this benefit is V43.3, organ or tissue replaced by other means; heart valve.

For services furnished on or after March 19, 2008, the applicable ICD-9-CM diagnosis codes for this benefit are:

- V43.3 (organ or tissue replaced by other means; heart valve),
- 289.81 (primary hypercoagulable state),
- 451.0-451.9 (includes 451.11, 451.19, 451.2, 451.80-451.84, 451.89) (phlebitis & thrombophlebitis),
- 453.0-453.3 (other venous embolism & thrombosis),
- 453.40-453.49 (includes 453.40-453.42, 453.8-453.9) (venous embolism and thrombosis of the deep vessels of the lower extremity, and other specified veins/unspecified sites)
- 415.11-415.12, 415.19 (pulmonary embolism & infarction) or,
- 427.31 (atrial fibrillation (established) (paroxysmal)).

Pub 100-4, 32, 60.4.2 – Healthcare Common Procedural Coding System (HCPCS) for Intermediaries

(Rev. 1562, Issued: 07-25-08, Effective: 03-19-08, Implementation: 08-25-08)

For services furnished on or after July 1, 2002, and prior to March 19, 2008, the applicable HCPCS codes for this benefit are:

G0248: Demonstration, at initial use, of home INR monitoring for patient with mechanical heart valve(s) who meets Medicare coverage criteria, under the direction of a physician; includes: demonstration use and care of the INR monitor, obtaining at least one blood sample, provision of instructions for reporting home INR test results and documentation of a patient ability to perform testing.

Short Description: Demonstrate use home INR mon

G0249: Provision of test materials and equipment for home INR monitoring to patient with mechanical heart valve(s) who meets Medicare coverage criteria. Includes provision of materials for use in the home and reporting of test results to physician; per 4 tests.

Short Description: Provide test material, equipment

For services furnished on or after March 19, 2008, the applicable HCPCS codes for this benefit are:

G0248: Demonstration, prior to initial use, of home INR monitoring for patient with either mechanical heart valve(s), chronic atrial fibrillation, or venous thromboembolism who meets Medicare coverage criteria, under the direction of a physician; includes: face-to-face demonstration of use and care of the INR monitor, obtaining at least one blood sample, provision of instructions for reporting home INR test results, and documentation of patient ability to perform testing prior to its use

Short Description: Demonstrate use home INR mon

G0249: Provision of test materials and equipment for home INR monitoring of patient with either mechanical heart valve(s), chronic atrial fibrillation, or venous thromboembolism who meets Medicare coverage criteria; includes provision of materials for use in the home and reporting of test results to physician; not occurring more frequently than once a week

Short Description: Provide INR test mater/equip

Pub 100-4, 32, 60.5 – Carrier Billing Instructions

(Rev. 1562, Issued: 07-25-08, Effective: 03-19-08, Implementation: 08-25-08)

Effective for claims with dates of service on and after March 19, 2008, the descriptors of HCPCS Codes G0248, G0249, and G0250 were changed to reflect revised coverage policy.

Pub 100-4, 32, 60.5.1 – Healthcare Common Procedural Coding System (HCPCS) for Carriers

(Rev. 1562, Issued: 07-25-08, Effective: 03-19-08, Implementation: 08-25-08)

For services furnished on or after July 1, 2002, and prior to March 19, 2008, the applicable HCPCS codes for this benefit are:

G0248 TOS (Type of Service): Demonstration, at initial use, of home INR monitoring for patient with mechanical heart valve(s) who meets Medicare coverage criteria, under the direction of a physician; includes: demonstration use and care of the INR monitor, obtaining at least one blood sample, provision of instructions for reporting home INR test results and documentation of a patient ability to perform testing.

Short Description: Demonstrate use home INR mon

G0249 TOS (Type of Service): Provision of test materials and equipment for home INR monitoring to patient with mechanical heart valve(s) who meets Medicare coverage criteria. Includes provision of materials for use in the home and reporting of test results to physician; per 4 tests.

Short Description: Provide test material, equipm

G0250 TOS (Type of Service): Physician review; interpretation and patient management of home INR testing for a patient with mechanical heart valve(s) who meets other coverage criteria; per 4 tests (does not require face-to-face service)

Short Description: MD review interpret of test

For services furnished on or after March 19, 2008, the applicable HCPCS codes for this benefit are:

G0248: Demonstration, prior to initial use, of home INR monitoring for patient with either mechanical heart valve(s), chronic atrial fibrillation, or venous thromboembolism who meets Medicare coverage criteria, under the direction of a physician; includes: face-to-face demonstration of use and care of the INR monitor, obtaining at least one blood sample, provision of instructions for reporting home INR test results, and documentation of patient ability to perform testing prior to its use

Short Description: Demonstrate use home INR mon

G0249: Provision of test materials and equipment for home INR monitoring of patient with either mechanical heart valve(s), chronic atrial fibrillation, or venous thromboembolism who meets Medicare coverage criteria; includes provision of materials for use in the home and reporting of test results to physician; not occurring more frequently than once a week

Short Description: Provide INR test mater/equip

G0250: Physician review, interpretation, and patient management of home INR testing for a patient with either mechanical heart valve(s), chronic atrial fibrillation, or venous thromboembolism who meets Medicare coverage criteria; includes face-to-face verification by the physician that the patient uses the device in the context of the management of the anticoagulation therapy following initiation of the home INR monitoring; not occurring more frequently than once a week

Short Description: MD INR test revie inter mgmt

Pub 100-4, 32, 60.5.2 – Applicable Diagnosis Codes for Carriers

(Rev. 1562, Issued: 07-25-08, Effective: 03-19-08, Implementation: 08-25-08)

For services furnished on or after July 1, 2002, the applicable ICD-9-CM diagnosis code for this benefit is V43.3, organ or tissue replaced by other means; heart valve.

For services furnished on or after March 19, 2008, the applicable ICD-9-CM diagnosis codes for this benefit are:

V43.3 (organ or tissue replaced by other means; heart valve),
289.81 (primary hypercoagulable state),
451.0-451.9 (phlebitis & thrombophlebitis),
453.0-453.3 (other venous embolism & thrombosis),
415.11-415.19 (pulmonary embolism & infarction), or,
427.31 (atrial fibrillation (established) (paroxysmal)).

Pub 100-4, 32, 60.6 – Carrier Claims Requirements

(Rev. 1562, Issued: 07-25-08, Effective: 03-19-08, Implementation: 08-25-08)

Note this test is not covered as durable medical equipment. Therefore, claims submitted to DMERCs will not be paid. It is covered under the physician fee schedule. Also note that the cost of the device and supplies is included in the payment for G0249 and therefore not separately billed to Medicare. G0249 continues to include materials for 4 tests. Additionally, G0250 continues to mean per 4 tests and should be billed no more frequently than once every 4 weeks.

Pub 100-4, 32, 60.7 – Carrier Payment Requirements

(Rev. 1562, Issued: 07-25-08, Effective: 03-19-08, Implementation: 08-25-08)

Payment and pricing information will be in the Medicare Physician Fee Schedule Database (MPFSDB). Pay for INR on the basis of the MPFS. Deductible and coinsurance apply.

Pub 100-4, 32, 60.8 – Carrier and Intermediary General Claims Processing Instructions

(Rev. 216, 06-25-04)

Pub 100-4, 32, 60.8.1 – Remittance Advice Notice

(Rev. 1562, Issued: 07-25-08, Effective: 03-19-08, Implementation: 08-25-08)

Use appropriate existing remittance advice reason and remark codes at the line level to express the specific reason for denying payment for PT/INR:

Remittance Advice Remark Code N386, "This decision was based on a National Coverage Determination (NCD). An NCD provides a coverage determination as to whether a particular item or service is covered. A copy of this policy is available at http://www.cms.hhs.gov/mcd/search.asp. If you do not have Web access, you may contact the contractor to request a copy of the NCD."

If denying services furnished after July 1, 2002, use ANSI X 12-835 claim adjustment reason code 50, "These are non-covered services because this is not deemed a 'medical necessity' by the payer."

Pub 100-4, 32, 60.8.2 – Medicare Summary Notice (MSN) Messages

(Rev. 1562, Issued: 07-25-08, Effective: 03-19-08, Implementation: 08-25-08)

If denying services furnished after July 1, 2002, use MSN message:

"The following policies [190.11] were used when we made this decision." (MSN Message 15.20)

Pub 100-4, 32, 70 – Billing Requirements for Islet Cell Transplantation for Beneficiaries in a National Institutes of Health (NIH) Clinical Trial

(Rev. 986, Issued: 06-16-06, Effective: 05-01-06, Implementation: 07-31-06)

For services performed on or after October 1, 2004, Medicare will cover islet cell transplantation for patients with Type I diabetes who are participating in an NIH sponsored clinical trial. See Pub 100-04 (National Coverage Determinations Manual) section 260.3.1 for complete coverage policy.

The islet cell transplant may be done alone or in combination with a kidney transplant. Islet recipients will also need immunosuppressant therapy to prevent rejection of the transplanted islet cells. Routine follow-up care will be necessary for each trial patient. See Pub 100-04, section

310 for further guidance relative to routine care. All other uses for islet cell services will remain non-covered.

Pub 100-4, 32, 70.1 – Healthcare Common Procedure Coding System (HCPCS) Codes for Carriers

(Rev. 261, Issued: 07-30-04, Effective: 10-01-04, Implementation: 10-04-04)

G0341 Percutaneous islet cell transplant, includes portal vein catheterization and infusion
Short Descriptor: Percutaneous islet cell trans
Type of Service: 2

G0342 Laparoscopy for islet cell transplant, includes portal vein catheterization and infusion
Short Descriptor: Laparoscopy islet cell trans
Type of Service: 2

G0343 Laparotomy for islet cell transplant, includes portal vein catheterization and infusion
Short Descriptor: Laparotomy islet cell transp
Type of Service: 2

Pub 100-4, 32, 70.2 – Applicable Modifier for Islet Cell Transplant Claims for Carriers

(Rev. 986, Issued: 06-16-06, Effective: 05-01-06, Implementation: 07-31-06)

Carriers shall instruct physicians to bill using the above procedure code(s) with modifier QR (Item or service provided in a Medicare-specified study) for all claims for islet cell transplantation and routine follow-up care related to this service.

Pub 100-4, 32, 70.3 – Special Billing and Payment Requirements for Carriers

(Rev. 261, Issued: 07-30-04, Effective: 10-01-04, Implementation: 10-04-04)

Payment and pricing information will be on the October 2004 update of the Medicare Physician Fee Schedule Database (MPFSDB). Pay for islet cell transplants on the basis of the MPFS. Deductible and coinsurance apply for fee-for-service beneficiaries.

Pub 100-4, 32, 70.4 – Special Billing and Payment Requirements for Intermediaries

(Rev. 1192, Issued: 03-02-07, Effective: 10-01-04, Implementation: 04-02-07)

This procedure (ICD-9-CM procedure code 52.85-heterotransplantation of islet cells of pancreas) is covered for the clinical trial in an inpatient hospital setting. The applicable TOB is 11X. A secondary diagnoses (diagnoses positions 2 – 9) of V70.7 (examination of participant or control in clinical research) must be present along with condition code 30 (qualifying clinical trial). V70.7 and condition code 30 alerts the claims processing system that this is a clinical trial. The procedure is paid under inpatient prospective payment system for hospitals with patients in the trial. Deductible and coinsurance apply for fee-for-service beneficiaries.

Inpatient hospitals participating in this trial are entitled to an add-on payment of $18,848.00 for islet isolation services. This amount is in addition to the final IPPS payment made to the hospital. Should two infusions occur during the same hospital stay, Medicare will pay for two add-ons for isolation of the islet cells, but never for more than two add-ons for a hospital stay.

Inpatient hospitals shall report charges for organ acquisition in Revenue Code 0810, 0811, 0812, 0813, or 0819. This includes charges for the pre-transplant items and services related to the acquisition and delivery of the pancreatic islet cell transplants. As is Medicare's policy with other organ transplants, Medicare contractors deduct acquisition charges prior to processing through the IPPS Pricer. Pancreata procured for islet cell transplant are not included in the prospective payment. They are paid on a reasonable cost basis. This is a pass-through cost for which interim payments may be made. Effective for services on or after May 1, 2006, contractors shall accept the QR modifier for islet cell transplantation follow up care when performed in an outpatient department of a hospital when the transplant was done in conjunction with an NIH-sponsored clinical trial, and when billed on type of bill 13X or 85X.

All other normal inpatient billing practices apply.

Pub 100-4, 32, 70.5 – Special Billing and Payment Requirements Medicare Advantage (MA) Beneficiaries

(Rev. 261, Issued: 07-30-04, Effective: 10-01-04, Implementation: 10-04-04)

CMS will make payment directly on a fee-for service basis for the routine costs of pancreatic islet cell transplants as well as transplantation and appropriate related items and services, for MA beneficiaries participating in an NIH-sponsored clinical trial. MA organizations will not be liable for payment for routine costs of this new clinical trial until MA payments can be appropriately adjusted to take into account the cost of this national coverage decision. Medicare contractors shall make payment on behalf of MA organizations directly to providers of these islet cell transplants in accordance with Medicare payment rules, except that beneficiaries are not responsible for the Part A and Part B deductibles. MA enrollees will be liable for any applicable coinsurance amounts MA organizations have in place for clinical trial benefits.

Pub 100-4, 32, 80 – Billing of the Diagnosis and Treatment of Peripheral Neuropathy with Loss of Protective Sensation in People with Diabetes

(Rev. 498, Issued: 03-11-05, Effective/Implementation: N/A)

Coverage Requirements – Peripheral neuropathy is the most common factor leading to amputation in people with diabetes. In diabetes, peripheral neuropathy is an anatomically diffuse process primarily affecting sensory and autonomic fibers; however, distal motor findings may be present in advanced cases. Long nerves are affected first, with symptoms typically beginning insidiously in the toes and then advancing proximally. This leads to loss of protective sensation (LOPS), whereby a person is unable to feel minor trauma from mechanical, thermal, or chemical sources. When foot lesions are present, the reduction in autonomic nerve functions may also inhibit wound healing.

Peripheral neuropathy with LOPS, secondary to diabetes, is a localized illness of the feet and falls within the regulation's exception to the general exclusionary rule (see 42 C.F.R. §411.15(l)(l)(i)). Foot exams for people with diabetic peripheral neuropathy with LOPS are reasonable and necessary to allow for early intervention in serious complications that typically afflict diabetics with the disease.

Effective for services furnished on or after July 1, 2002, Medicare covers, as a physician service, an evaluation (examination and treatment) of the feet no more often than every 6 months for individuals with a documented diagnosis of diabetic sensory neuropathy and LOPS, as long as the beneficiary has not seen a foot care specialist for some other reason in the interim. LOPS shall be diagnosed through sensory testing with the 5.07 monofilament using established guidelines, such as those developed by the National Institute of Diabetes and Digestive and Kidney Diseases guidelines. Five sites should be tested on the plantar surface of each foot, according to the National Institute of Diabetes and Digestive and Kidney Diseases guidelines. The areas must be tested randomly since the loss of protective sensation may be patchy in distribution, and the patient may get clues if the test is done rhythmically. Heavily callused areas should be avoided. As suggested by the American Podiatric Medicine Association, an absence of sensation at two or more sites out of 5 tested on either foot when tested with the 5.07 Semmes-Weinstein monofilament must be present and documented to diagnose peripheral neuropathy with loss of protective sensation.

Pub 100-4, 32, 80.1 – General Billing Requirements – Follow the general bill review instructions in §3604.

(Rev. 498, Issued: 03-11-05, Effective/Implementation: N/A)

The following providers of service may bill you for these services:

Hospitals;

Rural Health Clinic;

Free-Standing Federally Qualified Health Clinic (FQHC);

Outpatient Rehabilitation Facility (ORF);

Comprehensive Outpatient Rehabilitation Facility (CORF); and

Critical Access Hospitals

Pub 100-4, 32, 80.2 – Applicable HCPCS Codes

(Rev. 498, Issued: 03-11-05, Effective/Implementation: N/A)

G0245 – Initial physician evaluation and management of a diabetic patient with diabetic sensory neuropathy resulting in a loss of protective sensation (LOPS) which must include:

1. The diagnosis of LOPS;
2. A patient history;
3. A physical examination that consists of at least the following elements:
   (a) visual inspection of the forefoot, hindfoot, and toe web spaces,
   (b) evaluation of a protective sensation,
   (c) evaluation of foot structure and biomechanics,
   (d) evaluation of vascular status and skin integrity,
   (e) evaluation and recommendation of footwear, and
4. Patient education.

G0246 Follow-up physician evaluation and management of a diabetic patient with diabetic sensory neuropathy resulting in a loss of protective sensation (LOPS) to include at least the following:

1. a patient history;
2. a physical examination that includes:
   (a) visual inspection of the forefoot, hindfoot, and toe web spaces,
   (b) evaluation of protective sensation,
   (c) evaluation of foot structure and biomechanics,
   (d) evaluation of vascular status and skin integrity,
   (e) evaluation and recommendation of footwear, and
3. patient education.

G0247 Routine foot care by a physician of a diabetic patient with diabetic sensory neuropathy resulting in a LOPS to include if present, at least the following:

(1) local care of superficial (i.e., superficial to muscle and fascia) wounds;
(2) debridement of corns and calluses; and
(3) trimming and debridement of nails.

NOTE: Code G0247 must be billed on the same date of service with either G0245 or G0246 in order to be considered for payment.

The short descriptors for the above HCPCS codes are as follows:

G0245 INITIAL FOOT EXAM PT LOPS

G0246 FOLLOWUP EVAL OF FOOT PT LOP

G0247 ROUTINE FOOTCARE PT W LOPS

Pub 100-4, 32, 80.3 – Diagnosis Codes

(Rev. 498, Issued: 03-11-05, Effective/Implementation: N/A)

Diagnosis Codes.--Providers should report one of the following diagnosis codes in conjunction with this benefit: 250.60, 250.61, 250.62, 250.63, and 357.2.

Pub 100-4, 32, 80.4 – Payment

(Rev. 498, Issued: 03-11-05, Effective/Implementation: N/A)

- Hospital outpatient departments – OPPS
- Critical Access Hospital (CAH) – Method I -- Reasonable cost; Method II -- Technical – reasonable cost, Professional -- 115 percent of the fee schedule
- Comprehensive Outpatient Rehabilitation Facility – Medicare physician fee schedule (MPFS)
- Skilled Nursing Facility – MPFS
- Rural Health Clinics/Federally Qualified Health Centers (RHCs/FQHCs) – All inclusive rate.

Deductible and coinsurance apply.

Examples of Payment calculation:

Part B Deductible Met: $900 (MPFS allowed amount) x 20 percent (co-insurance) = $720 (Medicare reimbursement). Beneficiary is responsible for $180.

Part B Deductible Not met: $900 (MPFS allowed amount) – $100 (Part B deductible) = $800 x 20 percent (co-insurance) = $640 (Medicare reimbursement). Beneficiary is responsible for $260.

Part B Deductible Met: $800 (actual charged amount) x 20 percent (co-insurance) = $640 (Medicare Reimbursement), beneficiary is responsible for $160 co-insurance.

Part B Deductible Not Met: $800 (actual charged amount) – $100 (Part B deductible) = $700 x 20 percent (co-insurance) = $560 (Medicare reimbursement). Beneficiary is responsible for $240, ($100 Part B deductible and $140 co-insurance).

Services are paid at 80 percent of the lesser of the fee schedule amount or the actual charges.

This service, when furnished in an RHC/FQHC by a physician or non-physician, is considered an RHC/FQHC service. RHCs/FQHCs bill you under bill type 71X or 73X with revenue code 940 and HCPCS G0245, G0246, and G0247.

Payment should not be made for this service unless the claim contains a related visit code.

Therefore, install an edit in your system to assure payment is not made for revenue code 940 unless the claim also contains a visit revenue code (520 or 521).

Applicable Revenue Codes

The applicable revenue code is 940, except for hospitals.

This service can be performed in other revenue centers such as a clinic (510) for hospitals. Therefore, instruct your hospitals to report these procedures under the revenue center where they are performed.

Pub 100-4, 32, 80.5 – Applicable Revenue Codes

(Rev. 498, Issued: 03-11-05, Effective/Implementation: N/A)

The applicable revenue code is 940, except for hospitals.

This service can be performed in other revenue centers such as a clinic (510) for hospitals. Therefore, instruct your hospitals to report these procedures under the revenue center where they are performed.

Pub 100-4, 32, 80.6 – Editing Instructions for Fiscal Intermediaries (FIs)

(Rev. 498, Issued: 03-11-05, Effective/Implementation: N/A)

Edit 1

Implement diagnosis to procedure code edits to allow payment only for the LOPS codes, G0245, G0246, and G0247 when submitted with one of the diagnosis codes 250.60, 250.61, 250.62, 250.63, or 357.2. Deny these services when submitted without one of the appropriate diagnoses.

Use the same messages you currently use for procedure to diagnosis code denials.

Edit 2

Deny G0247 if it is not submitted on the same claim as G0245 or G0246.

Use MSN 21.21 – This service was denied because Medicare only covers this service under certain circumstances.

Use RA claim adjustment reason code 107 – Claim/service denied because the related or qualifying claim/service was not paid or identified on the claim.

Pub 100-4, 32, 80.7 – CWF General Information

(Rev. 498, Issued: 03-11-05, Effective/Implementation: N/A)

Though G0245 and G0246 have no technical or professional components, for these codes, CWF will post FI claims for bill types 13X, 74X, and 75X as technical, and carrier claims as professional. For bill type 85X with revenue code 940, CWF will post as technical. For 85X bill type with revenue code 98X, (Method II), CWF will post as technical and professional. This will allow both the facility and professional service payments to be approved by CWF for payment when the code and date of service match. Therefore, should a claim from a carrier and an FI be received with the same code and same date of service for the same beneficiary, the second claim submitted will not be rejected as a duplicate.

Medicare References

Due to the billing and payment methodology of Rural Health Clinics – bill type 71X and Federally Qualified Health Centers – bill type 73X, CWF will post these claims as usual, which will correctly allow claims from these entities that are billed to the FI to reject as duplicates when the HCPCS code, date of service, and beneficiary Health Insurance Claim number are an exact match with a claim billed to a carrier.

Carriers and FIs must react to these duplicate claims as they currently do for any other duplicates.

Pub 100-4, 32, 80.8 – CWF Utilization Edits

(Rev. 1742, Issued: 05-22-09, Effective: 06-08-09, Implementation: 06-08-09)

Edit 1 – Should CWF receive a claim from an FI for G0245 or G0246 and a second claim from a contractor for either G0245 or G0246 (or vice versa) and they are different dates of service and less than 6 months apart, the second claim will reject. CWF will edit to allow G0245 or G0246 to be paid no more than every 6 months for a particular beneficiary, regardless of who furnished the service. If G0245 has been paid, regardless of whether it was posted as a facility or professional claim, it must be 6 months before G0245 can be paid again or G0246 can be paid. If G0246 has been paid, regardless of whether it was posted as a facility or professional claim, it must be 6 months before G0246 can be paid again or G0245 can be paid. CWF will not impose limits on how many times each code can be paid for a beneficiary as long as there has been 6 months between each service.

The CWF will return a specific reject code for this edit to the contractors and FIs that will be identified in the CWF documentation. Based on the CWF reject code, the contractors and FIs must deny the claims and return the following messages:

MSN 18.4 – This service is being denied because it has not been __ months since your last examination of this kind (NOTE: Insert 6 as the appropriate number of months.)

RA claim adjustment reason code 96 – Non-covered charges, along with remark code M86 – Service denied because payment already made for same/similar procedure within set time frame.

Edit 2 – The CWF will edit to allow G0247 to pay only if either G0245 or G0246 has been submitted and accepted as payable on the same date of service. CWF will return a specific reject code for this edit to the contractors and FIs that will be identified in the CWF documentation. Based on this reject code, contractors and FIs will deny the claims and return the following messages:

MSN 21.21 – This service was denied because Medicare only covers this service under certain circumstances.

RA claim adjustment reason code 107 – The related or qualifying claim/service was not identified on this claim.

Edit 3 – Once a beneficiary's condition has progressed to the point where routine foot care becomes a covered service, payment will no longer be made for LOPS evaluation and management services. Those services would be considered to be included in the regular exams and treatments afforded to the beneficiary on a routine basis. The physician or provider must then just bill the routine foot care codes, per Pub 100-02, Chapter 15, §290.

The CWF will edit to reject LOPS codes G0245, G0246, and/or G0247 when on the beneficiary's record it shows that one of the following routine foot care codes were billed and paid within the prior 6 months: 11055, 11056, 11057, 11719, 11720, and/or 11721.

The CWF will return a specific reject code for this edit to the contractors and FIs that will be identified in the CWF documentation. Based on the CWF reject code, the contractors and FIs must deny the claims and return the following messages:

MSN 21.21 – This service was denied because Medicare only covers this service under certain circumstances.

The RA claim adjustment reason code 96 – Non-covered charges, along with remark code M86 – Service denied because payment already made for same/similar procedure within set time frame.

Pub 100-4, 32, 100 – Billing Requirements for Expanded Coverage of Cochlear Implantation

(Rev. 601, Issued: 07-01-05; Effective: 04-04-05; Implementation: 07-25-05)

Effective for dates of services on and after April 4, 2005, the Centers for Medicare & Medicaid Services (CMS) has expanded the coverage for cochlear implantation to cover moderate-to-profound hearing loss in individuals with hearing test scores equal to or less than 40% correct in the best aided listening condition on tape-recorded tests of open-set sentence recognition and who demonstrate limited benefit from amplification. (See Publication 100-03, chapter 1, section 50.3, for specific coverage criteria).

In addition CMS is covering cochlear implantation for individuals with open-set sentence recognition test scores of greater than 40% to less than or equal to 60% correct but only when the provider is participating in, and patients are enrolled in, either:

- A Food and Drug Administration (FDA)-approved category B investigational device exemption (IDE) clinical trial; or
- A trial under the CMS clinical trial policy (see Pub. 100-03, section 310.1); or

A prospective, controlled comparative trial approved by CMS as consistent with the evidentiary requirements for national coverage analyses and meeting specific quality standards.

Pub 100-4, 32, 100.1 – Intermediary Billing Procedures

Pub 100-4, 32, 100.1.1 – Applicable Bill Types

(Rev. 601, Issued: 07-01-05; Effective: 04-04-05; Implementation: 07-25-05)

11X, 12X (see note below), 13X, 83X, 85X

NOTE: Surgical procedures are not acceptable on 12x bill types.

Pub 100-4, 32, 100.1.2 – Special Billing Requirements for Intermediaries

(Rev. 601, Issued: 07-01-05; Effective: 04-04-05; Implementation: 07-25-05)

For inpatient billing:

- The second or subsequent diagnosis code must be V70.7 (examination of participant or control in clinical research). V70.7 alerts the claims processing system that this is a clinical trial.

For inpatient Part B and outpatient bills:

- For patients in an approved clinical trial with hearing test scores greater than 40% to less than or equal to 60% hearing, the QR modifier must be reported with the cochlear implantation device and all other related costs or; (see note below)
- For patients in an approved clinical trial under the clinical trial policy with hearing test scores greater than 60% hearing, the QV modifier must be billed for routine costs.

NOTE: The QR or QV modifier does not need to be applied to HCPCS 92601-92604 or any applicable audiology codes.

Pub 100-4, 32, 100.2 – Intermediary Payment Requirements

(Rev. 601, Issued: 07-01-05; Effective: 04-04-05; Implementation: 07-25-05)

There are no special payment methods. Existing payment methods shall apply.

Pub 100-4, 32, 100.3 – Carrier Billing Procedures

(Rev. 601, Issued: 07-01-05; Effective: 04-04-05; Implementation: 07-25-05)

Effective for dates of service performed on and after April 4, 2005, the following applies:

Carriers shall accept claims for cochlear implantation devices and services for beneficiaries with moderate-to-profound hearing loss with hearing test scores equal to or less than 40%.

Carriers shall accept claims for cochlear implantation devices and all related costs for beneficiaries with hearing test scores of greater than

40% to less than or equal to 60% hearing provided in an FDA-approved category B IDE clinical trial, a trial under the CMS Clinical Trial policy, or a prospective, controlled comparative trial approved by CMS that is billed with the QR modifier. The definition of the QR modifier is, "Item or service provided in a Medicare specified study."

Carriers shall accept claims for routine costs pertaining to beneficiaries with hearing test scores of greater than 60% hearing who are in a clinical trial under the clinical trial policy that is billed with the QV modifier. The definition of the QV modifier is, "Item or service provided as routine care in a Medicare qualifying clinical trial."

Carriers shall accept claims for evaluation and therapeutic services related to cochlear implantation.

NOTE: Modifiers QR or QV do not need to be applied to these services (92601– 92604 or any applicable audiology codes).

These services should be billed on an approved electronic claim form or a paper CMS Form 1500.

Pub 100-4, 32, 100.4 – Healthcare Common Procedural Coding System (HCPCS)

(Rev. 601, Issued: 07-01-05; Effective: 04-04-05; Implementation: 07-25-05)

The following HCPCS codes are some of those available for use when billing for cochlear implantation services and devices provided by audiologists or physicians, and for the services of 92506 and 92507, by speech language pathologists.

69930 – Cochlear device implantation, with or without mastoidectomy

L8614 Cochlear Device/System

L8619 Cochlear implant external speech processor, replacement

L7500 Repair of prosthetic device, hourly rate (excludes V5335 repair of oral laryngeal prosthesis or artificial larynx)

L7510 Repair of prosthetic device, repair or replace minor parts

92506 Evaluation of speech, language, voice, communication, auditory processing, and/or aural rehabilitation status

92507 Treatment of speech, language, voice, communication, and/or auditory processing disorder (includes aural rehabilitation); individual

92601 Diagnostic analysis of cochlear implant, patient under 7 years of age; with programming

(Codes 92601 and 92603 describe post-operative analysis and fitting of previously placed external devices, connection to the cochlear implant, and programming of the stimulator.

Codes 92602 and 92604 describe subsequent sessions for measurements and adjustment of the external transmitter and re-programming of the internal stimulator.)

92602 Diagnostic analysis of cochlear implant, patient under 7 years of age; subsequent programming. (Do not report 92602 in addition to 92601.)

92603 Diagnostic analysis of cochlear implant, age 7 years or older; with programming

92604 Diagnostic analysis of cochlear implant, age 7 years or older; subsequent reprogramming

A complete list of audiology codes can be found in Pub 100-4, chapter12, section 30.3.

Pub 100-4, 32, 110 – Coverage and Billing for Ultrasound Stimulation for Nonunion Fracture Healing

(Rev. 597, Issued: 06-24-05, Effective: 04-27-05, Implementation: 08-01-05)

An ultrasonic osteogenic stimulator is a non-invasive device that emits low intensity, pulsed ultrasound. This device is applied to the surface of the skin at the fracture site and ultrasound waves are emitted via a conductive coupling gel to stimulate fracture healing. The ultrasonic osteogenic stimulators are not to be used concurrently with other noninvasive osteogenic devices.

Pub 100-4, 32, 110.1 – Coverage Requirements

(Rev. 597, Issued: 06-24-05, Effective: 04-27-05, Implementation: 08-01-05)

Effective for dates of service on and after April 27, 2005, ultrasonic osteogenic stimulators are covered as medically reasonable and necessary for the treatment of nonunion bone fractures prior to surgical intervention. In demonstrating nonunion fractures, CMS expects:

- A minimum of 2 sets of radiographs, obtained prior to starting treatment with the osteogenic stimulator, separated by a minimum of 90 days. Each radiograph set must include multiple views of the fracture site accompanied with a written interpretation by a physician stating that there has been no clinically significant evidence of fracture healing between the 2 sets of radiographs.

For further coverage information, please refer to the National Coverage Determinations Manual, Pub. 100-03, chapter 1, section 150.2.

Pub 100-4, 32, 110.2 – Intermediary Billing Requirements

(Rev. 597, Issued: 06-24-05, Effective: 04-27-05, Implementation: 08-01-05)

The RHHIs will pay for ultrasonic osteogenic stimulators only when services are submitted on type of bills (TOBs) listed under Pub. 100-04, Medicare **Claims Processing Manual**, chapter 32, section 100.3.

Fiscal intermediaries (FIs) must educate hospitals that there are no covered services for Ultrasonic Osteogenic Stimulation for which hospitals can be paid by the FI.

NOTE: Hospitals can not bill for Ultrasonic Osteogenic Stimulators.

Pub 100-4, 32, 110.3 – Bill Types

(Rev. 597, Issued: 06-24-05, Effective: 04-27-05, Implementation: 08-01-05)

Only the following TOBs can bill for Ultrasonic Osteogenic Stimulators: 32X, 33X, 34X, which is payable under the DMEPOS Fee Schedule.

NOTE: Ultrasonic Osteogenic Stimulators must be in the patient's home health plan of care if billed on TOBs 32X or 33X.

Pub 100-4, 32, 110.4 – Carrier and Intermediary Billing Instructions

(Rev. 597, Issued: 06-24-05, Effective: 04-27-05, Implementation: 08-01-05)

Effective for dates of service on or after April 27, 2005, contractors shall allow payment for ultrasonic osteogenic stimulators with the following current procedural terminology (CPT) code:

20979 Low intensity ultrasound stimulation to aid bone healing, noninvasive (nonoperative)

Pub 100-4, 32, 110.5 – DMERC Billing Instructions

(Rev. 816, Issued: 01-20-06, Effective: 04-27-05, Implementation: 04-03-06)

Effective for dates of service on or after April 27, 2005, DMERCs shall allow payment for ultrasonic osteogenic stimulators with the following HCPCS codes:

E0760 for low intensity ultrasound (include modifier "KF")
E1399 for other ultrasound stimulation (include modifier "KF")

Pub 100-4, 32, 130 – External Counterpulsation (ECP) Therapy

(Rev. 898, Issued: 03-31-06; Effective/Implementation Dates: 03-31-06)

Commonly referred to as enhanced external counterpulsation, is a non-invasive outpatient treatment for coronary artery disease refractory medical and/or surgical therapy. Effective for dates of service July 1, 1999, and after, Medicare will cover ECP when its use is in patients with stable angina (Class III or Class IV, Canadian Cardiovascular Society Classification or equivalent classification) who, in the opinion of a cardiologist or cardiothoracic surgeon, are not readily amenable to surgical intervention, such as PTCA or cardiac bypass, because:

- Their condition is inoperable, or at high risk of operative complications or postoperative failure
- Their coronary anatomy is not readily amenable to such procedures
- They have co-morbid states that create excessive risk.

(Refer to Publication 100-03, section 20.20 for further coverage criteria.)

Medicare References

Pub 100-4, 32, 130.1 – Billing and Payment Requirements

(Rev. 898, Issued: 03-31-06; Effective/Implementation Dates: 03-31-06)

Effective for dates of service on or after January 1, 2000, use HCPCS code G0166 (External counterpulsation, per session) to report ECP services. The codes for external cardiac assist (92971), ECG rhythm strip and report (93040 or 93041), pulse oximetry (94760 or 94761) and plethysmography (93922 or 93923) or other monitoring tests for examining the effects of this treatment are not clinically necessary with this service and should not be paid on the same day, unless they occur in a clinical setting not connected with the delivery of the ECP. Daily evaluation and management service, e.g., 99201- 99205, 99211-99215, 99217-99220, 99241-99245, cannot be billed with the ECP treatments. Any evaluation and management service must be justified with adequate documentation of the medical necessity of the visit. Deductible and coinsurance apply.

Pub 100-8, 5, 5.3 – Certificates of Medical Necessity (CMNs) and DME Information Forms (DIFs)

(Rev. 242: Issued: 02-22-08; Effective/Implementation Dates: 03-01-08)

A Certificate of Medical Necessity (CMN) (see Table 1) or a DME Information Form (DIF) (see Table 2) is a form required to help document the medical necessity and other coverage criteria for selected DMEPOS items. CMNs contain Sections A through D. Section A and C are completed by the supplier and Section B and D are completed by the physician. A DIF is completed and signed by the supplier. It does not require a narrative description of equipment and cost or a physician signature.

The following forms below have been approved by the Office of Management and Budget (OMB). For the CMS- 484 form, the OMB# is 0938-0534. For the CMS forms-846, 847, 848, 849, 854, 10125 and 10126, the OMB# is 0938-0679.

Table 1 identifies the CMNs. The forms below can be accessed at: http://www.cms.hhs.gov/CMSForms/CMSForms/list.asp#TopOfPage

Table 1

**Beginning January 1, 2007, the new TENS CMN is for purchases only. A TENS CMN will no longer be necessary for rentals.*

DME FORM	CMS FORM	ITEMS ADDRESSED
484.03	484	Oxygen
04.04B	846	Pneumatic Compression Devices
04.04C	847	Osteogenesis Stimulators
06.03B	848	Transcutaneous Electrical Nerve Stimulators
07.03A	849	Seat Lift Mechanisms
11.02	854	Section C Continuation Form

Table 2 identifies the DIFs. The forms below can be accessed at: http://www.cms.hhs.gov/CMSForms/CMSForms/list.asp#TopOfPage

Table 2

DME FORM	CMS FORM	ITEMS ADDRESSED
09.03	10125	External Infusion Pumps
10.03	10126	Enteral and Parenteral Nutrition

For certain items or services billed to a DME MAC, the supplier must receive a signed CMN from the treating physician or a signed DIF from the supplier. For these items, a supplier must have a signed original, faxed, photocopied, or electronic CMN or DIF in their records before they can submit a claim for payment to Medicare. CMNs or DIFs have a DME form number (e.g., 01, 02, 03) and a revision number (e.g., .01, .02). Some forms also have an alpha suffix (e.g., A, B, C).

All CMNs and DIFs have a CMS form number in addition to the DME form number. (See the following listing of form numbers.) The CMS form number is in the bottom left corner of the form. CMNs and DIFs are referred to by their CMS form numbers. DME form numbers identify the CMN on electronic claims submitted to the DME MAC. For example, CMS Form 484 serves as the CMN for oxygen; CMS Form 10125 serves as the DIF for External Infusion Pump.

A signed original, faxed, photocopied, or electronic CMN or DIF must be maintained by the supplier and be available to the DME MACs, DME PSCs, or ZPICs on request. When hardcopy CMNs or DIFs are submitted to the DME MACs, DME PSCs, or ZPICs, the supplier must include a copy of only the front side. When CMNs are submitted electronically to the DME MAC, information from sections A and B are required.

The CMN sent to the physician must be two-sided with instructions on the back. If the CMN is mailed to the physician, the supplier must send the two-sided form. If the CMN is faxed, the supplier must fax both the front and back of the form. It is in the supplier's interest to maintain a copy of what they faxed to the physician. Suppliers must maintain a copy of the completed CMN or DIF in their records. However, if the physician only faxes the front of the completed CMN then the supplier is only required to maintain the front portion of the CMN. The DIF must be two-sided with instructions on the back and completed by the supplier.

However, when the CMN or DIF is submitted electronically and the supplier chooses to maintain a hard copy CMN or DIF, the font may be modified as follows:

- Pitch may vary from 10 characters per inch (cpi) to 17.7 cpi;
- Line spacing must be 6 lines per inch
- Each form must have a minimum 1/4 inch margin on all four sides.

Without exception, these modified hard copy forms must contain identical questions/wording to the CMS forms, in the same sequence, with the same pagination, and identical instructions/definitions printed on the back; and CMN question sets may not be combined.

The CMN can serve as the physician's detailed written order if the narrative description in section C is sufficiently detailed. This would include quantities needed and frequency of replacement for accessories and supplies. For items requiring both a CMN and a written order prior to delivery (seat lift mechanisms and TENS units) suppliers may utilize a completed and physician-signed CMN for this purpose. Otherwise, a separate order in addition to a subsequently completed and signed CMN is necessary.

The supplier may not complete the information in section B of the CMN. A supplier who knowingly and willfully completes section B of the form is subject to a civil monetary penalty up to $1,000 for each form or document so distributed. Any supplier who remains in non-compliance after repeated attempts by the contractor to get the supplier into compliance, refer to your RO (for DME PSCs and ZPICs, refer the supplier to the primary GTL or associate GTL and SME) as a potential civil monetary penalty case.

The fee schedule amount, narrative description of the items furnished and the supplier's charge for the medical equipment or supplies being furnished must be completed on a CMN by the supplier prior to it being furnished to the physician. A supplier who knowingly and willfully fails to include this information may be subject to a civil monetary penalty up to $1,000 for each form or document so distributed. Any supplier who remains in non-compliance, after repeated attempts by the contractor to get the supplier into compliance, refer to your RO (for DME PSCs and ZPICs, refer the supplier to the primary GTL or associate GTL and SME) as a potential civil monetary penalty case.

Do not modify the language or content when reprinted. Also, do not accept any CMN or DIF that has been modified in any way by any other party. In addition, do not accept any other certifications of medical necessity by other insurers or government agencies.

Suppliers and physician may choose to utilize electronic CMNs (e-CMNs) or electronic DIFs (e-DIFs). E-CMNs or e-DIFS must adhere to all privacy, security, and electronic signature rules and regulations promulgated by CMS and DHHS. Additionally, e-CMNs or e-DIFs must contain identical questions/wording to the CMS forms, in the same sequence, with the same pagination, and identical instructions/definitions as printed on the back of the hardcopy form.

If an item requires a CMN or a DIF and the supplier does not have a faxed, photocopied, an original hardcopy, or an electronic signed CMN or DIF in their records before they submit a claim to Medicare, the claim will be denied. If the CMN or DIF is used to verify that statutory benefit requirements have been met, then the claim will be denied as not meeting the benefit category.

In cases where two or more suppliers merge, the resultant supplier should make all reasonable attempts to secure copies of all active CMNs or DIFs from the supplier(s) purchased. This document should be kept on file by the resultant supplier for future presentation to the DME MACs, DME PSCs, or ZPICs.

When reviewing claims where the medical record contains a copied, faxed or electronically maintained CMN or DIF (any CMN or DIF created, modified, and stored via electronic means such as commercially available software packages and servers), the DME MACs, DME PSCs, or ZPICs must accept the copied, faxed or electronic document as fulfilling the requirements for these documents.

When a DME PSCs and ZPICs are investigating potentially fraudulent behavior by a supplier, it will be the supplier's responsibility to prove the authenticity/validity of the claim(s) under investigation. DME PSCs and ZPICs may require the supplier to prove the authenticity/validity of the signature on the CMN, DIF, order, or any other questionable portion of the claim(s) under investigation.

Upon request by the MACs, DME PSCs, and ZPICs, suppliers must provide the CMN or DIF, in a format that the DME MACs, DME PSCs, and ZPICs can accept, in a timely manner. Upon medical review, the DME MACs, DME PSCs, and ZPICs should not deny claims solely because the CMN or DIF is faxed, copied, or electronic. The DME MACs, DME PSCs, or ZPICs may request the supplier to download and print a hard copy of an electronic order, CMN or DIF if the DME MACs, DME PSCs, or ZPICs cannot access it electronically.

For items that require a CMN, and for accessories, supplies, and drugs related to an item requiring a CMN, the CMN may serve as the written order if the narrative description in Section C is sufficiently detailed (as described above). This applies to both hard copy and electronic orders or CMNs. A DIF does not contain a section for a narrative description and is not applicable.

A supplier must have a hard copied, faxed or electronic order, CMN or DIF in their records before they can submit a claim for payment to Medicare. Suppliers must ensure the security and integrity of electronically maintained CMNs or DIFs are in accordance with any regulations published by CMS.

The DME MACs or DME PSCs need not make any shared system changes to electronically accept e-CMNs or DIFS as CMS views e-CMNs or DIFs as a transaction between the physician and suppliers. Suppliers must continue to use current systems for transmitting claim information to the DME MAC or DME PSC.

Social Security Act

PAYMENT OF BENEFITS

SEC. 1833. [42 U.S.C. 13951] (a)

Except as provided in section 1876, and subject to the succeeding provisions of this section, there shall be paid from the Federal Supplementary Medical Insurance Trust Fund, in the case of each individual who is covered under the insurance program established by this part and incurs expenses for services with respect to which benefits are payable under this part, amounts equal to—

1 In the case of services described in section 1832(a)(1)—80 percent of the reasonable charges for the services; except that (A) an organization which provides medical and other health services (or arranges for their availability) on a prepayment basis (and either is sponsored by a union or employer, or does not provide, or arrange for the provision of, any inpatient hospital services) may elect to be paid 80 percent of the reasonable cost of services for which payment may be made under this part on behalf of individuals enrolled in such organization in lieu of 80 percent of the reasonable charges for such services if the organization undertakes to charge such individuals no more than 20 percent of such reasonable cost plus any amounts payable by them as a result of subsection (b), (B) with respect to items and services described in section 1861(s)(10)(A), the amounts paid shall be 100 percent of the reasonable charges for such items and services, (C) with respect to expenses incurred for those physicians' services for which payment may be made under this part that are described in section 1862(a)(4), the prosthetic devices and orthotics and prosthetics (as defined in section 1834(h)(4)), the amounts paid shall be the amounts described in section 1834(h)(1), the amounts paid shall be subject to such limitations as may be prescribed by regulations, (D) with respect to clinical diagnostic laboratory tests for which payment is made under this part (i) on the basis of a fee schedule under subsection (h)(1) or section 1834(d)(1), the amount paid shall be equal to 80 percent (or 100 percent, in the case of such tests for which payment is made on an assignment-related basis) of the lesser of the amount determined under such fee schedule, the limitation amount for that test determined under subsection (h)(4)(B), or the amount of the charges billed for the tests, or (ii) on the basis of a negotiated rate established under subsection (h)(6), the amount paid shall be equal to 100 percent of such negotiated rate, (E) with respect to services furnished to individuals who have been determined to have end stage renal disease, the amounts paid shall be determined subject to the provisions of section 1881, (F) with respect to clinical social worker services under section 1861(s)(2)(N), the amounts paid shall be 80 percent of the lesser of (i) the actual charge for the services or (ii) 75 percent of the amount determined for payment of a psychologist under clause (L), [(G) Stricken.] (H) with respect to services of a certified registered nurse anesthetist under section 1861(s)(11), the amounts paid shall be 80 percent of the least of the actual charge, the prevailing charge that would be recognized (or, for services furnished on or after January 1, 1992, the fee schedule amount provided under section 1848) if the services had been performed by an anesthesiologist, or the fee schedule for such services established by the Secretary in accordance with subsection (1), (I) with respect to covered items (described in section 1834(a)(13)), the amounts paid shall be the amounts described in section 1834(a)(1), and (J) with respect to expenses incurred for radiologist services (as defined in section 1834(b)(6)), subject to section 1848, the amounts paid shall be 80 percent of the lesser of the actual charge for the services or the amount provided under the fee schedule established under section 1834(b), (K) with respect to certified nurse-midwife services under section 1861(s)(2)(L), the amounts paid shall be 80 percent of the lesser of the actual charge for the services or the amount determined by a fee schedule established by the Secretary for the purposes of this subparagraph (but in no event shall such fee schedule exceed 65 percent of the prevailing charge that would be allowed for the same service performed by a physician, or, for services furnished on or after January 1, 1992, 65 percent of the fee schedule amount provided under section 1848 for the same service performed by a physician), (L) with respect to qualified psychologist services under section 1861(s)(2)(M), the amounts paid shall be 80 percent of the lesser of the actual charge for the services or the amount determined by a fee schedule established by the Secretary for the purposes of this subparagraph, (M) with respect to prosthetic devices and orthotics and (N) with respect to expenses incurred for physicians' services (as defined in section 1848(j)(3)), the amounts paid shall be 80 percent of the payment basis determined under section 1848(a)(1), (O) with respect to services described in section 1861(s)(2)(K) (relating to services furnished by physicians assistants, nurse practitioners, or clinical nurse specialists), the amounts paid shall be equal to 80 percent of (i) the lesser of the actual charge or 85 percent of the fee schedule amount provided under section 1848, or (ii) in the case of services as an assistant at surgery, the lesser of the actual charge or 85 percent of the amount that would otherwise be recognized if performed by a physician who is serving as an assistant at surgery, (P) with respect to surgical dressings, the amounts paid shall be the amounts determined under section 1834(i), (Q) with respect to items or services for which fee schedules are established pursuant to section 1842(s), the amounts paid shall be 80 percent of the lesser of the actual charge or the fee schedule established in such section, (R) with respect to ambulance services, (i) the amounts paid shall be 80 percent of the lesser of the actual charge for the services or the amount determined by a fee schedule established by the Secretary under section 1834(l) and (ii) with respect to ambulance services described in section 1834(l)(8), the amounts paid shall be the amounts determined under section 1834(g) for outpatient critical access hospital services (S) with respect to drugs and biologicals not paid on a cost or prospective payment basis as otherwise provided in this part (other than items and services described in subparagraph (B)), the amounts paid shall be 80 percent of the lesser of the actual charge or the payment amount established in section 1842(o), (T) with respect to medical nutrition therapy services (as defined in section 1861(vv)), the amount paid shall be 80 percent of the lesser of the actual charge for the services or 85 percent of the amount determined under the fee schedule established under section 1848(b) for the same services if furnished by a physician, and (U) with respect to facility fees described in section 1834(m)(2)(B), the amounts paid shall be 80 percent of the lesser of the actual charge or the amounts specified in such section;

2 In the case of services described in section 1832(a)(2) (except those services described in subparagraphs (C), (D), (E), (F), (G), (H), and (I) of such section and unless otherwise specified in section 1881)—

A) with respect to home health services (other than a covered osteoporosis drug) (as defined in section 1861(kk)), the amount determined under the prospective payment system under section 1895;

(B) with respect to other items and services (except those described in subparagraph (C), (D), or (E) of this paragraph and except as may be provided in section 1886 or section 1888(e)(9))—

(i) furnished before January 1, 1999, the lesser of—

(I) the reasonable cost of such services, as determined under section 1861(v), or

(II) the customary charges with respect to such services, less the amount a provider may charge as described in clause (ii) of section 1866(a)(2)(A), but in no case may the payment for such other services exceed 80 percent of such reasonable cost, or

(ii) if such services are furnished before January 1, 1999, by a public provider of services, or by another provider which demonstrates to the satisfaction of the Secretary that a significant portion of its patients are low-income (and requests that payment be made under this clause), free of charge or at nominal charges to the public, 80 percent of the amount determined in accordance with section 1814(b)(2), or

(iii) if such services are furnished on or after January 1, 1999, the amount determined under subsection (t), or

(iv) if (and for so long as) the conditions described in section 1814(b)(3) are met, the amounts determined under the reimbursement system described in such section;

C) with respect to services described in the second sentence of section 1861(p), 80 percent of the reasonable charges for such services;

D) with respect to clinical diagnostic laboratory tests for which payment is made under this part (i) on the basis of a fee schedule determined under subsection (h)(1) or section 1834(d)(1), the amount paid shall be equal to 80 percent (or 100 percent, in the case of such tests for which payment is made on an assignment-related basis or to a provider having an agreement under section 1866 of the lesser of the amount determined under such fee schedule, the limitation amount for that test determined under subsection (h)(4)(B), or the amount of the charges billed for the tests, or (ii) on the basis of a negotiated rate established under subsection (h)(6), the amount paid shall be equal to 100 percent of such negotiated rate for such tests;

E) with respect to—

(i) outpatient hospital radiology services (including diagnostic and therapeutic radiology, nuclear medicine and CAT scan procedures, magnetic resonance imaging, and ultrasound and other imaging services, but excluding screening mammography), and

(ii) effective for procedures performed on or after October 1, 1989, diagnostic procedures (as defined by the Secretary) described in section 1861(s)(3) (other than diagnostic x-ray tests and diagnostic laboratory tests), the amount determined under subsection (n) or, for services or procedures performed on or after January 1, 1999, subsection (t);

F) with respect to a covered osteoporosis drug (as defined in section 1861(kk)) furnished by a home health agency, 80 percent of the reasonable cost of such service, as determined under section 1861(v); and

G) with respect to items and services described in section 1861(s)(10)(A), the lesser of—

(i) the reasonable cost of such services, as determined under section 1861(v), or

(ii) the customary charges with respect to such services, or, if such services are furnished by a public provider of services, or by another provider which demonstrates to the satisfaction of the Secretary that a significant portion of its patients are low-income (and requests that payment be made under this provision), free of charge or at nominal charges to the public, the amount determined in accordance with section 1814(b)(2);

3 in the case of services described in section 1832(a)(2)(D), the costs which are reasonable and related to the cost of furnishing such services or which are based on such other tests of reasonableness as the Secretary may prescribe in regulations, including those authorized under section 1861(v)(1)(A), less the amount a provider may charge as described in clause (ii) of section 1866(a)(2)(A), but in no case may the payment for such services (other than for items and services described in section 1861(s)(10)(A)) exceed 80 percent of such costs;

4 in the case of facility services described in section 1832(a)(2)(F), and outpatient hospital facility services furnished in connection with surgical procedures specified by the Secretary pursuant to section 1833(i)(1)(A), the applicable amount as determined under paragraph (2) or (3) of subsection (i) or subsection (t);

5 in the case of covered items (described in section 1834(a)(13)) the amounts described in section 1834(a)(1);

6 in the case of outpatient critical access hospital services, the amounts described in section 1834(g);

7 in the case of prosthetic devices and orthotics and prosthetics (as described in section 1834(h)(4)), the amounts described in section 1834(h);

8 in the case of—

A) outpatient physical therapy services (which includes outpatient speech-language pathology services) and outpatient occupational therapy services furnished—

(i) by a rehabilitation agency, public health agency, clinic, comprehensive outpatient rehabilitation facility, or skilled nursing facility,

(ii) by a home health agency to an individual who is not homebound, or

(iii) by another entity under an arrangement with an entity described in clause (i) or (ii); and

B) outpatient physical therapy services (which includes outpatient speech-language pathology services) and outpatient occupational therapy services furnished—

(i) by a hospital to an outpatient or to a hospital inpatient who is entitled to benefits under part A but has exhausted benefits for inpatient hospital services during a spell of illness or is not so entitled to benefits under part A, or

(ii) by another entity under an arrangement with a hospital described in clause (i), the amounts described in section 1834(k); and

9 in the case of services described in section 1832(a)(2)(E) that are not described in paragraph (8), the amounts described in section 1834(k).

Prospective Payment System for Hospital Outpatient Department Services

Section 1833(t)

1 AMOUNT OF PAYMENT:

A) IN GENERAL:With respect to covered OPD services (as defined in subparagraph (B)) furnished during a year beginning with 1999, the amount of payment under this part shall be determined under a prospective payment system established by the Secretary in accordance with this subsection.

B) DEFINITION OF COVERED OPD SERVICES:For purposes of this subsection, the term "covered OPD services"—

(i) means hospital outpatient services designated by the Secretary;

(ii) subject to clause (iv), includes inpatient hospital services designated by the Secretary that are covered under this part and furnished to a hospital inpatient who (I) is entitled to benefits under part A but has exhausted benefits for inpatient hospital services during a spell of illness, or (II) is not so entitled;

(iii) includes implantable items described in paragraph (3), (6), or (8) of section 1861(s) ; but

(iv) does not include any therapy services described in subsection (a)(8) or ambulance services, for which payment is made under a fee schedule described in section 1834(k) or section 1834(l) .

2 SYSTEM REQUIREMENTS:Under the payment system—

A) the Secretary shall develop a classification system for covered OPD services;

B) the Secretary may establish groups of covered OPD services, within the classification system described in subparagraph (A), so that services classified within each group are comparable clinically and with respect to the use of resources and so that an implantable item is classified to the group that includes the service to which the item relates;

C) the Secretary shall, using data on claims from 1996 and using data from the most recent available cost reports, establish relative payment weights for covered OPD services (and any groups of such services described in subparagraph (B)) based on median (or, at the election of the Secretary, mean) hospital costs and shall determine projections of the frequency of utilization of each such service (or group of services) in 1999;

D) the Secretary shall determine a wage adjustment factor to adjust the portion of payment and coinsurance attributable to labor-related costs for relative differences in labor and labor-related costs across geographic regions in a budget neutral manner;

E) the Secretary shall establish, in a budget neutral manner, outlier adjustments under paragraph (5) and transitional pass-through payments under paragraph (6) and other adjustments as determined to be necessary to ensure equitable payments, such as adjustments for certain classes of hospitals;

F) the Secretary shall develop a method for controlling unnecessary increases in the volume of covered OPD services;

G) the Secretary shall create additional groups of covered OPD services that classify separately those procedures that utilize contrast agents from those that do not; and

H) with respect to devices of brachytherapy consisting of a seed or seeds (or radioactive source), the Secretary shall create additional groups of covered OPD services that classify such devices separately from the other services (or group of services) paid for under this subsection in a manner reflecting the number, isotope, and radioactive intensity of such devices furnished, including separate groups for palladium-103 and iodine-125 devices.".

For purposes of subparagraph (B), items and services within a group shall not be treated as "comparable with respect to the use of resources" if the highest median cost (or mean cost, if elected by the Secretary under subparagraph (C)) for an item or service within the group is more than 2 times greater than the lowest median cost (or mean cost, if so elected) for an item or service within the group; except that the Secretary may make exceptions in unusual cases, such as low volume items and services, but may not make such an exception in the case of a drug or biological that has been designated as an orphan drug under section 526 of the Federal Food, Drug and Cosmetic Act.

3 CALCULATION OF BASE AMOUNTS:

A) AGGREGATE AMOUNTS THAT WOULD BE PAYABLE IF DEDUCTIBLES WERE DISREGARDED: The Secretary shall estimate the sum of—

(i) the total amounts that would be payable from the Trust Fund under this part for covered OPD services in 1999, determined without regard to this subsection, as though the deductible under section 1833(b) did not apply, and

(ii) the total amounts of copayments estimated to be paid under this subsection by beneficiaries to hospitals for covered OPD services in 1999, as though the deductible under section 1833(b) did not apply.

B) UNADJUSTED COPAYMENT AMOUNT:

(i) IN GENERAL: For purposes of this subsection, subject to clause (ii), the "unadjusted copayment amount" applicable to a covered OPD service (or group of such services) is 20 percent of the national median of the charges for the service (or services within the group) furnished during 1996, updated to 1999 using the Secretary's estimate of charge growth during the period.

(ii) ADJUSTED TO BE 20 PERCENT WHEN FULLY PHASED IN: If the pre-deductible payment percentage for a covered OPD service (or group of such services) furnished in a year would be equal to or exceed 80 percent, then the unadjusted copayment amount shall be 20 percent of amount determined under subparagraph (D).

(iii) RULES FOR NEW SERVICES: The Secretary shall establish rules for establishment of an unadjusted copayment amount for a covered OPD service not furnished during 1996, based upon its classification within a group of such services.

C) CALCULATION OF CONVERSION FACTORS:

(i) FOR 1999:

(I) IN GENERAL: The Secretary shall establish a 1999 conversion factor for determining the medicare OPD fee schedule amounts for each covered OPD service (or group of such services) furnished in 1999. Such conversion factor shall be established on the basis of the weights and frequencies described in paragraph (2)(C) and in such a manner that the sum for all services and groups of the products (described in subclause (II) for each such service or group) equals the total projected amount described in subparagraph (A).

(II) PRODUCT DESCRIBED: The Secretary shall determine for each service or group the product of the medicare OPD fee schedule amounts (taking into account appropriate adjustments described in paragraphs (2)(D) and (2)(E)) and the estimated frequencies for such service or group.

(ii) SUBSEQUENT YEARS: Subject to paragraph (8)(B), the Secretary shall establish a conversion factor for covered OPD services furnished in subsequent years in an amount equal to the conversion factor established under this subparagraph and applicable to such services furnished in the previous year increased by the OPD fee schedule increase factor specified under clause (iii) for the year involved.

(iii) ADJUSTMENT FOR SERVICE MIX CHANGES: Insofar as the Secretary determines that the adjustments for service mix under paragraph (2) for a previous year (or estimates that such adjustments for a future year) did (or are likely to) result in a change in aggregate payments under this subsection during the year that are a result of changes in the coding or classification of covered OPD services that do not reflect real changes in service mix, the Secretary may adjust the conversion factor computed under this subparagraph for subsequent years so as to eliminate the effect of such coding or classification changes.

(iv) OPD FEE SCHEDULE INCREASE FACTOR: For purposes of this subparagraph, the "OPD fee schedule increase factor" for services furnished in a year is equal to the market basket percentage increase applicable under section 1886(b)(3)(B)(iii) to hospital discharges occurring during the fiscal year ending in such year, reduced by 1 percentage point for such factor for services furnished in each of 2000 and 2002. In applying the previous sentence for years beginning with 2000, the Secretary may substitute for the market basket percentage increase an annual percentage increase that is computed and applied with respect to covered OPD services furnished in a year in the same manner as the market basket percentage increase is determined and applied to inpatient hospital services for discharges occurring in a fiscal year.

D) CALCULATION OF MEDICARE OPD FEE SCHEDULE AMOUNTS: The Secretary shall compute a medicare OPD fee schedule amount for each covered OPD service (or group of such services) furnished in a year, in an amount equal to the product of—

(i) the conversion factor computed under subparagraph (C) for the year, and

(ii) the relative payment weight (determined under paragraph (2)(C)) for the service or group.

E) PRE-DEDUCTIBLE PAYMENT PERCENTAGE: The pre-deductible payment percentage for a covered OPD service (or group of such services) furnished in a year is equal to the ratio of—

(i) the medicare OPD fee schedule amount established under subparagraph (D) for the year, minus the unadjusted copayment amount determined under subparagraph (B) for the service or group, to

(ii) the medicare OPD fee schedule amount determined under subparagraph (D) for the year for such service or group.

4 MEDICARE PAYMENT AMOUNT: The amount of payment made from the Trust Fund under this part for a covered OPD service (and such services classified within a group) furnished in a year is determined, subject to paragraph (7) as follows:

A) FEE SCHEDULE ADJUSTMENTS: The medicare OPD fee schedule amount (computed under paragraph (3)(D)) for the service or group and year is adjusted for relative differences in the cost of labor and other factors determined by the Secretary, as computed under paragraphs (2)(D) and (2)(E).

B) SUBTRACT APPLICABLE DEDUCTIBLE: Reduce the adjusted amount determined under subparagraph (A) by the amount of the deductible under section 1833(b) , to the extent applicable.

C) APPLY PAYMENT PROPORTION TO REMAINDER: The amount of payment is the amount so determined under subparagraph (B) multiplied by the pre-deductible payment percentage (as determined under paragraph (3)(E)) for the service or group and year involved, plus the amount of any reduction in the copayment amount attributable to paragraph (8)(C).

5 OUTLIER ADJUSTMENT:

A) IN GENERAL: Subject to subparagraph (D), the Secretary shall provide for an additional payment for each covered OPD

Medicare References

service (or group of services) for which a hospital's charges, adjusted to cost, exceed—

(i) a fixed multiple of the sum of—

(I) the applicable medicare OPD fee schedule amount determined under paragraph (3)(D), as adjusted under paragraph (4)(A) (other than for adjustments under this paragraph or paragraph (6)); and

(II) any transitional pass-through payment under paragraph (6); and

(ii) at the option of the Secretary, such fixed dollar amount as the Secretary may establish.

B) AMOUNT OF ADJUSTMENT: The amount of the additional payment under subparagraph (A) shall be determined by the Secretary and shall approximate the marginal cost of care beyond the applicable cutoff point under such subparagraph.

C) LIMIT ON AGGREGATE OUTLIER ADJUSTMENTS:

(i) IN GENERAL: The total of the additional payments made under this paragraph for covered OPD services furnished in a year (as estimated by the Secretary before the beginning of the year) may not exceed the applicable percentage (specified in clause (ii)) of the total program payments estimated to be made under this subsection for all covered OPD services furnished in that year. If this paragraph is first applied to less than a full year, the previous sentence shall apply only to the portion of such year.

(ii) APPLICABLE PERCENTAGE: For purposes of clause (i), the term "applicable percentage" means a percentage specified by the Secretary up to (but not to exceed)—

(I) for a year (or portion of a year) before 2004, 2.5 percent; and

(II) for 2004 and thereafter, 3.0 percent.

D) TRANSITIONAL AUTHORITY: In applying subparagraph (A) for covered OPD services furnished before January 1, 2002, the Secretary may—

(i) apply such subparagraph to a bill for such services related to an outpatient encounter (rather than for a specific service or group of services) using OPD fee schedule amounts and transitional pass-through payments covered under the bill; and

(ii) use an appropriate cost-to-charge ratio for the hospital involved (as determined by the Secretary), rather than for specific departments within the hospital.

E) EXCLUSION OF SEPARATE DRUG AND BIOLOGICAL APCS FROM OUTLIER PAYMENTS.—No additional payment shall be made under subparagraph (A) in the case of ambulatory payment classification groups established separately for drugs or biologicals.".

6 TRANSITIONAL PASS-THROUGH FOR ADDITIONAL COSTS OF INNOVATIVE MEDICAL DEVICES, DRUGS, AND BIOLOGICALS:

A) IN GENERAL: The Secretary shall provide for an additional payment under this paragraph for any of the following that are provided as part of a covered OPD service (or group of services):

(i) CURRENT ORPHAN DRUGS: A drug or biological that is used for a rare disease or condition with respect to which the drug or biological has been designated as an orphan drug under section 526 of the Federal Food, Drug and Cosmetic Act if payment for the drug or biological as an outpatient hospital service under this part was being made on the first date that the system under this subsection is implemented.

(ii) CURRENT CANCER THERAPY DRUGS AND BIOLOGICALS AND BRACHYTHERAPY: A drug or biological that is used in cancer therapy, including (but not limited to) a chemotherapeutic agent, an antiemetic, a hematopoietic growth factor, a colony stimulating factor, a biological response modifier, a bisphosphonate, and a device of brachytherapy or temperature monitored cryoablation, if payment for such drug, biological, or device as an outpatient hospital service under this part was being made on such first date.

(iii) CURRENT RADIOPHARMACEUTICAL DRUGS AND BIOLOGICAL PRODUCTS: A radiopharmaceutical drug or biological product used in diagnostic, monitoring, and therapeutic nuclear medicine procedures if payment for the drug or biological as an outpatient hospital service under this part was being made on such first date.

(iv) NEW MEDICAL DEVICES, DRUGS, AND BIOLOGICALS: A medical device, drug, or biological not described in clause (i), (ii), or (iii) if—

(I) payment for the device, drug, or biological as an outpatient hospital service under this part was not being made as of December 31, 1996; and

(II) the cost of the drug or biological or the average cost of the category of devices is not insignificant in relation to the OPD fee schedule amount (as calculated under paragraph (3)(D)) payable for the service (or group of services) involved.

B) USE OF CATEGORIES IN DETERMINING ELIGIBILITY OF A DEVICE FOR PASS-THROUGH PAYMENTS [82]: The following provisions apply for purposes of determining whether a medical device qualifies for additional payments under clause (ii) or (iv) of subparagraph (A):

(i) ESTABLISHMENT OF INITIAL CATEGORIES:

(I) IN GENERAL: The Secretary shall initially establish under this clause categories of medical devices based on type of device by April 1, 2001. Such categories shall be established in a manner such that each medical device that meets the requirements of clause (ii) or (iv) of subparagraph (A) as of January 1, 2001, is included in such a category and no such device is included in more than one category. For purposes of the preceding sentence, whether a medical device meets such requirements as of such date shall be determined on the basis of the program memoranda issued before such date.

(II) AUTHORIZATION OF IMPLEMENTATION OTHER THAN THROUGH REGULATIONS: The categories may be established under this clause by program memorandum or otherwise, after consultation with groups representing hospitals, manufacturers of medical devices, and other affected parties.

(ii) ESTABLISHING CRITERIA FOR ADDITIONAL CATEGORIES:

(I) IN GENERAL: The Secretary shall establish criteria that will be used for creation of additional categories (other than those established under clause (i)) through rulemaking (which may include use of an interim final rule with comment period).

(II) STANDARD: Such categories shall be established under this clause in a manner such that no medical device is described by more than one category. Such criteria shall include a test of whether the average cost of devices that would be included in a category and are in use at the time the category is established is not insignificant, as described in subparagraph (A)(iv)(II).

(III) DEADLINE: Criteria shall first be established under this clause by July 1, 2001. The Secretary may establish in compelling circumstances categories under this clause before the date such criteria are established.

(IV) ADDING CATEGORIES: The Secretary shall promptly establish a new category of medical devices under this clause for any medical device that meets the requirements of subparagraph (A)(iv) and for which none of the categories in effect (or that were previously in effect) is appropriate.

(iii) PERIOD FOR WHICH CATEGORY IS IN EFFECT: A category of medical devices established under clause (i) or (ii) shall be in effect for a period of at least 2 years, but not more than 3 years, that begins—

(I) in the case of a category established under clause

(i), on the first date on which payment was made under this paragraph for any device described by such category (including payments made during the period before April 1, 2001); and

(II) in the case of any other category, on the first date on which payment is made under this paragraph for any medical device that is described by such category.

(iv) REQUIREMENTS TREATED AS MET: A medical device shall be treated as meeting the requirements of subparagraph (A)(iv), regardless of whether the device meets the requirement of subclause (I) of such subparagraph, if—

(I) the device is described by a category established and in effect under clause (i); or

(II) the device is described by a category established and in effect under clause (ii) and an application under section 515 of the Federal Food, Drug, and Cosmetic Act has been approved with respect to the device, or the device has been cleared for market under section 510(k) of such Act, or the device is exempt from the requirements of section 510(k) of such Act pursuant to subsection (l) or (m) of section 510 of such Act or section 520(g) of such Act.

Nothing in this clause shall be construed as requiring an application or prior approval (other than that described in subclause (II)) in order for a covered device described by a category to qualify for payment under this paragraph.

C) LIMITED PERIOD OF PAYMENT:

(i) DRUGS AND BIOLOGICALS: The payment under this paragraph with respect to a drug or biological shall only apply during a period of at least 2 years, but not more than 3 years, that begins

(I) on the first date this subsection is implemented in the case of a drug or biological described in clause (i), (ii), or (iii) of subparagraph (A) and in the case of a drug or biological described in subparagraph (A)(iv) and for which payment under this part is made as an outpatient hospital service before such first date; or

(II) in the case of a drug or biological described in subparagraph (A)(iv) not described in subclause (I), on the first date on which payment is made under this part for the drug or biological as an outpatient hospital service.

(ii) MEDICAL DEVICES: Payment shall be made under this paragraph with respect to a medical device only if such device—

(I) is described by a category of medical devices established and in effect under subparagraph (B); and

(II) is provided as part of a service (or group of services) paid for under this subsection and provided during the period for which such category is in effect under such subparagraph.

D) AMOUNT OF ADDITIONAL PAYMENT: Subject to subparagraph (E)(iii), the amount of the payment under this paragraph with respect to a device, drug, or biological provided as part of a covered OPD service is—

(i) in the case of a drug or biological, the amount by which the amount determined under section 1842(o) (or if the drug or biological is covered under a competitive acquisition contract under section 1847B, an amount determined by the Secretary equal to the average price for the drug or biological for all competitive acquisition areas and year established under such section as calculated and adjusted by the Secretary for purposes of this paragraph) for the drug or biological exceeds the portion of the otherwise applicable medicare OPD fee schedule that the Secretary determines is associated with the drug or biological; or

(ii) in the case of a medical device, the amount by which the hospital's charges for the device, adjusted to cost, exceeds the portion of the otherwise applicable medicare OPD fee schedule that the Secretary determines is associated with the device.

E) LIMIT ON AGGREGATE ANNUAL ADJUSTMENT:

(i) IN GENERAL: The total of the additional payments made under this paragraph for covered OPD services furnished in a year (as estimated by the Secretary before the beginning of the year) may not exceed the applicable percentage (specified in clause (ii)) of the total program payments estimated to be made under this subsection for all covered OPD services furnished in that year. If this paragraph is first applied to less than a full year, the previous sentence shall apply only to the portion of such year.

(ii) APPLICABLE PERCENTAGE: For purposes of clause (i), the term "applicable percentage" means—

(I) for a year (or portion of a year) before 2004, 2.5 percent; and

(II) for 2004 and thereafter, a percentage specified by the Secretary up to (but not to exceed) 2.0 percent.

(iii) UNIFORM PROSPECTIVE REDUCTION IF AGGREGATE LIMIT PROJECTED TO BE EXCEEDED: If the Secretary estimates before the beginning of a year that the amount of the additional payments under this paragraph for the year (or portion thereof) as determined under clause (i) without regard to this clause will exceed the limit established under such clause, the Secretary shall reduce pro rata the amount of each of the additional payments under this paragraph for that year (or portion thereof) in order to ensure that the aggregate additional payments under this paragraph (as so estimated) do not exceed such limit.

7 TRANSITIONAL ADJUSTMENT TO LIMIT DECLINE IN PAYMENT:

A) BEFORE 2002: Subject to subparagraph (D), for covered OPD services furnished before January 1, 2002, for which the PPS amount (as defined in subparagraph (E)) is—

(i) at least 90 percent, but less than 100 percent, of the pre-BBA amount (as defined in subparagraph (F)), the amount of payment under this subsection shall be increased by 80 percent of the amount of such difference;

(ii) at least 80 percent, but less than 90 percent, of the pre-BBA amount, the amount of payment under this subsection shall be increased by the amount by which (I) the product of 0.71 and the pre-BBA amount, exceeds (II) the product of 0.70 and the PPS amount;

(iii) at least 70 percent, but less than 80 percent, of the pre-BBA amount, the amount of payment under this subsection shall be increased by the amount by which (I) the product of 0.63 and the pre-BBA amount, exceeds (II) the product of 0.60 and the PPS amount; or

(iv) less than 70 percent of the pre-BBA amount, the amount of payment under this subsection shall be increased by 21 percent of the pre-BBA amount.

B) 2002: Subject to subparagraph (D), for covered OPD services furnished during 2002, for which the PPS amount is—

(i) at least 90 percent, but less than 100 percent, of the pre-BBA amount, the amount of payment under this subsection shall be increased by 70 percent of the amount of such difference;

(ii) at least 80 percent, but less than 90 percent, of the pre-BBA amount, the amount of payment under this subsection shall be increased by the amount by which (I) the product of 0.61 and the pre-BBA amount, exceeds (II) the product of 0.60 and the PPS amount; or

(iii) less than 80 percent of the pre-BBA amount, the amount of payment under this subsection shall be increased by 13 percent of the pre-BBA amount.

C) 2003: Subject to subparagraph (D), for covered OPD services furnished during 2003, for which the PPS amount is—

(i) at least 90 percent, but less than 100 percent, of the pre-BBA amount, the amount of payment under this subsection shall be increased by 60 percent of the amount of such difference; or

(ii) less than 90 percent of the pre-BBA amount, the amount of payment under this subsection shall be increased by 6 percent of the pre-BBA amount.

D) HOLD HARMLESS PROVISIONS:

(i) TEMPORARY TREATMENT FOR SMALL RURAL HOSPITALS: In the case of a hospital located in a rural area and that has not more than 100 beds, for covered OPD services furnished before January 1, 2004, for which the PPS amount is less than the pre-BBA amount, the amount of payment under this subsection shall be increased by the amount of such difference.

(ii) PERMANENT TREATMENT FOR CANCER HOSPITALS AND CHILDREN'S HOSPITALS: In the case of a hospital described in section clause (iii) or (v) of 1886(d)(1)(B), for covered OPD services for which the PPS amount is less than the pre-BBA amount, the amount of payment under this subsection shall be increased by the amount of such difference.

E) PPS amount defined.—In this paragraph, the term "PPS amount" means, with respect to covered OPD services, the amount payable under this title for such services (determined without regard to this paragraph), including amounts payable as copayment under paragraph (8), coinsurance under section 1866(a)(2)(A)(ii) , and the deductible under section 1833(b)

F) PRE-BBA AMOUNT DEFINED:

(i) IN GENERAL: In this paragraph, the "pre-BBA amount" means, with respect to covered OPD services furnished by a hospital in a year, an amount equal to the product of the reasonable cost of the hospital for such services for the portions of the hospital's cost reporting period (or periods) occurring in the year and the base OPD payment-to-cost ratio for the hospital (as defined in clause (ii)).

(ii) BASE PAYMENT-TO-COST-RATIO DEFINED: For purposes of this subparagraph, the "base payment-to-cost ratio" for a hospital means the ratio of—

(I) the hospital's reimbursement under this part for covered OPD services furnished during the cost reporting period ending in 1996 (or in the case of a hospital that did not submit a cost report for such period, during the first subsequent cost reporting period ending before 2001 for which the hospital submitted a cost report), including any reimbursement for such services through cost-sharing described in subparagraph (E), to (II) the reasonable cost of such services for such period.

The Secretary shall determine such ratios as if the amendments made by 4521 of the Balanced Budget Act of 1997 were in effect in 1996.

(G) INTERIM PAYMENTS: The Secretary shall make payments under this paragraph to hospitals on an interim basis, subject to retrospective adjustments based on settled cost reports.

(H) NO EFFECT ON COPAYMENTS: Nothing in this paragraph shall be construed to affect the unadjusted copayment amount described in paragraph (3)(B) or the copayment amount under paragraph (8).

(I) APPLICATION WITHOUT REGARD TO BUDGET NEUTRALITY: The additional payments made under this paragraph

(i) shall not be considered an adjustment under paragraph (2)(E); and

(ii) shall not be implemented in a budget neutral manner.

8 COPAYMENT AMOUNT [83]:

A) IN GENERAL: Except as provided in subparagraphs (B) and (C), the copayment amount under this subsection is the amount by which the amount described in paragraph (4)(B) exceeds the amount of payment determined under paragraph (4)(C).

B) ELECTION TO OFFER REDUCED COPAYMENT AMOUNT: The Secretary shall establish a procedure under which a hospital, before the beginning of a year (beginning with 1999), may elect to reduce the copayment amount otherwise established under subparagraph (A) for some or all covered OPD services to an amount that is not less than 20 percent of the medicare OPD fee schedule amount (computed under paragraph (3)(D)) for the service involved. Under such procedures, such reduced copayment amount may not be further reduced or increased during the year involved and the hospital may disseminate information on the reduction of copayment amount effected under this subparagraph.

C) LIMITATION ON COPAYMENT AMOUNT:

(i) TO INPATIENT HOSPITAL DEDUCTIBLE AMOUNT: In no case shall the copayment amount for a procedure performed in a year exceed the amount of the inpatient hospital deductible established under section 1813(b) for that year.

(ii) TO SPECIFIED PERCENTAGE: The Secretary shall reduce the national unadjusted copayment amount for a covered OPD service (or group of such services) furnished in a year in a manner so that the effective copayment rate (determined on a national unadjusted basis) for that service in the year does not exceed the following percentage:

(I) For procedures performed in 2001, on or after April 1, 2001, 57 percent.

(II) For procedures performed in 2002 or 2003, 55 percent.

(III)For procedures performed in 2004, 50 percent.

(IV) For procedures performed in 2005, 45 percent.

(V) For procedures performed in 2006 and thereafter, 40 percent.

D) NO IMPACT ON DEDUCTIBLES: Nothing in this paragraph shall be construed as affecting a hospital's authority to waive the charging of a deductible under section 1833(b) .

E) COMPUTATION IGNORING OUTLIER AND PASS-THROUGH ADJUSTMENTS: The copayment amount shall be computed under subparagraph (A) as if the adjustments under paragraphs (5) and (6) (and any adjustment made under paragraph (2)(E) in relation to such adjustments) had not occurred.

9 PERIODIC REVIEW AND ADJUSTMENTS COMPONENTS OF PROSPECTIVE PAYMENT SYSTEM:

A) PERIODIC REVIEW: The Secretary shall review not less often than annually and revise the groups, the relative payment weights, and the wage and other adjustments described in paragraph (2) to take into account changes in medical practice, changes in technology, the addition of new services, new cost data, and other relevant information and factors. The Secretary shall consult with an expert outside advisory panel composed of an appropriate selection of representatives of providers to review (and advise the Secretary concerning) the clinical integrity of the groups and weights. Such panel may use data collected or developed by entities and organizations (other than the Department of Health and Human Services) in conducting such review.

B) BUDGET NEUTRALITY ADJUSTMENT: If the Secretary makes adjustments under subparagraph (A), then the adjustments for a year may not cause the estimated amount of expenditures under this part for the year to increase or decrease from the estimated amount of expenditures under this part that would have been made if the adjustments had not been made. In determining adjustments under the preceding sentence for 2004 and 2005, the Secretary shall not take into account under this subpara-graph or paragraph (2)(E) any expenditures that would not have been made but for the application of paragraph (14).

C) UPDATE FACTOR: If the Secretary determines under methodologies described in paragraph (2)(F) that the volume of services paid for under this subsection increased beyond amounts established through those methodologies, the Secretary may appropriately adjust the update to the conversion factor otherwise applicable in a subsequent year.

10 SPECIAL RULE FOR AMBULANCE SERVICES: The Secretary shall pay for hospital outpatient services that are ambulance services on the basis described in section 1861(v)(1)(U) , or, if applicable, the fee schedule established under section 1834(l) .

11 SPECIAL RULES FOR CERTAIN HOSPITALS: In the case of hospitals described in clause (iii) or (v) of section 1886(d)(1)(B)

A) the system under this subsection shall not apply to covered OPD services furnished before January 1, 2000; and

B) the Secretary may establish a separate conversion factor for such services in a manner that specifically takes into account the unique costs incurred by such hospitals by virtue of their patient population and service intensity.

12 LIMITATION ON REVIEW: There shall be no administrative or judicial review under section 1869 , 1878, or otherwise of—

A) the development of the classification system under paragraph (2), including the establishment of groups and relative payment weights for covered OPD services, of wage adjustment factors, other adjustments, and methods described in paragraph (2)(F);

B) the calculation of base amounts under paragraph (3);

C) periodic adjustments made under paragraph (6);

D) the establishment of a separate conversion factor under paragraph (8)(B); and

E) the determination of the fixed multiple, or a fixed dollar cutoff amount, the marginal cost of care, or applicable percentage under paragraph (5) or the determination of insignificance of cost, the duration of the additional payments, the determination and deletion of initial and new categories (consistent with subparagraphs (B) and (C) of paragraph (6)), the portion of the medicare OPD fee schedule amount associated with particular devices, drugs, or biologicals, and the application of any pro rata reduction under paragraph (6).

13 MISCELLANEOUS PROVISIONS:

A) APPLICATION OF RECLASSIFICATION OF CERTAIN HOSPITALS: If a hospital is being treated as being located in a rural area under section 1886(d)(8)(E) , that hospital shall be treated under this subsection as being located in that rural area.

14 DRUG APC PAYMENT RATES

A) IN GENERAL.—The amount of payment under this subsection for a specified covered outpatient drug (defined in subparagraph (B)) that is furnished as part of a covered OPD service (or group of services)

(i) in 2004, in the case of

(I) a sole source drug shall in no case be less than 88 percent, or exceed 95 percent, of the reference average wholesale price for the drug;

(II) an innovator multiple source drug shall in no case exceed 68 percent of the reference average wholesale price for the drug; or

(III)a noninnovator multiple source drug shall in no case exceed 46 percent of the reference average wholesale price for the drug;

(ii) in 2005, in the case of—

(I) a sole source drug shall in no case be less than 83 percent, or exceed 95 percent, of the reference average wholesale price for the drug;

(II) an innovator multiple source drug shall in no case exceed 68 percent of the reference aver-age wholesale price for the drug; or

(III) a noninnovator multiple source drug shall in no case exceed 46 percent of the reference average wholesale price for the drug; or

(iii) in a subsequent year, shall be equal, subject to subparagraph (E)—

(I) to the average acquisition cost for the drug for that year (which, at the option of the Secretary, may vary by hospital group (as defined by the Secretary based on volume of covered OPD services or other relevant characteristics)), as determined by the Secretary taking into account the hospital acquisition cost survey data under subparagraph (D); or

(II) if hospital acquisition cost data are not available, the average price for the drug in the year established under section 1842(o), section 1847A, or section 1847B, as the case may be, as calculated and adjusted by the Secretary as necessary for purposes of this paragraph.

B) SPECIFIED COVERED OUTPATIENT DRUG DEFINED

(i) IN GENERAL.—In this paragraph, the term 'specified covered outpatient drug' means, subject to clause (ii), a covered outpatient drug (as defined in section 1927(k)(2)) for which a separate ambulatory payment classification group (APC) has been established and that is

(I) a radiopharmaceutical; or

(II) a drug or biological for which payment was made under paragraph (6) (relating to pass-through payments) on or before December 31, 2002.

(ii) EXCEPTION.—Such term does not include

(I) a drug or biological for which payment is first made on or after January 1, 2003, under paragraph (6);

(II) a drug or biological for which a temporary HCPCS code has not been assigned; or

(III)during 2004 and 2005, an orphan drug (as designated by the Secretary).

C) PAYMENT FOR DESIGNATED ORPHAN DRUGS DURING 2004 AND 2005.—The amount of payment under this sub-section for an orphan drug designated by the Secretary under subparagraph (B)(ii)(III) that is furnished as part of a covered OPD service (or group of services) during 2004 and 2005 shall equal such amount as the Secretary may specify.

(D) ACQUISITION COST SURVEY FOR HOSPITAL OUTPATIENT DRUGS.

(i) ANNUAL GAO SURVEYS IN 2004 AND 2005

(I) IN GENERAL – The Comptroller General of the United States shall conduct a survey in each of 2004 and 2005 to determine the hospital acquisition cost for each specified covered outpatient drug. Not later than April 1, 2005, the Comptroller General shall furnish data from such surveys to the Secretary for use in setting the payment rates under subparagraph (A) for 2006.

(II) RECOMMENDATIONS.—Upon the completion of such surveys, the Comptroller General shall recommend to the Secretary the frequency and methodology of subsequent surveys to be conducted by the Secretary under clause (ii).

(ii) SUBSEQUENT SECRETARIAL SURVEYS.—The Secretary, taking into account such recommendations, shall conduct periodic subsequent surveys to determine the hospital acquisition cost for each specified covered outpatient drug for use in setting the payment rates under subparagraph (A).

(iii) SURVEY REQUIREMENTS.—The surveys con-ducted under clauses (i) and (ii) shall have a large sample of hospitals that is sufficient to generate a statistically significant estimate of the average hospital acquisition cost for each specified covered outpatient drug. With respect to the surveys conducted under clause (i), the Comptroller General shall report to Con-gress on the justification for the size of the sample used in order to assure the validity of such estimates.

(iv) DIFFERENTIATION IN COST.—In conducting surveys under clause (i), the Comptroller General shall determine and report to Congress if there is (and the extent of any) variation in hospital acquisition costs for drugs among hospitals based on the volume of covered OPD services performed by such hospitals or other relevant characteristics of such hospitals (as defined by the Comptroller General).

(v) COMMENT ON PROPOSED RATES.—Not later than 30 days after the date the Secretary promulgated proposed rules setting forth the payment rates under subparagraph (A) for 2006, the Comptroller General shall evaluate such proposed rates and submit to Congress a report regarding the appropriateness of such rates based on the surveys the Comptroller General has conducted under clause (i).

E) ADJUSTMENT IN PAYMENT RATES FOR OVERHEAD COSTS.—
   (i) MEDPAC REPORT ON DRUG APC DESIGN.—The Medicare Payment Advisory Commission shall submit to the Secretary, not later than July 1, 2005, a report on adjustment of payment for ambulatory payment classifications for specified covered outpatient drugs to take into account overhead and related expenses, such as pharmacy services and handling costs. Such report shall include—
      (I) a description and analysis of the data available with regard to such expenses;
      (II) a recommendation as to whether such a payment adjustment should be made; and
      (III)if such adjustment should be made, a recommendation regarding the methodology for making such an adjustment.
   (ii) ADJUSTMENT AUTHORIZED.—The Secretary may adjust the weights for ambulatory payment classifications for specified covered outpatient drugs to take into account the recommendations contained in the report submitted under clause (i).

F) CLASSES OF DRUGS.—For purposes of this paragraph:
   (i) SOLE SOURCE DRUGS.—The term 'sole source drug' means
      (I) a biological product (as defined under section 1861(t)(1)); or
      (II) a single source drug (as defined in section 1927(k)(7)(A)(iv)).
   (ii) INNOVATOR MULTIPLE SOURCE DRUGS.—The term 'innovator multiple source drug' has the meaning given such term in section 1927(k)(7)(A)(ii).
   (iii) NONINNOVATOR MULTIPLE SOURCE DRUGS.- The term 'noninnovator multiple source drug' has the meaning given such term in section 1927(k)(7)(A)(iii).

G) REFERENCE AVERAGE WHOLESALE PRICE.—The term 'reference average wholesale price' means, with respect to a specified covered outpatient drug, the average wholesale price for the drug as determined under section 1842(o) as of May 1, 2003.

H) INAPPLICABILITY OF EXPENDITURES IN DETER-MINING CONVERSION, WEIGHTING, AND OTHER ADJUSTMENT FACTORS.—Additional expenditures resulting from this paragraph shall not be taken into account in establishing the conversion, weighting, and other adjustment factors for 2004 and 2005 under paragraph (9), but shall be taken into account for subsequent years.

15 PAYMENT FOR NEW DRUGS AND BIOLOGICALS UNTIL HCPCS CODE ASSIGNED.—With respect to payment under this part for an outpatient drug or biological that is covered under this part and is furnished as part of covered OPD services for which a HCPCS code has not been assigned, the amount provided for payment for such drug or biological under this part shall be equal to 95 percent of the average wholesale price for the drug or biological.".

16 MISCELLANEOUS PROVISIONS

A) APPLICATION OF RECLASSIFICATION OF CERTAIN HOSPITALS.—If a hospital is being treated as being located in a rural area under section 1886(d)(8)(E), that hospital shall be treated under this subsection as being located in that rural area.

B) THRESHOLD FOR ESTABLISHMENT OF SEPARATE APCS FOR DRUGS.—The Secretary shall reduce the threshold for the establishment of separate ambulatory payment classification groups (APCs) with respect to drugs or biologicals to $50 per administration for drugs and biologicals furnished in 2005 and 2006.

C) PAYMENT FOR DEVICES OF BRACHYTHERAPY AT CHARGES ADJUSTED TO COST.—Notwithstanding the preceding provisions of this subsection, for a device of brachytherapy consisting of a seed or seeds (or radioactive source) furnished on or after January 1, 2004, and before January 1, 2007, the payment basis for the device under this subsection shall be equal to the hospital's charges for each device furnished, adjusted to cost. Charges for such devices shall not be included in determining any outlier payment under this subsection.

USE OF CARRIERS FOR ADMINISTRATION OF BENEFITS

SEC. 1842 (o) [42 U.S.C. 1395u]

(o)

(6) In the case of an immunosuppressive drug described in subparagraph (J) of section 1861(s)(2) and an oral drug described in subparagraph (Q) or (T) of such section, the Secretary shall pay to the pharmacy a supplying fee for such a drug determined appropriate by the Secretary (less the applicable deductible and coinsurance amounts).

DEFINITIONS OF SERVICES, INSTITUTIONS, ETC.

SEC. 1861(n) [42 U.S.C. 1395x]

The term "durable medical equipment" includes iron lungs, oxygen tents, hospital beds, and wheelchairs (which may include a power-operated vehicle that may be appropriately used as a wheelchair, but only where the use of such a vehicle is determined to be necessary on the basis of the individual's medical and physical condition and the vehicle meets such safety requirements as the Secretary may prescribe) used in the patient's home (including an institution used as his home other than an institution that meets the requirements of subsection (e)(1) of this section or section 1819(a)(1)), whether furnished on a rental basis or purchased, and includes blood-testing strips and blood glucose monitors for individuals with diabetes without regard to whether the individual has Type I or Type II diabetes or to the individual's use of insulin (as determined under standards established by the Secretary in consultation with the appropriate organizations); except that such term does not include such equipment furnished by a supplier who has used, for the demonstration and use of specific equipment, an individual who has not met such minimum training standards as the Secretary may establish with respect to the demonstration and use of such specific equipment. With respect to a seat-lift chair, such term includes only the seat-lift mechanism and does not include the chair.

SEC. 1861(r) [42 U.S.C. 1395x]

For purposes of this title—

Physician

(r) The term "physician", when used in connection with the performance of any function or action, means (1) a doctor of medicine or osteopathy legally authorized to practice medicine and surgery by the State in which he performs such function or action (including a physician within the meaning of section 1101(a)(7)), (2) a doctor of dental surgery or of dental medicine who is legally authorized to practice dentistry by the State in which he performs such function and who is acting within the scope of his license when he performs such functions, (3) a doctor of podiatric medicine for the purposes of subsections (k), (m), (p)(1), and (s) of this section and sections 1814(a), 1832(a)(2)(F)(ii), and 1835 but only with respect to functions which he is legally authorized to perform as such by the State in which he performs them, (4) a doctor of optometry, but only for purposes of subsection (p)(1) with respect to the provision of items or services described in subsection (s) which he is legally authorized to perform as a doctor of optometry by the State in which he performs them, or (5) a chiropractor who is licensed as such by the State (or in a State which does not license chiropractors as such, is legally authorized to perform the services of a chiropractor in the jurisdiction in which he performs such services), and who meets uniform minimum standards promulgated by the Secretary, but only for the purpose of sections 1861(s)(1) and 1861(s)(2)(A) and only with respect to treatment by means of manual manipulation of the spine (to correct a subluxation) which he is legally authorized to perform by the State or jurisdiction in which such treatment is provided. For the purposes of section 1862(a)(4) and subject to the limitations and conditions provided in the previous sentence, such term includes a doctor of one of the arts, specified in such previous sentence, legally authorized to practice such art in the country in which the inpatient hospital services (referred to in such section 1862(a)(4)) are furnished.

MEDICAL AND OTHER HEALTH SERVICES

SECTION 1861(s)

The term "medical and other health services" means any of the following items or services:

1 Physicians' services;

2

A) Services and supplies (including drugs and biologicals which are not usually self-administered by the patient) furnished as an incident to a physician's professional service, of kinds which are commonly furnished in physicians' offices and are commonly either rendered without charge or included in the physicians' bills;

B) Hospital services (including drugs and biologicals which are not usually self-administered by the patient) incident to physicians' services rendered to outpatients and partial hospitalization services incident to such services;

C) Diagnostic services which are—

(i) Furnished to an individual as an outpatient by a hospital or by others under arrangements with them made by a hospital, and

(ii) Ordinarily furnished by such hospital (or by others under such arrangements) to its outpatients for the purpose of diagnostic study;

D) Outpatient physical therapy services and outpatient occupational therapy services;

E) Rural health clinic services and Federally qualified health center services;

F) Home dialysis supplies and equipment, self-care home dialysis support services, and institutional dialysis services and supplies;

G) Antigens (subject to quantity limitations prescribed in regulations by the Secretary) prepared by a physician, as defined in section 1861(r)(1) , for a particular patient, including antigens so prepared which are forwarded to another qualified person (including a rural health clinic) for administration to such patient, from time to time, by or under the supervision of another such physician;

H)

(i) Services furnished pursuant to a contract under section 1876 to a member of an eligible organization by a physician assistant or by a nurse practitioner (as defined in subsection (aa)(5)) and such services and supplies furnished as an incident to his service to such a member as would otherwise be covered under this part if furnished by a physician or as an incident to a physician's service; and

(ii) Services furnished pursuant to a risk-sharing contract under section 1876(g) to a member of an eligible organization by a clinical psychologist (as defined by the Secretary) or by a clinical social worker (as defined in subsection (hh)(2)), and such services and supplies furnished as an incident to such clinical psychologist's services or clinical social worker's services to such a member as would otherwise be covered under this part if furnished by a physician or as an incident to a physician's service;

I) Blood clotting factors, for hemophilia patients competent to use such factors to control bleeding without medical or other supervision, and items related to the administration of such factors, subject to utilization controls deemed necessary by the Secretary for the efficient use of such factors;

J) Prescription drugs used in immunosuppressive therapy furnished, to an individual who receives an organ transplant for which payment is made under this title;

K)

(i) Services which would be physicians' services if furnished by a physician (as defined in subsection (r)(1)) and which are performed by a physician assistant (as defined in subsection (aa)(5)) under the supervision of a physician (as so defined) and which the physician assistant is legally authorized to perform by the State in which the services are performed, and such services and supplies furnished as incident to such services as would be covered under subparagraph (A) if furnished incident to a physician's professional service; and but only if no facility or other provider charges or is paid any amounts with respect to the furnishing of such services,

(ii) Services which would be physicians' services if furnished by a physician (as defined in subsection (r)(1)) and which are performed by a nurse practitioner or clinical nurse specialist (as defined in subsection (aa)(5)) working in collaboration (as defined in subsection (aa)(6)) with a physician (as defined in subsection (r)(1)) which the nurse practitioner or clinical nurse specialist is legally authorized to perform by the State in which the services are performed, and such services and supplies furnished as an incident to such services as would be covered under subparagraph (A) if furnished incident to a physician's professional service, but only if no facility or other provider charges or is paid any amounts with respect to the furnishing of such services;

L) Certified nurse-midwife services;

M) Qualified psychologist services;

N) Clinical social worker services (as defined in subsection (hh)(2));

O) Erythropoietin for dialysis patients competent to use such drug without medical or other supervision with respect to the administration of such drug, subject to methods and standards established by the Secretary by regulation for the safe and effective use of such drug, and items related to the administration of such drug;

P) Prostate cancer screening tests (as defined in subsection (oo));

Q) An oral drug (which is approved by the Federal Food and Drug Administration) prescribed for use as an anticancer chemotherapeutic agent for a given indication, and containing an active ingredient (or ingredients), which is the same indication and active ingredient (or ingredients) as a drug which the carrier determines would be covered pursuant to subparagraph (A) or (B) if the drug could not be self-administered;

R) Colorectal cancer screening tests (as defined in subsection (pp));

S) Diabetes outpatient self-management training services (as defined in subsection (qq));

T) An oral drug (which is approved by the Federal Food and Drug Administration) prescribed for use as an acute anti-emetic used as part of an anticancer chemotherapeutic regimen if the drug is administered by a physician (or as prescribed by a physician)—

(i) For use immediately before, at, or within 48 hours after the time of the administration of the anticancer chemotherapeutic agent; and

(ii) As a full replacement for the anti-emetic therapy which would otherwise be administered intravenously;

U) Screening for glaucoma (as defined in subsection (uu)) for individuals determined to be at high risk for glaucoma, individuals with a family history of glaucoma and individuals with diabetes; and

V) Medical nutrition therapy services (as defined in subsection (vv)(1)) in the case of a beneficiary with diabetes or a renal disease who—

(i) Has not received diabetes outpatient self- management training services within a time period determined by the Secretary;

(ii) Is not receiving maintenance dialysis for which payment is made under section 1881 ; and

(iii) Meets such other criteria determined by the Secretary after consideration of protocols established by dietitian or nutrition professional organizations;

W) an initial preventive physical examination (as defined in subsection (ww));

(X) cardiovascular screening blood tests (as defined in subsection (xx)(1));

(Y) diabetes screening tests (as defined in subsection (yy)); and

Medicare References

(Z) intravenous immune globulin for the treatment of primary immune deficiency diseases in the home (as defined in subsection (zz));

3 Diagnostic X-ray tests (including tests under the supervision of a physician, furnished in a place of residence used as the patient's home, if the performance of such tests meets such conditions relating to health and safety as the Secretary may find necessary and including diagnostic mammography if conducted by a facility that has a certificate (or provisional certificate) issued under section 354 of the Public Health Service Act [350]), diagnostic laboratory tests, and other diagnostic tests;

4 X-ray, radium, and radioactive isotope therapy, including materials and services of technicians;

5 Surgical dressings, and splints, casts, and other devices used for reduction of fractures and dislocations;

6 Durable medical equipment;

7 Ambulance service where the use of other methods of transportation is contraindicated by the individual's condition, but only to the extent provided in regulations; [351]

8 Prosthetic devices (other than dental) which replace all or part of an internal body organ (including colostomy bags and supplies directly related to colostomy care), including replacement of such devices, and including one pair of conventional eyeglasses or contact lenses furnished subsequent to each cataract surgery with insertion of an intraocular lens;

9 Leg, arm, back, and neck braces, and artificial legs, arms, and eyes, including replacements if required because of a change in the patient's physical condition;

10

A) Pneumococcal vaccine and its administration and, subject to section 4071(b) of the Omnibus Budget Reconciliation Act of 1987, [352] influenza vaccine and its administration; and

B) Hepatitis B vaccine and its administration, furnished to an individual who is at high or intermediate risk of contracting hepatitis B (as determined by the Secretary under regulations);

11 Services of a certified registered nurse anesthetist (as defined in subsection (bb));

12 Subject to section 4072(e) of the Omnibus Budget Reconciliation Act of 1987 [353] , extra-depth shoes with inserts or custom molded shoes with inserts for an individual with diabetes, if—

A) The physician who is managing the individual's diabetic condition (i) documents that the individual has peripheral neuropathy with evidence of callus formation, a history of pre-ulcerative calluses, a history of previous ulceration, foot deformity, or previous amputation, or poor circulation, and (ii) certifies that the individual needs such shoes under a comprehensive plan of care related to the individual's diabetic condition;

B) The particular type of shoes are prescribed by a podiatrist or other qualified physician (as established by the Secretary); and

C) The shoes are fitted and furnished by a podiatrist or other qualified individual (such as a pedorthist or orthotist, as established by the Secretary) who is not the physician described in subparagraph (A) (unless the Secretary finds that the physician is the only such qualified individual in the area);

13 Screening mammography (as defined in subsection (jj));

14 Screening pap smear and screening pelvic exam; and

15 Bone mass measurement (as defined in subsection (rr)).

No diagnostic tests performed in any laboratory, including a laboratory that is part of a rural health clinic, or a hospital (which, for purposes of this sentence, means an institution considered a hospital for purposes of section 1814(d)) shall be included within paragraph (3) unless such laboratory—

16 If situated in any State in which State or applicable local law provides for licensing of establishments of this nature, (A) is licensed pursuant to such law, or (B) is approved, by the agency of such State or locality responsible for licensing establishments of this nature, as meeting the standards established for such licensing; and

17

A) Meets the certification requirements under section 353 of the Public Health Service Act; [354] and

B) Meets such other conditions relating to the health and safety of individuals with respect to whom such tests are performed as the Secretary may find necessary.

There shall be excluded from the diagnostic services specified in paragraph (2)(C) any item or service (except services referred to in paragraph (1)) which would not be included under subsection (b) if it were furnished to an inpatient of a hospital. None of the items and services referred to in the preceding paragraphs (other than paragraphs (1) and (2)(A)) of this subsection which are furnished to a patient of an institution which meets the definition of a hospital for purposes of section 1814(d) shall be included unless such other conditions are met as the Secretary may find necessary relating to health and safety of individuals with respect to whom such items and services are furnished.

DRUGS AND BIOLOGICALS

SECTION 1861(t)

1 The term "drugs" and the term "biologicals", except for purposes of subsection (m)(5) and paragraph (2), include only such drugs (including contrast agents) and biologicals, respectively, as are included (or approved for inclusion) in the United States Pharmacopoeia, the National Formulary, or the United States Homeopathic Pharmacopoeia, or in New Drugs or Accepted Dental Remedies (except for any drugs and biologicals unfavorably evaluated therein), or as are approved by the pharmacy and drug therapeutics committee (or equivalent committee) of the medical staff of the hospital furnishing such drugs and biologicals for use in such hospital.

2

A) For purposes of paragraph (1), the term "drugs" also includes any drugs or biologicals used in an anticancer chemotherapeutic regimen for a medically accepted indication (as described in subparagraph (B)).

B) In subparagraph (A), the term "medically accepted indication", with respect to the use of a drug, includes any use which has been approved by the Food and Drug Administration for the drug, and includes another use of the drug if—

(i) the drug has been approved by the Food and Drug Administration; and

(ii)

(I) such use is supported by one or more citations which are included (or approved for inclusion) in one or more of the following compendia: the American Hospital Formulary Service-Drug Information, the American Medical Association Drug Evaluations, the United States Pharmacopoeia-Drug Information, and other authoritative compendia as identified by the Secretary, unless the Secretary has determined that the use is not medically appropriate or the use is identified as not indicated in one or more such compendia, or

(II) the carrier involved determines, based upon guidance provided by the Secretary to carriers for determining accepted uses of drugs, that such use is medically accepted based on supportive clinical evidence in peer reviewed medical literature appearing in publications which have been identified for purposes of this subclause by the Secretary.

The Secretary may revise the list of compendia in clause (ii)(I) as is appropriate for identifying medically accepted indications for drugs.

EXCLUSIONS FROM COVERAGE AND MEDICARE AS SECONDARY PAYER

SEC. 1862. [42 U.S.C. 1395y]

(a) Notwithstanding any other provision of this title, no payment may be made under part A or part B for any expenses incurred for items or services—

1 A) which, except for items and services described in a succeeding subparagraph, are not reasonable and necessary for the diagnosis or treatment of illness or injury or to improve the functioning of a malformed body member,

B) in the case of items and services described in section 1861(s)(10), which are not reasonable and necessary for the prevention of illness,

C) in the case of hospice care, which are not reasonable and necessary for the palliation or management of terminal illness,

D) in the case of clinical care items and services provided with the concurrence of the Secretary and with respect to research and experimentation conducted by, or under contract with, the Medicare Payment Advisory Commission or the Secretary, which are not reasonable and necessary to carry out the purposes of section 1886(e)(6),

E) in the case of research conducted pursuant to section 1142, which is not reasonable and necessary to carry out the purposes of that section,

F) in the case of screening mammography, which is performed more frequently than is covered under section 1834(c)(2) or which is not conducted by a facility described in section 1834(c)(1)(B), in the case of screening pap smear and screening pelvic exam, which is performed more frequently than is provided under section 1861(nn), and, in the case of screening for glaucoma, which is performed more frequently than is provided under section 1861(uu),

G) in the case of prostate cancer screening tests (as defined in section 1861(oo)), which are performed more frequently than is covered under such section,

H) in the case of colorectal cancer screening tests, which are performed more frequently than is covered under section 1834(d), and

I) the frequency and duration of home health services which are in excess of normative guidelines that the Secretary shall establish by regulation;

2 for which the individual furnished such items or services has no legal obligation to pay, and which no other person (by reason of such individual's membership in a prepayment plan or otherwise) has a legal obligation to provide or pay for, except in the case of Federally qualified health center services;

3 which are paid for directly or indirectly by a governmental entity (other than under this Act and other than under a health benefits or insurance plan established for employees of such an entity), except in the case of rural health clinic services, as defined in section 1861(aa)(1), in the case of Federally qualified health center services, as defined in section 1861(aa)(3), in the case of services for which payment may be made under section 1880(e), and in such other cases as the Secretary may specify;

4 which are not provided within the United States (except for inpatient hospital services furnished outside the United States under the conditions described in section 1814(f) and, subject to such conditions, limitations, and requirements as are provided under or pursuant to this title, physicians' services and ambulance services furnished an individual in conjunction with such inpatient hospital services but only for the period during which such inpatient hospital services were furnished);

5 which are required as a result of war, or of an act of war, occurring after the effective date of such individual's current coverage under such part;

6 which constitute personal comfort items (except, in the case of hospice care, as is otherwise permitted under paragraph (1)(C));

7 where such expenses are for routine physical checkups, eyeglasses (other than eyewear described in section 1861(s)(8)) or eye examinations for the purpose of prescribing, fitting, or changing eyeglasses, procedures performed (during the course of any eye examination) to determine the refractive state of the eyes, hearing aids or examinations therefor, or immunizations (except as otherwise allowed under section 1861(s)(10) and subparagraph (B), (F), (G), or (H) of paragraph (1));

8 where such expenses are for orthopedic shoes or other supportive devices for the feet, other than shoes furnished pursuant to section 1861(s)(12);

9 where such expenses are for custodial care (except, in the case of hospice care, as is otherwise permitted under paragraph (1)(C));

10 where such expenses are for cosmetic surgery or are incurred in connection therewith, except as required for the prompt repair of accidental injury or for improvement of the functioning of a malformed body member;

11 where such expenses constitute charges imposed by immediate relatives of such individual or members of his household;

12 where such expenses are for services in connection with the care, treatment, filling, removal, or replacement of teeth or structures directly supporting teeth, except that payment may be made under part A in the case of inpatient hospital services in connection with the provision of such dental services if the individual, because of his underlying medical condition and clinical status or because of the severity of the dental procedure, requires hospitalization in connection with the provision of such services;

13 where such expenses are for—

(A) the treatment of flat foot conditions and the prescription of supportive devices there for,

(B) the treatment of subluxations of the foot, or

(C) routine foot care (including the cutting or removal of corns or calluses, the trimming of nails, and other routine hygienic care);

14 which are other than physicians' services (as defined in regulations promulgated specifically for purposes of this paragraph), services described by section 1861(s)(2)(K), certified nurse-midwife services, qualified psychologist services, and services of a certified registered nurse anesthetist, and which are furnished to an individual who is a patient of a hospital or critical access hospital by an entity other than the hospital or critical access hospital, unless the services are furnished under arrangements (as defined in section 1861(w)(1)) with the entity made by the hospital or critical access hospital;

15 (A) which are for services of an assistant at surgery in a cataract operation (including subsequent insertion of an intraocular lens) unless, before the surgery is performed, the appropriate utilization and quality control peer review organization (under part B of title XI) or a carrier under section 1842 has approved of the use of such an assistant in the surgical procedure based on the existence of a complicating medical condition, or

(B) which are for services of an assistant at surgery to which section 1848(i)(2)(B) applies;

16 in the case in which funds may not be used for such items and services under the Assisted Suicide Funding Restriction Act of 1997;

17 where the expenses are for an item or service furnished in a competitive acquisition area (as established by the Secretary under section 1847(a)) by an entity other than an entity with which the Secretary has entered into a contract under section 1847(b) for the furnishing of such an item or service in that area, unless the Secretary finds that the expenses were incurred in a case of urgent need, or in other circumstances specified by the Secretary;

18 which are covered skilled nursing facility services described in section 1888(e)(2)(A)(i) and which are furnished to an individual who is a resident of a skilled nursing facility during a period in which the resident is provided covered post-hospital extended care services (or, for services described in section 1861(s)(2)(D), which are furnished to such an individual without regard to such period), by an entity other than the skilled nursing facility, unless the services are furnished under arrangements (as defined in section 1861(w)(1)) with the entity made by the skilled nursing facility; or

19 which are for items or services which are furnished pursuant to a private contract described in section 1802(b);

20 in the case of outpatient occupational therapy services or outpatient physical therapy services furnished as an incident to a physician's professional services (as described in section 1861(s)(2)(A)), that do not meet the standards and conditions (other than any licensing requirement specified by the Secretary) under the second sentence of section 1861(p) (or under such sentence through the operation of section 1861(g)) as such standards and conditions would apply to such therapy services if furnished by a therapist; or

21 where such expenses are for home health services (including medical supplies described in section 1861(m)(5), but excluding durable medical equipment to the extent provided for in such section), furnished to an individual who is under a plan of care of the home health agency if the claim for payment for such services is not submitted by the agency.

Paragraph (7) shall not apply to Federally qualified health center services described in section 1861(aa)(3)(B).

CODE OF FEDERAL REGULATIONS

TITLE 42 – PUBLIC HEALTH

Section 410.62 [42CFR410.62]

Subpart B—Medical and Other Health Services

Sec. 410.62 Outpatient speech-language pathology services: Conditions and exclusions.

(a) Basic rule. Medicare Part B pays for outpatient speech pathology services if they meet the following conditions:

(1) They are furnished to a beneficiary while he or she is under the care of a physician who is a doctor of medicine or osteopathy.

(2) They are furnished under a written plan of treatment that-(i) Is established by a physician or, effective January 1, 1982, by either a physician or the speech pathologist who will provide the services to the particular individual;

(ii) Is periodically reviewed by a physician; and

(iii) Meets the requirements of Sec. 410.63.

(3) They are furnished by a provider as defined in Sec. 489.2 of this chapter or by others under arrangements with, or under the supervision of, a provider.

(b) Outpatient speech pathology services to certain inpatients of a hospital, CAH, or SNF. Medicare Part B pays for outpatient speech pathology services furnished to an inpatient of a hospital, CAH, or SNF who requires them but has exhausted or is otherwise ineligible for benefit days under Medicare Part A.

(c) Excluded services. No service is included as an outpatient speech pathology service if it would not be included as an inpatient hospital service if furnished to a hospital or CAH inpatient.

(d) Limitation. After 1998, outpatient speech-language pathology services are subject to the limitation in Sec. 410.60(e).

Medicare References

Appendix D

Jurisdiction List

The following is an updated list of the HCPCS codes for what has been known as Durable Medical Equipment Regional Carriers (DMERC) and local carrier jurisdictions. Under Section 911 of the *Medicare Prescription Drug, Improvement and Modernization Act* (MMA), Congress mandated the Secretary of Health and Human Services replace the current contracting authority under Title XVIII of the Social Security Act with the new Medicare Administrative Contractor (MAC) authority. Jurisdiction for these carriers will be referred to as DME MAC.

Claims for immunosuppressive drugs, inhalation drugs, oral anticancer drugs, oral antiemetic drugs or drugs administered in the patient's home through external infusion pumps should be submitted to the DME MACs. All other claims for drugs should be submitted to the local carriers. Claims for supplies (including dressings), accessories, and replacement parts for implanted DME or implanted prosthetic devices should be submitted to the local carriers. In addition, claims for repair of implanted DME or implanted prosthetic devices should be submitted to the local carriers.

It is not uncommon for CMS to update this list periodically, so it is important that you read your Medicare carrier, fiscal intermediary, or DME MAC bulletins for changes.

HCPCS	DESCRIPTION	JURISDICTION
A0021 – A0999	Ambulance Services	Local Carrier
A4206 – A4209	Medical, Surgical, and Self-Administered Injection Supplies	Local Carrier if incident to a physician's service (not separately payable). If other DME MAC.
A4210	Needle Free Injection Device	DME MAC
A4211	Medical, Surgical, and Self-Administered Injection Supplies	Local Carrier if incident to a physician's service (not separately payable). If other DME MAC.
A4212	Non Coring Needle or Stylet with or without Catheter	Local Carrier
A4213 – A4215	Medical , Surgical, and Self-Administered Injection Supplies	Local Carrier if incident to a physician's service (not separately payable). If other DME MAC.
A4216 – A4218	Saline	Local Carrier if incident to a physician's service (not separately payable). If other DME MAC.
A4220	Refill Kit for Implantable Pump	Local Carrier
A4221 – A4250	Medical, Surgical, and Self-Administered Injection Supplies	Local Carrier if incident to a physician's service (not separately payable). If other DME MAC.
A4252 – A4259	Diabetic Supplies	DME MAC
A4261	Cervical Cap for Contraceptive Use	Local Carrier
A4262 – A4263	Lacrimal Duct Implants	Local Carrier
A4264	Contraceptives	Local Carrier
A4265	Paraffin	Local Carrier if incident to a physician's service (not separately payable). If other DME MAC.
A4266 – A4269	Contraceptives	Local Carrier
A4270	Endoscope Sheath	Local Carrier
A4280	Accessory for Breast Prosthesis	DME MAC
A4281 – A4286	Accessory for Breast Pump	DME MAC
A4290	Sacral Nerve Stimulation Test Lead	Local Carrier
A4300 – A4301	Implantable Catheter	Local Carrier
A4305 – A4306	Disposable Drug Delivery System	Local Carrier if incident to a physician's service (not separately payable). If other DME MAC.

HCPCS	DESCRIPTION	JURISDICTION
A4310 – A4358	Incontinence Supplies/ Urinary Supplies	If provided in the physician's office for a temporary condition, the item is incident to the physician's service & billed to the Local Carrier. If provided in the physician's office or other place of service for a permanent condition, the item is a prosthetic device & billed to the DME MAC.
A4360 – A4434	Urinary Supplies	If provided in the physician's office for a temporary condition, the item is incident to the physician's service & billed to the Local Carrier. If provided in the physician's office or other place of service for a permanent condition, the item is a prosthetic device & billed to the DME MAC.
A4450 – A4456	Tape; Adhesive Remover	Local Carrier if incident to a physician's service (not separately payable). If other DME MAC.
A4458	Enema Bag	DME MAC
A4461 – A4463	Surgical Dressing Holders	Local Carrier if incident to a physician's service (not separately payable). If other DME MAC.
A4465 – A4466	Non-elastic Binder and Elastic Garment	Local Carrier if incident to a physician's service (not separately payable). If other DME MAC
A4470	Gravlee Jet Washer	Local Carrier
A4480	Vabra Aspirator	Local Carrier
A4481	Tracheostomy Supply	Local Carrier if incident to a physician's service (not separately payable). If other DME MAC.
A4483	Moisture Exchanger	DME MAC
A4490 – A4510	Surgical Stockings	DME MAC
A4520	Diapers	DME MAC
A4550	Surgical Trays	Local Carrier
A4554	Disposable Underpads	DME MAC
A4556 – A4558	Electrodes; Lead Wires; Conductive Paste	Local Carrier if incident to a physician's service (not separately payable). If other DME MAC.
A4559	Coupling Gel	Local Carrier if incident to a physician's service(not separately payable). If other DME MAC.
A4561 – A4562	Pessary	Local Carrier
A4565 – A4566	Sling	Local Carrier
A4570	Splint	Local Carrier

HCPCS	DESCRIPTION	JURISDICTION
A4575	Topical Hyperbaric Oxygen Chamber, Disposable	DME MAC
A4580 – A4590	Casting Supplies & Material	Local Carrier
A4595	TENS Supplies	Local Carrier if incident to a physician's service (not separately payable). If other DME MAC.
A4600	Sleeve for Intermittent Limb Compression Device	DME MAC
A4601	Lithium Ion Battery for Non-Prosthetic Use	DME MAC
A4604	Tubing for Positive Airway Pressure Device	DME MAC
A4605	Tracheal Suction Catheter	DME MAC
A4606	Oxygen Probe for Oximeter	DME MAC
A4608	Transtracheal Oxygen Catheter	DME MAC
A4611 – A4613	Oxygen Equipment Batteries and Supplies	DME MAC
A4614	Peak Flow Rate Meter	Local Carrier if incident to a physician's service (not separately payable). If other DME MAC.
A4615 – A4629	Oxygen & Tracheostomy Supplies	Local Carrier if incident to a physician's service (not separately payable). If other DME MAC.
A4630 – A4640	DME Supplies	DME MAC
A4641 – A4642	Imaging Agent; Contrast Material	Local Carrier
A4648	Tissue Marker, Implanted	Local Carrier
A4649	Miscellaneous Surgical Supplies	Local Carrier if incident to a physician's service (not separately payable) or if supply for implanted prosthetic device or implanted DME. If other DME MAC.
A4650	Implantable Radiation Dosimeter	Local Carrier
A4651 – A4932	Supplies for ESRD	DME MAC
A5051 – A5093	Additional Ostomy Supplies	If provided in the physician's office for a temporary condition, the item is incident to the physician's service & billed to the Local Carrier. If provided in the physician's office or other place of service for a permanent condition, the item is a prosthetic device & billed to the DME MAC.
A5102 – A5200	Additional Incontinence and Ostomy Supplies	If provided in the physician's office for a temporary condition, the item is incident to the physician's service & billed to the Local Carrier. If provided in the physician's office or other place of service for a permanent condition, the item is a prosthetic device & billed to the DME MAC.
A5500 – A5513	Therapeutic Shoes	DME MAC
A6000	Non-Contact Wound Warming Cover	DME MAC
A6010-A6024	Surgical Dressing	Local Carrier if incident to a physician's service (not separately payable) or if supply for implanted prosthetic device or implanted DME. If other DME MAC.
A6025	Silicone Gel Sheet	Local Carrier if incident to a physician's service (not separately payable) or if supply for implanted prosthetic device or implanted DME. If other DME MAC.
A6154 – A6411	Surgical Dressing	Local Carrier if incident to a physician's service (not separately payable) or if supply for implanted prosthetic device or implanted DME. If other DME MAC.

HCPCS	DESCRIPTION	JURISDICTION
A6412	Eye Patch	Local Carrier if incident to a physician's service (not separately payable) or if supply for implanted prosthetic device or implanted DME. If other DME MAC.
A6413	Adhesive Bandage	Local Carrier if incident to a physician's service (not separately payable) or if supply for implanted prosthetic device or implanted DME. If other DME MAC.
A6441 – A6512	Surgical Dressings	Local Carrier if incident to a physician's service (not separately payable) or if supply for implanted prosthetic device or implanted DME. If other DME MAC.
A6513	Compression Burn Mask	DME MAC
A6530 – A6549	Compression Gradient Stockings	DME MAC
A6550	Supplies for Negative Pressure Wound Therapy Electrical Pump	DME MAC
A7000 – A7002	Accessories for Suction Pumps	DME MAC
A7003 – A7039	Accessories for Nebulizers, Aspirators and Ventilators	DME MAC
A7040 – A7041	Chest Drainage Supplies	Local Carrier
A7042 – A7043	Pleural Catheter	Local Carrier
A7044 – A7046	Respiratory Accessories	DME MAC
A7501-A7527	Tracheostomy Supplies	DME MAC
A8000-A8004	Protective Helmets	DME MAC
A9150	Non-Prescription Drugs	Local Carrier
A9152 – A9153	Vitamins	Local Carrier
A9155	Artificial Saliva	Local Carrier
A9180	Lice Infestation Treatment	Local Carrier
A9270 – A9273	Noncovered Items or Services	DME MAC
A9274 – A9278	Glucose Monitoring	DME MAC
A9279	Monitoring Feature/Device	DME MAC
A9280	Alarm Device	DME MAC
A9281	Reaching/Grabbing Device	DME MAC
A9282	Wig	DME MAC
A9283	Foot Off Loading Device	DME MAC
A9284	Non-electric Spirometer	DME MAC
A9300	Exercise Equipment	DME MAC
A9500 – A9700	Supplies for Radiology Procedures	Local Carrier
A9900	Miscellaneous DME Supply or Accessory	Local Carrier if used with implanted DME. If other, DME MAC.
A9901	Delivery	DME MAC
A9999	Miscellaneous DME Supply or Accessory	Local Carrier if used with implanted DME. If other, DME MAC.
B4034 – B9999	Enteral and Parenteral Therapy	DME MAC
D0120 – D9999	Dental Procedures	Local Carrier
E0100 – E0105	Canes	DME MAC
E0110 – E0118	Crutches	DME MAC
E0130 – E0159	Walkers	DME MAC
E0160 – E0175	Commodes	DME MAC
E0181 – E0199	Decubitus Care Equipment	DME MAC
E0200 – E0239	Heat/Cold Applications	DME MAC
E0240 – E0248	Bath and Toilet Aids	DME MAC
E0249	Pad for Heating Unit	DME MAC
E0250 – E0304	Hospital Beds	DME MAC

HCPCS	DESCRIPTION	JURISDICTION
E0305 – E0326	Hospital Bed Accessories	DME MAC
E0328 – E0329	Pediatric Hospital Beds	DME MAC
E0350 – E0352	Electronic Bowel Irrigation System	DME MAC
E0370	Heel Pad	DME MAC
E0371 – E0373	Decubitus Care Equipment	DME MAC
E0424 – E0484	Oxygen and Related Respiratory Equipment	DME MAC
E0485 – E0486	Oral Device to Reduce Airway Collapsibility	DME MAC
E0487	Electric Spirometer	DME MAC
E0500	IPPB Machine	DME MAC
E0550 – E0585	Compressors/Nebulizers	DME MAC
E0600	Suction Pump	DME MAC
E0601	CPAP Device	DME MAC
E0602 – E0604	Breast Pump	DME MAC
E0605	Vaporizer	DME MAC
E0606	Drainage Board	DME MAC
E0607	Home Blood Glucose Monitor	DME MAC
E0610 – E0615	Pacemaker Monitor	DME MAC
E0616	Implantable Cardiac Event Recorder	Local Carrier
E0617	External Defibrillator	DME MAC
E0618 – E0619	Apnea Monitor	DME MAC
E0620	Skin Piercing Device	DME MAC
E0621 – E0636	Patient Lifts	DME MAC
E0637 – E0642	Standing Devices/Lifts	DME MAC
E0650 – E0676	Pneumatic Compressor and Appliances	DME MAC
E0691 – E0694	Ultraviolet Light Therapy Systems	DME MAC
E0700	Safety Equipment	DME MAC
E0705	Transfer Board	DME MAC
E0710	Restraints	DME MAC
E0720 – E0745	Electrical Nerve Stimulators	DME MAC
E0746	EMG Device	Local Carrier
E0747 – E0748	Osteogenic Stimulators	DME MAC
E0749	Implantable Osteogenic Stimulators	Local Carrier
E0755	Reflex Stimulator	DME MAC
E0760	Ultrasonic Osteogenic Stimulator	DME MAC
E0761	Electromagnetic Treatment Device	DME MAC
E0762	Electrical Joint Stimulation Device	DME MAC
E0764	Functional Neuromuscular Stimulator	DME MAC
E0765	Nerve Stimulator	DME MAC
E0769	Electrical Wound Treatment Device	DME MAC
E0770	Functional Electrical Stimulator	DME MAC
E0776	IV Pole	DME MAC
E0779 – E0780	External Infusion Pumps	DME MAC

HCPCS	DESCRIPTION	JURISDICTION
E0781	Ambulatory Infusion Pump	Billable to both the local carrier and the DME MAC. This item may be billed to the DME MAC whenever the infusion is initiated in the physician's office but the patient does not return during the same business day.
E0782 – E0783	Infusion Pumps, Implantable	Local Carrier
E0784	Infusion Pumps, Insulin	DME MAC
E0785 – E0786	Implantable Infusion Pump Catheter	Local Carrier
E0791	Parenteral Infusion Pump	DME MAC
E0830	Ambulatory Traction Device	DME MAC
E0840 – E0900	Traction Equipment	DME MAC
E0910 – E0930	Trapeze/Fracture Frame	DME MAC
E0935 – E0936	Passive Motion Exercise Device	DME MAC
E0940	Trapeze Equipment	DME MAC
E0941	Traction Equipment	DME MAC
E0942 – E0945	Orthopedic Devices	DME MAC
E0946 – E0948	Fracture Frame	DME MAC
E0950 – E1298	Wheelchairs	DME MAC
E1300 – E1310	Whirlpool Equipment	DME MAC
E1353 – E1392	Additional Oxygen Related Equipment	DME MAC
E1399	Miscellaneous DME	Local Carrier if implanted DME. If other, DME MAC.
E1405 – E1406	Additional Oxygen Equipment	DME MAC
E1500 – E1699	Artificial Kidney Machines and Accessories	DME MAC
E1700 – E1702	TMJ Device and Supplies	DME MAC
E1800 – E1841	Dynamic Flexion Devices	DME MAC
E1902	Communication Board	DME MAC
E2000	Gastric Suction Pump	DME MAC
E2100 – E2101	Blood Glucose Monitors with Special Features	DME MAC
E2120	Pulse Generator for Tympanic Treatment of Inner Ear	DME MAC
E2201 – E2397	Wheelchair Accessories	DME MAC
E2402	Negative Pressure Wound Therapy Pump	DME MAC
E2500 – E2599	Speech Generating Device	DME MAC
E2601 – E2625	Wheelchair Cushions	DME MAC
E8000 – E8002	Gait Trainers	DME MAC
G0008 – G0329	Misc. Professional Services	Local Carrier
G0333	Dispensing Fee	DME MAC
G0337 – G0365	Misc. Professional Services	Local Carrier
G0372	Misc. Professional Services	Local Carrier
G0378 – G9147	Misc. Professional Services	Local Carrier
J0120 – J3570	Injection	Local Carrier if incident to a physician's service or used in an implanted infusion pump. If other, DME MAC.
J3590	Unclassified Biologicals	Local Carrier
J7030 – J7130	Miscellaneous Drugs and Solutions	Local Carrier if incident to a physician's service or used in an implanted infusion pump. If other, DME MAC.
J7184 – J7195	Antihemophilic Factor	Local Carrier
J7196 – J7197	Antithrombin	Local Carrier

HCPCS	DESCRIPTION	JURISDICTION
J7198	Anti-inhibitor; per I.U.	Local Carrier
J7199	Other Hemophilia Clotting Factors	Local Carrier
J7300 – J7307	Intrauterine Copper Contraceptive	Local Carrier
J7308 – J7309	Aminolevulinic	Local Carrier
J7310	Ganciclovir, Long-Acting Implant	Local Carrier
J7311 – J7312	Intravitreal Implant	Local Carrier
J7321 – J7325	Hyaluronan	Local Carrier
J7330	Autologous Cultured Chondrocytes, Implant	Local Carrier
J7335	Capsaicin topical	Local Carrier
J7500 – J7599	Immunosuppressive Drugs	Local Carrier if incident to a physician's service or used in an implanted infusion pump. If other, DME MAC.
J7604 – J7699	Inhalation Solutions	Local Carrier if incident to a physician's service. If other, DME MAC.
J7799	NOC, Other than Inhalation Drugs through DME	Local carrier if incident to a physician's service. If other, DME MAC.
J8498	Anti-emetic Drug	DME MAC
J8499	Prescription Drug, Oral, Non Chemotherapeutic	Local carrier if incident to a physician's service. If other, DME MAC.
J8501 – J8999	Oral Anti-Cancer Drugs	DME MAC
J9000 – J9999	Chemotherapy Drugs	Local Carrier if incident to a physician's service or used in an implanted infusion pump. If other, DME MAC.
K0001 – K0108	Wheelchairs	DME MAC
K0195	Elevating Leg Rests	DME MAC
K0455	Infusion Pump used for Uninterrupted Administration of Epoprostenal	DME MAC
K0462	Loaner Equipment	DME MAC
K0552	External Infusion Pump Supplies	DME MAC
K0601 – K0605	External Infusion Pump Batteries	DME MAC
K0606 – K0609	Defibrillator Accessories	DME MAC
K0669	Wheelchair Cushion	DME MAC
K0672	Soft Interface for Orthosis	DME MAC
K0733	Power Wheelchair Accessory	DME MAC
K0738	Oxygen Equipment	DME MAC
K0739	Repair or Nonroutine Service for DME	Local Carrier if implanted DME. If other, DME MAC
K0740	Repair or Nonroutine Service for Oxygen Equipment	DME MAC
K0800 – K0899	Power Mobility Devices	DME MAC
L0112 – L2090	Orthotics	DME MAC
L2106 – L2116	Orthotics	DME MAC
L2126 – L4631	Orthotics	DME MAC
L5000 – L5999	Lower Limb Prosthetics	DME MAC
L6000 – L7499	Upper Limb Prosthetics	DME MAC
L7500 – L7520	Repair of Prosthetic Device	Local Carrier if repair of implanted prosthetic device. If other, DME MAC.
L7600	Prosthetic Donning Sleeve	DME MAC
L7900	Vacuum Erection System	DME MAC
L8000 – L8485	Prosthetics	DME MAC

HCPCS	DESCRIPTION	JURISDICTION
L8499	Unlisted Procedure for Miscellaneous Prosthetic Services	Local Carrier if implanted prosthetic device. If other, DME MAC.
L8500 – L8501	Artificial Larynx; Tracheostomy Speaking Valve	DME MAC
L8505	Artificial Larynx Accessory	DME MAC
L8507	Voice Prosthesis, Patient Inserted	DME MAC
L8509	Voice Prosthesis Inserted by a Licensed Health Care Provider	Local Carrier or dates of service on or after 10/01/2010, DMA MAC for dates of service prior to 10/01/2010
L8510 – L8515	Voice Prosthesis	DME MAC
L8600 – L8699	Prosthetic Implants	Local Carrier
L9900	Miscellaneous Orthotic or Prosthetic Component or Accessory	Local Carrier if used with implanted prosthetic device. If other, DME MAC.
M0064 – M0301	Medical Services	Local Carrier
P2028 – P9615	Laboratory Tests	Local Carrier
Q0035	Influenza Vaccine; Cardiokymography	Local Carrier
Q0081	Infusion Therapy	Local Carrier
Q0083 – Q0085	Chemotherapy Administration	Local Carrier
Q0091	Smear Preparation	Local Carrier
Q0092	Portable X-ray Setup	Local Carrier
Q0111 – Q0115	Miscellaneous Lab Services	Local Carrier
Q0138-Q0139	Ferumoxytol Injection	Local Carrier
Q0144	Azithromycin Dihydrate	Local Carrier if incident to a physician's service. If other, DME MAC.
Q0163 – Q0181	Anti-emetic	DME MAC
Q0478 – Q0506	Ventricular Assist Devices	Local Carrier
Q0510 – Q0514	Drug Dispensing Fees	DME MAC
Q0515	Sermorelin Acetate	Local Carrier
Q1003 – Q1005	New Technology IOL	Local Carrier
Q2004	Irrigation Solution	Local Carrier
Q2009	Fosphenytoin	Local Carrier
Q2017	Teniposide	Local Carrier
Q2026 – Q2027	Injectable Dermal FIllers	Local Carrier
Q2035 – Q2039	Influenza Vaccine	Local Carrier
Q3001	Radio Elements for Brachytherapy	Local Carrier
Q3014	Telehealth Originating Site Facility Fee	Local Carrier
Q3025 – Q3026	Vaccines	Local Carrier
Q3031	Collagen Skin Test	Local Carrier
Q4001 – Q4051	Splints and Casts	Local Carrier
Q4074	Inhalation Drug	Local Carrier if incident to a physician's service. If other, DME MAC.
Q4081	Epoetin	DME MAC for method II home dialysis. If other, Local Carrier.
Q4082	Drug Subject to Competitive Acquisition Program	Local Carrier
Q4100 –Q4121	Skin Substitutes	Local Carrier
Q5001 – Q5009	Hospice Services	Local Carrier
Q9951 – Q9954	Imaging Agents	Local Carrier
Q9955 – Q9957	Microspheres	Local Carrier
Q9958 – Q9968	Imaging Agents	Local Carrier

HCPCS	DESCRIPTION	JURISDICTION
R0070 – R0076	Diagnostic Radiology Services	Local Carrier
V2020 – V2025	Frames	DME MAC
V2100 – V2513	Lenses	DME MAC
V2520 – V2523	Hydrophilic Contact Lenses	Local Carrier if incident to a physician's service. If other, DME MAC.
V2530 – V2531	Contact Lenses, Scleral	DME MAC
V2599	Contact Lens, Other Type	Local Carrier if incident to a physician's service. If other, DME MAC.
V2600 – V2615	Low Vision Aids	DME MAC
V2623 – V2629	Prosthetic Eyes	DME MAC
V2630 – V2632	Intraocular Lenses	Local Carrier
V2700 – V2780	Miscellaneous Vision Service	DME MAC
V2781	Progressive Lens	DME MAC

HCPCS	DESCRIPTION	JURISDICTION
V2782 – V2784	Lenses	DME MAC
V2785	Processing--Corneal Tissue	Local Carrier
V2786	Lens	DME MAC
V2787 – V2788	Intraocular Lenses	Local Carrier
V2790	Amniotic Membrane	Local Carrier
V2797	Vision Supply	DME MAC
V2799	Miscellaneous Vision Service	DME MAC
V5008 – V5299	Hearing Services	Local Carrier
V5336	Repair/Modification of Augmentative Communicative System or Device	DME MAC
V5362 – V5364	Speech Screening	Local Carrier

contexo | media

CPT® Professional Edition

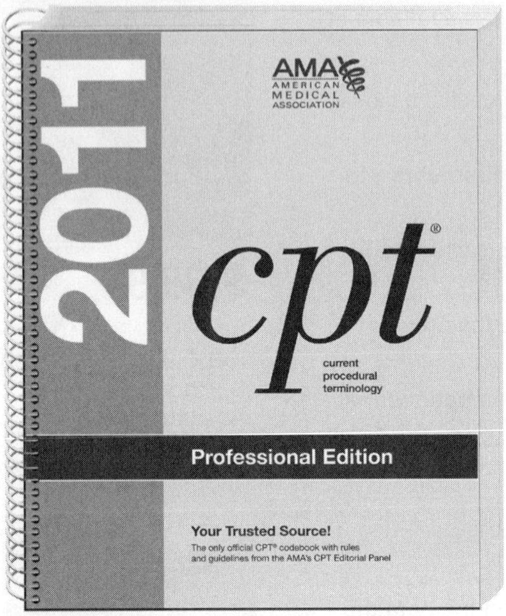

Contains the official CPT® coding rules and guidelines as well as hundreds of code, guideline and text changes, including extensive changes to the surgery section (e.g., Excision and Debridement subsection) for 2011 as well as:

- New! E/M reference tables have been added to summarize the requirements for reporting E/M services
- New! Coding tips added throughout—a select group of helpful tips added throughout to aid in better understanding of coding
- Section-specific table of contents—provide users with an efficient tool to navigate information relevant to the codes listed in each section
- Anatomical and procedural illustrations incorporated within the code sections
- Reference tables for quick identification of the codes—assist in understanding the definition and differentiation of key parameters in large families of codes
- Inclusion of *CPT® Assistant* newsletter citations in Appendix A

$107.95

Item ID: PCPT-11
ISBN: 978-1-60359-217-8
Spiralbound
Available October 2010

Promo Code: FOBA11

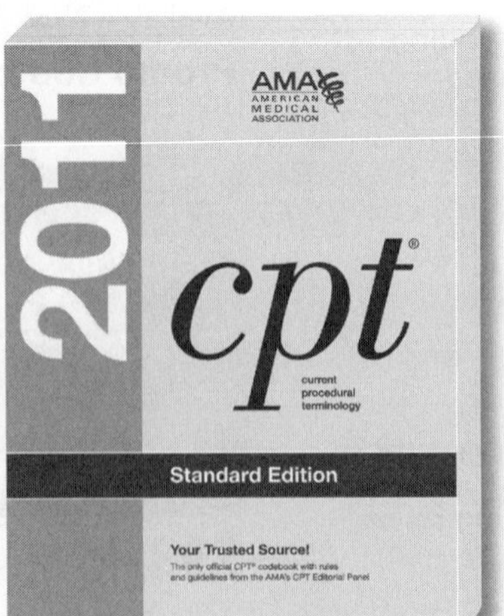

CPT® Standard Edition

The 2011 Standard Edition includes:

- A limited number of anatomical illustrations
- Summary of additions, deletions and revisions
- Extensive index helps you locate codes by procedure/service, organ/other anatomic site, condition, synonyms/eponyms, and abbreviations

$84.95

Item ID: CPT4-11
ISBN: 978-1-60359-216-1
Softbound
Available October 2010

Contexo Media
P.O. Box 25128
SLC, UT 84125-0128

FAX
801.365.0710

PHONE
800.334.5724

ONLINE
www.codingbooks.com